Cockburn Library, Yorkhill

T05119

616
02992
WOL
2011

174
WOL

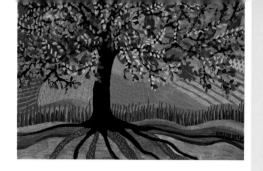

Textbook of Interdisciplinary Pediatric Palliative Care

Joanne Wolfe, MD, MPH

Division Chief, Pediatric Palliative Care Service
Department of Psychosocial Oncology and Palliative Care
Dana-Farber Cancer Institute
Director, Pediatric Palliative Care
Children's Hospital Boston
Assistant Professor of Pediatrics
Harvard Medical School
Boston, Massachusetts

Pamela S. Hinds, PhD, RN, FAAN

Director, Department of Nursing Research and Quality Outcomes
Children's National Medical Center
Professor of Pediatrics
The George Washington University
Washington, DC

Barbara M. Sourkes, PhD

John A. Kriewall and Elizabeth A. Haehl Director
Palliative Care Program
Lucile Packard Children's Hospital at Stanford
Associate Professor of Pediatrics
Stanford University School of Medicine
Stanford, California

ELSEVIER
SAUNDERS

ELSEVIER
SAUNDERS

1600 John F. Kennedy Blvd.
Ste 1800
Philadelphia, PA 19103-2899

TEXTBOOK OF INTERDISCIPLINARY PEDIATRIC PALLIATIVE CARE   ISBN: 978-1-4377-0262-0

Copyright © 2011 by Saunders, an imprint of Elsevier Inc.

No part of this publication may be reproduced or transmitted in any form or by any means, electronic or mechanical, including photocopying, recording, or any information storage and retrieval system, without permission in writing from the publisher. Details on how to seek permission, further information about the Publisher's permissions policies and our arrangements with organizations such as the Copyright Clearance Center and the Copyright Licensing Agency can be found at our website: www.elsevier.com/permissions.

This book and the individual contributions contained in it are protected under copyright by the Publisher (other than as may be noted herein).

Notices

Knowledge and best practice in this field are constantly changing. As new research and experience broaden our understanding, changes in research methods, professional practices, or medical treatment may become necessary.

Practitioners and researchers must always rely on their own experience and knowledge in evaluating and using any information, methods, compounds, or experiments described herein. In using such information or methods they should be mindful of their own safety and the safety of others, including parties for whom they have a professional responsibility.

With respect to any drug or pharmaceutical products identified, readers are advised to check the most current information provided (i) on procedures featured or (ii) by the manufacturer of each product to be administered, to verify the recommended dose or formula, the method and duration of administration, and contraindications. It is the responsibility of practitioners, relying on their own experience and knowledge of their patients, to make diagnoses, to determine dosages and the best treatment for each individual patient, and to take all appropriate safety precautions.

To the fullest extent of the law, neither the Publisher nor the authors, contributors, or editors, assume any liability for any injury and/or damage to persons or property as a matter of products liability, negligence or otherwise, or from any use or operation of any methods, products, instructions, or ideas contained in the material herein.

Library of Congress Cataloging-in-Publication Data

Textbook of interdisciplinary pediatric palliative care/ [edited by] Joanne Wolfe, Pamela Hinds, Barbara Sourkes.
    p. ; cm.
  Includes bibliographical references and index.
  ISBN 978-1-4377-0262-0 (hardcover : alk. paper) 1. Terminally ill children–Care. 2. Palliative treatment.
I. Wolfe, Joanne. II. Hinds, Pamela S. III. Sourkes, Barbara M.
  [DNLM: 1. Palliative Care. 2. Child. 3. Patient Care Team. 4. Professional-Family Relations.
5. Professional-Patient Relations. 6. Terminal Care. WB 310]
  RJ249.T49 2011
  362.17'5083–dc22
                                                                          2010027305

Acquisitions Editor: Pamela Hetherington
Publishing Services Manager: Anne Altepeter
Team Manager: Radhika Pallamparthy
Project Managers: Cindy Thoms/Vijay Antony Raj Vincent
Senior Book Designer: Ellen Zanolle
Cover and frontispiece art: Evelyn Berde

Printed in China

Last digit is the print number: 9 8 7 6 5 4 3 2 1

Working together to grow
libraries in developing countries

www.elsevier.com | www.bookaid.org | www.sabre.org

ELSEVIER   BOOK AID International   Sabre Foundation

With love for Sam, Hannah, Ben,
and Michael
JOANNE WOLFE

To Ron, Ben, and Adam Griffin for caring and believing,
and to Wayne L. Furman, Linda L. Oakes, and
Charles Pratt for having always known the essential
nature of pediatric palliative care and research
PAMELA HINDS

For Talia Jade
and
Eric & David
BARBARA SOURKES

And to the colleagues from whom we have
learned and the children and families
for whom we have had the privilege to care

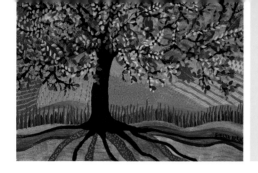

About the Artist

Evelyn Berde grew up in the old "West End" of Boston, a neighborhood of European, African-American, and Latin immigrants. Today, many of her images and colors reflect her passion for Native American, Southeast Asian, Latin American, and African art, but also, her paintings still somehow recall for her the world she lived in as a child in the West End. Evelyn brings much of her life experiences to each painting. Her work resembles the patchwork of her childhood and adult life, as an artist, mother, wife, and teacher. Evelyn incorporates her connection to people and their "stories," her surroundings in everyday life, inspirations, and dreams. Evelyn's artwork has been commissioned by Children's Hospital Boston for the Anesthesia Department Library, the Children's Hospital Chapel, and the patient family house at 241 Kent Street. In creating these works, Evelyn notes, "I try to talk with many patients, parents, and staff members before I create a piece of art. The colors, lights, textures, and lines of each painting hopefully reflect the thoughts and feelings of each person I have met."

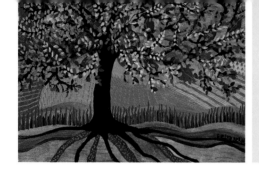

Contributors

Leslie Adams, MSW
PPC Consultant
CHPCC and former Pediatric Palliative Care Consultant
Seattle Children's Hospital
Seattle, Washington

Justin N. Baker, MD
Assistant Member
Department of Pediatric Medicine
Division of Palliative and End-of-Life Care
St. Jude Children's Research Hospital
Memphis, Tennessee

Charles B. Berde, MD, PhD
Division Chief, Pain Medicine
Senior Associate in Perioperative Anesthesia and Pain
    Medicine
Professor of Anaesthesia (Pediatrics)
Harvard Medical School
Children's Hospital Boston
Boston, Massachusetts

Myra Bluebond-Langner, PhD
Professor and True Colours Chair in Palliative Care for
    Children and Young People
Louis Dundas Centre for Children's Palliative Care
University College London
Institute of Child Health in Partnership with Great Ormond
    Street Hospital
London, United Kingdom

Elizabeth D. Blume, MD
Associate Professor
Harvard Medical School
Medical Director
Heart Failure/Transplant Program
Children's Hospital Boston
Boston, Massachusetts

Renee Boss, MD
Assistant Professor
Division of Neonatology
Department of Pediatrics
Johns Hopkins University School of Medicine
Baltimore, Maryland

Kimberly A. Bower, MD
Medical Director
San Diego Hospice and Palliative Care
San Diego, California

Debra Boyer, MD
Pediatric Pulmonologist
Children's Hospital
Boston, Massachusetts

Alberto Broniscer, MD
Associate Member
Department of Oncology
St. Jude Children's Research Hospital
Memphis, Tennessee

Janie Brooks, M Div BCC
Staff Chaplain
The Children's National Medical Center
Washington, DC

Michelle R. Brown, PhD
Clinical Associate Professor of Psychiatry
    Division of Child Psychiatry
Stanford University School of Medicine
Lucile Packard Children's Hospital at Stanford
Palo Alto, California

Susan Cadell, MSW PhD
Acting Dean
Faculty of Social Work
Wilfrid Laurier University
Kitchener, Ontario
Canada

Naimah Campbell, RN, BSN
Nurse Clinician
Circle of Life Children's Center, Inc.
The University of Medicine and Dentistry of New Jersey
    (UMDNJ)
New Jersey Medical School (NJMS)
Newark, New Jersey

Jean Marie Carroll, RN, MSN
Program Manager
NeuroCardiac Care Program
The Cardiac Care Center at The Children's Hospital of
    Philadelphia
Philadelphia, Pennsylvania

Colette Case, MA, CCLS, CTRS
Director, Child and Family Life Services
Lucile Packard Children's Hospital at Stanford
Palo Alto, California

Melanie Chan, Pharm.D.
Pharmacy Operations Manager
Lucile Packard Children's Hospital at Stanford
Palo Alto, California

Jody Chrastek, MSN RN
Pain and Palliative Care Coordinator
Children's Hospitals and Clinics of Minnesota
Minneapolis, Minnesota

Harvey J. Cohen, MD, PhD
Deborah E. Addicott - John A. Kriewall and Elizabeth
   A. Haehl Family Professor of Pediatrics, Stanford University
   School of Medicine
Katie and Paul Dougherty Medical Director
   Palliative Care Program
Lucile Packard Children's Hospital at Stanford
Palo Alto, California

John J. Collins, MB BS, PhD, FFPMANZCA, FAChPM, FRACP
Head of Department
Pain Medicine and Palliative Care
The Children's Hospital at Westmead
Sydney, Australia
Clinical Associate Professor
Discipline of Paediatrics and Child Health
Sydney Medical School
University of Sydney
Sydney, Australia

Nancy Contro, MSW, LCSW
Palliative Care Program
Lucile Packard Children's Hospital at Stanford
Palo Alto, California

Betty Davies, RN, PhD, FAAN
Professor and Chair
Department of Family Health Care Nursing
University of California, San Francisco
San Francisco, California

Dawn Davies, MD, FRCPC
Associate Professor, Department of Pediatrics
University of Alberta
Medical Director
Pediatric Palliative Care Program
Stollery Children's Hospital
Edmonton, Alberta
Canada

Pedro A. De Alarcón, MD
William H. Albers Professor and Chair
Department of Pediatrics
University of Illinois College of Medicine at Peoria
Peoria, Illinois

Elisabeth Potts Dellon, MD, MPH
Assistant Professor
Department of Pediatrics, Division of Pulmonology
North Carolina Children's Hospital
University of North Carolina School of Medicine
Chapel Hill, North Carolina

Deborah L. Dokken, MPA
Family Health Care Advocate
Former Associate Director
Initiative for Pediatric Palliative Care
Chevy Chase, Maryland

Helen Douglas, BSc, (Hons), MCSP
Clinical Specialist Pediatric Physiotherapist
Children's Hospital Oxford
Headington, Oxford
United Kingdom

Ross Drake, BSc, MBChB, FRACP, FChPM
Paediatric Palliative Care and Pain Specialist
Clinical Director Paediatric Palliative Care and Complex Pain
   Services
Starship Children's Hospital
Auckland District Health Board
Auckland, New Zealand

Sarah Dugan, MD
Clinical Geneticist
Children's Hospitals and Clinics of Minnesota
Minneapolis, Minnesota

Janet Duncan, RN, MSN, CPNP, CPON
Nursing Director
Pediatric Palliative Care Division
Children's Hospital Boston
Dana-Farber Cancer Institute
Boston, Massachusetts

Amy Durall, MD
Assistant in Critical Care
Department of Anesthesia
Perioperative and Pain Medicine
Children's Hospital Boston
Boston, Massachusetts

Reverend Kathleen Ennis-Durstine, BCC
Senior Chaplain
Manager of Pastoral and Spiritual Care
The Children's National Medical Center
Washington, DC

Elana E. Evan, PhD
Assistant Professor of Pediatrics
Department of Pediatrics
David Geffen School of Medicine at UCLA
Director, UCLA Children's Comfort Care Program, Pediatrics
Mattel Children's Hospital, UCLA
Los Angeles, California

Chris Feudtner, MD, PhD, MPH
Research Director, Pediatric Advanced Care Team
Director, Department of Medical Ethics
Stephen D. Handler Endowed Chair of Medical Ethics
The Children's Hospital of Philadelphia
Philadelphia, Pennsylvania

Mary B. Fleck, EdD, CT
Coordinator of Bereavement Services
Circle of Life Children's Center
University of Medicine and Dentistry of New Jersey (UMDNJ)
Newark, New Jersey

Onajovwe Fofah, MD, FAAP
Associate Medical Director
Circle of Life Children's Center of New Jersey
Assistant Professor
Attending Neonatologist
Division of Neonatology
Department of Pediatrics
Newark, New Jersey

Gerri Frager, MD
Medical Director Pediatric Palliative Care
IWK Health Centre
Professor, Faculty of Medicine
Director, Medical Humanities
Dalhousie University
Halifax, Nova Scotia
Canada

Lorry R. Frankel, MD, MBA
Professor Emeritus
Stanford University School of Medicine
Emeritus Medical Director
Critical Care and Palliative Care Services
Lucile Packard Children's Hospital
Chair of Pediatrics
Sutter/California Pacific Medical Center
San Francisco, California

Dawn Freiberger, RN, MSN
Lung Transplant Coordinator
Children's Hospital Boston
Boston, Massachusetts

David R. Freyer, DO, MS
Director
LIFE Cancer Survivorship and Transition Program
Childrens Center for Cancer and Blood Diseases
Childrens Hospital Los Angeles
Professor of Clinical Pediatrics
Keck School of Medicine
University of Southern California
Los Angeles, California

Sarah Friebert, MD
Director
Haslinger Family Center for Pediatric Palliative Care
Akron Children's Hospital
Associate Professor of Pediatrics
Northeastern Ohio Universities College of Medicine
Akron, Ohio

Stefan J. Friedrichsdorf, MD
Medical Director Pain Medicine and Palliative Care
Children's Hospitals and Clinics of Minnesota
Minneapolis, Minnesota

Judith A. Frost, RN, Dip Ed, MN
Clinical Nurse Consultant
The Children's Hospital at Westmead
Sydney, Australia

Michelle Frost, RN
Nurse Manager
Consultant
Pediatric Advanced Care Team
Seattle Children's Hospital
Seattle, Washington

Amanda Gamble, PhD, MClinPsych
Postdoctoral Research Fellow
Woolcock Institute of Medical Research
Sydney, Australia

Mary Jo Gilmer, PhD, MBA, CNLhD, MBA, CNS, CNL, RN-BC
Professor of Nursing
Professor of Pediatrics
Monroe Carell Jr. Children's Hospital at Vanderbilt
Co-Director, Pediatric Palliative Care Research Team
Nashville, Tennessee

Ann Goldman, MB, FRCP
Great Ormond Street Hospital for Children
London, United Kingdom

Michelle Goldsmith, MD, MA
Chief Fellow
Stanford Child and Adolescent Psychiatry
Stanford, California

Richard Goldstein, MD
Attending Physician
Division of Pediatric Palliative Care
Department of Psychosocial Oncology and Palliative Care
Dana-Farber Cancer Institute
Department of Medicine
Children's Hospital Boston
Harvard Medical School
Boston, Massachusetts

Angela Green, PhD, APN
Director of Nursing Research
John Boyd Family Endowed Chair in Pediatric Nursing
    Arkansas Children's Hospital
Clinical Associate Professor
University of Arkansas for Medical Sciences
College of Nursing
Little Rock, Arkansas

Shireen V. Guide, MD
Dermatologist
Saddleback Dermatology Laser Center
Lake Forest, California

Richard Hain, MBBS, MSc, MD, MRCP(UK), FRCPCH, DipPalMed
Lead Clinician in Paediatric Palliative Medicine
Senior Lecturer in Child Health
Cardiff University School of Medicine
Children's Hospital for Wales
Cardiff, Wales
United Kingdom

Julie Hauer, MD
Pediatric Palliative Care Physician
Children's Hospital Boston
Boston, Massachusetts

Ross M. Hays, MD
Professor
Departments of Rehabilitation Medicine, Pediatrics, and Bioethics and Humanities
University of Washington School of Medicine
Medical Director
PACT — Pediatric Palliative Care Program
Children's Hospital and Regional Medical Center
Seattle, Washington

Lynne Helfand, MSW, LICSW, MPH
Lung Transplant Social Worker
Children's Hospital Boston
Boston, Massachusetts

Anthony Herbert, MBBS, B Med Sc, FRACP, FAchPM
Staff Specialist in Paediatric Palliative Care
Oncology-Haematology Service
Royal Children's Hospital
Children's Health Services District
Melbourne, Australia

Joy Hesselgrave, MSN, RN, CPON
Clinical Specialist
Texas Children's Cancer Center and Hematology Service
Texas Children's Hospital
Houston, Texas

Kari Hexem, MPH
Clinical Research Associate
Children's Hospital of Philadelphia
Philadelphia, Pennsylvania

Marilyn Hockenberry, PhD, RN, PNP-BC, FAAN
Professor Hematology/Oncology Section
Department of Pediatrics
Baylor College of Medicine
Nurse Scientist
Texas Children's Hospital
Houston, Texas

Nancy Hutton, MD
Associate Professor and Medical Director
Harriet Lane Compassionate Care Team
General Pediatrics and Adolescent Medicine
Johns Hopkins University
Baltimore, Maryland

Shana S. Jacobs, MD
Assistant Professor
George Washington University
Attending Physician
Leukemia/Lymphoma Program and Pediatric Advanced Needs Assessment and Care Team (PANDA)
Center for Cancer and Blood Disorders
Children's National Medical Center
Washington, DC

Barbara L. Jones, PhD, MSW
Associate Professor
Co-Director
The Institute for Grief, Loss, and Family Survival
University of Texas Austin School of Social Work
Austin, Texas

Marsha Joselow, MSW, LICSW
Social Worker and Director Social Work Fellowship Program
Pediatric Advanced Care Team (PACT)
Children's Hospital Boston
Dana-Farber Cancer Institute
Boston, Massachusetts

Javier R. Kane, MD
Director
Division of Palliative and End-of-Life Care
Associate Member
Department of Pediatric Medicine
St. Jude Children's Research Hospital
Memphis, Tennessee

Karen Kavanaugh, PhD, RN, FAAN
Professor
Department of Women, Children, and Family Health Science
Co-Director
Center for End-of-Life Transition Research
University of Illinois at Chicago College of Nursing
Chicago, Illinois

Jeffrey C. Klick, MD
Assistant Professor of Pediatrics
University of Pennsylvania School of Medicine
Fellowship Director
Pediatric Hospice and Palliative Medicine
Division of General Pediatrics
Children's Hospital of Philadelphia
Philadelphia, Pennsylvania

Kathie Kobler, MS, RN
ELNEC-Core and ELNEC-Pediatric Palliative Care
Advocate Lutheran General Hospital
Park Ridge, Illinois

Robin Kramer, RN, MS, PNP
Co-Director, Compass Care
Pediatric Palliative Care Program
University of California at San Francisco Children's Hospital
San Francisco, California

Ulrika Kreicbergs, RN, PhD
Associate Professor
Nurse Scientist
Karolinska Institutet
Lecturer
Sophiahemmet University College
Stockholm, Sweden

Deborah A. Lafond, MS, PNP-BC, CPON
Nurse Practitioner
Neuro-Oncology and PANDA Care Team
Department of Hematology/Oncology
Children's National Medical Center
Washington, DC

John D. Lantos, MD
Professor of Pediatrics
University of Missouri at Kansas City
Director
Children's Mercy Bioethics Center
Children's Mercy Hospital
Kansas City, Missouri

Stephen Liben, MD
Associate Professor of Pediatrics
McGill University
Director
Pediatric Palliative Care Program
The Montreal Children's Hospital
Montreal, Quebec
Canada

Grace MacConnell, RN MN CHPCN(C)
Clinical Nurse Specialist
IWK Health Centre
Halifax, Nova Scotia
Canada

Jennifer W. Mack, MD, MPH
Assistant Professor of Pediatrics
Harvard Medical School
Division of Pediatric Hematology/Oncology
Dana-Farber Cancer Institute
Children's Hospital Boston
Boston, Massachusetts

Michael McCown, DO
Pulmonary Fellow
Children's Hospital Boston
Medical Corps
United States Army
Boston, Massachusetts

Gerit D. Mulder, DPM, MS
Associate Clinical Professor of Surgery
Associate Clinical Professor of Orthopedics
Director Wound Treatment and Research Center
University of California
San Diego, California

Anna C. Muriel, MD, MPH
Chief
Division of Pediatric Psychosocial Oncology
Dana-Farber Cancer Institute
Assistant Professor of Psychiatry
Harvard Medical School
Boston, Massachusetts

Linda Muro-Garcia, LCSW
Lead Social Worker
Jonathan Jaques Children's Cancer Center
Miller Children's Hospital
Long Beach, California

Amrita D. Naipaul, MSN, PCCNP
Professional Pain Practice Specialist
Children's National Medical Center
Washington, DC

Helen Wells O'Brien, M Ed, M Div, BCC
Staff Chaplain
Regions Hospital and Gillette Children's Specialty Healthcare
St. Paul, Minnesota

James Oleske, MD, MPH
François-Xavier Bagnoud Professor of Pediatrics
Director, Division of Pulmonary
Allergy, Immunology, and Infectious Diseases
Department of Pediatrics
University of Medicine and Dentistry of New Jersey (UMDNJ)
Newark, New Jersey

Stacy F. Orloff, Ed D, LCSW, ACHP-SW
Vice President
Palliative Care and Community Programs
Suncoast Hospice
Clearwater, Florida

Paulina Ortiz-Rubio, BA
Medical Student
Stanford Medical School
Palo Alto, California

Maryland Pao, MD
Clinical Director
National Institute of Mental Health
National Institutes of Health
Washington, DC

Danai Papadatou, PhD
Professor of Clinical Psychology
Faculty of Nursing
University of Athens
Athens, Greece

Jessica Parker-Raley, MA
Assistant Professor
Basic Course Director
University of Texas Pan American
Department of Communication
Edinburg, Texas

Philip A. Pizzo, MD
Dean of the School of Medicine
Carl and Elizabeth Naumann Professor
Professor of Pediatrics and of Microbiology and Immunology
Stanford University School of Medicine
Stanford, California

Gregory H. Reaman, MD
Chair, Children's Oncology Group
George Washington University
School of Medicine and Health Sciences
Washington, DC

Reverend Wilma J. Reichard, M Div, M A R
Chaplain
Lucile Packard Children's Hospital at Stanford
Palo Alto, California

Anke Reineke, PhD, BCIAC
Psychologist
Rady Children's Hospital
San Diego, California

Stacy S. Remke, MSW, LICSW
Children's Institute for Pain and Palliative Care
Pain and Palliative Care Program
Children's Hospitals and Clinics
Minneapolis, Minnesota

Walter M. Robinson, MD, MPH
Associate Professor of Pediatrics and Medical Ethics
Vanderbilt University
Division of Pediatric Pulmonary Medicine
Vanderbilt Children's Hospital
Nashville, Tennessee

Brian R. Rood, MD
Director of Clinical Neuro-Oncology
Children's National Medical Center
Assistant Professor of Pediatrics
George Washington University School of Medicine
Washington, DC

Mary Elizabeth Ross, MD, PhD
Assistant Professor of Pediatrics
University of Illinois College of Medicine at Peoria
Adjunct Member St. Jude Children's Research Hospital
St. Jude Midwest Affiliate at Children's Hospital of Illinois
Peoria, Illinois

Mary T. Rourke, PhD
Psychologist
The Children's Hospital of Philadelphia
Philadelphia, Pennsylvania

Sally Sehring, MD
Health Sciences Clinical Professor
Department of Pediatrics
Division of Neonatology
University of California San Francisco Children's Hospital
San Francisco, California

Chris Seton, MBBS, FRACP
Respiratory and Sleep Paediatrician
Department of Respiratory Medicine
The Children's Hospital at Westmead
Sydney, Australia

Richard J. Shaw, MB, BS
Professor of Psychiatry and Pediatrics
Department of Psychiatry and Behavioral Sciences
Stanford University School of Medicine
Medical Director
Pediatric Psychosomatic Medicine Service
Lucile Packard Children's Hospital at Stanford
Palo Alto, California

Harold Siden, MD, MHSc, FRCPC
Medical Director
Canuck Place Children's Hospice
Division of General Pediatrics
British Columbia Children's Hospital
Clinical Associate Professor, Pediatrics
University of British Columbia
Vancouver, British Columbia
Canada

Sandra Staveski, RN, MS, CPNP-AC, CNS, CCRN
Cardiovascular ICU Nurse Practitioner
Lucile Packard Children's Hospital at Stanford
Assistant Clinical Professor
University of California at San Francisco
Department of Family Health Care Nursing
Palo Alto, California

Rose Steele, RN, PhD
Professor
School of Nursing
Faculty of Health
York University
Toronto, Ontario
Canada

David M. Steinhorn, MD
Professor in Pediatrics
Children's Memorial Hospital
Chicago, Illinois

Lynn Straatman, MD, FRCPC
Assistant Clinical Professor
University of British Columbia
British Columbia Children's Hospital
Vancouver, British Columbia
Canada

Nancy Sydnor-Greenberg, MA
Coordinator
Learning Services Program
American University
Washington, DC

Renee Temme, MS, CGC
Genetic Counselor
Children's Hospitals and Clinics of Minnesota
Minneapolis, Minnesota

Christina Ullrich, MD, MPH
Attending Physician
Pediatric Hematology
Oncology and Hematopoietic Stem Cell Transplant
Pediatric Advanced Care Team
Dana-Farber Cancer Institute
Children's Hospital Boston
Harvard Medical School
Boston, Massachusetts

Tamara Vesel, MD
Director
Pediatric Palliative Fellowship
Instructor in Pediatrics
Harvard Medical School
Dana-Farber Cancer Institute and Children's Hospital
Boston, Massachusetts

Joetta Deswarte Wallace, MSN, RN, FNPC, CPON
Palliative Care Program Coordinator
Miller Children's Hospital
Long Beach, California

Sheila Lenihan Walsh, APRN, BC
Director of Program Services
Circle of Life Children's Center, Inc.
Newark, New Jersey

M. Louise Webster, MBChB, FRACP, FRANZCP
Child and Adolescent Psychiatrist
Clinical Director Paediatric Consultation Liaison Team
Starship Children's Hospital
Auckland District Health Board
Auckland, New Zealand

Kimberley Widger, RN, MScN
PhD Candidate
Lawrence S. Bloomberg Faculty of Nursing
University of Toronto
Toronto, Ontario
Canada

Lori Wiener, PhD
Head, Psychosocial Support and Research Program
Pediatric Oncology Branch
National Cancer Institute
National Institutes of Health
Bethesda, Maryland

Joseph L. Wright, MD, MPH
Senior Vice President
Child Health Advocacy Institute
Faculty, Emergency Medicine and Trauma
Principal Investigator, Children's Research Institute (CRI)
Children's National Medical Center
Professor, Pediatrics (Vice Chair)
Emergency Medicine
School of Medicine and Health Sciences
Professor, Health Policy, Prevention, and Community Health
School of Public Health and Health Services
George Washington University
Washington, DC

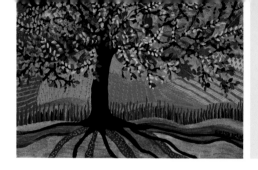

Foreword

I have been awed and inspired by the strength, resilience, and wisdom of children and parents facing life-threatening diseases. I have also been amazed by the insights that even young children have about end-of-life transitions – including the prospect of their own imminent death. Sadly, there are times when the awareness of children and their families is more realistic and transparent than that of those entrusted with their care and well-being. In part, this reflects the orientation of the health care professionals who enter the broad fields of pediatrics and child health. Most children, even those with serious illness, do survive. But when the prospects for life are challenged, many of those same providers are ill-equipped to engage in a supportive and caring role with the dying child and her or his family. Some find the possibility of a death during childhood too hard to cope with, but many have simply not been adequately trained to provide proactive palliative care.

The prospect and profiles for death in children are quite variegated. The neonatologist, for example, will often experience the death of an infant with whom a personal relationship never formed. The entire encounter is around acute illness measured in days to weeks. In contrast, the pulmonologist caring for a child with cystic fibrosis will forge a deep relationship with an infant or child that endures over many years or decades. This is now frequently coupled with passing the care of the patient to a adult care provider who may be less aware of the patient's long struggle for quality-of-life punctuated by a gradual decline toward death. For the pediatric oncologist the possibility of death is both acute and chronic and is sometimes clearly demarcated, but at other times can be associated with denial – by both the provider and the family.

I believe that all physicians entering medicine and pediatrics should be trained in palliative as well as therapeutic and preventive medicine. Importantly, physicians must be educated as members of the interdisciplinary team that also includes palliative-trained doctors, nurses, social workers, psychologists, pharmacists, and others who deliver modern palliative care. This will require reformation of education programs for medical students as well as those entering pediatric residencies and allied professions. The depth of this training can be tailored to the nature of the specialty and should be deep and comprehensive for those involved in the care of children with acute or chronic disorders that have likelihood for death. In addition, education and training is needed for those adult care specialists who assume the care of children with chronic disorders when they graduate from pediatric care. An important emphasis should be placed on team-based management. This is a difficult time for the patient and the family, and it is important that adult specialists approach these patients with sensitivity and awareness of the decades that the child and family have already expended in medical care.

Although it is the responsibility of all pediatric and adult care providers of childhood disease survivors to be knowledgeable in palliative care, it is also important to underscore that pediatric palliative care has emerged as a discipline that requires the coordination of a number of medical, nursing, psychological social work, and other specialties – in both ambulatory and hospital settings that are in communities as well as major pediatric centers. Not only do these palliative care experts and specialists provide direct support to children and families, but they also are the source for coordination of care and for the education of the broader pediatric community. It is for *all* these reasons and more that the *Textbook of Interdisciplinary Pediatric Palliative Care* by Joanne Wolfe, Pamela Hinds, and Barbara Sourkes is such a landmark. In fact, I would add an additional word that describes this book – "comprehensive."

Wolfe, Hinds, and Sourkes provide an authoritative compendium that defines the scope and programs needed for effective and compassionate care, the professionals who engage in this discipline, and the knowledge they require to support the child and family with a wide range of disorders. It is a resource for palliative care specialists as well as pediatric providers caring for high-risk children.

During my career I have personally cared for many children and families of children who have died because of cancer, AIDS, and other disorders. I would like to think that I served as a compassionate physician who offered knowledgeable end-of-life care. However, I must admit that my education and training in palliative care was empirical and experiential and not driven by data, defined principles, or guidelines. I doubt I am alone. Thankfully, with the *Textbook of Interdisciplinary Pediatric Palliative Care*, a resource exists to help and guide providers and, as an important and vital extension, to help children and families. For this I thank the authors and editors for their contributions as educators and providers of compassionate and comprehensive palliative care.

Philip A. Pizzo, MD

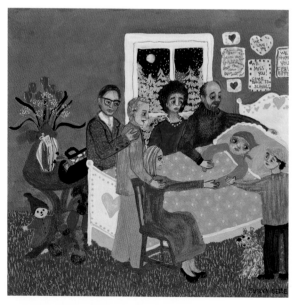

Holding the Moment by Evelyn Berde, (2007)

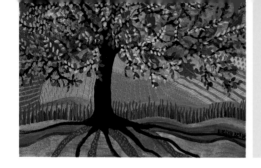

Preface

Pediatric palliative care is a new frontier in the comprehensive care of children. Children living with life-threatening conditions have always been part of the health care system; however, only now is an integrated vision toward their care emerging. Although the field of palliative care is based on the principle that an interdisciplinary team should care for patients (adult and pediatric) and their families throughout the illness trajectory, most clinical texts are specific to a single discipline. The *Textbook of Interdisciplinary Pediatric Palliative Care* is the first in the field to be written by and for interdisciplinary clinicians who care for children and adolescents living with life-threatening conditions. Our editorial team is interdisciplinary (medicine, nursing, psychology) and our discussions consistently speak to the essential and remarkable contributions to pediatric palliative care from all disciplines. These discussions reflect our shared belief that the highest quality pediatric palliative care is indeed, interdisciplinary. Most of the chapters in this textbook are co-authored by an interdisciplinary group. The organization and content of the textbook purposefully encompass perspectives across and between disciplines. Although the chapters address the specific needs and responsibilities of individual professions, we feel that the interwoven perspectives from many disciplines best convey the dynamism and creativity of our newly emerging field. We believe that the interwoven perspectives provide the basis for an effective care alignment with the ill child or adolescent and with the family.

Textbook of Interdisciplinary Pediatric Palliative Care highlights current concepts and interventions as well as future directions in pediatric palliative care. The underlying principles and ethics of palliative care are universal across the life span. However, as in all specialties, children bring with them unique issues and dilemmas. A child or adolescent with a life-threatening condition throws an assumed sequence out of order. A time of role reversal is expected, when children will care for dying parents. When parents instead find themselves watching their child face the threat of death—imminent or not any sense of order is shattered. There is little preparation for separation by death even before a child has passed through the separation that occurs in the sequence of normal development. The adolescent who is beginning to negotiate an independent existence is often especially hard to face when that "moving forward" is irreversibly halted, or at least disrupted. A child has not even had the chance to form life goals. In mirror image, and all too early in life, the healthy siblings also live the experience of illness and the threat or actuality of loss.

We will be honored and pleased if the *Textbook of Interdisciplinary Pediatric Palliative Care* proves valuable to students and new and senior clinicians who practice in multiple settings. Our overriding hope is that the book adds meaning for all clinicians in their experience of providing pediatric palliative care. We thank all of our authors and Pamela Hetherington, our editor, who has been a full partner in developing this text. We are grateful to Evelyn Berde for allowing us to reprint three pieces of her vivid artwork on the cover and the frontispiece pages. Finally, we thank Dr. Philip Pizzo for his insightful foreword.

Joanne Wolfe, MD, MPH
Pamela S. Hinds, RN, PhD, FAAN
Barbara M. Sourkes, PhD

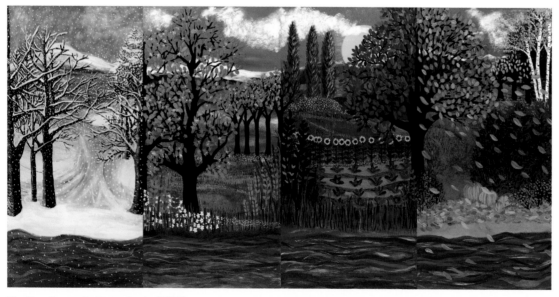

The Four Seasons by Evelyn Berde, (2008)

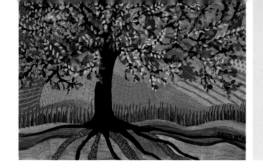

Contents

SECTION 4
Illness and Treatment Experience

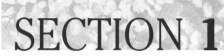

SECTION 1 Setting the Stage

Children are born with rainbows in their hearts and you'll never reach them unless you reckon with rainbows.
                                                                —Carl Sandburg

We hope that the lives of all children will be filled with possibility, with open horizons and rainbows into the future. Children with life-threatening illnesses, their families, and those who care for them, confront the realization that "not everything is possible," that despite dramatic scientific and medical advances, the lifespan of some children will be abbreviated. This threat of premature loss heightens the sense of time for children and families alike, and challenges clinicians to create new pathways of hope for them.

The interdisciplinary field of pediatric palliative care has emerged over the last two decades, with rapid development in clinical care, education, research, and policy. In this section, *"Setting the Stage,"* themes and constructs that encompass the spectrum of care provide a conceptual framework for the book.

Words define, clarify, and communicate experience; their potential impact is powerful, in both positive and negative ways. The importance of a common language cannot be underestimated when clinicians from many disciplines care for children and families who face extraordinary challenges. The opening chapter, "The Language of Pediatric Palliative Care" sets this foundation.

Who are these children? Who are the parents and families who care for them? The chapter on the epidemiology of pediatric palliative care portrays the distribution of conditions, their trajectories and symptoms, and trends in mortality. Families are discussed with regard to their structure, the "work of care" for the child, coping and financial issues. Overarching both the child and family variables are epidemiological factors in health care systems at regional, national, and international levels.

In "Children's Voices" these children and their siblings provide another type of portrait: through their own words and images they convey their experience of *living* with illness: their awareness of its life-threatening nature, the undercurrent of anticipatory grief and their role in decision-making. The next chapter focuses on the establishment of a therapeutic alliance between the interdisciplinary team and the family as a *sine qua non* of optimal care. Clear communication, trust, and non-judgmental understanding of the family's beliefs and values are critical factors. The meaning of hope in families is discussed with relation to anticipatory planning, decision-making and continuity of care. The themes of these two chapters weave together in "Anticipatory Grief and Bereavement."

Who cares for these children and families, and where? "The Team" provides the conceptual underpinnings of a dynamic interdisciplinary approach. In relationship-centered care, the subjective impact of caring for these children shapes the team's understanding of the patient and family's experience, and ultimately affects the quality of care. "Settings of Care" describes the distinctive cultures of the hospital, particularly the intensive care unit; emergency services; and community resources, including home hospice, palliative care and respite facilities, and schools. The crucial importance of a seamless transition between and among these settings is emphasized. "Program Development and Implementation" provides comprehensive guidelines to establishing a pediatric palliative care program. Although the focus is on the hospital setting, the underlying principles are relevant for any institution or agency that serves these children.

The acquisition and dissemination of knowledge is the subject of the following three chapters. How can the best research evidence be combined with clinical expertise to provide optimal care for these children and families? What are the complexities unique to research in the field of pediatric palliative care? What are the challenges and strategies in interdisciplinary education? The "pioneering" and creativity necessary in establishing a new field is a theme common to the chapters.

"Setting the Stage" closes with chapters on ethics and spirituality, both integral to the principles of pediatric palliative care. Ethics is an overlapping domain; spirituality is a thread that, in many forms, unites the experience of children, families, and teams. Both address profound questions of suffering, meaning, and hope.

1

The Language of Pediatric Palliative Care

JOANNE WOLFE | PAMELA S. HINDS | BARBARA M. SOURKES
WITH CONTRIBUTIONS FROM ALL CHAPTER AUTHORS

Words are deeds. The words we hear
May revolutionize or rear
A mighty state. The words we read
May be a spiritual deed
Excelling any fleshly one,
As much as the celestial sun
Transcends a bonfire, made to throw
A light upon some raree-show.
A simple proverb tagged with rhyme
May colour half the course of time;
The pregnant saying of a sage
May influence every coming age;
A song in its effects may be
More glorious than Thermopylae,
And many a lay that schoolboys scan
A nobler feat than Inkerman
   —William Charles Wentworth

Basic words such as palliative care, end-of-life care, and terminal care are often used interchangeably, yet they convey very different meanings to clinicians, patients, and families. Those different meanings can lead to unintentioned harmful consequences. As stated by Dr. Eric Cassell, "Similar to scalpels for surgeons, words are the palliative care clinician's greatest tools. Surgeons learn to use their tools with extreme precision, because any error can be devastating. So too should clinicians who rely on words." (Personal communication) A primary focus of the textbook is to promote consistent use of predefined terminology as a means of exemplifying this critical tenet of palliative care.

Definition of Terms

The definitions of words in this chapter were derived through consensus. Specifically, the list of terms were generated by the editors and distributed to all authors for review. Any suggested edits were then considered by the editors and if consensus agreement was reached, then the edit was incorporated. Additional terms were also suggested by chapter authors and the same process was used to determine whether such terms should be included in this overview.

LIFE-THREATENING OR LIFE-LIMITING?

Differences of opinion exist about whether the term *life-threatening* (where cure may be possible) or the term *life-limiting* (no realistic hope of cure) is more appropriate when defining palliative care conditions. In this textbook we use the broadest term, life-threatening, because we believe that most serious illnesses are characterized by prognostic uncertainty, with little consensus among experts regarding which conditions have "no reasonable hope for cure."

ILLNESS

The subjective experience of a patient with an underlying disease or medical condition.[1]

PALLIATIVE CARE

The term *palliative care* is from the Latin *palliare*, to cloak.[2]

Palliative care is an approach that improves the quality of life of patients and their families facing the problems associated with life-threatening illness, through the prevention and relief of suffering by means of early identification and impeccable assessment and treatment of pain and other problems, physical, psychosocial, and spiritual. Palliative care:

- Considers the patient and family as the center of the unit of care,
- Provides relief from pain and other distressing symptoms,
- Affirms life and regards dying as a normal process,
- Intends neither to hasten nor to postpone death,
- Integrates the psychological and spiritual aspects of patient care,
- Offers a support system to help patients live as actively as possible until death,
- Offers a support system to help the family cope during the patient's illness and in their own bereavement,
- Uses a team approach to address the needs of patients and their families, including bereavement counseling, if indicated,
- Aims to enhance quality of life, and may also positively influence the course of illness,
- Is applicable early in the course of illness, in conjunction with other therapies that are intended to prolong life, and includes those investigations needed to better understand and manage distressing clinical complications.

WHO Definition of Palliative Care for Children (Adapted)[2]

Palliative care for children represents a special, albeit closely related, field to adult palliative care. WHO's definition of palliative care appropriate for children and their families:

- Is the active total care of the child's body, mind, and spirit, and also involves giving support to the family,
- Begins when illness is diagnosed, and continues regardless of whether or not a child receives treatment directed at the disease,
- Demands that health providers evaluate and alleviate a child's physical, psychological, and social distress,
- Requires a broad interdisciplinary approach,
- Includes the family and makes use of available community resources; it can be successfully implemented even if resources are limited,
- Can be provided in tertiary care facilities, in community health and hospice centers, and in children's homes,
- Should be developmentally appropriate and in accordance with family values.

END-OF-LIFE CARE OR TERMINAL CARE

Unlike most of palliative care, which is often delivered in the context of prognostic uncertainty, the term *end-of-life care* or *terminal care* refers to the care delivered when the prognosis of death is almost certain and close in time. Examples include a patient with advanced refractory metastatic cancer who is expected to die within days or weeks, or a patient with end-stage lung disease who had been maintained on high ventilator settings when this technological support is withdrawn. Exceptions arise and patients can survive well beyond what was expected to be an earlier death. *Comfort care* is often used to describe the interdisciplinary care provided at this time. However, there is little consensus on what comprises comfort care, and as such, the term should be avoided.

HOSPICE

In the United States, *hospice* is a Medicare benefit[3] and is defined as a special way of caring for people who are *terminally ill*. Hospice care involves a team-oriented approach that addresses the medical, physical, social, emotional, and spiritual needs of the patient. Hospice provides support to the patient's family and/or caregiver as well. Hospice care is given by a public agency or private company approved by Medicare. It is for all age groups during a patient's final stages of life. The goal of hospice is to care for a terminally ill patient and family, not to cure the illness.

Outside the United States, hospice is a term used to describe a philosophy of care that focuses on the palliation of terminally ill patients. The term is also often used in association with a building, which may house patients receiving terminal care and/or a hospice program serving patients in the community.

DYING

Dying refers to the period when a patient is approaching death within days, hours, or moments. Though in conversations with patients clinicians may echo terms used by patients and/or family members such as "passing away" or "at life's end," these gentler terms should be avoided in this textbook unless being used as a communication example.

HOSPICE AND PALLIATIVE CARE

Hospice and Palliative care is the term used to denote the interdisciplinary field as a whole.

HOSPICE AND PALLIATIVE MEDICINE

Hospice and Palliative medicine is the term used by the American Board of Medical Subspecialties to denote the physician subspecialty established in 2006.

MULTIDISCIPLINARY

This is a collection of disciplines in which each retains its own methodologies and assumptions, without change or development from the others. It is a linear model in which the disciplines run parallel to one other.

INTERDISCIPLINARY

An integrative model wherein people from multiple disciplines work together in addressing a common challenge. This model can be seen as overlapping circles (as in a Venn diagram) where each specialty maintains its own identity while also sharing some common methodologies and assumptions with other disciplines in the web. This collaborative work is more typical of pediatric palliative care and is the underlying tenet of this text (as per the title).

TRANSDISCIPLINARY

A term used with increasing frequency that does not yet have a stable, consensus meaning. Usage suggests that a transdisciplinary approach dissolves boundaries between disciplines. In a newly emerging field, porous boundaries may create confusion and undercut the richness and uniqueness of each discipline.

MEDICAL PROVIDER, MEDICAL CAREGIVER, OR CLINICIAN? PSYCHOSOCIAL CLINICIAN?

The most general term we would recommend using to refer to a practitioner of palliative care would be clinician, no matter what the underlying discipline, including physician, nurse, pharmacist, etc. Medical provider may connote physician, and caregiver is often used in referring to a layperson such as a family member who cares for a patient. Other acceptable terms include healthcare provider and mental health provider for psychologists, social workers, etc. However, if referring to a skill set unique to one of these types of clinicians, then that discipline should be explicitly named.

CHILD LIFE SPECIALIST

Child life specialists provide both therapeutic play interventions and social recreation for children on an individual and group basis.

CHAPLAIN

A *chaplain* is typically, although not always, a member of the clergy who serves in specific settings such as hospitals, hospices, or the military. Chaplains carry out religious rituals for families in addition to providing spiritual guidance and counseling.

OPIOID

An *opioid* is a chemical substance that has a morphine-like action in the body. These agents work by binding to opioid receptors, which are found principally in the central nervous system and the gastrointestinal tract. The receptors in these two organ systems mediate both the beneficial effects and the undesirable side effects. Although the term opiate is often used as a synonym for opioid, it is more properly limited to the natural opium alkaloids and the semi-synthetics derived from them.

There are a number of broad classes of opioids:

- Natural opiates (alkaloids contained in the resin of the opium poppy including morphine and codeine),
- Semi-synthetic opiates, created from the natural opioids, such as hydromorphone, hydrocodone, oxycodone, oxymorphone, desomorphine, diacetylmorphine (heroin), nicomorphine, dipropanoylmorphine, benzylmorphine, and ethylmorphine,
- Fully synthetic opioids, such as fentanyl, methadone, and tramadol,
- Endogenous opioid peptides, produced naturally in the body, such as endorphins, enkephalins, dynorphins, and endomorphins.

The term *narcotic* is believed to have been coined by the Greek physician Galen to refer to agents that benumb or deaden, causing loss of feeling or paralysis. It is based on the Greek word for narcosis, the term used by Hippocrates for the process of benumbing or the benumbed state. Because the term is often used broadly, inaccurately, or pejoratively outside medical contexts and often instills fear in families, we prefer the more precise term opioid.

RESUSCITATION STATUS AND DO NOT RESUSCITATE

Resuscitation status refers to the outcome of a discussion, or a series of discussions, among a patient and family and a clinician regarding the potential use of certain medical interventions in the care of a patient with life-threatening illness. Most healthcare facilities have a specific order form, entitled *Do Not Resuscitate (DNR)*, used to denote the patient's resuscitation status. The exact content of a DNR order varies widely depending on legal jurisdiction and individual facility interpretation. Terms such as Do Not Attempt Resuscitation (DNAR) and Allow Natural Death (AND) have been proposed to replace DNR in order to emphasize differing qualities of such orders. For example, DNAR negates the underlying assumption that if an intervention is employed, the outcome will be successful and has been recommended as a more acceptable term from a patient perspective, although this has not been explicitly studied among families of children with life-threatening illness. The expression "the parents signed the DNR" is misleading because in most settings they are not required to do so. It is more accurate to state the parents agreed to the recommendations of the healthcare team regarding resuscitation status.

ADDITIONAL TERMS TO AVOID

Withdrawal or Withholding of Support

These frequently used terms result in the unintended message that all care is ending, rather than just the particular intervention that is being stopped. We would greatly prefer to model language such as "ventilator support will be stopped or forgone because it is no longer clinically indicated, and maximal supportive care will be continued."

Closure

The word closure is used all too often, especially around bereavement, to denote some completion of a psychological process. In the words of Peggy Broxterman who lost a son in the Oklahoma City bombing, scoffing at the idea that Timothy McVeigh's execution could bring closure, "you close on a house, you don't close on a death." If the word closure is used, it must be qualified carefully.[4]

The Child Failed

The expression "the child failed treatment" or "the child failed extubation attempts" implies that the child was at fault in the intervention not succeeding. Truly no one has failed anything or anyone (neither the child, nor the clinical team); rather, a treatment or procedure was unsuccessful. As such, the word "failure" should be avoided.

Labeling the Child with His/Her Disease

A frequently used shortcut is to label the child with the name of the underlying illness, for example, "the leukemic child" or "the hypoplast." A preferable approach, though slightly longer, is "the child with leukemia" or "with hypoplastic left heart syndrome."

"Mom" and "Dad"

These terms are frequently used when talking about or with parents. The only time "mom" and "dad" should be used is when the child talks to them or about them with another family member or friend. In written vignettes, we would recommend using "the mother," "the father," "the parents," an initial, or pseudonym.

"Noncompliance"

Unintentionally or not, this term has come to suggest a *willful* ignoring of instructions, although many factors often contribute to an inability to follow through with medical recommendations. As such, health care professionals prefer to talk about "adherence" to a regimen rather than "compliance."

Summary

There are many other words used by clinicians in the care of children with life-threatening illness which can relay unintended potentially harmful messages to children, families, and members of the interdisciplinary team. Even simple words can be harmful. For example, Macdonald and Murray describe in detail how the term "appropriate" has replaced "normal" to describe what is suitable for a particular person, situation, or place.[5] Its use is "appropriate" when being used as a descriptor for the physical condition of the patient; for example, "the child's growth was *appropriate* for his age."

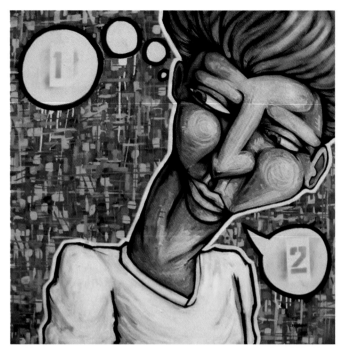

Fig. 1-1   Thinking Before Speaking, No.2, Painting by John Osgood. (Reprinted courtesy of the artist.)

However, they argue that the term is increasingly used to pass moral judgment; for example, "the mother's tears were *appropriate* given the news she had just received" or "the father's series of questions were *inappropriate*." From this example they conclude that there are many hidden values behind one's choice of words and phrases and eloquently state, "it is essential that we bring an awareness to our language. . . and reflect on what we mean, what messages we are [trying] to convey."[5] This emphasis on language is not intended to impart a heightened sense of anxiety around communication, rather to underscore the importance of, "thinking before speaking" (Fig. 1-1).

REFERENCES

1. Jennings D: The confusion between disease and illness in clinical medicine, *CMAJ* 135(8):865-870, 1986.
2. WHO Definition of Palliative Care: www.who.int/cancer/palliative/definition/en/. Accessed February 10, 2010.
3. Medicare Hospice Benefits: www.medicare.gov/publications/pubs/pdf/hosplg.pdf. Accessed February 10, 2010.
4. Newsweek: May 7, 2001, p 21. You close on a house. You don't close on a death. Peggy Broxterman, whose son was killed in the Oklahoma City bombing, commenting on the idea that Timothy McVeigh's execution could bring "closure."
5. Macdonald ME, Murray MA: The appropriateness of appropriate: smuggling values into clinical practice, *Can J Nurs Res* 39(4):58-73, 2007.

2 Epidemiology and the Care of Children with Complex Conditions

CHRIS FEUDTNER | KARI HEXEM | MARY T. ROURKE

The medical art consists in three things —
The disease, the patient, and the healer.

—Hippocratic *Epidemics*,

Book 1, Section 2

Epidemiology involves the science and art of comparison. While historically the ideas and tools of epidemiology were developed to study the distribution of health and disease in human populations and environmental factors associated with illnesses, modern epidemiologic concepts and methods can and are applied to a wide range of questions, from molecular to social epidemiology. Epidemiologic research can improve our understanding of how diseases and conditions affect various people in different places over time, and build evidence to either accept or reject certain cause-and-effect relationships. Increasingly, epidemiologic investigations also consider how human maladies are located in and affected by multilevel or hierarchical systems, such as families and communities or hospitals and health systems.

In this chapter, we apply an epidemiologic framework of investigation to the issues and challenges that we confront in pediatric palliative and hospice medicine. When people casually refer to the epidemiology of a particular illness or disease, they often mean the body of knowledge about the condition—who it affects and why, what happens to persons with the condition, and what is known about the effect of treatment for the condition—that has been built up through epidemiologic research. We try to encapsulate some of what is known about pediatric patients who receive palliative and hospice care, or more broadly children who die, while acknowledging that because these children suffer from a variety of conditions, ranging from acute trauma to complex and chronic, we must be. While presenting this information, we will also emphasize a systems-oriented perspective to the study of pediatric palliative and hospice care. While the Hippocratic practitioner of the medical art who authored the opening epigraph certainly emphasized core aspects of this systems perspective, we need to expand our practice and our science beyond the disease, patient, and a single healer. Many readers likely already consider the experience of individual children as best understood in the context of their family and healthcare, education, and other social services, as well as the systems of payment for services and laws and regulations that influence these other systems (Fig. 2-1). Our scheme is no more complicated than this common sense of the hierarchy of influences on the lives of children with life-threatening illness. Such a scheme provides not only an organized approach to the study of pediatric palliative and hospice care, but also provides insights as to how we can improve these systems. To make this

scheme as down-to-earth as possible, we will over the course of the chapter illustrate aspects of the different levels by tracing the profile of a single child.

Patients and Individual-Level Systems

Alex is a 3-year-old boy with a probable mitochondrial disorder. He has a nearly intractable seizure disorder, profound developmental disabilities, and recurrent respiratory illnesses that increasingly have culminated in hospitalizations, including a recent stay in the pediatric intensive care unit. Alex is on a slew of medications: three antiepileptic drugs, four stomach and bowel drugs, three respiratory drugs, and two drugs for spells of apparent discomfort. Alex also has a pulse oximeter and supplemental oxygen at home.

While each child receiving palliative care services is unique, there are discernable patterns of conditions and diseases, probabilities of mortality, symptoms and quality of life concerns, and receipt of specific palliative care pharmacologic treatments and other interventions.

CONDITIONS AND DISEASES

Not all children who die receive palliative care services, but national profiles of children who die provide the strongest epidemiological evidence to characterize the conditions and diseases of children receiving pediatric palliative care. Examining mortality data in the United States between 1999 and 2006 (Fig. 2-2), one notices immediately that infant deaths are due mostly to specific perinatal conditions, such as premature birth and congenital syndromes or chromosomal disorders, whereas older children are most likely to die from external causes, such as traumatic injury.

We can examine the number of children who die from complex chronic conditions (CCCs) as one statistic that can inform the field of pediatric palliative and hospice care by defining it as:

- Any medical condition that can reasonably be expected to last at least 12 months unless death intervenes,
- Any that involves either several organ systems or one organ system severely enough to require specialty pediatric care, with a likelihood of some period in a tertiary care center.

For children with CCCs, congenital and chromosomal abnormalities were associated with 5819 (20.3% of 28,527 total) infant and 1087 (4.4%) child deaths, diseases of the nervous system caused 373 (1.3%) infant and 1173 (4.8%) child deaths. Deaths from cancer, which is perhaps the condition most

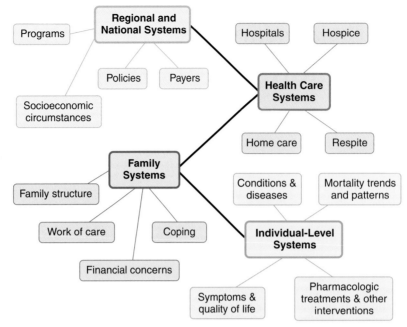

Fig. 2-1 Multi-level systems influencing experience of children receiving palliative or hospice care.

strongly associated with the imagery of palliative care in mind of the public and much of the medical profession, accounted for only 141 (0.5%) infant deaths and 2150 (8.9%) deaths past infancy. A few studies of patients enrolled in pediatric palliative care programs support the evidence of diverse conditions in this population. In a recent study of 8 pediatric palliative care programs in Canada, patients had as their primary diagnosis nervous system disorders (39.1%), cancer (22.1%), or perinatal-onset conditions or congenital anomalies (22.1%).[1]

TRENDS AND AGE-SPECIFIC PATTERNS OF MORTALITY

Over the past century, child mortality has been declining for both children suffering from trauma and from complex chronic conditions. Examining U.S. mortality data from 1979 to 2006, the rates of death attributed to CCCs as well as injury, sudden infant death syndrome, and other causes declined substantially (Fig. 2-3), with the corresponding numbers of deaths also declining but less so since 2000 (Fig. 2-4).

One published study focused on the interval between 1979 and 1997, when the annual death rate due to non-cancer and cancer-related CCCs declined for almost every age group (from a 7.1% decline for infants with cancer to a 49.9% decline for 1 to 4 year olds dying from non-cancer CCCs). The one exception to this decline was the mortality attributed to non-cancer CCCs among 20 to 24 year olds for whom the rate of death actually increased by 11.6% over this 18-year interval, which may be due to the longer lifespan of younger children with CCCs dying at later ages.[2] For this reason, studies of pediatric deaths and

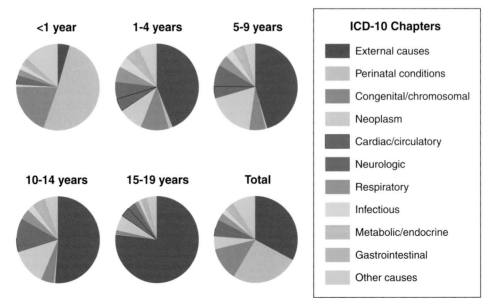

Fig. 2-2 Major causes of pediatric death in the United States, 1999-2006. (Data from National Center for Health Statistics.)

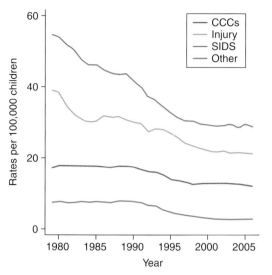

Fig. 2-3 Trends in the rates of pediatric death by causes, 1979-2006. (Data from National Center for Health Statistics.)

palliative care need to include the experiences of young adults, perhaps into their 20s or 30s, who die from conditions with congenital or childhood-onset.

SYMPTOMS AND QUALITY OF LIFE

The management of physical and psychological symptoms is of utmost importance in palliative care. Most studies published are on bereaved parents of children with cancer. In one such study, 96 bereaved Australian parents of children with cancer reported that, in the last month of life, 84% of children suffered from at least one physical symptom (pain, fatigue, poor appetite, constipation, dyspnea, nausea/vomiting, diarrhea, and seizures), with pain, fatigue, and poor appetite the most frequent.[3] Nearly half (43%) of children suffered from three or more physical symptoms. Parents also reported that 42% of children had been "more than a little sad," 38% experienced "little or no fun," and 21% were "often afraid." In a Swedish study of 449 bereaved parents of children with cancer, physical fatigue was the most frequently reported symptom

(86%) to have a higher or moderate impact on the child's well-being, with reduced mobility (76%), pain (73%), and decreased appetite (71%) also major concerns.[4] In this study, parents were more likely to report anxiety in children older than 9 years of age than in younger children (relative risk [RR] 1.8, 95% confidence interval [CI]: 1.2-2.6) and 16 years of age (RR 2.0, 1.3-2.9). Children also suffered from difficulties in swallowing, depression, reduced mobility, impaired speech, swelling, disturbed sleep due to anxiety, and urinary problems. Problems with breathing during the last day of life, and with loss of motor function in the last week of life, were also reported by 28 bereaved parents whose children had been enrolled in a pediatric hospice program in St. Louis.[5] Another study of 65 parents of 52 children reported similar symptoms, which did not differ according to patient gender, disease, or location of death, such as the ICU, elsewhere in hospital, or home.[6] A study of bereaved parents of 48 children who died from cancer also cited that their children suffered from anxiety, which was not treated effectively.[7] Given the prevalence of symptoms, and the nature of the child's condition, it is challenging to measure quality of life for children receiving palliative care services, especially using generalized instruments that may not be suitable for this population of children.[8] Nevertheless, much remains to be done in improving the treatment of symptoms in this population.

PHARMACOLOGIC TREATMENTS AND OTHER INTERVENTIONS

Medications are one of the mainstays of modern medicine. Polypharmacy is usually considered a problematic phenomenon among geriatric patients, but children admitted to children's hospitals are typically (median count) exposed to five different medications during their hospitalization, with 10% of the patients exposed to 14 or more medications. By the time pediatric patients have been hospitalized for a month or more, the 10% receiving the most medication have been exposed to 40 or more medications (unpublished data).

The drugs used to treat children who are receiving palliative or hospice care have not yet been well described. Among pediatric patients who died while hospitalized, the most common

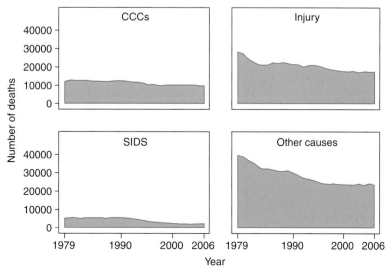

Fig. 2-4 Trends in the number of pediatric death by causes, 1979-2006. (Data from National Center for Health Statistics.)

exposures on the last day of life are to epinephrine (45%), dopamine (45%), fentanyl (42%), midazolam (33%), morphine (30%), vancomycin (29%), and ranitidine (26%); examining only oncology patients, the list and proportions are essentially the same (unpublished data). In a cohort of 834 pediatric patients enrolled in hospices across the United States, the most commonly used class of drug was opioids (72% of all patients), followed by hypnotics (60%), laxatives and other medications for the bowels (50%), antacids and other medications for the stomach (41%), and anti-epileptic drugs (38%) (unpublished data).

The use of specific medications appears to vary substantially across hospitals and hospices. For instance, in a study of 1466 pediatric oncology patients who died in children's hospitals, the proportion of patients who received opioids daily during their last week ranged across the hospitals from zero to 90.5%, a variation in practices that did not diminish substantially even after adjustment for patient characteristics (Fig. 2-5).

Medications are only one of many possible interventions used in palliative or hospice care or end of life situations to ameliorate symptoms or improve the quality of life. Much less is known about the epidemiology of other interventions, such as a child's exposure to complementary and alternative medical (CAM) practices. We do know that in one study of 92 parents of children with cancer in the United States, 49% reported that their children used at least one type of CAM and 20% used herbal remedies, homeopathy, or vitamins in the two months preceding the survey,[9] which suggests if any of these children died, some likely continued to receive CAM treatments at the end of life.

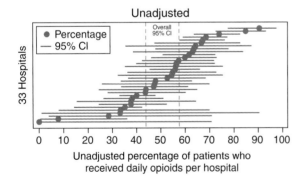

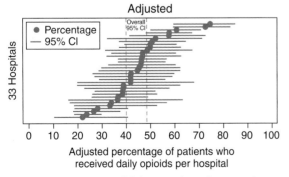

Fig. 2-5 Wide variation in opioid daily receipt by pediatric oncology patients who died in children's hospitals. (Data abstracted from Orsey AD, Belasco JB, Ellenberg JH, Schmitz KH, Feudtner C. Variation in receipt of opioids by pediatric oncology patients who died in children's hospitals. *Pediatr Blood Cancer.* 2009; 52(7): 749-50.)

Family Systems

Alex's parents, who have been married for seven years, readily speak of the strain that Alex's illness and care has placed upon the family, including Alex's sister who is now 6 years old, as well as the two surviving grandparents who often are pressed into helping out. The mother had to quit her job as a retail store manager in order to provide Alex's demanding care, and the father believes he has not been promoted due to the amount of time he has had to take off from work, but is thankful that his job does provide good health insurance coverage for the family, including Alex.

The experience of children receiving pediatric palliative care is clearly affected by a variety of specific aspects of their particular families. The structure and membership of a family as well as patterns of family organization and function, such as patterns of communication, cohesion among members, hierarchy, and adaptability to change, influences the care of children with complex chronic conditions.[10] Family structure shapes how tasks are divided and roles are assigned in caring for the child, whereby one parent often assumes primary physical care for the patient, and the other parent or other family members manage care of the household and siblings. Structure also dictates how families respond to and regulate their intense emotional reactions to a child's illness, which influence daily symptom management, soothing the ill child, and making critical end-of-life decisions. Family structure critically affects how care is performed, and is in turn affected by the family's finances, their social and cultural backgrounds or community, and their religious and spiritual beliefs and practices. To varying degrees, the medical literature provides useful data and knowledge about each of these topics.

FAMILY STRUCTURE

Families can have many different structures, and families of children with complex chronic conditions are no different. In two-parent married households, research has reported mixed results as to the effects on the marriage. Some studies, such as a case-control study of marital quality in mothers and fathers parenting children with spina bifida, report no difference in marital distress than in parents of healthy children.[11] Another study on the same disease reports marital breakdown.[12] Other studies, such as one on functioning in parents of children with cancer, suggest that while marital difficulties may occur, positive benefits such as feeling closer as a family and supporting each other may offset the stresses.[13] When parents are divorced, communication difficulties may exist, especially when the nonresidential parent has a different opinion about the child's care than that of the custodial parent.[14] Single-parent households have been less frequently studied,[15] but some evidence suggests that single mothers of children with cystic fibrosis may have higher stress-related symptoms and that their children may have higher hospitalization rates;[16] another study on handicapped children suggests that single mothers have greater difficulty with finances, but also were more flexible in adapting to new family roles and arrangements.[17] Step-parents in the home also alter the family structure.[18]

Siblings add another dimension. While the national percentage of children with complex chronic conditions who have siblings is unknown, meta-analyses investigating the effects of childhood chronic illness on siblings suggests a modest, negative effect on psychological functioning, peer activities, and cognitive development, with lower scores reported by parents than by the siblings themselves.[19,20] Recommendations for siblings include providing information about their brother's or sister's illness early on, group discussions, and informing school personnel.[21]

Another aspect of families that we can consider concerns other social and cultural characteristics. Various studies indicate that racial and ethnic minorities may have difficulties with trust and communication with the medical profession, poverty, and different belief systems and family structures.[22–25] Religion and spirituality are very important to families, but their impact is not uniform nor prescriptive.[26,27]

THE WORK OF CARE

The work of care consists of the effort, labor, and various tasks in which parents and other family members engage in to care for the child with a complex chronic condition and for the family system. Daily tasks include administering medications, feeding and bathing, providing emotional support, and monitoring any changes in the child's health.[28–32] Parents also are responsible for managing their child's medical care by arranging and bringing their child to appointments and filling out copious amounts of paperwork,[33] while creating an environment where their child can have as normal a life as possible.[34] These efforts can occupy a great deal of time.[35] One study of parents whose children had gastrostomy tubes, compared to parents whose children did not, found parents in the first group devoted more than 7 hours a day to technical and non-technical care of the child compared to 3 hours in the second group (Fig. 2-6).[36] How this work is organized, distributed, and completed likely varies across family structures, and some evidence also exists that stronger family function is related to better execution of disease management activities.[37–39]

COPING

Parents and siblings have been observed to suffer from an array of psychological and physical forms of distress: parents report depression, grief, guilt, and anxiety as well as problems such as insomnia, headaches, and musculoskeletal pain. One study of

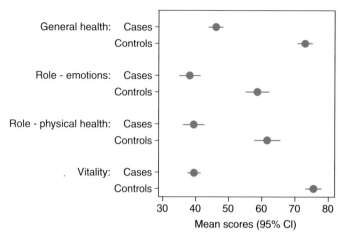

Fig. 2-7 Quality of life dimensions of parents of children with cardiac disease. (Data abstracted from Arafa MA, Zaher SR, El-Dowaty AA, Moneeb DE. Quality of life among parents of children with heart disease. *Health Qual Life Outcomes.* 2008; 6:91.)

parents of children with severe cardiac disease, compared to control parents of healthy children, found substantial decrements in the parents quality of life in general and specifically regarding emotions, physical health, and vitality (Fig. 2-7).[40] Siblings struggle with fears, traumatic reactions, isolation, difficulties in school and social settings, and the behavior problems that result.[41]

Few methodologically rigorous studies have examined the impact of a child's death on family members or the family structure. Much of what is known about parental reactions to a child's death is based on samples of those who present for psychological treatment; presumably, a much larger percentage of bereaved families experience essentially normal patterns of grief and other mental health consequences from the death of a child, without ever presenting for clinical care. Estimates of psychopathology in bereaved parents are therefore likely to be erroneously high.

FINANCIAL CONCERNS

Related to both the work of care and coping is a family's financial concerns. In particular, three areas of finances—

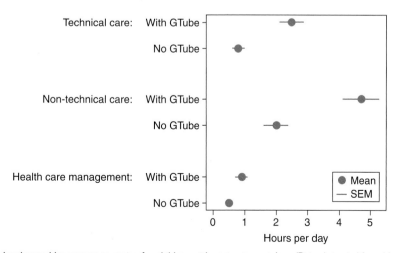

Fig. 2-6 Number of hours per day devoted by parents to caring for children with gastrostomy tubes. (Data abstracted from Heyman MB, Harmatz P, Acree M, Wilson L, Moskowitz JT, Ferrando S, et al. Economic and psychologic costs for maternal caregivers of gastrostomy dependent children. *J Pediatr.* 2004;145(4):511-516.)

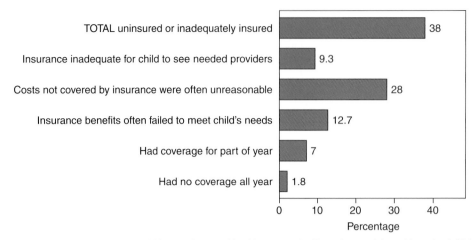

Fig. 2-8 Levels of inadequate health insurance among children with special healthcare needs. (Data abstracted from Newacheck PW, Houtrow AJ, Romm DL, Kuhlthau KA, Bloom SR, Van Cleave JM, et al. The future of health insurance for children with special health care needs. *Pediatrics.* 2009;123(5):e940-947.)

insurance, paid work, and out-of-pocket expenses—are affected by caring for a child with a complex chronic condition. Due to the high costs of care, families may have difficulty finding or keeping insurance coverage, and may find that certain services are not covered or caps on spending prevent other services from being used.[42] The result is that 38% of the U.S. population of parents of children with special health care needs are either uninsured or inadequately insured (Fig. 2-8),[43] a phenomenon that is especially pressing as the adolescents transition into adulthood.[44] Often in families caring for a child with a complex chronic condition, one family member, usually the mother, decides to stay at home, forsaking the income and benefits provided by paid work.[45,46] Out-of-pocket expenditures also are very high, and may further impoverish families.[47] Very poor families, however, may actually be at a slight advantage due to the infusion of additional resources and outside attention into the home.[48]

Healthcare Systems

Alex received an 8-hour shift of home care nursing a day, usually provided overnight to enable his parents to get some sleep, in the past year. Due to nursing shortages where he lives, about two shifts a week are not covered. After a recent stay in the intensive care unit, where Alex was intubated and mechanically ventilated for a week, conversations among the parents, Alex's neurologist and the hospital's palliative care team led to the decision to forgo cardiopulmonary resuscitation and to see if hospice services can be provided.

Encompassing both the child and the family is the level of healthcare systems, which can provide care in settings as varied as the child's own home to intensive care units.

CARE IN THE HOME

Pediatric palliative and hospice home care is intended to increase the quality of life of patients and families, and some, if not most, families prefer being at home to care for the child.[30] From 1989 to 1993, only 12.3% of children with CCCs died in the home; in 1999 to 2003, 17.7% of children with CCCs died in the home. In the same period, hospital deaths declined and deaths at all other sites and care institutions remained comparably stable.[49] This pattern of a rising proportion of pediatric deaths attributed to CCCs occurring at home is traceable to 1979 (Fig. 2-9). Over the same time periods, stark differences in the proportion of death that occurred at home are evident and persistent among patients classified on their death certificates as white, Hispanic, or black (Fig. 2-10).[49]

Home care usually involves the partnering of skilled nurses with the parents, who are able to share knowledge and divide tasks related to the work of care.[50] Issues to be considered in home care include the work of care, impact on the family, the likelihood of adverse events, and cost.[30,51-54] In a study of parents of 48 children who died from cancer, while only 41% of parents provided palliative care in the home and 48% of children died at home, 88% of parents chose "at home" as the most appropriate location of death in hindsight.[7]

HOSPICE CARE

While in general, little is known about the hospice care services that dying children receive, these services are generally thought to be simultaneously useful but underused. Research has demonstrated rare differences in the use of hospice services, but whether these differences arise due to differential access, eligibility, or other reasons remains unknown. A study of Florida

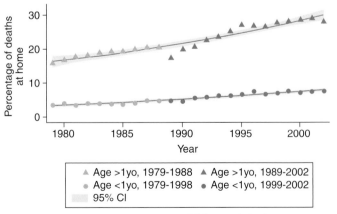

Fig. 2-9 Rising percentage of pediatric CCC-related deaths occurring at home, 1979-2002. (Data from National Center for Health Statistics.)

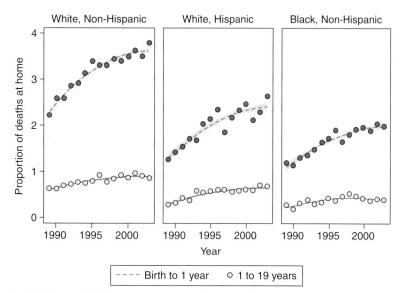

Fig. 2-10 Differences in proportion of CCC-related deaths occurring at home by race and/or ethnicity. (Data abstracted from Feudtner C, Feinstein JA, Satchell M, Zhao H, Kang TI. Shifting place of death among children with complex chronic conditions in the United States, 1989-2003. *JAMA*. 2007;297(24):2725-2732.)

Medicaid pediatric patients who died revealed that only 11% received any hospice services, but those who did were more likely to be non-Hispanic whites than non-Hispanic black, have chronic conditions, and longer Medicaid enrollment than non-hospice users.[55] In a study of pediatric oncologists, physicians with access to hospice that accepted patients receiving chemotherapy had more patients die at home, but not all hospices admit patients actively receiving chemotherapy.[56] A broader survey of pediatric medical providers experienced in end-of-life care reported that 86% of responders thought hospice was beneficial, especially in the provision of non-medical services.[57]

HOSPITALS

While there is a trend of increasing hospice and home-based pediatric palliative care, pediatric death still occurs mostly in the

hospital setting. From 1989 to 2003, 80.1% of childhood deaths resulting from CCCs occurred in the hospital (down from 85.7% in 1989 to 2003), with considerable variation in the location of death by CCC category.[49] The same study also demonstrated that infants and racial and ethnic minorities, were more likely to die in the hospital than older children and non-minorities.

Hospitalizations of children with CCCs who subsequently died were characterized by long lengths of stay (Fig. 2-11), mechanical ventilation during their terminal admissions, and death in the intensive care unit. In a study that linked information from death certificates to hospital use records from 1990 to 1996 in Washington state, 458 infants with CCCs who died under a week of age spent 92% of their lives in the hospital, and 286 infants with CCCs who died during the second to twelve months of life spent 41% of all their lives in the hospital.[58] For children and young adults with CCCs, the median number of days spent in the hospital in the year

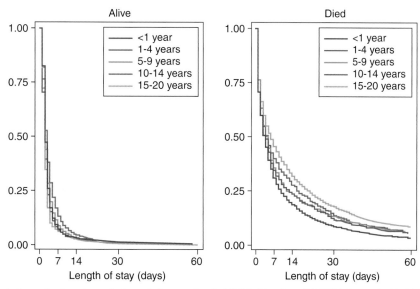

Fig. 2-11 Length of hospital stay for pediatric patients discharged alive or who died, 2006. (Data from KID 2006, Agency for Healthcare Quality and Research.)

preceding death was 18, and only a third of this group was hospitalized until the last week of life. Across all age groups, rates of hospital use increased closer to the child's death. Half of hospitalized infants and 19% of children and young adults with CCCs were mechanically ventilated during their terminal admission. Studies from hospitals in a range of countries (the United States, Australia, and the Netherlands), suggest that although a number of deaths take place in the operating room and emergency departments, most pediatric deaths occur in the intensive care unit.[59–62] In a study of a United Kingdom children's hospital, infants with congenital malformations and perinatal conditions were most likely to die in the ICU (OR 2.42, 95% CI 1.65 to 1.35) and older children with cancer were the most likely to die outside the ICU (OR 6.5, 95% CI 4.4 to 9.6).[63]

Over the past decade, hospital-based palliative care services have begun in many pediatric hospitals across the country. An evaluation of the impact of one such interdisciplinary program in Boston documented, after the program's establishment, an increased frequency of hospice discussions (76% vs. 54%, for an adjusted risk difference of 22%), earlier documentation of do-not-resuscitate orders (18 vs. 12 days), and fewer deaths in the intensive care unit or in other hospitals (decrease of 16%). Parents also reported that their child suffered less pain (adjusted risk difference of 19%), and that they felt more prepared during their child's last month of life and at the death.[64] In another study on the impact of a pediatric palliative care program in Germany, 69% of families preferred to have their child at home for the death compared to 18% of families before the program was instituted.[65]

RESPITE AND OTHER MODALITIES OF CARE

Beyond hospital and hospice care, other modes may also be useful for dying children. Broadening the definition of the population in need to encompass children with complex or special healthcare needs, respite care provides parents with time off from being in charge of the care. Respite care also has different meanings and purposes attributed to it by different families.[66] In a study among caregivers of children with cerebral palsy in Canada, 46% of caregivers reported using respite services in the past year, and 90% of caregivers indicated that respite was beneficial for both the child and family.[67] In another study of children with special healthcare needs, researchers demonstrated that a program in an emergency department setting to provide telephone advice and care coordination enhanced parental satisfaction with emergency care.[68]

Regional and National Systems

A dually licensed home healthcare and hospice agency that serves the adult patients in the eastern part of the state where Alex lives has developed a pediatric program over the past 3 years. Entitled Transitions, the program enables children such as Alex to receive both home care and hospice services, as permitted by a recently enacted state waiver program.

One can study programs, policies, or even payers as entities that exist at the regional or national level, much in the same way that we study children requiring pediatric pallia-

tive care services as individuals. How many programs exist? How are these programs evaluated? How do new programs come into being? What policies exist, at both the state and national levels? How do policies differ by state? What programs and services are covered by payers, how are these services reimbursed, and how do policies impact payments by both private and public insurers? While essentially none of these questions has been adequately studied, some pertinent data does exist.

PROGRAMS

In general, pediatric palliative and hospice care programs are characterized as being interdisciplinary and focused holistically on both the child and the family, with important functions being pain management, coordination of care, and decision-making support. For example, the Seattle Pediatric Palliative Care Project enrolled 41 patients over a 2-year period (1999 to 2001) whose ages ranged from infancy to 22 years old, with 31 specific diagnoses in the population and 34% cancer diagnoses.[69] Another program in Florida, the Partners in Care: Together for Kids (PIC:TFK) program, which uses government subsidies to create partnerships between state-employed care coordinators and home and community-based hospice staff, enrolled 468 children in the 3-year period between 2005 and 2008.[70] The PIC:TFK program was intended to provide supportive services to families beginning at diagnosis, and 92% of the children were either newly diagnosed or mid-stage. Services received in years 1 and 2 were support counseling, 46%; respite, 22%; nursing care, 15%; activity therapies, 14%; personal care, 2.5%; bereavement care, 0.8%; and pain and symptom management, 0.1%. While pain and symptom management services usage was very low, the study authors suggested that these services may have been provided by physicians who were not associated with the PIC:TFK program. The PIC:TFK was funded by Children's Hospice International in partnership with the U.S. government, other programs by the CHI partnership exist in Colorado, Kentucky, New York, Virginia, and Utah, and would benefit from being similarly profiled.

POLICIES

Both federal and state governments have been involved in crafting policies to address pediatric palliative care for families and providers. Federally, the best example remains the 1993 Family Medical Leave Act (FMLA), which protects parents who take time off to be with children receiving medical and psychiatric care from job loss. FMLA permits, among other things, both mothers and fathers to take unpaid leaves of absences from work while still receiving employer-provided health benefits. While the FMLA covers less than half of workers in the private sector, one study of employment statistics across the United States showed that the FMLA did increase leave coverage and usage without negatively impacting women's employment or wages overall.[71] In California, the "Nick Snow Children's Hospice and Palliative Care Act of 2005" created a pilot waiver program to address provision of palliative care through home health and hospice agencies, funded by a partnership between Medi-Cal and California Children's Services.

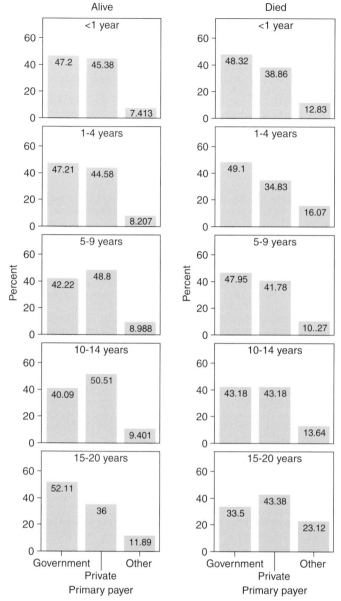

Fig. 2-12 Primary payers of hospital care for children. (Data from KID 2006, Agency for Healthcare Quality and Research.)

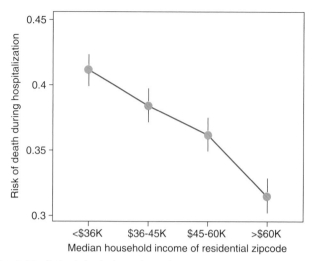

Fig. 2-13 Risk of death during hospitalization and neighborhood wealth. (Data from KID 2006, Agency for Healthcare Quality and Research.)

In the same U.S. hospitalization data, another economic aspect of childhood mortality is evident: the risk of dying during hospitalization is highest among patients from the poorest neighborhoods, and reduces across each step upward in median household income (Fig. 2-13). This observation, which accords with an extensive body of research connecting child wellbeing to socioeconomic circumstances,[72] reveals the connections between all the layers of the systems that we have outlined. Those layers are from individual risk of having a life-threatening medical condition, through the impact on family finances of having a child with a CCC, to access to and usage of healthcare system services, to the programs and policies that shape the availability of payers and services.

INTERNATIONAL PEDIATRIC PALLIATIVE CARE

Within the international setting, many national and multinational nonprofit organizations provide a support structure for independent programs based around the world by assisting with fundraising and advocacy. Multinational organizations such as Children's Hospice International and the International Children's Palliative Care Network link palliative care programs and hospices in South Africa, Zimbabwe, Uganda, India, Singapore, Argentina, Thailand, Indonesia, Costa Rica, and Belarus.[73] In Europe, the European Association for Palliative Care provides a similar program for pediatric palliative care and hospice programs in Norway, Sweden, the Netherlands, Germany, France, Spain, Italy, and other European countries. Within the United Kingdom, the Association for Children's Palliative Care (ACT) and the Association of Children's Hospices (ACH) network with individual programs and the British government to advocate for the best possible care.

Issues in pediatric palliative care differ by geopolitical regions in at least two major ways. First, causes of childhood mortality differ drastically around the globe. For example, in a study of death in children under 15 years in Mozambique between 1997 and 2006, 73.6% of deaths were attributable to communicable diseases, with 21.8% caused by malaria, 9.8% by pneumonia, and 8.3% caused by HIV/AIDS.[74] In Africa, the large number of children living with HIV are intended recipients of many palliative care services.[73,75] In a study on causes of mortality in children younger than 5 years of age in

PAYERS AND SOCIOECONOMIC CIRCUMSTANCES

The economics of health and healthcare have direct influences on the experiences of children and families receiving palliative and hospice care. According to data collected by the Agency for Healthcare Research and Quality for 2006 (Fig. 2-12), most children hospitalized in the United States who were discharged alive were insured either by government or private insurance, with less than 10% of patients having had no primary insurance (the slight exception being pediatric patients age 15 to 20 years, where 11.9% had no insurance). By contrast, among patients who died during their hospitalization, a larger percentage of patients in each age bracket had no primary insurance, and a smaller percentage had private insurance as their primary payer (with the exception again of the older adolescents, who upon reaching 18 years of age are no longer eligible for certain forms of government health insurance coverage).

Iraq, diarrhea was the leading cause of death in both infants (49.8%) and children 12 to 59 months (43.4%).[76] In the same study, researchers noted that cause of childhood death in Iraq often goes unreported when access to health services is limited, and most deaths occur at home. While causes of childhood mortality are certainly linked to broader geopolitical issues of overall morbidity and mortality, poverty, and health services availability and access, pediatric palliative care needs to adapt in each situation to meet the needs of local children.

Second, ethical perspectives about neonatal and childhood illness and death vary significantly around the world. The most obvious example concerns divergent views on euthanasia.[77,78] More broadly, variations in how societies and cultures conceptualize the nature of childhood, parental responsibility, the parent-child relationship, and death likely all affect how pediatric palliative care policies and decisions are framed, understood, and implemented.

Summary

Epidemiologic concepts and methods offer a rigorous and informative way to improve our understanding of the experiences of children receiving palliative and hospice care. These concepts and methods address questions regarding the distribution of conditions or symptoms, identify the causes of particular forms of suffering or different approaches to care, map trends over time in populations or typical illness trajectories within groups of patients, and determine the effectiveness of treatment interventions. Combining these analytic approaches with a multilevel systems-based perspective may reveal, if we are diligent and determined, the most effective path forward as we attempt to improve the care provided to these children and their families.

REFERENCES

1. Widger K, Davies D, Drouin DJ, Beaune L, Daoust L, Farran RP, et al: Pediatric patients receiving palliative care in Canada: results of a multicenter review, *Arch Pediatr Adolesc Med* 161(6):597–602, 2007.
2. Feudtner C, Hays RM, Haynes G, Geyer JR, Neff JM, Koepsell TD: Deaths attributed to pediatric complex chronic conditions: national trends and implications for supportive care services, *Pediatrics* 107(6):E99, 2001.
3. Heath JA, Clarke NE, Donath SM, McCarthy M, Anderson VA, Wolfe J: Symptoms and suffering at the end of life in children with cancer: an Australian perspective, *Med J Aust* 192(2):71–75, 2010.
4. Jalmsell L, Kreicbergs U, Onelov E, Steineck G, Henter JI: Symptoms affecting children with malignancies during the last month of life: a nationwide follow-up, *Pediatrics* 117(4):1314–1320, 2006.
5. Hendricks-Ferguson V: Physical symptoms of children receiving pediatric hospice care at home during the last week of life, *Oncol Nurs Forum* 35(6):E108–E115, 2008.
6. Pritchard M, Burghen E, Srivastava DK, Okuma J, Anderson L, Powell B, et al: Cancer-related symptoms most concerning to parents during the last week and last day of their child's life, *Pediatrics* 121(5):e1301–e1309, 2008.
7. Hechler T, Blankenburg M, Friedrichsdorf SJ, Garske D, Hubner B, Menke A, et al: Parents' perspective on symptoms, quality of life, characteristics of death and end-of-life decisions for children dying from cancer, *Klin Padiatr* 220(3):166–174, 2008.
8. Huang IC, Shenkman EA, Madden VL, Vadaparampil S, Quinn G, Knapp CA: Measuring quality of life in pediatric palliative care: challenges and potential solutions, *Palliat Med* 2009.
9. Martel D, Bussieres JF, Theoret Y, Lebel D, Kish S, Moghrabi A, et al: Use of alternative and complementary therapies in children with cancer, *Pediatr Blood Cancer* 44(7):660–668, 2005.
10. Patterson J: Integrating family resilience and family stress theory, *J Marriage Family* 64:349–360, 2002.
11. Cappelli M, McGarth PJ, Daniels T, Manion I, Schillinger J: Marital quality of parents of children with spina bifida: a case-comparison study, *J Dev Behav Pediatr* 15(5):320–326, 1994.
12. Martin P: Marital breakdown in families of patients with spina bifida cystica, *Dev Med Child Neurol* 17(6):757–764, 1975.
13. Barbarin OA, Hughes D, Chesler MA: Stress, coping, and marital functioning among parents of children with cancer, *J Marriage Family* 47(2):473–480, 1985.
14. Ganong L, Doty ME, Gayer D: Mothers in post divorce families caring for a child with cystic fibrosis, *J Pediatr Nurs* 18(5):332–343, 2003.
15. Brown RT, Wiener L, Kupst MJ, Brennan T, Behrman R, Compas BE, et al: Single parents of children with chronic illness: an understudied phenomenon, *J Pediatr Psychol* 2007.
16. Macpherson C, Redmond AO, Leavy A, McMullan M: A review of cystic fibrosis children born to single mothers, *Acta Paediatr* 87(4):397–400, 1998.
17. McCubbin MA: Family stress and family strengths: a comparison of single- and two-parent families with handicapped children, *Res Nurs Health* 12(2):101–110, 1989.
18. Zarelli DA: Role-governed behaviors of stepfathers in families with a child with chronic illness, *J Pediatr Nurs* 24(2):90–100, 2009.
19. Sharpe D, Rossiter L: Siblings of children with a chronic illness: a meta-analysis, *J Pediatr Psychol* 27(8):699–710, 2002.
20. Barlow JH, Ellard DR: The psychosocial well-being of children with chronic disease, their parents and siblings: an overview of the research evidence base, *Child Care Health Dev* 32(1):19–31, 2006.
21. Lähteenmäki PM, Sjöblom J, Korhonen T, Salmi TT: The siblings of childhood cancer patients need early support: a follow up study over the first year, *Arch Dis Child* 89(11):1008–1013, 2004.
22. Rehm RS: Cultural intersections in the care of Mexican American children with chronic conditions, *Pediatr Nurs* 29(6):434–439, 2003.
23. Elfert H, Anderson JM, Lai M: Parents' perceptions of children with chronic illness: a study of immigrant Chinese families, *J Pediatr Nurs* 6(2):114–120, 1991.
24. Williams HA: A comparison of social support and social networks of black parents and white parents with chronically ill children, *Soc Sci Med* 37(12):1509–1520, 1993.
25. McCubbin HI, Thompson EA, Thompson AI, McCubbin MA, Kaston AJ: Culture, ethnicity, and the family: critical factors in childhood chronic illnesses and disabilities, *Pediatrics* 91(5 Pt 2):1063–1070, 1993.
26. Feudtner C, Haney J, Dimmers MA: Spiritual care needs of hospitalized children and their families: a national survey of pastoral care providers' perceptions, *Pediatrics* 111(1):e67–e72, 2003.
27. Robinson MR, Thiel MM, Backus MM, Meyer EC: Matters of spirituality at the end of life in the pediatric intensive care unit, *Pediatrics* 118(3):e719–e729, 2006.
28. Canam C: Common adaptive tasks facing parents of children with chronic conditions, *J Adv Nurs* 18(1):46–53, 1993.
29. Monaghan MC, Hilliard ME, Cogen FR, Streisand R: Nighttime caregiving behaviors among parents of young children with Type 1 diabetes: associations with illness characteristics and parent functioning, *Fam Syst Health* 27(1):28–38, 2009.
30. Wang KW, Barnard A: Caregivers' experiences at home with a ventilator-dependent child, *Qual Health Res* 18(4):501–508, 2008.
31. Kirk S, Glendinning C, Callery P: Parent or nurse? The experience of being the parent of a technology-dependent child, *J Adv Nurs* 51(5):456–464, 2005.
32. Sullivan-Bolyai S, Deatrick J, Gruppuso P, Tamborlane W, Grey M: Constant vigilance: mothers' work parenting young children with type 1 diabetes, *J Pediatr Nurs* 18(1):21–29, 2003.
33. Osterlund CS, Dosa NP, Arnott Smith C: Mother knows best: medical record management for patients with spina bifida during the transition from pediatric to adult care, *AMIA Annu Symp Proc* 580–584, 2005.
34. Williams C: Alert assistants in managing chronic illness: the case of mothers and teenage sons, *Sociol Health Illn* 22(2):254–272, 2000.
35. Curran AL, Sharples PM, White C, Knapp M: Time costs of caring for children with severe disabilities compared with caring for children without disabilities, *Dev Med Child Neurol* 43(8):529–533, 2001.
36. Heyman MB, Harmatz P, Acree M, Wilson L, Moskowitz JT, Ferrando S, et al: Economic and psychologic costs for maternal caregivers of gastrostomy-dependent children, *J Pediatr* 145(4):511–516, 2004.
37. DeLambo KE, Ievers-Landis CE, Drotar D, Quittner AL: Association of observed family relationship quality and problem-solving skills with treatment adherence in older children and adolescents with cystic fibrosis, *J Pediatr Psychol* 29(5):343–353, 2004.

38. Fiese BH, Wamboldt FS, Anbar RD: Family asthma management routines: connections to medical adherence and quality of life, *J Pediatr* 146(2):171–176, 2005.

39. Lewin AB, Heidgerken AD, Geffken GR, Williams LB, Storch EA, Gelfand KM, et al: The relation between family factors and metabolic control: the role of diabetes adherence, *J Pediatr Psychol* 31(2):174–183, 2006.

40. Arafa MA, Zaher SR, El-Dowaty AA, Moneeb DE: Quality of life among parents of children with heart disease, *Health Qual Life Outcomes* 6:91, 2008.

41. Alderfer MA, Labay LE, Kazak AE: Brief report: does posttraumatic stress apply to siblings of childhood cancer survivors? *J Pediatr Psychol* 28(4):281–286, 2003.

42. Satchell M, Pati S: Insurance gaps among vulnerable children in the United States, 1999-2001, *Pediatrics* 116(5):1155–1161, 2005.

43. Newacheck PW, Houtrow AJ, Romm DL, Kuhlthau KA, Bloom SR, Van Cleave JM, et al: The future of health insurance for children with special health care needs, *Pediatrics* 123(5):e940–e947, 2009.

44. Lotstein DS, Inkelas M, Hays RD, Halfon N, Brook R: Access to care for youth with special health care needs in the transition to adulthood, *J Adolesc Health* 43(1):23–29, 2008.

45. Thyen U, Kuhlthau K, Perrin JM: Employment, childcare, and mental health of mothers caring for children assisted by technology, *Pediatrics* 103(6):1235–1242, 1999.

46. Porterfield SL: Work choices of mothers in families with children with disabilities, *J Marriage Family* 64:972–981, 2002.

47. Lukemeyer A, Meyers MK, Smeeding T: Expensive children in poor families: Out-of-pocket expenditures for the care of disabled and chronically ill children in welfare families, *J Marriage Family* 62:399–415, 2000.

48. Cohen MH: The technology-dependent child and the socially marginalized family: a provisional framework, *Qual Health Res* 9(5):654–668, 1999.

49. Feudtner C, Feinstein JA, Satchell M, Zhao H, Kang TI: Shifting place of death among children with complex chronic conditions in the United States, 1989-2003, *JAMA* 297(24):2725–2732, 2007.

50. McIntosh J, Runciman P: Exploring the role of partnership in the home care of children with special health needs: qualitative findings from two service evaluations, *Int J Nurs Stud* 45(5):714–726, 2008.

51. Leonard BJ, Brust JD, Nelson RP: Parental distress: caring for medically fragile children at home, *J Pediatr Nurs* 8(1):22–30, 1993.

52. Stevens B, Croxford R, McKeever P, Yamada J, Booth M, Daub S, et al: Hospital and home chemotherapy for children with leukemia: a randomized cross-over study, *Pediatr Blood Cancer* 47(3):285–292, 2006.

53. Leonard BJ, Brust JD, Sielaff BH: Determinants of home care nursing hours for technology-assisted children, *Public Health Nurs* 8(4):239–244, 1991.

54. Teague BR, Fleming JW, Castle A, Kiernan BS, Lobo ML, Riggs S, et al: "High-tech" home care for children with chronic health conditions: a pilot study, *J Pediatr Nurs* 8(4):226–232, 1993.

55. Knapp CA, Shenkman EA, Marcu MI, Madden VL, Terza JV: Pediatric palliative care: describing hospice users and identifying factors that affect hospice expenditures, *J Palliat Med* 2009.

56. Fowler K, Poehling K, Billheimer D, Hamilton R, Wu H, Mulder J, et al: Hospice referral practices for children with cancer: a survey of pediatric oncologists, *J Clin Oncol* 24(7):1099–1104, 2006.

57. Dickens DS: Comparing pediatric deaths with and without hospice support, *Pediatr Blood Cancer* 2010.

58. Feudtner C, DiGiuseppe DL, Neff JM: Hospital care for children and young adults in the last year of life: a population-based study, *BMC Med* 1:3, 2003.

59. Lantos JD, Berger AC, Zucker AR: Do-not-resuscitate orders in a children's hospital, *Crit Care Med* 21(1):52–55, 1993.

60. Ashby MA, Kosky RJ, Laver HT, Sims EB: An enquiry into death and dying at the Adelaide Children's Hospital: a useful model? *Med J Aust* 154:165–170, 1991.

61. van der Wal ME, Renfurm LN, van Vught AJ, Gemke RJ: Circumstances of dying in hospitalized children, *Eur J Pediatr* 158(7):560–565, 1999.

62. McCallum DE, Byrne P, Bruera E: How children die in hospital, *J Pain Symptom Manage* 20(6):417–423, 2000.

63. Ramnarayan P, Craig F, Petros A, Pierce C: Characteristics of deaths occurring in hospitalised children: changing trends, *J Med Ethics* 33(5):255–260, 2007.

64. Wolfe J, Hammel JF, Edwards KE, Duncan J, Comeau M, Breyer J, et al: Easing of suffering in children with cancer at the end of life: is care changing? *J Clin Oncol* 26(10):1717–1723, 2008.

65. Wolff J, Robert R, Sommerer A, Volz-Fleckenstein M: Impact of a pediatric palliative care program, *Pediatr Blood Cancer* 54(2):279–283, 2010.

66. MacDonald H, Callery P: Different meanings of respite: a study of parents, nurses and social workers caring for children with complex needs, *Child Care Health Dev* 30(3):279–288, 2004, discussion 289.

67. Damiani G, Rosenbaum P, Swinton M, Russell D: Frequency and determinants of formal respite service use among caregivers of children with cerebral palsy in Ontario, *Child Care Health Dev* 30(1):77–86, 2004.

68. Sutton D, Stanley P, Babl FE, Phillips F: Preventing or accelerating emergency care for children with complex healthcare needs, *Arch Dis Child* 93(1):17–22, 2008.

69. Hays RM, Valentine J, Haynes G, Geyer JR, Villareale N, McKinstry B, et al: The Seattle Pediatric Palliative Care Project: effects on family satisfaction and health-related quality of life, *J Palliat Med* 9(3):716–728, 2006.

70. Knapp CA, Madden VL, Curtis CM, Sloyer PJ, Huang IC, Thompson LA, et al: Partners in care: together for kids: Florida's model of pediatric palliative care, *J Palliat Med* 11(9):1212–1220, 2008.

71. Waldfogel J: The Impact of the Family and Medical Leave Act, *J Policy Anal Manage* 18(2), 1999.

72. Feudtner C, Noonan KG: Poorer health: the persistent and protean connections between poverty, social inequality, and child well-being, *Arch Pediatr Adolesc Med* 163(7):668–670, 2009.

73. Marston J, Germ RM, Granera Lopez DJ, Lowe P, Shaw R: Children's hospice and palliative care worldwide. In Armstrong-Dailey A, Zarbock S, editors: *Hospice care for children*, New York, 2009, Oxford University Press, pp 365–377.

74. Sacarlal J, Nhacolo AQ, Sigauque B, Nhalungo DA, Abacassamo F, Sacoor CN, et al: A 10 year study of the cause of death in children under 15 years in Manhica, Mozambique, *BMC Public Health* 9:67, 2009.

75. De Baets AJ, Bulterys M, Abrams EJ, Kankassa C, Pazvakavambwa IE: Care and treatment of HIV-infected children in Africa: issues and challenges at the district hospital level, *Pediatr Infect Dis J* 26(2):163–173, 2007.

76. Awqati NA, Ali MM, Al-Ward NJ, Majeed FA, Salman K, Al-Alak M, et al: Causes and differentials of childhood mortality in Iraq, *BMC Pediatr* 9:40, 2009.

77. Cuttini M, Casotto V, de Vonderweid U, Garel M, Kollee LA, Saracci R: Neonatal end-of-life decisions and bioethical perspectives, *Early Hum Dev* 85(Suppl 10):S21–S25, 2009.

78. Pignotti MS, Donzelli G: Periviable babies: Italian suggestions for the ethical debate, *J Matern Fetal Neonatal Med* 21(9):595–598, 2008.

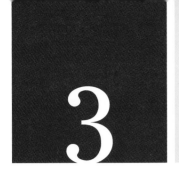

3 Children's Voices: The Experience of Patients and Their Siblings

ANNA C. MURIEL | COLETTE CASE | BARBARA M. SOURKES

Life is so strange. Sometimes you feel it's like a book with chapters to fill, never ending.

Sometimes it's like a chess game where you have to make each move so carefully.

Other times it's like a mystery where each hidden chamber reveals its secrets.

It is even a war where to live it is to win it.[1] (p. 131)

—Karen Beth Josephson, age 10

It's no privilege having someone with cancer in your family. Of all the things I ever could have chosen, having my brother get cancer is not one of them.[2] (p. 38)

—8-year-old sibling

As pediatric palliative care develops into an interdisciplinary field, it is crucial to further our understanding of children's psychological responses to life-threatening illness. In many ways, the patient and his or her siblings live the illness in mirror-image fashion: while the patient endures the physicality of the illness in all its relentless and insistent presence, the siblings are witness to its ravages. All the children must cope with great uncertainty, confronted with the threat, if not the actuality, of premature separation, loss, and death.

Although the healthy siblings live the illness experience with the same intensity as the patient and parents, historically, they have stood outside the spotlight of attention and care.[3–4] Many of these children demonstrate positive growth in their maturity and empathy. Yet their distress can be significant, including elevated rates of anxiety and depression; symptoms of post-traumatic stress; few peer activities; lower cognitive development scores and school difficulties; diminished parental attention and overall ratings of a poor quality of life.[5–6] Sibling relationships are a crucial axis within the family system and the children's mutual caring and devotion can be enhanced rather than overlooked (Figs. 3-1 and 3-2).

A group of siblings were asked: "Imagine that you are doing a campaign on behalf of siblings of seriously ill children. Draw a poster to illustrate your cause." The children drew an ill child in a hospital bed, surrounded by medical equipment, the parents at bedside. No siblings are present. They entitled their poster: "Don't brothers and sisters count too??"[7]

A six-year-old sibling of a child who had been hospitalized for months spontaneously drew a smiling person—then changed the smile into a downturned mouth and said: "This is me. I am crying because I want my brother to be with me."

Certain psychological themes that emerge are universal for both patients and siblings, although the mode of expression will depend on the child's level of cognitive and emotional development. These factors determine how he or she understands and integrates the illness itself as well as the responses of close family and friends. Also significant is the nature of the illness – its manifestations, its overall time course, and the particular phase at a given time.

This chapter provides a portrait, through the voices of both patients and siblings, of the experience of living with life-threatening illness. The words and images of children are essential touchstones for understanding pediatric palliative care. A conceptual overview of developmental considerations can frame the discussion of selected clinical themes: the impact of the illness itself, the children's awareness of their condition (or their sibling's), and anticipatory grief. The experiences of the children in this chapter are universal; however, the degree of openness and candor of their expression is a function of individual and family psychology, cognitive competence, and cultural background. The impact of culture emerges particularly in the discussion of the voice of the child in decision-making. The unique contributions of child psychology, psychiatry, and other mental health professions, as well as the specialty of child life, are delineated as they contribute to providing truly interdisciplinary pediatric palliative care.

Developmental Considerations

INFANTS AND TODDLERS (AGES 0-3)

The earliest years are crucial for children's development of attachment and trust through their relationship to the primary caregiver, usually the mother. At 6 to 12 months of age, infants go through a phase of stranger anxiety, mitigated by the proximity to the mother. Separation anxiety, which emerges between about ten and eighteen months, is a response to discrepancy: the more regular the presence of the mother, the earlier this anxiety manifests. By toddlerhood, the infant "becomes" a child with advances in motor, language, and social development.

The implications of serious illness, hospitalization, and pain for such young patients and siblings are enormous. At a critically formative time, the ill child may be overwhelmed with pain, strange people and situations, and separation. Nursing or feeding in infants is often disrupted, if not precluded. Parents caring for an ill child may be incapable of

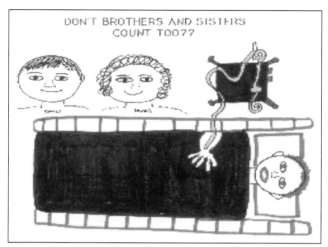

Fig. 3-1 Don't brothers and sisters count too?? (Reprinted from Sourkes B et al. Food, toys, and love: pediatric palliative care, *Curr Probl Pediatr Adolesc Health Care* 35(9):345–392, 2005.)

adapting to the cues of infant siblings. Toddlers, too young to fully comprehend verbal explanations, lack the means to make sense of crisis and unpredictability. Parents of such young children may be young themselves, or first-time parents. They are thrust into the medical world, often without experience of "normal" parenting. Much of the intervention with infants and toddlers (both patients and siblings) is to help the parents re-establish a secure routine and framework to enable the resumption of developmental progress.

Two-year-old Jimmy had been hospitalized for six months, and had undergone many traumatic medical procedures. He was withdrawn; fearful of noises, sudden movements, and new people who entered his room; and disinterested in food or toys. Prior to his discharge home, the parents requested strategies from the psychologist to "get him back" to his pre-morbid level of functioning. Recommendations to the parents included:

- *Take a gradual and consistent approach with Jimmy in all areas. The 6-month disruption in his development will not be righted overnight; he needs to re-familiarize himself with his family, room, house, and toys.*

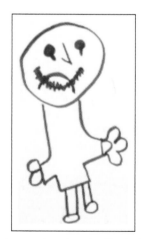

Fig. 3-2 I am crying because I want my brother to be with me. (Reprinted from Sourkes B et al. Food, toys, and love: pediatric palliative care, *Curr Probl Pediatr Adolesc Health Care* 35(9):345–392, 2005.)

- *It is fine if he wants you within sight at all times. After all the coming and goings of the hospital, he will crave your presence. The intensity will abate with time. Very gradually, once he re-engages with toys, try to move away from him as he plays (first in the same room, then out of the room). Initially, do so for only moments at a time.*
- *Jimmy has to re-learn how to play and have fun. Start with a few toys that he can get to know over the first few weeks, such as blocks to build up and knock down, a cloth for peek-a-boo, pull toys that encourage crawling, and cuddly stuffed animals. Keep the toys around him and do several play sessions with him each day.*
- *As much as possible, have him on the floor or in his playpen rather than in your arms. Put him into the playpen for as little as ten seconds and gradually increase the time. Reinforce him with hugs and verbal praise for being a "big boy." Put toys or food slightly out of reach to tempt him to crawl and to stand to reach them.*
- *Jimmy should eat all his meals in his high chair, always in the same location. Put only a bite of each kind of food out at a time. Because he seemed to eat more in the hospital when he was playing, use small toys as both distraction and enjoyment.*
- *It is important that Jimmy begin to use his words again. When he points to an object, give him its name and develop a back-and-forth language game with him.*

PRESCHOOL CHILDREN (AGES 3-5)

Natural egocentricity, magical thinking, and associative logic all characterize preschool children's thinking. They are therefore prone to interpret illness and suffering in terms of their own thoughts and actions, and to have misconceptions about the cause of the illness or the reasons for medical treatment. Temporal coincidences may be interpreted as causal, and they may experience illness or treatment as punishment. While most of these children cannot yet express abstract concepts of time or the permanence of death, they are acutely aware of the emotional climate around them, particularly separation from caregivers and changes in routine.

Young children's reporting of symptoms is usually situation-specific, and they rarely can report their experience of physical or emotional symptoms over time. Thus, for example, responses about how they feel today as compared with yesterday, or concepts of better or worse may not be accurate indicators. However, these young children can readily express, through words and actions, their fears or dislike of specific sensations and circumstances.

Irritability may be a generalized response to physical discomfort, or to the disruptions in routines. The behavior of a child with delays in language or cognitive development may appear particularly regressed and out of control, responses to distress and to frustration of expression.

Similarly, while brothers and sisters may not report their sibling's symptoms accurately, they often resort to catastrophic images, often involving themselves, to express that something is drastically wrong. Symbolic play, stories, and drawing may be the most accessible expression of their experiences.

Matthew, 4, who was receiving palliative care for a brain tumor, told the psychologist: "I'm not sick anymore" and adamantly denied any discomfort. His response to most queries by his parents or the medical team was "I'm OK" or "I'm fine" even when it was obvious that he was not. In fact, his non- or underreporting of symptoms made it difficult for his mother to administer pain medication effectively. The psychologist introduced Matthew to a rabbit puppet that he promptly named Donald Bunny. She used the puppet to model the reporting of symptoms (e.g., Donald Bunny has a headache, his eyes hurt when it is too bright, etc.). Matthew watched and listened with some interest. The psychologist left the puppet with him. At the next session, his mother said Matthew had begun reporting symptoms attributed "through the voice" of Donald Bunny. He still would not verbally acknowledge that he had any of these problems; however, his drawing of a dark and threatening "batman tunnel" connoted distress and pain (Fig. 3-3) and contrasted with his earlier bright image (Fig. 3-4). By the next session, while Matthew still would not initially mention any of what had been "bad" during the week, he did allow his mother to list some of his symptoms and would nod affirmatively to them. He then added spontaneously for the first time: "I don't like when I cough."[8]

A 3-year-old sibling manifested intense anxiety both at home and at preschool during his sister's long hospitalization. He drew a picture of the hospital with the following commentary: "A building with only three windows because some fell out and broke on the street. People have to be careful or their toes could get cut off. Nobody is in the hospital—they were all in a meeting. But you were there and were happy to see us and then everyone else came back. I was born and I got poison ivy and I died in the car. My sister was scared" (Fig. 3-5).

SCHOOL-AGE CHILDREN (AGES 6-12)

Children in these middle years are ordinarily consumed with mastering skills in a range of physical, intellectual, and social activities. They are invested in fitting in with peers and with the social norms of their immediate community. Children struggling with illness are set apart by virtue of physical changes and loss of bodily integrity, absence from their usual activities,

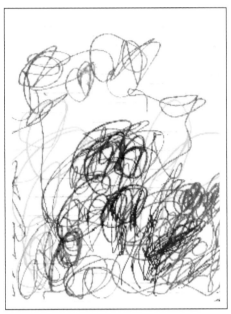

Fig. 3-4 **Untitled early image.** (Reprinted from Sourkes B: "Psychological impact of life-limiting conditions on the child." In Goldman, Haines, Liben [eds]. *Oxford Textbook of Palliative Care for Children* (2006). By permission of Oxford University Press.)

and overwhelmingly, the ramifications of the diagnosis. They may experience the loss of friends and changes in their relationships with family members. Thinking patterns are characterized by relatively concrete cause and effect with an interest in bodily functions and factual information. They have an understanding of the permanence of death, and yet may not always integrate that it is universal. There may be less direct expression of emotion and more coping by using cognition, activity, and distraction.

School-age children are aware of the impact of their illness and distress on others, and may amplify or minimize their communication based on others' reactions. These children may not consciously change their behavior or be aware of the interplay between their emotions and their physical experiences. While children in this age group may use words more effectively than younger children, they may also need encouragement and normalization of experiences to freely describe their physical symptoms or emotional experience. Drawing and displacement through play or storytelling may continue to be important methods for expression.

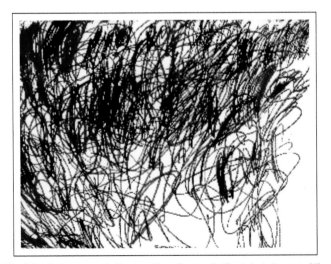

Fig. 3-3 **Batman tunnel.** (Reprinted from Sourkes B: "Psychological impact of life-limiting conditions on the child." In Goldman, Haines, Liben [eds]. *Oxford Textbook of Palliative Care for Children* (2006). By permission of Oxford University Press.)

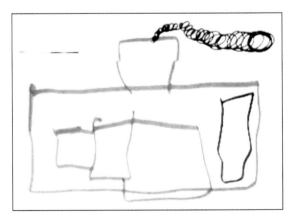

Fig. 3-5 **Hospital picture.**

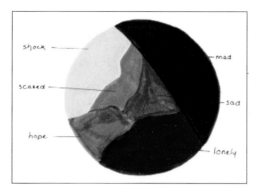

Fig. 3-6 How I felt when I heard that I had leukemia. (Reprinted and adapted from *Armfuls of Time: The Psychological Experience of the Child with a Life-Threatening Illness* by Barbara M. Sourkes, 1996, by permission of the University of Pittsburgh Press.)

Through a drawing (Fig. 3-6), an 8-year-old boy captured the immediacy of his response to the diagnosis of a life-threatening illness: "When I heard that I had leukemia, I turned pale with shock. That's why I chose yellow—it's a pale color. Scared is red—for blood. I was scared of needles, of seeing all the doctors, of what was going to happen to me. I was MAD [black] about a lot of things: staying in the hospital, taking medicines, bone marrows, spinal taps, IVs, being awakened in the middle of the night. I was sad [purple] that I didn't have my toys and that I was missing out on everything. I chose blue for lonely because I was crying about not being at home and not being able to go outside. Green is for hope: getting better, going home, eating food from home, and seeing my friends." He has articulated the shock; the fear of everything from the concrete medical procedures to the sudden possibility of an altered future ("what was going to happen to me"); the constellation of sadness, grief, and loneliness of separation; and the absence from his normal life. Accompanying all these feelings is a forthright statement of hope.[1] (p. 31)

Tim, an 11-year-old boy, had struggled with recurrent cancer since the age of 4. He was troubled by insomnia and anxiety during an inpatient stay in isolation for intensive treatment. Upon discharge, he continued to have significant anxiety, avoiding school and playing with friends. His medical team had cleared him for all activity, and he did not report pain or side effects of his medication. Tim had been using escalating doses of benzodiazepines at bedtime, as well as when needed during the day. When interviewed alone by the psychiatrist, he reported feeling "nervous and worried."
Psychiatrist: About what?
Tim: About dying.
Psychiatrist: Which part?
Tim: Just being dead.
When questioned further, Tim articulated specific worries about many issues: dying suddenly while away from his parents; wondering what dying will feel like and what the afterlife holds; not being able to "come back as a ghost" to visit his family if they were to move away from their current house. He denied worry about pain: "I have been sick so long and had lots of pain." The discussion continued on a spectrum from the current stable status of his illness to his feelings about God and spirituality. Following this session, Tim engaged in the most direct conversation with his medical team than ever before: about his illness, the stability of his scan results, and the fact that death was not imminent. The team reassured him that there would be time to talk more when death is closer at hand. Over

the next few months, Tim returned to active play with peers, engaged in video games and early romantic interests, prepared for the next school year, and articulated future plans to go to college and get a job.

Siblings also experience a sense of "apartness" of being different or stigmatized, by having a seriously ill brother or sister. These children often live in fear of becoming sick themselves, along with suffering a complicated mix of guilt at having escaped the illness and shame at feeling this relief. They are exceedingly conscious of the physical exigencies of the illness, as well as the impact on the child's functioning. Private theories about what caused the illness are common, and the siblings frequently implicate themselves in the explanation. They often express a fervent wish to understand and be more involved.[3-4]

Bobby, 10, reported his version of the sequence of events that led to his sister's diagnosis of osteosarcoma and amputation: "She hurt her leg on the chain of her bike. She didn't even notice it until I pointed it out to her. I don't even ride my bike anymore. One night I went out and broke the chain so I couldn't ride it. I told my mother it broke by itself, but I broke it."[3] (p. 55) He wrote a story: "This is my sister (drew a one-legged stick figure) and this is me (drew a two-legged stick figure). There is a difference. But I still think that this is the same Cindy and I know that she is not the same to you and I think that she is beautiful." He then drew a picture of Cindy, stressing her very short hair and her stump. He expressed much concern about how the stump would look.[3] (p. 57) (Fig. 3-7) In a subsequent session, Bobby admitted to nightmares of "the same thing" happening to him (Fig. 3-8).

A ten-year-old sibling spoke about her brother's diagnosis of a brain tumor: (Fig. 3-9) "I feel scared (green)—I feel as if I don't really know what is happening. Sad is blue—at first my parents just told me that my brother needed an operation. They didn't say it was cancer. Confused is yellow—just all mixed feelings—I don't know what to think. Hopeful is purple—bright—I don't really have a lot of hope, but maybe just a little. Angry is red because that is a mad color. Why him? What did it have to happen to him? My drawing is called 'Mixed Messages' because I have all of these different feelings and everyone is telling me different things. Like they say mostly that he is going to be okay, but they—and I—don't really believe it...."[9]

ADOLESCENTS (13-18 YEARS)

Adolescence is characterized by an evolving process of identity formation, appreciation of abstract concepts, and increasing sophistication in both intellectual and emotional understanding of situations and relationships. Future orientation is paramount in the areas of educational and career goals and the development of intimate relationships. Just as these young people are struggling to establish separation and autonomy from family, they must contend with the enforced dependence and vulnerability imposed by the illness. While adolescents understand the permanence and universality of death, they may still feel personally and emotionally invincible. Offering adolescents a role in decision-making is always important, whether or not they accept. They may need

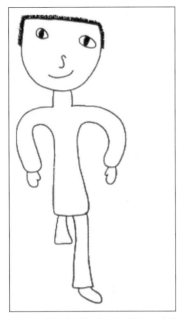

Fig. 3-7   Bobby's portrait of Cindy. (Reprinted with permission from Kellerman, J. *Psychological Aspects of Childhood Cancer.* (1980). Courtesy of Charles C. Thomas, Publisher, Ltd., Springfield, Illinois.)

assistance from the medical team or mental health clinician to distinguish their preferences from those of their family. Because many adolescents try to protect their parents from their own distress, it can be a frightening prospect to make their own needs known. Peer relationships and activities and self-directed symptom management are critical components of quality of life for adolescents. Written expression, music, media, and web-based activities can provide windows into the impact of the illness on their life and how it has impinged on their sense of self.

Younger children are not developed in themselves yet, in their own persons, in their own individualism. They can still be with their mother. Older people are away from their mother; they're detached, more adult. When you're in the middle, parents don't want to let you go. You want to be set free a little bit, but you want to be able to come back. I just felt that I was denied any sort of chance.... Instead, it was decided for me:

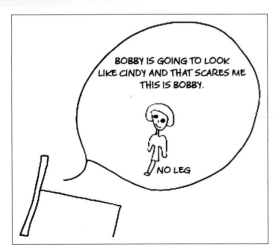

Fig. 3-8   Bobby's nightmare. (Reprinted with permission from Kellerman, J. *Psychological Aspects of Childhood Cancer.* (1980). Courtesy of Charles C. Thomas, Publisher, Ltd., Springfield, Illinois.)

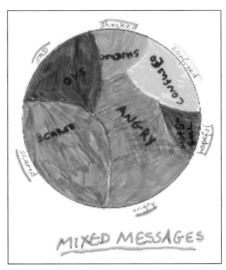

Fig. 3-9   Mixed messages. (Reprinted with permission from Pizzo, P. *Principles and Practice of Pediatric Oncology*, 5th Edition. Lippincott Williams, and Wilkins, 2006.)

"You are going to mature very fast right now. You have to make life and death decisions. You have to accept things that children who are young adults between the ages of thirteen and nineteen don't normally have to face." It's like: "Grow up right now and become what you have to become to deal with this." I never had the chance to be sweet sixteen. I never had the chance to be gay old seventeen. I had to automatically be an adult, and it was very hard."[2]

(Katherine, age 18) (p. 101)

Adolescent siblings are caught in a similar web: just as they are beginning to develop their individual identity and to negotiate their own independence, they are pulled back into the family. They are preoccupied and worried. These young people have difficulty sorting out their role and needs from that of being another parental figure.

Joanne fell on the stairs at school and split her lip open on the day before Cindy's amputation. Her explanation: "I was walking in flat heels on the stairs. I thought of Cindy's operation. That's why I fell."[3] (p. 63)

In response to the question: "What has been especially hard for you during your brother's illness?" an adolescent sibling responded: "Waiting while he is in the OR and worrying about what they are finding."

Clinical Themes

THE ILLNESS EXPERIENCE

The patient experiences the illness both physically and emotionally through symptoms, changes in appearance and body image, and also the intrusion of technology. These traumatic aspects reverberate for the siblings as well and may become a source of great distress because they often go unacknowledged.

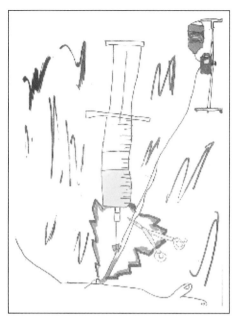

Fig. 3-10 IV exploding in my arm. (Reprinted from Sourkes B et al. Food, toys, and love: pediatric palliative care, *Curr Probl Pediatr Adolesc Health Care* 35(9):345–392, 2005.)

Psychologist: If you could choose one word to describe the time since your diagnosis, what would it be?

Patient: "PAIN—once I felt as if the IV was exploding in my arm!"

The child went on to describe the excruciating pain he had felt amidst the chaos of his IV pole falling over and crashing[7] (p. 365) (Fig. 3-10).

In response to the question: "What is the scariest feeling, thought, or experience you have had since your sister became ill?" a child drew her response: "Dreaming of my sister in pain." She depicted herself as a diminutive brown figure in a small bed, overwhelmed by the dream image of her sister in bright orange screaming "OW" (Fig. 3-11).

A 12-year-old child with end-stage renal disease depicted his absolute dependence on hemodialysis to live. He entitled his drawing "MY machine." One hand is literally plugged into the machine while the other is in a "thumbs up" gesture. His facial expression is ambiguous—triumph, horror, or a combination of the two (Fig. 3-12). A sibling's drawing of his brother hooked up to multiple wires and monitors communicates his fear at what he has witnessed (Fig. 3-13).

Concerns about sexuality can be quite pronounced in children living with serious illness. Sexuality in all its facets represents a life force, which is exactly the struggle in which these children are engaged. Furthermore, the body is the focus of illness and sexuality is an integral part of that same body. Sexual identity, functioning, and fertility—and the potential or actual losses thereof—loom particularly large for adolescents, although younger children may also harbor worries about immediate and long-term effects of illness and treatment.[10]

An 18-year-old boy who had had his leg amputated expressed fears about his sexual functioning and how his girlfriend would react. On a clinic visit shortly after surgery, he greeted the psychologist: "You'll be glad to know I still work! I was glad too!"[10]

A 12-year-old girl insisted on reading the informed consent for her bone marrow transplant. When she asked what "sterility" meant, her physician replied: "It means you can't have babies." She retorted quickly and with spirit: "Then I'll adopt!" However, following this discussion, she spoke frequently about her sadness at the loss of fertility.[10]

An 8-year-old sibling talked about her adolescent sister's hair loss secondary to chemotherapy. With some embarrassment, she admitted that she had glimpsed her sister in the shower and only then realized that she had lost her pubic hair as well. She was disturbed at seeing her sister's body looking like that of a young child again.

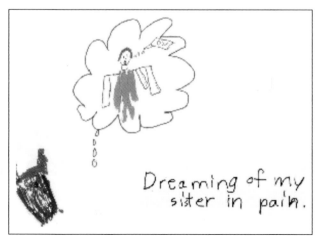

Fig. 3-11 Dreaming of my sister in pain.

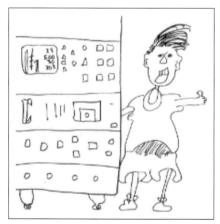

Fig. 3-12 MY machine.

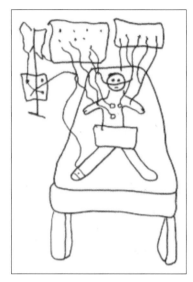

Fig. 3-13 My brother in the hospital.

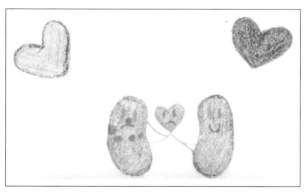

Fig. 3-14 My lungs.

An 8-year-old boy with muscular dystrophy was tripping and falling constantly, but adamantly refused to use a wheelchair, protesting that he did not need it. His older brother with the same disease was already severely compromised. In a family drawing, the child portrayed himself jumping and smiling; he drew his brother as an incomplete almost ghost-like figure at the computer. The extremities of all four family members are distorted or missing. This child's awareness—and attempted denial—of his own progressive deterioration as well as his brother's status (and thus his own in the future) are embedded in the drawing (Fig. 3-16).

A 14-year-old boy with hemophilia who had just been informed that he was HIV-positive graphically described the experience: "Before hearing the news, I was just thinking: I hope they are not going to tell me I have HIV" (on a "happy" purple background). After hearing the news, he depicted himself in a coffin against a black background saying: "I hope I'll be alive when they get the cure…" (Fig. 3-17).

An 8-year-old sibling said his biggest worry was that his brother might die of his illness. He drew a somber picture of two faceless black figures lowering a coffin into the ground, next to a tombstone inscribed "RIP" and a pile of dirt. Anxious scribbling filled part of the page (Fig. 3-18).

For all the children, their longing to return to their "normal life" or their "life from before" (or, in situations where a child has a congenital condition, "life without sickness") is counterbalanced by the recognition that the presence of illness in the family cannot be erased, nor its impact reversed.[1] Rather, the children are confronted with the extraordinary challenge of pursuing the developmental tasks of childhood and adolescence while negotiating the illness experience.

AWARENESS OF THE LIFE-THREATENING NATURE OF THE ILLNESS

Children's awareness is a fluid process not a static state, and depends on factors including: their current medical status and knowledge about the illness (or that of the sibling's), their "wisdom of the body," the urgency and intensity of treatment, the emotions of family and caregivers, the family communication style and encounters with other children who are ill.[1,11] These issues are particularly poignant when more than one child in the family has the illness. References to death may be somewhat veiled and allusive, or direct and explicit.

During a psychotherapy session in the last few months of her life, 13-year-old Evangeline drew a picture entitled "My Lungs." She portrayed herself as a heart with a sad face between (and connected to) two lungs: "One of my lungs is sad because it has disease in it; the other lung is smiling because it is still OK" (Fig. 3-14). Her use of the word "still" expressed her qualified confidence in its current state.

A 4-year-old child had always done medical play with a stuffed Curious George monkey, giving him shots and bandages. In a session close to her death, she methodically covered him with tissues and taped them in place. By the end of her play, he appeared to be buried under a shroud. She was very quiet during her activity and made no comment about her play[8] (Fig. 3-15).

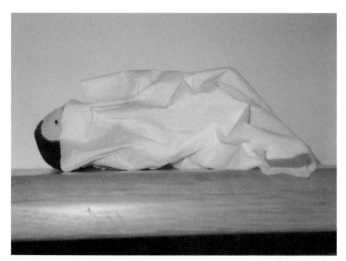

Fig. 3-15 Curious George under a shroud. Reprinted from Sourkes B: "Psychological impact of Life-Limiting conditions on the child." In Goldman, Haines, Liben [eds]. *Oxford Textbook of Palliative Care for Children* (2006). By permission of Oxford University Press.

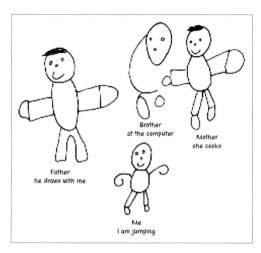

Fig. 3-16   I am jumping.

ANTICIPATORY GRIEF

Psychologist: "Are you in any pain? Does anything hurt?"
Jenny: "My heart."
Therapist: "Your heart?"
Jenny: "My heart is broken.... I miss everybody."[1] (p. 153)

Children's expressions of anticipatory grief—for many cumulative losses—accompany their awareness of the implications of the illness.[1-2,12] Patients grieve the loss of control over their body and disease, the loss of identity of what had been their roles and functions in the family and in the outside world,

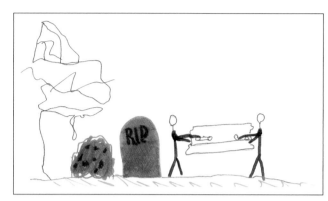

Fig. 3-18   Rest in peace.

and the foregoing of future goals. The children face the ultimate leave-taking, the departure from all that is familiar and loved. Loss of relationships—expressed through fears of separation, absence, and ultimately death itself—is paramount, and is the dimension shared with the siblings.

An interchange between Mariesa, 16, and Mikaela, her 10-year-old sister with a brain tumor:

Mariesa: "We've always been really close. I just hate to think of... just too many scary thoughts and too many feelings.... I just know one thing: I just want everything to be OK and everything to go away and hopefully it will work out."
Mikaela: "Same with me."
Mariesa: "And she knows that I love her no matter what."[13]

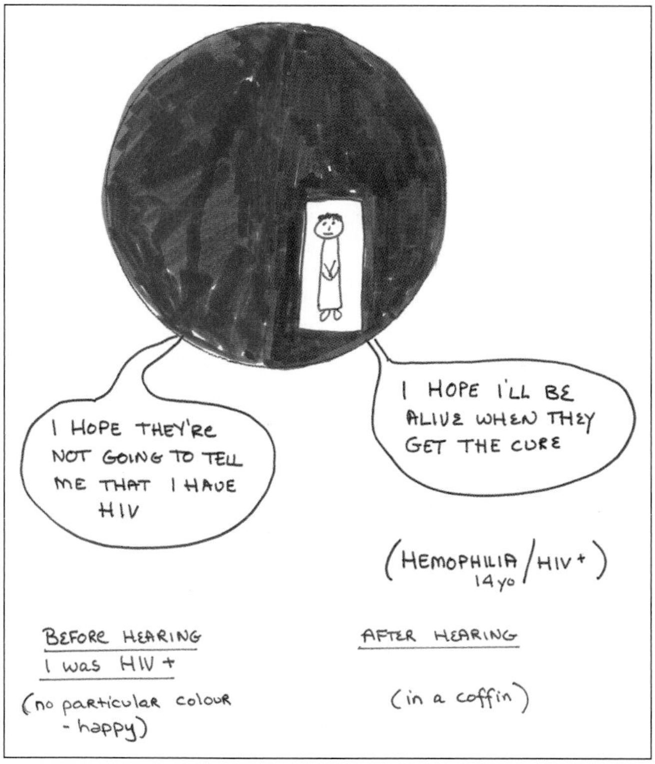

An adolescent with thalassemia, whose brother had died in infancy of the same disease, drew a cemetery image (Fig. 3-19). "My parents and friends are surrounding me [the large cross]. Others who passed away are buried there—especially my little brother—actually, he was my oldest brother. It's raining—sad and depressing. Rain means that something has happened or will happen. I would like people to remember who I am. I don't want any enemies around my grave—or to visit me."

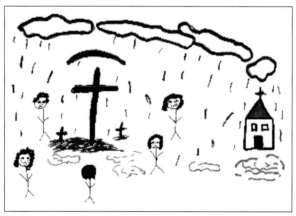

Fig. 3-17   Before and after.

Fig. 3-19   Cemetery.

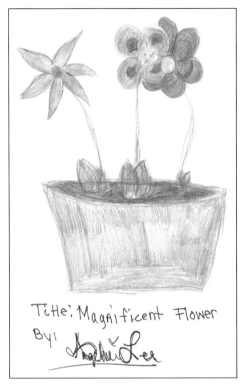

Fig. 3-20 Magnificent flower.

A few weeks before her death, Evangeline, age 13, spontaneously drew a pot of three flowers: two similar blooms nestled into one another, the other flower of a different kind leaning away. She was an only child who worried about how her parents would manage without her after her death (Fig. 3-20). She mused, "What will I call this drawing? 'Flowers on a Journey'… No… 'Flowers Forever'… No. I think I will call it 'Magnificent Flower.'" She moved away from the title that reflected her vulnerability and instead chose the least-threatening option.

A 7-year-old girl had a recurrent dream: "In the dream, I want to be with my mother, and I can never quite get to her." The girl recounted the dream in a joint psychotherapy session with her mother. Whereas the mother found the dream "excruciating," her daughter articulated that "even though the dream is very sad, it's not a nightmare." The dream eventually provided the focal image for mother and child to work through the anticipatory grief process[2] (p. 70).

The distillation of anticipatory grief to its essence marks the imminence of death. At times imperceptibly, at other times dramatically, children often turn inward as they pull back from the external world. Cognitive and emotional horizons narrow because all energy is needed simply for physical survival. A generalized irritability is not uncommon. Children may talk very little, and may even retreat from physical contact. Although such withdrawal is not universal, a certain degree of quietness is almost always in evidence. This behavior is a normal and expected precursor to death.[1]

The Voice of the Child in Decision-Making

Mikaela drew a picture entitled "This or This." (Fig. 3-21) when she found out that her disease had recurred. On one side of a doughnut she depicted tumor cells, on the other side she drew a needle for spinal taps. In the middle of the doughnut is a little stick figure of a person. At the time of drawing the picture, Mikaela said: "I hate needles and spinal taps, but I also don't want my tumor to come back. If I don't have all the needles, then more tumor cells will grow. So if I don't want them to grow, I have to have all those awful needles. That's why I feel as if I am stuck in the middle of a doughnut." Reflecting on the drawing months later, Mikaela elaborated more explicitly: "What I mean by 'I was stuck in a doughnut' is that I had two choices and I didn't want to take either of them. One of the choices was to get needles and pokes and all that stuff and make the tumor go away. My other choice was letting my tumor get bigger and bigger and I would just go away up to heaven…. My mom wanted me to get needles and pokes. But I felt like I just had had too much—too much for my body—too much for me…. So I kind of wanted to go up to heaven that time…. But then I thought about how much my whole entire family would miss me and so just then I was kind of like stuck in a doughnut…."[7]

A 10-year-old sibling whose sister was critically ill stated intensely: "I am mad at all the doctors. I think that they are giving up too soon. I KNOW that my sister will not die, I just know it. But I feel like it's only me who feels that way and no one listens to my opinion." She then drew a heart called "wants to burst" with a black dot of "depression, madness and sadness" (Fig. 3-22).

Over the last decade, there has been increased recognition of children's participation in making treatment decisions. Attention to children's experience of their illness is essential not only to enhance their quality of life, but also as a guide to clinical decisions and goals of care. This may become more challenging as an illness progresses, especially if the family and clinicians are reticent to discuss death with children. A landmark study[14] showed that bereaved parents who had talked with their child about death had no regrets about doing so, whereas those who had not engaged in such discussions were often left with regret. While younger children may not be able to take an abstract or time-based perspective, their expressed fears, concerns, and specific preferences can

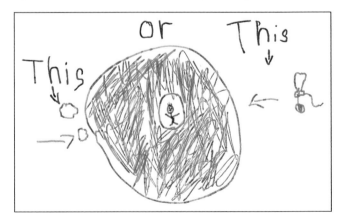

Fig. 3-21 **This or this.** (Reprinted from Sourkes B et al. Food, toys, and love: pediatric palliative care, *Curr Probl Pediatr Adolesc Health Care* 35(9):345–392, 2005.)

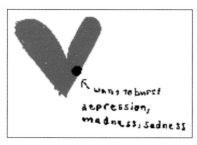

Fig. 3-22 A heart that wants to burst.

provide the basis for decisions. Older children and adolescents who have more capacity to plan over time can engage in complex end-of-life decisions that may be driven by interpersonal relationships.[15–16] However, because actual assessment tools are only in the early stages of development, clinicians are often left to rely on their own judgment to assess children's understanding of the contingencies they face.

Children are often aware of the diminishing curative or life-prolonging options available. It is at this time that they may ask anxiously: "What if this medicine doesn't work? What will you give me next?"[1] Input from members of the interdisciplinary team can be crucial at this juncture: children often express their understanding, awareness, and thoughts about treatment options and living or dying to individuals other than their parents or primary physician. Frequently, their most candid disclosures evolve within the context of psychotherapy.

The ethnic and spiritual culture of the family is a significant factor in how the child's voice is incorporated into the decision-making process. It is especially critical for clinicians to understand how a family's culture defines the construct of "childhood" in terms of protectiveness (e.g., if to tell, how much to tell a child, should a child be an active participant in planning?). A child's expressions about the illness experience must be understood within this framework. The current emphasis in mainstream American culture on the "rights" of children to have access to information and participate in decisions is far from universal. Furthermore, the zeal to include children may inadvertently create a burden on the child that he or she does not feel equipped to manage.

The following vignettes illustrate a spectrum of children's involvement in decision-making.

Child's voice is instrumental in determining plan:

A 7-year-old girl told her parents that she was too tired to fight anymore, and that she wanted to give up. She added: "If I have to continue suffering, I would rather be in heaven." She repeated this statement to the medical team. The parents acknowledged that their child's statements were major determinants in their shifting to a palliative care plan[1] (p. 156).

An adolescent is comfortable within his family culture of non-involvement in decision-making:

A 16-year-old boy from the Middle East had HIV disease secondary to hemophilia. His parents were adamant that he not be told his diagnosis of HIV or the prognosis: "No child of any age should be burdened with such things." The boy politely and repeatedly declined staff's queries about whether he wanted

more information about his condition or whether he had any opinions that he wished to express about treatment options. His knowledge, however "veiled" was nonetheless accurate: he stated that he had a serious immune condition in addition to the hemophilia, that he was aware of body fluid precautions including safer sex, and that he fully trusted his parents' decisions about treatment. He maintained active involvement in school and with friends until his death.

The inadvertent burden of decision-making on a child:

An 11-year-old child had been through many remission-relapse cycles, and had been informed and involved in all aspects of her treatment from the beginning. When she was offered radiation therapy for palliative symptom control, she confided to her psychologist: "I'm scared because I'm not so good at making decisions. My parents want me to have radiation, but a little voice in me tells me not to…. My mother always said that if I die, she wants me to die happy and at home. If I had radiation, I'd have to come into the hospital every day. And I don't know if radiation will really help, or if I would die anyway." Despite what had been her clear understanding of the reason for radiation therapy (exclusively for palliative symptom management), her intense emotion and hope overrode her intellectual grasp as she wondered whether the radiation would help her to live longer ("or would I die anyway")[1] (p. 156).

Role of the Mental Health Professions and Child Life

Palliative care clinicians of all disciplines must rely on many sources to understand and relieve children's distress. The etiology of psychological symptoms in children are multifactorial, and responsive to a host of physical and situational variables. For younger children, physical complaints and irritable or withdrawn behavior may be the most common expressions of emotional distress. The differential for depression or anxiety syndromes includes delirium and encephalopathy, medication side effects, and pain or other physical symptoms such as dyspnea or fatigue. Anxiety may be generalized or specific to separation, procedures, or the anticipation of pain. Medical trauma and terror can also present in a variety of ways in both children and their parents. (See Chapter 26.) Uncertainty around the illness, misconceptions, and lack of communication or secrets surrounding the illness can also fuel distress and changes in behavior. Mental health clinicians, and the entire medical team, need to pay close attention to the history provided by the parents. They also have a specific role, in the course of an evaluation or psychotherapy, to uncover the individual child or adolescent's perceptions of the illness and its implications.

Because children's experiences are so intertwined with those of their parents and the professional team, it is essential to clarify whose distress is being reported. There are often discrepancies in parent and child assessment of symptoms of depression, for example, with parents both over- and underreporting as compared with their child's self-reports.[17] Children and adolescents in particular, try to protect their parents from the extent of their distress.[18] Clinicians who care for these children must be vigilant about the influence of past personal or professional experiences, especially those involving loss, on their assessment of a particular situation.

Mental health professionals and child life specialists focus on children's subjective experience of the illness. Their expertise lies in eliciting and understanding children's language, images, and play. As such, they often serve as interpreters of the child's experiences and needs to the medical team and the parents.

PSYCHOLOGICAL TREATMENT

"I felt much better because I knew that I had somebody to talk to all the time. Every boy needs a psychologist! To see his feelings!"[1] (p. 3).

6-year-old child

"You don't look at me like other people do and judge my behavior. Instead you analyze my behavior and try to get to the root of it. Mostly you helped <u>me</u> get to the root of it, and helped me handle it on my own. You can ask for your family's support, wisdom, experience; but it's not fair to burden them. I have an older sister whom I talk to, but at the same time, I don't want to upset her. I don't want to make her cry for me, I know that when I first met you, I didn't want to talk about it. I wanted to handle it on my own. But that faded so quickly because you're so helpless. You really do need somebody that can come in and help you"[2] (p. 113).

Ideally, the psychological status of each child receiving palliative care should be evaluated in order to plan for optimal care, in the same way that medical and nursing assessments are carried out. The contribution of child psychology and psychiatry, as well as other mental health disciplines, provides specialized knowledge and skills. The specific and unique interventions include: evaluation of the child's psychological status, diagnosis of psychological/psychiatric symptoms and disturbance, psychotherapy and psychotropic medication, and consultation to families and the team. The healthy siblings are included within this network of care.[8]

Reasons for referral for psychological treatment include:

- Diagnosis of depression, anxiety, or traumatic responses in the child or sibling,
- Generalized distress in coping with the exigencies of the illness, as perceived by the child, parents, and/or team,
- Pre-existent stressors or vulnerabilities in the child's life that are now exacerbated by the illness (e.g., psychiatric history in child or family member; recent geographical move, loss of employment, divorce, death of family member),
- Dilemmas in decision-making,
- Requests by parents who want their child to have all possible avenues of intervention and support.[19]

Children and their families respond best to referrals for psychological intervention when key team members explain it as recommended and routine and something that "other families we have treated have found helpful." Children's anxiety can be allayed when they hear the simple, non-threatening explanation: "All children who are ill, or who have siblings who are ill, have worries." Terms such as the "talking doctor"

or the "feelings doctor" provide a functional description that clearly distinguishes the mental health clinician from others on the team. The concept of confidentiality, or privacy, should be introduced early, with a definition of its meaning and boundaries. Over time, even if not articulated, children come to understand the mental health clinician's role in their care. For older children and adolescents, the concept of the "psych person" as a team member, albeit with special bounds of confidentiality, helps to diminish any sense of stigma.

Psychotherapy is the treatment modality unique to the mental health clinician and can add a crucial dimension to a child's comprehensive care. It facilitates psychological adjustment by providing a protected framework for the expression of profound grief, and for the integration of all that he or she has lived, albeit in an abbreviated lifespan. The child conveys the experience of living with uncertainty and the threat of loss through words, drawings, and play and transforms the essence of his or her reality into expression. Furthermore, even for a young child, considerations about remaining quality of life may be discussed.[1,7] Psychotherapy may be the sole intervention, or may be combined with psychotropic medication and behavioral symptom-management techniques.

With the intrusion of the illness, the relationship between children and their parents organizes around the pivot of potential loss. Thus, it is critical that the mental health clinician not intercede as a divisive wedge between them. From the outset, an ongoing alliance diminishes this threat, and optimizes the outcome of the work. Such collaboration is an essential part of the process. Because the parents must sustain the therapeutic work in the child's day-to-day encounters with both physical and emotional stresses, their role cannot be underestimated.[1]

The availability of psychological consultation in pediatric palliative care is often limited. While it is true that psychological treatment is not universally necessary, the opportunity to identify "high-risk" children and intervene in a timely fashion is often missed. The challenge, under these circumstances, is to provide thoughtful emotional support for the child in a carefully planned manner. Such support comes in many forms, from a willingness to listen and answer questions, to regular visits at expected times, to creative art and play that allows the child to express feelings and concerns. If a child has demonstrated particular comfort or closeness with one particular individual on the team, that person may be designated as a resource for the child, with efforts to ensure consistent contact between them. On a cautionary note, there are risks when unskilled or inadequately trained personnel attempt to undertake a psychotherapeutic role. These risks include: opening up too much vulnerability in the child and then not knowing how to contain the emotion; interpreting – beyond simply clarifying – the child's disclosures; promising confidentiality that may set up competition, rather than collaboration, with the parents; and becoming involved with the child beyond appropriate boundaries.[8]

CHILD LIFE INTERVENTION

Child life specialists play a vital role in reducing the impact of stressful and traumatic events on children in medical settings.[20] They work with children and adolescents individually and in groups and develop the programs in the hospital playrooms. They provide both therapeutic intervention and social recreation, framed by their understanding of children's responses to illness. Their insights are integral to the team's understanding of a child's adjustment to the overall experience. They are often a source of emotional support to the siblings and parents as well.

Child life specialists use developmentally appropriate and enjoyable techniques with patients and their siblings to familiarize children with aspects of the medical experience and to provide outlets for their feelings. They prepare the children for medical procedures and teach them coping techniques to alleviate distress, while at the same time enhancing their sense of control and mastery. Their encouragement of children's social interaction, both in the hospital and at home, as well as their liaison with school re-entry programs, mitigates the children's sense of isolation. Importantly, child life specialists assist children in the process of decision making by encouraging and facilitating communication with their parents and with their medical team. Guiding parents in helping the child live as fully as possible, even when close to death, as well as in talking with and involving the siblings during the illness and in bereavement, is another aspect of the child life specialist's role. They are also often instrumental in initiating "legacy activities" with children, siblings, and parents to create lasting memories.

A 5-year-boy who could not have visits from his little sister because he was being prepared for transplant missed her intensely. When it turned out that the transplant could not be done, plans were put in motion to transfer him to home hospice. During that week, he refused to get out of bed or play. When discharge was imminent, his mother asked the child life specialist how to engage him in play at home with his sister. The child life specialist gave the mother many suggestions and also put together a bag including fun objects such as silly string and serious materials including a handprint kit. The family was deeply appreciative and reported that the ideas and the materials had helped them interact and play as well as build memories.

A 16-year-old girl who spoke only Vietnamese was hospitalized for a long period. The week before she died, a nurse asked the child life specialist to bring in a project that would be enjoyable for the child and that the mother could then keep as a memory. The child life specialist brought an example of spin art into the girl's room, and through an interpreter asked whether she wanted to do it. The girl nodded. She had engaged in very little over the past few weeks. The child life specialist returned later in the day with the spin art materials and demonstrated how to do it. It was a magical moment: the child and her mother laughed together as she grabbed the paints and glitter. The child life specialist kept asking her if she wanted to make another, and she nodded yes over and over again. At the end of the afternoon, the mother showed the grandmother all the pictures that were lined up on display. The art project had brought enjoyment to the girl in the company of her mother, gave a sense of control as she wielded the spinner, and left good memories for the family.

Summary

The children who speak in this chapter articulate the concerns of patients and siblings who live in the shadow of life-threatening illness. Children who are not, or who are no longer verbal, or who are developmentally delayed also experience many of these issues, albeit in different ways. As children and families negotiate an illness through its progressive losses and the anticipation of death, palliative care clinicians, in their individual roles and as a team, are their unique companions.

Portions of page 23 in this chapter are reprinted with permission from Brandell, J. *Countertransference in Psychotherapy with Children and Adolescents.* Jason Aronson Publishing Company, 1992. Additional portions of this chapter are reprinted with permission from Sourkes, B. *The Deepening Shade: Psychological Aspects of Life-Threatening Illness*, University of Pittsburgh Press, 1992.

REFERENCES

1. Sourkes B: *Armfuls of time: the psychological experience of the child with a life-threatening illness*, Pittsburgh, 1995, University of Pittsburgh Press.
2. Sourkes B: *The deepening shade: psychological aspects of life-threatening illness*, Pittsburgh, 1982, University of Pittsburgh Press.
3. Sourkes B: Siblings of the pediatric cancer patient. In Kellerman J, editor. *Psychological aspects of childhood cancer*, Springfield, Ill, 1980, Charles C. Thomas, pp 47–69.
4. Sourkes B: Siblings of the child with a life-threatening illness, *J Child Contemp Soc* 19:159–184, 1987.
5. Sharpe D, Rossiter L: Siblings of children with a chronic illness: a meta-analysis, *J Pediatr Psychol* 27(8):699–710, 2002.
6. Alderfer MA, Long KA, et al: Psychosocial adjustment of siblings of children with cancer: a systematic review, *Psychooncology* 27 Oct 2009 Epub.
7. Sourkes B, Frankel L, Brown M, Contro N, et al: Food, toys, and love: pediatric palliative care, *Curr Probl Pediatr Adolesc Health Care* 35(9):345–392, 2005.
8. Sourkes B: The psychological impact of life-limiting illness. In Goldman A, Haines R, Liben S, editors: *Oxford textbook of pediatric palliative care*, London, 2006, Oxford University Press.
9. Wolfe J, Sourkes B: Palliative care for the child with advanced cancer. In Pizzo P, Poplack D, editors. *Principles and practice of pediatric oncology*, ed 5, Philadelphia, 2006, Lippincott, pp 1531–1555.
10. Sourkes B: The child with a life-threatening illness. In Brandell J, editor. *Countertransference in child and adolescent psychotherapy*, New York, 1992, Jason Aronson, pp 267–284.
11. Bluebond-Langner M, editor. *The private worlds of dying children*, Princeton, NJ, 1978, Princeton University Press.
12. Sourkes B: The broken heart: anticipatory grief in the child facing death, *J Palliat Care* 12(3):56–59, 1996.
13. Kuttner L: *Making every moment count: pediatric palliative care.* Documentary film, 2003, National Film Board of Canada.
14. Kreicbergs U, Valdimarsdóttir U, Onelöv E, Henter J, Steineck G: Talking about death with children who have severe malignant disease, *JAMA* 351(12):1175–1186, 2004.
15. Hinds PS, Schum L, Baker JN, Wolfe J: Key factors affecting dying children and their families, *J Palliat Med* 8(Suppl 1):S70–S78, 2005.
16. Hinds PS, Drew D, Oakes LL, Fouladi M, Spunt SL, Church C, Furman WL: End-of-life preferences of pediatric patients with cancer, *J Clin Oncol* 23(36):9146–9154, 2005.
17. DeJong M, Fombonne E: Depression in pediatric cancer: an overview, *Psychooncology* 15:553–566, 2006.
18. Stuber ML, Gonzalez S, Benjamin H, et al: Fighting for recovery: group interventions for adolescents with cancer and their parents, *J Psychother Pract Res* 4(4):286–296, 1995.
19. Sourkes B, Kazak A, Wiener L: Psychotherapeutic interventions. In Kazak A, Kupst M, Pao M, Patenaude A, Weiner L, editors: *Quick reference for pediatric oncology clinicians: the psychiatric and psychological dimensions of pediatric cancer symptom management*, Charlottesville, Va, 2009, International Psycho-Oncology Society Press.
20. Munn E, Robison K: Palliative care and the role of child life, *Child Life Council* 22(3):4–6, 2004.

4 Understanding the Illness Experience and Providing Anticipatory Guidance

JAVIER R. KANE | MARSHA JOSELOW | JANET DUNCAN

Matthew was a red-haired little boy suffering from congenital microvillus inclusion disease, an autosomal recessive disorder that is characterized by intestinal failure and often treated with multivisceral organ transplantation. This patient and his family experienced a great deal of suffering. When he was 5 years old, after a year-long hospitalization and careful consideration of prognosis and establishment of realistic goals of care, his family decided to bring him home despite concerns for the complexity of his care. He was discharged on multiple medications including continuous opioid infusion and parenteral nutrition under the care of the local hospice and palliative care team. Medical care continued at home as an integral aspect of a normal family life. His last months included a trip to a Nascar race, visits by a local fireman, and a full array of school services. Most importantly he was wrapped in the love of his two sisters, parents, and grandparents through his death (Figs. 4-1 to 4-3).

Establishing a Therapeutic Alliance

The relationship between clinicians and families is the cornerstone of quality care for the child with a life-threatening illness and his or her family. The bond of trust that exists among clinicians, pediatric patients, and their families is vital to the process of caring. The development of this relationship is greatly promoted if the clinician has knowledge of the person and family who are the focus of his or her care. Healthcare providers must create an open, nonjudgmental atmosphere in which vulnerable persons can feel free to share their experiences. Demonstrating empathy and a personal interest in the well-being of the patient and their family leads to a sense of connection and provides the foundation for an effective therapeutic alliance.

Understanding the patient's and family's beliefs, values, hopes, wishes, expectations, fears, and worries is crucial for clinicians who strive to create a plan of care with their patients. Clinicians must be willing to listen, empathize, solve problems, and encourage life-affirming events with patients and families as they face the challenges associated with a life-threatening illness. Misunderstandings and frustrations more often occur when clinicians offer treatment options without understanding the feelings, thoughts, and underlying themes that guide the patient's and family's decision-making process. A sample of exploratory responses that may be used in communicating with children and families is included in Table 4-1.

An essential part of establishing a therapeutic alliance is regular meetings with the patient and his or her family in which issues outlined in this chapter are discussed. Such discussions

should be planned with care. For example, adequate time for in-depth conversation should be allotted, a private setting should be arranged, and the presence of both parents and/or others who are identified as primary supporters should be ensured. By listening respectfully and building on the parents' knowledge, the interdisciplinary team (IDT)—which is typically composed of doctors, nurses, social workers, child life specialists, chaplains, and psychologists—can tailor information and educate the family about treatment options and other issues of relevance. Recommendations may be made based on the existing evidence, on realistic goals, and within the child's and family's psychosocial and spiritual context. Elements of anticipatory guidance in the palliative care setting are discussed in the following section and suggested themes are presented in Box 4-1.

Understanding the Illness Experience

BELIEFS AND VALUES

To understand the patient's and family's illness experience, the IDT must actively listen and question to gain insight about the family's core beliefs and values. Values are the personal beliefs that the patient and/or family consider important and to which they are emotionally attached. Values are subjective, may evolve over time as a result of life experiences, and can influence specific behaviors and personal goals. Values that develop during childhood often are derived from the experiences a person has in his or her family, culture, religion, or community. They can also evolve from unchallenged or unexplored assumptions. All of these values make up an individual's belief system.

Beliefs and values give meaning to a person's life. They influence the patient's and family's perceptions about how things are and how things should be. Values may dictate preferences in some circumstances. Patients with life-threatening conditions and their parents apply a set of values to guide decisions about medical care.[1,2] Decisions made by patients and families about whether a certain treatment is desirable are often based on their determination of the treatment's positive or negative qualities and whether it is perceived as beneficial. For those dealing with a progressive or incurable illness, these judgments may occur in the context of values that reflect the dual goal of seeking disease-directed therapies and comfort-directed care.[3]

Identifying and understanding the patient's and family's beliefs and values is an important palliative care skill that helps direct efforts toward improving the quality of end-of-life care. Having open and thoughtful conversations about the patient's and family's goals of care can be an effective approach to understanding their values and priorities. These conversations may also help patients and families who

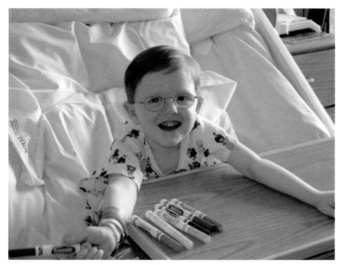

Fig. 4-1   Matthew enjoying an art project in the hospital.

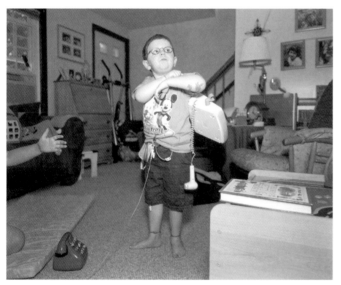

Fig. 4-2   Matthew at home.

are not fully aware of the values they hold deeply and which may guide decisions about their care. In a study examining end-of-life care preferences, parents of seriously ill children identified the following as important end-of-life priorities: honest and complete information, ready access to staff,

communication and care coordination, emotional expressions and support by staff, preservation of the integrity of the parent-child relationship, and faith.[4] Moreover, when considering withdrawal of artificial life-sustaining support, parents placed the highest priorities on prognosis, quality of life, and their child's level of comfort.[5,6] Honoring these personal values may facilitate the family's ability to maintain a sense of dignity and integrity.

An important universal value shared by seriously ill patients and their families is the presence of consistent and meaningful relationships within the family unit and with the care team.[7] Relationship-based value judgments consistently inform patients' preferences and decision making.[8] Sometimes the expressed values of patients and families differ from those of their healthcare providers. In a study to ascertain parents' and physicians' assessments of quality of end-of-life care for children dying from cancer, Mack et al, found that for parents, doctor-patient communication is the principal determinant of high-quality physician care.[9] Communicating with honesty and sensitivity about what to expect at the end of their child's life, communicating directly with the child when appropriate, and preparing the parent for circumstances surrounding the child's death were all cited by parents as high-quality care. In contrast, physicians' ratings of high-quality end-of-life care depended on biomedical variables such as less pain and fewer days in the hospital rather than relational parameters. Consequently, clinicians are advised to think about what they consider important in the care of a patient at the end of life and acknowledge the risk of imposing their own value system in the context of a therapeutic alliance with a patient and family facing end-of-life care issues.

HOPES AND WISHES

In talking with patients and their families about hope, it is important for clinicians to distinguish being hopeful from wishful thinking, having unrealistic expectations, or feeling optimistic.[10] Palliative care clinicians can help patients, families, and their healthcare providers by listening without judgment to their experiences and helping to solidify a deeper understanding of these concepts as they evolve in the context of serious illness. Ultimately, hope influences the decisions made by patients and families facing a life-threatening illness.

Hope is a response to severe distress that allows a person to adapt to a situation, such as the realization that their child has an incurable illness that cannot be controlled. Hope presupposes an accurate assessment and acknowledgment of the reality of a situation, as determined by the evidence made

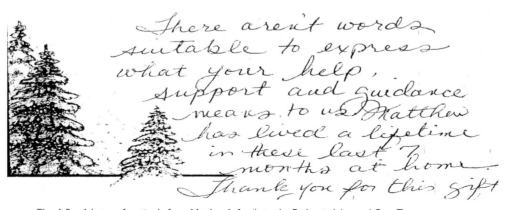

Fig. 4-3   A letter of gratitude from Matthew's family to the Pediatric Advanced Care Team.

TABLE 4-1 Exploratory Questions Useful in Communicating with Children and Families

Lila is 10 years old and has a progressive neurodegenerative disorder leading to severe developmental delay, blindness, feeding intolerance, poor swallowing coordination, recurrent aspiration pneumonias, and spastic quadriplegia (Fig. 4-4). Lila is an integral member of her family and enjoys toys and activities that provide tactile, visual, and auditory stimulation. Lila lives with her parents, Dana and Robert, and her older brother, Joe (Fig. 4-5).

Communication theme	Exploratory questions	Illness experience	Parental responses
Beginning the conversation	Tell us about your child before she became sick. What types of things does your child enjoy? How has this illness impacted your child? Your family? What is most bothersome to your child today? Pain, shortness of breath, fatigue, nausea, constipation, anxiety, sadness?	Lila's parents are most concerned about her worsening respiratory condition and the possible need for frequent hospital admissions in the winter. They have questions about placement of a tracheostomy tube and whether it would be beneficial. Parents want to maintain normalcy for the older brother. Parents are exhausted and questioning how to continue caring for their daughter and son.	Dana: "I worry that she will have a bad winter and have to come back to the hospital often." Robert: "Some doctor told me that she might need a tracheostomy at some point, I just don't think I want my baby girl to go through that." Dana: "Lila's brother, Joe, is doing well in school but he does worry about Lila. Lila has been in the hospital so many times, I wish I could spend more time with Joe." Robert: "Having a nurse at home would help. Right now it is either my wife or me taking care of Lila during the night and we do not get much sleep."
Beliefs and values	Do you have particular beliefs that guide you? What is most important for you and your family right now? Given your understanding of your child's illness, what are your priorities and goals for Lila and your family right now? What gives you strength as you face this adversity?	Lila's parents are struggling with how to decide/deciding when enough is enough. Lila's mother values comfort and quality of life. She believes that her daughter has suffered a great deal. She would like to avoid invasive painful procedures. The family would prefer to limit hospital visits and to stay at home as much as possible. The family has many friends and a community that supports them. Lila's mother gathers strength from the support of her friends and family. Lila's father values his spirituality and relationship to God.	Dana: "Lila hates being in the hospital, and I worry she will get sick there. Is there a way we can keep her at home but still keep her comfortable?" Robert: "We used to go to church. I still pray,…but truthfully I am kind of mad at God."
Hopes and wishes	What are you expecting from the treatment/medical interventions that your child is receiving? Given your understanding of your child's illness, what are you hoping for?	Lila's parents understand the serious nature of her condition. They want to maintain her quality of life by treating illnesses she will most likely recover from. They want her to be comfortable and able to participate in family activities.	Dana: "We know there is no cure. We hope to have her for as long as possible, as healthy as possible."
Sadness and depression	How has your child's illness impacted your own life? Please share with me the emotional changes you have noticed in your child. Tell me about what helps you get through these days.	Lila's mother gets teary as she relates how difficult it is for her to watch her daughter in pain with multiple medical procedures. She describes how settling it is for her daughter to be in the hospital. Lila's condition has had a significant impact on her family's life.	Dana: "When she is in the hospital, my husband has to work and I have to run back and forth from home to check on Joe and the pets and house. I know Lila gets scared when I am not with her." Dana: "Having Lila has made me a better and stronger person but has put a strain on our marriage."
Fear and anxiety	What worries you the most right now? For your child, your family and yourself? Would it be helpful to talk about what to expect if your child's illness gets worse?	Her family believes that Lila's previous surgery was associated with onset of further neurological decline and for that reason they deferred recommended hip surgery for years.	Dana: "If Lila had the surgery would she be able to come off the breathing machine? They told us she probably wouldn't live past 2 years old. I wonder how much longer she will live. I just do not want to put her at risk for complications that could make her dependent on machines."

available through thoughtful conversations about prognosis. A hopeful person understands the present reality but is open to a future full of possibilities, rendering him or her less likely to take a position of certainty about what the future will bring. The psychological benefit of hope may be derived from the person's openness to possible alternatives in the presence of uncontrollable forces, a sense of connection to someone or something beyond himself or herself, and the ability to surrender control to a higher being or force (that is, generalized, unconditional hope). For instance, parents may hope for a miracle cure while making medical decisions guided by the expectation that their

child will die, the basis of which is previous conversations about the child's poor prognosis for survival.

Hope is also the belief that there will be a positive outcome related to circumstances in the patient's and family's lives. A hopeful state arises from having a sense that what is desired will indeed happen. Here, the psychological benefit of hoping during times of trouble and uncertainty may result from the expectation that what is hoped for will be fulfilled (i.e., specific, conditional hope). For example, the parent of a child whose death is imminent may hope for a miracle, and the expectation of its fulfillment may facilitate personal coping but prevent

BOX 4-1 Suggested Themes of Effective Anticipatory Guidance of Patients and Families in Need of Pediatric Palliative Care

Advanced Illness Care Planning

- Engage in effective communication with members of the care team
- Ask about cultural, ethnic, religious, familial beliefs and values
- Establish realistic expectations during conversations with parents about the patient's prognosis
- Identify distress and discuss the need for support in making difficult decisions about care
- Establish goal-directed treatment options, such as cure, prolongation of a good quality life, and comfort at the end of life
  - Benefit vs. burden of invasive procedures, including mechanical ventilation, tracheostomy, cardiopulmonary support, cardiopressors, aimed at prolonging life artificially in an intensive care unit setting
  - Use of other interventions aimed at prolonging life artificially, such as chemotherapy, transfusion of blood products, antibiotics, artificially provided hydration and nutrition, CPAP and BIPAP
  - Escalation of comfort medications, such as morphine, benzodiazepines, antiemetics
  - Personal goals that may influence decision making and plan of care—comfort, suffering, quality of life
- Recognize and convey that there may be no realistic chance of cure early in the illness trajectory or that there may be continued uncertainty of the illness trajectory
- Assist in reaching a consensus as a family about crucial decisions
- Identify in advance those issues that may need clarification by the treating physician
- Offer to talk with patients and their siblings about dying and death
- Help patients and families make informed decisions and avoid decisional regret. Provide medical recommendations as appropriate
- Support parents in their goal of being the best parents possible

Ethical and Legal Considerations

- Ethical and legal considerations about the following should be discussed:
  - Do Not Resuscitate orders
  - Advanced directives and other care-planning documents
  - Appointment of a healthcare agent
  - Appointment of a surrogate decision-maker
- Balance the legal presumption of incompetence of minors with the mature adolescent patient's moral right to participate in care decisions
- Address questions about withholding or withdrawing treatment with curative intent for reasons of conscience
- Formulate a consistent response from physicians and the institution to requests for treatment considered to be medically inappropriate
- Provide access to the institutional Ethics Committee to help resolve conflict

Symptom Control

- Alert the care team to the patient's comfort needs and level of function
- Identify and address the symptoms of most concern to the patient and family
- Inform the family about the child's physical and psychological symptom burden at the end of life and what to expect
- Provide access to expert symptom control, including pain or palliative care teams, if needed
- Provide comfort medications and access to a symptom control kit for home use
- Address opioid myths of physical dependence, tolerance, addiction, and pseudo-addiction, decreased respirations equated with hastening of death
- Address questions about alternative and complementary therapies

Emotional, Social, and Spiritual Care

- Discuss the family's emotional, social, and spiritual needs with the care team
- Make available interdisciplinary psychosocial and spiritual support to the family
- Provide culturally sensitive care
- Inform families about community resources and help access these resources
- Discuss death and dying with members of the care team

Care Coordination and Continuity

- Provide coordinated services and promote collaboration among members of the IDT
- Provide continuity of information and relationships throughout the illness trajectory and across care settings
- Discuss the option of hospice care early during the course of the illness
- Conduct family care conferences and IDT meetings

Care of the Imminently Dying Child

- Provide access to expert symptom control
- Provide access to interdisciplinary psychosocial and spiritual support
- Allow the child and family to participate in the decision-making process
- Discuss with the family end-of-life care preferences including the desired location of death
- Discuss the patient's right to die in a familiar setting that is as free of burdens as possible
- Query the family about funeral arrangements and possible autopsy and organ tissue donation
- Help the family build the child's legacy

Bereavement Care

- Reinforce positive role of parents and participation of child in leading the way in the journey of the illness
- Focus on the child's and family's goals and comfort at the end of life
- Encourage self-care of parents and attention to any sibling issues
- Provide access to psychosocial and spiritual support
- Participate in staff debriefing and support

---

decisions about withholding potentially harmful treatment with curative intent. In this scenario, additional guidance may be needed to help reframe the focus of the parents' hope and transition them to a more realistic stance, such as hope for comfort at the end of life.

Within a patient's or family's construct of hope, they may have wishful thinking and optimism that helps them find meaning in the situation and allows them to face each day with some purpose and balance. Wishful thinking identifies a desire for more concrete objects, actions, or goals and may or may not be based on an accurate interpretation of reality. Wishful thinking involves personal determination, effort, and the need for control, all of which may result in experiencing a sense of distress. For instance, parents may wish for one more family vacation, or a teen may dream about his or her first car. However, in the presence of a hopeless situation such as imminent death, a person's expressed desire for treatment with curative intent, even if considered medically inappropriate, would be more consistent with wishful thinking rather than possessing hope. The expression "to hope against hope" is used to describe a hope for something that is not likely to be fulfilled.

Families facing the end of a life often hope for a miracle and sometimes ask clinicians if they believe in miracles. This question is most often meant in a global sense, as they are simply seeking reassurance that anything is possible. It may be useful for the family to articulate perceived differences between the hope that they obtain from having a sense of connection with a higher power and the expectation of any benefit resulting from a specific medical intervention. Expressions of optimism by patients and parents may also seem unrealistic to healthcare providers when verbalized in the midst of dire circumstances. Expressions of optimism differ from hope in that they are often a reflection of the mood of the patient or family member and involve self-assertive statements such as, "I'm OK!" Such comments are often in contrast with the perceptions of others who wonder how that can be true.

It is not uncommon to hear staff members worry that parents are not "getting it," have not been told about the child's prognosis, or are in denial when the parents make hopeful, optimistic, or wishful statements. A communication schism may occur, and the therapeutic alliance can be severely compromised, if parents are denied the opportunity to express their hopes

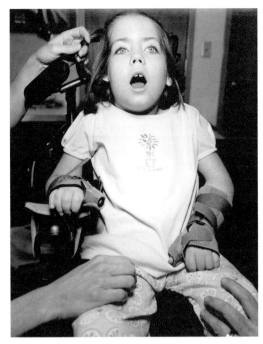

Fig. 4-4   Lila.

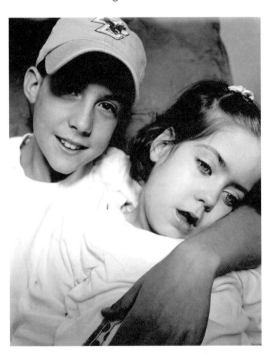

Fig. 4-5   Lila and her older brother, Joe.

and wishes. Patients and families may express their hopes and wishes interchangeably, and many use the language of hope in a religious or spiritual context. In the presence of progressive illness, hope can be a powerful coping mechanism, and caregivers must be careful not to strip it away through careless confrontation or premature conversations. It is difficult, however, to differentiate between expressions of wishful thinking and those of hope, and in practice, patients and families often experience a combination of the two. Although helping the patient or family to reframe hope may be appropriate in some circumstances, clinicians must do so only in the context of a relationship based on trust and always remain respectful

of the patient's and family's overall experiences. A clinician's responsibility is to acknowledge hope and gently reframe the patient's and family's expectations by providing relevant clinical data. In a study to evaluate the relationship between prognostic disclosure and hope, Mack et al. found that parents who received more information about the patient's prognosis and had high-quality communication were more likely to report communication-related hope, even when the likelihood of a cure was low.[11] Such conversations may allow for a balanced perspective of hope for cure and expectations of benefit from treatment.

SADNESS AND DEPRESSION

The experience of serious illness is always deeply emotional. Intense feelings greatly influence patients' and families' sense of hope and affect how they make decisions about their medical care.

Expressions of hopelessness are often accompanied by profound sadness, defined as an emotional state of varying intensity characterized by feelings of unhappiness.[12] Sadness, sorrow, or desolation are normal responses when individuals face a threat to meaningful relationships, a loss of their personal values, or feelings of loneliness and isolation. Sadness in children may be their mourning the loss of the life they previously had (e.g., interacting with friends, playing, attending school) as well as their threatened future; parents mourn the loss of the dreams they held for their child.

Learning to distinguish between sadness and depression is important in palliative care. Depression is a mood disorder characterized by the loss of self-esteem, feelings of guilt, anger, and despair, and negative views about one's own future. A profound sense of hopelessness at times may be accompanied by suicidal ideation.[10] Symptoms of depression include fatigue, insomnia, decreased performance at school or work, loss of appetite, loss of interest in activities previously enjoyed, and social withdrawal. In general, the source of sadness is more specific than that of depression, and a sad person is usually able to experience pleasure and happiness about other aspects of his or her life. For a depressed person, sadness and hopelessness are broader and more pervasive. Although encouraging patients and families to openly share their feelings and reconnect with loved ones may alleviate their sadness, concerns about depression may warrant a psychiatric consult, counseling, and pharmacotherapy.[13,14]

FEAR AND ANXIETY

Fear and anxiety are reactions to the vulnerability and lack of control inherent in the presence of serious illness and to the anticipation of an uncertain future. Although they are normal and expected responses, they may impair parents' abilities to think clearly and communicate effectively with the clinical team. Fear is an emotional reaction to a specific threat or the expectation of danger. Anxiety is a state of uneasiness and distress in response to a vague and less specific threat and may be manifested as apprehension or worry.[12] Anxiety is considered normal when it is in proportion to the source of distress and the person is able to adapt and function once the anxiety has run its course. When anxiety becomes pathological, as in generalized anxiety disorder, phobias, or panic attacks, the degree of anxiety is not proportional to the event that generated the distress, and the person is rendered incapable of functioning effectively (see Chapter 25).

Factors that contribute to parental anxiety include guilt about their inability to protect the child, a sense of meaninglessness, and feelings of isolation from family and friends. Overwhelming anxiety may interfere with a parent's ability to cope effectively and lead to withdrawal from the child, extreme anger, avoidance of the medical team, or inappropriate and threatening comments. When parents present with intense anxiety, it is important to help them identify resources, such as spiritual practices and nurturing relationships, that have helped them in the past when they have felt overwhelmed and threatened. A joint effort of the palliative care clinician and primary care team is essential to provide increased support for the parents. This support may be in the form of assuring the team's consistent presence, encouraging the parents to take a break and scheduling regular (or more frequent) family meetings. It is also important that the team identify and understand particular triggers and circumstances in the medical setting, including the child's transfer to the ICU, initiating opioids, or discharge home that increase anxiety in order to guide families through these transitions with less distress.

Referrals to a mental health clinician for psychotherapy or evaluation for pharmacotherapy are essential when anxiety compromises a parent's ability to function. Some people benefit from cognitive behavioral therapy,[15] benzodiazepines, or selective serotonin reuptake inhibitors,[16] physical activity,[17] hypnosis, or guided imagery.[18] Others have used complementary therapies including massage or herbs such as Kava or Valerian.[19,20]

ASSESSMENT OF NEEDS

High-quality palliative and end-of-life care requires interdisciplinary patient- and family-centered assessments of physical, emotional, social, and spiritual needs.[21,22] Assessment of the effect of the illness on practical aspects of daily life such as eating, sleeping, playing, performing at school or work, housing, transportation, family dynamics, and finances is also important. This assessment can identify what the ill child, adolescent, or parents consider important and provide information on what is needed to optimize comfort and quality of life.[23] The family's values may also reflect a cultural understanding of illness and its treatment.[24] The response of the IDT to the patient's and family's needs in the presence of progressive illness is considered an ethical imperative.[25] Ongoing, regular assessment of these needs allows the team to jointly formulate a care plan with the family that incorporates interventions, practices, and support services that enhance comfort, facilitate care coordination, and optimize quality of life.[26] Instruments for assessing pain and other symptoms[27] and guidelines for psychosocial assessment and support are available elsewhere.[28,29]

Providing Anticipatory Guidance

SHARING RELEVANT INFORMATION

Anticipatory guidance in pediatric palliative care is challenging for many reasons: the complexity of the issues encountered and their sensitive natures, the uniqueness of each patient's and family's experience, the limited time available for relevant conversations, and the natural resistance that some families have in confronting such difficult and threatening issues. To facilitate communication with patients and families, one must take into consideration their physical, emotional, social, and spiritual needs, their need for support in the process of making difficult decisions, and anticipatory guidance. As discussed in previous sections, two important components of anticipatory guidance in pediatric palliative care are learning about the child and the illness experience from his or her perspective and establishing a therapeutic alliance. The third component of anticipatory guidance is sharing relevant information, which may include information learned from other families in similar circumstances. This process helps patients and families to feel a sense of control and comfort in the knowledge that they have made the best decisions possible throughout the illness trajectory.

ADVANCED ILLNESS CARE PLANNING

Care of children with life-threatening conditions is characterized by difficult communication and sensitive information sharing. Establishing a prognosis is part of the therapeutic alliance; patients and families have the right to be informed about the prognosis, and these conversations must occur within the context of a comprehensive, individualized, patient-centered approach.[30] Children suffer from the disease and the symptoms that it produces, as well as from the pain and discomfort that result from the procedures and therapies. To empower families to effectively participate in treatment decisions, clinicians must have open and honest conversations about the patient's prognosis to guide the family's expectations and identify realistic goal-directed treatment options.[21,31,32] Having these conversations and setting realistic goals of care in the context of planning for advanced illness care is an important and effective way to ensure that all of the family's decisions are made with their child's well-being and best interests in mind.[25] Families can be taught to recognize specific events in the child's care as markers for the need to revisit his or her prognosis and goals.[33] The integration of palliation into the continuum of care may help the family to optimize the child's comfort and quality of life.[26]

In general, clinicians recognize that the participation of patients and families in the decision-making process has many benefits, and they are willing to engage in conversations about advanced illness care planning. This is best done as a longitudinal process that is initiated soon after the diagnosis and maintained throughout the illness.[34,35] Anticipatory guidance when a child is not in crisis may be better tolerated. For instance, the family may be more receptive to discussing resuscitation recommendations before the child is facing imminent death. An unspoken, but common, fear of parents is that the search and hope for curative therapies will be abandoned or that their child's care will be compromised. Families will need to know in advance that the team is willing to talk about difficult issues, including the topics of death and dying.[36] The team should offer parents the opportunity to think and talk about their worst fear—the possibility that their child may not survive the illness.

Clinicians must recognize that communication, care planning, and establishing realistic care goals are important components of high-quality medical care.[37] Clinicians may help parents achieve peace of mind in the presence of a life-threatening illness by providing appropriate medical information.[38] Factors perceived by parents to facilitate communication and decision making include trust, confidence, building relationships, demonstrating effort, availability of the team and feeling supported by it, the exchange of information on the health and disease status of the child, an appropriate level of child and parent involvement, and the knowledge that all curative options have been attempted.[39,40] Consideration of these factors is particularly important at the end of life when patients and families face the challenges of deciding whether to participate in Phase I clinical studies, maintain or withdraw artificial life support, receive further disease-directed therapy, or agree to a Do Not Resuscitate order, which are some of the most difficult decisions parents have to make.[41]

Anticipatory guidance for patients with a progressive illness and their families includes helping parents recognize that a cure is no longer possible and helping them to deal with the child's impending death.[42] Physicians usually recognize that a child does not have a realistic possibility of a cure months before the child's parents do, and earlier recognition of this prognosis by physicians and parents is associated with a stronger emphasis on treatment directed at lessening suffering and greater integration of palliative care.[43] Parents also learn the importance of reaching a consensus as a family about critical decisions. Interestingly, the mother's and father's goals are often in agreement with each other at the time of diagnosis but can differ at the end of life, and their level of parental agreement about lessening suffering at the end of life may influence their decisions and perceptions about the child's suffering.[44]

Finally, parents often worry about making the best decision for their child. Families must be supported during this process to help avoid decisional regret during their bereavement. In a recent study, many bereaved parents indicated that they would not recommend the last course of chemotherapy for children with incurable cancer, mostly because they felt their own children suffered as a result of such therapy.[45] Clinicians should aim to understand parents' perceptions about their own roles in the care of their seriously ill child and assist them in their goal of being the best parents they can be. Parents may blame themselves for the child's illness or suffering. They may feel guilty because they cannot alleviate suffering. They may also think that they have failed as parents, because they could not protect their child or save him or her from the illness. It is essential that the team reassure parents of their strengths, reframe their perceived deficiencies, and support their decisions.

ETHICAL AND LEGAL CONSIDERATIONS

Sometimes families need additional information about ethical and legal considerations (also see Chapter 13). Issues that may be appropriate for anticipatory guidance include the legal aspects of Do Not Resuscitate orders, advanced directives, appointment of a healthcare agent or designation of surrogates, and possible responses of emergency medical professionals if 911 is called. Parents of teenaged children may welcome further education on the need to balance the legal presumption of incompetence of children younger than 18 years with the moral right of a mature adolescent to participate in making decisions about his or her own medical care.[46] Some parents may need counsel on the legality of withholding or withdrawing artificial life-sustaining therapies during the last stages of illness because they fear being accused of medical neglect of their child.[47,48] Others may need information on legal considerations related to foregoing treatment for religious reasons.[49]

The use of life-sustaining or invasive interventions may cause harm in patients who are in a persistent vegetative state or in those whose death is imminent. Families can benefit from guidance about what constitutes futility. Physicians and institutions need to have in place a process that aims to enhance deliberation and resolution of conflict when families request therapies considered medically inappropriate.[50] Regardless of the clinical scenario, families need to be assured that all treatment options have been explored. In addition, they may benefit from assistance in arranging a second opinion. In situations of conflict, anticipatory guidance may also include helping parents access the institutional Ethics Committee to assist them and their care team in the process of making difficult decisions.[51]

SYMPTOM CONTROL

Families often worry that their child will suffer as the disease progresses or suffer at the end of life.[52,53] Informing families about what they may face in caring for their child is helpful. Families need to know the nature of the child's underlying condition and the symptoms that can be expected.[54] For example, severe pain occurs more commonly in children with solid tumors, and neurological symptoms are more common in children with brain tumors or other disorders of the central nervous system. The integration of palliative care adds healthcare resources designed to optimize physical comfort. Families need to know that integrating such services during the early stages of the illness does not represent premature access to end-of-life care.[55] Families can be alerted about the possibility of thoughtful and creative pharmacologic and nonpharmacologic management of symptoms such as pain, seizures, anxiety, gastrointestinal distress, insomnia, and dyspnea across the spectrum of the child's illness. Furthermore, families may need additional counseling on the uses of alternative and complementary therapies such as massage, meditation, Reiki, healing touch, or music thanatology.[56] Finally, families should receive information to dissipate fears about the use of opioids and their association with respiratory depression and addiction and understand the differences between physical dependence, tolerance, addiction, and pseudo-addiction.[57]

EMOTIONAL, SOCIAL, AND SPIRITUAL CARE

Chronic, life-threatening, and incurable illness in a child is emotionally challenging and tragic. Anticipatory guidance in psychosocial and spiritual care includes helping families know that they are not alone in these experiences and that there are many resources and strategies for coping and gaining some sense of control.[58] Acknowledging the risk for physical and emotional fatigue, recognizing the benefit of communicating their needs to clinicians, and having access to consistent care and support in solving problems may decrease a family's sense of isolation and despair. The team should provide options to enhance coping such as referrals for grief counseling and financial advice, Web-based support groups and resources, the opportunity to speak to other families who have had a similar experience, and access to relevant books and reading materials. The team should also facilitate access to hospital and/or community supports such as chaplains, art and music therapists, child life specialists, psychologists, psychiatrists, and social workers.

Anticipatory guidance should also include education about community resources.[59] This may be even more relevant upon the child's discharge from the hospital. Parents often experience fear about not having access to the services they perceive as necessary to satisfy the home-based needs of their seriously ill child. Knowing that resources and additional support are available if needed is comforting and stress-relieving.[7] Particularly important in this regard is guidance on the use of hospice services for children. Many families have incorrect perceptions about what hospice is and the kind of services that these agencies provide. Presenting hospice as a possible resource at least 12 months prior to expected death has been suggested as a preferred practice for quality care.[22] Families also need guidance in accessing hospital, community, local, state, and federal resources.[58] Anticipating current and future needs and providing hands-on assistance in accessing these resources is necessary to maximize family function and minimize additional stress. Such needs may include supplemental health insurance, respite care, transportation, financial resources, school and community programs, and home and vehicle modifications.

CARE COORDINATION AND CONTINUITY

Families encounter a multitude of clinicians and may be given different opinions or recommendations, and those clinicians may not know of the child's and family's goals.[39] In these situations, families must ask clinicians for greater transparency and continuity of information among the members of the team and their medical home.[60,61] Families who receive services from healthcare professionals representing a variety of specialties and disciplines may ask for greater care coordination and collaboration in the form of an interdisciplinary care team meeting, or request to meet with healthcare providers as a group, as in a family care conference. Bringing together clinicians to build a consensus based on the shared knowledge of the family's perspectives allows for consistent communication and works toward mutual goals. Identifying a case manager or advanced practice nurse as the point person to assist the parents may help alleviate stress and confusion.[62,63]

Provision of continuity of care, including trusting relationships and information, throughout the illness and across the hospital, clinic, and home settings may best convey the principles of nonabandonment.[64] Indeed, for patients with chronic conditions, care continuity may be associated with fewer care-related problems.[65] This concept presupposes that the therapeutic relationship established among patients, families, and their clinicians will be maintained throughout the illness, particularly when the illness progresses. Barriers imposed by a fragmented healthcare delivery system may threaten this therapeutic bond. Parents need to know that their child's team will not abandon the patient or family as their goals of care place greater emphasis on comfort and quality of life than on provision of curative therapies. As the illness progresses and more home-based resources are used, families often seek to maintain the close bonds established with clinicians in tertiary care centers, where the child received most of his or her care. Families should know of their right to access a flexible care-coordination approach rooted in ongoing communication, trust, and continuity of care that incorporates understanding of the family's values, goals, and their religious, cultural, and spiritual beliefs.

CARE OF THE IMMINENTLY DYING CHILD

Anticipatory guidance at the end of life includes helping parents recognize that their child has an incurable illness and when their child is showing signs and symptoms of imminent death.[22] Having delicate discussions about what parents hope and expect for their child may help guide care planning for end of life and facilitate the availability of services to enhance comfort and quality of life.[43] Conversations about imminent death may also allow clinicians to ensure adequate pain relief and provide the guidance that families need to attend suffering, and allow the family enough time to grieve.[66] Anticipatory guidance during this time includes the participation of the child and family in the decision making, identification of symptoms that cause the most distress, strategies for managing escalating symptoms, enhanced focus on comfort and quality of life, access to interdisciplinary psychosocial and spiritual support, and minimizing medical technology or artificial means of prolonging life.[22] Furthermore, raising questions about funeral arrangements and the possibility of autopsy or tissue donation can be helpful, because it lets parents know that these difficult topics can be discussed openly before death.

Identifying and addressing the patient's symptoms that cause the most concern at the end of life is particularly important. This may include parental concerns about pain, weakness, and fatigue and changes in behavior, appearance, or breathing. Parents also report additional benefit from spending time with clinicians, receiving advice about these issues, and having access to appropriate symptom management.[67] Depending on the location and needs of the child, home-based services may be provided by a visiting nurse association or hospice agency. If the child transitions home, it is important to consider what measures are practical and possible in the hospital vs. the home setting, where parents may feel a lack of immediate access to healthcare professionals and treatment. Prescription of medications that are potentially useful in the home setting and guidance about how to use those drugs in the event of distressful symptoms empowers parents and offers them a practical and immediate response to their child's distress at home.

Parents often are conflicted about whether to discuss the likely possibility of death with their child. In a study of bereaved parents whose child had died of cancer, none of the parents who talked to their child about death regretted it, but as many as 27 percent of parents who did not talk to their child about death regretted not having done so, particularly when they sensed that the child was aware of his or her imminent death.[68] Parents also struggle with how to talk to their healthy children about their ill sibling's imminent death. Parents may benefit from counseling on the cognitive and developmental understanding of the concepts of illness and death.[69] Conversations in advance that allow parents to formulate or even role play can help alleviate parental distress. Encouraging parents to verbalize and incorporate their family's communication style and beliefs about death and afterlife into the conversation can lead to authentic and effective communication with their children. Guidelines to help parents and clinicians communicate with children about death have been suggested by Beale et al.[70] Members of the IDT may have additional experience and resources to counsel parents through this difficult process.

Finally, anticipatory guidance about the patient's and family's preferences for the location of death may represent a better marker of quality palliative care than the actual location of death.[71] Planning where the child will die correlates with an increased number of children dying at home, fewer children dying in the critical care unit or undergoing endotracheal intubation, and less parental regret about the location of death.

Bereavement Care

The death of a child is one of the most devastating events in the life of a parent, and for a child, the death of a sibling may be equally traumatic. Counseling on the need for self care during the bereavement process is of utmost importance. Bereaved parents, for example, experience high rates of anxiety, depression,[72] and psychiatric hospitalizations.[73] The death of a child is also associated with an overall increased mortality among bereaved parents.[74] Factors that complicate the bereavement process include whether the parents perceived the child to be in pain or that the child experienced a difficult time at the moment of death.[75] Access to psychosocial support and guidance prior to or at the time of death may ease bereavement.[76] Families may benefit from knowing that bereavement is highly individual with no timetable and that there is no right or wrong answer on how one should grieve.

Bereaved parents should be counseled on the possibility of experiencing feelings of disbelief, yearning, anger, and sadness.[77] These feelings are normal, and parents may struggle with them for years after the death of their child.[76] Parents may also benefit from sharing their burden with others, particularly supportive family members.[78] Some bereaved family members need guidance about the struggle to resume living, continue working, caring for siblings, and/or relating within the couple. Being aware of prior stressors and how these may further complicate an individual's bereavement experience may help guide appropriate clinical interventions. Counseling may also include information about ways for families to navigate their grief, such as normalizing their desire to stay connected to the child after his or her death and maintaining the child's legacy. During the bereavement process, parents should be informed of the availability of specialized counseling if the intensity of their grief interferes with their ability to function normally.

Summary

The care of vulnerable patients struggling with serious illness demands a comprehensive approach that includes the need for clinicians to understand the illness experience from the perspective of the sick child and family. It also demands the formation of a therapeutic alliance with the goal of attending to those needs and optimizing comfort and quality of life. Although this chapter provides some sample questions and information that can be used in guided conversations with families, such conversations must flow naturally in the context of a relationship founded on mutual trust and respect of the child as a unique person and member of a family unit. The aspects of care described in this chapter often do not happen sequentially; thus, being in the moment, maintaining a willingness to listen to the patient's and family's experiences, and trusting one's inner voice are essential. Ultimately, the competent and compassionate presence of each clinician on the team remains the single most important element of optimal care.

REFERENCES

1. Hinds PS, Oakes L, Furman W, et al: Decision making by parents and healthcare professionals when considering continued care for pediatric patients with cancer, *Oncol Nurs Forum* 24(9):1523–1528, 1997.
2. Robinson MR, Thiel MM, Backus MM, Meyer EC: Matters of spirituality at the end of life in the pediatric intensive care unit, *Pediatrics* 118(3):e719–e729, 2006.
3. Bluebond-Langner M, Belasco JB, Goldman A, Belasco C: Understanding parents' approaches to care and treatment of children with cancer when standard therapy has failed, *J Clin Oncol* 25(17):2414–2419, 2007.
4. Meyer EC, Ritholz MD, Burns JP, Truog RD: Improving the quality of end-of-life care in the pediatric intensive care unit: parents' priorities and recommendations, *Pediatrics* 117(3):649–657, 2006.
5. Meyer EC, Burns JP, Griffith JL, Truog RD: Parental perspectives on end-of-life care in the pediatric intensive care unit, *Crit Care Med* 30(1):226–231, 2002.
6. Michelson KN, Koogler T, Sullivan C, Ortega MP, Hall E, Frader J: Parental views on withdrawing life-sustaining therapies in critically ill children, *Arch Pediatr Adolesc Med* 163(11):986–992, 2009.
7. Kane JR, Hellsten MB, Coldsmith A: Human suffering: the need for relationship-based research in pediatric end-of-life care, *J Pediatr Oncol Nurs* 21(3):180–185, 2004.
8. Hinds PS, Drew D, Oakes LL, et al: End-of-life care preferences of pediatric patients with cancer, *J Clin Oncol* 23(36):9146–9154, 2005.
9. Mack JW, Hilden JM, Watterson J, et al: Parent and physician perspectives on quality of care at the end of life in children with cancer, *J Clin Oncol* 23(36):9155–9161, 2005.
10. *Dictionary of Pastoral Care and Counseling*, Nashville, Tenn, 2009, Abingdon Press.
11. Mack JW, Wolfe J, Cook EF, Grier HE, Cleary PD, Weeks JC: Hope and prognostic disclosure, *J Clin Oncol* 25(35):5636–5642, 2007.
12. *The American Heritage Dictionary*, Second College Edition, Boston, Mass, 2009, Houghton Mifflin.
13. Burns BJ, Hoagwood K, Mrazek PJ: Effective treatment for mental disorders in children and adolescents, *Clin Child Fam Psychol Rev* 2(4):199–254, 1999.
14. Campbell M, Cueva JE: Psychopharmacology in child and adolescent psychiatry: a review of the past seven years. Part II, *J Am Acad Child Adolesc Psychiatry* 34(10):1262–1272, 1995.
15. Cartwright-Hatton S, Roberts C, Chitsabesan P, Fothergill C, Harrington R: Systematic review of the efficacy of cognitive behaviour therapies for childhood and adolescent anxiety disorders, *Br J Clin Psychol* 43(Pt 4):421–436, 2004.
16. Seedat S, Stein MB: Double-blind, placebo-controlled assessment of combined clonazepam with paroxetine compared with paroxetine monotherapy for generalized social anxiety disorder, *J Clin Psychiatry* 65(2):244–248, 2004.
17. Parfitt G, Eston RG: The relationship between children's habitual activity level and psychological well-being, *Acta Paediatr* 94(12):1791–1797, 2005.
18. Huynh ME, Vandvik IH, Diseth TH: Hypnotherapy in child psychiatry: the state of the art, *Clin Child Psychol Psychiatry* 13(3):377–393, 2008.
19. Burden B, Herron-Marx S, Clifford C: The increasing use of reiki as a complementary therapy in specialist palliative care, *Int J Palliat Nurs* 11(5):248–253, 2005.
20. Beaubrun G, Gray GE: A review of herbal medicines for psychiatric disorders, *Psychiatr Serv* 51(9):1130–1134, 2000.
21. Kane JR, Primomo M: Alleviating the suffering of seriously ill children, *Am J Hosp Palliat Care* 18(3):161–169, 2001.
22. A National Framework and Preferred Practices for Palliative and Hospice Care Quality: *National Quality Forum*, 2006. Available at www.qualityforum.org.
23. Freyer DR, Kuperberg A, Sterken DJ, Pastrynak SL, Hudson D, Richards T: Multidisciplinary care of the dying adolescent, *Child Adolesc Psychiatr Clin North Am* 15(3):693–715, 2006.
24. De TM, Kovalcik R: The child with cancer. Influence of culture on truth-telling and patient care, *Ann NY Acad Sci* 809:197–210, 1997.
25. Wolfe J: Suffering in children at the end of life: recognizing an ethical duty to palliate, *J Clin Ethics* 11(2):157–163, 2000.
26. Baker JN, Hinds PS, Spunt SL, et al: Integration of palliative care practices into the ongoing care of children with cancer: individualized

care planning and coordination, *Pediatr Clin North Am* 55(1):223–250, xii, 2008.

27. Collins JJ, Devine TD, Dick GS, et al: The measurement of symptoms in young children with cancer: the validation of the Memorial Symptom Assessment Scale in children aged 7–12, *J Pain Symptom Manage* 23(1):10–16, 2002.

28. Kazak AE, Rourke MT, Alderfer MA, Pai A, Reilly AF, Meadows AT: Evidence-based assessment, intervention and psychosocial care in pediatric oncology: a blueprint for comprehensive services across treatment, *J Pediatr Psychol* 32(9):1099–1110, 2007.

29. Kazak AE, Cant MC, Jensen MM, et al: Identifying psychosocial risk indicative of subsequent resource use in families of newly diagnosed pediatric oncology patients, *J Clin Oncol* 21(17):3220–3225, 2003.

30. Maltoni M, Caraceni A, Brunelli C, et al: Prognostic factors in advanced cancer patients: evidence-based clinical recommendations—a study by the Steering Committee of the European Association for Palliative Care, *J Clin Oncol* 23(25):6240–6248, 2005.

31. Baker JN, Barfield R, Hinds PS, Kane JRA: Process to facilitate decision making in pediatric stem cell transplantation: the Individualized Care Planning and Coordination Model, *Biol Blood Marrow Transplant* 13(3):245–254, 2007.

32. Kane JR, Himelstein BP: Palliative care for children. In Berger AM, Shuster JL, Von Roenn JH, editors: *Principles and practice of palliative medicine and supportive oncology*, ed 3, Philadelphia, 2007, Lippincott Williams & Wilkins.

33. Walling A, Lorenz KA, Dy SM, et al: Evidence-based recommendations for information and care planning in cancer care, *J Clin Oncol* 26(23):3896–3902, 2008.

34. Mack JW, Wolfe J: Early integration of pediatric palliative care: for some children, palliative care starts at diagnosis, *Curr Opin Pediatr* 18(1):10–14, 2006.

35. Wharton RH, Levine KR, Buka S, Emanuel L: Advance care planning for children with special health care needs: a survey of parental attitudes, *Pediatrics* 97(5):682–687, 1996.

36. Levetown M: Communicating with children and families: from everyday interactions to skill in conveying distressing information, *Pediatrics* 121(5):e1441–e1460, 2008.

37. Hui D, Con A, Christie G, Hawley PH: Goals of care and end-of-life decision making for hospitalized patients at a Canadian tertiary care cancer center, *J Pain Symptom Manage* 38(6):871–881, 2009.

38. Mack JW, Wolfe J, Cook EF, Grier HE, Cleary PD, Weeks JC: Peace of mind and sense of purpose as core existential issues among parents of children with cancer, *Arch Pediatr Adolesc Med* 163(6):519–524, 2009.

39. Hsiao JL, Evan EE, Zeltzer LK: Parent and child perspectives on physician communication in pediatric palliative care, *Palliat Support Care* 5(4):355–365, 2007.

40. Hinds PS, Oakes L, Furman W, et al: End-of-life decision making by adolescents, parents, and healthcare providers in pediatric oncology: research to evidence-based practice guidelines, *Cancer Nurs* 24(2):122–134, 2001.

41. Hinds PS, Oakes L, Furman W, et al: Decision making by parents and healthcare professionals when considering continued care for pediatric patients with cancer, *Oncol Nurs Forum* 24(9):1523–1528, 1997.

42. Kars MC, Grypdonck MH, de Korte-Verhoef MC, et al: Parental experience at the end-of-life in children with cancer: 'preservation' and 'letting go' in relation to loss, *Support Care Cancer* 2009.

43. Wolfe J, Klar N, Grier HE, et al: Understanding of prognosis among parents of children who died of cancer: impact on treatment goals and integration of palliative care, *JAMA* 284(19):2469–2475, 2000.

44. Edwards KE, Neville BA, Cook EF Jr, Aldridge SH, Dussel V, Wolfe J: Understanding of prognosis and goals of care among couples whose child died of cancer, *J Clin Oncol* 26(8):1310–1315, 2008.

45. Mack JW, Joffe S, Hilden JM, et al: Parents' views of cancer-directed therapy for children with no realistic chance for cure, *J Clin Oncol* 26(29):4759–4764, 2008.

46. Committee on Bioethics, American Academy of Pediatrics: Informed consent, parental permission, and assent in pediatric practice, *Pediatrics* 95(2):314–317, 1995.

47. Ridgway D: Court-mediated disputes between physicians and families over the medical care of children, *Arch Pediatr Adolesc Med* 158(9):891–896, 2004.

48. American Academy of Pediatrics Committee on Bioethics: Guidelines on foregoing life-sustaining medical treatment, *Pediatrics* 93(3):532–536, 1994.

49. Mercurio MR, Adam MB, Forman EN, Ladd RE, Ross LF, Silber TJ: American Academy of Pediatrics policy statements on bioethics: summaries and commentaries: part 1, *Pediatr Rev* 29(1):e1–e8, 2008.

50. Medical futility in end-of-life care: report of the Council on Ethical and Judicial Affairs, *JAMA* 281(10):937–941, 1999.

51. Committee on Bioethics: Institutional ethics committees, *Pediatrics* 107(1):205–209, 2001.

52. Wolfe J, Grier HE, Klar N, et al: Symptoms and suffering at the end of life in children with cancer, *N Engl J Med* 342(5):326–333, 2000.

53. Collins JJ, Byrnes ME, Dunkel IJ, et al: The measurement of symptoms in children with cancer, *J Pain Symptom Manage* 19(5):363–377, 2000.

54. Goldman A, Hewitt M, Collins GS, Childs M, Hain R: Symptoms in children/young people with progressive malignant disease: United Kingdom Children's Cancer Study Group/Paediatric Oncology Nurses Forum survey, *Pediatrics* 117(6):e1179–e1186, 2006.

55. Duncan J, Spengler E, Wolfe J: Providing pediatric palliative care: PACT in action, *MCN Am J Matern Child Nurs* 32(5):279–287, 2007.

56. Horowitz S: Complementary therapies for end-of-life care, *Alternative Complementary Therapies* 15(5):226–230, 2009.

57. Levetown M, Frager G: *UNIPAC Eight: The hospice/palliative medicine approach to caring for pediatric patients*, Glenview, Ill, 2003, American Academy of Hospice and Palliative Medicine.

58. Jones BL: Pediatric palliative and end-of-life care: the role of social work in pediatric oncology, *J Soc Work End Life Palliat Care* 1(4):35–61, 2005.

59. Ziring PR, Brazdziunas D, Cooley WC, American Academy of Pediatrics, et al: Committee on Children with Disabilities. Care coordination: integrating health and related systems of care for children with special health care needs, *Pediatrics* 104(4 Pt 1):978–981, 1999.

60. Care coordination in the medical home: integrating health and related systems of care for children with special health care needs, *Pediatrics* 116(5):1238–1244, 2005.

61. Stille CJ, Antonelli RC: Coordination of care for children with special health care needs, *Curr Opin Pediatr* 16(6):700–705, 2004.

62. Antonelli RC, Stille CJ, Antonelli DM: Care coordination for children and youth with special health care needs: a descriptive, multisite study of activities, personnel costs, and outcomes, *Pediatrics* 122(1):e209–e216, 2008.

63. Meier DE, Beresford L: Advanced practice nurses in palliative care: a pivotal role and perspective, *J Palliat Med* 9(3):624–627, 2006.

64. Christakis DA, Wright JA, Zimmerman FJ, Bassett AL, Connell FA: Continuity of care is associated with well-coordinated care, *Ambul Pediatr* 3(2):82–86, 2003.

65. Mack JW, Co JP, Goldmann DA, Weeks JC, Cleary PD: Quality of health care for children: role of health and chronic illness in inpatient care experiences, *Arch Pediatr Adolesc Med* 161(9):828–834, 2007.

66. Shinjo T, Morita T, Hirai K, et al: Care for imminently dying cancer patients: family members' experiences and recommendations, *J Clin Oncol* 28(1):142–148, 2010.

67. Pritchard M, Burghen E, Srivastava DK, et al: Cancer-related symptoms most concerning to parents during the last week and last day of their child's life, *Pediatrics* 121(5):e1301–e1309, 2008.

68. Kreicbergs U, Valdimarsdottir U, Onelov E, Henter JI, Steineck G: Talking about death with children who have severe malignant disease, *N Engl J Med* 351(12):1175–1186, 2004.

69. Schum LN, Kane JR: Psychological adaptation of the dying child. In Walsh D, editor: *Palliative medicine*, 2009, Saunders, Elsevier, pp 1085–1093.

70. Beale EA, Baile WF, Aaron J: Silence is not golden: communicating with children dying from cancer, *J Clin Oncol* 23(15):3629–3631, 2005.

71. Dussel V, Kreicbergs U, Hilden JM, et al: Looking beyond where children die: determinants and effects of planning a child's location of death, *J Pain Symptom Manage* 37(1):33–43, 2009.

72. Kreicbergs U, Valdimarsdottir U, Onelov E, Henter JI, Steineck G: Anxiety and depression in parents 4–9 years after the loss of a child owing to a malignancy: a population-based follow-up, *Psychol Med* 34(8):1431–1441, 2004.

73. Li J, Laursen TM, Precht DH, Olsen J, Mortensen PB: Hospitalization for mental illness among parents after the death of a child, *N Engl J Med* 352(12):1190–1196, 2005.

74. Li J, Precht DH, Mortensen PB, Olsen J: Mortality in parents after death of a child in Denmark: a nationwide follow-up study, *Lancet* 361(9355):363–367, 2003.

75. Kreicbergs U, Valdimarsdottir U, Onelov E, Bjork O, Steineck G, Henter JI: Care-related distress: a nationwide study of parents who lost their child to cancer, *J Clin Oncol* 23(36):9162–9171, 2005.

76. Kreicbergs UC, Lannen P, Onelov E, Wolfe J: Parental grief after losing a child to cancer: impact of professional and social support on long-term outcomes, *J Clin Oncol* 25(22):3307–3312, 2007.

77. Maciejewski PK, Zhang B, Block SD, Prigerson HG: An empirical examination of the stage theory of grief, *JAMA* 297(7):716–723, 2007.

78. Laakso H, Paunonen-Ilmonen M: Mothers' experience of social support following the death of a child, *J Clin Nurs* 11(2):176–185, 2002.

5 Anticipatory Grief and Bereavement

NANCY CONTRO | ULRIKA KREICBERGS |
REVEREND WILMA J. REICHARD | BARBARA M. SOURKES

*I didn't know what 'metachromatic leukodystrophy' meant.
I asked for an explanation and when they told us it was
something to do with his brain I just kind of panicked and
freaked out… His mental abilities are going to be changing
and I think having the mental aspect going in his life is going
to be a big situation in our lives… When he's not going to
acknowledge or know who we are is going to be a big issue.
[tears]. We know he's going to die and his life expectancy is
a lot shorter, which makes it very hard. I'm not ready for that.
I don't think I'll ever be ready for that but I'm going to do
my best.[1]* —Mother of a 6-year-old child

*Imagine—I was only eight years old when my brother died!
Now I have to live with this for the rest of my life.[2]*

—10-year-old sibling

*When my son died, visitors offering their condolences, thinking
to comfort me, said: 'Life goes on.' What nonsense, I thought, of
course it doesn't. It's death that goes on. My child is dead now
and will be dead tomorrow and next year and forever. There's
no end to that. But perhaps there will be an end to the sorrow
of it. Sorrow has rushed over the world like the waters of the
Deluge, and it will take time to recede.[3]*

Anticipatory grief and bereavement—the before and after of
loss—comprise physical, psychological, spiritual, social, and
cultural facets. Webster's Dictionary defines "bereaved" as "a
word derived from 'reaved' or 'reft' meaning: to deprive and
make desolate, especially by death."[4] (Fig. 5-1). Bereavement is
a process that ebbs and flows over a lifetime. At its core is the
child, surrounded by concentric circles of family, friends, members of the professional team, and the wider community and
culture.

Over the past decade of research, the perspectives of
bereaved parents have proved to be an invaluable resource for
the development of pediatric palliative care.[5-7] Such research
has explored the care provided to the child and family throughout the illness and into bereavement, rather than an exclusive
focus on the loss itself.[8-9] Approaching bereaved families for
research purposes had been questioned in terms of the risk
of inflicting psychological harm or distress.[10] Yet several studies have shown that parents find participation to be a positive and therapeutic experience—more so than non-bereaved
parents.[11-13]

This chapter focuses on the interplay between the universality of the grief experience and the uniqueness of each
individual and family's response. The phenomenon of anticipatory grief in the family is described, followed by a discussion of bereavement (Box 5-1). Particular emphasis is on the
role of assessment in bereaved families and the implications
for intervention, including cultural and spiritual dimensions.
Clinical vignettes of bereaved families highlight the themes of
the chapter. The grief of the palliative care clinicians who care
for these children and families is also addressed.

The Family Unit

In modern times, the definition of family has expanded to
encompass many diverse constellations. From the outset, a
family's own definition of their family unit and the role of each
member should be elicited. Without such information, clinicians' assumptions of inclusion or exclusion may be faulty,
and valuable sources of support overlooked. The nuclear family of child, siblings, and parents is at the core, surrounded by
the extended family. In particular, grandparents frequently
play a major role. Close friends may be indistinguishable from
family, especially in palliative care situations. With the changing structure of the family, latitude must be made for alternative and complicated arrangements. These include divorced
and reconstituted (blended) families, with their inherently conflicted histories and new alliances; single-parent families; and
children of gay parents.[14] The composition of the family frames
many other factors, including developmental level; psychological history, particularly coping with past losses and trauma;
sources of support; and cultural and spiritual beliefs.

The developmental level of the family unit is frequently a
salient dimension in the impact of a child's illness and death.[15-18]
Young parents are often just learning how to incorporate children into their relationship as they begin to expand their definition of family. The premature death of a young child can send
parents reeling into uncertainty about their identity: Are they
still parents? Are they still a family? Furthermore, with little
prior experience of negotiating loss or death as a couple, they
may experience confusion and fear about each other's reactions. These families often need more structured guidance than
an older family that has already negotiated previous losses.

A universal phenomenon in the bereavement process is
that individuals in the same family grieve in different ways and
on different schedules.[15-18] Despite mourning the same child,
family members are often out of sync with one another in their
experience and expressions of grief. Misunderstanding, guilt,
anger, and resentment, and a profound loneliness, often arise
when this phenomenon is not understood.

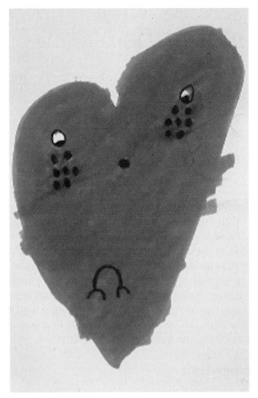

Fig. 5-1 A heart weeping. (Reprinted from Sourkes, B. et al. Food, toys, and love: pediatric palliative care. *Curr Probl Pediatr Adolesc Health Care* 35(9): 345–392, 2005.)

BOX 5-1 Anticipatory Grief and Bereavement: Key Concepts

Anticipatory grief and bereavement—the before and after of loss—begin at the time of the child's diagnosis and extend years after his or her death.

Anticipatory Grief
- Grief expressed in advance when a loss is perceived to be threatening or inevitable
- Child grieves for everyone and everything in his or her life
- Family faces cumulative losses leading up to the child's death and then bereavement
- The child and family may feel overwhelmed by the intensity of their emotions, not recognizing that underlying their sadness is the even deeper phenomenon of anticipatory grief. Clarifying this distinction can be of relief and comfort
- The death of another patient engenders powerful grief—and anticipatory grief—for ill children and their families

Bereavement
- A process that ebbs and flows over a lifetime. No absolute timeframe for its resolution
- Families often express a sense of double loss: of their child as an individual and a member of the family and community, and of their professional family, the team who cared for the child, often over months and years
- Bereavement follow up is an integral part of comprehensive pediatric palliative care and assuages the family's sense of abandonment
- Bereavement assessment, and re-assessment over time, is both prevention and intervention; in particular for those families judged to be at risk
- Despite mourning the same child, individuals in the family grieve in different ways and on different schedules. Being out of sync with one another is a normal phenomenon
- Siblings grieve deeply for their brother or sister. However, because children's modes of expressing grief may differ substantially from that of adults', their mourning may be underestimated or missed entirely

---

It is crucial to recognize the impact of background, culture, and language on the family's experience of the child's illness and treatment, how they make decisions along the way, and on the grief process.[19] Cultural perceptions may challenge the use of language. For instance, in English, compassion connotes a deep caring. In some Spanish traditions, however, the word is primarily connoted with care for the dying. Thus, compassion may communicate an unintended message to the family. Deepening the awareness of such nuances and differences enables bereavement care to begin where the family is cuturally.

As for children, their modes of expressing grief may differ substantially from adults' and thus their grief's meaning and depth are often underestimated or even missed completely (Fig. 5-2). All too often, siblings become disenfranchised grievers,[20] their loss is minimized compared to that of their parents'. They are often admonished to be strong for their parents with little acknowledgment of their own mourning process.[2]

Current Research

Research in the field of anticipatory grief and bereavement is only now emerging; until recently, most studies have been descriptive or conceptual in nature. Thus caution must be exercised in making overarching assumptions from such new data. Rather, the research provides a context within which the characteristics of an individual family may be viewed.

PARENTS

The loss of a child is described as one of the most stressful life events possible.[21] The grief is more intense and longer lasting than that following any other type of loss.[22] Some studies suggest it may take at least four to six years to "work through" the death of a child[23] (Fig. 5-3). The loss itself is compounded when parents have witnessed their child's protracted physical and emotional suffering throughout the illness.[24–26] Despite the traumatic nature of the experience, and the fact that bereaved parents are at increased risk of physical and psychological morbidity,[27–29] most individuals are able to come to terms with the loss over time. Two types of factors have been studied for their impact on bereavement outcome in parents: those that can be managed (modified or avoided) in the current health care setting, and those that cannot.

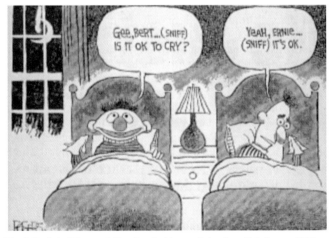

Fig. 5-2 Is it OK to cry? (Reprinted with permission from Rob Rogers: © The Pittsburgh Post Gazette/Dist. by United Feature Syndicate, Inc.)

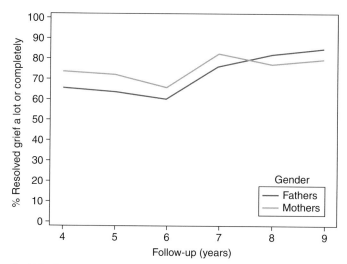

Fig. 5-3 Bereaved parents' reports of their grief following the loss of a child to cancer 4 to 9 years earlier: Although fewer fathers than mothers have worked through their grief at four to six years after the death of the child, they have come to terms with their loss to a greater extent at seven to nine years.

Factors that lie beyond the scope of the healthcare setting include a family's history of previous losses, pre-morbid conditions, and financial problems. Even the age and gender of the child has been found to affect parental bereavement outcome.[27,30,31] For fathers, the risk of anxiety and depression is greater after the death of a child older than 8, nearly twice as high as those fathers whose younger child died.[27] No such relationship to the child's age is seen in mothers. Gender of the child also affects mothers and fathers differently. The risk of morbidity in mothers is higher when a daughter dies.[31] Although such factors are not changeable, it is extremely important for clinicians to be aware of them in their daily work with families.

Factors that can be modified within the healthcare setting are all related to the quality of palliative care. For example, the absence of clinicians at the moment of a child's death increases the likelihood of parents reporting unrelieved pain, as well as an intensely difficult death.[8] Location of the child's death is another factor in bereaved parents' morbidity: fathers are less likely to suffer from depression if the child dies at home.[32] It must still be determined whether the significant factor is the actual location of the child's death—or the planning of it.[33]

Open and honest communication has been emphasized as crucial in pediatric palliative care.[34–36] It has been found that providing psychological support to parents from the healthcare team, even in the last month of their child's life, facilitates their grieving process. Informing families about the evolving nature of a child's illness and prognosis is always challenging. Communication about the child's prognosis has proved valuable for the bereavement outcome.[23] Although most parents want to be fully informed of their child's status, many clinicians continue to avoid this type of communication. Parents who have been informed that their child's death is imminent are, not surprisingly, more likely to be aware of the pending death.[37] Their awareness impacts the opportunity for them to tailor the child's care according to their wishes. Bringing the child home, as well as planning for a death at home, is more likely to be considered if parents are cognizant of the imminence of death.[38] Furthermore, these parents are more likely to talk about death with their child, even more so when they perceive the child also to be aware, which is an approach that has been shown to reduce the risk of psychological morbidity in bereavement.[39] However, many children in pediatric palliative care are unable to engage in any type of communication because of age, developmental delay or the nature of the illness. Mothers of children who had severe malignancy and were unable to communicate in their last week of life were more likely to think that death would be best for the child; this finding was not consistent for the fathers.[40]

Assisting bereaved families is an integral part of pediatric palliative care, beginning with the issues around anticipatory grief at the child's diagnosis. However, research on bereavement intervention is still in its early stages, and the efficacy of counseling has not yet been well validated.[41] Several studies have shown that both professional and social support is beneficial for parents' grief outcomes, although not all parents find it helpful. Some parents choose to cope on their own, with or without support from family or friends. Over the long term, the social network has proved to be particularly valuable for many bereaved parents. Fathers talk mainly with their spouse, while mothers confide in family, friends, and other bereaved parents. Both types of sharing have a beneficial impact on the grief outcome.[23] The identification of parents at risk for pathological grief reactions, and designing optimal intervention for them, remains a critical topic for future research. Emerging from the research are the following recommendations in caring for bereaved parents:

- Alleviate the child's suffering during the illness through optimal symptom management,
- Communicate openly and honestly with parents,
- Be present at the time of child's death,
- Inform parents about the demonstrated value of open communication with and support from family and friends,
- Recommend that parents seek professional psychological support during the child's illness and following the death, particularly when there are risk factors in the family.

Although long-term consequences often refer to sequelae one or two years following a loss, a time frame for parental bereavement has not been established in the literature.[42] Hospitalization for psychological morbidity and an elevated incidence of death have been reported as long-term consequences following the death of a child.[28,43] In a Danish study, it was found that both natural and unnatural deaths are more likely among bereaved parents than in a matched sample who were not bereaved. Bereaved mothers had an increased risk throughout the study period of 3 to 18 years, while for fathers the risk was limited to the first 3 years. Unresolved grief emerges as a specific risk factor for the psychological and physical health of both mothers and fathers in the long term. Bereaved fathers with unresolved grief are seven times more likely to report sleep disturbances,[44] with the ensuing impact on their capacity for work and overall well-being. A common, and damaging misconception, is that the incidence of separation or divorce is elevated in couples whose child has died. Yet a recent study on long term marital status shows the opposite: bereaved parents actually are less likely to divorce or separate than non-bereaved.[45]

SIBLINGS

Research on bereaved siblings is extremely limited; their long-term adjustment has yet to be explored in a systematic fashion. However, certain issues have emerged in both clinical observations and empirical studies.[46–51] Siblings are often referred to as being invisible because of the parents' intense involvement in the care of their ill child.[52,53] During the illness, the siblings desire open and honest communication within the family, adequate information from clinicians, involvement in the care of the sick child, and support to continue their own interests and activities.[52–54] Parents often try to protect the siblings from involvement in the child's illness, particularly end-of-life care, thinking that it will shelter them from trauma. Yet this well-intentioned approach instead leads the siblings to feel abandoned and excluded from the family tragedy,[55] with these feelings persisting long into bereavement. Findings suggest that after the death, siblings perceive their life to change, not only within the family but also in relationships with others outside the family. Clinicians can play an important role in communicating directly with siblings whenever possible and educating the parents about the importance of addressing their needs.

Anticipatory Grief

Anticipatory grief is the process that links everyone who is facing the loss of the child. It is catapulted into being at the time of diagnosis, and wends its way through the illness trajectory until the moment of death. Anticipatory grief initially resembles the grief that immediately follows a death: emotions are alternately raw and numb, and very much in evidence.[56] The classic definition of anticipatory grief is "grief expressed in advance when the loss is perceived as inevitable."[57] A broader definition includes loss that is threatened, with the implication of a much longer time frame. Experientially the process reflects the emotional response to the pain of separation before the actuality of loss. The child grieves multiple losses: of his or her healthy self, of function and role, of separation from loved ones. (For discussion of anticipatory grief in the child, see Chapter 3.) The family members face anticipatory grief, and then bereavement after the child dies. They move from the realization that "Our child is going to die" to an even more anguished dawning that "We are going to lose our child."[56] It is at this juncture that the recognition of an inevitable separation has begun. The ebb and flow of anticipatory grief charts an individual course for each family, dependent on the nature and length of the illness trajectory, as well as psychological and cultural factors.

Katy, a 7-year-old girl, had a recurrent dream: "I want to be with my mother, and I can never quite get to her." The girl recounted the dream in a joint psychotherapy session with her mother. Whereas the mother found the dream "excruciating," her daughter articulated that "even though the dream is very sad, it's not a nightmare." The dream eventually provided the focal image for mother and child to work through the anticipatory grief process.[56,p. 70]

The child and family may feel overwhelmed by their intense emotions, not understanding the source. Often they do not recognize that below the sadness lies the deeper and more complex phenomenon of anticipatory grief. Articulating this distinction can be a powerful therapeutic intervention. It is also important to explain that grief arises not only around the finality of death, but also in an ongoing way for the cumulative losses that occur over the course of an illness.

A mother berated herself: "I can't understand why I cry all the time. My daughter is doing reasonably well right now. It makes me feel guilty when I cry like this – I feel as if I am burying her before she actually dies." When the psychologist explained the concept of anticipatory grief, she experienced enormous relief at being able to attribute a meaning to her tears.

A certain degree of disengagement from the child on the part of family members, or from one another, may be part of the anticipatory grief process. In a self-protective move against loss and further pain, the family may seem "to leave before being left." Such disengagement may be seen in a general emotional withdrawal from the child, or it may take specific forms: for example, parents may begin to focus on the sibling nearest in age to the patient in a type of "replacement"; or one member of the couple begins an extramarital affair; or a sibling may distance him or herself from the family.

These phenomena are neither inevitable, nor, when they occur, irreversible. However, they do signify a family's difficulty in negotiating a phase of the anticipatory grief process. It is crucial that the family not feel chastised for their distancing maneuvers. Rather, this is often a time for a referral to a mental health clinician for individual, marital, or family therapy.[56]

The sense of exhaustion that accompanies a remission-relapse cycle in an illness is inordinate. The family may find it increasingly difficult to know whether to prepare for loss or for life—and how to apportion their emotional energy. A similar discomfort may occur when a patient lives beyond his or her prognostic expectancy. The family is jubilant at having more time with the child but they may also wonder how they will continue to manage the ongoing threat of death.

Three healthy siblings complained to the psychologist: "Every holiday our parents say: 'Let's make this holiday perfect for your brother, since it may be his last.' Meanwhile, he has lived for four years. How long are we supposed to keep this up?"[56,p. 73]

Enormous grief and anticipatory grief are engendered by the death of another patient. The reverberations are particularly intense when the children have the same disease. On one level, the child and family grieve the loss of their acquaintance or friend. On a deeper level, they are struck with the awareness: "This could have been me/our child … and will I/our child be next?"[56] This close sense of identification provides an opening for the child and family to address their own sadness and fear. It is a time for the clinician to be actively present and reassuring until the acute anxiety and grief abate.

Because there are no social rituals to mark anticipatory grief, as there are in bereavement, people not directly involved are often confused as to what the family is experiencing, or how to help. Family members frequently describe a profound sense of loneliness and separateness from others as they live the illness experience.

"Right now we are living in a different world … Our friends in the 'outside world' care about us, but they can't really understand what we are living through. Our closest people right now are the other families at the hospital and our team."

Therapeutic interventions by the palliative care team, in addition to identifying and explaining anticipatory grief, include facilitating family dialogue about their ongoing shared sadness, suggesting legacy-building activities such as (filming or scrap-booking) and encouraging interaction with other families who are going through a similar experience. Most important through "the long haul" of prolonged illness is the accessibility and avail-ability of the clinicians who best know the child and family.

With the approach of the child's death, the family confronts the full intensity of anticipatory grief. The child faces the ultimate leave-taking from everyone and everything; the family stands at the brink of their new life ahead, facing the specter of life without the child. This sequence of anticipatory grief and then bereave-ment is represented metaphorically (in Fig. 5-4): desperate, pow-erless and ultimately unsuccessful pleas to prevent the death of a loved one followed by ensuing sadness and attempts at solace.

Bereavement

Death ends a life, but it does not end a relationship. . .
Robert Anderson[58, p. 77]

Parenting is a permanent change in the individual. A person never gets over being a parent. Parental bereavement is also a permanent condition. The bereaved parent, after a time, will cease showing the… symptoms of grief, but the parent does not "get over" the death of a child.[59, p. 178]

Bereavement follow-up by the professional team is an intrin-sic component of comprehensive pediatric palliative care. Without such continuity, many families express anguish over the experience as a double loss. Primary is the death of their child, of an individual, and of a member of the family and the greater community. Compounding this grief, they mourn the loss of their professional family – the treatment team whom they have known and trusted, often over months and years.[5–7,9,60]

Contact from a team member after the child's death not only assuages the family's sense of abandonment, but it can also serve a crucial preventive role by identifying families at risk for serious physical, psychological, and social sequelae.

In many circumstances, the opportunity for ongoing face-to-face assessment and follow-up does not exist. Other means of communication, including periodic phone calls or notes, can provide some evaluation and serve as a springboard for referring a family to local resources. Events such as an annual hospital memorial service provide valuable and natural opportunities to assess a family's functioning: those who attend are eager to reconnect with staff, and often quite spon-taneously describe their life since the child's death.

ASSESSMENT

Under ideal circumstances, a mental health clinician carries out a comprehensive bereavement assessment. However, other scenarios are possible. If a family feels more comfortable with another team member, that person can function as a bridge by introducing and supporting the importance of the assessment. Bereavement assessments can be effectively done by an inter-disciplinary duo: one with a medical background, the other with psychological expertise. When a mental health clinician is not available for direct clinical involvement, another team member may do the evaluation and then seek consultation about the family's status, risk, and needs.

A bereavement assessment[61] is often done over several ses-sions, beginning in some instances in the immediate after-math of the child's death, and then followed up over weeks or months. The clinician must carefully monitor the pace of the assessment, both within meetings and in scheduling sub-sequent times, always based on the family's cues. "Plowing through" an interview for the sake of completing the assess-ment frequently results in distress and the loss of important information (Box 5-2).

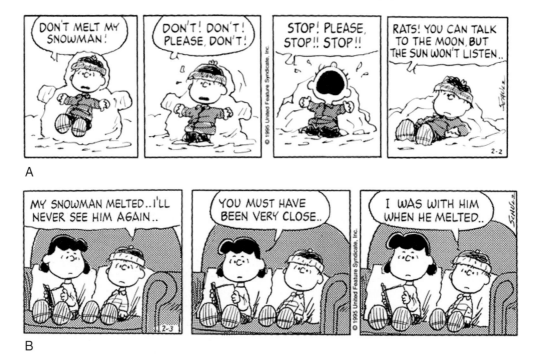

Fig. 5-4 **Linus and the Snowman.** (Reprinted with permission of PEANUTS. Copyright United Feature Syndicate, Inc.)

BOX 5-2 Fundamentals of Bereavement Assessment*

- Allow for time, without interruption, to speak with the family in a manner that conveys your complete attentiveness
- Provide a comfortable and confidential physical setting, with items such as tissues and water available. If children are included, set out toys, books, and drawing or writing materials
- Welcome the family, express your condolences, and acknowledge the enormity of their loss
- Refer to the deceased child by name. Be open to looking at photographs of the child if the family offers them. Use clinical judgment about initiating a request to see pictures
- Approach the family in an open and nonjudgmental manner to facilitate trust and reduce any sense of intimidation
- Pose questions in a way that reflects the family's cognitive, developmental, and educational levels and cultural background
- Always ask, never assume
- Before focusing on the child's illness and death, allow time for the family to describe and reminisce about the child
- Invite families to tell the story of their child in their own way and at their own pace. It is common for bereaved individuals to repeat details of the illness and death numerous times as they move through the grief experience
- Pace the assessment. Avoid overwhelming the family; use clinical judgment as to whether it is time to take a break or end the session. Plowing through an interview for the sake of completing the assessment frequently results in unnecessary distress and the loss of important information
- Let the family express their feelings and opinions, whether or not you agree. Refrain from interrupting or trying to fill silences
- Verify your impressions with the family. When necessary, ask explicitly if your understanding is accurate. If you make a mistake or misunderstand something, apologize and continue. Families tend to be very forgiving
- If red flags emerge in the assessment, consult with a mental health clinician
- Bereavement interviews elicit the expression of intense emotions. Closely monitor your own reactions during and after the session. Just as all families are different, each clinician brings his or her background and vulnerabilities to the setting

*Although only the word family is used in the box, these points apply to individual assessment as well.

In the immediate aftermath of the child's death, it is important to assess each family member's response and determine what is needed to carry the family through the crisis, including referrals for medical or mental health issues. Initial discussions often include their wishes for a funeral and/or memorial service and burial and, in some instances, the clarification of logistical issues around transporting the body. If the family has not made advance arrangements, they often need assistance in sorting through their options. This initial assessment also may include sensitive inquiry into the family's financial resources and identification of people who can help them in the days and weeks ahead. Questions about the course of the child's illness and death, or unresolved issues with the medical team, can usually wait until after the service has taken place. Other major areas of bereavement assessment include developmental level of the individual and the family; family composition, relationships, and background; significant medical issues; psychological history, particularly coping with past losses or trauma; ethnicity, culture, and spiritual beliefs; available support within the family and community; and access to professional services. A "loss history" encompasses loss in its broadest sense;[56] for example, through illness and death, trauma, change in relationships (e.g., divorce); loss of employment and/or financial security; geographical moves. A critical dimension of the loss history includes the experience of immigrant or refugee families: in addition to the loss of their home country, many have suffered unspeakable trauma in their journey to their new home. Given the extreme sensitivity of these issues, which may include fear of legal repercussions if disclosed, utmost care must be exercised in any inquiry.

The heart of the bereavement assessment is the family's experience of the child's illness and death. In broaching this segment of the interview, the family should be invited first to describe and reminisce about their child. Hearing the family's story as they choose to recount it is essential, both for its content and for how it is told. The following issues, both the facts and the accompanying emotions, are important to listen for or elicit as the family relates their experience.

- How was information about your child communicated to you?
- How did you and the staff share information with your child? What did he or she know or understand?
- Did you and your child participate in decisions about treatment?
- Was there any staff member with whom you felt especially comfortable or uncomfortable?
- When and how did you realize, or when and how were you told, that your child was going to die?
- Were you given information about home and hospice options and comfort measures for your child?
- Were you prepared for what to expect at the time of death?
- Did the child seem to be suffering before he or she died? If so, how?
- Was your family alone with your child before his or her death? Was everyone there that you wanted to be present? Did you have the support you needed from staff?

"Red flags" in the family that may indicate a predisposition to a particularly complicated bereavement period include a history of multiple losses or trauma, psychiatric disturbance (especially suicidal ideas or behavior), and addictions. Family relationships that were already fragile or stressed before the child's death are at risk for further deterioration. If the individual or family has an existing relationship with a mental health clinician, the team may seek permission to contact that individual to ensure timely follow up. For others, it is crucial to have an emergency plan, including access to immediate psychiatric assessment at the child's death. The importance of helping a family to create a "safety net" of extended family and friends *before* the child's death cannot be overestimated.

An underlying premise of the assessment process is "always ask, never assume." Assumptions about behavior based upon gender, ethnic or cultural background, age or even the type of loss suffered must be evaluated against the information provided by the individual. Furthermore, while the assessment marks a starting point for working with a bereaved family, the process of evaluation continues. Periodic checking in with the family provides ongoing supportive contact as well as a lens for monitoring changes in emotion or behavior that might otherwise be missed. For example, a parent may go through periods of seeming "almost normal," only to be followed by incapacitating grief when he or she is unable to leave the house or even get out of bed. Another example may be a sibling who appears to be functioning well who is suddenly stricken with nightmares, becomes inconsolable and fearful, and withdraws from friends and activities.

Exploring a family's ethnic and cultural background—and degree of acculturation in immigrant families—is essential for assessment and formulation of an optimal bereavement care plan. Family members may vary considerably in their attachments to beliefs and customs from their home country; as a consequence, individual beliefs and needs can be quite different. Critical issues include:

- What are the family's beliefs and values related to childhood illness and death?
- Is it considered appropriate to talk about death with, or around, children?
- What are their expectations of medical care and their own involvement?
- What are the unique and expected roles of family members and the community?
- Are different levels of acculturation causing friction among family members?

Through sensitive and thorough inquiry, important information can be gleaned to frame the family's psychological responses within the context of their own cultural background. The clinician's effort to understand these factors promotes respect and candor within the therapeutic relationship (Box 5-3).

INTERVENTION

Universally accepted standards for bereavement follow-up do not yet exist in pediatric palliative care. In their absence, the role of individual and family assessment is paramount in

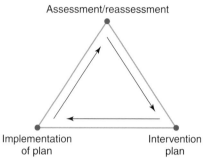

Fig. 5-5 Assessment/intervention triangles.

providing optimal clinical care, as well as in developing effective protocols that can be empirically tested. The ongoing assessment and/or reassessment process guides the clinician as to what type of intervention would be most valuable at a given time (Fig. 5-5). To achieve the best "fit," a referral must be based on astute clinical judgment in combination with the unique needs and wishes of the individual or family. It is not uncommon for these needs to fluctuate over time, and thus a variety of support and treatment modalities may be accessed concurrently or sequentially in the bereavement process. Many families turn to their community for support. For example, a deeply religious family may find solace through their spiritual organization. Others turn to self-help bereavement groups at local agencies that rely on volunteers and trained peer counselors. Some people choose more intensive intervention in the form of individual, marital, or family psychotherapy to examine the enduring impact of the child's illness and death on their lives.

Psychotherapy can be critical for those individuals or families who have pre-existing or current vulnerabilities in addition to, or inextricable with, the child's death. While there is much debate about the precise characterization of "pathological grief," inextricable with features include extremes of emotion in both adults and children that persist over time, such as consuming rage that envelops the individual and alienates the family, or the total suppression of any sign of feeling. Psychotherapy permits the unfolding of the grief process within a well-contained and safe context. It can play a pivotal role in rebuilding, strengthening and sustaining the individual's and family's resources as they move forward into the future.

The exigencies of bereavement demand that mental health clinicians have a solid base in psychopathology, evaluation, and psychotherapy. In addition, for those who work with bereaved siblings, knowledge of child development and psychotherapy is critical. Without a broad foundation, clinicians lack a context in which to place the intense issues of bereavement, and their ability to intervene effectively may be severely compromised.

Working with families through death and bereavement can be treacherous ground for inexperienced or unsupported clinicians from any discipline. Throughout the process, it is critical that clinicians keep constant check on their own reactions and expressed beliefs and withhold judgment about the way a family grieves. Consultation with a colleague from a mental health discipline can be valuable in maintaining perspective when working with families in crisis. Furthermore, while many families feel honored and moved at witnessing professionals' grief for their child, this compassion must be demonstrated without taking over and superseding the family's own intensity. Clinicians can judge the appropriateness of their involvement

---

BOX 5-3 Bereavement Assessment: Topics to Address

In the Immediate Aftermath of a Child's Death
- Reactions of each individual in the family
- What the family needs to carry them through the immediate crisis, including referrals
- Funeral planning and arrangements
- Available supports, both emotional and financial

Background
- Developmental level of each individual and the family as a whole
- Family composition
- Family relationships
- Ethnic, cultural, and spiritual or religious background
- Significant medical conditions
- Psychological history
- "Loss history," which encompasses loss in its broadest sense, that is, through illness and death, trauma, change in relationships such as divorce, loss of employment and/or financial security, geographical moves
- Experience of immigrant or refugee families and degree of acculturation

The Child's Illness and Death
- Course of the illness beginning at diagnosis
- How the medical team communicated information about the child
- The child's knowledge and understanding of his or her situation
- Child's and family's participation in decision making about treatment
- Relationship with members of the team; any individual with whom the family was especially comfortable or uncomfortable
- How and when the family realized that the child was going to die
- Adequacy of information about home and hospice options and comfort measures for the child
- Preparation for what to expect at the time of death
- The child's death: description of the death and child's level of suffering, time for family to be alone with the child, staff support of the family
- Any unresolved issues with the medical team that the family wishes to address

Red Flags
- History of multiple losses or trauma
- Psychiatric disturbance, especially suicidal ideas or behavior
- Alcohol or substance abuse
- Fragile or stressed family relationships
- Extremes of emotion that persist over time, or the suppression of any sign of feeling

in response to the question: "Whose needs are being served?" The answer is unequivocally, "The family's."[56] This balanced perspective is an absolute of effective bereavement intervention.

The effect of a child's death expands in waves from the family to the broader community, including the child's school and extra-curricular activities, neighborhood, work site, and religious community. These organizations are deeply affected by the child's death and often need guidance to cope with their collective grief. Although palliative care clinicians cannot be expected to meet all of these needs, they can play a key role in identifying them and suggesting avenues for care.

SPIRITUAL DIMENSIONS

"I was brought up to believe that life is a gift. God gives life as a gift with no strings attached. It should be a given, just to live. Then if you want to work to be different things, you work for that. But you shouldn't have to struggle just to live."
—Adolescent [62, p. 265]

The experience of a child's illness and death challenges one's understanding of God's presence and power. It is difficult to one's understand the meaning of a young person's suffering. As part of the "meaning-making" process, it forces many to reconsider what they believe or to believe in something greater than themselves. As the Rev. Carl Howie wrote, "Faith, though subjective, engenders hope and provides meaning for life."[63] To foster such belief requires active listening as individuals describe and define their faith or values, and explore the ways in which their faith can support possibilities and hopes. The process of spiritual assessment and reassessment is ongoing for many children and their families throughout the illness, and afterward.

As spiritual care is provided, the task is to offer emotional and spiritual support to persons of many faiths, cultures, and practices without absolutes but within perimeters.[64] For example, some people find more comfort within their own tradition, while others may seek or accept prayer, or supportive listening from persons outside of their own tradition. An important aspect of spiritual assessment is exploring with children and the family which spiritual needs can be met by a newcomer, and which are better met by a known spiritual caregiver. A mitigating factor is often geographical distance, in that the primary spiritual and religious supports may be unavailable for many families. Having to make new spiritual connections is another of the adjustments and losses that accompany the new normal of having an ill child.

Mark, a 12-year-old Catholic adolescent, was newly confirmed, and communion represented that rite of passage to him. Receiving daily communion was a resource for his faith and his sense of self. It provided a way to incarnate his faith, as well as his passage into young adulthood, even as he was hospitalized and losing his independence in many domains. Although the chaplain was not a Catholic, both Mark and his mother were open to and grateful for receiving communion from her. In fact, this ritual became the centerpiece of his spiritual care and conversations during his five-month hospitalization. When Mark died, the family requested that this Protestant chaplain offer the eulogy at his funeral Mass.

A Muslim boy had a life-threatening kidney disease and without a transplant would require ongoing dialysis, with all its risks and complications. The mother was a match for transplant and said that she would do anything to avoid losing her son. Her husband expressed fear at losing both his ill son and his wife, the mother of his children. The father requested that the chaplain, who was not a practitioner of Islam, pray for his family. The fact that the chaplain represented faith was sufficient for the family to make her part of their hopes and fears.

Although notions of retributive justice are rarely taught, people of many faiths try to link a person's illness to the actions of the child, parent, or another significant individual. With some children, this link can be almost magical or mythical in nature, as their minds struggle to understand what is happening. In addition, sacred stories in many cultures and traditions connect the acts of one generation to the next. As children and their families seek to make sense of the suffering and illness, such intergenerational lore can be particularly poignant. The search for meaning becomes primary, regardless of the context selected for explanation. If the spiritual or religious tradition focuses on punishment, the child's illness becomes the ultimate punishment. Consequently, there is enormous guilt wrapped into the anticipatory grief process from the beginning. In the words of one mother, "What if I put him through all this – and he still dies?" The role of the chaplain is to help individuals describe and work through their fear of retribution from a theological perspective.

In most spiritual practices, prayer is a demonstration of faithfulness. In some of these traditions, the belief is that prayers are answered if they are asked properly and with faith. When prayers go unanswered, and children become sicker, the notion of punishment looms large for the family. Doubt about both God's and human faithfulness can be a painful part of unanswered prayers and unfulfilled hopes.

A sixteen-year-old boy explained that he no longer prayed because God did not listen to him, but if the chaplain prayed for him, God might hear his prayers. This disclosure led to a series of conversations about how to know whether God listens or hears.

The frustration of unanswered prayers in combination with the loss of hopes and dreams for a child intersect sadly. A mother who grieved that her daughter would never grow into a woman; a father who grieved that his son would never learn to ride a bicycle; a sibling who hoped that his brother would be his best man one day; a child who wished she could live to have her first kiss: each of these was expressed in the context of having prayed for healing.

Cecilia, a 7-year-old girl, asked her mother over several nights if she could see the angel outside her hospital window. Though the mother could not see anything, she explained that the angel must be Cecilia's and that was why she alone could see her. A few days later, when Cecilia died, her mother believed that this angel had come to take her to heaven. In her tradition, children have guardian angels, and this belief comforted her from the time of Cecilia's diagnosis through her death.

The grief of the children who are ill has its own immediacy.[65–67] Being in the hospital for an extended period separates them from the family and friends they love—at home, school and in other activities, the neighborhood and their faith community. The children often address their longing for these interrupted, if not suspended, relationships. Awareness of the siblings' needs is also paramount.

An older brother of an eight-year-old child with mitochondrial disorder was able, because of the bedside nurse's advocacy, to be present when her ventilatory support was removed. He reassured his sister with the words: "Everything will be OK."

Although the chaplain was not present, the nurse sought her out afterward, along with other staff members, to share the experience. The team had cared for this child since she was six months old. Over the years, the family had repeatedly said to the chaplain "We are not religious, but please keep her in your prayers." They invited the chaplain to preside over the family's memorial service for her, as well as a remembrance ceremony at the hospital.

A chaplain's involvement with a family during the illness can lead to a continuing relationship beyond the child's death, even for years and decades. For many families, birthdays, holidays, other important events and the date of death are all reminders of the loss of their hopes for the child who died.

In our interfaith chapel in the hospital, there is a book in which family members can write their own prayers. On numerous occasions, someone who has written a prayer returns months and years later to find the entry. Their inscribed prayer is an enduring way to honor and remember the child.

SIBLINGS' EXPERIENCES

When we first went to the psychologist, my little brother thought she was a checkup doctor. But I explained to him "You know how we lost our older sister? This doctor tries to get the sadness out of your heart." —7-year-old child

Bereaved children face inordinate psychological challenges that test their resilience to the utmost.[68] At home, there are two central issues during the acute bereavement period. First is the question of the siblings' attendance at the funeral. If the parents discuss the issue with the siblings, they can usually make a decision based upon the child's direct and indirect cues. Ideally, an adult who is close to the child (other than a parent) can keep a close eye on the child during the service, and take the child out or leave early if necessary. No child should ever be forced to attend. Secondly, while it is important to talk about the deceased child, the here-and-now life focus of the well siblings must not be forgotten in the intensity of immediate grief. This is a critical period to ensure the prevention of insidious comparisons with the idealized deceased child, or the beginning of a replacement child process.[46]

With the death of the patient, the siblings suffer multiple losses: their brother or sister, and then all the roles that were inherent in the relationship.[46–51] Siblings must negotiate this permanent loss while feeling the temporary, although often prolonged, psychological loss or distance of their parents who are immersed in their own grief. Siblings struggle with issues, including overwhelming sadness, that are strikingly similar to those faced by bereaved adults.[68] Children often report previous losses; thus a "loss history" is crucial in understanding their strengths and vulnerabilities. Young children's past experience with death, if any, is typically the loss of a grandparent or a pet. They may also talk about objects that they have lost, especially if they are associated with their brother or sister. Children report traumatic memories and fears for the future. Frightening images tend to focus on the illness itself, such as how the person looked, visible symptoms, medical technology, or on the funeral or burial. Worries include: the threat of other losses; loss of a specific aspect of the sibling relationship; religious concerns; harm befalling the child himself or herself; contagion and familial risk of illness; sleep and somatic disorders; and school difficulties. Adolescents often mention sadness about the future (e.g., my brother or sister will never know my children). Anger at the injustice of the loss, as well as at the pain that they must now suffer, takes on many shapes: verbal outbursts; physical aggression and other forms of acting out; and somewhat paradoxically, in withdrawal from others, especially the family.

One of the most painful—and common—aspects of bereavement is a child's sense of guilt. The guilt may focus on an act, word, or thought that was committed or omitted, real or imagined, rational or irrational. Whatever the source, its existence may sharply exacerbate the loss and carry with it a weight of depression that complicates grief resolution. The frequent and intense intrusion of traumatic thoughts, or an unrelenting sense of guilt, often signals the need for psychological treatment. Children also grapple with the fact that their loss reverberates throughout the social environment, often bearing a combination of both positive and negative consequences, such as the outpouring of support vs. stigmatization.

STAFF: CYCLES OF ATTACHMENT AND LOSS

"One runs the risk of weeping a little, if one lets himself be tamed." —Saint Exupery: The Little Prince[69]

Clinicians who work with these children and families experience repeated cycles of attachment and loss. They must cope with the cumulative impact of loss over time and find a way to balance their suffering and grief with their ongoing commitment to the work.[70–74] (See Chapter 18.) A pediatric hospice nurse described her experience as artwork (Fig. 5-6).

I always feel challenged (green) in the work—it surrounds everything and keeps my commitment going. Commitment (purple) is the core and affects all the other feelings. Feeling hopeful (yellow) and in control (orange) are important if you are going to keep doing this work. Anger (red) is the only feeling that doesn't touch on commitment in my drawing—so that it does not impinge on it. I have the anger embedded in control. Frustration is there (brown)—you always wish you could do more. And fear (black) …. Hospice forces me to confront and come to terms with death. As children I work with go, I know that I will go too …. Sadness (blue) is there, but it does not take over all my other feelings.

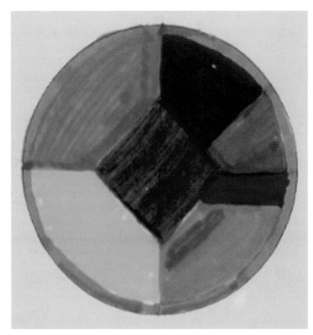

Fig. 5-6 As children I work with go, I know that I will go, too. . . .

Mental health clinicians and chaplains can play an important role in supporting staff members in preparation for the loss of a child and then in bereavement.

> *In the words of a hospital chaplain, "I've had Jewish and Hindu doctors, Catholic and Muslim nurses, Protestant and secular social workers, Christian and non-believing child life specialists, Buddhist and Bahai respiratory therapists (and almost every other combination of belief and profession within the interdisciplinary team!) seek spiritual support for themselves—not only for the children and families they care for."*

A particularly poignant occurrence is when staff members are confronting loss simultaneously in both their personal and professional lives. To remain open and empathic with the children and families while immersed in one's own deep grief is an almost indescribable challenge. Frequent check-ins with the mental health clinician or chaplain on the team can be crucial to the individual's balance and self-preservation in the work. A referral for psychotherapy may also be indicated.

Memorial services to commemorate the children who have died are also a tribute to the staff members who cared for them. These events can be a time both for grieving and for the renewal of professional commitment.

> *"It is my pleasure to help out and to meet these families again. The spirit of this gathering is so beautiful, and I love to feel shaken by emotions and let the emotions overwhelm me, instead of restraining them as we need to when working in the hospital."*
>
> —*Social Worker*

Clinical Vignettes

The following vignettes, along with their clinical implications, illustrate some of the key themes that emerge in assessment and intervention with bereaved families.

MICHAEL'S FAMILY

Michael died of a brain tumor at the age of 15. He, his parents and younger brother, Andrew, 12, had lived with the uncertainty of his prognosis through several years of intensive treatment. Andrew had spent a great deal of time with Michael during his last months. During particularly difficult periods, Andrew would retreat to a computer fantasy game that featured castles and knights slaying dragons. His maternal grandmother had been very involved with the family, and particularly with Michael, in the last year of his life. Michael's best friend throughout childhood was at his side daily over the last several weeks of his life. Present at the time of Michael's death were all of the members of his family, his best friend, the hospice nurse, and the oncology social worker. Although the local hospice team had taken over most of Michael's care at home in his last two months, the hospital social worker as well as the nurse practitioner from the palliative care team had visited often.

Michael's father was born in the United States; his mother had emigrated from England as a teenager. After Michael's death, his parents found themselves at odds in their styles of grieving. Coming from a traditional British upbringing, Michael's mother was uncomfortable with the public expression of strong emotion. She tended to keep her feelings to herself and spent much of her time in a garden creating a special memorial area. Michael's father found it helpful to share his deep sadness with family and friends. When he would try to engage his wife in conversation about Michael, she listened attentively but usually remained quiet and composed. Andrew was talkative and often tearful when alone with the social worker, but around his parents, he was reserved and avoided any discussion of Michael other than happy memories.

The social worker and the hospice bereavement counselor met with the family, including the grandmother, both individually and as a family shortly after Michael's death. Michael's father expressed interest in attending a bereaved parents group at a local agency; his mother wanted nothing to do with it. The social worker maintained weekly contact with the family for the first few months and monthly thereafter, for both individual and family therapy sessions. Over time, the family members learned to understand and respect that each had unique needs and paths in bereavement. Andrew was gradually able to share more of his private world with his parents and used writing to express many of the feelings that he had been harboring.

The parents appreciated the ongoing connection to the medical team and the hospital afforded them by the meetings with the social worker. They often asked about Michael's primary physician and were very grateful when she called. At the suggestion of the social worker, Andrew agreed to meet with the school psychologist whom he had met earlier in the year when he was having difficulty completing his homework. His connection to the psychologist provided a safety net for him at school. The grandmother stated that her role was to "keep a stiff upper lip" and to support her daughter by helping with the household tasks and driving Andrew to his activities. She found solace in her church community.

The nurse practitioner had talked to Michael's best friend at the funeral. She asked him whether she could call in a few weeks to see how he was doing. He agreed and when they spoke, he told her he could not stop thinking about Michael—especially the day of his death. He agreed to consider joining a teen group at the same agency that Michael's father attended, but did not want to commit to it yet. When the nurse called him again a week later, the boy had decided against contacting the group. However, he promised to call the nurse if he continued to feel so preoccupied with Michael's death. A few months later, the high school principal contacted the nurse and asked her to meet with the students to discuss the impact of their peer's illness and death.

Implications:

- The "family" may include extended family members and significant friends,
- A child's death affects both the immediate family and wider community,
- Individuals in the same family experience a death differently, and thus a variety of interventions should be considered,
- It is common for family members to feel perplexed and at times distressed about differences in individual styles of coping. The clinician plays an important role in helping to clarify these differences, as well as to point out the commonalities in the grief,
- A single assessment of a family in the bereavement process is not sufficient. Rather, ongoing check-ins, with the family's agreement, can provide a more accurate picture of the family's needs, as well a safety net for them,
- Siblings often hide their feelings from parents to avoid causing them additional pain,
- Continuity with the care team after the death helps lessen feelings of abandonment and loss of the "hospital family."

ANDREA'S FAMILY

Andrea was born with multiple congenital anomalies to Mexican-American parents. She was the youngest of five children (ages 12, 8, 6, 5); all but the oldest were born in the United States. Both parents spoke only spanish. When Andrea was born, the mother left her job to spend most of her time at the hospital. The father worked as a dishwasher in a local restaurant and took on extra shifts to compensate for the loss of income. The children's aunt arrived from Mexico, where the entire extended family still lived, to help care for the other children. Without the mother's income, the family experienced extreme financial hardship, including the loss of electric and water service because of their inability to pay the bills. The social worker from the palliative care team met the mother during Andrea's admissions, and followed up with family therapy sessions in their home after her death.

The children rarely saw Andrea during her months-long stay in the neonatal intensive care unit. The hospital was more than two hours away from the family's home; they did not own a car and public transportation was extremely limited in their rural community. The children were given little information about the severity of Andrea's condition. The aunt would respond to any questions by saying that Andrea was "in God's hands and only He knows what her fate would be." The mother explained that neither the parents nor the aunt talked to any of the children about the severity of Andrea's condition because they feared it would scare them. When Andrea was discharged home for about two months, José, the 8-year-old, was especially involved with her. He said, "I helped take care of her and I made her smile and hugged her."

Andrea was readmitted to the hospital at six months of age and died there three weeks later. All the children were shocked because neither their parents nor their aunt had talked about the possibility of death. They all attended their sister's funeral; José commented that it was "scary" because he didn't know that his sister would feel so cold and be so still when he touched her. He visited the cemetery often, both with the family and on his own. The family spoke openly of Andrea, but not of her death. As part of their tradition, the family created an altar made up of her special belongings, pictures and religious symbols on a shelf in the main room of the house. Every morning before school, José would speak to Andrea's picture, sharing his thoughts about the day ahead. "I always tell her goodbye and that I loved her." He said Andrea was like an angel who watched over him all the time. Although tearful when telling the story of his sister to the social worker, he also said he felt happy to talk about her. Prior to this conversation, he had not told the story of Andrea to anyone, not even his closest friends.

According to the mother, the oldest son, age 12, was extremely quiet and stoic. During the social worker's visits, he would stand in the doorway listening attentively to the conversation, at times tearful, but never joining in. Clearly he took the lead from his father, who was deeply sad, but reluctant to talk about his feelings. Such stoicism is a highly valued trait in Mexican culture, especially in men, and is perceived as a way to protect others from added pain. In the first few months after Andrea's death, the marital relationship was somewhat strained. Although the mother understood her husband's emotional stance, she longed for more sharing in their grief. As a result of several family therapy meetings, he began to be more open. The two youngest children, both girls, were eager to be part of every meeting, and frequently added their own comments while drawing pictures of their baby sister.

In the months following Andrea's death, the aunt, who stayed on with the family, expressed surprise and concern about how little community support was offered. She stated that friends and neighbors would have been much more involved in Mexico. In particular, the children were somewhat "invisible" in the turmoil after Andrea's death. Because their visits to the hospital had been infrequent, the siblings had never met with anyone from child life, social work, or psychology/psychiatry. The palliative care social worker referred José to a local support agency, but he did not want to go, saying that he did not want to talk with a stranger and that he just needed to be strong. However, when the mother reported feeling severely depressed months after the baby's death, she followed up a referral to a local agency for individual therapy, recommended both by the Spanish-speaking chaplain who called regularly and the social worker, and found it helpful.

Implications:

- The parents' and aunt's reticence to disclose the dire nature of Andrea's condition reflected a strong cultural value about protecting children from talk of death. Clinicians must be aware of and respect this belief, while also gently offering ideas about more open sharing with their children,
- José's mother believed that it was important for her children to be involved in the funeral and to visit the cemetery. In contrast to the prohibition about discussing death ahead of time, children of all ages partake in these rituals in her culture. It is important to understand these customs as bereavement interventions in the family's natural setting,

- The altar represents one culture's tradition of maintaining ties with the deceased. It is therapeutic and respectful for clinicians to inquire about such traditions; often the question opens discussion about the family's bereavement process in general,
- Certain traits, such as stoicism, represent both individual psychology and cultural forces and must be understood within both contexts,
- José, as the most expressive child, illustrates some of the unique experiences of a bereaved sibling attempting to cope with his loss. The death of his baby sister was clearly an ongoing thread in his life that he wrestled with daily. José's focus on the sensory perception of Andrea's body "feeling cold" at the funeral is a typical response of children and is often a graphic illustration of their fear. His altar conversations with Andrea were a way for him to maintain an ongoing connection with her. Such avenues are crucial for bereaved children as well as adults,
- Had the family lived in Mexico during their time of hardship, the community would have been much more involved. In the absence of such support, particularly for immigrant families, the palliative care team must be proactive in helping families find and connect with support through local resources. Simply offering the name of an individual or an agency is often inadequate; the family may need help in making the contact, or even be accompanied for an initial visit,
- Siblings are often invisible to the team at the hospital, even more so when language, culture, and distance are factors. For truly comprehensive family-centered palliative care, the siblings' needs must be recognized and addressed by the clinical team, both during the illness and in bereavement.

FRANK, 4, SIBLING OF KATY, 8[46]

When Frank was told of Katy's death from leukemia (see earlier section about Katy under Anticipatory Grief), he immediately said he wished he had had the chance to say goodbye. Over the next few days he asked many questions: Why was Katy dead, what does dead mean, what does she look like now? The parents told him that although Katy could no longer talk to him, he could still tell her things if it would make him feel better. During the first month after Katy's death, Frank asked to go to the cemetery several times. At the grave he would pose questions to Katy through his mother, such as: "Ask Katy if she really loved me." He would recount anecdotes to Katy about his daily life. When the family dog was found after being lost for a day, Frank insisted on going to the cemetery with the dog so that Katy would know about his return. At school, Frank attached himself to a little girl in his class, and would panic on days that she was absent. About a month after Katy's death, while Frank was in the bathtub, he suddenly burst into sobs about how much he missed taking a bath with Katy. Bath time continued to be difficult for about six months, after which it became a time for happy memories. Almost a year later, Frank still woke up some mornings saying that he felt sad because he missed Katy.

Implications:

- Even very young children can grasp the absolute finality of death. Frank alternates between conventional verbal reminiscence and the more concrete working through of grief,
- Intellectual questions about death are children's attempts to cognitively master a highly abstract concept,
- Through his "talking to Katy," Frank came to understand that his relationship with her continued even though she was no longer alive. The parents' initiation and support of these conversations was pivotal in Frank's grieving and solace,
- Frank's immediate attachment to the girl at school represents the concrete attempts at replacement so often seen in young children, along with their heightened sensitivity to the threat of loss,
- Frank's reminiscences at bath time are similar to adult grieving, when memories are stirred up by activities once shared,
- Frank's expressed sadness on waking some mornings is a spontaneous form of grieving, in no way induced by adult probing.

BOBBY, 10, AND JOANNE, 17, SIBLINGS OF CINDY, 14[46]

After the death of Cindy at age 14 of osteosarcoma, her two siblings were followed in psychotherapy for several months. During Cindy's illness, Bobby had expressed much fear of his leg being amputated (see Figs. 3-7 and 3-8). His identification with her physical illness and suffering continued into bereavement. When asked how he was feeling, Bobby responded, "I feel like a bug is just eating me up." He then drew a picture of a bald boy with bugs "in the leg and chest only"—the sites of his sister's cancer (Fig. 5-7). Even more significant was the fact that his asthma, previously mild, became quite severe during this period.

In Joanne's sessions with the psychologist, she reviewed the process of Cindy's illness and death (see Chapter 3, p. 22) and reminisced about their relationship. She initially expressed a

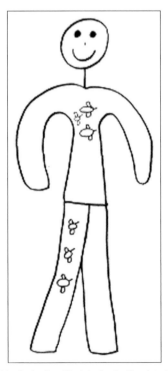

Fig. 5-7 How Bobby feels after Cindy's death. (Reprinted with permission from Kellerman, J. *Psychological Aspects of Childhood Cancer.* (1980). Courtesy of Charles C. Thomas, Publisher, Ltd. Springfield, Illinois.)

great deal of guilt about not being able to protect her younger sister, as well as regret for some of her past actions and thoughts. "I feel so selfish. I always used to tell Cindy that I wanted my own room. And now I have it—two twin beds—and I am so lonely." Over the next few months, Joanne did a school project on the cancer center, with the following prologue: "This project is dedicated to my beloved little sister Cindy. At the age of fourteen, my little sister and closest friend departed... Because of my very personal involvement, I chose the cancer institute as my assignment for Urban Studies."

Implications:

- Somatic reactions are common indices of distress in bereaved siblings. Particular attention must be paid to symptoms that in some way mirror the illness of the child who died. These symptoms tend to be more resistant to abating on their own, and may require more intensive psychological—as well as medical—treatment,
- Adolescents' grief often closely resembles that of adults, often with a strong need to commemorate their sibling.

Summary

These clinical vignettes attest to parents' and siblings' wide range of responses, in both content and intensity, to a child's death. Bereavement is a process of converting presence into absence, actuality into memory. Families must construct a framework for memories of the child that can endure over a lifetime.[68] Most individuals, adults and children alike, demonstrate remarkable resilience in their emergence from the child's death. They derive strength from the deep commitment of the clinicians who care for them.

Portions of this chapter are reprinted with permission from Sourkes, B. *The deepening shade: psychological aspects of life-threatening illness,* University of Pittsburgh Press, 1992.

REFERENCES

1. Kuttner L: *Making every moment count: pediatric palliative care,* documentary film. National Film Board of Canada, 2003.
2. Sourkes B, Frankel L, Brown M, Contro N, et al: Food, toys and love: pediatric palliative care, *Curr Probl Pediatr Adolesc Health Care* 35(9):345–392, 2005.
3. Shaffer MA, Barrows A, editors: *The Guernsey Literary and Potato Peel Pie Society,* New York, 2008, Random House.
4. Webster's College Dictionary. *Random House,* New York, 2000.
5. Contro N, Larson J, Scofield S, et al: Family perspectives on the quality of pediatric palliative care, *Arch Pediatr Adolesc Med* 156:14–19, 2002.
6. Field MJ, Behrman RE, editors: *When children die: improving palliative and end-of-life care for children and their families,* Washington, DC, 2003, National Academy Press.
7. Contro N, Larson J, Scofield S, et al: Hospital staff and family perspectives regarding the quality of pediatric palliative care, *Pediatrics* 113:1248–1252, 2004.
8. Kreicbergs U, Valdimarsdottir U, Onelov E, et al: Care-related distress: a nationwide study of parents who lost their child to cancer, *J Clin Oncol* 23:9162–9171, 2005.
9. D'Agostino NM, Berlin-Romalis D, Jovcevska V, et al: Bereaved perspectives on their needs, *Palliat Support Care* 6:33–41, 2008.
10. Hynson JL, Aroni R, Bauld C, et al: Research with bereaved parents: a question of how not why, *Palliat Med* 20:805–811, 2006.
11. Scott DA, Valery PC, Boyle FM, et al: Does research into sensitive areas do harm? Experiences of research participation after a child's diagnosis with Ewing's sarcoma, *Med J Aust* 177:507–510, 2002.
12. Kreicbergs U, Valdimarsdottir U, Steineck G, et al: A population-based nationwide study of parents' perceptions of a questionnaire on their child's death due to cancer, *Lancet* 364:787–789, 2004.
13. Dyregrov K: Bereaved parents' experience of research participation, *Soc Sci Med* 58:391–400, 2004.
14. Sourkes B: *Armfuls of Time: The psychological experience of the child with a life-threatening illness,* Pittsburgh, 1995, University of Pittsburgh Press.
15. Raphael B: *The anatomy of bereavement,* New York, 1983, Basic Books.
16. Rando T: *Parental loss of a child,* Champaign Ill, 1986, Research Press Company.
17. Rosen E, editor: *Families facing death,* San Francisco, 1990, Jossey-Bass.
18. Rosof BD, editor: *The worst loss,* New York, 1994, Henry Holt.
19. Crawley LM: Racial, cultural, and ethnic factors influencing end-of-life care, *J Palliat Med* 8(1):S58–S67, 2005.
20. Doka K, Tucci A, editors: *Living with grief: children and adolescents,* Washington, DC, 2008, Hospice Foundation of America.
21. Wheeler I: Parental bereavement: the crisis of meaning, *Death Stud* 25:51–66, 2001.
22. Whittam EH: Terminal care of the dying child: psychosocial implications of care, *Cancer* 71:3450–3462, 1993.
23. Kreicbergs UC, Lannen P, Onelov E, et al: Parental grief after losing a child to cancer: impact of professional and social support on long-term outcomes, *J Clin Oncol* 25:3307–3312, 2007.
24. Jalmsell L, Kreicbergs U, Onelov E, et al: Symptoms affecting children with malignancies during the last month of life: a nationwide follow-up, *Pediatrics* 117:1314–1320, 2006.
25. Wolfe J, Grier HE, Klar N, et al: Symptoms and suffering at the end of life in children with cancer, *N Engl J Med* 342:326–333, 2000.
26. Hendricks-Ferguson V: Physical symptoms of children receiving pediatric hospice care at home during the last week of life, *Oncol Nurs Forum* 35:E108–E115, 2008.
27. Kreicbergs U, Valdimarsdottir U, Onelov E, et al: Anxiety and depression in parents 4–9 years after the loss of a child owing to a malignancy: a population-based follow-up, *Psychol Med* 34:1431–1441, 2004.
28. Li J, Precht DH, Mortensen PB, et al: Mortality in parents after death of a child in Denmark: a nationwide follow-up study, *Lancet* 361:363–367, 2003.
29. Li J, Laursen TM, Precht DH, et al: Hospitalization for mental illness among parents after the death of a child, *N Engl J Med* 352:1190–1196, 2005.
30. Sirki K, Saarinen-Pihkala UM, Hovi L: Coping of parents and siblings with the death of a child with cancer: death after terminal care compared with death during active anticancer therapy, *Acta Paediatr* 89:717–721, 2000.
31. Shanfield SB, Benjamin AH, Swain BJ: Parents' reactions to the death of an adult child from cancer, *Am J Psychiatry* 141:1092–1094, 1984.
32. Goodenough B, Drew D, Higgins S, et al: Bereavement outcomes for parents who lose a child to cancer: are place of death and sex of parent associated with differences in psychological functioning? *Psychooncology* 13:779–791, 2004.
33. Dussel V, Kreicbergs U, Hilden JM, et al: Looking beyond where children die: determinants and effects of planning a child's location of death, *J Pain Symptom Manage* 37:33–43, 2009.
34. Masera G, Spinetta JJ, Jankovic M, et al: Guidelines for assistance to terminally ill children with cancer: a report of the SIOP Working Committee on psychosocial issues in pediatric oncology, *Med Pediatr Oncol* 32:44–48, 1999.
35. Mack JW, Hilden JM, Watterson J, et al: Parent and physician perspectives on quality of care at the end of life in children with cancer, *J Clin Oncol* 23:9155–9161, 2005.
36. Mack JW, Wolfe J, Grier HE, et al: Communication about prognosis between parents and physicians of children with cancer: parent preferences and the impact of prognostic information, *J Clin Oncol* 24:5265–5270, 2006.
37. Valdimarsdottir U, Kreicbergs U, Hauksdottir A, et al: Parents' intellectual and emotional awareness of their child's impending death to cancer: a population-based long-term follow-up study, *Lancet Oncol* 8:706–714, 2007.
38. Surkan PJ, Dickman PW, Steineck G, et al: Home care of a child dying of a malignancy and parental awareness of a child's impending death, *Palliat Med* 20:161–169, 2006.
39. Kreicbergs U, Valdimarsdottir U, Onelov E, et al: Talking about death with children who have severe malignant disease, *N Engl J Med* 351:1175–1186, 2004.
40. Hunt H, Valdimarsdottir U, Mucci L, et al: When death appears best for the child with severe malignancy: a nationwide parental follow-up, *Palliat Med* 20:567–577, 2006.
41. Stroebe W, Schut H, Stroebe MS: Grief work, disclosure and counseling: do they help the bereaved? *Clin Psychol Rev* 25:395–414, 2005.

42. Davies R: New understandings of parental grief: literature review, *J Adv Nurs* 46:506–513, 2004.
43. Li J, Laursen TM, Precht DH, et al: Hospitalization for mental illness among parents after the death of a child, *N Engl J Med* 352:1190–1196, 2005.
44. Lannen PK, Wolfe J, Prigerson HG, et al: Unresolved grief in a national sample of bereaved parents: impaired mental and physical health 4 to 9 years later, *J Clin Oncol* 26:5870–5876, 2008.
45. Ellegard A, Kreicbergs U: Risk of parental dissolution of partnership following the loss of a child to cancer: a population-based long-term follow-up, *Arch Pediatr Adolesc Med* 164(1):100–101, 2010.
46. Sourkes B: Siblings of the pediatric cancer patient. In Kellerman J, editor: *Psychological aspects of childhood cancer*, Springfield, Ill, 1980, Charles C. Thomas, pp 47–69.
47. Sourkes B: Siblings of the child with a life-threatening illness, *J Child Contemp Soc* 19:159–184, 1987.
48. Rosen H: *Unspoken grief: coping with sibling loss*, Lanham, Md, 1990, Lexington Books.
49. Davies B: *Shadows in the sun: the experience of sibling bereavement in childhood*, Philadelphia, 1999, Brunner-Mazel.
50. Bluebond-Langner M: *In the shadow of illness: parents and siblings of the chronically ill child*, Princeton, NJ, 2000, University Press.
51. DeVita-Raeburn E: *The empty room: surviving the loss of a brother or sister at any age*, New York, 2004, Scribner Press.
52. Nolbris M, Hellstrom AL: Siblings' needs and issues when a brother or sister dies of cancer, *J Pediatr Oncol Nurs* 22:227–233, 2005.
53. Wilkins KL, Woodgate RL: A review of qualitative research on the childhood cancer experience from the perspective of siblings: a need to give them a voice, *J Pediatr Oncol Nurs* 22:305–319, 2005.
54. Alderfer MA, Labay LE, Kazak AE: Brief report: does posttraumatic stress apply to siblings of childhood cancer survivors? *J Pediatr Psychol* 28:281–286, 2003.
55. Ballard KL: Meeting the needs of siblings of children with cancer, *Pediatr Nurs* 30:394–401, 2004.
56. Sourkes B: *The deepening shade: psychological aspects of life-threatening illness*, Pittsburgh, 1982, University of Pittsburgh Press.
57. Aldrich CK: Some dynamics of anticipatory grief. In Schoenberg B, Carr A, Kutscher A, et al, editors: *Anticipatory grief*, New York, 1974, Columbia University Press.
58. Anderson R: Notes of a survivor. In Troup SB, Greene WA, editors: *The patient, death and the family*, New York, 1974, Scribner.
59. Klass D: *Parental grief: solace and resolution*, New York, 1988, Springer.
60. deCinque N, Monterosso L, Dadd G, et al: Bereavement support for families following the death of a child from cancer: practice characteristics of Australian and New Zealand pediatric oncology units, *Journal of Pediatrics and Child Health* 40(2):1–5, 2004.
61. Contro N, Scofield S: The power of their voices: child and family assessment in pediatric palliative care. In Goldman A, Haines R, Liben S, editors: *Oxford textbook of pediatric palliative care*, London, 2006, Oxford University Press, pp 143–153.
62. Sourkes B: Psychotherapy with the dying child. In Chochinov H, Breitbart W, editors: *Psychiatric dimensions of palliative care*, New York, 2000, Oxford University Press, pp 265–272.
63 *Science, art and theology: a call for dialogue by Dr. Carl G. Howie*, Richmond, Va, Union Theological Seminary.
64. Mitchell K, Anderson H: *All our losses, all our griefs: resources for pastoral care*, Philadelphia, 1983, Westminster Press.
65. Huntley T: *Helping children grieve when someone they love dies*, Minneapolis, 1991, Augsburg.
66. Komp D: *Children are… images of grace: a pediatrician's trilogy of faith, hope and love*, Grand Rapids Mich, 1996, Zonderman Publishing.
67. Grossoehme D: *The pastoral care of children*, Oxford, 1999, Haworthe Press.
68. Hanus M, Sourkes B: *Les enfants en deuil: portraits du chagrin [Bereaved children: portraits of grief]*, Paris, 1997, Frison-Roche.
69. Saint-Exupery A. de: *The little prince*, 1971, Harcourt, Brace and World.
70. Rashotte J, Fothergill-Boourbonnais F, Chamberlain M: Pediatric intensive care nurses and their grief experiences: a phenomenological study, *Heart Lung* 26(5):372–386, 1997.
71. Rushton C: The other side of caring: caregiver suffering. In Carter B, Levetown M, editors: *Palliative care for infants, children and adolescents: a practical handbook*, Baltimore, 2004, Johns Hopkins Press, pp 220–243.
72. Serwint J, Rutherford L, Hutton N: Personal and professional experiences of pediatric residents concerning death, *J Palliat Med* 9(1):70–79, 2006.
73. Swinney R, Yin L, Lee A, et al: The role of support staff in pediatric palliative care: their perceptions, training and available resources, *J Palliat Care* 23(1):44–50, 2007.
74. Papadatou D, editor: *In the face of death: professionals who care for the dying and the bereaved*, New York, 2009, Springer.

6

The Team

DANAI PAPADATOU | MYRA BLUEBOND-LANGNER |
ANN GOLDMAN

It takes a village to raise a child. —Igbo Proverb[1]

This well-known Igbo proverb highlights the key role played by the community in the healthy development of its members. Such a community takes an active role in the transmission of its beliefs, values, priorities, and practices. It provides the conditions that help infants, toddlers, children, and adolescents develop into responsible, emotionally healthy adults who form respectful and collaborative relationships with others, cope with adversities, and are mindful of the well-being of their community. The quality of life of an individual within such a society is directly related to the quality of life of the entire community.

In the case of children with life-threatening illness and their families one could paraphrase, "It takes a team to care for a child with a life-threatening illness." Such a team relies on the close collaboration of its members to address the needs of the ill child as well as those who are part of the child's larger network, including parents, grandparents, siblings, peers, and teachers. For many of these significant people in the ill child's life, this is the first time they are confronted with the possibility, and in some cases the eventuality, of a child's death.

The team's role is to accompany the child and family during the course of the illness and through bereavement. In so doing the team pursues an active and comprehensive approach to care, with the goal of helping the child and family cope with the challenges of the disease and treatment. The team acts to alleviate the patient's physical discomfort and endeavors to temper the suffering caused by the uncertainties of the prognosis and outcomes of treatment. The team works with the child and family in their quest for a life worth living, that is, a life characterized by quality and meaning regardless of whether or not the child lives. When a child dies, the team offers or recommends services to those who had been involved with the child's life that are aimed at facilitating their adjustment to the death.

In this chapter we focus on the development and structure of teams, a major feature of the care that is provided to children with life-threatening illnesses and their families. We do so with the caveat that the literature on teamwork in pediatric palliative care is rather limited.[2,3] Conspicuously absent are systematic empirical studies of how teams develop and operate and their effects on team members, patients, families, institutions, and communities.[4,5] The literature that does exist is descriptive and of varying depth and breadth.[4] Articles that deal with teams focus on the educational background of professionals who make up the team, their roles, and responsibilities.[6] With few exceptions little attention is given to team development, team functioning, and team support in the face of serious illness and death.[7–10] The purpose of this chapter is to draw attention to these issues in order to enhance our understanding of the team's role in the care of children with life-threatening illnesses and determine what is needed to ensure the highest quality of care. Also, we hope to point the way toward further research and training.

Our discussion and recommendations are rooted in a relationship-centered approach that focuses on relationships among children, adolescents, and families who receive care services, and professionals who offer them. Such an approach recognizes the reciprocal influence between children and families on the one hand, and professionals, teams, and organizations on the other. These professionals, affected by their interactions, seek creative ways to contain, reduce, or transform suffering, and in so doing enhance the quality of care for a child who may never grow into adulthood.[9,11,12] In other words, the relationship-centered approach is concerned with the establishment of relations that are potentially enriching, and are rewarding for all involved. Achievement of this goal requires understanding not only the patient's and family's subjective views and experiences so as to provide them with appropriate care, but also the professionals' and team's subjectivity, which shapes interactions with children and parents, and affects the quality of services.

This view perceives care-giving as a social affair that is determined by the relations among care seekers and care providers. All of them are inevitably affected by the serious illness and death of the child, and as a result, their relationships are impacted by feelings that must be recognized and addressed as they affect the process and quality of care.

Team Development

A DYNAMIC, NON-LINEAR PROCESS

For a group of people to become a team they must share a common purpose, be strongly committed to the achievement of specific tasks, and value teamwork through which they expect to accomplish more by cooperating. Setting a clear task that is owned by each member and sharing outcomes are central to the transition from a group to a team.[13]

Another characteristic that distinguishes groups from teams is their size and leadership.[13] While groups vary in size, teams contain no more than a few members who share leadership in clinical practice, although at an administrative level they are led by a senior member. Depending on a child's condition and family's situation, for example, different professionals may take the lead at any time and make a special contribution in order to achieve the team's goal and tasks.

Regardless of whether the team uses a manager to facilitate the coordination of actions or it chooses to be self-managed, the importance is that responsibility for outcomes be shared. By contrast, in a group, leadership is assigned to one person who imposes his or her leadership style that usually remains unchanged despite the changing focus or work activity.[14]

We view teams as dynamic systems that have the potential to evolve, grow, and function with increasing degrees of openness, communication, and collaboration among care providers. A team's development is not linear. It is characterized by cycles of forward vs. regressive movement, as well as by periods of stability, disorganization, being stuck, and growth. What determines a team's level of development is related to the ability of its members to establish and maintain collaborations that ensure quality care and are enriching to both families and team members.

Among the available models for understanding team development, and especially applicable to palliative care, are those proposed by Papadatou and Morasz.[9,15] They take the position that over the course of development, team members experience periods of co-existence, mutual acknowledgment and parallel collaboration, and of collaborative alliance with concomitant changes in disciplinary boundaries[7,9,15,16] (Fig. 6-1).

When functioning in the *mode of co-existence*, professionals work more as a group than as a team. Goals are generally shared, specific roles are identified, and tasks are divided among care providers who provide services that are fragmented and compartmentalized. Not infrequently a predetermined package of medical, nursing, psychological, social, and spiritual services is offered to families of seriously ill children, who are then introduced or referred to different experts. Transactions among professionals tend to be rigid and communication limited. They rarely report to their colleagues about the nature and outcomes of their intervention or observations—information that could be useful to others in their interactions with the families. Each care provider is focused on his or her field of expertise and communicates achievements through brief reports that are usually included in the patient's file.

In the *mode of parallel collaboration*, care providers begin to work as a team. They acknowledge each other's knowledge and skills, and work in parallel yet independent ways toward shared goals and tasks. Transactions are richer and communication is more open, but it remains superficial. The team members accomplish their job, but lack the ability to integrate the richness of existing services into an explanatory and comprehensive framework.

In parallel collaboration, teamwork is often multidisciplinary and team members do not necessarily adapt their roles and responsibilities to those of other professionals. Information is usually communicated via the patient's file or in staff meetings where each provider reports his or her work that is added rather than integrated into the plan of care that is offered to a child and family.

In the *mode of collaborative alliance*, emphasis is placed on effective and open communication among professionals who plan, offer, and evaluate their collective services. Information circulates and team members learn from each other, broaden their horizons of understanding, and critically review their work by acknowledging their strengths and limitations. A reflective process is central to their collaboration and evaluation is periodic both with regard to the outcomes as well as to the process by which services are provided and goals are achieved.

Teamwork now becomes interdisciplinary in nature and is based upon the close collaboration among professionals who set clear goals, decide upon a course of action, and assume the responsibility of care as a team—not as individuals. Team members are characterized by a high degree of interconnectedness and a sense of belonging. The identity of the team is set above their personal identities. Mutual support becomes essential in the pursuit of collective goals and in coping with challenges and difficulties that are inherent in care. Leadership, responsibility, and accountability in interdisciplinary teams are usually shared.

In well-balanced and experienced teams, teamwork often takes the form of a transdisciplinary alliance. Care providers train one another in some domains of their expertise to broaden the horizon of knowledge and skills and become competent in assessing and responding to a wide range of needs without necessarily duplicating their services. This is particularly important when caring for children who are terminally ill and whose families choose to limit the number of relationships with professionals, and focus on the dying child and themselves.

For a collaborative alliance to develop, care providers must spend time working together, sharing experiences, exploring different points of views, and developing a common language that does not exclude any member. Interdisciplinary and transdisciplinary teamwork require interdependent collaboration and are possible only if the team functions as an open system that makes use of relevant information. Relevant information is any information that helps members to understand how they operate as a system, how they manage suffering and adversities, and how they make use of their resources.[9,17] Such information helps team members learn from experience, consider alternative ideas and coping patterns, embrace new initiatives, take risks, implement changes, and grow as a team. Unless there is opportunity to share information about *what* is happening in the day-to-day work, *how* things are accomplished, and *how* professionals think, feel and behave, team members cannot be in control of the quality of services they provide, and the system cannot be self-correcting.[18] Such openness is not simply limited to the disclosure and airing

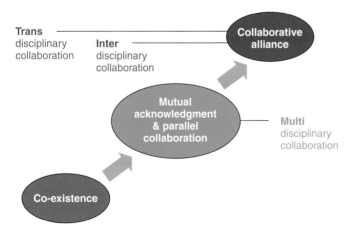

Fig. 6-1 **Dynamics of Team Development.** Redrawn from Papadatou, D. In the Face of Death: Professionals Who Care for the Dying and the Bereaved, New York, Springer Publishing; 2009.)

of feelings and thoughts, but demands a reflective openness that enables team members to challenge their own and others' thinking, suspend a sense of certainty, and share experiences with a receptiveness to having them challenged or changed.[16,19]

In such a team, care providers derive satisfaction from both the provision of services that are helpful and meaningful to patients and families, as well as from their collaborations with one another in the pursuit of a common purpose.

ORGANIZATIONAL CULTURE AND CONTEXT

A team's development is not solely determined by its members.[9,20] The social and organizational context in which it provides services has a major impact on how it develops and functions. For example, in some places pediatric palliative care services are delivered by teams in the community through home, respite, or hospice programs.[21-24] In others, they are introduced in the hospital and offer consultation services to professionals, families, and other teams.[4,25] In many countries that lack resources or are reluctant to acknowledge the needs of dying children and grieving families, palliative care teams are either non-existent or encounter major social, institutional, and legal obstacles in the provision of interdisciplinary services. Even in resource-rich countries that acknowledge the needs of dying children and grieving families, provision of interdisciplinary and palliative care services may be hampered by the country's healthcare system.

The value system of a given social context affects the culture of the organization or service to which a team belongs, which, in turn, influences the services it provides. The organization's culture plays a major role in how seriously ill children are perceived, how they are cared for, and how they are integrated into the organization or service. Organizational culture also has an impact on how suffering is regulated, hope is instilled, and time is managed when a child's life is threatened.

Some organizations that assume a cure-oriented approach tend to dismiss or downplay the role of palliative care services, and instead adopt a protective approach by concealing the possibility of death from the child and occasionally from parents. Other organizations strive to integrate curative, life-prolonging and palliative care services and create a space for mutual collaborations among several teams and family members who are actively involved in the decision-making process.

Hence, the culture of an organization or service may promote or hinder different forms of teamwork, depending on its philosophy of care, its values, goals, and priorities. This does not mean that teams do not shape their own course of development, rather, some are helped and supported through this process, while others have to work harder to fully develop and pioneer their approach through the healthcare system.

Teams at Work

INDICATORS OF TEAM DEVELOPMENT, FUNCTIONALITY, AND EFFECTIVENESS

We take the position that teams are active and dynamic systems with potential to change, develop, and grow. Teams, like the individuals who compose them, are not passive agents. Teams, like their members, are active agents who both shape and are shaped by their individual and collective responses to life-threatening illnesses, loss, suffering, and those whom they encounter in their work. Teams, like their members, are both subject to and react to internal and external stressors associated with the care of seriously ill patients and their families. Affected by the wider social and organizational context of work, team members, consciously or unconsciously, decide how to operate and collaborate with each other in order to meet the challenges of life-and-death situations. The team's development, functionality and effectiveness are reflected in the patterns by which its members manage team boundaries and team operations as well as suffering and time.[9]

Team Boundaries

Teams with defined but flexible and permeable boundaries facilitate interdisciplinary collaborations and promote open teamwork. In contrast, teams with rigid boundaries tend to function as closed systems in which transactions are tightly controlled and collaboration is limited. In a parallel way, teams with diffused or blurred boundaries expose their members to intrusions and invasions from within or outside the team, and sustain chaotic transactions that render intra- and inter-team relationships a source of constant distress. This compromises their development because they become more absorbed by their conflicts than by opening up to opportunities for learning, collaborating, and expanding.

Team Operation

Teams that set clear and realistic goals, sustained by a holistic and comprehensive approach to care, foster open communication and mutual collaboration that benefit both families and professionals. In such teams, care providers agree upon a mode of operation that is periodically evaluated and adapted to new situations and emerging needs. Losses, traumas, and achievements are openly addressed instead of being avoided, and team resources are effectively used to manage a crisis or challenging situation. By contrast, teams with unclear or unrealistic goals, or blurred roles and functions, tend to diffuse responsibility among members who compartmentalize their services and work independently from each other. They are unable to cooperate in the management of a crisis or traumatic event, which then tends to be silenced, buried, or acted upon. The team's mode of functioning is rarely reviewed, leading to the development and perpetuation of dysfunctional patterns.

Management of Suffering

Teams are repositories for the suffering of the children and families, as well as that of their own members. When they recognize and address the suffering caused by the threat upon a child's life, team members can integrate painful experiences into their daily functioning without being disabled or consumed by them. The acknowledgment of suffering motivates them to establish a safe environment in which families, as well as team members, can openly express, explore, accept, and eventually transform their suffering. By contrast, teams that strive to eliminate, hide, or suppress suffering, perceiving it as a sign of weakness and incompetence, are likely to develop distant or enmeshed relationships that compromise meaningful collaborations with children, families, and colleagues and forestall the team's development.

Experience and Management of Time

When a child's life is threatened by a serious condition, time is perceived and experienced in unique ways by families and by care providers.[26] A team that paces its work encourages children and their families not only to reflect on and work through their grief, but also to live a life that is meaningful to them. Such a team also takes the time to process work-related experiences that evoke anxiety in team members. The team learns from the past, integrates knowledge into the present practice, and strives toward future goals that aim at increasing the quality of the services it provides. In contrast, teams that avoid difficult subjects and experiences stagnate. Those teams become unable to take action, make decisions, and effect interventions. They delve into apathy and inertia. They become frozen in time. Some teams act as if time could be eliminated. They do too much; perhaps to avoid difficult issues such as case overload, loss, or death. Time is experienced as event-full. Work is driven by events or crises. An ongoing over-agitation prevents the team from slowing down in order to process its experiences and use relevant information for learning, changing, and growing.[9,17]

Teams and Families

A PARTNERSHIP IN CARE

Most parents want to assume a central and active role in the care of their ill child. They acquire in-depth knowledge of the child's condition and treatments, and develop appropriate skills in order to meet their complex needs.[27,28] Parents of seriously ill children are faced with challenges and crises that are different from anything they have ever encountered in their lives.[27] In their desire to be effective in this new parenting role, they have to interact with the professionals who can help them develop strategies and skills in order to manage present situations and anticipate future needs in both their sick and healthy children.[27,28] This close involvement often leads to the erroneous assumption that parents are members of the team. Contrary to some clinicians who have written about teams and palliative care, we take the position that parents and patients are not members of the team.[8,29]

To speak of a patient or parent as a member of the team works best at a metaphorical level, and even then it is misleading. No parent or child can ever be a member of a multidisciplinary or interdisciplinary team in any real sense. They do not share the team's history, its achievements and failures, its traumas and successes, or its trajectory through time. Nor do they necessarily have the same goals, values, and priorities that a team holds for itself and the families it serves. And not insignificantly, to view parents and patients as members of the team is to demean the unique relationship not only between ill children and their parents, but also between teams and those they serve.

A more appropriate way of conceptualizing the patient and parents' place with and around the team is to consider that all share a symbolic space in which care is offered and received. This space belongs neither to the family nor to the team, but to their unique relationship.

It is hoped the relationship develops into a partnership. As partners, professionals and families define goals of care, which may change over the course of the illness, and rely upon each other in order to achieve them. While team members assume the responsibility of providing information, guidance, advice, and specialized care, family members are responsible for participating in decisions and communicating their needs, concerns, values, and preferences. The family's responsibility should be taken into consideration when developing a care plan.

In this partnership, children's views, concerns, and desires must be considered and approached with sensitivity and skill. This requires awareness of the differences in the ways children express both directly and symbolically, their physical, psychosocial and spiritual needs, preferences, and concerns; children and parents' positions in the family; the rights, duties, and obligations each has to the other; and the impact of team's actions on the patient's and parents' futures.[30]

Teams that are well-balanced and well-developed function as open systems. They have flexible yet stable boundaries that enable families of seriously ill children to move in and out, according to need. Team members are not threatened by becoming overwhelmed by the family's grief, confusion, disorganization, despair, or suffering. They are able to contain these experiences. They assist parents and children in acknowledging, expressing, and accepting their feelings as well as in assimilating their experiences, and adjusting to a reality that is often filled with challenges, uncertainty, and surprises. They accompany families in their trajectory through the child's illness, cure, or death and in some instances maintain enduring bonds throughout the long period of bereavement.

Teams that experience difficulties with various aspects of boundary maintenance, goal setting, or time management are more likely to establish enmeshed or avoidant relationships with the patient and family.[9] An enmeshed relationship develops when both the team and the family are unable to contain suffering, as well as the threat or reality of death. They become one, and remain undifferentiated, sometimes even after the child's cure or death. For example, a team may need families that adore and glorify it, while at the same time some families need the team to maintain the memory of their deceased child to avoid moving on with life. An avoidant relationship between a team and a family, on the other hand, transforms their partnership into a strictly bureaucratic affair, a consumer-provider business that aims to manage practical issues without addressing the emotional and spiritual aspects of living with a life-threatening illness. Avoidant or enmeshed relationships are often reflective of the team's and family's inability to effectively manage the challenges of living with or dying from a life-threatening illness.

Teams Working Together

PRINCIPLES, PRACTICES AND PARTICULAR CHALLENGES

It is common for pediatric palliative care teams to collaborate with a range of other professionals and teams. These include teams who specialize in specific disease-directed intervention (such as cystic fibrosis team, oncology team, neuro-muscular team), those that perform organ transplantations, or critical care interventions, and also those involved in day-to-day care such as home care teams, community care teams, hospice and educational teams. Palliative care teams also work closely with mental health and bereavement specialists who provide counseling services to family members. These parallel collaborations with other professionals, teams, organizations and services are vital to pediatric palliative care, however they require good communication, planning, mutual respect, and an approach that has been described by Payne as "open teamwork," discussed below.[31]

Although all of these teams may recognize that other teams are also necessary for meeting the complex needs of children with life-threatening illnesses and their families, the particular problems that each addresses and the roles that each assumes may overlap. Exactly who delivers which aspects of care may also vary over the course of the child's illness. For example, the oncology team may include in their domain issues of pain and symptom control as well as the child's and family's social and emotional needs during treatment with curative intent. However, as the disease progresses and the possibility of death emerges, the oncology team may see the responsibility for pain and symptom control as well as meeting the social and emotional needs of the child and family as falling more within the purview of the palliative care team. The child and parents may not perceive or desire this dichotomy at all, and want the services that each team offers to continue simultaneously.[28,32] Hence, it is essential that all teams involved in the care of these children and families be committed to an agreed-philosophy, which also acknowledges the families' choices. Often families' preferences are for an approach that integrates disease-directed care along with treatment of symptom-directed and supportive care.[28,33,34]

For children with life-threatening illnesses and their parents the possibility of recurrence, further deterioration, and death are never far from their thoughts. These thoughts often emerge at those times when critical decisions need to be made about further disease-directed care and treatment. The challenge is intensified not only by the nature of the decisions to be made, but also by the variety of people who are involved and affected by such decisions. Teams have a shared responsibility in guiding patients and families through the decision-making process.

Like families, all teams caring for children with life-threatening illnesses are confronted with the possibility of the children dying. While disease-directed teams may spend more of their energy against death, it would be wrong for these teams to proceed as if the possibility were not an eventuality for many of the patients they treat. Similarly, while palliative care teams accept childhood mortality as inevitable in some cases, and acknowledge their limitations in reversing a terminal disease, they cannot proceed as if battling the disease is not present in the minds of some team members, other teams they work with, or the patients and families. All must resist declarations such as "Things may get better tomorrow," or "There is nothing we can do." Instead, teams need to work with families to contain a suffering that is inevitable when life is seriously threatened and death becomes imminent, to address their needs and concerns during the most stressful period of their lives and to accept the reality before them.[9]

While the alleviation of suffering remains a priority, it can never be eradicated. At diagnosis, at each relapse of the disease, with each sign of physical deterioration, and particularly during the terminal phase, the family experiences a grieving process that is intense and often chronic.[35] All teams who work with these families must acknowledge that suffering cannot be fixed with quick solutions and pre-determined interventions. Patients and families must be assisted in coping with their losses and grief, and in building resources and resilience that will enable them to live through the disease as well as after the child's death.

The Team's Ability to Function with Competence

All teams confront a number of challenges in the uncertainty and grief that mark the experiences of the children and families. Teams mobilize various patterns to cope with the anxiety and suffering these realities evoke. Functional patterns are most likely to occur when three basic conditions are present. These are a *commitment* to clearly define goals and tasks and to a team member's co-workers, a *holding environment* for children, adolescents, families, and care providers, and *open teamwork* through interdisciplinary collaborations.[9]

COMMITMENT

Working in a field that causes increased distress requires a high degree of commitment from care providers who perceive their services to seriously ill children and families as meaningful and valuable. These professionals must recognize both the possibilities as well as the limitations of science in the treatment of life-threatening diseases, and facilitate conditions that promote quality of life. Their commitment in this field of work has two components: a commitment to a philosophy of care with clear, realistic, and well-defined goals and tasks, and a commitment to co-workers and to the team.

These goals and tasks promote the welfare and quality of life of children, adolescents, families, and of people who are significant to them. They help delineate the team members' roles, responsibilities, and methods by which to achieve them. When goals and tasks are vague or conflicting, professionals are less likely to be committed to them and tend to assume responsibilities that are off-task or transgress role boundaries.

One of the challenges in caring for children with life-threatening illnesses is that teams strive to achieve ideal or unrealistic goals of excellence.[36] Realistic goals acknowledge the limitations of what care providers and teams can offer. For example, sometimes death cannot be avoided, nor life prolonged. At times, despite the best efforts of all involved, the dying trajectory is painful. There are also times when death occurs under traumatic conditions or the impending reality of death is not being dealt with by the family. Even though it is crucial for a team to work toward ensuring a dignified life for the entire family, and a dignified death for the patient, in reality there is only one thing that care providers can promise: the availability of a relationship. In that relationship, they will remain present, available, and able to introduce continuity in the midst of loss, separation, and suffering.

A commitment to co-workers and to the team is necessary to achieve the desired goals and to form an ethos of collaboration and of mutual support among team members. Professionals often experience grief and suffering while working with children with life-threatening illnesses. Acknowledging the professionals' pain, and doing something about it, implies the sharing of personal experiences among team members who assume the responsibility to care for themselves as well as for each other. When committed to co-workers, they display care and concern through holding behaviors and mutual support.[9,36-39]

Holding behaviors involve acts of care, kindness, and support. Examples include listening to a colleague's experiences and pain, offering feedback instead of advice and therapy, or standing by a co-worker during distressing times. Such behaviors are essential in establishing a culture of mutual support. Mutual support is marked by:[9,37]

- *Informational support:* the exchange of information about patients and families, as well as about the team's operations through feedback that is conducive to quality care, change, or adaptation,
- *Practical support:* the provision of practical advice, help, or assistance in the process of completing specific tasks,
- *Emotional support:* the establishment of opportunities for sharing personal feelings and thoughts in a safe environment where team members feel heard, understood, valued, and appreciated,
- *Support in the construction of meaning:* the provision of opportunities for reflection and processing of work-related experiences so as to attribute meaning and integrate them into the team's history.

It is important to note that while all types of mutual support are essential, the form that the support takes must be responsive to the needs and preferences of care providers, which vary at different times. Mutual support has been found to be a factor that determines professionals' degree of job satisfaction.[40–42] Studies indicate that one of the primary factors that contributes to professional burnout and turnover is not the team's confrontation with multiple child deaths, however distressing, but rather the team's inability to support its members.[40–42] Committed care providers are devoted to meaningful goals and tasks, and rely upon one another to achieve the goals while providing mutual support through the process of care giving.

HOLDING ENVIRONMENT

The concept of holding environment was first proposed by Donald Winnicott, an English pediatrician and psychoanalyst who described the significant role played by parents in providing their infant with effective care, which contributes to the child's psychosocial development.[43] Parents create an environment with safe boundaries that provides the infant with a sense of protection from the external world. In this environment parents cultivate a sense of order, continuity, and predictability that eventually helps the child to move from the safety of the parental relationship to the external world, which is gradually assimilated and to which the child adjusts.

In a parallel way, the team cultivates in families a sense of safety, order, predictability, and continuity, all of which are critical in times of crisis, ambiguity, uncertainty, and loss. However, such a team must also provide its members with a similar environment by creating a safe organizational space in which stresses, conflicts, suffering, and hopes associated with the challenges of caring for children with life-threatening illnesses can be worked out. This is important, because professionals can more effectively hold children and families through a serious illness when they are themselves held by their team and organization.[44]

Repeated encounters with death can deplete a team's resources and leave professionals alone to manage their pain and suffering.[39,42] When a holding environment is in place, care providers can feel safely overwhelmed by experiences, acknowledge, and accept their suffering as natural, and lean temporarily upon others who understand, validate their feelings, and have faith in their abilities to manage

work challenges. In a paradoxical way, being securely attached and held by others enables team members to be self-reliant.[38] Intra-team relationships are characterized by mature dependence, and are marked by a collective healthy respect for autonomy and for relatedness.[39]

A holding environment does not disempower care providers by overprotecting them, nor does it excuse their shortcomings. Instead, it provides a shelter in which they can retreat when they feel distressed, anxious, angry, sad, or frightened and offers a secure base from which they can work through their experiences and move toward, rather than away from difficulties and anxiety-provoking situations.

A holding environment fulfils five important functions for team members:[9]

- *A sense of safety* creates boundaries that protect team members from destructive interferences from outside sources such as organizational, bureaucratic, and financial restrictions, or from intra-team sources including gossip or misapplied blame. In a safe environment, care providers feel free to express feelings, thoughts, frustrations, and concerns, without the fear of being judged or criticized.
- *The containment of experiences* is an ability to empathically understand and hold within experiences that are painful or threatening without dismissing, repressing, masking, distorting, or dividing them into parts. Rather than moving away from distressing feelings and experiences, the team moves toward them and openly addresses the anxiety, pain, or distress.
- *The elaboration of experiences* involves exploring and assimilating difficult experiences, losses, and frustrations. It prevents immobilization, especially in situations that are traumatic or cause increased anxiety. It requires circulating information among team members who explore the underlying dynamics of a given situation, and use this information to develop as individuals and as a team. Elaboration helps them adopt alternative perspectives in an anxiety-provoking situation, reframe painful events, reconstruct meaningful narratives, and develop a better understanding of self, others, and of the team.
- *The regulation of distress and transformation of suffering* provide team members with opportunities to pace their work, prioritize tasks and minimize chaos, confusion, and distress. The goal is not to eliminate the stressors that are inherent in caring for children with life-threatening illnesses, but rather to manage them, and transform the inevitable suffering caused by loss and dying in meaningful ways. In this way the team builds upon its resources and develops its resilience.
- *Fostering interconnectedness, interdependence and a sense of belonging* prevents care providers from feeling alone, and teach them to hold others while being held by them. Mutual respect and shared responsibility are at the core of effective collaborations, which cultivate interdependence and promote autonomy.

The development of a holding environment always contains a risk for the team: to be directly confronted with the fear, anxiety, despair, powerlessness, and other aspects of personal and collective suffering elicited by uncertainty, loss, and death, which are often perceived as too threatening. Such confrontation, although painful, is necessary because it allows experiences to be processed and integrated into the team's story, and enhances a forward movement. However, there are teams that are not willing to take this risk and sabotage every conscious effort toward building a holding environment by preventing members from reflecting and elaborating difficult experiences or distressing emotions. They reinforce a culture of invulnerability and omnipotence that compromises the team's competence. While a holding environment allows the emergence of pain, it also serves as an antidote to the distress and suffering that is associated with the care of seriously ill children.

INTERDISCIPLINARY COLLABORATION AND OPEN TEAMWORK

Competence is reflected in the team's capacity to promote interdisciplinary collaboration among professionals with different expertise, who do not simply co-exist or juxtapose their services but integrate them into a comprehensive framework of care. Such integration is at the core of a relationship-centered approach that responds, in appropriate ways, to the needs of a network of significant people who affect, and are affected by, the life of a seriously ill child.

Integration of services into a comprehensive framework requires open teamwork. The team develops relations and collaborations with other professionals, teams, organizations, or services within the larger organization or community. The team maintains permeable yet flexible boundaries, thereby allowing the circulation of information within and beyond its boundaries. Open teamwork is facilitated when the team provides a secure base for its members, who temporarily leave their base to form coalitions with different groups and teams, which are subsequently drawn into the team. This process helps the team respond in a comprehensive way to the multiple and complex physical, psychosocial, and spiritual needs of children and families, which emerge over the course of the illness in various settings. Open teamwork is also vital when the team must facilitate the transition of patient care from pediatric experts to adult experts—a consequence of the number of children diagnosed with life-threatening illnesses in childhood who live well into adulthood.

Overall, open teamwork promotes initiatives and developments, and integrates different approaches and services into a plan of care that benefits the entire family as well as the individuals who are significant to them. Another positive outcome of open teamwork is that it enables care providers to see how others perceive their services, and aids in assessing the impact they have upon a community by realizing what society gains from their contribution.

Assessing the Team's Ability to Function with Competence

Teams are systems that are constantly changing and evolving. Acknowledging that their competence is enhanced by working conditions that promote commitment, a holding environment and open teamwork, can help professionals determine which among these conditions are well-developed and which require the team's attention and further enhancement. Ideally, the development of all three conditions form an equilateral triangle with a base representing commitment to a philosophy of care, to clearly defined goals and tasks, and to each other. According to Ketchum and Trist, "commitment to work is central to people's lives."[45]

The more solid the commitment, the more likely team members are to trust each other in creating a holding environment, which can contain their experiences and emotions, and the more willing they are to take risks and collaborate with other professionals and teams for the benefit of their patients. In a parallel way, the more reliable a holding environment is in providing team members with a sense of safety, order, predictability, and continuity in times of distress, then the more committed they remain to shared goals and co-workers. Similarly, the more open care providers are to interdisciplinary collaborations within and beyond the team, the more likely they are to become enriched, to grow and value their work that further reinforces their commitment to their job and team.

It becomes obvious that the described conditions are closely interrelated, and that the development of one enhances the development of the others (Fig. 6-2, *A*).

The following figures represent difficulties experienced by two teams in developing work conditions that ensure competence. In one pediatric palliative care team (Fig. 6-2, *B*), the professionals are committed to well-defined goals and tasks, and are supported in a holding environment in which they feel relatively secure to share cases and talk openly about their emotional responses, misgivings, or mistakes. Rather than going through suffering alone, team members draw on the experience and feedback of their colleagues. However, in the team described here, there is a gap between the need for nurturing and mutual support and the existing holding environment which, although in place, is not fully developed. As a result, team members engage in limited risk-taking because they feel uncertain that their team will hold them in times of high distress or crisis. The shorter line of open teamwork reflects the team's tendency to avoid or restrict collaborations with other professionals in the larger organization and community. This

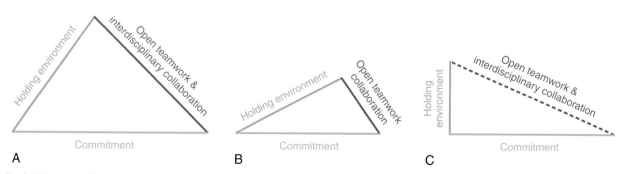

Fig. 6-2 **A,** Working conditions of a team that functions with competence. (Adapted from Papadatou D. *In the Face of Death: Professionals Who Care for the Dying and the Bereaved*, New York, NY: Springer Publishing 2009.) **B,** Working Conditions of a Team That Functions Without Full Competence. **C,** Second Example of Working Conditions of a Team That Functions Without Full Competence.

affects families, who are deprived of valuable services, and care providers, who rely solely on their resources, with both becoming secluded into a cocoon-like environment. While this environment provides them with a relative sense of safety and protection, it concurrently marginalizes them from the rest of society.

Fig. 6-2, *C*, illustrates the working conditions of another pediatric care team, which remains too open and too permeable to collaborations with other professionals and teams without securing the boundaries of a holding environment, as indicated by the dotted line. This hampers the team's ability to process experiences, frustrations, conflicts, and emotions resulting from its members' interactions with others. Information that goes out from the team and information that is introduced into it is not used effectively to benefit families and team members. If team goals, tasks, and practices are not reviewed, enhanced, or changed, commitment to them, although strong, remains rigid. Concurrently, commitment to colleagues and co-workers is circumstantial and depends from the nature of collaborations that develop within or outside the team, at a given time.

The internal space of the triangles in Figs. 6-2, *B*, and 6-2, *C*, is limited by comparison to the space in Fig. 6-2, *A*, and graphically represents the limited opportunities of these teams to develop and use their resources in order to develop their competence.

Directions for Research, Education, and Practice

There is not a single professional who can meet the myriad needs of children and families dealing with life-threatening illnesses. Care of children with life-threatening illnesses requires a large and varied tool kit and knowledge base as well as a deep and abiding appreciation of the children's and families' struggles and triumphs; it is greater than any one individual can possess or indeed even muster. Simply assembling a group of highly qualified, highly trained compassionate professionals will not ensure that the children's and families' needs are met either. The provision of quality care for these children and families requires the development and maintenance of team competency. Achieving and sustaining team competence requires attention not only to how the team cares for the children and families, but also to how it cares for itself and its members.

There is a dearth of literature both on how teams care for patients and families and on how they care for themselves and their members. In an effort to fill this gap we would suggest a research agenda that includes the systematic study of the experiences of care providers and of teams. More specifically, we need to consider:

- How teams develop, with attention to the professional, interpersonal, and institutional challenges and opportunities for teamwork and the skills and abilities necessary for the achievement and maintenance of team competency,
- What is the nature of various models of service delivery (e.g., palliative care teams, hospice teams, disease-directed teams, integrated palliative care and disease-directed teams), their costs; effectivenes; and patient and family outcomes. Such studies could serve as part of evi-

dence-based recommendations for the provision of care in settings of various communities; as well as for various illness conditions and trajectories. What is the nature of relationships that develop between individuals, the care providers, patients, and family members, as well as between the teams and families with particular attention to issues of trust, decision making, transition, and continuity of care—all found to be important consequences of professional, patient, and parent relationships,
- How professionals and the teams of which they are a part, affect and are affected by the care they provide. These studies need to include both the positive effects of caregiving, such as personal growth, acquisition of leadership skills, and the negative impacts of their experience, which may include anxiety, burnout, or compassion fatigue,
- What is the impact of the culture and societies in which these teams work on their abilities to develop and meet the needs of patients and families.

There is also a need for more training in effective team practice. While there has been an increase in the number of training opportunities and programs in palliative care, there is very little offered in the way of training in team dynamics, functioning and growth in the face of serious illness, and death. We would urge program organizers to take advantage of the presence of individuals from different professional backgrounds, skills, and experiences and include sessions that address issues in teamwork.

In addition, we would also suggest the development of materials and programs that model and teach collaboration among clinicians with different scientific and professional backgrounds. Of critical importance is the development of materials and programs that offer techniques for:

- Eliciting and discussing responses to difficult situations and relationships,
- Discussion of difficult issues, both clinical and managerial,
- Team self-monitoring and reflection during provision of services.

Useful resources for the development of materials and programs include: Children's Project on Palliative/Hospice Services (The ChiPPS Project) sponsored by the National Hospice and Palliative Care Association; IPPC (The Initiative for Pediatric Palliative Care) sponsored by the Education Development Center, Inc.; and End of Life Education for Nurses-Pediatric Palliative Care.[4,46–48]

Educational and training programs, like teams themselves, need to be evaluated. Tools for assessing palliative care curricula are starting to be developed, but work needs to expand to other disciplines and other types of programs.[4] We would recommend instruction in methods for evaluating the team's role in service delivery that could be used by teams in the course of their work with one another.

These methods also could be used to evaluate the short-term and long-term effects of new or current team practices, such as support groups, debriefing, and away days. They could also provide an evidence base of the sustainability or termination of such practices. The need for research on interventions that aim to prevent compassion fatigue and burnout has been underscored by a variety of researchers and clinicians.[4]

Summary

Caring for children whose lives are threatened and attending to the needs of grieving family members is important, strenuous, enriching, and rewarding work.[4,42,49-52] Attending to how we care for families and for each other, can only enhance our practice, our lives, and the lives for whom we care.

REFERENCES

1. Hron M: *Oran a-azu nwa*: the figure of the child in third-generation Nigerian novels, *Res African Lit* 39:27–48, 2008.
2. McCulloch RE, Comac M, Craig F: Paediatric palliative care: Coming of age in oncology? *Med* 44:1139–1145, 2008.
3. Morgan D: Caring for dying children: assessing the needs of the pediatric palliative care nurse, *Pediatr Nurs* 35:86–90, 2009.
4. Liben S, Papadatou D, Wolfe J: Paediatric palliative care: challenges and emerging ideas [see comment], *Lancet* 371:852–864, 2008.
5. Holleman G, Poot E, Mintjes-de Grot J, van Achterberg T: The relevance of team characteristics and team directed strategies in the implementation of nursing innovations: a literature review, *Int J Nurs Stud* 2009. 10.101/j.ijnurstu.01:005.
6. Hubble RA, Ward-Smith P, Christenson K, et al: Implementation of a palliative care team in a pediatric hospital, *J Pediatr Health Care* 23:126–131, 2009.
7. Connor S: *Hospice and palliative care: the essential guide*, New York, 2009, Routledge.
8. Jassal SS, Sims J: Working as a team. In Goldman A, Haines R, Liben S, editors: *Oxford textbook of palliative care for children*, Oxford, 2006, Oxford University Press.
9. Papadatou D: *In the face of death: professionals who care for the dying and the bereaved*, New York, 2009, Springer.
10. Rushton CH: A framework for integrated pediatric palliative care: being with dying, *J Pediatr Nurs* 20:311–325, 2005.
11. Beach MC, Inui T, the Relationship-Centered Care Research Network: relationship-centered care: a constructive reframing, *J Gen Intern Med* 21:53–58, 2006.
12. Report of the Pew-Fetzer Task Force on Advancing Psychosocial Health Education. *Health Professions Education and Relationship-Centered Care*, San Francisco, Calif, 2000, Pew Health Professions Commissions.
13. Speck P: Team or group—spot the difference. In Speck P, editor: *Teamwork in palliative care*, Oxford, 2006, Oxford University Press, pp 7–23.
14. Belbin RM: *Beyond the team*, Buttersworth-Heinemann, Oxford, 2000, Oxford University Press.
15. Morasz L: *Le Soignant Face a la Souffrance*, Paris, 1999, Dunod.
16. Larsen D: *The helper's journey: working with people facing grief, loss, and life-threatening illnesses*, Champaign, Ill, 1993, Research Press.
17. Ausloos G: *La Compétence des Familles: Temps, Chaos, Processus*, Ramonville, Saint-Agne, 2003, Érès.
18. Steele F: *The open organization: the impact of secrecy and disclosure on people and organizations*, Reading, Mass, 1975, Addison-Wesley.
19. Senge P: *The fifth discipline: the art and practice of the learning organization*, New York, 1990, Doubleday.
20. Kaës R: Réalité psychique et souffrance dans les insitutions. In Kaës R, Bleger J, Enriquez E, Fornari F, Fustier P, Roussillon R, Vidal J.-P, editors: *L'Instituiton et Les Institutions: Études Psychanalytiques*, Paris, 2003, Dunod.
21. Burne S, Dominica F, Baum JD: Helen House: a hospice for children: analysis of the first year, *BMJ Clin Res Ed* 289:1665–1668, 1984.
22. Davies B, Collins JB, Steele R, Cook K, Brenner A, Smith S: Children's perspectives of a pediatric hospice program, *J Palliat Care* 21:252–261, 2005.
23. Steele R, Davies B, Collins JB, Cook K: End-of-life care in a children's hospice program, *J Palliat Care* 21:5–11, 2005.
24. Davies B, Steele R, Collins JB, Cook K, Smith S: The impact on families of respite care in a children's hospice program, *J Palliat Care* 20:277–286, 2004.
25. Rushton CH, Reder E, Hall B, et al: Interdisciplinary interventions to improve pediatric palliative care and reduce health care professional suffering, *J Palliat Med* 9(4):922–933, 2006.
26. Sourkes B: *Armfuls of Time: The psychological experience of the child with a life-threatening illness*, New York, 1996, Taylor & Francis.
27. Bluebond-Langner M: *In the shadow of illness: parents and siblings of the chronically ill child*, Princeton, NJ, 1996, University Press.
28. Bluebond-Langner M, Belasco JB, Goldman A, Belasco C: Understanding parents' approaches to care and treatment of children with cancer when standard therapy has failed, *J Clin Oncol* 25:2414–2419, 2007.
29. Egan K: *Patient-family value based end-of-life care model*, Lergo, 1998, Hospice Institute of the Florida Suncoast.
30. Bluebond-Langner M, DeCicco A, Belasco JB: Involving children with life-shortening illnesses in decisions about participation in clinical research: a proposal for shuttle diplomacy and negotiation. In Kodish E, editor: *Ethics and research with children: a case based approach*, New York & London, 2005, Oxford University Press.
31. Payne M: *Teamwork in multiprofessional care*, New York, 2000, Palgrave.
32. Wolfe J, Wolfe J, Klar N, Grier HE, et al: Understanding of prognosis among parents of children who died of cancer: impact on treatment goals and integration of palliative care, *JAMA* 284:2469–2475, 2000.
33. Foster TL: Pediatric palliative care revisited, *J Hosp Palliat Nurs* 9:212–219, 2007.
34. Field MJ, Behrman RE: *When children die: improving palliative and end-of-life care for children and their families*, Washington, DC, 2003, National Academic Press.
35. Monterosso L, Kristjanson LJ: Supportive and palliative care needs of families of children who die from cancer: an Australian study, *Palliat Med* 22:59–69, 2008.
36. Marquis S: Death of the nursed: burnout of the provider, *Omega, Special Issue on Death, Distress, and Solidarity* 17–34, 1993.
37. Papadatou D, Papazoglou I, Petraki D, Bellali T: Mutual support among nurses who provide care to dying children, *Illness, Crisis & Loss* 71(1):37–48, 1999.
38. Kahn W: Holding environments at work, *J Appl Behav Sci* 37:260–279, 2001.
39. Kahn WA: *Holding Fast: The struggle to create resilient caregiving organizations*, New York, 2005, Brunner-Routledge.
40. Vachon M: *Occupational stress in the care of the critically ill, the dying and the bereaved*, New York, 1987, Hemisphere Publishing.
41. Vachon M: Recent research into staff stress in palliative care, *Euro J Palliat Care* 4:99–103, 1997.
42. Papadatou D, Martinson IM, Chung PM: Caring for dying children: a comparative study of nurses' experiences in Greece and Hong Kong, *Cancer Nurs* 24:402–412, 2001.
43. Winnicott DW: *The maturational process and the facilitating environment: studies in the theory of emotional development*, London, 1990, Karnac Book. (Originally published 1960.)
44. Papadatou D: Care providers' response to the death of a child. In Goldman A, Hain R, Liben S, editors: *Oxford textbook of palliative care for children*, Oxford, 2006, Oxford University Press.
45. Ketchum LT, Trist E: *All teams are not equal*, London, 1992, Sage.
46. The ChiPPS Project (Children's Project on Palliative/Hospice Services) sponsored by the National Hospice and Palliative Care Association. www.nhpco.
47. IPPC (The Initiative for Pediatric Palliative Care) sponsored by the Education Development Center, Inc. www.IPPCweb.org.
48. End of Life Education for Nurses—Pediatric Palliative Care. www.aacn.nche.edu/ELNEC/Pediatric.htm. Accessed July 9, 2010.
49. Clarke-Steffen L: The meaning of peak and nadir experiences of pediatric oncology nurses: secondary analysis, *J Pediatr Oncol Nurs* 15:25–33, 1998.
50. Davies B, Clarke D, Connaughty S, et al: Caring for dying children: nurses' experiences, *Pediatr Nurs* 22(6):500–507, 1996.
51. Olson MS, Hinds PS, Euell K, et al: Peak and nadir experiences and their consequences described by pediatric oncology nurses, *J Pediatr Oncol Nurs* 15:13–24, 1998.
52. Wooley H, Stein A, Forrest GC, Baum JD: Staff stress and job related satisfaction at a children's hospice, *Arch Dis Child* 64:114–118, 1989.

7 Settings of Care

JEAN MARIE CARROLL | JOSEPH L. WRIGHT | LORRY R. FRANKEL

In thinking about where your child will die, at home or in the hospital, you have to contemplate something that is utterly heart-breaking. Recognize that you are doing the hardest, most selfless, and most loving work a parent ever could do. Take credit for that.[1]

—Joanne Hilden and Daniel Tobben

This chapter explores the settings in which children with life-threatening conditions and their families receive palliative care. It is not uncommon that at different points in the illness trajectory, patients may be treated at different sites such as hospitals, home care facilities and agencies, chronic care facilities, with different teams of clinicians in each setting. Care also extends to respite, schools and other community venues where the children continue to live their lives. The medical home, as described by the American Academy of Pediatrics[2] has particular relevance for these children. It is a model of delivering primary care that is accessible, continuous, comprehensive, family-centered, coordinated, compassionate, and culturally effective. The aim of the medical home is to support the needs of children in the home through collaboration among families, clinicians, and community providers. There are statewide initiatives for developing and implementing the medical home model throughout the country.

This chapter addresses:

- Epidemiological factors in death in children,
- Hospital settings: the intensive care unit and the emergency department,
- Community settings: home hospice, freestanding palliative and respite facilities, school,
- The impact of reimbursement on pediatric palliative care.

Epidemiological Factors in Death in Childhood

Despite significant advances in medicine, and the ensuing reduction in mortality rates in children over the past 25 years, children still die (Figs. 7-1 and 7-2). This is attributed to a number of improvements and advances in pediatric health care, including:

- Child safety laws, such as bicycle helmets, seat restraints, childproof caps on medicine containers,
- Pediatric Advanced Life Support, intensive care, surgery, and anesthesia,
- Therapy for neonatal, cardiac, and oncologic disorders,
- Emphasis on anticipatory guidance in general pediatrics.

A 2003 Institute of Medicine report[3] estimates that there are approximately 55,000 deaths of children younger than 18 years per year, compared to more than 2 million adult deaths per year in the United States. Approximately, 51 percent of those children die in the first year of life (34 percent in the neonatal period and 17 percent from one month to 12 months of age), 10 percent from 1 year to 4 years of age, 14 percent from 5 years of age to 14 years, and 25 percent from 15 to 19 years of age. In addition there is a large group of young adults (ages 20 to 24), who succumb to chronic debilitating pediatric diseases.

The causes of death vary and are age-dependent: birth defects, low birth weight, maternal complications, respiratory distress, and sepsis account for the majority of deaths in the first year of life. Unintentional injuries, homicide, suicide, cancer, heart disease, and sudden infant death syndrome account for more than 51 percent of pediatric deaths. There still remains a large category of other causes, accounting for 18 percent of pediatric deaths.[3]

Conditions appropriate for pediatric palliative care fall into one of the following groups:

1. Children with diseases, such as cancer or complex congenital heart disease, in which attempts at cure may fail.
2. Children who have life-threatening diseases, such as cystic fibrosis and HIV, for whom treatment may significantly extend life.
3. Children with progressive diseases, such as spinal muscular atrophies, metabolic and genetic disorders, for whom palliative care may be the only treatment.
4. Children who have severe non-progressive neurologic disabilities, such as cerebral palsy, that may result in premature death from recurrent respiratory difficulties or sepsis.
5. Previously healthy children who have a sudden and totally unanticipated death, such as trauma, severe infections, or an adverse event in the hospital.[4–6]

The Hospital

As children live for longer periods, the need for complex services also escalates.[3,6–9] In addition to multiple visits to subspecialty clinics, many of these children have prolonged and repeated hospital admissions. Whatever the nature and duration of the admission, hospitalization exerts extraordinary psychological demands. The child's physical distress, and the parents' witnessing of that distress, is compounded by the implications of the illness that necessitate hospitalization, and by the separation from normal life and from other family members, especially siblings or other children.[10] Counterbalancing these stressors, particularly for children with illnesses who have required frequent and prolonged admissions, is the sense that the hospital clinicians become a second family who understand and share in the family's experiences. Hospitals

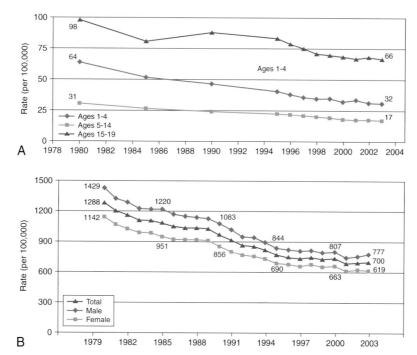

Fig. 7-1 A, Death rates for children ages 1-19 (deaths per 100,000), 1980-2003. **B,** Death rates for infants (deaths per 100,000), by gender, 1980-2003. (Data for 1980-1999 ages 1-14 from National Center for Health Statistics (2002). Health United States, 2002 with Chartbook on Trends in the Health of Americans. Table 36; Data for 1990-1999 ages 15-19 from Federal Interagency Forum on Child and Family Statistics. America's Children Key National Indicators of Well-Being, 2002. Washington, DC; Data for ages 15-19 for 1999 from Hogert DL, Arias E, Smith BL, Murphy SL, Kochanek KD. "Deaths: Final Data for 1999." National Vital Statistics Reports 49(8), Hyattsville, Md: National Center for Health Statistics, 2002; Data for ages 15-19 for 2000 from Minino AM, Arias E, Kochanek KD, Murphy SL, Smith BL. "Deaths: Final Data from 2000." National Vital Statistics Reports 50(15), Hyattsville, Md: National Center for Health Statistics, 2002; Data for 2000 from Arias E, Smith BL. "Deaths: Preliminary Data for 2001." National Vital Statistics Reports 51(5), Hyattsville, Md: National Center for Health Statistics, 2003, Table 1; Data for 2001 from Arias E, Anderson R, Kung H, Murphy SL, and Kochanek KD. (2003). "Deaths: Final Data from 2001." National Vital Statistics Reports 52(3), Hyattsville, Md: National Center for Health Statistics, Tables 3 and 4. Estimates for ages 5-14 total and gender are based on Childs Trends calculations using July 1, 2001, population estimates based on the 2000 census. Race population estimates for ages 5-14 are based on population estimates from National Center for Health Statistics; Data for 2002 from Kochanek KD, Murphy SL, Anderson RN, Scott C. "Deaths: Final Data for 2002." National Vital Statistics Reports 53(5), Hyattsville, Md: National Center for Health Statistics, Table 4. Estimates for ages 5-14 are based on Childs Trends calculations using July 1, 2002, population estimates based on the 2000 census, as presented in Table 1 in the same report. Data for 2003 from Hogert DL, Heron MP, Murphy SL, Kung H. (2006). "Deaths: Final Data for 2003." National Vital Statistics Reports 54(13), Hyattsville, Md: National Center for Health Statistics.)

are a place where many children with life-threatening illnesses and families *live,* often for prolonged periods.

The Intensive Care Unit

The majority of children (more than 56 percent) die in hospitals and more than 85 percent of these deaths occur in the ICU.[3,7] These ICU settings include neonatal (NICU), pediatric (PICU) and more recently created cardiovascular (CVICU) units. Exceptions include tertiary children's hospitals with end-of-life programs that work collaboratively with community resources.[11] A retrospective analysis of deaths in a Canadian tertiary care children's hospital over a 2½ year period studied children who were hospitalized for at least 24 hours prior to their deaths and those who were hospitalized for at least 7 days prior to their deaths.[12] Acutely ill children who were previously healthy were excluded. Demographic data included age, gender, primary diagnosis, location of death, pain and symptom management, communication at end of life including CODE status, family preference for location of death, and the child's involvement. Of the 236 deaths, only 86 met study criteria. Neonates accounted for 56 percent of the deaths; in 8, death was unexpected. The ICU saw 83 percent of the

deaths and 78 percent of those children were intubated at the time of death. More than half, 57 percent, were medically paralyzed and 3 were on extra-corporeal membrane oxygenation (ECMO). Opioids were administered, mostly by continuous infusion, in 84 percent of the children for pain, dyspnea, discomfort related to mechanical ventilation, or post-operative pain. Acetaminophen, non-steroidal anti-inflammatory drugs and complementary medications were also used, as well as non-pharmacologic therapy, including relaxation and imagery.

A retrospective analysis reviewed the hospital care required for 9000 children and young adults with complex chronic conditions (CCCs) during their last year.[8] Children with these conditions accounted for one-fourth of all pediatric deaths. More than 84 percent were hospitalized at death and 50 percent received mechanical ventilation during their terminal admission. Neonates who were less than 7 days of age spent 92 percent of their lives in the hospital; those aged 7 to 28 days spent 85 percent; and infants between one month and 1 year of age spent 41 percent of their lives in the hospital. In the non-neonates, 55 percent were hospitalized at death, with 19 percent mechanically ventilated. The rate of hospital use increased overall as death approached.

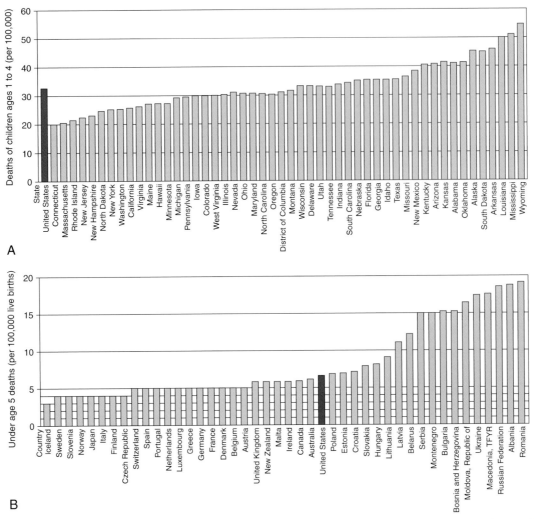

Fig. 7-2 **A,** Deaths of children, ages 1-4, by state. **B,** Under age 5 deaths, (by country, per 100,000). (Data adapted from Field MJ and Behrman RE, eds. "Patterns of Childhood Deaths in America," *Institute of Medicine of the National Academy of Sciences,* the National Academy of Press:2003, pp 41-71.)

This study[8] also found variability as to whether children's code and resuscitation status had been addressed. Discussion about code status was documented only for 79 percent of patients. Results demonstrated that multiple discussions with families were required regarding resuscitation and an actual Do Not Resuscitate (DNR) order. Once a DNR decision was obtained, the majority of children died within one day, although some children lived as long as 30 days. In charts without documentation of DNR status, cardiopulmonary resuscitation was initiated but was unsuccessful.

The mode of death in a number of PICUs has been well described.[13–18] A decision to forgo life-sustaining treatments was made in only 20 to 55 percent of critically ill children who eventually died. Diverse cultural, religious, philosophical, legal, and professional attitudes often affect these decisions. Despite the children's grave prognoses, CPR was initiated and had a failure rate that varied from 16 percent to as high as 73 percent. Full life support at the time of death varied from 18 to 55 percent of the patients. A DNR order was found in less than 25 percent of the patient's charts. Withdrawal or limitation of life-sustaining therapy, including extubation, occurred in 43 percent of the patients. More than 90 percent of these children died within 24 hours; the rest died on the second day.

The Intensivist's Role

The intensivist must engage the family in ongoing discussions about end-of-life issues and repeatedly address and evaluate the goals of care.[5] This role continues long after decisions to forgo life-sustaining treatments have occurred, as families look to the attending intensivist throughout the dying process. The ICU team assures the family that the child's care is undertaken with a focus on quality of life, dignity, and comfort.[19,20] The ICU nurses play a central role; at the bedside, families often call upon them for explanations of the child's care and the existing options as well for emotional sharing.[21] This is also where the social workers, psychologists, child life specialists, and chaplains of the interdisciplinary team can play pivotal roles. Studies have shown that when the ICU staff spends time conversing and providing bereavement resources, the families experience less stress, anxiety, and depression after the child's death.[22]

Decision-Making in the ICU Setting

The decision-making process is often extremely difficult and may require many meetings and interdisciplinary care conferences with the family. The process may be divided into three steps: deliberation, eventually leading to the decision and goal setting; implementation; and evaluation of the decision and its application.[23-25] During the deliberation, the family's decision makers and the clinical teams must weigh the benefits and burdens of various options in terms of survival, long-term outcomes, and quality of life for the child. The concept of shared decision making allows for a consensus to be reached by all active participants once the pertinent information has been shared. It should enable the family to make a truly informed consent.

CARDIO-PULMONARY RESUSCITATION

The use of cardio-pulmonary resuscitation (CPR) has had enormous impact on children's care. Unfortunately, providing CPR for both acutely and terminally ill patients is not as beneficial as had been hoped, because less than 27 percent of children who arrest in the hospital survive to discharge. Some advocate CPR should be reserved only for those children with truly reversible medical conditions.[26] Nonetheless, with the use of more invasive procedures in critical care, more children may be resuscitated onto an ECMO circuit following a cardio-pulmonary arrest. This intervention may indeed improve survival, but is associated with the high risk of neurologic injury.[27,28] Clinicians should inform families about the risks and benefits of CPR. It is also crucial that the family be reassured that a Do Not Resuscitate order does not mean the cessation of care for the child. Rather, it indicates a shift in priorities, toward the implementation of more comfort interventions for the child.[29-31]

WITHHOLDING OR WITHDRAWING LIFE-SUSTAINING SUPPORT

The decision to withhold or withdraw life-sustaining treatment is always difficult. While they are considered to be ethically equivalent, physicians seem to be more comfortable with withholding; withdrawing may increase a sense of responsibility for a patient's death. The minimizing and eventual withdrawal of technology increases opportunities for the family to hold the child. Parents may hold and cuddle their child, or lie in bed and comfort the child during this transitional period. The process of withdrawal of technological intervention requires a team effort and an environment that is supportive for the family. A room that provides privacy for the family, while also shielding other patients and families in the intensive care unit, is beneficial.[5,13,32,33]

COMPASSIONATE EXTUBATION

Families' questions about what to expect when a terminal, or compassionate, extubation is planned revolve around whether the child will feel pain or suffer, be conscious, or breathe. Liberal use of sedatives, analgesics, and anxiolytics should prevent most negative symptoms. Families must be prepared for different scenarios that could unfold; however, no sure predictions can nor should be made regarding when their child will die. Certain children will die shortly after extubation, including those who are brain dead, in severe refractory shock, or in severe respiratory failure with refractory hypercarbia and hypoxia. Children who are not brain dead

may linger for hours, days or longer, with variable respiratory patterns. If the parents or nurses perceive the child to be uncomfortable, then opioids and/or benzodiazepines should be given; for children who are difficult to sedate, propofol or pentobarbital may be used. Pain and suffering should be treated aggressively, even if this results in a foreseen unintended hastening of death. This principle is referred to as the "doctrine of double effect."[33-35]

WITHHOLDING OR WITHDRAWING MEDICALLY PROVIDED NUTRITION AND HYDRATION

Although not a frequent issue in the ICU, pediatricians often have a difficult time with this aspect of terminal care and benefit from team discussion. Arguments that have been made for continued hydration and nutritional support are that children have a remarkable ability to recover, infants need assistance with feedings, and very little is known about whether or not a child at the end of life willfully refuses food and water. The American Academy of Pediatrics concluded in 2009 that the withdrawal of medically administered fluids and nutrition for pediatric patients is ethically acceptable in certain circumstances.[19]

AUTOPSY

Although it is often difficult to request an autopsy, it may provide the parents and clinicians with more information about the child's illness and death. An autopsy may be all-inclusive or limited to those organs most involved in the disease process. Many clinicians have found the request for autopsy to be more successful if the subject is broached during end-of-life discussions with the family before the child has died. Parents may be too distraught to consent if they are approached for the first time in the immediate aftermath of the child's death. When an autopsy is performed, it is imperative that one of the physicians who cared for the child review the results with the parents when they feel emotionally ready.[36] In addition to providing information, this meeting provides a valuable opportunity for follow-up with the family. If the death is a coroner's case, then the coroner will make the determination about the post-mortem exam and the potential for organ and tissue donation.

ORGAN AND TISSUE DONATION

Most ICUs work closely with an Organ Procurement Organization (OPO), whose professionals are trained to counsel families. In the past, brain death criteria had to be met in order to be a donor. Now, all hospitals must have a Donation after Cardiac Death (DCD) policy. This allows organs to be donated after life-sustaining interventions are discontinued, even when criteria for brain death have not been met. In these instances, it is anticipated that the patient will have a cardiac death within 2 hours in the operating room, and then have the appropriate organs retrieved for transplantation. Although the procedure is designed to increase the number of organs available, it is a cumbersome process and involves many additional steps and significant waiting times. If the patient does not sustain a cardiac death in the requisite time for donation, the child must be returned to the ICU or another in-patient area for ongoing care.[32-34]

Emergency Medical Services

Unintentional injury remains the leading cause of mortality among children age 1 to 19 years, accounting for 44 percent of deaths.[40,41] Thus, from an epidemiologic perspective, the dominant trajectory of childhood death is sudden and unexpected.[42] An estimated 20 percent of childhood deaths actually occur in the emergency medical services (EMS) environment.[43,44] Myriad pediatric palliative care issues face clinicians in the EMS, a setting where all trajectories of pediatric life-threatening conditions may intersect. As a result of biomedical, procedural and technologic advances, many children with complications of prematurity, congenital malformations, complex chronic, and life-threatening diseases are surviving longer and living in community-based settings such as sub-acute care facilities or at home. Physiologic exacerbation of an underlying disease state, intermittent infection risk and/or mechanical complications of technology dependence all require immediate attention, and present a spectrum of palliative care challenges to staff. This section will focus on sudden and unexpected death in childhood, and elucidate:

- The organization of emergency medical services for children (EMSC) in the United States as it relates to palliative care,
- The incorporation of a family-centered approach with the family present during end-of-life care for the child in the emergency department.

ORGANIZATION OF EMERGENCY MEDICAL SERVICES FOR CHILDREN

EMSC are organized around the premise that childhood is a relatively healthy time of life and that the death of a child is a relatively rare event. The overwhelming majority of children who present for emergency care are initially seen close to home at community hospital emergency departments (EDs). Only 3 percent of seriously ill or injured children initially present to pediatric tertiary, critical care, or trauma centers.[45,46] More so than for adults, EMSC are highly regionalized, with scarce subspecialty and multidisciplinary services strategically concentrated in a hub-and-spoke wheel model in population centers. The more extensive the anatomic or physiologic derangement and the higher the clinical acuity, the greater is the need for care of the child to flow centrally to the hub. Especially for life- or limb-threatening conditions of sudden onset, the goal is to get the right patient to the right place in the right time. This often necessitates bypassing local community resources to access more sophisticated levels of care. The EMSC system is an integrated continuum of care model, such that patient care flows seamlessly from the local community response through pre-hospital transport and on to hospital-based definitive care (Fig. 7-3). Implementation of this model necessitates a minimum level of expertise and readiness by multiple professionals, including basic emergency medical technicians, paramedics, nurses, and physicians at every step to ensure that timely and appropriate care is rendered.

Among the unique challenges of such an approach are:

- Separation of a child from the family in order to expeditiously accomplish transport, such as air medevac from the scene or inter-facility transfer to definitive care at a distant referral center,
- Families are displaced from existing support systems and clinicians with whom they are familiar. A high likelihood

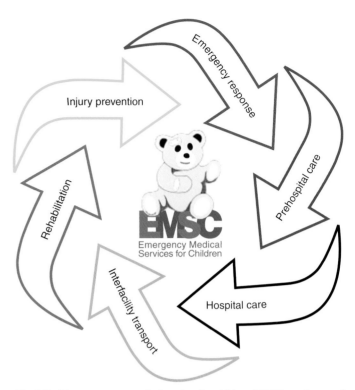

Fig. 7-3   The emergency medical services for children (EMSC) continuum of care. Seriously ill and injured children interface with many health care personnel as they move through the EMSC system.

of the absence of pre-existing clinical relationships with patients and their families is germane to most scenarios in the EMSC environment,

- Extraordinary, non-systematic behaviors and interventions on the part of clinicians, including the provision of futile care, as part of a family-centered approach to the dying child in the ED.

The following hypothetical example illustrates a typical system response pattern, as well as the complex responsibility for managing sudden and unexpected death that often occurs in EDs of tertiary care centers. These challenging circumstances notwithstanding, end-of-life care principles must be systematically incorporated into the EMSC model.

ND is a 6-year-old girl with a neurodegenerative illness. Her disease is characterized by a slow deterioration punctuated by acute complications such as aspiration pneumonia. ND lives at home with her family in a midsized community where her pediatrician, the rescue squad and emergency department personnel are all familiar with her clinical baseline and the nuances of her condition, including her inability to mount a fever in response to a brewing inflammatory process. Of late, ND has become less mobile and disruption of skin integrity secondary to pressure lesions increases her risk of infection. One evening, ND's parents note decreased alertness and an unusual flushed appearance. They call 911 and are transported, as they have numerous times before, to the local community hospital ED. This time, however, the staff immediately recognizes that ND's bounding pulses and worsening skin perfusion signal a problem beyond their capabilities and will require critical care intervention to manage her evolving septic shock. As the local team struggles to stabilize ND, a helicopter is dispatched to transport her to the tertiary care pediatric facility 50 miles away in another state. The family is instructed to begin driving to the definitive care facility, as they will be unable to accompany their daughter in the helicopter. ND is placed aboard the helicopter in clinical extremis. Although experienced, the flight paramedics have never cared for a patient with her underlying condition, complicated by uncompensated shock and impending vascular collapse. Upon arrival at the tertiary care center, ND is immediately taken to the resuscitation bay. After several minutes it is evident that despite extraordinary measures there will be no return of spontaneous circulation; she has succumbed to overwhelming sepsis. However, the code team leader, aware that the family is still en route, orders now-futile resuscitative efforts to continue. The team also begins to plan how best to receive and support the inbound family.

FAMILY-CENTERED CARE

A growing body of evidence attests to the benefits of family-centered care in the ED. Such an approach focuses on effective, culturally sensitive communication and close interaction with parents.[47] A number of institutions have formally incorporated practices for parental presence during invasive procedures, even when a child is in full arrest and requires resuscitation in a code room or trauma bay. Family presence involves their attendance in a location that affords visual or physical contact with the patient. This topic has generated strong debate. The most compelling and frequently cited argument against family presence is based on surveys that presented a hypothetical situation. Respondents thought that the event might be so traumatic that families could lose emotional control, and as a result compromise the functioning of the medical team and the care of the child. Another issue that emerged is providers' fears that family presence could intensify the risk of litigation, unsettle clinicians such that their technical skills would decline, and infringe upon the patient's confidentiality and privacy rights. However, no evidence exists to support any of those arguments.[48] Thus the time-honored practice of banning families from the bedside during resuscitation and other emergency procedures appears to be grounded in tradition, rather than in evidence of beneficial or adverse outcomes.

For the purpose of illustration, the hypothetical case presented in the preceding section is repeated here with an alternate ending:

ND is a 6-year-old girl with a neurodegenerative illness. Her disease is characterized by a slow deterioration punctuated by acute complications such as aspiration pneumonia. Each successive bout has been more difficult to clear, requiring multiple courses of antibiotics and aggressive pulmonary toilet. Despite the occasional need for supplemental oxygen at night, ND has never required mechanical ventilation. The family understands that were she ever to be intubated, she would never be able to be extubated. However, advance directives are not in place. After an unusually stubborn bout of pneumonia, ND appeared to be on the road back to her clinical baseline, when she acutely developed severe respiratory distress. Her family rushed her to the emergency department where, based

on her clinical appearance, she was triaged directly to a resuscitation bay. By all objective measures, including oxygen desaturation via pulse oximetry and rising carbon dioxide on arterial blood gas, she was in impending respiratory failure and in need of endotracheal intubation and mechanical ventilation. ND's parents were initially directed to a designated private waiting area near the resuscitation area. A social worker from the ED accompanied them as their liaison and clinical interpreter. As the personnel, equipment and medications were gathered to perform the intubation procedure, the social worker brought ND's parents into the resuscitation bay. They were positioned just outside the perimeter of the activity surrounding their daughter. They were able to touch her and she acknowledged their presence through eye contact. The lead physician briefly explained what they would see as their daughter underwent rapid sequence administration of sedative and paralytic agents prior to the intubation. As the procedure progressed, including two unsuccessful attempts interspersed by bag-valve-mask ventilation, the social worker provided ongoing commentary about what was being done. The interaction among the medical team members was uncensored and seemingly unaffected by the parental presence. Despite full knowledge that this was likely the last time they would see their daughter without life support dependence, the parents expressed gratitude at being present during the procedure. ND's deterioration had advanced to the point where she could no longer support her own ventilation and after a short period of being intubated in the intensive care unit, she died comfortably and peacefully with family present.

Invasive, technical procedures typically accompany resuscitation and stabilization of critically ill children in the emergency care setting. It is crucial that the team be clinically transparent, especially in circumstances where the child's death may be imminent. While family presence certainly should not be undertaken lightly, responsible, evidence-based approaches and protocols will offer confidence for clinicians and parents alike in the future.

The Community

While sitting at a particularly lengthy and detailed family meeting, a nurse was struck by the family's lack of focus, as if they had checked out of the discussion. When she asked them, "What do you wish for your child?" their response was straightforward: to take her home and make her comfortable.

Transitioning the child from the acute care setting to the community involves challenges not only for the child and family, but also for the clinical team and the institution. The decision to leave the hospital and receive care at home usually reflects a shift in treatment from life-prolonging therapy to comfort measures and quality of life.[1] This change requires advanced planning and coordination of care amongst many stakeholders: the family, the hospital team, the hospice home care team, and the third-party payer. It is essential that one member of the team be identified as a coordinator, that a social worker or case manager participate in the discussion, and that a well-organized plan for care and communication be in place.[49] Additionally, in finalizing the discharge plans, it is extremely beneficial to have representation from the community-based agency and, when possible, the third-party payer. The effort to include these stakeholders upfront is well worth the end result of smooth coordination. The team must advocate that:

- The family have the appropriate services to support the child's needs,
- The goals and wishes of the end-of-life care plan are clearly communicated,
- The healthcare benefits can be maximized.

The team must facilitate conversation with the family to dispel their fears and misconceptions about hospice, particularly their sense of taking their child home to die and giving up hope.[1] While their child may ultimately die at home, families need reassurance that the focus is to maximize the quality of their child's life and provide all possible comfort measures. They also need to know that returning to the hospital is always an option. This entails having a plan for a seamless transition back to the hospital should that become preferable or advisable.

The fact that most children still die in the hospital is related to many factors. On an affirmative note, the comfort that many families feel with the hospital staff is often a reason for choosing the hospital as the setting for a child's end-of-life care and death. Other reasons include:

- A completely unanticipated death such that the child is admitted to the hospital and the family has not had the opportunity to plan for end-of-life care until very late in the disease,
- The family was never referred to hospice because the hospital staff was not knowledgeable about the community's options,
- The parents have the perception that the hospice agency has inadequate pediatric expertise,
- Socioeconomic factors can play a role in the decision to have the child die in the hospital, including that a family living in poverty may not have a house that is comfortable or equipped for adequate care for the child,
- Psychological and cultural beliefs also contribute to the decision.

Home-Based Hospice Services

In the United States, the most common setting for providing palliative care to children in the community occurs through hospice-based home-care programs. The majority of children die in hospitals, except where tertiary children's hospitals have palliative care programs that work collaboratively with community resources.[11] Although some adult hospices and programs have an interest and willingness to care for pediatric patients, adult-focused programs and staff are typically unprepared to respond to infrequent pediatric referrals and also lack connections to pediatric providers to assist them in providing safe, appropriate hospice care.[50]

Adult hospices vary in the amount of experience staff has had with children.[1] One study indicated that of the palliative and hospice programs in the United States that admit children, 40 percent care for an average of 3 or fewer children per year.[51] The Children's Project on Palliative/Hospice Services (ChiPPS) conducted a survey of the more than 3,000 hospice programs in the United States in 2001. These results showed that only 450, or 15 percent, of those hospices

---

BOX 7-1   Evaluating Home Hospice Agencies

Information to obtain from home hospice agencies when considering referral of a child
- What experience has the agency had in pediatric palliative care?
- If the agency has had experience with children and their families, what did they learn about working with this patient population?
- Does the agency have personnel that are trained in pediatric end-of-life care?
- Will attendants from the agency be available to meet with the child, family and staff prior to discharge from the hospital?
- What is the agency's capacity to provide continuing bereavement support for the family?
- Does the agency have a provision for respite care for the caregivers?

Carroll JM, Torkildson C, Winsness JS. Issues related to providing quality pediatric palliative care in the community. *Pediatr Clin North Am*. 2007 Oct;54(5):813-827, xiii.

---

surveyed indicated that they were prepared to offer hospice services to children.[52] In a 2005 report from The National Hospice and Palliative Care Organization (NHPCO), it is noted that of the 4,100 hospice and palliative care programs in the United States that year, only about 738, or 18 percent, provided any pediatric services.[53]

Many physicians are unaware of or uncomfortable with the specialized services that pediatric hospice and palliative care programs can provide and thus are reluctant to make referrals.[54,55] Inadequate training in pediatric palliative care[56–59] can in turn have clinical ramifications in the children and may not receive services that would enhance their quality of life. Parents whose child had died at home with palliative or hospice care reported a calm and peaceful last month of life.[58]

There are practical steps to facilitate the process of transitioning the child to the home. Acquiring information about the hospice home care agencies in the family's area is essential prior to the transition (Box 7-1, 7-2).

Free-Standing Palliative and Respite Care Facilities

There are only two facilities that offer inpatient palliative and end-of-life care services for children and their families: the George Mark Children's House in San Leandro, California and Exceptional Care for Children in Newark, Delaware. Both of these programs also offer respite support.

BOX 7-2   Guidelines for Coordinating Community-Based Palliative and Hospice Services

The following are guidelines for coordinating community-based palliative and hospice services for the child and family:
- Meet with the family to identify their goals and wishes for their child's care, including provision of antibiotics, oxygen, nutrition and hydration, resuscitation, and blood transfusions as well as other treatment modalities. A form such as the Physician Orders for Life-Sustaining Treatment (POLST), at www.caPOLST.org, can serve as a valuable basis for discussion and explanation of options. Furthermore, the family can bring the form with them across settings so that their wishes are communicated with clarity and consistency.
- Verify insurance plans and benefits. Identify the available provider network for home hospice agencies and respite facilities.
- Clarify the treatment plan with the third-party payer in order to assure both authorization and reimbursement of services.
- Make a referral to the home hospice agency best able to meet the child's and family's needs.
- Provide a detailed treatment plan, including medications for comfort in emergency situations at the end of life.

The concept of respite care[59] is to provide temporary relief or rest to the caregivers of the seriously ill child, either in or outside the home, whether for hours or weeks at a time. Respite care is designed to give parents and other caregivers the opportunity to recharge their batteries so that they can better manage the challenges of caring for the child. Respite care may be offered voluntarily or on a fee-for-service basis, as a benefit with some insurance plans. A case manager or care coordinator can assist the family in accessing this essential service.

School

Appreciating the context of the child's life, understanding what makes it meaningful, and respecting the relationships that are central to it are essential.[60] For the child who wishes to attend school, many crucial issues must be considered in preparation. Does the school have a nurse or other designated personnel available to accommodate the child's medical needs? Is there a need for an out-of-hospital DNR order? What is the plan for managing issues in the child's care that might arise during the school day? What is the responsibility of the administration to the other students regarding the possibility of a child dying at school? Frequently parents decide that it is easier to have their child home-schooled rather than deal with these many and often controversial issues. However, under the Education for All Handicapped Children Act (Public Law 94-142), all children are guaranteed the right to be in the classroom. The question of "What is in the best interest of the individual child?" must be balanced against the interests of others in the situation, such as the school community.

In 2000, the American Academy of Pediatrics (AAP) Committees on Bioethics and School Health issued the policy statement that "parents have a legal right to forego cardiopulmonary resuscitation and to ask the school to respect that decision." Rushton[60] says DNR orders are simply an extension of the right of families to make decisions about medical treatment or non-treatment. However, school officials argue that medically untrained staff may misinterpret a DNR order, thereby doing more harm than good for the child. Administrators are concerned that failing to act could make the school and/or school district liable.

The DNR order is usually honored without reservation in the hospital or hospice setting, but is rarely supported for children in school or other community settings. Although 43 out of 50 states and the District of Columbia have enacted out-of-hospital DNR orders, only five would extend legal protection to school personnel for honoring such decisions.[61] Only 17 of these states and D.C. permit advance healthcare decisions for minors. These ill-defined laws obviously create problems for parents and legal guardians of children who choose to attend school.

Hospital teams and community agencies can collaborate with the school for the child's care. Establishing a relationship with the school team early and sorting out dilemmas prior to the child's return to class will assure a better outcome. The school team should be included in discharge planning discussions, particularly about an out-of-hospital DNR. In anticipation of a life-threatening event occurring at school, the parents, school administrators, and clinicians, in conjunction with the local EMS system, need to delineate a plan that would invoke comfort care for the child, rather than life-sustaining measures. The school nurse is a crucial part of this collaborative effort to assure that the best interests of the child are upheld. A proactive, coordinated plan that is communicated to the appropriate school personnel can go a long way in relieving their anxiety.

Reimbursement Issues

The reasons for woeful treatment of dying children and grieving families is due in large part to the healthcare system's inability to recognize the need for palliative care even when children are receiving curative care.[62]

Reimbursement issues are a major obstacle to children and families receiving palliative care services for the following reasons:

- Criteria used to determine reimbursement for pediatric palliative care are only partly applicable to children,
- Eligibility restrictions related to life expectancy frequently make it difficult for families to choose palliative care for their children,
- Different systems of payments between the government and private insurers affect both reimbursement and the types of services provided.

A significant barrier is that state Medicaid hospice benefits are based on the federal Medicare model. Hospice eligibility criteria restrict care to individuals who will die within six months. Furthermore, concurrent treatment to prolong life cannot be pursued while receiving palliative care. Additionally, within the 2010 regulations and reimbursement structure, families risk the loss of benefits such as dietary supplements or skilled home nursing care if they accept hospice. These criteria prevent families and clinicians from integrating both aspects of care.[63] It is also important to note that private insurers model their hospice benefits along Medicare guidelines. There are multiple payers and financial sources for pediatric palliative care, versus one payer source, Medicare, for adult palliative care.

The Institute of Medicine report[1] states: "Approximately two-thirds of children are covered by employment-based or other private health insurance; about one-fifth are covered by state Medicaid or other public programs, but some 14 to 15 percent of children under age 19 have no health insurance." Some of these uninsured children receive services based on safety-net providers, grants, or private donations. However, there remain children who do not receive necessary services. The IOM report further states that "for insured children and families, coverage limitations, provider payment methods and rules, and administrative practices can discourage timely and full communication between clinicians and families and restrict access to effective palliative and end-of-life care."

The IOM report's recommendations are based on the premise that the hospice benefit be restructured to better meet the needs of children. These recommendations include:

- Elimination of eligibility restrictions related to life expectancy,
- Elimination of the requirement to discontinue all curative treatment,
- Addition of an outlier payment category for children whose care is unusually costly.

The IOM also warns that the hospice healthcare delivery model for adults and children in 2010 can create "incentives for under treatment, overtreatment, inappropriate transitions between settings of care, inadequate coordination of care, and poor overall quality of care."[3]

In an effort to counterbalance the inequities created by the Medicare hospice model, Children's Hospice International (CHI) developed the Program for All-Inclusive Care for Children (PACC) and their Families. This program provides an alternative to the existing barriers regarding referral and reimbursement to obtaining palliative care for children. The PACC model is an innovative program, which provides access to care for all children diagnosed with life-threatening conditions. It allows for reimbursement by all payers including private insurance, workplace coverage, managed care, and Medicaid. CHI PACC permits states to receive federal reimbursement for more coordinated services than are usually provided under Medicaid.[64]

Congressional appropriations through the Centers for Medicare and Medicaid Services (CMS) initially funded pilot programs in Colorado, Florida, Kentucky, New York, New England, Utah, and Virginia.[64,65] Florida and Colorado have been fully approved for CMS waivers.[65-67] Florida received its waiver approval in July 2005 for a 5-year, statewide demonstration project of the PACC program.[66] In January 2007, Colorado received approval of their request for a CMS waiver. They will implement a 3-year renewable demonstration project for pediatric palliative care.[67] Based on legislation mandated in the fall of 2006, California began a 3-year pilot program in 2009 under the Children's Hospice and Palliative Care waiver.[68] Other states interested in implementing CHI PACC and are submitting requests for waivers include Arkansas, Illinois, Louisiana, Maryland, New Mexico, Pennsylvania, Ohio, Tennessee, Texas, Utah, West Virginia, and the District of Columbia.[64] The myriad issues that surround reimbursement for palliative and end-of-life care, both for adults and children, are trigger topics for challenge and reform.

Summary

At the diagnosis of a life-threatening condition, it is important to offer an integrated model of palliative care that continues throughout the course of illness, regardless of outcome.[63]

Significant and lasting improvements and reform in the delivery of pediatric palliative care involve innovations in research, education, funding, and program development. Healthcare providers must assume not only the role of clinician, but also of advocate, communicator, coordinator, and facilitator to ensure the provision of these essential services for children and their families.

REFERENCES

1. Hilden J, Tobin D: *Shelter from the storm: caring for a child with a life-threatening condition*, Cambridge, 2003, Perseus, p 164.
2. American Academy of Pediatrics: *AAP National Center of Medical Home Initiatives for Children with Special Needs*, www.medicalhomeinfo.org/. Accessed January 19, 2010.
3. Field MJ, Behrman RE, editors: *Patterns of childhood death in America, Institute of Medicine of the National Academy of Sciences*, 2003, the National Academy of Press, pp 41–71.
4. ACT (Association for Children with Life-threatening and Terminal Conditions and their Families), National Council for Hospice and Specialist Palliative Care Services and SPAPCC (Scottish Partnership Agency for Palliative and Cancer Care): *Palliative care for young people: ages 13–24*. London, 2001.
5. Frankel LR: Pediatric palliative care: the role of the intensivist, current concepts in pediatric critical care, *Soc Crit Care Med* 103–110, 2007.
6. Sourkes B, Frankel LR, Brown M, et al: Food, toys, and love: pediatric palliative care, *Curr Probl Pediatr Adolesc Health Care* 35:350–386, 2005.
7. Feudtner C, Feinstein JA, Satchell M, et al: Shifting place of death among children with complex chronic conditions in the United States, 1989–2003, *JAMA* 297:2725–2732, 2007.
8. Feudtner C, DiGiuseppe DL, Neff JM: Hospital care for children and young adults in the last year of life: a population-based study, *BMC Med* 1:1–9, 2003.
9. Liben S, Lissauer T: Intensive care units. In Goldman A, Hain R, Liben S, editors: *Oxford textbook for palliative care for children*, 2006, Oxford University Press, pp 549–556.
10. Sourkes B: *Armfuls of time: the psychological experience of the child with a life-threatening illness*, Pittsburgh, 1995, University of Pittsburgh Press.
11. National Center for Health Statistics: www.cdc.gov/nchs/. Accessed May 4, 2010.
12. McCallum DE, Byrne P, Bruera E: How children die in hospital, *J Pain Symptom Manage* 20:417–423, 2000.
13. Devictor D, Latour JM, Tissieres P: Forgoing life-sustaining or death-prolonging therapy in the pediatric ICU, *Pediatr Clin North Am* 55(3):791–804, 2008.
14. Burns JP, Mitchell C, Outwater KM, et al: End-of-life care in the pediatric intensive care unit after the forgoing of life-sustaining treatment, *Crit Care Med* 28(8):3060–3066, 2000.
15. Devictor DJ, Nguyen DT: Forgoing life-sustaining treatments; how the decision is made in French pediatric intensive care units, *Crit Care Med* 29(7):1356–1359, 2001.
16. Garros D, Rosychuk RJ, Cox PN: Circumstances surrounding end of life in a pediatric intensive care unit, *Pediatrics* 112(5):e371, 2003.
17. Althabe M, Cardigni G, Vassallo JC, et al: Dying in the intensive care unit: collaborative multicenter study about forgoing life-sustaining treatments in Argentine pediatric intensive care units, *Pediatr Crit Care Med* 4(2):163–169, 2003.
18. Zawistowski CA, DeVita MA: A descriptive study of children dying in the pediatric intensive care unit after withdrawal of life sustaining treatment, *Pediat Crit Care Med* 6(3):258–263, 2004.
19. Diekema DS, Botkin JR: Clinical report: forgoing medically provided nutrition and hydration in children, *Pediatrics* 124:813–822, 2009.
20. Riling DA, Hofmann KH, Deshler J: Family-centered care in the pediatric intensive care unit. In Fuhrman B, Zimmeran J, editors: *Pediatric critical care*, ed 3, Philadelphia, 2006, Mosby Elsevier, pp 106–116.
21. Latour JM, Haines C: Families in the ICU: do we truly consider their needs, experiences and satisfaction? *Nurs Crit Care* 12(4):173–174, 2007.
22. Hov R, Hedelin B, Athlin E: Being an intensive care nurse related to questions of withholding or withdrawing curative treatment, *J Clin Nurs* 16(1):203–211, 2007.
23. Burns JP, Rushton CH: End-of-life in the pediatric intensive care unit: research review and recommendations, *Crit Care Clin* 20(3):467–485, 2004.
24. Solomon MZ, Sellers DE, Heller KS, et al: New and lingering controversies in pediatric end-of-life care, *Pediatrics* 116(4):872–883, 2005.
25. Sharman M, Meert K, Sarnaik A: What influences parents' decisions to limit or withdraw life support? *Pediatr Crit Care Med* 6(5):513–518, 2005.
26. Ralston M, Hazinski MF, Zaritsky AL, et al: *PALS Provider Manual*, American Heart Association, 2006, p 3.
27. Tajik M, Cardarelli MG: Extracorporeal membrane oxygenation after cardiac arrest in children: what do we know? *Eur J Cardiothorac Surg* 33:409–417, 2008.
28. Barrett CS, Bratton SL, Salvin JW, et al: Neurological injury after extracorporeal membrane oxygenation use to aid pediatric cardiopulmonary resuscitation, *Pediatr Crit Care Med* 10(4):445–451, 2009.
29. Levy M, Curtis R: Improving end-of-life care in the intensive care unit, *Crit Care Med* 34(Suppl):S301, 2006.
30. Truog RD, Meyer ED: Toward interventions to improve end-of-life care in the pediatric intensive care unit, *Crit Care Med* 34(Suppl):S3739, 2006.
31. Morrison W, Berkowitz I: Do not attempt resuscitation orders in pediatrics, *Pediatr Clin North Am* 54(5):757–771, 2007.
32. Mathers LH, Whitney SN: Letting go: a study in pediatric life-and-death decision-making. In Frankel LR, Goldwirth A, Rorty MV, Silverman WA, editors: *Ethical dilemmas in pediatrics*, Cambridge, 2005, Cambridge Univeristy Press, pp 89–112.
33. Munson D: Withdrawal of mechanical ventilation in pediatric and neonatal intensive care units. *Pediatr Clin North Am* 54(5):773–785, 2007.

34. Frankel LR, Randle CJ, Goldwirth A: Complexities in the management of a brain-dead child. In Frankel LR, Goldwirth A, Rorty MV, Silverman WA, editors: *Ethical dilemmas in pediatrics*, Cambridge, 2005, Cambridge University Press, pp 135–155.

35. Davidson JE, Powers K, Hedayat KM, et al: Clinical practice guidelines for support of the family in the patient-centered intensive care unit: American College of Critical Care Medicine Task Force 2004–2005, *Crit Care Med* 35(2):605–622, 2007.

36. Riggs D, Weibley RE: Autopsies and the pediatric intensive care unit, *Pediatr Clin North Am* 41(6):1383–1393, 1994.

37. Antommaria AH, Trotochaud K, Kinlaw K, et al: Policies on donation after cardiac death at children's hospitals: a mixed-methods analysis of variation, *JAMA* 301(18):1902–1908, 2009.

38. Pleacher KM, Roach ES, Van der Werf W, et al: Impact of a pediatric donation after cardiac death program, *Pediatr Crit Care Med* 10(2):166–170, 2009.

39. Hamilton TE: Improving organ transplantation in the United States: a regulatory perspective, *Am J Transplant* 8:2503–2505, 2008.

40. Heron M, Sutton PD, Xu J, et al: Annual summary of vital statistics, *Pediatrics* 125:4–15, 2010.

41. Michelson KN, Steinhorn DM: Pediatric end-of-life issues and palliative care, *Clin Pediatr Emerg Med* 8:212–219, 2007.

42. Lunney JR, Lynn J, Foley DJ, et al: Patterns of functional death at the end of life, *JAMA* 289:2387–2392, 2003.

43. Wright J, Johns C, Joseph J: End-of-life care in EMS for children. In Field M, et al: *When children die*, Institute of Medicine, Washington, 2003, National Academy Press, pp. 580–589.

44. Knapp J, Mulligan-Smith D, the Committee on Pediatric Emergency Medicine: Death of a child in the emergency department, *Pediatrics* 115:1432–1437, 2005.

45. Wright J, Krug S: Emergency Medical services for children. In Kliegman R, et al, editors: *Nelson textbook of pediatrics*, ed 19, Philadelphia, 2010, Elsevier (in press).

46. Gausche-Hill M, Krug S, the AAP ED Preparedness Guidelines Advisory Council: Guidelines for Care of Children in the ED—Policy Statement, *Pediatrics* 124:1233–1243, 2009.

47. O'Malley PJ, Brown K, the Committee on Pediatric Emergency Medicine: Patient and family-centered care of children in the emergency department: technical report, *Pediatrics* 122:e511–e521, 2008.

48. Guzzetta C, Clark A, Wright J: Family presence in emergency medical services for children, *Clin Pediatr Emerg Med* 7:15–24, 2006.

49. Kang T, Hoehn S, Licht D, et al: Pediatric palliative, end-of-life and bereavement care, *Pediatr Clin North Am* 52:1029–1046, 2005.

50. Sumner L: Pediatric care: the hospice perspective. In Ferrell B, Coyle N, editors: *Textbook of Palliative Nursing*, ed 2, New York, 2006, Oxford University Press, p. 916.

51. Maxwell T, Reifsnyder J, Davis C, et al: *Our littlest patients: a national description of pediatric hospice patients*. Paper presented at the American Academy of Hospice and Palliative Medicine annual assembly. Nashville, Tenn, 2006.

52. Levetown M, Barnard M, Hellston M, et al: *A call for change: recommendations to improve the care of children living with life-threatening conditions*. A white paper produced by the Children's International Project on Palliative/Hospice Services (ChIPPS) Administrative/Policy workgroup of the National Hospice and Palliative Care Organization. Alexandria, Va, 2001, NHPCO.

53. *National data set—NHPCO's facts and figures 2005 findings*, 2006, NHPCO.

54. Carroll JM, Torkildson C, Winsness JS: Issues related to providing quality pediatric palliative care in the community, *Pediatr Clin North Am*, 54(5):813–827, 2007.

55. Armstrong-Daily A, Zarbock S, editors. *Hospice care for children*, ed 3 New York, 2008, Oxford University.

56. Contro NA, Larson J, Scofield S, et al: Hospital staff and family perspectives regarding quality of pediatric palliative care, *Pediatrics* 114(5):1248–1252, 2004.

57. Drake R, Frost J, Collins JJ: The symptoms of dying children, *J Pain Symptom Manage* 26(1):594–603, 2003.

58. Wolfe J, Grier HE, Klar N, et al: Symptoms and suffering at the end of life in children with cancer, *N Engl J Med* 342(5):326–333, 2000.

59. American Academy of Pediatrics: Committee on bioethics and committee on hospital care: palliative care for children, *Pediatrics* 106 (2 Pt 1):351–357, 2000.

60. Rushton CH, Will JC, Murray MG: To honor and obey: DNR orders and the school, *Pediatr Nurs* 20(6):581–585, 1994.

61. Kimberly MB, Forte AL, Carroll JM, Feudtner C: Pediatric do-not-attempt-resuscitation orders and public schools: a national assessment of policies and laws, *Am J Bioeth* 2005.

62. Texas Cancer Council: *End-of-life care for children*, Houston, 2000, Texas Children's Cancer Center, Texas Children's Hospital.

63. AAP: Palliative care for children, *Pediatrics* 106(2):351–357, 2000.

64. *Children's Hospice International program for all-inclusive care for children and their families (CHI PACC)*, www.chionline.org/programs/. Accessed July 30, 2009.

65. CHI: *CHI PACC model: The Colorado, Florida, Kentucky, Utah and New York experience. Children's Hospice International*, www.chionline.org/programs/. Accessed May 4, 2010.

66. *The Florida CHI PACC model: partners in care, together for kids*, www.chionline.org/states/fl.php. Accessed May 4, 2010.

67. *The butterfly program: a Children's Hospice International program for all-inclusive care for children and their families (CHI PACC)*, www.chionline.org/states/co. Accessed May 4, 2010.

68. *The Nick Snow Children's Hospice & Palliative Care Act of 2006—Assembly Bill 1745*, http://childrenshospice.org/coalition/ab-1745-the-nick-snow-childrens-hospice-palliative-care-act-of-2006/. Accessed May 4, 2010.

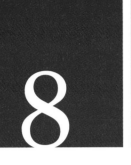

8 Program Development and Implementation

ROBIN KRAMER | STACY S. REMKE | SALLY SEHRING

Culture does not change because we desire to change it. Culture changes when the organization is transformed; the culture reflects the realities of people working together every day.

—Frances Hesselbein, The Key to Cultural
Transformation, Leader to Leader, Spring 1999

The field of pediatric palliative care has evolved over the past decade in response to an escalating acknowledgment of need and a call to action by the Institute of Medicine (IOM) Report: When Children Die.[1] A report from the First Forum for Pediatric Palliative Care in 2007[2] indicated that 31 children's hospitals in the United States had pediatric palliative care programs and many more were developing them. Developing and implementing a palliative care program requires not only an understanding of the principles and practice of good pediatric palliative care, but also a familiarity with techniques to bring about change within an institution.

Palliative care program development is not a fixed, linear process; rather, it unfolds and takes shape over time. There are opportunities to address needed changes in organizations in each phase of program evolution. The necessity of attending to the interests of all stakeholders over time cannot be underestimated. The goal of program development is to change the culture of the healthcare organization in order to anticipate and provide for palliative care needs of children, ideally from the time of their diagnosis.

The majority of children with life-threatening conditions are referred to a regionalized medical center with expertise in complex pediatric health problems. Most childhood deaths occur in hospitals. These same hospitals may provide care for an additional estimated ten-fold number of children who have chronic, complex conditions that may limit life. It is crucial for these institutions to make palliative care available to children and their families.

This chapter outlines phases of program development, including suggestions for tasks or important work to be done; challenges; and strategies to promote buy-in and generate small successes that facilitate bigger change. Change is an ongoing process that requires focused, consistent efforts and responsiveness to emerging obstacles and needs. Shifting the culture of an institution requires both flexibility and tenacity in achieving the goal of excellent interdisciplinary palliative care for children.

Although this chapter focuses on development of a pediatric palliative care program in the hospital, the phases of growth and the challenges of each stage share commonalities across

diverse settings. The strategies offered here can be extrapolated and adapted to other circumstances. No hospital-based program would be complete without the ability to coordinate with the community resources that serve these same children and their families. It is only through such reciprocal relationships that continuity of care can occur.

The phases of program development described are neither rigid nor self-contained. Certain tasks, such as ensuring alignment with institutional goals and priorities, should be repeated in each phase. Some tasks that drive organizational change may prove too difficult to be completed within one phase and thus stages may blur. Nevertheless, it is useful to have a structure that facilitates planning the requisite steps for change and addresses challenges proactively as the program evolves.

Phase I: Planning

Comprehensive planning from the earliest stages is essential (see Table 8-1). An early start-up strategy often involves convening an interdisciplinary task force. Five to seven members, representing different medical specialties, can identify needs and delineate a plan toward improving the institution's provision of palliative care. The first task is to collect institution-wide information about practices, policies, and procedures related to palliative care. It is also critical to identify the many ways in which children with life-threatening conditions move through the organization. Early on, raising others' awareness of the deficits in care delivery arouses a sense of need or urgency to make improvements.[3,4] Identifying the many issues, barriers, and concerns related to the provision of care helps define the problem that the planning group is organizing to improve.

IDENTIFY EARLY CHAMPIONS

Based on this preliminary information, the task force must communicate a cohesive and consistent message that substantiates the need for improved palliative care at the institution. Initial task force members are selected for their ability to articulate this need, as well as to gain support as the planning team moves forward. Fostering interdisciplinary leadership from the start is fundamental to creating a balanced program. It is strategic to include a well-respected physician who will advocate for inclusion of the interdisciplinary team. Whether or not this individual eventually assumes the medical directorship, he or she can help advance early planning efforts. In many settings, particularly within an academic hospital, a physician and a clinician from another discipline share leadership responsibilities. The leader or leaders should be clearly defined for the planning group as well as for the larger hospital community.

TABLE 8-1 Program Development Phase 1: Planning

Marshall resources for change	Define and promote the Program	Educate
• Carefully select task force/ planning committee members • Engage stakeholders • Identify partners for collaboration • Investigate start up funding possibilities • Create an action plan to initiate change	• Align mission & goals with those of the organization • Solicit input from proponents & antagonists • Uncover strengths & weaknesses • Convey clear, consistent program message • Communicate needs & plans	• Hone expertise & skill of planning committee • Use every opportunity, formal & informal • Extend awareness of PPC principles • Reinforce the message

The task force should expand over the first several months to include respected champions[5]—staff members who have demonstrated a special interest and expertise in palliative care. The central work of this group is to communicate what is needed, to generate institutional support, to identify possible solutions, and to organize improvements in the delivery of care. To succeed at transformative program development,[3] it is critical to assemble individuals who are respected as achievers, experts, innovators, and leaders. They will be key spokespeople in creating a coalition for change.[3,4] Recruitment focuses on individuals who have power within the institution through their influence and reputation; the skill to leverage organizational resources; and the clinical expertise to advance program development effectively.

CREATE A VISION AND ACTION PLAN

Within the first few months, the task force must begin to articulate the program goals,[6] which will eventually lead to a mission or vision statement.[3,4,7] A well-articulated statement clearly defines pediatric palliative care[7] and reveals core objectives that guide program planning. It will be necessary to explain the range of services that the program plans to offer. The start-up paths of programs can vary. For example, programs have begun with a primary focus on staff support and education,[8] on advanced care planning and care coordination,[9] or on services within the pediatric oncology population.[10]

Building a program is a daunting endeavor. It is fundamental to outline small, manageable steps; to use resources that already exist; and to establish a realistic timeline. The Center to Advance Palliative Care (CAPC) has designed a training methodology for programs at any stage of development. Expert guidance and written worksheets are combined with yearlong mentoring.[11] The CAPC website, www.capc.org, also offers extensive program development resources.

EDUCATION AS A DEVELOPMENT TOOL

During this early phase, it is essential to provide pediatric palliative care interdisciplinary education for the planning committee. This education increases the confidence of the task force members in their clinical skills, as well as gives them an understanding of the steps involved in program development. The dual focus helps to steer program efforts in a productive direction while developing collegial relationships for networking and mentorship. In addition, educating the entire hospital community raises awareness of the need and benefits of palliative care and conveys how best to use the nascent services. Capitalizing on existing venues for communication and education, such as Grand Rounds, staff meetings, and resident conferences, is a successful way to reach staff without asking them to attend extra meetings. Participating in these educational initiatives fosters group cohesion and promotes consistency of the pediatric palliative care vision among the planning members as well as throughout the organization.

Systems Assessment: Align with Institutional Goals

A systems assessment examines how the palliative care program will fit into the organization, and whether its goals are compatible with the overall mission of the institution. The receptivity of hospital administrators is enhanced not only through adherence to organizational priorities, but also through meeting national standards of excellence for palliative care. These standards are recommended by influential organizations such as the American Academy of Pediatrics (AAP), the Joint Commission, the National Hospice and Palliative Care Organization (NHPCO), the American Academy of Hospice and Palliative Medicine (AAHPM), the Center to Advance Palliative Care (CAPC), and the National Quality Forum.

A helpful assessment activity is the Strengths, Weaknesses, Opportunities, and Threats (SWOT) analysis,[12] which can reveal the overt and covert power dynamics of the organization. This type of introspection can prepare the team for difficulties that may arise in program implementation, and it allows them to develop proactive strategies to avoid or minimize barriers.

A systems assessment also determines how existing resources within the institution and community might interface with the pediatric palliative care program. The task force can contact those in charge of pertinent departments, clinical services, committees, or community agencies, proposing collaboration to improve efficiency and standardize practice.

SECURE STAKEHOLDER SUPPORT

Key administrative and clinical stakeholders should be consulted for their opinions and also recruited for support. Every informal or formal opportunity to influence stakeholders can be seized to publicize the program's vision while building collegiality around a common purpose.[3,4] The task force should be ready to communicate a compelling case for the program within the context of an informed understanding of the organization. Ultimately, the goal is to obtain endorsement of the endeavor; doing so secures essential stakeholder buy-in and paves the way for access to tangible resources needed to establish the program.

Creating a small advisory council of administrative and clinical stakeholders can foster their ongoing investment in the program. This group's involvement validates the importance of pediatric palliative care and helps sanction quality improvement efforts in this area. It is also important to solicit constructive feedback from potential antagonists, as well as from staunch supporters. Individuals from both groups can be recruited as advocates for the program, and they should be given options for their involvement.

ESTABLISH WORKGROUPS

As the task force grows, smaller work groups can tackle specific projects such as systems and needs assessments, educational training sessions, and PowerPoint presentations for stakeholders. This is also the time, perhaps for a designated group, to secure start-up funding, write grants for specific projects and investigate options for ongoing financial support. The institution's development office can be helpful in obtaining seed money to fund early program planning and educational efforts. It is important to find out about any rules or procedures that may effect applying for grants, soliciting funds from the community, and gaining publicity. Knowing these guidelines ahead of time can save time and frustration, and may even help to identify existing resources within the organization. The development office staff can also direct funds to the pediatric palliative care program if they have been given a good understanding of the program's vision and goals. Involving these resource people early opens doors, provokes curiosity, raises awareness, and influences future stakeholders' interest.

CONDUCT A NEEDS ASSESSMENT

A formal needs assessment can uncover the concerns of patients, families, and staff, in addition to the circumstances and practices that affect the provision of care. It describes current clinical metrics, such as the documentation of pain scores and the numbers and locations of hospital deaths, that can validate the program's necessity and scope. The data identify strengths and weaknesses, as well as challenges and opportunities for quality improvement initiatives—all critical for program development. The needs assessment also serves as a baseline for comparison once the program is established: what progress is being made, where changes are still needed, and whether services are making a difference. Thus, planning efforts are designed to integrate data, service delivery strategies, and goals from the outset, facilitating an ongoing process of evaluation and improvement.

There are several avenues to pursue in developing a needs assessment, including reviewing the literature; contacting other institutions for advice; sharing tools that can be modified to address unique institutional questions; and enlisting the assistance of other departments within the organization. The Quality Improvement (QI) staff may already have relevant information or may be able to help with data collection. Other areas, such as strategic support, may be able to analyze pertinent hospital statistics including length of stay (LOS) in intensive care settings prior to death, days on the ventilator, and costs associated with the last days of life. Needs assessments may also include a chart audit, a staff survey, a parent survey, focus groups with providers or family members, or the results from applicable metrics already collected at the institution, such as Press Ganey Satisfaction with Care scores. A broad-based understanding of organizational issues and opinions is important. Clinicians and administrators surveyed should represent various disciplines and levels of experience; families should represent different backgrounds and have children with different ages and diagnoses. A needs assessment can turn into a labor-intensive endeavor, so adequate time and resources should be allocated. A realistic option is to pilot a needs assessment in one or two areas (such as the PICU, NICU or Hematology Oncology service), and then eventually expand to other areas.

A representative appraisal also seeks opinions from clinicians who may be less receptive to program development efforts. Resistance may come from those who are uncomfortable with limiting aggressive medical interventions for personal or moral reasons, or from those who lack familiarity with clinical practice standards in pediatric palliative care. Others are concerned about redundancy of services or that their relationships with children and families will be compromised by another team stepping in. The needs assessment often uncovers the belief that a separate program for pediatric palliative care is unnecessary because it is already done well enough within the institution. A better understanding of the principles of pediatric palliative care can mitigate many of these objections, and staff education is often a result of the assessment itself.

Comparing the institution's palliative care program efforts with those of other local, regional, and national institutions is also valuable. Ultimately, the data from benchmarking, the systems assessment, and the needs assessment will comprise the evidence that makes a solid case for program support to the institution and potential funding sources. The information also contributes to the development of a strategic business plan, and focuses clinical resources where they are most needed.[13]

Strategies should be well-thought out for communicating the assessment results, together with program recommendations, to all leadership groups. Emotionally charged, real-life clinical stories, both positive and negative, can highlight critical points and carry the important message of family-centered care. All of this initial information identifies a clear direction for the program's development and promotes the acceptance necessary to move into the next phase.

Phase II: Creating the Foundation: Program Implementation

The tasks during this phase are to delineate both the scope and components of the pediatric palliative care services that will be offered, and to elucidate the logistics involved in service delivery and program marketing (see Table 8-2). Helpful steps include making a site visit to learn from other successful programs and building collaborative relationships with key personnel from departments within the hospital. Take time to learn the options; carefully consider what may work well in the organization, what may present unforeseen barriers, and how internal resources might be used to support program efforts. Throughout this phase, it will also be important to constantly analyze services given ongoing needs, gaps, strengths, and priorities, culminating in a multiyear business plan to ensure sustainability. Building a comprehensive program also includes developing expertise at interfacing effectively with community agencies, optimizing palliative care services across settings.

As this program building and implementation phase rolls out, it is helpful to note the following intersecting elements that all go into a strong program:

- Scope of Services: The particular set of services and interventions that the team will offer in the setting in which they work. This may include interdisciplinary assessment, interventions and referrals, direct care, crisis intervention, and advanced care planning. This may also be defined by specific patient populations, such as oncology patients or those with neuro-developmental disorders. Careful consideration of the scope of services can assist the team

TABLE 8-2 Program Development Phase II: Program Implementation

Find & create allies	Build team & define function	Show your worth
• Identify early clinical supporters & pilot services in receptive area • Cultivate strategic partners necessary for implementation • Draft a strategic business plan	• Delineate team roles, expectations, & needs • Promote team visibility & choose a name • Foster flexibility & efficacy • Affirm & support patient/family relationship with primary providers • Facilitate & model communication • Set priorities in sync with resources/limitations • Solicit feedback • Proactively plan for growth	• Demonstrate "value added" • Establish cooperative relationships with hospital providers & community • Contribute to organizational operations • Track data re: program's impact & communicate it • Educate re: standard of excellence

in managing program activities by avoiding unrealistic expectations, excessive workloads, and program growth at a pace that outstrips resources.

- Standards: In the area of pediatric palliative care, NHPCO has identified standards for pediatrics[18] that incorporate the key elements from adult standards, the National Quality Forum[13a] and the National Consensus Project.[34] In addition, several groups, including CAPC and the American Academy of Pediatrics[14] have outlined essential service standards and begun to define the expectations that need to be met in order to offer a quality program.
- Core Competencies: Extensive expertise in specifically defined skill sets that pediatric palliative care team members demonstrate, enabling them to be highly effective practitioners. These core competencies have begun to be delineated by several groups, including CAPC and ACGME (www.acgme.org). Discipline-specific competency guidelines are also emerging as the field advances, for example, in social work.[15] Although these competencies will overlap with those of colleagues who practice in other specialty areas, they also include certain skills and perspectives that particularly belong to pediatric palliative care. This combination of strengths will help establish the value added by the palliative care service to their colleagues and to patient and family consumers.

After the most pressing initial needs are met, these standards and competencies should continue to be used to establish goals to guide further program development over a planned trajectory. For example, in order to meet standards for child development expertise in talking with a child about the possibility of death, a team may establish educational programs to help build that knowledge base. There would be an anticipated outcome that expertise is available from the team within a specified time. In another situation, perhaps the team will link new staff to specified volume indicators so that the expectations for a practitioner's caseload are well communicated and understood by all parties.

It can also be helpful to consider how these program elements can help set the work of the team apart from customary practice of the institution. Is there greater skill or knowledge in some areas? Is there more experience with certain situations? Does the pediatric palliative care program offer an assurance that certain resources and skill sets are brought into a complex situation? What's the value added by the pediatric palliative care team? These kinds of program issues and questions are challenging to address because the field is so new. Nonetheless, it is useful to consider these aspects of successful service delivery in order to establish expectations, manage clinical tasks, and plan for interdisciplinary team growth.

Create an Identity: Choosing a Program Name

The program's name should be selected by the time Phase II begins. Consistently using a name helps brand and market the program within the institution and the community. It is important for administrators and clinicians, as well as patients and their families, to be able to identify the program and to understand the focus for services. Clear identification makes it easier for those who need help to seek assistance from the program, and for those who appreciate the program's efforts to give credit where credit is due. Some programs have chosen succinct, medical based names, with or without reference to palliative care, such as PACT: Pediatric Advanced Care Team, PACCT: Pediatric Advanced Comfort Care Team, and Pain and Palliative Care Team. Others have chosen a name that is associated with metaphoric imagery such as Footprints, Compass Care, and The Butterfly Program. Parents in particular have emphasized how an identified program name improves access to services. Some believe, however, that including palliative care in the name can be associated with diminished hope[16,17] and associated with hospice. Other opinions focus on the importance of calling it what it is, and then working to dispel misunderstandings in the broader community. Be prepared for the ongoing challenge of addressing misperceptions around the term palliative care until the term is better understood by society.[16]

FUNDAMENTAL PROGRAM COMPONENTS

There are fundamental program components that serve as the building blocks of pediatric palliative care program development. The specific characteristics and infrastructure for implementation may vary considerably from program to program.

Service Delivery

THE TEAM

The current state of the art of pediatric palliative care requires effective, collaborative efforts of an interdisciplinary team, which includes the child, as appropriate, and the family.[1,14,18] Team members may be selected from the original planning group. However, these individuals will need approval from their departments and the organization to allocate time in their current roles to provide palliative services throughout the hospital. Once assembled, the interdisciplinary pediatric palliative care team will work closely with a larger advisory group and/or task force to continue to direct the program's growth.

Including representation from core disciplines—medicine, nursing, social work, psychology or psychiatry, child life, and spiritual care—is necessary for promoting interdisciplinary leadership, planning, practice, and acceptance. "The team approach ensures that the stresses and responsibilities of this work are shared."[19] Collaboration among various disciplines ensures a holistic approach to providing pediatric palliative care to patients and their families. The palliative care team may look different from one organization to another, depending on the size, resources, fiscal constraints, and culture of the institution. Hospital-based teams are often led by physicians. Additional staff may include an advanced practice nurse (APN) and a chaplain, and then rely on unit-based staff from child life, social work, case management, and pharmacy to round out interdisciplinary input as needed. Other models involve dedicated staff time for pediatric palliative care from the outset. The composition of the initial team is often a function of passionate interest, expertise, availability, budgetary constraints, and fit within the organizational structure.

Over time, the team's composition may change to accommodate lessons learned, as well as availability of specialists. It is important to start and then to grow the team, and to not become stalled by an inability to staff the ideal team configuration. Resource pressures, the startup strategy, unclear utilization patterns, and other limitations may preclude dedicating a team of practitioners solely to palliative care at the outset. New staff can be added as emerging needs, program acceptance, and financial support are demonstrated. Other, more established programs can provide guidance in planning team membership and expansion. The CAPC website also has resources to help calculate staffing requirements, including projected needs based on program growth over the next several years.[20]

Members of the team will need to be highly visible and receptive to a wide range of staff, patients, and families. When feasible, consider selecting team members who represent practice areas where specific needs have been uncovered or where program receptivity is anticipated, such as pediatric oncology or pediatric intensive care. Clinical proficiency, leadership abilities, excellent interpersonal and diplomacy skills, and a capacity to influence others are qualities desired in each team member.

Although it may be easier to start with a dedicated pediatric palliative care physician and nurse while using unit or subspecialty staff to round out interdisciplinary participation, there can be limitations of this model. As a case in point, a medical director of a two-year-old program that began using unit-based ancillary staff said he now recommends using dedicated staff from the beginning to accelerate skill acquisition and to enhance cohesion as a team. A social worker or chaplain focused exclusively on palliative care is likely to develop greater expertise than someone who practices palliative care as only a part of their clinical assignment. Teams that learn and grow together often develop greater capacity than a group of individual practitioners operating in parallel.

PRACTICE MODEL

Once the interdisciplinary team has been established, it is time to consider the following:

- What types of services can the team provide?
- How will providers and families within the institution find out about these services?
- When should patients be referred and how can the team be contacted?
- Will a formal consult be obtained, and is there a mechanism for billing?
- Will there be resistance to making appropriate referrals, and how will this resistance be countered?
- How will these requests and services be tracked and validated for the institution's administration?
- How will the program be structured to address these demands?

Achieving a feasible structure depends upon the availability of funding and personnel, as well as the extent of institutional acceptance for the program. Many programs use a structure that resembles a medical consultation service model, wherein a formal consult request is made to the pediatric palliative care team. Institutional protocols for a formal consult often require that a physician make the request and specify a reason for the referral, and that the consult be completed within a specific time frame. In some institutions, this request may be for a particular problem such as pain control or for transfer to the palliative care team for end of life management. The consult team, generally led by a physician or an APN, is typically identified as a distinct service having additional training, skills, and, in an increasing number of programs, formal credentialing or certification in palliative care appropriate to their discipline.

In the consultative model, the primary team acknowledges a need for outside assistance. Without the primary team's acknowledgment of need and request for services, pediatric palliative care may not be available to all children and families who would benefit, or access may come only at the end of life. Ongoing provider education, which reiterates the principles of palliative care and clarifies the distinction between palliative, end of life, and hospice care, is crucial for promoting provider acceptance and the timely initiation of services.

An alternative to a consultative model is an integrated structure, where the interdisciplinary team supports and educates providers in developing basic competencies in pediatric palliative care appropriate to their disciplines. This approach helps incorporate palliative care as a core value throughout the institution. The primary team, guided by the pediatric palliative care team, ensures the delivery and continuity of palliative care through recovery or death. Policy and procedure guidelines may be needed in this model to facilitate buy in from the larger system. The team may also help units develop communication tools or care algorithms that optimize care throughout the hospital. In individual cases, the team may provide resources to help with difficult symptom management and may facilitate consensus-building among providers. They may offer their services in mentoring the primary team in having difficult conversations if needed. The pediatric palliative care team can also identify helpful practices being used in some parts of the hospital that could be more widely disseminated for the benefit of patients in other areas.

An integrated approach can help transition palliative care into the institution when either funding or hospital support precludes hiring a separate consult team, or when a full complement of providers are unavailable. The integrated model also has the advantage that it maintains continuity with familiar and trusted care providers at the most trying times for families and can support the primary team in introducing palliative care resources early in the illness. The pediatric palliative care team's involvement could come via suggestions at interdisciplinary unit rounds, through the charge or bedside nurse, or when the social worker from the primary team requests additional resources or clinical support. This model helps to raise the bar of clinical practice in the hospital by providing ongoing education at the bedside. The primary team invites pediatric palliative care involvement and participates with them in direct patient and family contact. In either model, the presence of both teams helps maintain consistency of message and improves communication. In this way the pediatric palliative care team and primary team learn from and enhance each other's work.

Consultative and integrated models are not mutually exclusive. In practice, features of both models are often found together in institutions with successful programs. The goal is to couple broad-based institutional understanding and acceptance with the expertise of the interdisciplinary palliative care team to address the most complex needs. As in any other specialty, providers get better and more efficient as they practice. This capacity development sets the skills of the pediatric palliative care team apart over time, and helps define their expertise to the organization.

COVERAGE AND REFERRAL CONSIDERATIONS

Ideally, regardless of the program model, team members with training in palliative care should be available to provide round-the-clock assistance to hospital staff.[13,14] Program size, demand, and allocated resources will dictate team availability. It is important to plan coverage realistically to both manage expectations and avoid burnout. Many programs provide on-site consults Monday through Friday, and offer phone consultation during off-hours. This model can help staff contend with patient needs, while protecting team members' time off. With a consult model, the practical aspects of staffing require a larger, more formal commitment of dedicated physician or APN FTE to fulfill the clinical demands of a separate service. This expense can be partially offset by billing for eligible clinical services. State agencies, and even the institution itself, can have different rules specifying who can bill for care, so it is important to know these rules. However, at this time, it is not feasible for pediatric hospital-based programs in the United States to meet program costs through consult-billing reimbursements. Philanthropy and hospital support remain important sources for funding the pediatric palliative care program's operations. (See Business Plan and Funding.)

As programs begin to announce their services, it will be important to address the referral process. The benefits of introducing palliative care as early as possible, such as at the time of diagnosis with a life-threatening condition, are widely advocated.[1,14,21,22] From a practical standpoint, the biggest challenges are initiating these discussions and gaining entry from providers or family members for early palliative care team involvement. Marketing materials can address myths and misunderstandings that equate palliative care with giving up, taking away hope, or certainty that the child is dying. Teams need to prepare consistent responses to these types of concerns.

More often than not, a palliative care team may find that its involvement is requested late in the trajectory of a life-threatening event or when death is imminent. Ongoing education at multiple levels throughout the hospital will be necessary to effect culture change. Until there is a universal understanding

of pediatric palliative care in hospitals, it will be necessary to reinforce two cardinal principles: curative or life prolonging therapies and palliative treatments can coexist; and this concurrent approach maximally benefits the family and child if it is implemented soon after the life-threatening condition is recognized. Likewise, pediatric palliative care programs need to recognize that the kinds of services needed at the time of diagnosis may differ considerably from the services required at the end of life.[23]

A number of resources offer suggestions as to how and when palliative care should be discussed.[9,24] These guides often identify significant medical events or diagnoses, such as the need for a bone marrow transplant or the placement of a non-urgent tracheostomy, that serve as automatic triggers for a consult. With these triggers in place, clinicians may be more inclined to initiate pediatric palliative care earlier, thereby conforming to best practice standards.

In addition to the timing of the team's involvement, the mechanism by which its input is requested should be defined. The palliative care team will need to decide if a formal order from a physician is required to initiate services, or if any staff or family member can request assistance. How a request for team involvement is initiated may be dictated in part by hospital policy and by whether the services will be billed to insurance, as in a formal consult.

PROGRAM OPERATIONS AND INTERNAL MARKETING

Referral intake and tracking forms for salient clinical data should be created and revised over time. In one common model, a nurse triages the request for assistance and involves other team members as needed. Other practical operational aspects include securing consultation and office space; setting up program contact information, and disseminating this information throughout the institution to promote access. (See program brochure examples at www.expertconsult.com.) These are essential marketing tactics that integrate the pediatric palliative care program into the hospital system.

When marketing the program to administrators, clinicians, foundations, and the community, it is imperative that the team be able to clearly describe the various services it can provide. The range of services (see Box 8-1) may change as resources are added and programs become more established. Services may expand to include outpatient pediatric palliative care consults, co-management for hospice care, perinatal palliative care, or a chronic pain clinic. The marketing aim is to effectively communicate the value added for accessing both palliative care resources and team members to help with the time-intensive, challenging care. The message to clinicians is that these extra measures enhance interdisciplinary care while continuing to involve the primary team(s).[14,25]

In addition to responding to referrals, the team should take advantage of the many different ways to influence care. For example, team members can conduct educational sessions at staff or division meetings and participate on the hospital pain or ethics committee. Another approach is to offer pilot activities in clinical areas where greater acceptance is anticipated, relying on the support of the so-called early adopters. Many units have routine, interdisciplinary meetings to review important patient issues, and perhaps certain pediatric palliative care team members might be able to attend.

BOX 8-1 Pediatric Palliative Care Program Scope of Services

Provide assistance with:
- Pain and symptom management
- Care coordination and continuity
- Ethical dilemmas
- Goals of care meetings with providers and/or families
  - Decision making regarding quality of life issues
  - Decision making regarding treatment options and recommendations
- Patient/family education and support around all aspects of care: physical, psychosocial, spiritual, and practical
- Consensus building when there are differing views
- Preparation of advanced directives
- Anticipatory guidance for end-of-life symptoms and care during the dying process
- Discharge planning for palliative and end-of-life care
- Anticipatory grief counseling
- Delivery of end-of-life or after-death bedside care
- How to talk with siblings or other children and involve them in a sensitive, age-appropriate manner
- Planning for post-death care: care of body, memento making, organ donation, autopsy, mortuary selection, burial, cremation, funeral planning
- Bereavement follow-up support and counseling
- Community referrals
  - Home/hospice care identification, liaison and/or co-management
  - Psychosocial, spiritual, financial, and practical care
- Staff education
- Staff support and debriefings
- School re-entry or bereavement visits
- Situations when it is not clear how to proceed or intervene when there are not straightforward answers[10]
- Transition from pediatric care to adult medical care

Increased visibility is an effective method for marketing the program. Take every opportunity to talk to staff members from various units, disciplines, departments, and community agencies about the new services. Trust and acceptance will evolve as staff and families experience positive collaborative relationships with palliative care team members.

Resource Development

CONTRIBUTING TO THE SYSTEM

Resource development and implementation to improve the overall level of palliative care in a hospital also raises the awareness among generalist and subspecialty teams that they already provide services under the domain of palliative care.[25] This awareness and use of pediatric palliative care resources raises the profile of the program, and thus becomes an effective internal marketing strategy. Efforts to establish a range of clinical care and educational resources should be directed at making "the right way the easy way."[7] This includes responding to the everyday practice needs of busy clinical staff and managers. It also requires a cooperative approach when redesigning operations so that these resources can incorporate palliative care practices into daily routines.[7] For example, because most Pediatric Intensive Care Unit (PICU) deaths involve withdrawal of life-sustaining treatments, it may be useful to collaborate on Compassionate Extubation Guidelines with staff in the intensive care areas. Make a point to investigate the tension points or gaps that develop around policies and procedures, which are difficult and confusing to staff.

Clinical care resources, which make a difference at the point-of-care, may also include such tangible items as a comfort care room or comfort care cart, and baskets of non-perishable food delivered to a child's room during family vigils at the end of life. End of life bedside practices can be standardized throughout the hospital by providing each unit with disposable cameras, memory boxes, and keepsake supplies to make handprints or footprints, to clip a lock of hair, and to measure the child's height using decorative ribbon (Fig. 8-1). Many programs maintain resource libraries of anticipatory grief and bereavement literature for staff to give to families. Promoting varied resources and providing the necessary educational support puts consistent palliative care into action throughout the institution.

Rather than attempting to create resources from scratch, staff can seek examples from colleagues that can be adapted to program needs. This will save time, money, and frustration as established tools will be more readily implemented.

THE ROLE OF EDUCATION

Interdisciplinary education takes on importance early in pediatric palliative care program evolution and continues to be an integral function of the team as it champions best practices within the institution. Ongoing, institution-wide education will be essential to improve knowledge, attitudes, skills and behavior of all health professionals. These clinicians need to be fully versed about the need for high-quality palliative care, the indications for initiating palliative or end of life treatments, and the services provided by palliative care specialists.[13]

Not all members of the interdisciplinary team, especially in the early days of program development, will have completed a comprehensive, formal training program in pediatric palliative care. They will, however, come to the team with expertise and commitment born of experience in related fields. It will be pivotal to assess the needs of each member of the core team and address any deficits in discipline-specific or interdisciplinary palliative care knowledge. (See Chapter 11.)

Beyond the more clinically focused training, the core team must also acquire program-building skills including managing program operations, creating a business plan, philanthropic fundraising, and developing quality improvement projects.

Pediatric palliative care curricular content, including national practice standards, must be widely disseminated both in the institution and in the wider health care community. Teaching must also include program information on appropriate criteria for referrals, as well as what services can and will be provided to patients, families, and staff by the team and other clinicians at the institution. Perhaps most importantly, education initiatives can highlight how good pediatric palliative care helps the institution meet its goals.

The quality of the program as an interdisciplinary effort will be enhanced if collaborative education begins early and the process is embedded in the team's day-to-day functions. When this occurs, the full potential for using all of the heterogeneous and complementary perspectives of a team approach is realized. It is necessary for all members of the core group to acquire skills in working as an interdisciplinary team, respecting and using each other's skills rather than working as parallel, non-collaborating agents. (See Chapter 16.) Team effectiveness can be strengthened by using input from various disciplines to craft program educational goals and by modeling interdisciplinary teamwork at every teaching opportunity, especially at the bedside.

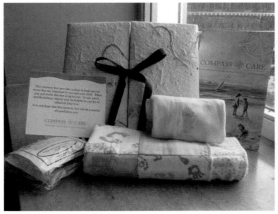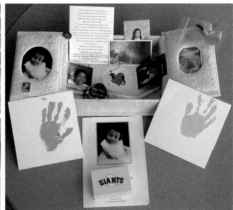

Fig. 8-1 Examples of keepsake and memory box collections.

Clinicians are not the only group that should be targeted for education. Hospital administrators, including those responsible for financial decisions, institutional strategic development, quality improvement, information systems, philanthropic or grant fundraising, and community relations, will all need to understand palliative care. Ongoing conversations help administrators understand that death, or the possibility of death, is a significant aspect of providing care to children with complex medical problems and as such, palliative care is an obligation of the institutions that provide care to these children and their families.

THE ROLE OF COMMUNICATION

Effective, collaborative communication is indispensable when striving for the highest quality of palliative care and has been described as one of the most common procedures in medicine. When performed well, communication conveys both reciprocal information and compassion, justifying its importance as a core competency for the pediatric palliative care team. Effective communication is also paramount to building a cohesive team and promoting positive, collaborative exchanges with referring staff, which ultimately facilitates both continuity and quality of care. Its role and importance have been emphasized in the literature in multiple research studies demonstrating key features and implications.[17,26–31]

A core function of the pediatric palliative care program is to structure opportunities that foster better interdisciplinary and family communication. In this way, team members help staff develop greater skill in timing important discussions that involve delicate matters. Examples of these conversations include:

- Discussing prognosis, signs of progressive disease, and treatment options,
- Anticipatory guidance in preparation for end-of-life care,
- Discussing family goals and wishes,
- Discussing, in a non-judgmental manner, end-of-life issues such as resuscitation, withdrawal of artificial life support, place of death, organ donation, and autopsy,
- Talking with the sick child and siblings as appropriate,
- Compassionately pronouncing the child's death.

Many palliative care teams introduce documentation tools to facilitate communication, decision making, and continuity of care. Examples include the Five Wishes advanced illness/directive booklets (available at www.agingwithdignity.org/index.php),[32] the Seattle Decision Making Tool,[33] and Palliative Care Summary Plans[9] that are distributed among various inpatient and community teams providing care. These communication tools, shared between the family and all providers, facilitate a mutual understanding of the goals of care and the treatment plan in the context of the child's changing needs.

Effective communication also includes consistent documentation of palliative care team consults or involvement; information discussed with providers, patients, and/or family members; and recommendations. Consult forms, checklists, and summary or discharge forms may be helpful in disseminating information. The quality, coordination, and continuity of care will be compromised without proper documentation. Charting needs to specify what has been addressed, what gaps in care remain, the family's preferences and wishes, and what medical, psychosocial, and spiritual interventions are in agreement with the goals of care.[17]

Routine interdisciplinary palliative care team meetings, adapted from the hospice model of care, have come to be regarded as an essential requirement for team communication and program functioning. Meeting agendas are focused on reviewing cases, solving problems, collaborating on quality improvement initiatives, and handling important administrative issues. These meetings most often occur weekly or bi-weekly and serve not only to accomplish clinical work but also to build team cohesiveness. Adding a formal educational component, even having guest speakers, can provide mentoring and support for the core team.

THE ROLE OF PAIN AND SYMPTOM MANAGEMENT

Developing pain and symptom management skills are a pivotal component of building a successful pediatric palliative care program.[18,34] Established best practices have advanced a trend in pediatrics to merge pain and palliative care programs in the United States and abroad.[35] From an economical and practical standpoint, this kind of joint program may be advantageous particularly for smaller institutions, where sharing resources allows for increased continuity, productivity, and efficiency while conserving program costs. Integrating pain and palliative care programs, or at minimum establishing a formal, collaborative working relationship between them, helps ensure relief of suffering and optimizes quality of life throughout the continuum of care.[35]

Many institutions have a separate pain service and perhaps even a separate integrative medicine service that can be consulted to help with symptom management. However, not all pain or integrative medicine services, especially if they are primarily focused on adults, are equipped to address the range of needs commonly found in pediatrics. For example, it is not unusual for the pediatric palliative care team to manage issues specific to pain and symptom management across the developmental spectrum, from premature newborns to young adults. Every effort should be made to proactively address how to prevent territorial issues when services overlap, how to work together in a coordinated manner, and how to educate staff about accessing assistance from various programs to prevent or alleviate patient's distress. Over time, better understandings will evolve, contributing to the formation of beneficial collegial relationships in response to the patients and their families.

Even if the institution has a separate pain service, it is still crucial that pediatric palliative care team members receive rigorous training to acquire specialist-level proficiency in symptom identification and management. Within the team, each person will have his or her individual, discipline-specific contribution to effective child and family-centered pain and symptom management. The team should be able to articulate these distinct clinical skill sets, and the goals for each team member's involvement. The team's approach to symptom control combines clinical competence with education to dispel the myths and misconceptions around symptom management. In this way, the team promotes effective care for the patient and improves care for future patients. This contribution in turn raises the standards for pain and symptom management throughout the hospital.

THE ROLE OF BEREAVEMENT CARE

Services to help ill children and their families cope with anticipatory grief, the end-of-life experience, and the ensuing bereavement are integral to pediatric palliative care and hospice programs. (See Chapter 5.) A growing body of literature suggests that the grief experienced when a child dies is more protracted and complex than the grief associated with adult death.[36–38] Providing bereavement care is unique among hospital services rendered because much of the support offered occurs when the actual patient is deceased. The family then becomes the focus of care.

When building bereavement services, programs should start simple, plan realistically, and access community organizations, collaborating whenever possible and expanding as resources allow. In the hospice model of care, bereavement support is built into the payment structure. However, this is not the case for hospitals and funding for their services can be limited. Many hospitals rely on philanthropy to fund bereavement support, which may be administered through the spiritual care department, the social work department, or the pediatric palliative care program. In some settings, bereavement services may be a separate program within the hospital. Establishing a collaborative relationship, even allocating a portion of the pediatric palliative care team's time and funding, enhances the spectrum of interventions that includes care through death and bereavement.

Recognizing the significant impact that a child's death has on families, it becomes the program's responsibility to provide the materials and training for staff to work with families to create meaningful end-of-life experiences. Families can draw upon these positive experiences as they cope with grief. Ideally, programs will also be able to offer routine follow-up with bereaved families, staying in touch via newsletters, condolence cards, and telephone calls at anniversary dates. Hosting memorials, scrapbooking events, and bereavement retreats are other effective ways to reach out to families who may feel isolated in their communities. Pediatric palliative care programs can contribute staff time to bereavement support groups sponsored by the hospital, or team members may even join forces with a local hospice agency, which allows the families access to a broader range of bereavement support. The program needs to be familiar with resources and expertise in the community to ensure effective partnerships are developed and duplicate services are avoided in an environment of limited resources. All of these programming pieces can fall into place only if the strategic planning process has not overlooked budgeting for staff time, supplies, publications, space requirements, and other bereavement support resources.

THE ROLE OF STAFF SUPPORT

Addressing staff support and team wellness is widely recognized as an essential endeavor.[1,13,14] The intensity of care and emotional demands experienced by staff places them at risk for compassion fatigue, moral distress and burnout. Promoting staff support and self-care measures is vital in preserving effective functioning for the palliative care team, as well as for the staff who provide bedside care. Taking the time to process the intense and highly emotional clinician-patient-family experiences recognizes the humanistic and compassionate nature of this work.

The impact of services to support staff in their caregiving role may be difficult to accurately measure with quantitative data (such as turnover, sick days, apathy) but it is an inherent function of a palliative care program. Ongoing staff-support activities, offered by the palliative care team, also helps build trusting relationships with clinicians, which can ultimately facilitate program acceptance, collaboration, and referrals. For the team itself, both formal and informal mechanisms for reflection and renewal are advised. Annual retreats, "project time" as breaks from direct care, flex-time and periodic memorial observances are practices that programs have employed. Administrative acknowledgment of this important area, coupled with policy-level planning for staff support, can go a long way toward developing a strong and stable workforce.

Creating a Business and Financial Plan

A business plan is a formal document that makes a solid case for program operations and strategic propositions. Producing a business plan can be instrumental in securing administrative support for dedicated resources allocated to pediatric palliative care services. Some hospital-based programs have initiated a business plan early on in their evolution while others launched the program, collected data, and then developed a business plan. The timing reflects a combination of factors, including attention to planning, institutional politics, financial considerations, and the level of strategic guidance provided at the institution. Because most clinicians do not have experience writing a business plan, it will be important to identify resources or partners within the institution, including senior leadership and finance staff for help. Several programs have also turned to the community to enlist business skills, recruiting local business school students to help collect pertinent data and formulate their business plans.

There are core elements included in a business plan that can be tailored to meet specific needs at various stages of program development (see Box 8-2). The introduction provides supporting background information, outlining the needs and rationale for the program. For this section, the team carefully selects and expands on the data from the systems and needs assessments. The document explains how the program cooperatively shares and builds upon existing resources. A central message emphasizes the value added to the institution, and the breadth and depth of services provided by the pediatric palliative care program. The Center to Advance Palliative Care (CAPC) has outlined compelling points that are useful in justifying program development (see Box 8-3). These points can be personalized to address institution-specific data when presented to hospital administrators.

It is essential to include a detailed, multi-year program budget, indicating direct program expenses: salaries with benefits; marketing costs; equipment and supplies; staff education; and specific program resources (e.g., memorials, educational literature, and comfort carts). In addition, the financial analysis includes revenue streams, such as medical center support for salaries and/or operations, as well as income from consult billing, philanthropy, and grants. The business plan also presents

---

BOX 8-2 Business Plan Components

- Executive summary: synthesizes content of overall plan
  - Context for the proposal
  - Identified need to be addressed; how proposed plan will create improvements
  - Key program features
  - Funding requirements
  - Expected impact and measures
- Statement of need and rationale for proposed program
  - System and needs assessment data
  - Pertinent clinical patient data: number and locations of deaths; average LOS, pain scores: current or improved with pediatric palliative care involvement
  - Family and staff input/satisfaction with care data
  - Financial implications as appropriate
  - Competing local/regional initiatives
- Operational plan for implementation
  - Description of program goals and services
  - Program model and structure; clinical care, education, research, community involvement
  - Collaboration with other programs in the hospital and community
  - Target patient population, estimated patient volume, and capacity projections over time
  - Staffing requirements and roles
  - Space and equipment needs; additional operational resources requested
  - Basic policies and procedures for program operations
  - Evaluation plan and expected impact: clinical, operations, financial metrics
- Marketing plan
- Financial/budget summary with projections over multiple years
- Appendices
  - Documents, data, and other supporting information

Adapted from CAPC resources on business plan development: The Business Plan (Level I): Worksheets; Appendix 3.6: PowerPoint - Business Plan Basics; Module 2: Creating Compelling Business and Financial Plan; http://www.capc.org/building-a-hospital-based-palliative-care-program/designing/presenting-plan/index_html (Building a Palliative Care Program-Presenting the Business Plan)

BOX 8-3 Making the Case for a Hospital Based Palliative Care Program

- Coordinates services from diverse hospital departments for safe, effective, and efficient family-centered care of patients with life-threatening, advanced and complex illnesses
- Facilitates high quality, well-planned treatments that address current needs, as well as anticipated needs
- Advances quality of care and pain management standards used to accredit and/or evaluate services by the Joint Commission and *U.S. News and World Report* annual rankings
- Facilitates care coordination, case management, and referrals to appropriate care settings as indicated
- Improves quality of care and services, which can help strengthen ratings of family satisfaction with care
- Provides staff support to ease the stress in caring for the most emotionally and time intensive patients and their families, which can strengthen staff satisfaction and retention
- Increases visibility of the institution in the community as being innovative and responsive to the holistic needs of patients with advanced illness and their families
- Maintains or increases capacity by matching resources to needs and preferences
- Promotes goals of care discussions, honoring the needs and wishes of patients and/or families, which can help avoid futile and burdensome treatments when medically advisable.

Adapted from "The Case for Hospital-Based Palliative Care" Center to Advance Palliative care. Accessed online 8.10.2010.
http://www.capc.org/building-a-hospital-based-palliative-care-program/case/hospitalbenefits/
www.capc.org/support-from-capc/capc_publications/making-thecase.pdf

---

outcome data that the team tracks to demonstrate quality of care and program impact. Typical categories include operational, customer, clinical, and financial metrics.[13,39]

Ultimately, the business plan needs to speak the language of those who are running the institution. It should reflect their goals and their priorities, be fiscally responsible and sustainable, and promote the necessary changes to fuel the growth of good interdisciplinary palliative care.[25] It is prudent to present the plan in such a way that it does not appear to be asking for unlimited resources and financial support but rather places the program in partnership with the institution.[25] The business plan presents evidence that makes a case for action, clearly stating what is needed from the institution to develop or expand the palliative care program.[40] Be careful to match expected workload to allocated resources, avoiding the precedent of giving away services without adequate institutional support. A business plan is not a static document and will need to be revised repeatedly as the program changes and expands.

Building a business case with cost-saving financial metrics is a significant challenge for pediatric palliative care programs trying to start, grow, or sustain their services.[41] It is widely recognized that pediatric programs have not been able to directly apply the same financial model of cost neutrality and cost avoidance that exists in the Diagnostic Related Groups driven adult healthcare environment. Although similar work is being done in pediatrics to create reliable cost accounting methods and templates to calculate appropriate staffing, volume, and projected income, pediatric programs are still forced to secure financial support from their institutions and from outside sources.[41]

A strong argument about generating or saving money may not be the best strategy for garnering institutional support. Rather, the most compelling value proposition lies in aligning with the priorities, needs, and challenges of the institution.[41] For example, if ICU bed capacity is an issue, work with the administration to identify throughput issues and then direct program efforts toward relieving ICU bottlenecks, preventing ICU diversions, and making room for elective surgeries. Also, institutions place great value on improving patient and family satisfaction scores, pain scores, and staff retention. Palliative care programs become more valuable to the institution when they can demonstrate how the program might help these areas and increase opportunities for marketing the institution within the community.

Programs need to work closely with finance staff, including billers and coders, to understand how to maximize revenues given the constraints and payer mix at the institution. See if other specialty services bill for symptom management; if they are not, the pediatric palliative care team should do so whenever appropriate. Learn about billing from other adult and pediatric palliative care programs, as well as from educational resources for understanding finances.[42] Explore how and where the institution loses revenue, as well as the circumstances where it maximizes revenue. For example, Children's of Minnesota conducted a quality study and found that the pediatric palliative care team's involvement saved money, and reduced hospital admits and days, as well as Emergency Department (ED) visits.[43] Realistically though, pediatric palliative care often involves aggressive and expensive therapy, which may continue for weeks, months, or years. Pediatric palliative care programs can demonstrate their roles in maximizing efficient, coordinated care that optimizes quality of life despite intense medical and practical needs.[41] More analysis needs to be done within the pediatric community to find the financial impact of providing pediatric palliative care and end-of-life services to children in the hospital and home.

Because reimbursement for the time clinicians spend with patients and families is sub-optimal, it is critical to solicit other funding for the program's survival. Philanthropic donations and grants provide not only direct payment to the institution, but also recognition and valuable community public relations. Most administrations look favorably on these contributions to the overall budget[25] and to the institution's reputation. The challenge here is to allocate time to work closely with the development office, ensuring its understanding of program objectives and services, and advocating fundraising for specific aspects of the program. Prepare program talking points, fundraising proposals, patient impact stories, and a wish list of both small and large program items so that both development officers and pediatric palliative care team members are always ready to meet with potential donors.

Part of a program's fiscal responsibility includes participation in regional and state efforts with other healthcare institutions to improve access and reimbursement for quality pediatric palliative and hospice care services. Efficient use of resources and the delivery of quality care are valued as contributions to the bottom line in the modern healthcare system.

Interfacing with Community Partners

UNDERSTANDING UNIQUE CONSTRAINTS

Children with complex, life-threatening conditions have spent significant amounts of time in hospitals because of limitations in community-based services. Children and their families can feel an immense sense of support from hospital clinicians,

often believing that the hospital represents a safe haven. That said, the hospital remains an unnatural and distorted place to live out one's childhood. Research and practice experience validate that a child's development and the family's coping are best served at home with adequate resources.[44] It is therefore important that pediatric palliative care teams develop strategic partnerships to enable safe, coordinated, and continuous care between the hospital and community.

Advanced science and technology, along with children's resiliency, mean that children are living longer with complex therapies that mimic ICU care at home. However, it can be extremely difficult to find this level of pediatric technology support and clinical expertise needed, particularly in rural areas. The reality is that parents usually have the primary responsibility for around the clock complex care at home. In these cases, respite care is an important consideration. While families initially may not be comfortable using community-based options, especially if they have not had the opportunity to establish trust in alternative caregivers, they will need encouragement to make long-term plans and to develop relationships with respite providers. Those relationships are very important, and underscore the importance of effective collaboration between home-based and hospital-based services.

Overall, the number of children requiring pediatric palliative care is significantly less than the number of adults using home care and hospice services. The challenge to community agencies is to acquire adequate experience to develop and sustain the knowledge, skills, and confidence necessary for providing care to children. Some adult providers describe the emotional burden of caring for children as prohibitive. With expert help, many adult home care or hospice programs have been open to pediatric training, consultative support, and education to help develop competencies and greater comfort in caring for pediatric patients and their families.

One of the more challenging goals of an in-patient pediatric palliative care program is to develop a seamless interface with community-based home care and hospice programs who serve these same children. For home-based pediatric palliative and end of-life care programs to be truly successful, they need to embrace a concurrent model of care. Philosophically, this concurrent approach is more acceptable to families who are not focused on end-of-life care, but who are still interested in receiving supportive measures focused on enhancing quality of life, such as expert symptom management and psychosocial care. These kinds of services have traditionally been available in the home through community hospice programs. However, the hospice movement has developed around a different philosophy of care based on the more predictable disease trajectories of many common adult diseases with an emphasis on end-of-life care for patients expected to live six months or less. The adult hospice model typically abides by rules and regulations that require patients to give up curative or life-prolonging treatments. Financial reimbursement tied to these restrictions is usually based upon Medicare guidelines, which leads to a philosophy and practice not suitable for children with life-threatening conditions.

Providers who focus on hospice care may not be comfortable with the prognostic uncertainty and complex care plans characteristic of pediatric palliative care patients. Costs for pediatric palliative care can be much greater than those of the typical adult hospice patient; children often receive life-prolonging therapies such as home TPN, repeated transfusions, palliative chemotherapy, and home IV antibiotics, which are not conventionally allowed under the hospice benefit. Most hospices, which operate on daily reimbursement, cannot provide this costly care unless they have sufficient philanthropic funds to offset expenses associated with pediatric cases. Significant financial and resource limitations cause many community-based providers to pursue both home care and hospice licensure, allowing greater flexibility for reimbursement based on patient acuity. A fee-for-service billing model, used by home care agencies, can offer a more financially solvent approach, particularly when caring for pediatric palliative care patients. Additionally, some hospices are willing to work with insurance companies to develop individual agreements to carve out a fee for service for certain therapies in order to be able to provide concurrent care. Understanding these intricacies allows the pediatric palliative care team to be more effective in discharge planning and advocating with payers.

Advocacy: Demand Driving Resource Development

In recent years, regional and state coalitions have formed to work with private insurance companies, and public and state medical assistance programs to improve reimbursement for home-based medical and psychosocial services. These groups have brought together hospital- and community-based clinicians, as well as parents and other family members, to establish collaborative partnerships. They have generated pressure on payers and service agencies to create more effective, family-centered models of care while responding with more cost-efficient solutions. In addition, they have joined forces to link organized responses for advocacy at local, state, and national levels. California's Children's Hospice and Palliative Care Coalition for Pediatric Palliative Care and the Ohio Pediatric End-of-life Network (OPPEN) are successful examples of this kind of effort. An ongoing advisory committee can foster creative collaboration with the pediatric palliative care program to ensure successful partnerships in providing seamless care across settings.

Given financial constraints and limited staffing expertise, it makes sense to create cooperative networks among pediatric palliative care consultants, inpatient hospitals, and home-based service providers.[8] Many children travel to regional specialty centers, and then are also seen at local hospitals and clinics for routine care. Networking with potential agencies can help identify the kinds of services available, barriers to overcome, and limitations to be considered before planning for a specific child's urgent needs. Effective coordination of services can go a long way toward reducing the stress on children and their families, while also creating efficiencies that benefit organizations which provide or pay for this complex level of care.

Some hospitals and community agencies opt to offer both home care and hospice services under an umbrella organization. This model requires complex licensure as hospital, hospice, and home-care regulatory agencies monitor care and determine standards for each setting. The benefits of this model include improved care coordination and continuity, allowing staff easier access to information between settings and agencies. The home-care department may not have the clinical expertise in hospice or palliative care, but the pediatric palliative care team can develop a consultative relationship with the staff. Based on identified gaps in knowledge and skill, the pediatric palliative care team will provide training to address the immediate, practical needs of the patient and family and support staff as they manage unfamiliar situations.

In response to these various constraints, community-based home care agencies most often work closely with pediatric hospices and/or palliative care specialists, or through adult-oriented hospice agencies that have been willing to extend their services to include pediatrics. Each group may have a different set of skills and expertise as their standard. Collaborative relationships with other providers can help wrap around these core services and create a competent network of comprehensive care. In addition, partnerships with key staff at the identified children's hospital are also important. The goal is to create a service delivery system that successfully connects hospital and community providers, enabling the child access to coordinated care in each setting that shares common treatment goals. (See clinical vignette.)

Phase III: Ensuring Sustainability

During Phase 3, program development is focused on embedding, strengthening, and sustaining the program, ultimately to make it indispensable to the organization. Sustainability requires ongoing goal setting, not just for program startup, but also for mid- and long-term program development. Anticipating growth, changes in resources, and staffing needs all assist program-planning efforts over the long haul (see Table 8-3).

Critical features of a successful, sustainable pediatric palliative care program include cultivating a highly functional team; fostering attitudes of acceptance among referring providers, families and the community; acquiring ongoing financial support; ensuring efficient use of resources; and promoting expert skill development throughout the institution.

As programs mature, teams encounter developmental issues in clinical expertise, collaboration, and productivity. Individual practitioners come into the team with variations in their knowledge, skills, and practice abilities. Over time, each develops greater capacity to manage patient volume efficiently and with proficiency. This phenomenon also occurs for the team as a whole, which can accomplish more than the sum of its parts. Teams eventually establish a common set of terms and practices, allowing a groupthink to take hold. When a consistent practice occurs across the team's members, an interdisciplinary approach emerges. Programs need to nurture the teams' growth curve by carefully planning for continual team development.

When volume grows and staff attrition occurs, it becomes necessary to bring on new team members. The team should re-evaluate training and mentorship needs regularly so that the newest staff members have time and support to become successful on the team. Effective team functioning can improve staff recruitment and retention, and facilitates greater capacity to address patient care needs. Encouraging staff to participate in non-clinical activities such as marketing, education, and research allows intermittent respite from the intensity of care delivery.

Referring clinicians need to recognize that the pediatric palliative care service is helpful to them as well as to patients

TABLE 8-3   Program Development Phase III: Ensuring Sustainability

Improve services & quality	Take care of what you have	Address long-term needs
• Utilize feedback to refine services • Adjust to changing needs • Enhance clinical skills through evidenced based practice • Demonstrate depth & breadth of services/skills available • Enhance communication with providers • Periodically reassess SWOT: Strengths, Weaknesses, Opportunities, & Threats	• Prevent compassion fatigue & burnout • Promote efficient use of human & financial resources • Foster team building	• Plan for staff development • Identify emerging issues & offer assistance • Revise business plan • Secure funds to match growing program needs

and their families. In this sense, clinicians too are clients of the pediatric palliative care team. If the team does not support and affirm the relationship the primary provider has with the child and family, or if the primary clinician feels challenged or criticized by the team's actions, then future referrals can be threatened. By taking time to address the needs of all parties, the team demonstrates effectiveness and becomes an important part of the care delivery system. Aligning interventions to the stated goals of referring physicians, families, and others invested in the outcomes is important to program survival. This intricate communication process also serves the palliative care program by inviting ongoing feedback that helps refine and re-focus the team's efforts.

A mature team takes feedback seriously, reflects upon its practice and makes the necessary changes. Provider and family satisfaction surveys provide metrics indicative of program impact. If the team considers that all stakeholders are clients from the outset, then the customer service attitude has the added benefit of creating allies and reducing potential conflict.

Re-evaluation of priorities and adjustment to new needs point to areas for expansion. The team must determine if it is meeting its own, as well as the institution's, expectations and goals. Additional information may be gained through focus groups with clinicians and/or family members. Chart audits comparing patients with similar diagnoses who have and who have not had pediatric palliative care team consultation may also be valuable, as could identifying reasons for patient readmissions within a week after discharge.

Another approach the team can take to embed itself in the system is to adopt tasks important to the organization's mission or operational requirements. For example, it can take a lead role in policy and procedure development, such as revising Withdrawal of Artificial Life Sustaining Therapy or Patient Controlled Analgesia. Team members might also serve on ethics, residency training, or family advisory committees. Pediatric palliative care teams may also be able to identify emerging patterns or trends, and so address potential problems before they escalate. Helping the organization meet its regulatory requirements, quality standards, and other tasks validates the team's breadth of expertise and worth. The presence of a strong pediatric palliative care program presents marketing opportunities for the institution, particularly if community or regional organizations do not have similar programs serving seriously ill children.

Many programs start with funding for a limited time, receiving small grants from organizations or philanthropic sources. Over time, that funding may dry up, or new criteria for continuation

Clinical Vignette: Interfacing with Community Partners

An identified children's hospital has formed formal partnerships with several home-based adult hospice programs that cover different geographic areas. These hospice programs have agreed to care for children with support from the hospital staff. Hospital physicians are available to consult with the agency staff around unexpected clinical challenges. The hospital pediatric palliative care team provides education, case consultation and training to the home-based team quarterly. Standardized communication forms between the two agencies have been created to facilitate transfer of healthcare information and treatment plans. Families are asked to sign Releases of Information to enable effective coordination of care. A Discharge Checklist accompanies the child when they go home from the hospital. A Home Update Form accompanies the child to all outpatient clinic appointments and admissions to the hospital to document changes in the treatment plan. An Advanced Care Planning Form describes child and family preferences and goals for care, and is shared with the child's team. The inpatient team appreciates improved communication about what is going on at home, and the home-based team's work benefits from improved communication around changes in the child's condition, orders, and updates from the hospital team. The hospice team is challenged by the need to be more flexible about procedures and interventions, which are not usually authorized within a strict hospice plan of care. It has taken some time to come to understand what each partner can expect from another.

may be established. It is very important to consider these initial sources of support and consider how the program's activities meet the funder's expectations. However, it is critical that each revision of the business plan addresses the need for ongoing funding that keeps up with expanding program demands. Philanthropic goals are necessary to achieve sustainability. Fundraising events and corporate contributions engage community support and increase institutional visibility, as does inviting the input of community representatives as advisory council members. Families who appreciated the care their children have received can be wonderful spokespeople for the program. When one home-base hospice program cared for a child in their community, they operated at a loss during the acute care phase of providing end-of-life care. The community responded with significant donations because they applauded the agency's

TABLE 8-4 Program Development Phase IV: Surviving Success

Strive for continued excellence	Maintain professional vitality
• Analyze areas still in need of improvement • Implement strategies to achieve new goals • Report needs, challenges & contributions to administration • Establish a mechanism to keep up with advances in pediatric palliative care • Incorporate structure for ongoing program evaluation	• Balance professional demands with self care • Celebrate accomplishments • Support educational growth of staff & palliative care team • Create regular opportunities for self reflection

willingness to care for children. Over time, philanthropy, grants, patient-care revenue, and cost-saving or cost-avoiding formulas can assist programs in developing a financial argument that supports their operations. Broad-based financial support can help programs move from start-up to self-sustaining.

It is vital that the pediatric palliative care team routinely provides formal and informal program updates to the administrative and clinical leadership. Being able to demonstrate involvement in multiple quality improvement initiatives that have advanced more efficient, effective, consistent, and coordinated care helps to integrate the program within the institution. Sources of data for quality improvement should include measurements of patient outcomes and activities that reflect organizational priorities, including:

- numbers of referrals changing over time,
- pain and symptom management needs identified and successfully treated,
- improved patient satisfaction scores,
- improved practices at the end of life.

During this phase, the program achieves credibility, accomplishes good work, and is well accepted by administrative, clinician, and family stakeholders.[45] The program has matured in its capability to offer services with depth of knowledge, skills, and resources, serving needs in many if not all areas where children and families are cared for within the organization. By the end of this phase, the program clearly will be able to validate that it makes a significant difference in many arenas, that successful practices have been adopted throughout the institution, and that palliative care has been woven into the fabric of the institution.

Phase IV: Surviving Success

Surviving success requires effective and forward-thinking management of program growth, increased patient care volume, and competing priorities (see Table 8-4). As experience grows, staff members and the team develop expertise, economies of scale, and greater efficiency. With this increased capacity the same number of staff members can provide more services—up to a point.

How many providers does it take to deliver excellent care, especially as programs mature? The Center to Advance Palliative Care has developed some formulas to address this question, but setting and practice patterns are likely to affect these numbers. It is important not to promise more than can be delivered, and to communicate barriers to achieving goals as this information becomes apparent. As the field evolves, patterns of practice and expectations for productivity need to be studied so that benchmarks can be developed.

Monitoring growth while planning for current and future needs requires not only attention to data but also attention to how the team is functioning. In such a stressful area of practice,

personal coping, and team effectiveness go hand in hand. Self-care practices translate into healthy work habits and positive contributions to the team. Conversely, when burnout begins to surface, it can become increasingly difficult to deliver the quality of care desired. Each individual has his or her own needs and capacities, so formulaic responses are likely to have only limited success. Yet members of well established, seasoned teams agree that they have succeeded, at least in part, by managing the personal stresses associated with their work, which helps maintain professional vitality.

One of the challenges of having a successful program is recognizing that the work is never done. A program that does not evolve will not continue to be successful, or at the least, it risks sliding into mediocrity without periodic readjustment. Research contributes to new knowledge and therapies. There are always areas that could be improved or new services that would address unmet needs. The sense of never being finished is real and adds a compelling motive to incorporate reflection and development of new goals into the team's plans. At the same time, acknowledging past accomplishments can lend a heartening perspective on the great strides that have been made and an appreciation for the distance already traveled.

REFERENCES

1. Field MJ, Behrman RE, editors: *For the Institute of Medicine Committee on Palliative and End-of-Life Care for Children and their Families. "When Children Die: Improving Palliative and End-of-Life Care for Children and their Families."* Washington, DC, 2003, National Academies Press.
2. Children's Hospitals and Clinics of Minnesota: www.childrensmn.org/services/painpalliativecare.
3. Kotter J: Leading change: why transformation efforts fail, *Harv Bus Rev* 1–10, 2007.
4. Periyakoil VS: Change management: the secret sauce of successful program building, *J Palliat Med* 12(4):329–330, 2009.
5. Meier DE: Ten steps to growing palliative care referrals, *J Palliat Med* 8(4):706–708, 2005.
6. Radwany S, Mason H, Clarke JS, et al: Optimizing the success of a palliative care consult service: how to average over 110 consults per month, *J Pain Symptom Manage* 2008.
7. Byock I, Twohig JS, Merriman M, et al: Promoting excellence in end-of-life care: a report on innovative models of palliative care, *J Palliat Med* 9(1):137–151, 2006.
8. Meier DE, Beresford L: Pediatric palliative care offers opportunities for collaboration, *J Palliat Med* 10(2):284–289, 2007.
9. Toce S, Collins MA: The FOOTPRINTS model of pediatric palliative care, *J Palliat Med* 6(6):989–1000, 2003.
10. Duncan J, Spengler E, Wolfe J: Providing pediatric palliative care: PACT in action, *Am J Matern Child Nurs* 32(5):279–287, 2007.
11. www.capc.org/palliative-care-leadership-initiative/overview/curriculum/pclc_peds/;last accessed 5.27.10.
12. Learned EP, Roland Christiansen C, et al: *Business Policy, Text and Cases*, Homewood, Ill, 1969, RD Irwin, Publisher.
13. Weissman DE, Meier DE: Operational features for hospital palliative care programs: consensus recommendations, *J Palliat Med* 11(9):1189–1194, 2008.
13a. *A National Framework and Preferred Practices for Palliative and Hospice Care Quality: A Consensus Report*, Washington, DC, 2006, National Quality Forum.

14. American Academy of Pediatrics: Committee on Bioethics and Committee on Hospital Care. Palliative care for children, *Pediatrics* 106(2 Pt 1):351–357, 2000.

15. Gwyther LP, Altilio T, Blacker S, Christ G, Csikai EL, Hooyman N, et al: Social work competencies in palliative and end-of-life care, *J Soc Work End Life Palliat Care* 1(1):87–120, 2005.

16. Morstad Boldt A, Yusuf F, Himelstein BP: Perceptions of the term palliative care, *J Palliat Med* 9(5):1128–1136, 2006.

17. Zhukovsky DS, Herzog CE, Kaur G, et al: The impact of palliative care consultation on symptom assessment, communication needs, and palliative interventions in pediatric patients with cancer, *J Palliat Med* 12(4):343–349, 2009.

18. Standards of Practice for Pediatric Palliative Care and Hospice: *National Hospice and Palliative Care. Organization*, Virginia, 2009, Alexandria, pp 1–31.

19. The Case for Hospital Palliative Care Improving Palliative Care. Reducing Costs. p. 15. Interview with Diane Meier, MD, Director, Center to Advance Palliative Care. http://www.capc.org/support-from-capc/capc_publications/making-the-case.pdf/file_view.

20. www.capc.org/building-a-hospital-based-palliative-care-program/implementation/staffing/;last accessed 5.27.10.

21. Frager G: Pediatric palliative care: building the model, bridging the gaps, *J Palliat Med* 12(3):9–12, 1996.

22. Mack JW, Wolfe J: Early integration of pediatric palliative care: for some children, palliative care starts at diagnosis, *Curr Opin Pediatr* 18(1):10–14, 2006.

23. Thompson LA, Knapp C, Madden V, et al: Pediatricians' perceptions of and preferred timing for pediatric palliative care, *Pediatrics* 123(5):e777–e782, 2009.

24. Friebert S, Osenga K: Pediatric Palliative Care Referral Guide. www.capc.org/tools-for-palliative-care-programs/clinicaltools/;last accessed 5.27.10.

25. Portenoy R, Heller KS: Developing an integrated department of pain and palliative medicine, *J Palliat Med* 5(4):623–633, 2002.

26. Mack JW, Hilden JM, Watterson J, et al: Parent and physician perspectives on quality of care at the end of life in children with cancer, *J Clin Oncol* 23:9155–9161, 2005.

27. Contro N, Larson J, Scofield S, et al: Family perspectives on the quality of pediatric palliative care, *Arch Pediatr Adolesc Med* 156(1):14–19, 2002.

28. Contro NA, Larson J, Scofield S, et al: Hospital staff and family perspectives regarding quality of pediatric palliative care, *Pediatrics* 114(5):1248–1252, 2004.

29. Meyer EC, Ritzholz MD, Burns JP, et al: Improving the quality of end-of-life care in the pediatric intensive care unit: parents and priorities and recommendations, *Pediatrics* 117:649–657, 2006.

30. Hinds PS, Drew D, Oakes LL, et al: End-of-life care preferences of pediatric patients with cancer, *J Clin Oncol* 23(36):9146–9154, 2005.

31. Hsiao JL, Evan EE, Zeltzer LK: Parent and child perspectives on physician communication in pediatric palliative care, *Palliative Support Care* 5(4):355–365, 2007.

32. Five Wishes advanced illness/directive booklets: www.agingwithdignity.org/five-wishes-resources.php. Accessed May 27, 2010.

33. Hays RM, Valentine J, Haynes G, et al: The Seattle Pediatric Palliative Care Project: effects on family satisfaction and health-related quality of life, *J Palliat Med* 9(3):716–728, 2006.

34. National Consensus Project for Quality Palliative Care: *Clinical Practice Guidelines for Quality Palliative Care*, ed 2, 2009. www.nationalconsensusproject.org/;last accessed 5.27.10.

35. Friedrichsdorf SJ, Remke S, Symalla B, et al: Developing a pain and palliative care programme at a US children's hospital, *Int J Palliat Nurs* 13(11):534–542, 2007.

36. Rando TA: *Parental Loss of a Child*, Champaign, Il 1986, Research Press.

37. Davies R: New understanding of parental grief: a literature review, *J Adv Nurs* 46:506–513, 2004.

38. Kreicbergs U, Lannen P, Onelov E, et al: Parental grief after losing a child to cancer: impact of professional and social support on long term outcomes, *J Clin Oncol* 25(22):3308–3314, 2007.

39. http://www.capc.org/building-a-hospital-based-palliative-care-program/measuring-quality-and-impact/; last accessed 5.27.10.

40. Spragens LH: *Creating Compelling Business and Financial Plans*, 2003. Accessed online at www.capc.org/support-from-capc/capc_presentations/ca-2003/module-2.ppt.

41. Friebert S: *Making the Financial Case for Pediatric Palliative Care*, CAPC web seminar, July 30, 2009.

42. http://capc.org/tools-for-palliative-care-programs/billing/overview-claims-payment/20090611.ppt/;Date accessed 5.27.10.

43. Friedrichsdorf SJ et al: Making the case for pediatric palliative care: one example, *J Palliat Med* 13(2):129–138, 2010.

44. Dussel K, Hilden W, Moore C, Turner BG: Looking beyond where children die: determinants and effects of planning a child's location of death, *J Pain Symptom Manage* 37(1):33–43, 2009.

45. Bruera E: The development of a palliative care culture, *J Palliat Med* 20(4):316–319, 2004.

SUGGESTED READINGS

Bruce A, Boston P: The changing landscape of palliative care: emotional challenges for hospice and palliative care professionals, *J Hosp Palliat Nurs* 10(1):49–55, 2008.

Dabbs D, Butterworth L, Hall E: Tender mercies: increasing access to hospice services for children with life threatening conditions, *MCN Am J Matern Child Nurs* 32(5):311–319, 2007.

Dickens DS: Building competence in pediatric end-of-life care, *J Palliat Med* 12(7):617–622, 2009.

Feudtner C: Collaborative communication in pediatric palliative care: a foundation for problem solving and decision making, *Pediatr Clin North Am* 54:583–607, 2007.

Feudtner C, Christakis DA, Connell FA: Pediatric deaths attributable to complex chronic conditions: a population-based study of washington state, 1980–1997, *Pediatrics* 106(1 Pt 2):205–209, 2000.

Feudtner C, Christakis DA, Zimmerman FJ, et al: Characteristics of deaths occurring in children's hospitals: implications for supportive care services, *Pediatrics* 109(5):887–893, 2002.

Gale G, Brooks A: Implementing a palliative care program in a newborn intensive care unit, *Adv Neonatal Care* 6(1):37–53, 2006.

Gerhardt CA, Grollman JA, Baughcum AE, et al: Longitudinal evaluation of a pediatric palliative care educational workshop for oncology fellows, *J Palliat Med* 12(4):323–328, 2009.

Golan H, Bielorai B, Grebler D, et al: Integration of a palliative and terminal care center into a comprehensive pediatric oncology department, *Pediatr Blood Cancer* 50(5):949–955, 2008.

Harper J, Hinds PS, Baker JN, et al: Creating a palliative and end-of-life program in a cure-oriented pediatric setting: the zig-zag method, *J Pediatr Oncol Nurs* 24(5):246–254, 2007.

Hatzmann J, Heymans HS, Ferrer-i-Carbonell A, et al: Hidden consequences of success in pediatrics: parental health-related quality of life—results from the care project, *Pediatrics* 122(5):e1030–e1038, 2008.

Homer CJ, Marino B, Cleary PD, et al: Quality of care at a children's hospital: the parents' perspective, *Arch Pediatr Adolesc Med* 153:1123–1129, 1999.

Hubble RA, Ward-Smith P, Christenson K, et al: Implementation of a palliative care team in a pediatric hospital, *J Pediatr Health Care* 23(2):126–131, 2009.

Johnston DL, Nagel K, Friedman DL, et al: Availability and use of palliative care and end-of-life services for pediatric oncology patients, *J Clin Oncol* 26(28):4646–4650, 2008.

Knapp CA, Thompson LA, Vogel WB, et al: Developing a pediatric palliative care program: addressing the lack of baseline expenditure information, *Am J Hosp Palliat Care* 26(1):40–46, 2009.

Linton JM, Feudtner C: What accounts for differences or disparities in pediatric palliative and end-of-life care? A systematic review focusing on possible multilevel mechanisms, *Pediatrics* 122(3):574–582, 2008.

Long T, Hale C, Sanderson L, et al: Evaluation of educational preparation for cancer and palliative care nursing for children and adolescents in England, *Eur J Oncol Nurs* 12(1):65–74, 2008.

Mack JW, Joffe S, Hilden JM, et al: Parents' views of cancer-directed therapy for children with no realistic chance for cure, *J Clin Oncol* 26(29):4759–4764, 2008.

McCallum DE, Byrne P, Bruera E: How children die in hospitals, *J Pain Symptom Manage* 20:417–423, 2000.

Meier DE, Beresford L: The palliative care team, *J Palliat Med* 11(5):677–681, 2008.

Michelson KN, Ryan AD, Jovanovic B, et al: Pediatric residents' and fellows' perspectives on palliative care education, *J Palliat Med* 12(5):451–457, 2009.

O'Connor M, Fisher C, Guilfoyle A: Interdisciplinary teams in palliative care: a critical reflection, *Int J Palliat Nurs* 12(3):132–137, 2006.

Rushton CH, Reder E, Hall B, et al: Interdisciplinary interventions to improve pediatric palliative care and reduce health care professional suffering, *J Palliat Med* 9(4):922–933, 2006.

Tan GH, Totapally BR, Torbati D, et al: End-of-life decisions and palliative care in a children's hospital, *J Palliat Med* 9(2):332–342, 2006.

Ward-Smith P, Korphage RM, Hutto CJ: Where health care dollars are spent when pediatric palliative care is provided, *Nurs Econ* 26(3): 175–178, 2008.

Ward-Smith P, Linn JB, Korphage RM, et al: Development of a pediatric palliative care team, *J Pediatr Health Care* 21(4):245–249, 2007.

Wolfe J, Grier HE, Klar N, et al: Symptoms and suffering at the end of life in children with cancer, *N Engl J Med* 342(5):326–333, 2000.

Wolfe J, Klar N, Grier HE, et al: Understanding of prognosis among parents of children who died of cancer: impact on treatment goals and integration of palliative care, *J Am Med Assoc* 284(19):2469–2475, 2000.

9 The Evidence Base

DEBORAH A. LAFOND | NANCY HUTTON

If we listen closely, children who are dying and their families will tell us everything we need to know to care for them: they want to be loved, to be cared for and cared about, to know that their lives have meaning and purpose, to be remembered as the special people they are. Most of all, they want the people caring for them to appreciate and celebrate their lives. —Cindy Stutzer

Definition of Evidence-Based Practice

The term *evidence-based practice* was coined in the 1990s and has been widely embraced by most healthcare disciplines.[1] Evidence-based practice (EBP) integrates the best scientific research evidence with clinical expertise of healthcare practitioners and patient and/or family preferences to facilitate clinical decision making.[2] Decisions are based upon factors from each domain: the clinical situation, the patient and family preferences, and the research evidence, and individualized to the circumstances. There are multiple models of EBP between and within healthcare disciplines. The conceptual model described by Satterfield et al is a interdisciplinary model based upon the strengths of EBP models and processes from medicine, nursing, psychology, social work, and public health[1] (Fig. 9-1). The strength of pediatric palliative care practice stems from the interdisciplinary collaboration of multiple healthcare disciplines. EBP is an approach to problem solving that addresses the needs of the organization, the individual practitioner, the patient, and the family to promote high-quality healthcare. Organizational experiences of quality improvement and financial data, combined with clinical research, clinical experience, and patient and/or family preferences promote shared decision making based upon all contextual factors.[3] Palliative care is a relatively young discipline and pediatric palliative care is even younger. The evidence base in palliative care is not robust and there is a paucity of evidence specific to pediatrics.[4]

Evidence-based practice is a process as well as a practice descriptor.[5] The process involves defining a practice issue, searching the literature for current research, critically appraising the evidence, synthesizing the evidence to make recommendations for changes in practice, implementing the recommended changes, and evaluating the outcomes. EBP relies on a holistic approach to decision making based less upon expert opinion. Translation of the domains of EBP, scientific research, clinical expertise, and patient and/or family preferences into practice produces products such as changes in clinical practice, clinical guidelines, organizational standards of practice, and opportunities for fostering a research agenda in pediatric palliative care.

The healthcare professions involved in pediatric palliative care, including medicine, nursing, psychology, social work, child life and others, are a science and applied professions with equal contributions to the art and science of clinical practice. The perceived value of evidence may vary depending upon the discipline of practice. Traditional evidence-based medicine relies heavily on randomized clinical trials, yet this approach to generations of evidence is not as practical for pediatric palliative care, where a vulnerable patient population is often excluded from clinical research.[6] Most palliative care research is adult-focused and this is one of the challenges to creating pediatric palliative care evidence-based guidelines (Table 9-1). The narrow scope of pediatric palliative care may be too focused for most standard literature search engines. The value of expert clinicians within and between disciplines is unclear and often underestimated in determining EBP recommendations. Evidence must be defined broadly and considered within the context of the specific clinical issue. Evidence is published in a wide variety of journals pertinent to a spectrum of diseases.

Levels of Evidence Used in Practice Guideline Development and Implications for Pediatrics

The development of clinical practice guidelines for the management of a variety of diseases and conditions brings together experts to review and summarize current evidence, evaluate the quality of the evidence, and make recommendations for practice. The National Consensus Project for Quality Palliative Care (NCP) brought together leaders of five national organizations representing hospice and palliative care. This task force followed a rigorous process of evidence review and consensus development to produce the Clinical Practice Guidelines for Quality Palliative Care in 2003, with an update in 2009.[7] The National Quality Forum, a private, nonprofit membership organization recognized for its national leadership in healthcare quality improvement, reviewed and adopted the NCP guidelines as the basis for its Framework for Palliative and Hospice Care Quality Measurement and Reporting. Clinicians and clinical organizations identified 38 best practices for implementation.[8] Quality indicators are being developed to evaluate the impact of those practices.

All clinical recommendations are not equivalent. Their importance will vary with the likelihood of significant benefit or harm avoidance to the patient. The evidence and experience that provides the foundation for the

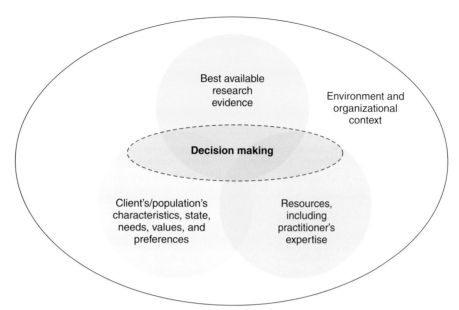

Fig. 9-1   **The interdisciplinary model of evidence-based clinical decisions.** (Adapted from Satterfield et al. Toward a transdisciplinary model of evidence based practice. Milbank Quarterly, 2009; 87(2), 368–390.)

recommendation will also vary in quality depending on the methods used to produce the results. Frameworks have been developed to rate these factors within a set of clinical guidelines. These frameworks use a letter designation for how strongly the practice recommendation is made or how uniform the consensus is for the recommendation, and a numeral designation for the quality of the evidence supporting that recommendation (Tables 9-2 and 9-3).

The randomized controlled trial (RCT) is considered the gold standard for evaluating the effect of treatment interventions. The RCT study design minimizes the likelihood that bias in the selection of research participants or in the evaluation of the study outcomes will influence the results. RCTs are prospective interventions, providing evidence of cause and effect.

Other research designs that generate evidence include prospective non-randomized trials and observational cohorts; retrospective record reviews, interviews, or surveys; cross sectional studies; qualitative, ethnographic research; and case series or reports. Observational studies may yield associations

but cannot determine cause and effect; hence, they are rated lower than RCTs for quality of evidence to support a particular clinical intervention. Similarly, qualitative studies are considered a source of credible evidence but are considered less informative about cause and effects than RCTs.[9] Expert consensus is the least-rigorous level of evidence but recognizes the knowledge accumulated through serial observations by experts in the field. It is therefore possible to have strong recommendations that are supported only by expert opinion.

The Working Group on Antiretroviral Therapy and Medical Management of HIV-Infected Children is made up of experts from different disciplines. This group is rating their clinical recommendations in the manner described above. However, they recognized that some of their strongest recommendations were based on the adoption of practices proved efficacious in rigorous, well-powered clinical trials of adult patients with minimal supporting evidence in a pediatric population. Following the framework above would result in a rating the supporting evidence as Level III—Expert Opinion. Yet this did not adequately

TABLE 9-1   Assumptions and Challenges of Evidence-Based Practice in Pediatric Palliative Care

Assumptions	Challenges
1. The healthcare professions involved in pediatric* palliative care, including medicine, nursing, psychology, social work, child life and others, are a science and an applied profession with equal contribution to the art and science of clinical practice.	1. Most palliative care evidence found in the literature is adult-focused. There is a paucity of pediatric specific evidence.
2. Evidence is the synthesis of scientific knowledge, clinical expertise and patient and family preferences to guide shared decision making.	2. Pediatric* patients represent a vulnerable population who are often excluded from research trials (Lorenz, et al., December 2004).
3. Evidence must undergo critical appraisal prior to recommendations for practice changes.	3. The scope of practice may be too narrow for standard literature search engines.
4. Evidence-based practice influences clinical outcomes.	4. Much of palliative care research is qualitative or descriptive in nature.
5. Resources and contextual factors in pediatric palliative care practice must be considered.	5. Multiple models exist for critical appraisal and synthesis of the evidence.
6. Pediatric palliative care is a transdisciplinary practice for which a common language must be defined.	6. The value of expert clinicians within and between disciplines is unclear and often underestimated in determining EBP recommendations.
7. The perceived value of evidence may vary depending upon the discipline of practice.	7. Evidence must be defined broadly and considered within the context of the specific clinical issue.
	8. Evidence is published in a wide variety of journals pertinent to a spectrum of diseases.

*(Pediatrics is defined as the care of children, adolescents and young adults.)
Adapted from Satterfield, JM, Spring, B, Brownson, RC, Mullen, EJ, Newhouse, RP, Walker, BB, et al. (2009). Toward a transdisciplinary model of evidence-based practice. *The Milbank Quarterly*, 87 (2), 368-390; and Newhouse, RP, Dearholt, SL, Poe, SS, Pugh, LC, & White, KM (2007). *Johns Hopkins Nursing Evidence-Based Practice Model and Guidelines*. Indianapolis: Sigma Theta Tau International.

TABLE 9-2 Framework for Rating Recommendations for Clinical Practice

Strength of recommendation	Quality of evidence for the recommendation	Modified coding for pediatrics
A: Strong recommendation **B:** Moderate recommendation **C:** Optional recommendation	**I:** One or more randomized controlled trials with clinical outcomes and/or validated laboratory endpoints	**I:** One or more randomized trials in children* with clinical outcomes and/or validated laboratory endpoints **I*:** One or more randomized trials in adults with clinical outcomes and/or validated laboratory endpoints with accompanying data in children* from one or more well-designed, nonrandomized trials or observational cohort studies with long-term clinical outcomes
	II: One or more well-designed, nonrandomized trials or observational cohort studies with long-term clinical outcomes	**II:** One or more well-designed, nonrandomized trials or observational cohort studies in children* with long-term clinical outcomes **II*:** One or more well-designed, nonrandomized trials or observational cohort studies in adults with long-term clinical outcomes with accompanying data in children* from one or more smaller nonrandomized trials or cohort studies with clinical outcome data
	III: Expert opinion	**III:** Expert opinion

*Studies that include children or children and adolescents but not studies limited to post-pubertal adolescents.
Adapted from Panel on Antiretroviral Guidelines for Adults and Adolescents: Guidelines for the use of antiretroviral agents in HIV-1 infected adults and adolescents; Guidelines for the Use of Antiretroviral agents in Pediatric HIV Infection. http://aidsinfo.nih.gov/Guidelines/GuidelineDetail.aspx?MenuItem=Guidelines&Search=Off&GuidelineID=7&ClassID=1, and http://aidsinfo.nih.gov/Guidelines/GuidelineDetail.aspx?MenuItem=Guidelines&Search=Off&GuidelineID=8&ClassID=1. Department of Health and Human Services. Published August 16, 2010.

reflect the high quality and compelling results of the evidence that could and should be applied to children with the same life-threatening condition. Therefore the Working Group has modified its rating system to recognize the application in pediatrics of evidence developed in studies of adult patients. An asterisk is added to the numeral to designate that the primary evidence is taken from adult studies and that there is evidence in smaller and more focused pediatric studies that support its application in children.[10]

Ideally, strong evidence underpins all treatment decisions, yet many clinical situations still demand that clinicians use their best professional judgment in the absence of conclusive evidence. This is precisely the definition of evidence-based practice: the integration of individual clinical expertise with the best available external clinical evidence in the care of individual patients.[11]

There are several reasons why a conclusive level of evidence is difficult to obtain in pediatric palliative care. First, designing and conducting randomized trials with seriously ill or dying patients of any age requires meticulous attention to the treatment alternatives, the burden of outcome assessment,[12] and the need for short-term outcome measures given the likelihood that patients may die early in the study. Second, many important questions in palliative care are not answerable through randomized clinical trial design. Finally, the questions that can be answered through RCT, such as comparing two medications for treatment of a specific symptom, are more difficult to conduct in pediatric populations due to a smaller sample of eligible patients, the wide variation in physical development associated with age, and the diversity of disease conditions.[13] Although not ideal, pediatric clinicians must sometimes make treatment decisions based on strong evidence obtained in adult trials and the presumption that there is likelihood of similar benefit in children.[14]

Searching the Palliative Care Literature

Palliative care is a broad category of clinical practice, crossing disciplines, diseases, and ages from prenatal to geriatrics. Thus, literature specific to pediatric palliative care is difficult to identify. Defining a search filter for evidence is essential. Medical Subject Headings (MeSH) terms may not elucidate the true intent of palliative care due to the diffuse nature of the subject area. Using a medical librarian skilled in database searches will help clinicians narrow the focus and screen articles quickly for inclusion or exclusion in review. Hand searches will often be necessary to augment electronic database searches. Multiple text words and phrases are needed in addition to traditional MeSH terms[15] (Table 9-4). In a 2007 study,

TABLE 9-3 National Comprehensive Cancer Network Categories of Evidence and Consensus

Category 1: The recommendation is based on high level evidence (e.g., randomized controlled trials) and there is uniform NCCN consensus.

Category 2A: The recommendation is based on lower level evidence and there is uniform NCCN consensus.

Category 2B: The recommendation is based on lower level evidence and there is non-uniform NCCN consensus (but no major disagreement).

Category 3: The recommendation is based on any level evidence but reflects major disagreement.

All recommendations are category 2A unless otherwise specified.

National Comprehensive Cancer Network Clinical Practice Guidelines in Oncology. NCCN categories of evidence and consensus. Available at http://www.nccn.org/professionals/physician_gls/f_guidelines.asp.

TABLE 9-4 Key MeSH and Text Terms for Searching the Palliative Care Literature

exp advance care planning/or	palliat$.tw. or
exp attitude to death/or	hospice$.tw. or
exp bereavement/or	terminal care.tw. or
death/or	physician-patient relations/or
hospices/or	prognosis/or
life support care/or	quality of life/or
palliative care/or	survival rate/or
terminal care/or	treatment outcomes/or
terminally ill/or	attitude to health/

Adapted from Sladek RM, Tieman J, Currow DC (2007): Improving search filter development: a study of palliative care literature. *BMC Medical Informatics and Decision Making*, 7 (18), 1-7.

use of this search strategy provided 64.7 percent sensitivity, 92 percent specificity, and 91.1 percent accuracy.[16] Information pertinent to searches specific to pediatric palliative care are lacking. However, using the key terms listed in Table 9-4 does yield inclusion of pediatric literature. It is encouraging that the number of clinical trials found in the literature is increasing, although still limited. In a recent systematic review, only 7.22 percent of palliative care literature was noted to be clinical trials.[4] Most palliative care research is qualitative or descriptive in nature, thus placing the level of evidence at Level III.[3] Clinicians are then challenged to use this level of evidence in conjunction with clinical expertise and patient and/or family preferences to optimize decision making.[17]

Examples of EBP in Pediatric Palliative Care

As stated earlier, the science of pediatric palliative care is emerging and critiquing the pediatric palliative care literature is challenging often due to the lack of randomized, controlled trials. Non-randomized clinical studies, cohort studies and even expert opinion provide a base of evidence upon which to plan care. An exemplar is an outstanding example of skilled practice leading to increased knowledge of a subject area.[18] Several exemplars exist in pediatric palliative care that demonstrate the commitment to improve the quality of care through the use of evidence-based practice, although not randomized controlled trials. These include use of symptom control, coping strategies, and outcomes of competence, confidence, and the ability to deal with personal grief when caring for dying children with interdisciplinary palliative care. As is the case with much of the palliative care literature, the following three exemplars are retrospective or cross-sectional cohort studies and qualitative or descriptive case studies that provide valuable evidence to influence practice changes.

EASING OF SUFFERING IN CHILDREN WITH CANCER AT END OF LIFE: IS CARE CHANGING?[19]— LEVEL II, A

This retrospective cohort study was undertaken at a large pediatric institution to investigate changes in patterns of care, advanced care planning, and symptom management by comparing an initial cohort from 1997 with one from 2004 in light of national and local efforts to increase awareness and education surrounding pediatric palliative care. Retrospective chart review and parent surveys were conducted with 102 patients and families from the initial cohort and 119 from the new cohort. This study documented several significant findings in the new cohort as compared to the initial cohort, including: discussions of hospice more often (p < .001) and earlier in the trajectory of illness (p = .002), earlier documentation of Do Not Resuscitate orders (p = 0.31), and a decrease in the number of deaths in an ICU or inpatient setting (p = .024). A decrease in suffering from pain (p = .018) and dyspnea (p = .020) was also reported. Parents also reported feeling more prepared for the medical issues in the last month of life (p < .001) and circumstances surrounding the time of death (p = .002). The investigators concluded that care had changed over time with better emphasis on optimal palliative care and less suffering perceived by parents.

LOOKING BEYOND WHERE CHILDREN DIE: DETERMINANTS AND EFFECTS OF PLANNING A CHILD'S LOCATION OF DEATH[20]—LEVEL II, A

This cross-sectional study of 140 bereaved parents from two tertiary pediatric hospitals in the United States examined factors that influenced the planning by parents of the location of a child's death and its effect on patterns of care and the parents' experience. The investigators documented that 88 percent of parents made a plan and 97 percent were able to accomplish that plan. For those families who had made a plan, more deaths at home with fewer hospitalizations were noted (p < .001). Parents felt more prepared during their child's end of life (p < .007) and were very comfortable with their choice of the location of death (p < .001). More deaths occurred in the ICU or inpatient setting for those patients who did not have a plan for location of death (p < .001). In those same patients, less intubation was noted (p = .029). Comprehensive communication and education by the healthcare team and adequate home care support are essential to improving coping for parents of children at the end-of-life stage.

INTERDISCIPLINARY INTERVENTIONS TO IMPROVE PEDIATRIC PALLIATIVE CARE AND REDUCE HEALTHCARE PROFESSIONAL SUFFERING[21]—LEVEL II, B

This prospective, descriptive study of a quality improvement project investigated the impact of interdisciplinary healthcare team education and support on competence, confidence, and the ability to deal with personal grief when caring for dying children. During a 19-month period, 100 sessions were conducted for 950 healthcare professional participants. The investigators documented that this model of a combination of an open forum for interdisciplinary team networking and communication, palliative care rounds, and patient care conferences improved self reports of competence and confidence in caring for children at the end of life. They also found improved self-coping strategies for grief and bereavement through education and improved communication.

Efforts to Build the Evidence Base in Pediatric Palliative Care

Pediatric palliative care investigators are building the body of evidence using a variety of research designs in single- and multiple-site studies. Multicenter clinical trials evaluating treatments for serious and life-threatening disorders in children, such as the Children's Oncology Group (COG) and the International Maternal, Pediatric, and Adolescent AIDS Clinical Trials (IMPAACT) Network, offer important opportunities to answer palliative care questions. Primary or secondary study objectives can include incidence and severity of symptoms by treatment group or the impact on health-related quality of life of the treatment under investigation. Substudies or nested studies provide opportunities to ask additional questions within the framework of the larger study. For instance, a smaller sample of adolescent study subjects might participate in an interview about their understanding of the informed consent process for deciding to enroll in the clinical trial.

Research specifically designed to answer pediatric palliative care questions may benefit from this multicenter approach.

The collaboration of several palliative care programs helps to achieve the necessary sample size and to increase the generalization of the study results. Study design can range from RCT to observational cohort studies to cross-sectional surveys. Although single-site studies may be limited by the available sample of eligible patients, specific types of questions, such as the pharmacokinetics of a new medication, may be answered through intensive evaluation of fewer subjects. Other study designs might generate new hypotheses or questions to be answered in future larger, multicenter studies. The "n-of-1 clinical trial" is recognized as an important method for determining the optimum regimen for an individual patient.[22] It too may generate hypotheses for larger studies.

Secondary data analysis and the use of public databases takes advantage of information already gathered to answer questions relevant to palliative care. For instance, the use of particular health services or specific prescription drugs may be investigated using insurance databases. Vital records provide data regarding causes of death by age and geographic region.

Limitations of Evidence in Pediatric Palliative Care

Each child and family receiving palliative care is unique. The usefulness of evidence must be viewed in light of both the individual and specific contextual factors surrounding the clinical practice decisions. Randomized controlled clinical trials are few in palliative care and even less common for pediatrics. Qualitative evidence is valuable and should be considered as appropriate. Clinicians must be skilled at critical appraisal of the evidence. Many models of EBP exist and should be examined for appropriateness to goals of the clinician, the institution, and the patient and family. EBP should not be used as mandatory practice standards but should be guidelines for clinical decision making in light of these goals. The practice of pediatric palliative care is broad but the evidence is often from a narrow focus of a specific symptom or issue. A holistic perspective is required for optimal decision making in pediatric palliative care and isolated evidence must be evaluated in the context of the broad picture. Decisions must be individualized and reassessed throughout the continuum of care. Efficacy of treatment must be evaluated at regular intervals and the treatment plan adjusted as the patient's condition changes and/or new evidence emerges.[23] Education of clinicians, patient, and families is paramount to success of any EBP initiative.

Summary

There is a variety of sources and breadth of knowledge in the palliative care literature. Little of this literature is specific to pediatrics. Opportunities for research within the domains of pediatric palliative care exist to expand the evidence base. The search strategies are cumbersome and time-consuming, requiring refinement. The development of pediatric palliative care specialty journals would improve efficiency and provide a platform for peer review. Growth is expansive in palliative care literature in general and within the discipline of pediatrics as well. Unfortunately, the need for clinical practice guidelines and tools for evidence-based practice are rising at a faster rate than the evidence base. The provision of pediatric palliative care is best provided within the context of the interdisciplinary team through which those collaborative efforts may generate and evaluate evidence, particularly evidence related to culturally sensitive pediatric palliative care. The knowledge and backgrounds of the interdisciplinary team members from medicine, nursing, psychology, social work, pastoral care, child life, and others provide unique opportunities to not only generate research inquiry but also to assess the strength of peer-reviewed evidence as it relates to their practice domains and patients.

REFERENCES

1. Satterfield JM, Spring B, Brownson RC, Mullen EJ, Newhouse RP, Walker BB, et al: Toward a transdisciplinary model of evidence-based practice, *Milbank Q* 87(2):368–390, 2009.
2. DiCenso A, Ciliska D, Guyatt G: Introduction to evidence-based nursing. In DiCenso A, Guyatt G, Ciliska D, *Evidence-Based Nursing: A Guide to Clinical Practice*, St Louis, 2005, Elsevier Mosby, pp 3–19.
3. Newhouse RP, Dearholt SL, Poe SS, Pugh LC, White KM: *Johns Hopkins Nursing Evidence-Based Practice Model and Guidelines*, Indianapolis, 2007, Sigma Theta Tau International.
4. Tiemann J, Sladek R, Currow D: Changes in the quantity and level of evidence of palliative and hospice care literature: the last century, *J Clin Oncol* 26(35):5679–5683, 2008.
5. Rutledge DN, Bookbinder M: Processes and outcomes of evidence-based practice, *Semin Oncol Nurs* 18(1):3–10, 2002.
6. Lorenz K, Lynn J, Morton SC, Dy S, Mularski R, Shugarman L, et al: *End-of-life Care and Outcomes, Evidence Report/Technology Assessment No 110*, Prepared by the Southern California Evidence-based Practice Center, under Contract No 290–02–0003. Rockville, Md, 2004, Agency for Healthcare Research and Quality.
7. National Consensus Project for Quality Palliative Care: *Clinical Practice Guidelines for Quality Palliative Care*, ed 2, 2009. Available at www.nationalconsensusproject.org. Accessed May 28, 2010.
8. National Quality Forum: *A National Framework and Preferred Practices for Palliative and Hospice Care Quality*, Washington, DC, 2006, National Quality.
9. Powers BA: Critically appraising qualitative evidence. In Melnyk BM, Fineout-Overholt E, editors: *Evidence-Based Practice in Nursing & Healthcare: A Guide to Best Practice*, Philadelphia, 2005, Lippincott Williams & Wilkins, pp 127–167.
10. Working Group on Antiretroviral Therapy and Medical Management of HIV-Infected Children: *Guidelines for the Use of Antiretroviral Agents in Pediatric HIV Infection*. In press. Available at http://aidsinfo.nih.gov/ContentFiles/PediatricGuidelines.pdf. Accessed May 28, 2010.
11. Sackett DL, Rosenberg WM, Gray JA, Haynes RB, Richardson WS: Evidence-based medicine: what it is and what it isn't, *BMJ* 312:71–72, 1996.
12. AAHPM: *Statement on Palliative Care Research Ethics*, 2007, Available at http://www.aahpm.org/positions/researchethics.html. Accessed February 6, 2010.
13. American Academy of Pediatrics, Committee of Drugs: guidelines for the ethical conduct of studies to evaluate drugs in pediatric populations, *Pediatrics* 95(2):286–294, 1995.
14. Food and Drug Administration. *Guidance for Industry: General considerations for pediatric pharmacokinetic studies for drugs and biological products*, November 30, 1998, Available at www.fda.gov/downloads/Drugs/GuidanceComplianceRegulatoryInformation/Guidances/ucm072114.pdf. Accessed February 10, 2010.
15. Sladek R, Tieman J, Fazekas BS, Abernathy AP, Currow DC: Development of a subject search filter to find information relevant to palliative care in the general medical literature, *J Med Libr Assoc* 94(4):394–401, 2006.
16. Sladek RM, Tieman J, Currow DC: Improving search filter development: a study of palliative care literature, *BMC Med Inform Decis Mak* 7(18):1–7, 2007.
17. Whitney SN, Holmes-Rovner M, Brody H, Schneider C, McCullough LB, Volk RJ, et al: Beyond shared decision making: an expanded typology of medical decisions, *Med Decis Making* 28:699–705, 2008.
18. Giordano BP: Clinical exemplars demonstrate perioperative nurses' courage and commitment to quality patient care, *AORN* 63(1):15–18, 1996.

19. Wolfe J, Hammel JM, Edwards KE, Duncan J, Comeau M, Breyer J, Aldridge SA, Grier HE, Berde C, Dussel V, Weeks JC: Easing of suffering in children with cancer: is care changing? *J Clin Oncol* 26(10): 1717–1723, 2008.

20. Dussel V, Kreicburgs U, Hilden JM, Watterson J, Moore C, Turner BG, Weeks JC, Wolfe J: Looking beyond where children die: determinents and effects of planning a child's location of death, *J Pain Symptom Manage* 37(1):33–43, 2009.

21. Rushton CH, Reder E, Hall B, Comello K, Sellers DE, Hutton N: Interdisciplinary interventions to to improve pediatric palliative care and reduce health care professional suffering, *J Palliat Med* 9(4): 922–933, 2006.

22. Evans CH, Ildstad ST, editors: *Small clinical trials: issues and challenges,* 2001, Available at http://www.nap.edu/openbook.php?record_id=10078&page=155. Accessed Feb. 10, 2010.

23. American College of Physicians & American Society of Health-System Pharmacists. Principles of Palliative Care Practice. In *ACP PIER & AHFS DI® Essentials™.* 2009, http://online.statref.com/titleinfo/fxid-92.html. Accessed Nov. 14, 2009.

Research Considerations in Pediatric Palliative Care

BETTY DAVIES | KIMBERLEY WIDGER | ROSE STEELE |
SUSAN CADELL | HAROLD SIDEN | LYNN STRAATMAN

No one can whistle a symphony. It takes an orchestra to play it.
— Halford E. Luccock

While the actual number of patients in pediatric palliative care is small relative to the number of adults, the scope of the field is vast. There are many areas and opportunities for research with the children, parents, siblings, extended family members, and peers, as well as the teachers, clinicians, and volunteers who work with the children and their families. There is diversity in the types of diseases, illness trajectories, biopsychosocial and spiritual facets of illness, developmental aspects of childhood, and care at diagnosis, end-of-life, and into bereavement. There also is a need to explore how to best translate completed research into improving care for children and families and a need to better support those who provide the care.

The opportunities, joys, and rewards of conducting research in any of these areas are many, but there also are challenges or pitfalls to be overcome or avoided. While many of the joys and challenges are not unique to pediatric palliative care, some of the distinct aspects of the field bring an additional level of complexity to the associated research. In this chapter, we review priority areas of research in pediatric palliative care. We also identify and explore various methodological and ethical issues inherent in research in this field and suggest methods to address them, including conducting research as a team. Our own research team, Transitions in Pediatric Palliative and End-of-life Care (PEDPALNET), was created following a call for proposals by the Canadian Institutes of Health Research (CIHR) to develop collaborative, multidisciplinary research teams organized around particular areas of study in palliative care. Of the nine teams funded across Canada, our team was the only one with a particular focus on pediatrics. Some of the examples we use in this chapter are from our experiences conducting research as a team over the last five years.

Priority Areas for Research

The Institute of Medicine (IOM) report on improving palliative and end-of-life care for children and their families highlighted the lack of research and systematic data on which to base their recommendations.[1] The authors identified a critical need for research in all aspects of pediatric palliative and end-of-life care and recommended focusing research activities on "the effectiveness of: clinical interventions including symptom management; methods for improving communication and decision-making; innovative arrangements for delivering,

coordinating, and evaluating care, including interdisciplinary care teams and quality improvement strategies, and different approaches to bereavement care."[1]

Others also have worked to identify research priorities. The four top questions identified from a Delphi survey with pediatric palliative care researchers and clinicians in Canada were: What matters most for patients and parents receiving pediatric palliative care? What are the bereavement needs of families in pediatric palliative care? What are the best practice standards in pain and symptom management? What are effective strategies to alleviate suffering at the end of life?[2] In pediatric oncology, the areas of palliative and end-of-life care have been identified as research priorities. Recommendations include a focus on: decision making and communication, characteristics of death and profiles of bereaved family members and health professionals, trajectories of dying, a comparison between the care provided and the care that was desired by families, financial cost of death after cancer, and outcomes from symptom management and bereavement support.[3,4]

The identified priority areas are broad enough to leave opportunities for exploring a wide range of specific research questions. Experience suggests that researchers need to identify the questions that keep them up at night. The questions need to be exciting and interesting enough to researchers so that they will keep going despite the inevitable challenges. Given the current lack of research in the field, it is likely that initial studies are needed to develop appropriate indicators or measures and to more fully understand the experiences and needs of a particular population. Initial studies should be completed before the most burning questions can be answered with designs such as randomized controlled trials (RCT) of interventions.

It has historically been challenging to obtain funding for pediatric palliative care research, partly because the major government funding agencies have agendas and limited resources that may not be supportive of this type of research. In Canada, the government recognized the importance of creating a health agenda that incorporated palliative care into the spectrum of care provided to its citizens. Therefore, in 2004 Canada took a leadership role in funding palliative care research through the CIHR, which is one of the three major research funding agencies in the country. Palliative care was identified as a priority and a targeted competition was held to create interdisciplinary teams (IDT) to facilitate the development of programs of research. Our own team was funded as a result of this competition and we remain the largest funded team in pediatric palliative care in Canada. However, we work in collaboration with colleagues from across the country who also may have their own more local teams. Subsequent funding for our work was obtained through operating fund competitions, but no further resources have been allocated specifically for palliative care let alone for pediatric palliative care. In the United States, the seminal work of the IOM on Approaching Death, published in 1997, explicated gaps in scientific knowledge. In response, the director of the National Institutes of Health (NIH) designated the National Institute for Nursing Research (NINR) to serve as the lead Institute at NIH for end-of-life research. To coordinate this effort, NINR has established the Office of Research on End-of-Life Science and Palliative Care, Investigator Training, and Education (OEPC) and offered numerous Program Announcements (PA) that solicit research pertaining to end-of-life care. The one PA that specifically addressed pediatrics (Improving Care for Dying Children and Their Families – PA 04-57) is inactive although pediatric proposals can be submitted in response to other PAs.

Methodological Challenges

When considering the development of a study in the area of pediatric palliative care, researchers need to be aware of potential impediments to their success. Some of the methodological challenges include research design, outcome measures, recruitment and sampling, and research teams. While ethical challenges are alluded to in this section, they will be discussed more fully later in the chapter.

RESEARCH DESIGN

Though the gold standard for research remains the RCT with the highest level of evidence being systematic reviews of multiple RCTs, primarily qualitative designs and descriptive methods may be more appropriate to address the research priorities and knowledge in pediatric palliative care.[1] Further, RCTs are difficult to conduct in both adult and pediatric palliative care. The heterogeneity of diseases, illness trajectories, and ages of participants are difficult to accommodate in a design that requires a homogeneous group of participants and testing of simple standardized interventions.[5] Bensink et al.[6] made two attempts to use an RCT to test videophones as a support for families receiving pediatric palliative care, but all families approached refused to participate. When the research team changed the design to an acceptability study, without randomization or any measures to be completed by the family, they had a participation rate of more than 90%. These researchers suggested that a clinical trial is overwhelming for families when initiated at the transition to palliative care. Kane, Hellsten, and Coldsmith[7] discussed the interpersonal relationships at the heart of palliative care and the need for understanding complex interactions among humans in order to identify the social and spiritual interventions needed to address human suffering. It may be that these interactions are not amenable to the quantified measurement and standardization needed for an RCT. Levels of evidence that may be more relevant for palliative care include quasi-experimental studies, qualitative studies, and consensus opinions of palliative care experts.[8]

Longitudinal studies in pediatric palliative care have been uncommon, but are useful in expanding the evidence base. Researchers who embark on longitudinal work need to design their studies in ways that will minimize attrition. Though families in pediatric palliative care often participate in research as a way of helping others, even when they find it challenging practically or emotionally,[9] researchers need to pay attention to keeping families involved in a study over time. A number of effective strategies have been reported in the literature,[10–13] and we are using some of them in our longitudinal study with families where a child has a progressive metabolic, neurological, or chromosomal condition and in our parent caregiver study. Development of a solid relationship with families is crucial. An initial face-to-face visit, telephone contact at prescribed intervals, and letters to thank families for their participation are useful for building and maintaining relationships. Continuity of research assistants or other personnel involved in the study is important and will contribute to the trusting relationship that is needed to help participants feel more connected to and interested in the study over time. Efforts should be made to respect families' time and to recognize the value of their contribution. Researchers should schedule data collection at the family's convenience and should regularly express verbal and written appreciation for their participation in the study. In addition, providing a monetary or other gift as a token of appreciation along with a letter thanking them for participation may encourage families to remain in a study, because families feel valued when their time and effort is recognized. Strategies that limit attrition will result in the type of high quality data needed to provide solid, evidence-based care.

Parent Participation

Parents in all of the studies we have undertaken as a team have given us feedback about what they see as being the value of their participation. In some cases this feedback was solicited and in others it was offered by the parents without our invitation. Our parent caregiver study has provided several touching examples. Many of the 273 participants took the time to do more than simply answer a survey. They wrote comments on the forms or sent letters to accompany their returning questionnaires. One mother wrote five pages about her story and added questions that she thought should be asked in the research. Another mother wrote a note about her depression, her partner leaving her, and the need to keep moving forward with a smile for her daughter who did not ask to be born as she was. Other parents have called the toll-free number to give us updates on their situations or thank us for the research. Some of our studies include or are solely comprised of qualitative interviews. Parents have commented on their desire to participate in research in order to make the difficult situations that they have experienced less difficult for someone else. Many parents want to participate in research. They also want the opportunity to decide for themselves if a study is right for them.

OUTCOME MEASURES

Science can progress no further than the measurement of its key variables.— ATTRIBUTED TO J. NUNNALLY, 1994

Unfortunately, in pediatric palliative care the most important variables or outcomes to be measured are not well defined, and there are few valid measures. Outcomes usually involve a change in the health status of the individual, but also can include increased knowledge of health conditions, changes in behavior related to health, or patient and family satisfaction with the care received and its outcomes.[14] The expected outcome for the child in pediatric palliative care is death, which cannot be changed. However, one can improve the quality of that death[15] and the family's satisfaction with the care provided. One also may be able to improve health outcomes for the family including reduction in the incidence and severity of depression, anxiety, post traumatic stress, guilt, and complicated grief.

Research in adult palliative care is more advanced than that of pediatrics; however, that field of research is still relatively recent and similar issues about the difficulty of identifying and measuring important outcomes have been reported. There has been some research in adult palliative care asking patients and family members to identify components of quality care and of a good death.[16–18] A number of measures have been developed and used with adult palliative care patients and their families (Mularski et al[19]). However, for multiple reasons, including the developmental level of children, the variables and/or outcomes and measures used in research with adults cannot simply be taken and applied to children. For example, one outcome deemed indicative of quality care for adults is that death occurs at home.[20] In children, this outcome may not be as indicative of quality end-of-life care. Dussel, Kreicbergs, Hilden et al.[21] found that the opportunity to plan the location of death was more important to parents than where the death actually occurred. Satisfaction is another outcome that has been identified as a component of quality care.[14] However, satisfaction has not been well conceptualized in the literature and may be influenced by demographic variables.[22] In end-of-life care, there is a concern that families have very low levels of expectation and therefore are easily satisfied with care.[23] In pediatric palliative care, there is evidence that parents tend to report high levels of satisfaction even when high levels of distressing symptoms are reported.[24] Thus, satisfaction may not be a good indicator of the actual quality of care.

Given that research in adult palliative care is more prevalent than in pediatric palliative care, pediatric researchers can learn from their adult-researching counterparts about possible instruments, methods, and research designs that might be useful. However, this information must be critically examined to see how instruments might need to be altered to fit the pediatric population. Any alterations must be based on clinical expertise and done with an intimate understanding of the population to be studied. This speaks to the need for researchers and clinicians to work together to conduct appropriate research in pediatric palliative care.

Given that there is no single instrument encompassing all of the dimensions of care in pediatric palliative care, researchers must choose among several to measure the specific domains of interest. Those domains will include tools that are specific to areas such as pain and other symptoms, the child's emotional well-being, family issues, and spiritual support. There is no single instrument in these fields that answers all questions. For example, in studying families one may want to know about marriage and relationship stability, personal growth, family stress and functioning, or the health of individuals.

The Team for Research with Adolescents and Children in Palliation and Grief (TRAC-PG) at Toronto's Hospital for Sick Children (SickKids) has compiled a list of instruments that some of its members have used with children, adolescents, and adults in pediatric palliative and end-of-life care research. This list is available on TRAC-PG's website at www.tracpg.ca/index. pho/researchers/instruments_measures_scales, but caution should be used when reviewing these instruments for future research. As previously noted, few measures have been specifically validated for use in pediatric palliative care. Many of the measures have also been used with parents in the months or years after their child's death.

RECRUITMENT AND SAMPLING

There are several challenges in identifying, accessing, and recruiting a sample to take part in a study related to pediatric palliative care. The number of children who die each year is small relative to the number of adults. However, small numbers at any one center may make it difficult to access a large enough sample to fit with particular research designs. As well, many children have rare illnesses where there may be very few in one country or around the world, let alone within a particular institution. Two possible methods to increase the size of the accessible population are to use disease groupings rather than single diseases or to conduct multicenter research.

Disease Groupings

The Association for Children with Life Threatening or Terminal Conditions and their Families (ACT) and the Royal College of Paediatrics and Child Health identified four distinct groups, or quadrants, of conditions (Table 10-1) seen in children who may not live until adulthood and who require palliative care.[25] Though there is some fluidity regarding which quadrant a condition fits into, conditions in a quadrant are similar to each other in terms of the expected trajectory and time course of the illness. Therefore, when planning a study, rather than only including children with a particular neurodegenerative condition, it may be possible, depending on the type of research questions being asked, to increase the available population by including children with any condition that fits into Quadrant 3.

Multicenter Research

Recruiting participants through a number of centers is another way to increase the size of the research population and to broaden the racial, ethnic, and geographic diversity of the sample.[26] However, multicenter research may raise other

TABLE 10-1 Association for Children with Life-Threatening or Terminal Conditions and Their Families and the Royal College of Paediatrics and Child Health Quadrants of Conditions That May Require Palliative Care

Quadrant 1	Quadrant 2
Conditions that can be cured but have a possibility of death (e.g., cancer)	Conditions requiring intensive medical therapy but are ultimately terminal (e.g., cystic fibrosis, HIV/AIDS)

Quadrant 3	Quadrant 4
Conditions that have no cure but whose symptoms can be managed (e.g., neurodegenerative, metabolic disease)	Severe neurological impairments where complications may lead to early death (e.g., anoxic brain injury)

challenges. The need for ethical approval at each site may add an additional six months or more to the time required to start a study.[27] Additional associated costs must be factored in to grant proposals. A great deal of negotiation may be needed to ensure that recruitment strategies at each site will meet the requirements of local ethics boards, but are similar enough to each other to not threaten the validity of the study findings.

Participatory action research (PAR) is one method that may help to overcome some recruitment challenges. PAR involves extensive collaboration between the researchers and those affected by the issue that is being studied.[28,29] In pediatric palliative care research, PAR has been used to some extent with both clinicians and families. For example, one study involved collaboration between a group of researchers and a group of clinicians who were providing hospice care. This collaboration included design and implementation of a project to evaluate the care provided by the clinical team. Trust between the two groups and active involvement of the clinicians in all aspects of the research facilitated recruitment of families as participants, as well as increased the uptake of study findings by the clinician group.[30] In a similar project designed to evaluate a hospice program, the research team used PAR with the families. This collaboration ensured project objectives and methods used for data collection were sensitive to family needs and issues and were meaningful to participants.[31]

The positive outcomes from such studies suggest that using PAR with clinicians and families in pediatric palliative care may assist with some of the challenges to recruitment. Even if all of the principles of PAR are not followed, some evidence that a research protocol has been developed with direct input of families may be helpful in receiving ethics approval as well as funding for pediatric palliative care studies. We have found that including families' input early as we design our studies, for example, asking families about the suitability of the potential instruments or piloting the accrual process with families, has contributed to an increased success rate for our funding proposals. It has also smoothed the process of conducting research, from receiving funding to ethical approval to recruitment.

Accessing Families

Once approval for a study has been obtained from the appropriate ethics boards, researchers generally need to rely on clinicians for assistance in recruiting participants. Clinicians who are not part of the research team or who have little experience with palliative or end-of-life care research may add to recruitment challenges if they act as gatekeepers to potential participants, especially if they are reluctant to identify potential participants.[32] Yet, parents often want to make the decision themselves about whether they participate, rather than have clinicians make that decision for them.[32] Tomlinson and colleagues highlighted the important impact that clinicians can have on recruitment.[33] Hinds[34] found that up to 8.6% of potential parent participants for a study that took place months to years after a child's death were placed in a "do not approach" category by clinicians. The proportion deemed not approachable by clinicians rose to 26.8% in studies where the child was still alive, but where an end-of-life decision had been made. Hinds also reported that 54.9% of potentially eligible families in an end-of-life decision-making study were not referred to the study team, often because of the rush to transfer the child home once this type of decision was made.

The urgency of the situation meant that clinicians sometimes forgot to make the referral or believed that the timing was inappropriate. As noted above, the use of PAR with clinicians may help to address their concerns about approaching families and may facilitate recruitment. As well, sharing existing evidence about the benefits of research for families and the ability of families to make their own choices may help to allay concerns. (This type of evidence is discussed later in this chapter under ethics.) Researchers should track the numbers of eligible participants who are not approached to participate in a study because the final sample may not be representative of the population under study. The findings of a study must be interpreted with this possibility in mind.

It is worth noting that once a researcher gains access to families, response rates are relatively good so long as it is easy for them to take part.[34] Our own experience in a recent study about parental caregiving (CIHR – MOP89984; S. Cadell, PI) when a child has a life-limiting illness illustrates the high response rate. Of the 367 potential participants who called our toll-free number, only 4 declined to participate after hearing about the study. After eliminating ineligible parents and a few who could not be contacted, a total of 339 survey packages were sent out. The return rate was 82.6% ($n = 280$ packages), but seven packages were unusable so the final sample size was 273. In another study exploring fathers' experiences, only two of the 70 fathers who agreed to participate in the study were unavailable for a second interview. Families who choose to participate in pediatric palliative care research tend to be committed to following through on their participation.

Involving Children

Another issue in sampling is the inability of children to participate in research because of developmental and cognitive limitations associated with their young age or as a result of their illness. However, researchers must make special efforts to listen to children themselves whenever possible so that their points of view are also taken into account in the development of knowledge in pediatric palliative care.[35] Creative ways of collecting data, such as video diaries, may be a useful complement to traditional ways of obtaining information.[36]

Gender and Diversity Challenges

Much of the research in pediatric palliative care in North America is based on English-speaking mothers who are Caucasian. In a recent review of 45 papers reporting on research about parents' perspectives on pediatric palliative care, only 25% of the total sample was made up of fathers.[37] Yet, there is some evidence of gender differences that may impact the types of interventions that should be offered to parents.[38] An NIH-funded study is currently examining fathers' experiences in pediatric palliative care (1R01 NR009430-01A1 [B. Davies, PI]). Similarly, a review of the prevalence of different languages and cultures in North American pediatric palliative care research found very few studies with greater than 20% non-Caucasian participants and only two that offered interviews or instruments in languages other than English.[39] Work is needed to translate validated tools into languages other than English. Careful planning and use of novel study designs, methods of recruitment, and data collection may be needed to ensure that the voices of children, fathers, and families from various cultural backgrounds are included in research in pediatric palliative care.[37,40,41]

RESEARCH TEAMS

Embedded in valuing the various perspectives that different disciplines bring to care, pediatric palliative care is usually delivered by an IDT. Similarly the conduct of research can be enhanced by working with an interdisciplinary research team. Though interdisciplinary research teams predominate in pediatric palliative care, one-discipline teams also have contributed to the field. For example, there has been work by physicians in symptom control, such as Joanne Wolfe[24] and her team in the United States and John Collins with his team in Australia.

Given that children who receive palliative and end-of-life care can be found in many areas of the hospital and community, a team of researchers who come from several care areas may facilitate recruitment. Conducting research as a team can assist in overcoming some recruitment challenges, but it also can create others. A multidisciplinary research approach and multicenter studies may bring together a team of researchers with a different set of philosophies, which can be challenging to accommodate. Yet finding ways to learn from one another can lead to uncovering new and better ways of conducting research and contributing to quality care for children and families.

Research Team Functioning

We knew from the literature and our clinical experiences that we needed to study the trajectories of children requiring palliative care. So we met face to face to lay the groundwork for developing a proposal. Everyone had really good ideas, but our discussion went in circles for a time. We were getting frustrated because we seemed to be at cross-purposes and we could not zero in on the central issue. We stopped to reflect on the process, and then it hit us—we were talking about the same topic, but from very different perspectives. A couple of us were focused on children's symptoms in orphaned diseases; another was imagining a study about the psychosocial aspects of children with cancer and other conditions; and others wanted to focus on the needs of families with children of varying diagnoses. Once we understood where we were all coming from, we could clearly identify and appreciate our varying points of view. It then became easy to name the paths of discovery that could be incorporated into our proposed study and to see how they fit with one another. Given our commitment to a non-hierarchical approach and to having a consensus in decisions, no single point of view took priority. Rather we combined all perspectives, including our various clinical and research backgrounds, and this approach resulted in a proposal for a much more comprehensive study than any one of us alone imagined or would have written. The synergy produced a longitudinal study, which was funded by CIHR and is in progress, that is innovative and opportune. It focuses on a population that is under-researched and not well-understood and will provide information about the symptoms of 300 children across Canada. These children have progressive metabolic, neurological, or chromosomal conditions and the study will include their family's associated emotional, social, physical, and spiritual experiences. None of us separately would have seen the whole picture that was developed by the team.

Effective teams are built on respect, flexibility, and shared goals, and behaviors such as communication, continuous assessment of progress on goals, and taking time to have fun together. It also needs to have efficient and effective support

from staff members who also are valued team members. Each member needs to work on understanding the views of others and must strive to respect and accept the differences that can arise when people come from various disciplines and philosophical and/or theoretical perspectives. It is not uncommon for members of two disciplines to use the same term, but to hold it to different meanings. Communication is essential so that misunderstandings and differing interpretations are recognized, discussed, and resolved to the greatest extent possible. Even something as simple as an acronym can cause confusion. For example, a physician or social worker may not understand a nurse who introduces herself as a CNS, because to them that term means central nervous system. The nurse, however, is a Clinical Nurse Specialist.

For a research team to be effective and productive, it is essential to lay a solid foundation where team functioning is detailed and formalized at the beginning, such as through a charter. The charter may include a process for decision making, inter-researcher relations, researcher-staff relations, researcher-collaborator relations and management roles, frequency of communication, roles and responsibilities of team members, guidelines for authorship, and so on (see Box 10-1 for a section of the PEDPALNET Charter on decision-making). Time spent in getting to know each other, and laying out expectations, including time commitment, and goals for the team at the start will enhance team functioning help get the team off to a good start. If team members are separated geographically, both face-to-face and frequent virtual meetings are essential to keep the team connected and allow for ongoing development. We recommend regularly scheduled teleconferences, as well as a web-based system to share files and develop and refine proposals and manuscripts, as ways of maintaining needed contact amongst members.

A research team may be from a single institution or from multiple institutions. The team may come together for a single study or it may work multiple studies around a particular theme. Other collaborators may be involved on specific projects as needed. Teams that come together for a single study can certainly be effective; however, a team that comes together for multiple studies will have more opportunities to develop truly collaborative relationships within the team.

One of the challenges of conducting team research is the varied interests of each member. It may be difficult to include all members on every project. We have found it helpful to rotate the person responsible for each project, so it fits well with the leader's interests and experience. In terms of authorship for the various publications that result from each project, we have found the International Committee of Medical Journal Editors (ICMJE) guidelines most useful.[42] It also is best to discuss potential authors and the author order prior to writing. Finally, though collaborative research is valued in many areas, academic institutions may favor individual authorship. It is incumbent on researchers to familiarize their academic settings with

BOX 10-1   PEDPALNET Process for Decision Making

The PEDPALNET will use a modified "shades of agreement" approach where there are classes of agreement. Result is one of five classes: unconditional agreement, agreement with minor modifications, agreement with major modifications, agreement with strong reservations, such as "disagree, but will not stop the decision," and full veto. In the case of full veto, discussion continues until one of the other four levels is reached.

the importance of collaborative research in an interdisciplinary field. Researchers also need them to be aware that a study from a multidisciplinary team is more likely to be applied to practice and thus to meet the knowledge translation requirements of major funding agencies.

Ethics

Even with the best research team assembled and a population available to meet the requirements of the research design, there may still be challenges to starting a study. These challenges may begin with an institutional ethics review board, which may include members reluctant to approve studies related to palliative, end-of-life, or bereavement care. Challenges also may come from the clinicians involved with families, who are reluctant to identify eligible participants even if the study has been ethically approved. Clinicians not familiar with pediatric palliative care research may have concerns about overburdening families during a difficult time, and they may try to protect families from these perceived burdens.

Children are under-represented in many areas of health research. They are considered to be inherently vulnerable due to their cognitive development, inability to understand the risks and benefits of taking part in research, and power differentials between the researcher and the child.[1,43] When the child is also dying, a second layer of vulnerability is added. Dying persons are considered vulnerable because of: perceived mental and physical frailty, the risks of imposing additional psychological distress, the burden of spending time in research rather than with loved ones or enjoying activities, the concern that patients may feel an obligation to participate in research conducted by their clinicians.[44]

Proxy reports by parents about their child's experience have frequently been used because of the ethical and methodological difficulties of including children in palliative and end-of-life research. Researchers comparing adult patients' and their family members' assessments of care quality found that the greatest congruence was between patients and the family members they lived with or saw every day.[45] In pediatric care, parents generally spend a great deal of time with the ill child and so it is likely that they are the best proxy for the child. Given that children may be non-verbal due to age, their illness, or too weak to participate in research at end-of-life, it is likely that parent reports will continue to be an important component of pediatric palliative care research. However, a skilled clinician or researcher can work directly with children as young as six years.[46] Based on the ethical principle of justice,[47] it is important that children be given more opportunities to share in both the burdens and benefits of the research that has the potential for the greatest impact on meeting their needs and improving the quality of their lives and care.

Another ethical concern about conducting research with dying persons is that the principle of beneficence is difficult to meet—the patient generally does not receive direct benefit from taking part in the research.[47] This concern holds particularly true in pediatric palliative care research, where most studies are qualitative or descriptive and are primarily designed to gain knowledge that will improve the care provided in the future.[48] However, adult patients facing death who participate in research have identified benefits of research participation, such as giving the opportunity for social interaction, making a contribution to society, and discussing their experiences.[49]

Similarly, there is some evidence that adolescents with cancer nearing death take part in research for altruistic reasons, hoping to help others and bring some meaning to their illness.[50] Bereaved parents who have participated in research identify personal benefits including being able to express feelings; revisiting, reflecting on, and making sense of their experiences; and bringing some meaning to the child's life and death.[51] From our experiences, many families in pediatric palliative care identify benefits of research participation and want to decide for themselves about participating in research. The majority of study participants are willing to be contacted about future research. For example, in our recent caregiving study previously discussed more than 90% of the 273 parents indicated their interest in future research and wanted us to contact them if we developed a suitable study.

Family-centered care is the norm in pediatrics and is based on the recognition that there are, in effect, two patients – the child and the family.[52] In addition to acting as proxies for the child, parents are an important group to be included in research to better understand their experiences and need for support. Similarly, research with siblings is important. Ethical concerns about involving siblings in research are similar to those outlined previously because the sibling is usually a child and, therefore, considered inherently vulnerable. Yet, it could be considered paternalistic if siblings are not asked about their experiences. Further, who better to report on their experiences than the siblings themselves?

There is some concern from health professionals and ethics boards that interviewing bereaved families may cause them further pain. However, some studies have highlighted parents' eagerness to share the story of their child's death and to provide input to help other families[53–55] and a few have included a component to systematically examine the emotional impact of participating in research. In the majority of studies, there were no parent reports of negative impact or distress caused by participation.[34,51,56,57] Parents in other studies have reported some degree of negative impact,[58] emotional difficulty,[59] or stress[60] as a result of taking part. However, in one of these studies 99% of parents reported that they thought the research was valuable.[58] Parents also have reported that even though they became tearful or very emotional while talking about their child, it did not mean they wanted or needed to end the interview.[56,61,62]

Hinds et al.[34] provided details from a number of studies related to end-of-life care in pediatric oncology and discussed the challenges faced in obtaining study approval from ethics review boards. Their research also offered methods for overcoming the challenges. It is important to include evidence about the benefits of pediatric palliative care research in grant and ethics proposals. As well, it may be useful to include a component within new studies to assess the participants' perspectives of the benefits and burdens of taking part in the study. We have added a few questions about impact of participation to a longitudinal study we recently started (CIHR – MOP79526, R. Steele & H. Siden, Co-PIs). Parents of children with life-limiting conditions who complete surveys every six months for 18 to 48 months, depending on when they are accrued, will provide information about impact after one year and at the end of participation. Most studies to date have assessed the impact on bereaved parents of taking part in cross-sectional studies that use interviews or written surveys. Little is known about the burdens on parents associated with focus groups, longitudinal studies, and prospective designs, or the burdens of research that may be placed on the ill child or siblings. However, our experiences are that perceived burden by clinicians and ethics board members may not be the same as actual burden.

The risk of inflicting harm on participants in research about pediatric palliative care is certainly a real one. However, this risk does not mean that research should not be done. Families have clearly indicated that research is valuable even when it may be emotionally difficult for them.[56,58] There is growing evidence that children and parents can have their autonomy preserved in being given choices about if, when, and how to take part in research and that they may experience direct benefit from participation even when the study design is primarily meant to benefit future families. Researchers are encouraged to use and expand on this body of evidence, but also to be cognizant of the risks. A good research proposal will identify the areas for potential harm or risk and have plans to prevent, minimize, or address it should it occur. These plans should include careful training and ongoing support for those involved in recruiting or collecting data from participants, lists of easily accessible support services, and availability of emergency supports if a participant becomes severely upset during the research.[26]

Dissemination and Knowledge Exchange

Though still limited, the knowledge base in pediatric palliative care is growing. The new challenge is to translate this knowledge into improved care for children and their families. Traditional dissemination methods, such as publications in peer-reviewed journals, can be difficult because the field remains relatively small, so an editor may not be willing to report results that will not be used by the majority of the journal's readers. Further, trying to publish descriptive and qualitative research in high-impact journals may pose a challenge. There is no specific pediatric palliative care journal, so reaching the right audience can be difficult. In addition, while pediatric and palliative care journals are useful vehicles for publication, there is a tendency to target specific audiences though the knowledge needs to be shared among the professionals who provide interdisciplinary, pediatric palliative care. Yet, given the nature of the field, the development of a specific journal faces its own challenges, such as finding qualified reviewers, attracting sufficient contributors, and obtaining funds to support a journal. In the meantime, potential authors are encouraged to target the mainstream journals and to find other ways of sharing their work.

Most funding agencies now require a knowledge translation plan that goes beyond the traditional venues of conference presentations and publications. In Canada, the CIHR encourages interaction between researchers and the public by funding Café Scientifiques. These CIHR Cafés are designed for the general public and are advertised through various media outlets. Everyone is welcome to attend and there is no admission fee. Our team has held two successful Cafés in coffee shops where we gave short presentations related to pediatric palliative care and then held a question and answer period. The public was very enthusiastic about the format and strongly supported more of these events. They also enjoyed the refreshments that were provided as an integral part of the Café. CIHR also funds some end-of-grant dissemination workshops for researchers, clinicians, and policy makers to meet and facilitate uptake of research into practice. Funding for such innovative dissemination strategies is crucial and researchers need to lobby funding agencies so that support in this burgeoning field of pediatric palliative care is forthcoming.

Researchers in pediatric palliative care need to build capacity in order to address the research priorities. Clinicians who want to conduct their own studies may need to seek additional training and mentorship. Beginning researchers also may need to work with more established researchers or teams to gain experience before leading large projects. For clinicians in particular, there may be opportunities to be involved as a site collaborator in multicenter projects conducted by experienced researchers or to take a lead role in a small part of a much larger study. These experiences may act as stepping stones to developing their own studies. There also is a role for clinicians to translate research that has been done by others into best practices in their own institutions.

Summary

The rewards and joys of conducting research that can improve the life and death of a child and the experience of family members and caregivers are well worth the care and effort required. This effort includes gaining research knowledge, skills, and experience; selecting important research questions; designing rigorous but sensitive studies; and overcoming the inevitable challenges that all researchers face but that may be particularly difficult in pediatric palliative care.

Acknowledgments

This work was supported by Canadian Institutes of Health Research (CIHR) grant, New Emerging Team (NET) *Transitions in Pediatric Palliative Care* (PET-69769). Kimberley Widger received a PhD Research Trainee Award related to this grant, a TD Meloche Monnex Scholarship from the Canadian Nurses Foundation, and a University of Toronto Fellowship.

REFERENCES

1. Institute of Medicine [IOM]: *When Children Die: Improving Palliative and End-of-Life Care for Children and Their Families.* Washington, DC, 2003, The National Academies Press.
2. Steele R, Bosma H, Fletcher-Johnston M, et al: Research priorities in pediatric palliative care: a delphi study, *J Palliat Care* 24(4):229–287, 2008.
3. Hare ML: Comparing research priorities for pediatric oncology from two panels of experts, *Semin Oncol Nurs* 21(2):145–150, 2005.
4. Hinds PS, Pritchard M, Harper J: End-of-life research as a priority for pediatric oncology, *J Pediatr Oncol Nurs* 21(3):175–179, 2004.
5. Aoun SM, Kristjanson LJ: Challenging the framework for evidence in palliative care research, *Palliat Med* 19(6):461–465, 2005.
6. Bensink ME, Armfield NR, Pinkerton R, et al: Using videotelephony to support paediatric oncology-related palliative care in the home: from abandoned RCT to acceptability study, *Palliat Med* 23:228–237, 2009.
7. Kane JR, Hellsten MB, Coldsmith A: Human suffering: the need for relationship-based research in pediatric end-of-life care, *J Pediatr Oncol Nurs* 21(3):180–185, 2004.
8. Aoun SM, Kristjanson LJ: Evidence in palliative care research: how should it be gathered? *Med J Aust* 183(5):264–266, 2005.
9. Steele R: Strategies used by families to navigate uncharted territory when a child is dying, *J Palliat Care* 21(2):103–110, 2005.
10. Given BA, Keilman LJ, Collins C, et al: Strategies to minimize attrition in longitudinal studies, *Nurs Res* 39(3):184–186, 1990.
11. Janus M, Goldberg S: Factors influencing family participation in a longitudinal study: comparison of pediatric and healthy samples, *J Pediatr Psychol* 22(2):245–262, 1997.
12. Sherman DW, McSherry CB, Parkas V, et al: Recruitment and retention in a longitudinal palliative care study, *Appl Nurs Res* 18(3):167–177, 2005.

13. Steinhauser KE, Clipp EC, Hays JC, et al: Identifying, recruiting, and retaining seriously-ill patients and their caregivers in longitudinal research, *Palliat Med* 20:745–754, 2006.
14. Donabedian A: The quality of health care: how can it be assessed? *JAMA* 260:1743–1748, 1988.
15. Wallston KA, Burger C, Smith RA, et al: Comparing the quality of death for hospice and non-hospice cancer patients, *Med Care* 26:177–182, 1998.
16. Emanuel EJ, Emanuel LL: The promise of a good death, *Lancet* 351:S21–S29, 1998.
17. Heyland DK, Dodek P, Rocker G, et al: What matters most in end-of-life care: perceptions of seriously ill patients and their family members, *CMAJ* 174(5):627–633, 2006.
18. Steinhauser KE, Clipp EC, McNeilly M, et al: In search of a good death: observations of patients, families, and providers, *Ann Intern Med* 132(10):825–832, 2000.
19. Mularski RA, Rosenfeld K, Coons SJ, et al: Measuring outcomes in randomized prospective trials in palliative care, *J Pain Symptom Manage* 34:S7–S19, 2007.
20. Grunfeld E, Lethbridge L, Dewar R, et al: Towards using administrative databases to measure population-based indicators of quality end-of-life care: testing the methodology, *Palliat Med* 20(8):768–777, 2006.
21. Dussel V, Kreicbergs U, Hilden JM, et al: Looking beyond where children die: determinants and effects of planning a child's location of death, *J Pain Symptom Manage* 37(1):33–43, 2009.
22. Aspinal F, Addington-Hall J, Hughes R, et al: Using satisfaction to measure the quality of palliative care: a review of the literature, *J Adv Nurs* 42(4):324–339, 2003.
23. Teno JM: Putting patient and family voice back into measuring quality care for the dying, *Hospice J* 14(3/4):167–176, 1999.
24. Wolfe J, Grier HE, Klar N, et al: Symptoms and suffering at the end of life in children with cancer, *N Engl J Med* 342(5):326–333, 2000.
25. Association for Children with Life-Threatening or Terminal Conditions and their Families, Royal College of Paediatrics and Child Health: *A Guide to the Development of Children's Palliative Care Services*, Bristol, UK, 2003, Author.
26. Meert KL, Eggly S, Dean JM, et al: Ethical and logistical considerations of multicenter parental bereavement research, *J Palliat Med* 11(3):444–450, 2008.
27. Cadell S, Ho G, Jacques L, et al: Considerations for ethics in multisite research in paediatric palliative care, *Palliat Med* 23(3):274–275, 2009.
28. Wells K, Jones L: "Research" in community-partnered, participatory research, *JAMA* 302(3):320–321, 2009.
29. Christopher S, Watts V, McCormick A, et al: Building and maintaining trust in a community-based participatory research partnership, *Am J Public Health* 98(8):1398–1406, 2008.
30. Mongeau S, Champagne M, Liben S: Participatory research in pediatric palliative care: benefits and challenges, *J Palliat Care* 23(1):5–13, 2007.
31. Davies B, Collins JB, Steele R, et al: The impact on families of a children's hospice program, *J Palliat Care* 19(1):15–26, 2003.
32. Davies B, Steele R: Challenges of identifying children for palliative care, *J Palliat Care* 12(30):5–8, 1996.
33. Tomlinson D, Bartels U, Hendershot E, et al: Challenges to participation in paediatric palliative care research: a review of the literature, *Palliat Med* 21:435–440, 2007.
34. Hinds PS, Burghen EA, Pritchard M: Conducting end-of-life studies in pediatric oncology, *West J Nurs Res* 29(4):448–465, 2007.
35. Morrow V, Richards M: The ethics of social research with children: an overview, *Children & Society* 10(2):90–105, 1999.
36. Buchwald D, Schantz-Laursen D, Delmar C: Video diary data collection in research with children, *IJOM* 8(1):12–20, 2009.
37. MacDonald ME, Chilibeck G, Affleck W, Cadell S: Gender imbalance in pediatric palliative care research samples, *Palliat Med* (in press).
38. Schneider M, Steele R, Cadell S, Hemsworth D: Differences on psychosocial outcomes between male and female caregivers of children with life-limiting illnesses, Manuscript accepted with minor revisions, *J Pediatr Nurs* 2009.
39. Davies B, Contro N, Larson J, et al: Information sharing by health care providers with Mexican American and Chinese American parents in need of pediatric palliative care, *Pediatrics* 125: e859–e865, 2010.
40. Davies B, Larson J, Contro N, et al: Conducting a qualitative culture study of pediatric palliative care, *Qual Health Res* 19:5–16, 2009.
41. Carnevale FA, MacDonald ME, Bluebond-Langner M, et al: Using participant observation in pediatric health care settings: ethical challenges and solutions, *J Child Health Care* 12:18–32, 2008.
42. International Committee for Medical Journal Editors: *Uniform requirements for manuscripts submitted to biomedical journals*: *Writing and editing for biomedical publication*. Available at: www.icmje. org/#author. Accessed June 23, 2009.
43. Carter B: Tick box for child? The ethical positioning of children as vulnerable, researchers as barbarians and reviewers as overly cautious, *Int J Nurs Stud* 46:858–864, 2009.
44. Karim K: Conducting research involving palliative patients, *Nurs Stand* 15(2):34–36, 2000.
45. Larsson BW, Larsson G, Carlson SR: Advanced home care: patients opinions on quality compared with those of family members, *J Clin Nurs* 13(2):226–233, 2004.
46. Davies B, Steele R, Collins J, et al: Children's perspectives of a pediatric hospice program, *J Palliat Care* 21(4):252–261, 2005.
47. Beauchamp TL, Childress JF: *Principles of Biomedical Ethics*, ed 6, New York, 2009, Oxford University Press.
48. Casarett D: Ethical considerations in end-of-life care and research, *J Palliat Med* 8:S148–160, 2005.
49. Pessin H, Galietta M, Nelson CJ, et al: Burden and benefit of psychosocial research at the end of life, *J Palliat Med* 11(4):627–632, 2008.
50. Hinds PS, Drew D, Oakes LL, et al: End-of-life care preferences of pediatric patients with cancer, *J Clin Oncol* 23(36):9146–9154, 2005.
51. Hynson JL, Aroni R, Bauld C, et al: Research with bereaved parents: a question of how not why, *Palliat Med* 20(8):805–811, 2006.
52. Homer CJ, Marino B, Cleary PD, et al: Quality of care at a children's hospital: the parents' perspective, *Arch Pediatr Adolesc Med* 153(11):1123–1129, 1999.
53. Collins JJ, Stevens MM, Cousens P: Home care for the dying child: a parent's perception, *Aust Fam Physician* 27(7):610–614, 1998.
54. Contro N, Larson J, Scofield S, et al: Family perspectives on the quality of pediatric palliative care, *Arch Pediatr Adolesc Med* 156(1):14–19, 2002.
55. Woodgate RL: Living in a world without closure: reality for parents who have experienced the death of a child, *J Palliat Care* 22(2):75–82, 2006.
56. Dyregrov K: Bereaved parents' experience of research participation, *Soc Sci Med* 58(2):391–400, 2004.
57. Scott DA, Valery PC, Boyle FM, et al: Does research into sensitive areas do harm? Experiences of research participation after a child's diagnosis with Ewing's Sarcoma, *Med J Aust* 177:507–510, 2002.
58. Kreicbergs U, Valdimarsdottir U, Steineck G, et al: A population-based nationwide study of parents' perceptions of a questionnaire on their child's death due to cancer, *Lancet* 364(9436):787–789, 2004.
59. Meyer EC, Burns JP, Griffith JL, et al: Parental perspectives on end-of-life care in the pediatric intensive care unit, *Crit Care Med* 30(1):226–231, 2002.
60. Taneja GS, Brenner RA, Klinger R, et al: Participation of next of kin in research following sudden, unexpected death of a child, *Arch Pediatr Adolesc Med* 161:453–456, 2007.
61. Widger K, Picot C: Parents' perceptions of the quality of pediatric and perinatal end-of-life care, *Pediatr Nurs* 34(1):53–58, 2008.
62. Kavanaugh K, Ayres L: "Not as bad as it could have been:" Assessing and mitigating harm during research interviews on sensitive topics, *Res Nurs Health* 21:91–97, 1998.

11 Interdisciplinary Education and Training

GERRI FRAGER | TAMARA VESEL |
GRACE MACCONNELL | STACY F. ORLOFF

You're a song,

a wished-for song.

Go through the ear to the center

where sky is, where wind,

where silent knowing.

Put seeds and cover them

blades will sprout

where you do your work. —Rumi

This chapter delves into interdisciplinary education and training in pediatric palliative care, both its basis in the underlying principles of adult education and its creative initiatives specific to the field. The chapter explores:

- Principles of adult education,
- Principles of interdisciplinary education as a framework for pediatric palliative care,
- The unique pedagogy of pediatric palliative care, including suggestions for creative initiatives in training.

In order to optimally tailor the teaching approach, the following factors must be considered: the background, perspective, and experience of the intended audience; the skills they bring; and the most likely and/or most significant gaps in their knowledge.

Principles of Adult Education

Learners seeking increased competency in pediatric palliative care are generally those with a large amount of experience, so the assumptions of andragogy (adult learning) are an integral part of curriculum development. These assumptions as defined by Malcolm Knowles include:

- Adults have a self -concept of being responsible for their learning,
- Adults become ready to learn what they need to know.[1]

These attributes lead to highly pragmatic learners who are likely to be motivated when the material is relevant. They are able to be critical about the value of what they learn. When adult learners feel respected by the teachers, they can actively test what they learn in the real world, integrating new learning into their professional roles[1] (Box 11-1).

Principles of Interdisciplinary Education

The World Health Organization (WHO) says "Interaction is the important goal, to collaborate in providing preventive, curative, rehabilitative, and other health-related services"[2] regarding interdisciplinary education. Other goals include "enhancing" or "improving" both collaboration and quality of care[3] (Table 11-1).

There is a mantra in palliative care circles that interdisciplinary teamwork and learning are beneficial. However, the supporting research and literature is limited, and where available, remains controversial. A review of the general and academic literature on interdisciplinary education identifies some of the salient qualities, benefits, and challenges[4] (Table 11-2).

The Pedagogy of Pediatric Palliative Care

UNIQUE DYNAMICS OF PEDIATRIC PALLIATIVE CARE

The unique dynamics of pediatric palliative care compound the challenges of educating clinicians of different disciplines and varied expertise levels. These cognitive and emotional complexities include:

- The life-threatening and life-limiting illnesses facing infants and children vary widely compared to illnesses impacting adults receiving palliative care. The adult population is far less heterogeneous: cancer and chronic cardio-respiratory illnesses are the usual conditions for adult recipients of palliative care. The illnesses that cause children to be very ill are frequently rare with poorly documented symptoms and an uncertain prognosis.
- Comprehensive assessment of pain and non-pain symptoms in the pediatric population is a challenge because of the spectrum of developmental capacity and frequent inability to self-report.
- Clinicians prescribe medications for pain and symptom relief in the pediatric population with inadequate or even absent pharmacokinetic and pharmacodynamic evidence.
- The care of infants and children have cure as a notable focus, often even when accompanied by compromise of quality for their remaining lives.
- Clinicians share that the emotional impact of caring for a critically ill child is experienced as exponentially greater compared to caring for an adult.

Core Curriculum

Although communication is listed equally among the components below, enhanced communication with patients, families, and colleagues is a priority and an intrinsic part of all the topics. Pediatric residents wished for "aspects of communication" as 4/5 of their top choices for additional education.[5] Core educational components include:

- Needs assessment of participants
- An overview of pediatric palliative care (demographics, philosophy)
- How to conduct a psychosocial assessment of patient and family

BOX 11-1   Necessary Ingredients of Adult Learning

- Choice
- Customization
- Authenticity
- Interaction
- Team reflection
- Educators trained in interdisciplinary facilitation
- Mentoring by expert clinicians
- Time for formal and informal learning
- A comfortable environment
- Access to food, drink, and washrooms
- Experiential and practical hands-on learning[6]
- Reflection on personal and professional interdisciplinary educational experiences[7,8]
- Social activities within the interdisciplinary learning format[9,10]

- Developmental considerations of children
- Comprehensive pain assessment
- Understanding pain pathophysiology
- Basic and complex pain management
- How to relieve nausea, vomiting, anorexia, fatigue, breathlessness, excess secretions, bleeding, depression, anxiety, delirium, disturbed sleep, seizures, spasticity, etc.
- Spiritual assessment and care of the patient
- Communication with children and their parents
- How to discuss tissue and organ donation and autopsy
- Ethical considerations
- Consideration and integration of ethnic and cultural perspectives
- Enhancing interdisciplinary team communication and collaboration
- Anticipatory grief and bereavement
- How to perform reflective practice, including self-care
- Finding and using resources
- ***Performing evaluation and feedback***

TEAM INTERDISCIPLINARY EDUCATION AND TRAINING

A dynamic mix of clinicians, from different disciplines and with varied skills, requires training in pediatric palliative care (Fig. 11-1).

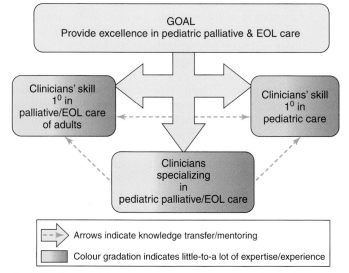

Fig. 11-1   Patterns of skill acquisition in clinicians training in pediatric palliative care.

TABLE 11-1   Core Competencies for Every Clinician

Institute of Medicine—IOM[11]	Interprofessional Education Consortium—IPEC[12]
Provide patient-centered care	Family-centered practice
Work in interdisciplinary teams	Integrated services through collaboration and/or group process
Employ evidence-based practice	
Apply quality improvement	
Use informatics	Assessment and outcome
	Social policy issues
	Communication
	Leadership

TABLE 11-2   Interdisciplinary Education: Benefits and Challenges

Benefits	Challenges and/or disadvantages
• Generally well received	• Variation by individual teacher and learner, compounds the challenge of also being from different disciplines
• Enables learning the necessary knowledge/skills for collaborative work	• Attitudes and perceptions remain less impacted than knowledge and/or skills
• Every learner embodies values reflective of themselves and others	• Faculty development is necessary for effective education and can be a challenge to deliver[14]
• All participants access core content components at the same time	• Discipline-specific content requires additional allocation of time, space, and educators
• Teaching that genuinely reflects practice is effective	• There can be a disconnect between what is taught and what is practiced
• Education can be a quality improvement measure, resulting in practice/service enhancement	• The physical and temporal hurdles involving space and coordination of varied schedules[15]
• Participant quotes: "I cannot imagine working again without the interdisciplinary team." "I will feel naked without the team members."[13]	• The necessary component of involving participants to learn from one another in social as well as academic situations can present a challenge

Interdisciplinary groups provide an opportunity to share information from each individual and discipline's perspective. Because each discipline has unique educational preparation, philosophy, and standard of practice, a common forum lends a richness and diversity to the group's knowledge. Furthermore, it fosters respect and appreciation for each individual's contribution. Research suggests that the earlier students from different disciplines are paired, the better their perceived understanding of roles.[16] Medical student participants shared what they perceived as institutional support or the lack thereof in interprofessional interventions.[17] Both within and outside the formal teaching session, the frequent and ongoing modeling of interdisciplinary practice must be considered in curricula implementation.[18,19] The evaluation of these initiatives is also crucial because trainees' perceptions of the importance of educational material is strongly linked to such data.[20]

It is helpful to plan the curriculum according to the skills to be imparted and acquired, rather than by discipline-specific teaching. Although each interdisciplinary team member has a particular scope of practice, a common knowledge base is often required. For example, consider a clinician who enters a room where the child appears to be in pain. The mother expresses concern about her child's discomfort and about how analgesia may affect him. Every attending nurse, physician, or psychosocial clinician coming into contact with the child and family should have the basic skills to address the child's pain and provide reassurance to the child and family.

Emerging research identifies the educational needs of the support staff on the pediatric palliative care team. A recent study pointed out that professional, educational, and emotional needs were notably unmet in this heterogeneous community of care providers. Although they had significant and direct contact with dying children and their families, none of them had received training in coping strategies and grief.[21]

Informal focus groups of trainees in pediatric palliative care rated respect of one another's disciplines as the most important outcome of an interdisciplinary educational initiative.[13] An integral component described by Health Canada is the development of mutual understanding for the contributions of various disciplines.[18] In this emotionally difficult field, such respect may help prevent and reduce staff distress, communication obstacles, and conflict. Furthermore, the sharing of experiences and perceptions across disciplines leads to the recognition of universal reactions and emotions. An Australian interdisciplinary education palliative care model involved 537 participants, whose feedback requested more group sharing.[22] Pediatric hematology-oncology and critical-care physicians noted that observing senior physicians in difficult conversations with families was the most helpful aspect of their palliative care training.[14] It bodes well for interdisciplinary education that respondents also requested that team members from disciplines other than medicine be involved in teaching of communication skills.

Clinicians from each discipline bring their own perspectives and share unique interactions with patients and families, resulting in significant clinical learning among team members. One individual or discipline cannot be an expert in every component of care; rather a collective team expertise is necessary.

Setting the stage for a level playing field within the group is essential within interdisiplinary education. For example, although nurses are often the most numerous of the participants, their input may be dismissed if there is a real or imagined power differential between them and the physicians present. On the other hand, the number of nurses may intimidate individuals from less well-represented disciplines. A study evaluating interdisciplinary workshops found that male participants and physicians tended to take over in role play and discussion formats.[23]

STRATEGIES

Despite the challenges in providing educational opportunities for an audience of diverse disciplines, there can be significant rewards. Advance knowledge about the audience and its learning goals ensures a targeted presentation. It is incumbent upon the educator or facilitator to create an environment that supports sharing ideas without judgment. A stated common goal or focus engages participants from all disciplines. Introductions that highlight each person's discipline and contribution facilitate the understanding of different perspectives and meaning of others' life work. With this groundwork, individual concerns during the training can be better addressed and are less likely to be discounted. Throughout the session, it is important to pose questions that relate these different perspectives to the common focus.

Suggested questions for an interdisciplinary audience include:

- Describe an ideal scenario of caring for a palliative care patient. This demonstrates the contributions and priorities of the many disciplines.
- Tell us about your team. How do you work together? What has worked well for your team in the past?
- Do you have a well-defined structure to your team? Do you have well-defined roles within your team?
- How does each person on your team contribute to the care of a patient? This can be explored through a patient-based discussion.
- What do you see as your team's strengths in caring for a pediatric palliative care patient?
- Have team members ever taken on different duties? Describe those situations, how did it work, were there any surprises?
- Would you change how you work together?
- Small group discussions can be very effective when participants from different disciplines are distributed within each group. Strategies to foster interaction include:
  - Each person describes the discipline-specific contribution of each team member, as well as the contributions that might be shared by all team members. A variation is to provide descriptions of specific practices and ask participants to match the practice with the team member/discipline.
  - Each participant describes what is needed to care for a child in pediatric palliative care. A flip chart can be used to graphically identify which discipline could perform each role. This encourages thinking in broader terms than how their teams may currently function.
  - Ask participants to describe what is most rewarding and most difficult about one's work in pediatric palliative care in regards to their specific discipline. A blackboard or flipchart may be used to document the responses. Ask which discipline experiences each item, there will likely be considerable overlap.

It is often the informal opportunities to learn within the interdisciplinary team that yield the richest treasures. Each observation or piece of information shared from one individual frequently reminds another person of further details about the patient and/or family. Teleconferencing sessions that connect the tertiary care center with remote sites provides a valuable mutual learning opportunity.

There are differences in approach depending on the kind of education and training being offered: is this a general session about palliative care that is focused on one particular component, or is it specific to the needs of a particular patient and family? Providing information that is ready when it's needed is more likely to be heard, integrated, and remembered when illustrated by relevant examples from patients and families. Web-based resources can provide practical material by those with pediatric palliative care expertise. List-servs are excellent venues to vet questions, teach difficult aspects of care and share educational tools, and share policies with the collective expertise of clinicians from a variety of disciplines.

PARENTS AND FAMILIES AS TEACHERS

Listen. Just listen and just dig deeply what they're saying... That's the kind of doctor to be. Not just a doctor that understands big words—doctor talk—whatever....Because they got to meet all kinds... like me. They got to understand me... I'm the one here with my child. I could read her face... You got to listen to what I'm saying about my child.
— INITIATIVE FOR PEDIATRIC PALLIATIVE CARE

The eloquence of stories recounted by parents and families has enormous impact on professional training and development, as attested to by the clinicians themselves. Hospitals have begun including family members in new resident orientation, grand rounds presentations, and advisory councils. Palliative care programs and hospices are creating novel ways to involve families in educational initiatives, institutional trainings, and conferences. Some curricula are also encouraging clinicians to involve family members in institutional change.

The core of pediatric palliative care is the relationship between the clinical team and the family. The involvement of the child and family in ongoing professional development may enhance that relationship. Family members have described the importance of continuous care coordinated through the efforts of an interdisciplinary team.[24] It is possible to train clinicians to be effective members of this team. Family members, including the child, can be interviewed or play roles in vignettes. Some programs have used innovative techniques such as developing scripts based on real situations with input from families. Actors then play the role of the patient or family with the clinicians acting as themselves.[25] Clinicians may gain a deeper understanding of parents' decision-making processes upon hearing their accounts firsthand.[26] The teaching provided by families provides a unique perspective, and the team should be advised to heed carefully what they hear, and consider these messages in the evolution of their own practice.

Clinicians are responsible for protecting the emotional integrity of families who participate in educational initiatives. Careful selection of individuals, as well as the identification of a clinical team member who is available for support and follow-up to the family, are essential.

The "Voice of the Child" as Teacher

The following drawing and description by Mikaela, a ten-year-old girl with a brain tumor, provides an example of teaching from the child's images and words, as well as valuable insight into the child's understanding of illness, capacity, decision-making and autonomy (Fig. 11-2). Mikaela shows her picture about cancer-related treatment decisions, and says "I feel like I'm stuck in the middle of a doughnut"[27] not knowing which option to choose. As described by her psychologist, Mikaela drew tumor cells on one side and a lumbar puncture needle on the other.[27]

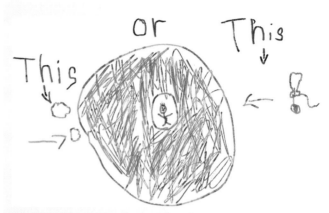

Fig. 11-2   This or this. (Reprinted from Sourkes B et al. Food, toys, and love: Pediatric Palliative Care, Curr Probl Pediatr Adolesc Health Care 35(9): 345-392, 2005.)

Mikaela describes her picture to her psychologist by saying: "What I mean by 'I was stuck in a doughnut' is that I had two choices and I didn't want to take either of them. One of the choices was to get needles and pokes and all that stuff and make the tumor go away ... even perhaps, it might have came back. My other choice was letting my tumor get bigger and bigger and I would just go away up to heaven.... My mom wanted me to get needles and pokes. But I felt like I just had too much. Too much for my body, too much for me.... so I kind of wanted to go up to heaven that time.... But then I thought about how much my whole entire family would miss me and so just then I was kind of like stuck in a doughnut."[27]

Prompts for discussion include:

Can you share some of your thoughts after hearing from Mikaela?

Do you think Mikaela understands the implications of her illness?

Do you think Mikaela understands the decisions related to her illness?

What are your thoughts about capacity? Do you think Mikaela has capacity?

Do you think Mikaela is able to decide about the treatment of her illness?

What are your thoughts about patient autonomy when you hear Mikaela talk about her family?

INTEGRATION OF THE MEDICAL HUMANITIES

Medical humanities have long been used to enhance the education of healthcare professionals. Consider the mission statement from the Medical Humanities program at New York University School of Medicine:

"We define the term 'medical humanities' broadly to include an interdisciplinary field of humanities (literature, philosophy, ethics, history, and religion), social science (anthropology, cultural studies, psychology, sociology), and the arts (literature, theater, film, and visual arts) and their application to medical education and practice. The humanities and arts provide insight into the human condition, suffering, personhood, our responsibility to each other, and offer a historical perspective on medical practice. Attention to literature and the arts helps to develop and nurture skills of observation, analysis, empathy, and self-reflection—skills that are essential for humane medical care. The social sciences help us to understand how bioscience and medicine take place within cultural and social contexts and how culture interacts with the individual experience of illness and the way medicine is practiced."[18]

The incorporation of the arts to illustrate a concept, a child's or parent's perspective, or a staff member's reflection on the personal impact of a professional experience, is invaluable. The performing arts are particularly excellent vehicles for illustration when followed by discussion opportunities.

Family stories that are shared publically may be effectively incorporated as interdisciplinary teaching tools. For example, newspaper journalist Ian Brown chronicles his experience of parenting Walker, his 12-year-old son with a complex chronic illness,[29] in *The Boy in the Moon*.

One of his reflections, reprinted from the *Globe and Mail*, could be incorporated into a curriculum about the issues that face these children and their families:

I took my 14-year-old daughter, Hayley, to the ballet. She's a dancer herself; it's my favourite evening out—I wear a bow tie and she wears a dress. Jerome Robbins had choreographed music by Philip Glass: row after row of evenly spaced dancers, pacing across the stage in identical time to Mr. Glass's rhythmic score. Only an occasional couple broke step to perform a pas de deux. A ballet about the life of a great city, in other words, with its armies of people doing the same things in the same impersonal place to the same rhythms—save when they break away from the pack and just as quickly slip back into position. A work of art that lets you see the crisp shape of your own existence, even while you are immersed in your repetitive, blinkered life. A generous, hopeful gesture. It brought thick tears to my eyes. Walker makes people cry too. It can happen any time and to almost everyone who meets him, eventually. They aren't tears of loss, or pity. I think they're tears of gratitude.

EVALUATIVE TOOLS

Some components of a pediatric palliative care curriculum are best shared in an interdisciplinary format; others require a more discipline-specific focus. Interdisciplinary groups will vary appropriate to community need, funding, service provision, and goals for training. Several palliative care organizations have defined hospice and palliative care competencies specifically for medicine, nursing, and social work. Delineation of such competencies provides a framework for evaluating quality indicators and best practice interventions. Some to consider:

- The American Academy of Hospice and Palliative Medicine (AAHPM) Task Force has identified competencies for physicians (www.aahpm.org).
- The American Association of Nursing Colleges developed an End-of-Life Nursing Education Consortium (ELNEC) with a Pediatric component (www.aacn.nche.edu/ELNEC). In Canada, competencies for palliative care, includimg pediatrics, have been developed for nurses and national certification in palliative care under the auspices of the Canadian Nurses Association (CNA).

- Social work competencies in end-of-life care with links to the published literature are available at: www.socialworkers.org/research/naswResearch/EndofLifeCare/default.asp

Pharmacy, child life, psychology, and occupational and physiotherapy disciplines are integral to interdisciplinary education; however, competencies in pediatric palliative care have not yet been developed.

In addition to discipline-specific competency evaluation, researchers of pedagogy have some tools to evaluate interdisciplinary education. However, little is published relating to palliative care, and even less that is specific to pediatric palliative care. For example, although the Readiness for Interprofessional Learning Scale (RIPLS) is available, it has not yet been applied to palliative care-related education.[30] However, some tools can be extrapolated and modified. For example, medical and social work students who received interdisciplinary education demonstrated a significantly better ability to lead family conferences in palliative care than the control group.[31]

Clinical Vignette

The following narrative of Riley elucidates the comprehensive care that a competent palliative care team can provide. This narrative may be used to expand participants' perceptions of who the recipients of care are, as well as timelines for involvement. Ideally, referrals for pediatric palliative care should match the demographics of childhood illnesses that are significantly life threatening: that is, one-third from oncology, and the balance varied with neurologic, cardiac, renal, and gastro-intestinal diagnoses as the primary condition. Participants may be encouraged to share their experiences through examples from their own practices.

The Pediatric Palliative Care Service was consulted when Riley was 4½ months old (Fig. 11-3). He had been awaiting a neurologic consultation for hypotonia when he was admitted with pneumonia and severe respiratory compromise. He was diagnosed with Spinal Muscular Atrophy, a progressive, life-threatening, neurodegenerative illness. The following quotes

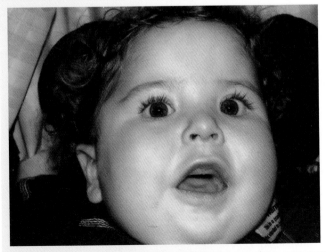

Fig. 11-3 Riley's story elucidates the comprehensive care that a competent palliative care team can provide.

are taken from a note written to members of the palliative care team, following Riley's death at 14 months of age. Riley's parents wrote: "We are so thankful for all the time you spent with us when Riley was diagnosed. Those hours you spent with us engaging us in productive, honest conversation were very positive for us. It helped us frame our hopes and wishes for Riley; how far we'd go with his care and his end of life care. Without our conversations I'm afraid we would have avoided thinking about those 'hard' things until we were in a critical, emotional time. I'm sure those decisions would have been much harder and not always thought through at those times."

This provides a poignant description of how the palliative care team ensures:

- *Patients and families receive the information they need to understand their child's condition and treatment options*
- *Values and goals are elicited over time, with sensitivity to relevant cultural issues*
- *Benefits and burdens of treatment are regularly reassessed and the decision-making process about the care plan remains sensitive to changes in the patient's condition*

Riley's parents continued: "We are also thankful for your visits on subsequent trips to the hospital and for your assistance and willingness to discuss Riley's care with his care team here (a distant rural community). As well, all the literature you offered us, the girls, and our parents. My parents were thrilled with the grandparents' book you sent."

This serves to reinforce how:

Care needs are addressed with the patients, families, and other clinicians through coordination and collaboration, ensuring continuity across varied settings at different times of transition and changing needs

Care is provided within the context of a trusting and respectful clinician-patient relationship

Riley's story speaks to the benefit of early involvement

Support is extended to siblings and extended family as part of the unit of care

To identify resources that are applicable, appropriate, and individualized to the child's and family's circumstances, needs, and wishes. Riley's story and his family's note provide a natural introduction to discussion of anticipatory grief and bereavement support, and resources.

With thanks to Riley's parents for sharing this narrative with their permission.

REFERENCES

1. Wlodkowski RJ: *Enhancing adult motivation to learn. A comprehensive guide for teaching all adults,* 2008, John Wiley and Sons Inc.
2. *Learning together to work together for health,* Report of a WHO study group on multiprofessional education of health personnel: the team approach. World Health Organization Technical Report Series. Geneva, 1988, *World Health Organization* 769:1–72.
3. Centre for Advancement in Interprofessional Education (CAIPE): *Interprofessional education – a definition,* 2002. Retrieved April 5, 2007, from http://www.caipe.org.uk/.
4. Hammick M, Freeth D, Koppel I, Reeves S, et al: A best evidence systematic review of interdisciplinary education, *Med Teach* 29:735–751, 2007.
5. Kolarik LK, Walker G, Arnold RM: Pediatric resident education in palliative care: a needs assessment, *Pediatrics* 117:1949–1954, 2006.
6. Dickens DS: Building competence in pediatric end-of-life care, *J Palliat Med* 12:617–622, 2009.
7. Reeves S, Freeth D: The London training ward: an innovative interprofessional learning initiative, *J Interprof Care* 16:41–52, 2002.
8. Mu K, Chao C, Jensen G, et al: Effects of interprofessional rural training on students' perceptions of interprofessional health care services, *J Allied Health* 33:125–131, 2004.
9. Nash A, Hoy A: Terminal care in the community: an evaluation of residential workshops for general practitioner/district nurse teams, *Palliat Med* 7:5–17, 1993.
10. Reeves S: Community-based interprofessional education for medical, nursing and dental students, *Health Soc Care Community* 4:269–276, 2000.
11. Institute of Medicine: *Crossing the quality chasm: a new health system for the 21st century,* Washington, DC, 2001, National Academies Press.
12. Interprofessional Education Consortium (IPEC): *Creating, Implementing, and Sustaining Interprofessional Education, volume III of a series* [Electronic version]. San Francisco, June, 2002, Stuart Foundation.
13. Vesel T: Personal Communication, Dana Farber Cancer Institute and Children's Hospital Boston - Pediatric interdisciplinary palliative care fellowship.
14. Kersun L, Gyi L, Morrison WE: Training in difficult conversations: a national survey of pediatric hematology-oncology and pediatric critical care physicians, *J Palliat Med* 12:525–530, 2009.
15. Tucker K, Wakefield A, Boggis C, et al: Learning together: clinical skills teaching for medical and nursing students, *Med Educ* 37:630–637, 2003.
16. Fineberg IC, Wenger NS, Forrow L: Interdisciplinary education: evaluation of palliative care training for pre-professionals, *Acad Med* 79:769–776, 2004.
17. Carpenter J, Hewstone M: Shared learning for doctors and social workers: evaluation of a programme, *Br J Soc Work* 26:239–257, 1996.
18. Health Canada: Interprofessional Education on Patient Centered Collaborative Practice (IECPCP): Available at http://hcsc.gc.ca/english/hhr/research-synthesis.html. Accessed April 15, 2007.
19. Morey JC, Simon R, Jay GD, et al: Error reduction and performance improvement in the emergency department through formal teamwork training: evaluation results of the MedTeams project, *Health Serv Res* 37:1553–1581, 2002.
20. Morison S, Boohan M, Jenkins J, et al: Facilitating undergraduate interprofessional learning in healthcare: comparing classroom and clinical learning for nursing and medical students, *Learn Health Soc Care* 2:92–104, 2003.
21. Swinney R, Yin L, Lee A, et al: The role of support staff in pediatric palliative care: their perceptions, training and available resources, *J Palliat Care* 23:4–50, 2007.
22. Quinn K, Hudson P, Ashby M, et al: Palliative care: the essentials. Evaluation of a multidisciplinary education program, *J Palliat Care* 11:1122–1129, 2008.
23. Kilminster S, Hale C, Lascelles M, et al: Learning for real life: patient-focused interprofessional workshops offer added value, *Med Educ* 38(7):717–726, 2004.
24. Heller K, Solomon MZ: Continuity of care and caring: what matters to parents of children with life-threatening conditions, *J Pediatr Nurs* 20(5):335–346, 2005.
25. Browning D: To show our humanness: relational and communicative competence in pediatric palliative care, *Bioethics Forum* 18(3–4):23–28, 2002.
26. Bluebond-Langer M, Belasco JB, Goldman A, Belasco C: Understanding parents' approaches to care and treatment of children with cancer when standard therapy has failed, *JCO* 25(27):2414–2419, 2007.
27. Sourkes B, Frankel L, Brown M, et al: Food, toys, and love: pediatric palliative care, *Curr Probl Pediatr Adolesc Health Care* 35(9):350–386, 2005.
28. Web-site New York University School of Medicine - Medical Humanities Program: http://medhum.med.nyu.edu/.
29. Globe and Mail Web-site with Ian Brown's Boy in the Moon Series: http://v1.theglobeandmail.com/boyinthemoon/. Last accessed November 12, 2009.
30. McFadyen AK, Webster VS, Maclaren WM: The test-retest reliability of a revised version of the Readiness for Interprofessional Learning Scale (RIPLS), *J Interprof Care* 20:633–639, 2006.
31. Fineberg IC: Preparing professionals for family conferences in palliative care: evaluation results of an interdisciplinary approach, *J Palliat Med* 8:857–866, 2005.

SUGGESTED RESOURCES

Pediatric Pain Master Class: www.childrensmn.org/services/PainPalliative Care

The Association for Children's Palliative Care: www.act.org.uk/

The Initiative for Pediatric Palliative Care: www.ippcweb.org

National Hospice and Palliative Care Organization: www.nhpco.org

ChIPPS curriculum: www.nhpco.org/i4a/pages/index.cfm?pageid=3409

The Canadian Network of Palliative Care for Children: www.cnpcc.ca

End of life/Palliative Education Resource Center: www.eperc.mcw.edu.

The Ian Anderson Continuing Education Program in End of Life Care: www.cme.utoronto.ca/endoflife

The Canadian Virtual Hospice: www.virtualhospice.ca

Education for Palliative and End-of-Life Care (EPEC): www.epec.net

St. Jude Children's Research Hospital: www.cure4kids.org

American Association of Colleges of Nursing/End of life Education Consortium: www.aacn.nche.edu/elnec/curriculum.htm

Texas Cancer Council/Texas Children's Hospital: www.childendof-lifecare.org

Harvard Medical School: Center for Palliative Care: www.hms.harvard.edu/pallcare/pcep.htm

Griefworks: www.griefworks.com

Centering Corporation: www.centeringcorp.com

List-serv or discussion of topics related to pediatric palliative care

List-serv or discussion of topics related to pediatric palliative care: paed-palcare@act.org.uk

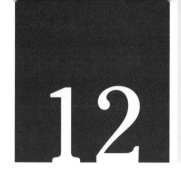

12

Faith, Hope, and Love: An Interdisciplinary Approach to Providing Spiritual Care

JANIE BROOKS | REVEREND KATHLEEN ENNIS-DURSTINE

I want to know if you will stand in the center of the fire with me and not shrink back....

I want to know if you can sit with pain–mine or your own–without moving to hide it, or fade it, or fix it. I want to know if you can be with joy–mine or your own; if you can dance with wildness and let the ecstasy fill you to the tips of your fingers and toes without cautioning us to be careful–be realistic–to remember the limitations of being human.

— Oriah Mountain Dreamer, Selections from "The Invitation"

Providing spiritual care to a person with a life-threatening illness involves standing, sitting, and dancing with that person through his or her unique experience. If we are careful, if we are realistic, if we recognize the limitations, then we can surely know joy.

The first half of this chapter is devoted to a review of the literature on the subject of faith and spirituality in children, especially children who are seriously ill, looking at faith, spirituality, and worldview, and examining the differences between screening and assessment. Much of what has been written begins from the perspective of data; while data is helpful to providing quality, interdisciplinary palliative care, it is not enough. The approach of this chapter places narrative and theology at the heart of the process and understanding. It will highlight the work of all the interdisciplinary team and examine the unique role of the professional chaplain.* The second part of the chapter will look at various case scenarios and the many ways the interdisciplinary team can participate in faith and/or spiritual care of the pediatric palliative care patient.

For the purposes of this chapter, *palliative care* is defined as addressing both the physical and emotional and/or spiritual distress from the moment of diagnosis through death.

A review of the literature suggests that there is much work to be done in addressing the spiritual needs of pediatric palliative care patients. A survey conducted in 2008 by the Pew Forum on Religion and Public Life polled 36,000 Americans concerning their religious and spiritual beliefs. The results revealed that 92 percent of American adults believe in "God or a universal spirit."[1] Although this poll was limited to American adults, the findings support the idea that spirituality is an inherently universal aspect of human beings. While the importance of spirituality seems to be of increasing concern, there are few articles on the subject and most identify significant challenges in providing spiritual care in a healthcare setting. Most articles on the topic are written by nursing professionals and are intended for nurses. There is little information regarding the role of the interdisciplinary team in meeting the spiritual needs of children, although a few writers emphasize the need for collaboration.[2]

Writers in the field agree that spirituality is important to children and that spiritual concerns are particularly significant during times of serious illness.[3] It is recognized that the distinction between spirituality and religious belief is important yet often overlooked,[4] and that developmentally appropriate assessment is necessary but there is a lack of validated tools in addition to some confusion about who is best equipped to make these assessments.[5] It is also clear that nurses, physicians, and chaplains are aware that spiritual needs are not adequately addressed.[6] Among the identified barriers to optimal spiritual care are inadequate staffing of pastoral care departments, lack of training on the part of clinical staff, discomfort due to lack of knowledge or skill, and priority being given to medical concerns at the expense of holistic care.[7] The general conclusion is that addressing spiritual needs in the child with a life-threatening illness is "an area that deserves continued exploration and attention."[7]

Spirituality and World View

Spirituality is often defined as pertaining to religious beliefs and values. This narrow understanding overlooks the reality that all human beings, religious or not, are spiritual beings. Spirituality must be described rather than defined, as it has to do with our search for meaning; it is a connection to something greater than ourselves that helps us to make sense of our world. This sense of sacred connection may denote a relationship with a divine Being such as God or Allah, or may be experienced in the context of family or community.

Spiritual needs change throughout our lives, according to our development and the circumstances we encounter. Our world view develops in relationship to our values, culture, tradition, and experience. As we grow and learn we are influenced by parents, faith communities, teachers, and peers, and what we see on television or learn from books and stories. These and many other factors contribute to our faith, our trust, and our hopes for how we will be in the world, for what will become our own life stories. Even very young children have a need to attach meaning to their lives and are working out their personal view of how the world works.

---

*Board Certified Professional Chaplain: This individual possesses a Master's Degree in Theology/Divinity, is ordained or endorsed by a particular faith/spiritual community, has completed a minimum of 1600 hours of clinical training under supervision, demonstrates clinical proficiency through written materials and interview with a board of Certified Chaplains from either the Association of Professional Chaplains, the National Association of Catholic Chaplains, or the National Association of Jewish Chaplains. Maintaining professional certification requires 50 continuing education hours per year and scheduled peer reviews to assure competency.

The diagnosis of a serious illness is a life changing event that not only interrupts[8] our day-to-day activities but may also disrupt our world view. Children who have been cared for by loving parents know the world as a safe place and trust that they can rely on their family to provide for their safety. The onset of a serious illness changes that understanding. The role of the parent shifts as doctors become the most powerful figures in the child's life, and parents may now feel unable to protect their son or daughter from pain and discomfort.

A child growing up in a traditional Christian home may have been taught that God protects and loves us, especially when we obey God's laws. Being hospitalized with a life-threatening illness can lead that child to blame herself for getting sick, or to doubt that God really exists at all. The same child might also discover that the God she has known all her life is present to her throughout her experience of illness in a powerful and reassuring way.

The African mother whose child is hospitalized in the United States may not have the opportunity to perform traditional cultural and religious practices that would bring her comfort and healing in her own community.

Michael's mother was very preoccupied with chanting and praying in her son's room. She had difficulty listening to medical team members when they came to update her about the daily plan of care, and was insistent that none of her extended family be allowed to visit Michael during his hospital stay. The chaplain, noticing that she did not seem to be experiencing any solace from her endless hours of praying, gently asked what she might do differently if she and Michael were back home. She began crying and admitted that she was carrying a heavy burden of guilt about a sin she had committed. She believed that God was punishing her by afflicting Michael with cancer. In Africa, she would have gone before her religious community and confessed her transgression, thereby receiving absolution from her priest and forgiveness from God. Having no access to this rite of penitence, she believed that God would not act on her behalf and there could be no miracle for Michael. Fearing judgment from her family, she isolated herself and her son from the support they needed.

The teenager with a troubled home life who has already experienced the world as a difficult and confusing place may consider his serious illness a reinforcement: life is hard and not very hopeful, and he cannot expect things to get much better.

Spirituality is a very personal and complex part of our lives, and every seriously ill child and his or her family will undoubtedly have unique spiritual needs.

If the interdisciplinary team is to address spiritual and cultural needs adequately, a thorough and thoughtful understanding of spiritual development and a quality spiritual assessment of the patient and family is critical.

THE QUESTION OF FAITH AND/OR SPIRITUAL DEVELOPMENT

The task of human beings is to grow and learn. Development is a given on many levels and, unless limited by neurological, biological, or psychosocial factors, will follow recognizable patterns. All development is influenced by the many cultures[9] in which an individual is embedded, perhaps none more so than the development of spiritual and/or faith concepts and needs. We cannot, with any certainty, describe specific faith development in children; we can only generalize about the ways faith development is related to human development. Each child, and each family system, must be understood as a unique entity. Exploring the cultures, which give each family its sense of meaning and purpose and upon which they will base much of their decision-making, is a vital process for the professional.

Developmental models are inclined to focus on stages. The human mind extrapolates that progress through these stages is success. Yet Erik Erikson, the progenitor of modern developmental theory (The Child and Society), cautioned his readers to be aware that all persons carry within themselves the potential future stages as well as the resources and unresolved issues of former stages. A person is never statically in one stage. Faith development, per James Fowler (Stages of Faith) is aligned with other psychosocial and biological development (Table 12-1). However, progress through faith-development stages does not tell us that a person's faith is better, more developed, or better able to support them through

TABLE 12-1 Comparisons Among Human and Faith Development

Erik Erikson	Jean Piaget	James Fowler	Dominant faith-development issues
Trust vs. mistrust	Sensorimotor	Undifferentiated (infancy): Seeds of trust, courage, hope and love are fused and contend with sensed threats of abandonment, inconsistencies, and deprivations	Building on experiences of basic trust Experiencing mutuality in relationship Experiencing a nascent sense of autonomy
Autonomy vs. shame and doubt, and initiative vs. guilt	Sensorimotor and preoperational	Intuitive projective: (toddler—early childhood) Language, consciousness of self, persistence of memory. Fluid thought patterns easily influenced by stories, actions, moods of others. Experiencing much newness	Building a sense of reality beyond one's self Learning basic rituals of community such as bedtime prayers, grace "Imagining" God/gods and faith stories
Industry vs. inferiority	Concrete operational	Mythic-literal: (childhood and beyond) Sense of belonging to family, culture, community. Literal interpretation. Observation of others. Building a sense of justice/fairness	Stories of the faith community become stories about me Religious symbols become concrete and literal Justice is absolute; moral values are absolute Heroes are cosmic and anthropomorphic
Identity vs. role confusion	Formal operational	Synthetic conventional: (Adolescence and beyond) World is larger than family. Belonging to different groups becomes important. Identity issues abound—developing personal myth. Incorporating past and projecting future	Faith and values become very personal and a uniting factor to others with similar beliefs and/or values. Faith and values are part of identity and not available for objective examination. Differences with others regarding faith and values are experienced as differences in the sort of person one is.

crises. The development stage of one's faith is influenced by culture and world view and frequently chosen because it assists the individual in making sense out of his or her life.

There is a distinction between faith and spiritual development, although they significantly overlap. Faith development refers to the tenets of any particular group, how and when they are taught and/or experienced by the child within her or his cultural milieu. Spiritual development refers to the ways in which children make meaning, feel connected (or disconnected) to something unseen, but experienced, that gives them a sense of being cared for and the ability to care for others. This experienced awareness of the holy assists children in developing their capacity for trust, for gratitude, for remorse or sorrow, and for their vitality in participating in life. We should never mistake not belonging to a faith community that has a particular story and language for a lack of spirituality.

Have you been with a 10 month old whose eyes grow as big as saucers at the sight of his first Christmas tree? Or shared a moment with a 6 year old who, with tears in her eyes and a huge smile, holds a butterfly on the tip of her finger? Or cared for a 90 year old whose last request is to watch the sunrise? That is awe, and it is the beginning, middle, and end of spirituality.

As human beings, one of our first tasks is to trust and to explore who we are in relationship to those we trust. The child who goes to sleep in a crib, in a dark room, is not only expressing trust in his parent, but also communicating a basic trust in the creation. As we grow and become more discerning and articulate, we begin to choose what it is in which we will have faith. A child makes choices about how open or closed she is to the world around her, to others, and to various concepts and practices offered by her family and communities. Children then begin to notice that what they receive is not to be taken for granted; they are able to express gratitude and desire the gratefulness of others. As trust and relationship are confirmed in the events of a child's life, the child experiences and articulates what loss means, what regret and sorrow are, and how she or he is connected to, and a participant in, what the child believes to be the expectations and promises of living.[10]

Where trust and communion, being cared for, and caring for others are disrupted, every other aspect of the child's psychosocial and spiritual development is also disrupted. A life-threatening injury or illness calls into question the intent or reality of something other or holy that is watching over the child. Every other concept which the child has integrated into his or her personal identity to this point will undergo some re-examination. What was easy, and practiced without much thought, such as gratitude, becomes difficult and problematic. Depending upon the cultures of the child's community, the child may become more focused on remorse or responsibility. Children often return to earlier stages of psychosocial coping when feeling exposed and unsure; this may or may not be true of children and their faith-based, or spiritual, perspectives. Erikson emphasized that development is process not progress, at least not entirely, and that each stage holds the following ones in potential and the past ones as resource and unresolved issues. There are children of all ages who need the more concrete, me-oriented concepts and ideals. However, there are other children of all ages for whom concepts or symbols become transparent,[11] the universe suddenly coherent, and vision transformed. Neither is better.

The work of faith, or spiritual, development happens along two fronts. One is the cultures in which the child is embedded, and the other includes all the experiences and relationships which the child internalizes as her or his own particular world view. It is never enough to know the tenets of a child's cultural and/or faith environment, one must know the child (Table 12-1).

Faith and/or Spiritual Screening and Assessment

Since faith and spirituality have become important aspects in the awareness of healthcare providers, the words screening and assessment have been used in various and often synonymous ways. This chapter encourages a separation of these very specific concepts. Screening can be done by any one of the interdisciplinary team members to identify a patient's and the family's relationship to their faith community, the beliefs and practices that they would like to continue and to have respected by the healthcare team; and any special needs for food, space, and male or female caregivers. Screening may also identify the need for additional support structures or personnel such as the professional chaplain. Assessment, however, is a much more abstract concept. A faith or spiritual assessment is ideally about describing a sense of self in relationship to the holy, in whatever way that is understood, the ways of making meaning and making decisions, what people understand to be community, and how they access their strengths and resources. Results of an assessment are unique. Assessments should always be completed by trained, professional chaplains.

Healthcare professionals should complete an appropriate spiritual screening with the patient upon admission to the clinical setting. Based on that information, clinicians can identify the presence of a spiritual issue and make the appropriate referrals to chaplains who will complete more thorough spiritual assessments. Clinicians should distinguish when the patient presents with emotional, psychosocial, spiritual issues, or a combination, and make the appropriate referral.

This model is based on a generalist-specialist model of care in which board-certified chaplains are considered the trained spiritual care specialists. Detailed assessment and complex diagnosis and treatment are the purview of the board-certified chaplains working with the interdisciplinary team as the spiritual-care experts.[12]

In short, screening answers the question, "Are there religious or spiritual issues or needs for this patient or family?" Assessment by the professional chaplain addresses the questions, "What are the religious and spiritual needs of this patient and family? How do they impact the living, the relationships, and the decisions of this family system? What are appropriate interventions to assist this patient and family?"

SCREENING TOOLS PRESENTLY AVAILABLE

There are several competent screening tools. One of the most familiar is the Faith and Belief, Importance, Community, and Address in Care (FICA) tool developed by Christina Puchalski, director of the George Washington University Institute for Spirituality and Health. There are two forms of this tool, one for use as a self-assessment the other for use by physicians. The patient and physician apply the answers to these questions to assist them in their partnership of care:

- F: Do I/you have a belief that helps in coping? If not, what gives my/your life meaning?
- I: Is this important to me/you? Does it influence healthcare decisions?

- C: Do I/you have a community that is important? Should I/you do more with this community? If I/you do not belong to a community should I/you find one?
- A: What is my action plan; what do I need to change/develop?/ How would you like me to address these issues in your healthcare?

A second familiar screening is HOPE, developed by Gowri Anandarajah, Professor of family medicine (clinical) and residency director for the Brown Family Medicine Program at the Warren Alpert Medical School of Brown University, and Ellen Hight, of the Brown University School of Medicine. HOPE stands for:

- H: identify sources of hope, strength, comfort, meaning and peace
- O: organized religion's role
- P: identifies personal spirituality and practices
- E: explores the effects on medical care and end-of-life decisions

The Spiritual Competency Resource Center has a lengthier Spiritual Assessment Interview that covers religious background and beliefs, six questions, spiritual meaning and values, two questions, and prayer experiences, three questions. (This interview technique was instituted by David Lukoff at The Institute of Transpersonal Psychology, Palo Alto, California.) These questions are primarily focused toward the quantifiable, but several yield more descriptive information such as "What have been important experiences about God/higher power? How has prayer worked in your life?"

Many professionals, chaplains, and other clinicians have attempted to create a succinct and effective assessment tool. Evidence, particularly in the field of pediatric care, is that these continue to rely heavily on data instead of narrative. This may be why there is no effective validated tool. Each individual's story and needs are unique. The most effective assessment is the narrative. The questions are not "do you go to church, synagogue, or mosque, and how often?" but "Can you tell me what you like the best or least about going to church, synagogue, mosque, or other?" The more open-ended the inquiry, the more one can learn about those things in the life and experience of the patient, and the patient's family, that assist them in making meaning, decisions, and assessing resources.

It is also important to emphasize that the most effective assessment is not a form or checklist that can be completed in one visit by the professional chaplain. If we take it seriously as narrative, then it requires being both told, and heard, over a period of time. The telling occurs in differing chapters to various members of the interdisciplinary team. As the patient and family tell the story of their faith and/or spirituality as it is rooted in their existence, they hear it again themselves as a defining aspect of their being and living. They may even uncover some facets of it which are no longer as vital, perhaps even troubling. As the interdisciplinary team member listens, he or she encourages the telling, demonstrates respect for the value system of the patient and his or her family, and skillfully learns more about how all of the interdisciplinary team may provide important services and support for the family.

The system of collecting a formal spiritual assessment or narrative that works best is the one which the professional chaplain on the interdisciplinary team uses most effectively. The process of spiritual and/or faith assessment is also just that, a process. While the child and family are receiving palliative care services, collecting the narrative is ongoing. This continues to be the most important role of the professional chaplain on the team. Unfortunately, care delivery systems frequently do not provide budgetary support for a full-time professional chaplain, and also frequently underestimate the services this person can provide not only to the patient and family, but also to the interdisciplinary team.

The chaplain on the interdisciplinary care team does not replace the religious clergy with whom a family has a personal relationship, but is one of the value-added personnel who assists the patient and the family and other staff determine what services are needed, when they are needed, and why.

There is another characteristic of the faith and/or spiritual assessment when the patient in palliative care is a child. In almost all other health care situations, patients are the primary decision-makers as long as they are competent to make informed decisions. This is not true for pediatric patients. Not only are children not their own primary decision makers, but also they, or their hopes, wishes, and concerns, may fall far down the family's list of what is important. This refers not only to the child's parents, but also to extended family members, and/or community members depending on the culture and/or ethnicity of the patient/family. Therefore, the effective faith and/or spiritual assessment is one that takes into account the entire family system.[13] It weakens the effectiveness of the child's narrative as a means to assist the child if we do not understand how other family members narratives may either subvert or overpower the child's. As the team gathers the narratives, the chaplain, team members, and perhaps the family's personal clergy, can evaluate where there may be power struggles in the family, whether keeping secrets may impact how the child understands his or her circumstances, and if this will affect the care being provided by the interdisciplinary team. Many other aspects of how the family functions, or does not function, may also be instrumental in planning appropriate care. Ideally, for work in pediatric palliative care, the professional chaplain should have some training in family systems theory across cultures, child, and spiritual development so that her or his evaluation is grounded and not merely guesswork. To provide this training could be an important commitment of a palliative care program.

USING THE FAITH/SPIRITUAL ASSESSMENT

As a member of the interdisciplinary team, the professional chaplain provides insight to other team members about the strengths, weaknesses, and values of the patient and the patient's family that will assist them in coordinating care. One's faith and/or spiritual perspective, which provides a context for making meaning, is of paramount influence to decision-making. It is the way by which persons assess risk versus benefit; it shapes the understanding of quality of life. All members of the interdisciplinary team can provide spiritual care.

Providing Spiritual Care: A Theological Concept

The word theology comes from the Greek *theos*, God, and *logos*, word—therefore, words about God. For our purpose we focus on God as the being, or the concept, which assists humans in making meaning of their lives, believing that there is purpose in life, and encourages relationship to others individually, and to community. For some children and their families

God may be very real: present, experienced, and holy. For others, presence, experience of the holy, providence, and other theological concepts are found in the midst of human relationships and events. Both are spiritual.

Spiritual care is provided by every member of the interdisciplinary team according to his or her own expertise. Following are some descriptions of the spiritual needs of children, and their families, in palliative care. Case examples highlight interventions that can be offered by many members of the care team. There is an emphasis on the importance with which the care team should consistently involve, as an equal partner in planning, the board-certified professional chaplain who has been trained in pediatric care. This person can not only provide support and service to the child and family, but also will be an important guide for the care team in assessing and addressing spiritual care. Every member of the interdisciplinary team brings her or his own particular authority to the relationship. Typically, families want to hear medical details from the physician, concrete support and strategies from the social worker, and faith and/or spiritual perspectives from one trained and vested with the authority of the faith or spiritual community. The professional chaplain also may assist the family's own clergy in assessing and providing care. We emphasize that a family's relationship with their personal clergy is to be respected and supported. However, the community clergy is not a member of the interdisciplinary team. A community clergyperson may not be familiar with medical processes or language and may not be comfortable in the clinical environment; in addition, he or she is not authorized to access medical records.

The list of spiritual needs is extensive. Children and adults need to receive, and share with others, the gifts of faith, hope, and love that are the heart of spirituality. Faith describes the need for safety, protection, and trust, as well as the desire for an experience of the Holy. Hope brings the ability to dream, to wish, and to make meaning out of one's life story. Love encompasses the relationships we cultivate, the value that we feel as unique individuals, and the legacy we leave with those whose lives we touch. The list includes, but is never limited to:

- Making meaning in the context of one's own value and/or religious system,
- Experiencing the world as a safe place,
- The need for protection or to protect others,
- Legacy making,
- Need for others to bear witness,
- Finding a place in community,
- Reconciliation or making amends,
- The many forms of ritual,
- Presence or accompaniment,
- Parenting,
- Sharing fear,
- Evidence of the Holy,
- Fulfilling wishes and hopes,
- Staying in the ambivalence.

The care team participates in all of these areas by interacting with the child and the family. In an extremely important way, the care team *is* the community for this child and his or her family. Children who are sick may have lost their sense that the world is a safe and caring place. Bearing witness to the unfairness of suffering is perhaps the single most important spiritual act that any caregiver can provide. All caregivers need to eliminate the phrase "I understand" from their vocabulary. Each one

must know, for themselves, what they are willing and not willing to do. For instance, a caregiver may be uncomfortable with the family's definition of miracle and their language of prayer. Admit it, but only to one's self. However, take seriously how this is assisting the child or family in making sense of the senseless. The presence of the caregiver is vital. Presence is not merely showing up to perform tasks. It is being able and willing to learn about the values, needs, and feelings of this particular child and family. Sit down. Listen. Use touch gently and compassionately. Illness is isolating and a patient's pain sometimes discourages family members from touching for fear of distressing the child. But being touched is a deep human need. Interdisciplinary care team members can model touching and/or holding, which decreases pain and anxiety. If caregivers communicate a willingness to stay, to be a compassionate and constant presence, they will have provided important spiritual care.

Children faced with serious illness have a need to express the powerful emotions that they may not be able to articulate. They also may not feel comfortable talking with their parents. In order to feel safe, children need to know that they are parented, that someone particular puts them first. If the parent is unable to care for the child because of his or her own distress, then the child will, at the least, experience fear. Yet children need to express what troubles them.

Sally,[14] 14, expressed to a nurse; "I know I'm dying, but, please, don't tell my mom, 'cause she can't handle it." Sally and her mother never had a conversation about what Sally wanted for her death, although the case team attempted to facilitate it. Sally's mother was intent on protecting her daughter; Sally was intent on protecting her mother. Sally, fortunately, was able to talk with one nurse and the social worker about her beliefs, her fears, and what she wanted for herself. Her mother excluded herself from that gift. However, the team respected Sally's mother's values, which was essential to her being able to cope. For patients who have difficulty talking about their feelings, art, music, and play therapy can provide powerful outlets for creative expression. Therapists and psychologists, in providing therapeutic interventions, become spiritual caregivers (Figs. 12-1 and 12-2).

Children want to know that their lives mattered. Constructing a legacy that expresses the child's values can be aided by any member of the care team. Children may want to make a video of them reading their favorite story, talking about their favorite family experiences, sharing how they hope they will be

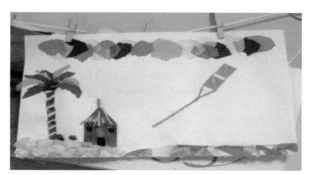

Fig. 12-1 Tissue Paper Collage by a 12-year-old girl who was not able to talk with her mother about dying. Children's National Medical Center (CNMC), Washington, DC.

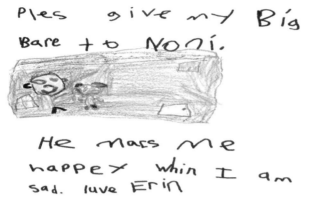

Ples give my Big
Bare to Noni.

He macs me
happey whin I am
sad. luve Erin

Fig. 12-2   An example of a child's will, this one belonging to a 7-year-old at Children's National Medical Center (CNMC), Washington, DC.

remembered. Children may also want to make their own will, leaving their special treasures to the people who have been important to them. Perhaps instead of one video, the child makes his own movie involving everyone in the family. A child can also write letters to each family member to be delivered on the family member's birthday, a special holiday, or the child's birthday and/or the anniversary of his or her death day. Child-life specialists have particular training in making legacies, and can assist the family in working together to create memories.

The need to feel the presence of a power greater than ourselves, an experience of the Holy, is as important to a child as it is to an adult. Prayer, sacraments, and other familiar religious practices can provide reassurance and peace for many children. For concrete thinkers, a symbol or ritual may represent the presence of the Divine.

Amy, 12, had end-stage osteosarcoma and went home with hospice care. Before she left the hospital, the chaplain came and said prayers at Amy's request, and anointed her with special oil. Amy asked if she could take the oil home with her. She knew that she was nearing death and had been asking many questions about the Christian tradition in which she had been raised. She also asked the chaplain, "How do I believe in God?" The chaplain told Amy that she didn't have to work at believing because faith was a gift she already had been given. A few days later the chaplain spoke to Amy by telephone. "Can you send me some more of that oil?" Amy asked. "When I rub it on my leg, it makes the pain go away. I know that God is with me.... I do believe!" For Amy, the ritual of anointing herself with oil and experiencing a relief from her pain was the evidence that she needed to realize God's presence.

Rituals and sacraments are extraordinarily important when patients and families are facing life-threatening or life-limiting situations. The rituals assist not only in making meaning, but also in making decisions. These rituals are the purview of religious professionals such as the chaplain. Other rituals such as bedtime stories, afternoon snacks, playing games, decorating the room, tea parties, using social media websites, involve many individuals and maintain familiar context and content for the child.

It is vital that every member of the interdisciplinary care team tries to comprehend what defines quality of life for the child and the family. The religious, spiritual, and ethical values of a family will dictate much. At a time when families are asked to make decisions about changing the course of treatment from aggressive cure to compassionate care, their core beliefs about death, salvation, the afterlife, and punishment and sin are as authoritative as medical information and advice. Families will frequently resort to theological language to express their hopes and fears. The team's chaplain brings theological expertise to these discussions.

Jimmy's mother asked the chaplain, "If I remove the ventilator, will I go to hell for killing my son?" The chaplain assured the mother that her decisions, based in love, would be understood by her God. Only the chaplain brings the authority of the religious community during these times. The physician, who may be an individual of faith, does not represent the theological establishments that have endorsed the chaplain.

Other members of the care team can assist the many individuals in the family in describing what they want most for themselves and for the child. The team members can ask questions such as, "Tell me what good living means to you?" and "What do you hope for most?"

In the late 1990s, a family had a 1-year-old boy in the hospital's Pediatric Intensive Care Unit (PICU) with spinal muscular atrophy. He was without any muscle tone, he could not even blink his eyes. Yet the family insisted on intensive interventional care. They asserted that "God is merciful." This was not quality of life according to the medical staff, but it was for the family. The child smiled with his eyes. He experienced loving care, and is still alive—tended by a family who still asserts that "God is merciful."

Theologians often avow that there is a significant difference between hopes and wishes. Hopes, they maintain, have to do with the transcendent and eternal; while wishes are worldly and refer to one's particular desires. This chapter asserts that, for children, wishes are just as important as hopes. Everyone wants to experience a full life, and a child's wishes are about filling up his or her life with every possible experience. Clearly, the Make-a-Wish Foundation has taken this seriously. Care team members can also assist a child in making real some long-held wishes.

Karl, 17, was in a clinical trial for a very aggressive cancer. One of his wishes was to have a California beach party. The 3000 mile trip was impossible, but one of the care team members brought in an inflatable child's pool, a bag of sand, a container of Pacific Ocean water (courtesy of a colleague and the UPS), a sun lamp, virgin piña coladas, a video of the Pacific coast, and a CD of the Beach Boys. Other members of the staff got in on the party. The attending physician dropped by wearing flip-flops and a Hawaiian shirt. What a wonderful time they had all one long afternoon.

Children also need permission to die. This is often something families have difficulty granting.

Andi, 4, was dying from acute sickle cell crisis. Her mother would stand at the side of the bed and watch the monitor. As Andi's blood pressure dropped, her mother would say, "Andi, get that blood pressure up! You're not going to leave me alone here." And Andi's blood pressure would climb. This went on for days. Some of the care team tried to press Andi's mother into telling the girl that it is all right to die. But Andi's mom angrily resisted, saying, "It's not all right!" Finally a nurse who had known Andi and her mom a long time sat down quietly at the bedside.... She agreed that it was not "all right" for Andi to die, no one wanted that. But she wondered aloud with Andi's mom what it might be "all right" for Andi to hear from her mother. Could mom say, "It's all right for you not to hurt anymore"? Or could she say, "I'll always love you, you never have to be afraid"? The nurse left and Andi's mother sat for a while watching Andi instead of the monitor. A few minutes later the mother asked the chaplain to come and say a prayer. Andi's mom bent over her and whispered to her daughter, and Andi died.

Tommy, 10, was hospitalized while waiting for a liver transplant. It was clear to the care team that he was very frightened, although he did not want to talk about how he was feeling. His mother was a single parent and could not spend the night with him very often. Tommy had trouble sleeping and would often wake from nightmares. These behaviors reflect the spiritual needs and/or distress of feeling secure, having agency, and trusting in a world that has a purpose for one's self and others. Tommy came from a very religious Christian family and enjoyed going to church and saying prayers. He was also a talented and creative artist, and a bright and gifted student. One of his favorite activities in the hospital was playing video games. The care team met to discuss how they might best support Tommy during his hospital stay (Table 12-2).

TABLE 12-2   Care Plan for Addressing Spiritual Needs

Discipline	Role In providing spiritual care
Physicians	Encourage Tommy to ask questions about his medical condition. Spend a few extra minutes playing video games with him when possible.
Nursing	Spend time sitting with Tommy at bedtime reading a favorite story when possible.
Social work	Connect Tommy and his family with a former transplant patient who is doing well. Offer emotional support for Tommy's mother through supportive counseling. Be a supportive presence for Tommy by regular visits.
Psychology	Provide play therapy for emotional expression. Practice relaxation techniques.
Art therapy	Provide a variety of art materials and work with Tommy in creating art for enjoyment and emotional expression.
Music therapy	Provide quiet meditative music on CD for Tommy to listen to when he is feeling distressed. Sing some of his favorite Sunday School songs with him.
Child life	Provide age-appropriate information about medical procedures, including pictures and dolls.
Pastoral care	Offer to pray with Tommy, provide appropriate religious materials such as music and bedtime prayers. Learn, through family spiritual assessment, about experience and beliefs surrounding illness and death in order to facilitate conversations with Tommy and to equip other team members to do the same.

Meeting spiritual needs is never about fixing anything. Caregivers cannot, and should not, attempt to fix another's value system. That system which gives patients and their families meaning and purpose, alleviates fear and anxiety, and provides a sense of belonging. But each caregiver can consistently respect, ask about and listen to what motivates another and helps that person make sense of their world, be present, be creative, participate as we are comfortable and engage others when we are not, and acknowledge that our value system may not harmonize with those for whom we are caring.

When we offer palliative care to a child and his or her family it is always, in some sense, theological: Faith, hope, love, trust. Believing in something, anticipating some good, being cared for and caring for others, relying upon something or someone is somewhat theological. Medicine and spirituality walk hand in hand. The book known now as Sirach, or Ecclesiasticus, begins Chapter 38 with "Honor the physician with the honor due him, according to your need of him, for the Lord created him; for healing comes from the Most High, and he will receive a gift from the king. The skill of the physician lifts up his head, and in the presence of great men he is admired. The Lord created medicines from the earth, and a sensible man will not despise them." Neither can the physician or care team "despise," or in other words, scorn, the spiritual, religious and moral values –that are the foundation of a child's and family's life. Caregivers can stand, sit, and dance with others during the most intimate moments of living. Each member of the interdisciplinary team can offer care which leads to healing, if not always to life.

REFERENCES

1. Salmon J: *Most Americans Believe in Higher Power, Poll Finds*, The Washington (DC) Post, Section A, p 2, June 24, 2008.
2. Fina D: The spiritual needs of pediatric patients and their families, *AORN J* 62(4):556–564, 1995.
3. Bluebond-Langner M: *The private worlds of dying children*, Princeton, 1978, Princeton University Press.
4. Heilferty C: Spiritual development and the dying child: the pediatric nurse practitioner's role, *J Pediatr Health Care* 18(6):271–275, 2004.
5. Hart D, Schneider D: Spiritual care for children with cancer, *Semin Oncol Nurs* 13(4):263–270, 1997.
6. Feudtner C, Haney J, Dimmers M: Spiritual care needs of hospitalized children and their families: a national survey of pastoral care providers' perceptions, *Pediatrics* 111(1):e67–e72, 2003.
7. McSherry W, Smith J: How do children express their spiritual needs? *Paediatr Nurs* 19(3):17–20, 2007.
8. Frank A: *The wounded storyteller: body, illness, and ethics*, Chicago and London, 1995, University of Chicago Press.
9. Ting-Toomey S: *Communication across cultures*, New York, 1999, Guilford Press.
10. Pruyser PW: *Personal problems in pastoral perspective: the minister as diagnostician*, Philadelphia, 1976, The Westminster Press.
11. Coleridge ST: The "transparent" symbol is a theme of the work as a whole, *Biographia Literaria*.
12. Puchalski C, et al: Improving the quality of spiritual care as a dimension of palliative care: the report of the Consensus Conference, *J Palliat Med* 12(10):2009.
13. The Professional Chaplains at The Children's National Medical Center have developed a Family System Assessment "tool." It includes a page that assists the chaplain in documenting various family strengths and weaknesses. We emphasize this is not a "one visit" tool, but a process of gathering faith/spiritual narrative. Available upon request to Rev. Kathleen Ennis-Durstine, BCC at kennisdu@cnmc.org.
14. All names are pseudonyms and details have been conflated between several similar cases.
15. McSherry M, Kehoe K, Carroll J, et al: Psychosocial and spiritual needs of children living with a life-limiting illness, *Pediatr Clin North Am* 54:609–629, 2007.
16. Cole R: *The spiritual life of children*, Boston, 1990, Houghton Mifflin.

17. Sommer D: The spiritual needs of dying children, *Issues Compr Pediatr Nurs* 12:225–233, 1989.
18. Sourkes B: *Armfuls of time*, Pittsburgh, 1995, Pittsburgh University Press.
19. Stuber M, Houskamp B: Spirituality in children confronting death, *Child Adolesc Psychiatr Clin* 13:127–136, 2003.
20. Hufton E: Parting gifts: the spiritual needs of children, *J Child Health Care* 10(3):240–249, 2006.

SUGGESTED READINGS

Bull A, Gillies M: Spiritual needs of children with complex healthcare needs in hospital, *Paediatr Nurs* 19(9):34–38.

Bluebond-Langner M: *The private worlds of dying children*, Princeton, 1978, Princeton University Press.

Cole R: *The spiritual life of children*, Boston, 1990, Houghton Mifflin.

Davies B, Brenner P, Orloff S, et al.: Addressing spirituality in pediatric hospice and palliative care, *J Palliat Care* 18(1):59–67, 2002.

Erikson E: *Childhood and society*, New York, 1950, WW Norton.

Fina D: The spiritual needs of pediatric patients and their families, *AORN J* 62(4):556–564, 1995.

Fochtman D: The concept of suffering in children and adolescents, *J Pediatr Oncol Nurs* 3(2):92–102, 2006.

Ford G: Hospitalized kids: spiritual care at their level, *J Christ Nurs* 24(3):135–140, 2007.

Feudtner C, Haney J, Dimmers M: Spiritual care needs of hospitalized children and their families: a national survey of pastoral care providers' perceptions, *Pediatrics* 111(1):e67–e72, 2003.

Frank A: *The wounded storyteller: body illness, and ethics*, Chicago, 1995, University of Chicago Press.

Fowler J: *Stages of faith: the psychology of human development*, New York, 1981, Harper Collins.

Hart D, Schneider D: Spiritual care for children with cancer, *Semin Oncol Nurs* 13(4):263–270, 1997.

Heilferty C: Spiritual development and the dying child: the pediatric nurse practitioner's role, *J Pediatr Health Care* 18(6):271–275, 2004.

Hufton E: Parting gifts: the spiritual needs of children, *J Child Health Care* 10(3):240–249, 2006.

McEvoy M: An added dimension to the pediatric health maintenance visit: the spiritual history, *J Pediatr Health Care* 14:216–220, 2000.

McSherry M, Kehoe K, Carroll J, et al: Psychosocial and spiritual needs of children living with a life-limiting illness, *Pediatr Clin North Am* 54:609–629, 2007.

McSherry W, Smith J: How do children express their spiritual needs? *Paediatr Nurs* 19(3):17–20, 2007.

Salmon J: Most american believe in higher power, poll finds, Washington Post [Washington, DC] June 24, 2008.

Sommer D: The spiritual needs of dying children, *Issues Compr Pediatr Nurs* 12:225–233, 1989.

Stuber M, Houskamp B: Spirituality in children confronting death, *Child Adolesc Psychiatr Clin* 13:127–136, 2003.

Quinn J: Perspectives on spiritual development as part of youth development, *New Dir Youth Dev* 118:73–78, 2008.

13 The Interface of Ethics and Palliative Care

JOHN D. LANTOS

Today, the road all runner's come,
Shoulder high, we bring you home,
And set you at the threshold down,
Townsman of a stiller town.
  —A.E. Housman.

Ethics committees and consultation in pediatrics are both relatively recent phenomena. In the 1970s, only a few hospitals had ethics committees.[1] By the end of the 1980s, most hospitals did. The stimulus for the development of ethics committees was the Baby Doe controversy of the early 1980s in which a baby with Down syndrome and esophageal atresia was allowed to die without routine surgery. This led the federal government to promulgate controversial guidelines for end-of-life decisions, guidelines that were challenged and eventually struck down by the U.S. Supreme Court.[2] In the aftermath of that controversy, the American Academy of Pediatrics (AAP) formed a task force to define the role of ethics committees.[3] The early committees focused almost exclusively on newborns and the controversies surrounding decisions to withhold or withdraw life-sustaining treatment. Later, ethics committees broadened the scope of their concerns.

According to the AAP, ethics committees (or "infant care review committees") were to have three purposes. First, they were to provide an educational resource to hospital personnel and families of seriously ill infants. Second, they were to recommend institutional policies and guidelines. Finally, they could offer ethics consultation and review treatment decisions regarding critically ill infants. This original guiding document suggested that the term "infant" refer to any person less than 2 years old.

Over the years, ethics committees and consultants have taken on more diverse roles. They broadened their mandates to include children of any age.[4] Some even began considering cases involving fetuses and perinatal decisions.[5] They also broadened the scope of their concern from clinical decisions to cases involving organizational ethics.[6] Organizational issues of concern include matters of informal organizational culture, especially when that informal culture leads to practices that conflict with organizational policy, communication problems, and issues of resource allocation that are built into but not explicitly addressed by organizational policy.[7]

Pediatric palliative care programs developed over the same time period as pediatric bioethics committees. Their development was not fueled by a political controversy so they had a somewhat slower start.[8] The field of palliative care gained legitimacy with the creation of a national board of hospice and palliative care medicine in 1995.[9] In 2003, the Institute of Medicine report "*When Children Die*," helped define the field of pediatric palliative care.[10] The first freestanding pediatric hospice and respite care facility, the George Mark Children's House, opened in California in 2003.

Most tertiary care children's hospitals now have both ethics committees and palliative care services. There are many ways in which these two entities can and should work together. There are also ways in which they might come into conflict. This chapter will outline some of the domains of overlap and discuss the implications of the different goals and missions of bioethics and palliative care.

The Overlapping Domains of Bioethics and Palliative Care

The field of bioethics addresses many issues that have nothing to do with death, dying, symptom management, life-threatening illness, or end-of-life care. These include, for example, ethical issues of resource allocation, issues in the development of use of stem cells, ethical issues in research, or the ethics of enhancement therapies. For decades, however, issues surrounding end-of-life decision making have been among central issues of clinical bioethics. Analysis of these issues has led to thousands of peer-reviewed publications, many books, numerous legal cases, and a few statutes, as well as to movies and novels. Underlying all these discussions is a central fact of medical progress—medical technology has advanced to the point where patients in hospitals rarely die without a decision to withhold or withdraw some form of life-supporting therapy. Thus, what used to happen without an explicit decision now requires one. Such decisions are sometimes morally ambiguous, often emotionally draining, and may be legally complex. Not surprisingly, they sometimes lead to disagreements among various parties who are involved in the care of the critically ill or dying patient. Bioethical analysis focuses upon the underlying principles that should guide such decisions.

Over the past 25 years, bioethics has developed fairly robust and widely accepted ethical guidelines for making such decisions. Those guidelines define three domains of clinical decisions:

- Where treatment is ethically obligatory because it is clearly beneficial for the child,
- Where treatment is clearly futile and should never be provided (an ever-shrinking but never entirely disappearing domain),
- Where treatment outcomes are ambiguous or uncertain and in which doctors, parents, and children, if they are capable, must together make decisions about whether or not life-sustaining treatment should be provided.

Many pediatric palliative care cases are not ethically controversial. Often, it is clear that a child is dying. If the child's parents understand this and, in discussion with doctors, they choose palliative care rather than or along with life-prolonging therapy, there may be no ethical controversy. Instead, the expertise of palliative care will be used to maximize the efficacy of palliative interventions in order to make the dying process as pain-free as possible. Such cases can be fraught with medical and moral uncertainty, but often they are not marked by conflict between providers and families of the type that lead to bioethics consultation. In such cases, the palliative care that is provided by skilled practitioners is as morally unproblematic as any other medical care, such as cardiology, nephrology, nursing, or chaplaincy services. That is, while there are certainly ethical issues that must be addressed in each of these fields, they are the sorts of ethical issues that are at the core of medical practice. They do not require consultation or collaboration with bioethicists.

Ethical issues arise in palliative care, as in other specialties, when there is conflict between patient and family, patient and professionals, among professionals, or when any or all of the parties consider treatment that may be in conflict with law or hospital policy. In such cases, reasonable people might disagree about what is the right thing to do. The most common of such disagreements focus on two issues: the appropriateness of withholding or withdrawing potentially life-sustaining therapy, and the appropriate use of analgesics or sedatives that could hasten the dying process. When such cases arise, the boundary between issues that might be called ethical and those that are deemed the sole and proper domain of palliative care may become indistinct.

Such blurry boundaries between bioethics and a clinical specialty are not unique to palliative care. They arise in neonatology, oncology, intensive care, pulmonology, and many other specialties. When that occurs, clinicians must decide when and whether to consult an outside expert. Such consultation is often appropriate. After all, the care of children with complex chronic conditions, life-threatening illnesses, or children who are terminally ill is and ought to be an endeavor that requires teamwork, expertise from many different disciplines, and openness to discussion, questioning, insight, and critique of clinical decisions. This teamwork is difficult to build into clinical algorithms for care. It takes time. More importantly, it requires an ethos of humility about the nature of the work that we do and the sorts of dilemmas that we confront. Today, however, clinicians in these other specialties who face complex decisions about end-of-life care may wonder when they should consult bioethics or when they should consult palliative care.

The Nature of the Work

The care of children with life-threatening illnesses is a moral experiment. We keep children alive today who have conditions that, until just a few decades ago, were routinely fatal. Our technologic ability has now reached the point where there are very few conditions that can be unambiguously deemed to be incompatible with life.[11] These technologies allow us to take children and their families into domains where, to paraphrase science fiction, nobody has ever gone before.

What does it mean to the parents and family of a baby born at 23 weeks of gestation to be told the odds of survival, the likelihood of disability, and then given the choice of treatment or non-treatment? What does it mean to give the family that choice or to take the decision away from them? What will the implications be if they choose treatment and their baby survives for months in the neonatal intensive care unit, undergoing numerous painful procedures, and is left with chronic illnesses or impairments? What does it mean to the family of a 5 year old with cancer to be told that the best hope for survival is a bone marrow donation from a sibling, and the best way to do that is a drug that has not been approved or studied for this indication? What does it mean for the families of children with hypoplastic left heart, or multiple congenital anomalies, or a traumatic brain injury, to be offered the options of treatments that can sustain life, but not cure the underlying disease? The only truthful answer is that we really don't know. Yet we must choose. In that sense, what we are doing is truly an expedition into unknown worlds.

We are beginning to map out those worlds. The maps are no doubt imperfect, as are the maps of all early explorers. We are beginning to understand the long-term outcomes for premature babies born at various gestational ages,[12] and to refine our prognostic estimates using other medical and demographic factors.[13] We are beginning to learn how to have conversations with parents in which we both deliver bad news and try to help them understand the choices that must be made.[14] We are beginning to understand a bit more about parents' experiences when faced with such choices.[15,16] We are untangling some of the quirky contradictions in the way both clinicians and families think about particular choices.[17]

The Future

In the brave new world of twenty-first century pediatrics, there will be fewer and fewer conditions that are fundamentally incompatible with life. That is not to say that there won't be children who die as a result of their medical conditions, in spite of receiving all available medical technology. It is only to say that there will always be options about treatments that might prolong the lives of those children. Thus, all parents of children with life-threatening illnesses will face decisions about what to withhold or withdraw. Doctors, too, will face those decisions in each and every case in which a child is critically ill or dying.

In this world, too, we will be able to diagnose disease much more accurately and much earlier in life, often before birth. But we will not be able to prognosticate as accurately because medical progress will so alter the natural history of disease that past studies will be dated and irrelevant. We will have more and more that we can do, with less knowledge of the consequences. Decisions will take place under conditions of significant uncertainty.

These coming changes to pediatrics will challenge the process by which parents and doctors make decisions together. We are just starting to understand how parents deal with these challenges. Payot, et al, have described the differences between parents and neonatologists facing decisions about resuscitation.[18] They write, "While neonatologists focus on the management of the unborn baby, parents have yet to fully conceptualize their infant as a distinct entity since they are in a process of grieving their pregnancy and their parenthood project." Hinds and colleagues analyzed a similar phenomenon in parents of children with cancer.[19] Although it was important to parents to make "informed, unselfish decisions in the child's best interest," it was equally important for them to "remain at the child's side, show the child that he is cherished, teach the child to make good decisions, advocate for the child with the staff, and promote the child's health." Parents are and want to be active participants in their child's care and in the decisions that are made about that care. Many do not see a sharp distinction between palliative care and life-prolonging care. They want both. They don't want to choose. They want them to be seamlessly intertwined.[20] Some parents reject any discussion of palliative care or the withholding of life-prolonging treatment.[21] The lessons that we've learned allow us to speculate about the future of the interface between pediatric palliative care and pediatric bioethics.

Three types of situations increasingly present occasions for collaboration between bioethics and palliative care. The first is in the management of conditions in which death is inevitable in a relatively short period of time. Such situations include metastatic cancer for which there is no further chemotherapy, multisystem organ failure in patients who are not candidates for transplantation, or degenerative metabolic diseases for which there is no curative therapy. In those cases, questions arise more and more frequently about the boundaries between appropriate palliative care and euthanasia. Such questions have already been raised in other countries and in other age groups. In the Netherlands, for example, the Groningen protocol defines certain conditions for which euthanasia is permissible.[22] The protocol has led to much debate,[23] which will continue and intensify.[24] In particular, controversies arise in the gray zone between active euthanasia and intensive palliative sedation at the end of life.[25]

A second common situation that calls for collaboration between bioethics and palliative care is where doctors think palliative care without continued disease-directed care is the best option for a child, and parents reject palliative care. This is a variation of the long-running debate about medical futility, but with a twist. In debates about futility, the choice is usually between continuing a burdensome life-sustaining treatment and discontinuing that treatment. Discontinuation usually leads quickly to death. Currently, the question is more philosophical than practical, what do we do when parents reject symptom-oriented treatment because they fear it signals a shift in the goals of therapy? Focusing solely on symptom-directed care today is largely offered only to patients whose parents accept it. That is not the case for most other clinical interventions. They are provided because doctors think that they are in the child's best interest. As the field of palliative care matures, there will certainly be more cases in which doctors think only palliative care is in the child's interest and parents reject it. The question that will arise more frequently is whether parents can refuse palliative interventions for their child.

A third situation is that in which better symptom management and better analgesia make it more acceptable to continue intensive and burdensome life-prolonging treatments. We commonly see this in oncology, surgery, and intensive care. Better management of pain and symptoms allows for more intensive care in the PICU. As Stoddard and colleagues noted, "Treating children who are critically ill with psychotropic drugs is an integral component of comprehensive pediatric critical care in relieving pain and delirium; reducing inattention or agitation or aggressive behavior; relieving acute stress, anxiety, or depression; and improving sleep and nutrition."[26] Better management of surgical and post-operative pain allows children to undergo many surgical procedures. Better symptom management in oncology allows more disease-directed chemotherapy. In all these cases, palliative care specialists may find themselves facing new sorts of ethical dilemmas.

Why might palliative care professionals call for ethics consults? As pediatric palliative care services take on larger and more complex case loads they no doubt discover more moral gray zones. For example, are there differences in withdrawing fluid and nutrition in a case involving a cognitively intact child with short gut syndrome and liver failure, a child with complex congenital heart disease and intractable congestive heart failure, or a child with a massive intracranial bleed? The ethics consult service might help analyze the moral differences between a child with an intact brain but multisystem organ failure and a child with an intact body but neurologic devastation. Reflection on valid and invalid moral distinctions in such cases will help inform the palliative care clinicians and enhance the moral foundation of end-of-life care.

EXAMPLES OF ETHICAL ISSUES IN PALLIATIVE CARE

A few cases illustrate how this works in practice:

> *A newborn was diagnosed with severe epidermolysis bullosa. The neonatologists and the dermatologists discussed with the parents various treatment options. After consideration, the parents requested comfort care. The baby was having trouble drinking a bottle because of blisters and sores in his mouth. The dermatologist had never been involved in a case in which he withheld fluid and nutrition. He called for an ethics consult and a palliative care consult. Both ethics and palliative care met with physicians and parents, and arranged for a hospital-based palliative care plan that included no fluid or nutrition, fentanyl as needed, and spiritual support for the parents. The baby died the next day.*

> *A newborn was diagnosed with congenital nephrotic syndrome of unknown etiology. He was also noted to have contractures of the upper and lower extremities. A genetics consultant recommended a complete genetic work-up. Nephrologists suggested dietary supplements of protein, calcium, magnesium, and vitamin D and discussed with the parents the possibility of dialysis if the baby's renal failure should worsen. The parents decided that they wanted no further testing and no further intervention. Instead, their preference was for comfort care only. An ethics consultation reviewed the standards of care and outcomes for babies with end-stage renal disease. There was no consensus in the expert community—some did not offer dialysis, some offered it, and some strongly recommended it. The ethics team could find no cases in which doctors sought a court order for neonatal dialysis. Ethics recommended that the parents' wishes be followed. Palliative care was consulted and arranged for home hospice. The baby went home on oral morphine and midazolam. He died two days later.*

What, exactly, do ethics consultants do when asked to consult on such cases? Generally, they use a number of well-established frameworks for ethics consultation in order to clarify the ethical dilemmas and to develop permissible responses. One such framework was developed by McCullough and Ashton.[27] They ask the following questions:

- What are the facts of the case?
- What are our obligations to your patient?
- What are our obligations to third parties?
- Do our obligations converge or conflict?
- What is the strongest objection that could be made to a convergence of obligations? How can this objection be effectively countered?
- Could the ethical conflict have been prevented?

An alternative four-box approach was developed by Jonsen, Siegler, and Winslade. Their four boxes are: medical indications, patient preferences, quality of life, and external factors.[28] In their book, *Clinical Ethics*, they argue that these four boxes provide a framework for identifying and resolving moral conflicts in particular cases.

Summary

Pediatric bioethics and pediatric palliative care have both come of age in the past two decades. The next two decades will present both fields with new challenges. Palliative care providers will no doubt find themselves asked to address many of the dilemmas in end-of-life decision making that were once addressed to bioethics consultants. Bioethicists may find themselves asked to analyze new sorts of dilemmas that arise as palliative care becomes more widely accepted. Careful attention to the ways in which palliative care creates ethical dilemmas and to the ways in which some ethical dilemmas can be solved by the availability of high-quality palliative care will improve the lot of children with life-threatening conditions.

REFERENCES

1. Michaels RH, Oliver TK Jr: Human rights consultation: a 12-year experience of a pediatric bioethics committee, *Pediatrics* 78:566–572, 1986.
2. Mahowald MB: Baby Doe committees: a critical evaluation, *Clin Perinatol* 15:789–800, 1988.
3. American Academy of Pediatrics Infant Bioethics Task Force and Consultants: Guidelines for infant bioethics committees, *Pediatrics* 74:306–310, 1984.
4. Mitchell C, Truog RD: From the files of a pediatric ethics committee, *J Clin Ethics* 11:112–120, 2000.
5. Bliton MJ: Ethics: "life before birth" and moral complexity in maternal-fetal surgery for spina bifida, *Clin Perinatol* 30(3):449–464, 2003.
6. Opel DJ, Wilfond BS, Brownstein D, et al: Characterisation of organisational issues in paediatric clinical ethics consultation: a qualitative study, *J Med Ethics* 35:477–482, 2009.
7. Magnus D: Organizational needs versus ethics committee practice, *Am J Bioeth* 9:1–2, 2009.
8. Corr CA, Corr DM: What is pediatric hospice care? *Child Health Care* 17:1, 1988.
9. von Gunten CF, Sloan PA, Portenoy RK, Schonwetter RS: Trustees of the American Board of Hospice and Palliative Medicine. Physician board certification in hospice and palliative medicine, *J Palliat Med* 3(4):441–447, 2000.
10. Institute of Medicine: *When children die: improving palliative and end-of-life care for children and their families*, Washington, DC, 2003, National Academies Press. www.nap.edu/catalog.php?record_id=10390. Accessed May 17, 2010.
11. Koogler TK, Wilfond BS, Ross LF: Lethal language, lethal decisions, *Hastings Cent Rep* 33(2):37–41, 2003.
12. Johnson S, Fawke J, Hennessy E, et al: Neurodevelopmental disability through 11 years of age in children born before 26 weeks of gestation, *Pediatrics* 124(2):e249–e257, 2009.
13. Tyson JE, Parikh NA, Langer J, Green C, Higgins RD; National Institute of Child Health and Human Development Neonatal Research Network: Intensive care for extreme prematurity: moving beyond gestational age, *N Engl J Med* 358:1672–1681, 2008.
14. Meyer EC, Sellers DE, Browning DM, et al: Difficult conversations: improving communication skills and relational abilities in health care, *Pediatr Crit Care Med* 10(3):352–359, 2009.
15. Forman V: This Lovely Life, 2000, Mariner Books.
16. Farlow B: Misgivings, *Hastings Cent Rep* 39(5):19–21, 2009.
17. Janvier A, Leblanc I, Barrington KJ: The best-interest standard is not applied for neonatal resuscitation decisions, *Pediatrics* 121(5):963–969, 2008.
18. Payot A, Gendron S, Lefebvre F, et al: Deciding to resuscitate extremely premature babies: how do parents and neonatologists engage in the decision? *Soc Sci Med* 64(7):1487–1500, 2007.
19. Hinds PS, Oakes LL, Hicks J, et al: "Trying to be a good parent" as defined by interviews with parents who made phase I, terminal care, and resuscitation decisions for their children, *J Clin Oncol* 27(35):5979–5985, 2009.
20. Mack JW, Wolfe J: Early integration of pediatric palliative care: for some children, palliative care starts at diagnosis, *Curr Opin Pediatr* 18(1):10–14, 2006.
21. Baergen R: How hopeful is too hopeful? Responding to unreasonably optimistic parents, *Pediatr Nurs* 32(5):482, 485–486, 2006.
22. Verhagen E, Sauer PJ: The Groningen protocol: euthanasia in severely ill newborns, *N Engl J Med* 352:959–962, 2005.
23. Lindemann H, Verkerk M: Ending the life of a newborn: the Groningen Protocol, *Hastings Cent Rep* 38(1):42–51, 2008.
24. Manninen BA: A case for justified non-voluntary active euthanasia: exploring the ethics of the Groningen Protocol, *J Med Ethics* 32:643–651, 2006.
25. Postovsky S, Moaed B, Krivoy E, et al: Practice of palliative sedation in children with brain tumors and sarcomas at the end of life, *Pediatr Hematol Oncol* 24(6):409–415, 2007.
26. Stoddard FJ, Usher CT, Abrams AN: Psychopharmacology in pediatric critical care, *Child Adolesc Psychiatr Clin North Am* 15(3):611–655, 2006.
27. McCullough LB, Ashton CM: A methodology for teaching ethics in the clinical setting, *Theoretical Med* 15:39–52, 1994.
28. Jonsen A, Siegler M, Winslade W: *Clinical ethics: a practical approach to ethical decisions in clinical medicine*, 2006, MacGraw Hill.

SECTION 2 Relationships: Structure and Communication

Be gentle with yourself, learn to love yourself, to forgive yourself, for only as we have the right attitude toward ourselves can we have the right attitude toward others.
—Wilfred Peterson

The chapters in this section of our text provide content and wisdom about the human connection that is the essence of pediatric palliative care. The human connection – or in pediatrics, perhaps more accurately described as the web of human relationships because of its density – is so profound that it endures across time and locations, during palliative sedation and after death, and occurs between intimates (such as child to parent) and strangers (one family to another, family to clinician). Critical elements of the human connection in pediatric palliative care as described in these chapters include: the intent to relieve or prevent human suffering; the use of words, silence, and presence to comfort; the intentional efforts to respect hope while helping others to prepare for likely sad outcomes; making honest efforts to have clearly defined care objectives; the honoring of child and family preferences for care; understanding parents' absolute longing for their child; and being attentive to the health of a palliative care team as a whole and to one's own health as a clinician. The latter critical element derives from a simple truth: we bring more to a human connection if we take good care of our own health.

Families, clinicians, and entire palliative care teams come in very different flavors. It is through the human connection that these very different flavors blend and harmonize over a shared experience, an idea, or an ideal. With each blending of the different flavors, care is individualized for each child and each child's family. It is quite likely that the exact palliative care provided for the individual child within the specific family cannot be replicated ever again. The human connection, then, is one-of-a-kind for each child and family. Components of pediatric palliative care can be standardized but the actual human connection cannot be.

There are threats to the human connection in pediatric palliative care, chief amongst them having the time to be present, to listen, to touch, to be silent, and in general, to be available. In the web of nearly infinite relationships in pediatric palliative care that undergird the human connection, there are multiple opportunities to experience conflict in any one or more of the connections. Conflict, too, can occur over a shared experience, idea, or ideal. For example, the idea of doing right by a seriously ill child could result in conflict between family members and clinicians over the possibility of shifting goals of care when the child's condition worsens. A conflict is, after all, a human connection. According to the chapters in this section, the human connection is hard to do, hard to maintain, and hard to bring to an end. Conflict will always be a risk of the human connection in pediatric palliative care.

As described in these chapters, our words and our presence are repeatedly relied on as the tools to use to avoid confusion, antagonism, and fear in pediatric palliative care. These are also the tools to support others and ourselves in the web of relationships, to provide hope, and to acknowledge feelings which are universally present in a human connection. The human connection in pediatric palliative care involves striking complexities: a unique developing child experiencing a life-threatening illness that can change quickly, a family also in development acutely experiencing the child's illness within its own culture and conditions that can change, and interacting in a highly interdependent way with clinicians who practice in ways influenced by their own respective cultures. All of this takes place across the diverse care settings where a seriously ill child spends time (home, school, clinic, inpatient, and community agencies). Further, the human connection does not necessarily take place face to face, and the focus of the connection may not be in the present but instead may be futuristic, aimed at the potential of a future benefit for as yet undiagnosed children and their families. Despite all of these complexities, the human connection at any point of intersection continues to be influenced by the two tools of our words and our presence.

Finally, any human connection in pediatric palliative care needs thoughtful attention over time and conditions. Even in a well established human connection, we need to be invited by the other members of the web of relationships to initiate the focus on a serious topic. This includes an invitation from ill children to talk about the seriousness of their clinical situation. Forgiveness – asking for it and giving it – is a part of the attention a human connection needs. These chapters provide the content to guide us in the real essence of pediatric palliative care – the human connection.

14 Child Relationships

ELANA E. EVAN | HARVEY J. COHEN

The tide recedes, but leaves behind bright seashells in the sand.
The sun goes down, but gentle warmth still lingers in the land.
The music stops, and yet echoes on in sweet refrains. For every
joy that passes, something beautiful remains. — Unknown

The Relationship with the Child

When first meeting a child with a life-threatening illness, there are many unknowns. From your introduction to the patient until the day goodbyes are said, the dynamic nature of this relationship can inspire pediatric palliative care clinicians to continually learn and investigate optimal methods of caring for their patients. Your relationship, as the clinician, with a pediatric patient is of the utmost importance in promoting the best quality of life possible for this child. The development of this relationship will also facilitate treatment decision-making for the family and prevent the brunt of future hardship, such as complicated grief, that family members can experience if and when the child dies.

BUILDING RAPPORT WITH PEDIATRIC PATIENTS

Children need to trust that an adult has a genuine concern for them, rather than a superficial interest, in order to disclose the very vulnerable nature and emotional or psychological issues related to their illness. When this genuine interest is experienced by the child, a foundation for rapport can be achieved. There are elements to rapport building that occur naturally, through mere chance and chemistry, and other elements that require some preparation. Using what is known regarding patient history, allowing time for communication, such as through the child's or your narratives, and building trust are key elements in developing rapport and establishing a solid relationship with a young patient coping with a life-threatening illness.

To the degree possible, having advance knowledge regarding the child's medical and psychosocial history can facilitate not only the first interaction with the pediatric patient, but also with the rapport building necessary for subsequent interactions. Along these lines, bridging what is known and/or familiar to the child with new situations can be an effective strategy for building rapport. Bridging the familiar to the less familiar can be accomplished using kinetic conversations. which promote the child to act naturally within his or her environment.[1] If clinicians consistently behave in the same way as other friendly adults who approach children and talk about pleasant things such as likes, dislikes, friends, or home, these types

of conversations can help the clinician be associated with the good emotions these topics elicit until he or she becomes a more familiar, positive figure to the child.[2]

Specific communication strategies to foster rapport building include using a personal line of questioning for the patient, providing rapport building statements, and opening up conversations. Inquiries reflecting a personal line of questioning demonstrate the professional's interest in the pediatric patient beyond the disease. These types of questions regarding topics such as favorite basketball teams, games, hobbies, increase the child's level of comfort and encourage the child to remember pleasant times and places and re-experience these pleasant situations.[2,3] Rapport-building statements, such as "let's figure this out together"[4] and using general supportive comments along with open-ended questions[5] can facilitate making a connection with the older child. Younger children and those pediatric patients who are less verbal can draw pictures and write stories to express themselves when interacting with healthcare staff.[6]

Opening up lines of communication by reframing[2] negative experiences to shine light on what is more hopeful and possible regarding the child's quality of life is another method that can be used to establish rapport. Using allegory and storytelling, both from the healthcare provider's perspective and by asking the pediatric patient to tell his or her story[7] are other ways to proceed. Arthur Frank wrote of the importance for allowing patients time to tell their stories in a narrative fashion, without interruption, and just being present for the patient.[8] Being present without having an immediate agenda, such as taking a history or conducting a physical exam, can be a powerful tool in building trust and establishing rapport.

Other trust-building strategies reflect not only how the clinician presents him or herself, but also depend on the child's own expectancies of rapport with the clinician. Pediatric patient's expectancies of rapport play a role in how they experience their relationship with the clinician. Children tend to feel more comfortable with newly acquainted adults when they experience them in predictable ways. For example, children meeting a clinician may feel more ready to establish rapport with the adult when they first present themselves demonstrating typical adult behavior, such as reviewing the patient's chart rather than with atypical adult behavior, such as playing with toys. Promoting a sense of autonomy while still acting in a supportive way for the child will yield greater rapport than a controlling style.[9–11] This can be achieved by respecting the child's perspective, that is validating the child's experience and granting the patient decision-making power where appropriate, as his or her initial perceptions affect the relationship. Even when acting in a supportive manner, if the child expects otherwise, such as a more authoritative approach, then the initial relationship may suffer. Clinicians should encourage children's openness to the relationship, by asking what their expectations are and dispelling myths regarding the role of the clinicians.[12] Trust-building can sometimes be helped along if a parent is initially present or if the clinician uses a distraction technique such as play or props.[3]

Daniel, 12, had multiple relapsed Hodgkin lymphoma. He was seen by the pediatric palliative care team to work primarily on establishing a quality-of-life plan while in treatment. Upon the clinician's arrival, Daniel said he didn't need another person trying to help him out. He told the palliative care clinician that he had managed to be in charge of his life since diagnosis and just felt that there was no need to have someone in charge of his quality of life in addition to his treatment. The clinician later discovered that Daniel thought the palliative care team became involved because his primary oncology team perceived him as not being responsible enough for his treatment. It took a couple more visits with Daniel by the palliative care team for him to realize that the palliative care clinicians were there for what he needed. The primary rapport-building strategy that the team used related to understanding Daniel's expectations and allowing him the opportunity to be autonomous and in control of his quality of life while the palliative care team acted as a consultant in a supportive role.

Influence of Familial Relationships

The child is part of a larger unit, the family. When considering how, what, where, when and if to speak with the child about palliative care and end-of-life issues, the history, and familial mechanisms and extents of communication must be appreciated. Acknowledging the individual child's role in the larger family unit, while taking into account the generational attitudes that affect issues, such as treatment decision-making and paying heed to how the course of illness influences family roles, can assist the clinicians in caring for their pediatric patients. It can be helpful to understand the extent of how protective parents have been in discussing aspects of the child's illness or other traumatic events that have occurred in the past. This will have a major influence on how they feel about communicating information and its implications to the child in the current situation. Therefore, it is important to assess the willingness for parents to share information early in the course of the child's illness, and to try to assist the parents in being as open and as truthful as they can in a developmentally appropriate fashion. It is often helpful to discuss with the parents how the child's sense that being told the truth can allay their child's fears, and that attempting to hide certain aspects of the disease and its consequent therapy may increase fears, and lead to the child no longer trusting the parents.[13]

In many families it is not only the parents that deserve consideration in healthcare care related discussions. Often, families include at least three generations, and attitudes of the grandparents toward discussing issues with children also influence the approach to the parents. With the additional stressors of life-threatening and life-limiting disease, the clinicians caring for the child can take into account the complexity of the prior and current intra- and inter-family interactions and psychological issues, including divorce, and how these may affect discussion with the child.

The role of the child in the family and the ability of the clinician to help guide the family is a dynamic process that can be dependent on the stage of disease. Often, early after the diagnosis, protecting the child seems most important, and because there has not as yet been the opportunity to establish a relationship with the clinicians, the ability to guide families may not be optimal. With time, especially if the family feels more comfortable that the clinicians care for their child and his/her overall well-being, increased trust may develop, and guidance by the healthcare provider is much more accepted by the family. However, when the disease trajectory changes, and issues related to palliative rather than curative care are being discussed, there may again be reluctance to burden the child with information or choices.[14,15] It is important both to respect the feelings and needs of the family and at the same time try to help them speak with their child and permit you to do the same.[16] Determine if the family is willing to allow these discussions to occur only in their presence, or permit private discussions between the clinicians and the child. It is often helpful to tell parents that sometimes children try to protect parents in the same way that parents try to protect children, and that their child might feel more comfortable discussing his or her concerns without them present.

For adolescents with life-threatening illnesses, it is even more important to determine how the family affects them and the ability of the clinicians to discuss important issues. While it might seem as if families would be more willing to allow discussions relating to palliative and end-of-life care with teenagers, again, the history of communication within the family and the decision-making processes need to be examined. In part, because the concept of death and its finality is more developed in adolescence, some families are even more uncomfortable in having clinicians discuss these issues. Establishing good and open relationships with both the parents and child can have a major impact in how accepting the parents are in having these conversations occur.

There are times, such as in the case of Maria, however, when family and cultural issues can have profound effects on the ability to communicate with the child about important issues.

Maria, 16, had advanced soft tissue sarcoma and came to the hospital from Greece for experimental therapy. She was a bright and highly interactive young woman. She had not been told that she had cancer, but had been told by her mother that she had tuberculosis and needed special therapy. One of the conditions the physician agreed to in caring for this child was that he would not tell her about her condition.

Maria's cancer initially responded to the therapy, but after a year, in which the doctor established a good relationship with both Maria and her family, there was concern about disease recurrence. A lung biopsy was recommended to diagnose the problem. Again, the physician approached the family and asked if he could discuss the nature of Maria's condition with her before they spoke about surgery. Because they now trusted him, they said that he could have that discussion. He then met with Maria, alone, and mentioned that he had been treating her for over a year, and asked whether she would like to know what disease she had. Despite coming to an oncology clinic, and being transported in a van from the American

Cancer Society, Maria said that she did not want to know. The biopsy showed recurrent disease, and Maria and her family returned to Greece, where she died a few months later. The family was extremely grateful for the care Maria received and the respect they received regarding their familial and cultural mores.

Clearly Maria knew what the disease was, but based on the messages she had received from her family, not talking about the nature of her disease was part of the family coping. This demonstrates how cultural and family relationships can greatly influence how and what is communicated to the child. The complexities of family relationships do affect all aspects of communication with children and adolescents, but they do not make these interactions impossible. Understanding and respecting family structures and values by the clinicians are necessary for establishing the best approach to discussing palliative and end-of-life care with the child, and thoughtful and caring guidance of the family during the illness can optimize the potential for effective discussions.[17]

Communication Across the Disease Course

Communicating with a child who has a life-threatening illness is often a very daunting and heart-wrenching task, even for pediatric clinicians with years of experience. Little training is offered on how to approach end-of-life communication with children.[18] In addition to dealing with the pediatric patients, healthcare providers must deal with the emotions of parents. Sharing information at the beginning of the illness with the child can establish trust; however, end-of-life issues should be discussed only if the clinician has already developed trust and a rapport with the patient.[19]

Frank discussions about death with children still remain relatively uncommon in most acute pediatric settings. Unfortunately medical staff tend to comply with parents' well-intentioned, but potentially detrimental requests, for non-disclosure regarding the child's prognosis. Staff members find themselves worrying that any confrontation with parents may harm the fragile trust that has taken a long time to develop with the family. While aiming to respect parental decision-making authority, communication obstacles regarding disclosure to the child can cause clinicians to feel despair and grief about the impending loss of their pediatric patients. They can also incur a sense of moral distress if they are unprepared to provide sufficient support for the dying child.[20] Published guidelines stress the importance of open, honest communication with dying children, but there is relatively little information available regarding concrete suggestions and practical help regarding disclosure discussions and post-disclosure support.[21,22]

At diagnosis, the healthcare team sets the groundwork for trust and honesty in their relationships with parents and patients, so parents will feel comfortable to allow independent clinician-child interactions. The best approach is a flexible one that adapts to the child's and family's needs. In adolescents, the approach also needs to foster personal growth of the patient throughout his or her experience with illness. Clinicians should take opportunities to promote decision-making in simple choices, such as allowing the child to choose the flavoring for oral medication.[23]

Assessing for communication barriers occurring within the family while asking open-ended questions in order to establish a framework for communication with the child throughout the disease course can be accomplished using strategies such as Beale's[19] 6 Es for communicating with the dying child. These 6 Es are:

1. Establish agreement with the child early in the relationship that open communication is critical to the relationship.
2. Engage the child at an appropriate time. A newly diagnosed serious illness or a moment during the disease course when a child's physical or emotional health may be taking a turn for the worse, are opportunities for initiating discussions.
3. Explore what the child already knows and wants to know about the illness. This allows the clinician an opportunity to correct misunderstandings about the medical facts and to provide information according to how the child wishes for information to be given.
4. Explain medical information according to the child's needs and age.
5. Empathize with the child's emotional reactions. When the clinician empathizes, "It seems like you are really worried about this," it validates, "we really care that you've been upset," and clarifies, "what have you been thinking about?" Then the child is given permission to be upset and express his or her feelings, that will allow for opportunities for discussion of more concrete concerns.
6. Encourage the child by reassuring him or her that you will be there to listen and be supportive. Anxiety regarding a child's family and friends and worries about symptoms such as pain are the major concerns for children who are dying. Being present and genuinely acknowledging these concerns is helpful for the child.

Communication strategies such as the 6 Es can also be helpful in eliciting information to create a preliminary quality-of-life plan for when the child is first diagnosed with a life-threatening illness. This important element to the plan of care will allow for all members of the child's team to have clear expectations of who is accountable for what elements of the child's care and will also promote clear communication for future care coordination.[24]

During the treatment phase, the clinician must be clear in his or her communications with the child regarding the nature and course of the illness and possible treatments. If age appropriate, helping the child weigh important treatment decisions can be accomplished through "what if questions," such as "what if a clinical trial is available to you, but it means feeling extreme nausea and fatigue for many months—would this be something you would like to consider?" Communicating choices that offer a degree of independence, such as time away from the clinician and hospital, is also something that can provide empowerment to the child during the treatment phase.[23]

Children have discussed their preferences for interpersonal relationships with their healthcare team. In multiple studies that queried the child directly, their main concerns revolved around communication. Overall, they appreciated openness and honesty; expressed needs for reassurance, support, and empathy, as well as to be taken seriously; while having sufficient time to talk, explain, and come to terms with their illness and treatment.[25,26]

TABLE 14-1 Communication Strategies for Use with the Child Across the Disease Course

Diagnosis
- Build rapport
- Assess any family barriers in communicating directly with the child
- Open-ended questions to assess child's role in family, current lifestyle, definition of quality of life
- Establish framework for open communication with the child across disease course

Treatment
- Clarify child's understanding of illness and course of treatment
- Depending upon age, ask "what if" questions to present possible prognostic scenarios and determine child's wishes
- Use empowering statements to help child tailor own quality of life plan

End of Life
- Use multimodal methods (drawing, written, verbal) to discuss end-of-life care plan
- Allow silence and space for reflection
- Offer comforting words and create moments for legacy-building activities

Regarding information exchange preferences, a group of seven Dutch cancer patients, ages 8 to 17 years, participating in a study stressed their rights to be fully informed about their illness and treatment, but this varied slightly depending on the individual child's survival rates and prognosis. Clarity on information about illness and treatment, age-appropriate language, and content of information were also identified as important. However, they wanted only general information during diagnosis, and then more detail in subsequent consultations. They commented that the majority of information was lost due to the shock at diagnosis, thus repeating explanations and answering questions were key elements to meetings with the healthcare team. At times, this group of patients preferred to use their parents to facilitate communication with their physician; however, they wished to be able to reach their healthcare provider, themselves, at all times. Preferences included wanting to collaborate in making decisions, but they admitted that sometimes they were prevented from doing so.[25]

At end-of-life, communications regarding physical issues (such as symptom management) as well as discussions around more existential issues (such as what they wish to leave behind for people to remember them by) are critical to the well-being of the child. It is important, once again, to assess the child's awareness and how much knowledge the child would like to have regarding his or her stage of disease. Clinicians can use multimodal methods, such as simple drawings, other visual aids, play, and/or written materials that include verbal communication to provide pediatric patients with information about end stage disease. During end-of-life care, clinicians, listening to fears and praising strength, and pausing for silent reflection, can help patients achieve peace of mind despite a terminal prognosis.[27] Often, just hearing that their clinician will be there for them allowed patients to feel comforted and not abandoned[27,28] (Table 14-1).

Developmental Issues in Speaking with Children about Palliative Care and Death

Developing an understanding of life, death, illness, and how one sees relationships with parents and others in light of this knowledge is a process that occurs in childhood and adolescence. These changes are important for clinicians to understand so that they may guide children to comprehend and respond to information regarding their illness and its implications. This is especially true for discussing death and palliative care with a child who is terminally ill.

Questions typically arise regarding whether the child should be told that he or she is dying, who should discuss this with the child, and how should the child be told. The answers to these questions require individual assessments as to the readiness of both the child and family to hear the information, and the additional issues of children's and adolescents' changing concepts of death that occur with development.

While there is not much known about what the child senses, even without discussions, it has been reported that young children who were terminally ill displayed greater anxiety than children who did not have a life-threatening illness.[13] What was also clear from this study was that even though the terminally ill children were not told they were dying, many were aware of it, as demonstrated by the tales they told involving death.[29]

There are a number of myths concerning children in terms of their grief and their awareness of their situation. Children do grieve loss although they may express it differently, they grieve as much as adults, they cannot be protected from death, and grief in children has no time limits. Despite belief to the contrary, terminally ill children typically know they are dying, thus adults' denial can be ineffective in protecting children from this knowledge.[29]

While there are definite stages of development that children and adolescents go through, when, how, and what affects this development may be variable and influenced by having a chronic, life-threatening illness. The guidelines described below are important to understand, but it is equally important to realize that individuals mature at different rates and not all aspects of development occur together.[30]

An overview of children's concepts of death as a function of age is presented in Table 14-1.[29] While each child may be different, these guidelines are very helpful in aiding the clinician in knowing what the child understands about death and what finality might be, and this information can be used to help the clinician approach the child and help guide the family in their discussions. The clinician needs to keep in mind when thinking about the developmental issues that despite their age, many children know they are dying, even if they don't know exactly what that means.[19,27,31] Also, depending on the age, forms of communication besides oral discussions can be very helpful. These include play, art, and writing. Often the use of these alternative forms of communication makes it possible for the child to start discussing his or her fears and understanding of the nature of the illness.[32,33] In addition, depersonalizing the discussion may make it easier to learn what the child is thinking about the nature of death. Speaking about friends or family members who have died may help the clinician learn where in the developmental path their patient is. Children do grieve differently from adults. They often grieve intermittently, and the grieving can change as they begin to get a better understanding of death.[34-36] There are also books available that discuss the deaths of animals, which can be used to begin the discussion of what death means in an age-appropriate manner. Examples include *The Dead Bird*, by Margaret Wise-Brown, which is appropriate for children ages 3 to 5, and *When Dinosaurs Die: A Guide to Understanding Death*, by Laurene and Marc Brown which can be useful for children between the ages 4 and 8 (Table 14-2).

TABLE 14-2 Overview of Children's Concepts of Death

Age range (years)	Concept
0 to 2	Death is perceived as separation or abandonment
	Protest and despair from disruption in caretaking
	No cognitive understanding of death
>2 to 6	Death is reversible or temporary
	Death is personified and often seen as punishment
	Magical thinking that wishes can come true
>6 to 11	Gradual awareness of irreversibility and finality
	Specific death of self or loved one difficult to understand
	Concrete reasoning with ability to see cause-and-effect relationships
Older than 11	Death is irreversible, universal, and inevitable
	All people and self must die, although latter is far-off
	Abstract and philosophical reasoning

Adapted from: Himelstein BP, Hilden JM, Boldt AM, Weissman D: Pediatric palliative care, *N Engl J Med* 350(17):1752-1762, 2004.

Cultural Issues

Culture acts as the framework that directs human behavior in many situations. Cultural backgrounds influence families' preferences and needs about discussing illness, decision making, and death. This is especially true in dealing with medical illness in their children. It is broadly believed that cultural values, beliefs, and practices play a critically important role in determining how families care for their children, interact with clinicians, and discuss disease and end-of-life issues. Reluctance to disclose information about a serious illness to a terminally child is not uncommon in many cultures, and discussions about dying and death may be avoided entirely.[37] Several studies highlight the underlying values that determine the communication patterns among children, parents, and families in different cultural contexts. For example, studies with Chinese,[38] Greek,[39] and Japanese parents[40] have shown that in these cultures, parents try to protect terminally ill children and their siblings from any knowledge regarding the disease and the likely outcome of the illness.

In order to both aid the family in coping and determine what might be the best mechanism to discuss the illness and its trajectory with the child, clinicians need to consider the family's culture. Assessment needs to include the culture-based health beliefs and practices, religious rites, thoughts about how and why illnesses occur, and meanings attributed to childhood suffering and death, in addition to how their culture and family feel about speaking with their child about illness and death. For example, in Chinese families there is a belief that bad news or sadness should not be discussed with children.[38] By respecting this particular cultural belief and other family values, professionals can avoid burdening families with their own cultural models of healthcare because professional models may not necessarily promote quality near the end of life for a given patient and family. In order to know what the cultural issues are for that family as they may affect communication with the child, the clinician should use respectful and open-ended questions about how the family wants the issues related to palliative and end-of-life care addressed to the child. While it is not unreasonable for the clinician to provide information as to how children can benefit from honest and caring discussions, if the culture of the family is such that these discussions would be seen as counter-productive, the wishes of the family should not be ignored.

As discussed in the previous section on how family issues affect communication with the child, it is crucial to realize that how the family responds to communication issues is often culturally driven. The description of 16-year-old Maria, who elected not to be given the name of the disease she was being treated for, is as much related to the culture of her family, as to the family itself. Given Maria's background with her individual preferences, providing her with the diagnosis she did not wish to receive would have only closed lines of communication further among her, her family and her physician. This was acknowledged by the physician, and led him to not press the matter. As a result, he was much more effective in helping both the child and family during the difficult terminal phases of the illness.

In some cultures, medical decision making is done with religious or social leaders, and how and what is told to the child is in large part decided on their advice.[41] Because these individuals can be very helpful to the family during the stressful times related to their child's illness and death, respectful conversations may need to include these cultural or religious leaders.

Both verbal and non-verbal language barriers between caregivers and parents often are very challenging when trying to communicate to them the desire to speak honestly with their children. While most children speak the language of the country they reside in, often parents do not speak this language fluently, if at all. Medical interpreters are important in helping families hear the reasons why the caregiver thinks it is important to speak with the child.

The following observation describes the importance of culturally-driven, non-verbal communication with children. As part of the process to determine how a pediatric palliative care program should be established, a needs assessment was performed. A Spanish-speaking social worker discovered that Latino families often mentioned that the display of affection toward their child by the professional not only made them feel better but also affected their view of the competence of that individual.

This type of non-verbal communication, while embraced by individuals of most cultures, seemed to have a greater impact on the effectiveness of the clinician in being able to develop trust with the aforementioned family. When certain culturally specified non-verbal communication is absent from a scenario, it becomes a barrier to trust and confidence in the medical team. The families often report being confused, isolated, and distrustful of the hospital system.[17] The role that culture plays on the ability to communicate with children of various ethnic backgrounds is only now emerging, and investigations on the impact of culture and language in communication with terminally ill children needs to occur if we are to be most effective in making palliative and end-of life care available to the diverse group of children under our care.[42,43]

Boundaries—Where the Relationship with the Child Begins and Ends

Interactions between clinicians and their patients, by their very nature, result in the establishment of a relationship. These relationships differ in intensity depending on the individual caregiver, child, family, and situation. While it had been thought in the past that involvement by a clinician in the personal life of a patient was to be strictly avoided because it may interfere with the professional relationship, this is no longer believed to be true by most clinicians working with children with life-threatening illnesses. In fact, it is generally believed that optimal care of a patient with chronic, life-threatening disease is enhanced when the clinician and patient have established strong bonds.

Children respond better to, and are more at ease with, clinicians who they sense have an interest in them as individuals.[2] Thus, there are great therapeutic benefits to children and their families when providers form meaningful relationships with their patients.[44,45] There are, however, risks associated with relationships that could deleteriously affect the role of the clinician with the child or family.

These boundary issues become potentially more problematic when the stresses of end-of-life care are added to the relationships. Boundaries between clinicians and patients need to be mutually understood in terms of the physical and emotional limits on the nature of the relationship.[46] When they are not understood or adhered to, unnecessarily harmful effects can occur to the patient, and enhanced stressors can develop for the professional. Appropriate boundaries can help ensure that not only will the patients suffer less, but also that equity in dealing with all patients will be enhanced and perceived.[47]

Two overarching principles must be kept in mind for the professional in terms of interactions with the child and family. First, while it is unavoidable and actually helpful when the relationships between patients and clinicians result in the professional benefiting from the interactions, it must always be kept in mind that this benefit must never be at the expense of the child or family. Second, while serving as a caregiver for the child and family, these relationships need to be such that they do not negatively impact the role of the clinician as a professional caregiver. If the relationship becomes more personal, and the clinician begins to assume the role of a friend or family member, it can have negative impact on the care of the child and family. It is the effect of the personal relationship, rather than the relationship itself, that needs to be considered. The clinician, while grieving for the child and family, should not allow this to affect his or her professional role, and should not be looking for comfort from the family at their expense.

Relationships with the family may continue after the death of the child. It is necessary for the clinician to decide whether he or she is still in a professional relationship with the family[48] and acting as a caregiver, or whether the relationship has changed and the clinician is no longer part of a therapeutic team, but has become a friend or colleague. The effect of not addressing this issue is that the clinicians become uncertain of their role, and this can add stress to both them and the family. For the clinician of an adolescent, the proximity in age with young clinicians can sometimes make boundary issues problematic. Identification of the clinician with the patient, or the patient's need and desire to have someone to relate to of a similar age, can lead to involvement in the private lives of each other, which results in an increased risk of overstepping professional boundaries, and for the professional being less effective as a clinician. When the sexes of the patient and clinician are different, there is an additional danger of fantasizing by the adolescent patient that the clinician might be a sexual partner. Excessive involvement of the clinician in the life of the adolescent patient may enhance these thoughts, and need to be considered by the professional to ensure that appropriate boundaries are not crossed.[49]

Boundary issues can occur for multiple reasons. Consideration must be given to the fact that the child and family come into the diagnosis of a life-limiting disease with a prior history. While for most individuals, it is the situation that produces the need for closeness, there are some individuals with certain personality types or who have psychiatric disorders, in which they may not be able to recognize or respect normal boundaries.[50] While this is uncommon with children, it still can occur with their parents, and can complicate pediatric care. Cultural differences between patients and clinicians might lead to misunderstandings of the relationships that are developing between patients and their clinicians. What one culture interprets as appropriate professional-patient interactions, may be seen as inappropriately close in other cultures. In some of the Asian cultures, touching or holding patients and family members is seen as intrusive, while among some Latino communities, *not* showing affection to children decreases the sense of the value of the clinician.[17] The stresses and burnout experienced by clinicians can lead to them crossing boundaries for their own needs. Clinicians often do not give themselves permission to deal with the effects of their patients' illnesses on themselves, and this can result in them not realizing when they are crossing appropriate boundaries.

Indications that appropriate boundaries are being blurred may occur when either accepting or giving gifts, when patients want to know personal information about their clinicians, or when the clinician shares personal information with the child or family. While these phenomena in and of themselves may not cross appropriate boundaries, they are of concern if they lead to the clinician losing therapeutic effectiveness in the care of the child or in the interactions with the family. Not all of these boundary issues are harmful to the therapeutic relationship between the clinicians and the patients and families, and some may even enhance care and serve to reinforce the caring interactions. However, it is important that the clinicians question whether these boundary-blurring activities result in some children and families being treated differently than others, whether the feelings these interactions elicit impact clinical decision-making, and whether the need for these interactions are the result of his or her own stresses or burnout.[45]

Managing boundary issues are important for the care provider if he or she is going to be optimally effective and not harm the child or family. If appropriate, it might be important to set clear expectations with the role of the professional in the care of the child. If the clinician is concerned about the effects of boundary blurring on the child and family, it can be very helpful to seek the advice of a mental health professional that is not directly involved in the patient's care. If these options do not prove to be effective, another path might be to find another healthcare provider to take one's place in caring for the patient.

An example of how assistance by a colleague can help clinicians when faced with boundary issues is demonstrated in the following case.

Jonathan was a 5-year-old boy with multiply relapsed acute lymphoblastic leukemia who was on experimental therapy. The physician had established a close relationship with both parents, but had especially made himself very available to the mother. At a critical part of the treatment regimen, the physician had to be out of town. When he returned, the mother yelled at him for not being around. He felt awful, and wondered what his role should be. He consulted a social worker who was not involved in the care of this child. She helped him realize that, although it was understandable that the mother was upset, his role as a physician was not the same as that of a parent, that she did not have the right to treat him that way, and that such behavior could damage the effectiveness of the child's care. He met with the mother and explained his concerns with her behavior, and they were able to establish a more appropriate relationship recognizing what his ongoing role would be. He remained close to the family, and was able to help them through the terminal part of the child's care, and beyond.

Close relationships can have positive therapeutic effects both for the child and family, and may be sources of solace to the family even years after the death of the child. Thus, the issues related to boundaries should not prevent these relationships from occurring.

The following case is an example of a relationship with a child and family that, while close, never interfered with the role of the clinician with the child or family, and continued years after the child died. This has resulted in positive consequences for both the child and family, and enrichment in the life of the physician.

Debra, 18, had stage IV Hodgkin disease and multiple recurrences. Her physician had cared for her for over three years, was invited to and attended her high school graduation, and helped her complete the first year of college by modifying the times for her chemotherapy. Her clinical situation then deteriorated, and the physician worked closely with the teen and family during the terminal phase of the illness. The physician went to the funeral, which was in the child's home state, and was invited to sit with the family in the front pew. For the past thirty years, the family and physician have been in contact on a yearly basis, and although they have shared many life changes, the mother continues to call the physician and has periodically asked his professional opinion on family health matters. Recently, the physician visited the family at their home, where he saw a picture of Debra and himself on the family's bureau. This relationship, while close and meaningful to both the physician and the child and family, never interfered with the ability of the physician to do and recommend the appropriate treatment for the child.

The closeness of relationships, by themselves, are not necessarily good or bad, but always need to be considered in terms of whether they benefit the child and family, and not just how meaningful it is to the clinician.

Saying Goodbye

The finality of any death is a reality difficult to imagine. This finality can appear even more incredulous when dealing with the impending death of a child. Saying "good-bye" to a child can be done directly, by saying the actual words, and indirectly, by discussing the history of the relationship and using other words to close the relationship, depending on the nature of the relationship that has been established. If a healthcare provider is not given or does not make use of an opportunity to say good-bye to a child, this can create a long-lasting impact on the clinician both from an emotional standpoint as well as from a professional perspective.[51] Not saying goodbye denies the clinician the opportunity to say final words, and/or from relaying messages in order to fully close the circle of the relationship. Not having the moment to say goodbye may trigger doubts in the clinician about whether the child knew the extent of the clinician's commitment to his or her care.

The importance of this act cannot be understated, but often, clinicians are unsure of when and how to say goodbye. Timing for when it might be appropriate to say goodbye can be challenging as the following questions may arise when ultimately deciding how and when to express oneself: Is the child ready to hear a goodbye? Will the parents want me to say goodbye? What will the emotional reaction be like for the child? Will saying goodbye be too difficult for me as the clinician? Will I say goodbye in the right way?

Preparation and timing is needed for this to occur in a way that is helpful for the child, his or her family, and the clinician. The timing and exact words are ultimately determined on a case-by-case basis.

Very little information has been described regarding timing, along with the words and discussions that occur during the closing moments between a clinician and the pediatric patient at the end of life. What has been described are the emotional reactions of the healthcare team following the death of their pediatric patients.[51,52] With the scant amount of information on this topic, clinicians are left with little direction for how to proceed in this important clinical situation.

For parents, it takes longer to become emotionally aware of the impending death of their child than it does for them to become intellectually aware of it. Not being emotionally and intellectually aware of the impending death can lead to anxiety and depression.[53] Parents who were given the time to process their child's impending death felt better able to prepare.[54] In many ways, this important paradigm can be extended to the clinician, such that the emotional component of saying goodbye to a pediatric patient may take time to be fully realized even though the intellectual component is what the clinician is operating under most of the time. Thus, taking the time to prepare for saying goodbye will be an important step for the clinician.

In other clinician-patient relationship paradigms, such as in psychotherapy, the end of the professional relationship or what is termed as termination needs to be a planned process that starts from the beginning of the therapeutic relationship.[55,56] In order to prevent the adult or child client from feeling abandonment or anxiety, the clinician can set goals regarding his or her working relationship so that as the end of that relationship nears, the client feels a sense of mastery or fulfillment. In the case of pediatric palliative care, where death can be the final outcome for the child, a sense of mastery and fulfillment can still be reached at the end of the therapeutic relationship when the clinician and child say goodbye to one another. Using developmentally appropriate language, the clinician can emphasize the strengths of the child, how he or she coped courageously with all medication changes, and the positive changes made, such as how he or she learned to communicate effectively.

Goodbye rituals such as a celebration of life, a closing letter, or another activity that is meaningful to both the clinician and child can also be a significant way to close the relationship.[55] Clinicians can create a goodbye book similar to a yearbook that professionals can sign, and while creating this book, children can express themselves with pictures and words.[56] Parents can also be a source of support by helping the child process the goodbye from the clinician.

While there have been more opportunities for clinicians to communicate their commitment, meaning of their relationship with the child, and final words to their pediatric patients, there are still many areas needed for continued growth. Progress and new knowledge in this field will not take away from the fact that the death of a child will be a sad experience for all those involved.

REFERENCES

1. Irwin LG, Johnson J: Interviewing young children: explicating our practices and dilemmas, *Qual Health Res* 15(6):821–831, 2005.
2. Fosson A, de Quan MM: Reassuring and talking with hospitalized children, *Child Health Care* 13(1):37–44, 1984.
3. MacDonald K, Greggans A: Dealing with chaos and complexity: the reality of interviewing children and families in their own homes, *J Clin Nurs* 17(23):3123–3130, 2008.
4. Ducharme JM, Harris KE: Errorless embedding for children with on-task and conduct difficulties: rapport-based, success-focused intervention in the classroom, *Behav Ther* 36:213–222, 2005.
5. Hershkowitz I: Socioemotional factors in child sexual abuse investigations, *Child Maltreat* 14(2):172–181, 2009.
6. Lambert V, Glacken M, McCarron M: "Visible-ness": the nature of communication for children admitted to a specialist children's hospital in the Republic of Ireland, *J Clin Nurs* 17(23):3092–3102, 2008.
7. Curtis K, Liabo K, Roberts H, Barker M: Consulted but not heard: a qualitative study of young people's views of their local health service, *Health Expect* 7(2):149–156, 2004.
8. Frank AW: You can't use plywood: the perilous success of spirituality and medicine, *Explore (NY)* 1(2):142–143, 2005.
9. Avery RR, Ryan RM: Object relations and ego development: comparison and correlates in middle childhood, *J Pers* 56(3):547–569, 1988.
10. Boggiano AK, Klinger CA, Main DS: Enhancing interest in peer interaction: a developmental analysis, *Child Dev* 57(4):852–861, 1986.
11. Deci EL, Eghrari H, Patrick BC, Leone DR: Facilitating internalization: the self-determination theory perspective, *J Pers* 62(1):119–142, 1994.
12. Gurland ST, Grolnick WS: Building rapport with children: effects of adults' expected, actual, and perceived behavior, *J Soc Clin Psychol* 27(3):226–253, 2008.
13. Waechter EH: Children's awareness of fatal illness, *Am J Nurs* 71:1168–1172, 1971.
14. Meert KL, Eggly S, Pollack M, Anand KJ, Zimmerman J, Carcillo J, Newth CJ, Dean JM, Willson DF, Nicholson C: Parents' perspectives on physician-parent communication near the time of a child's death in the pediatric intensive care unit, *Pediatr Crit Care Med* 9(1):2–7, 2008.
15. Levetown M: Communicating with children and families: from everyday interactions to skill in conveying distressing information, *Pediatrics* 121(5):e1441–e1460, 2008.
16. Korones DN: Talking to children who are dying: confessions from the trenches, *Am Acad Hospice Palliative Med Bull* 5:2, 2004.
17. Contro N, Larsen J, Scofield S, Sourkes B, Cohen H: Family perspectives on the quality of pediatric palliative care, *Arch Pediatr Adolesc Med* 156:14–19, 2002.
18. Liben S: Enlightening medical students, *CMAJ* 168(11):1390, 2003.
19. Beale EA, Baile WF, Aaron J: Silence is not golden: communicating with children dying from cancer, *J Clin Oncol* 23(15):3629–3631, 2005.
20. Lee KJ, Dupree CY: Staff experiences with end-of-life care in the pediatric intensive care unit, *J Palliat Med* 11(7):986–990, 2008.
21. Masera G, Spinetta JJ, Jankovic M, Ablin AR, D'Angio GJ, Van Dongen-Melman J, Eden T, Martins AG, Mulhern RK, Oppenheim D,

Topf R, Chesler MA: Guidelines for assistance to terminally ill children with cancer: a report of the SIOP Working Committee on psychosocial issues in pediatric oncology, *Med Pediatr Oncol* 32(1):44–48, 1999.
22. Goldberg A, Frader J: Holding on and letting go: ethical issues regarding the care of children with cancer, *Cancer Treat Res* 140:173–194, 2008.
23. Freyer DR: Care of the dying adolescent: special considerations, *Pediatrics* 113(2):381–388, 2004.
24. Hays RM, Valentine J, Haynes G, Geyer JR, Villareale N, McKinstry B, et al: The Seattle Pediatric Palliative Care Project: effects on family satisfaction and health-related quality of life, *J Palliat Med* 9(3):716–728, 2006.
25. Zwaanswijk M, Tates K, van Dulmen S, Hoogerbrugge PM, Kamps WA, Bensing JM: Young patients', parents', and survivors' communication preferences in paediatric oncology: results of online focus groups, *BMC Pediatr* 7:35, 2007.
26. Hsiao JL, Evan EE, Zeltzer LK: Parent and child perspectives on physician communication in pediatric palliative care, *Palliat Support Care* 5(4):355–365, 2007.
27. Sahler OJ, Frager G, Levetown M, Cohn FG, Lipson MA: Medical education about end-of-life care in the pediatric setting: principles, challenges, and opportunities, *Pediatrics* 105(3 Pt 1):575–584, 2000.
28. Hinds PS, Drew D, Oakes LL, Fouladi M, Spunt SL, Church C, et al: End-of-life care preferences of pediatric patients with cancer, *J Clin Oncol* 23(36):9146–9154, 2005.
29. Himelstein BP, Hilden JM, Boldt AM, Weissman D: Pediatric palliative care, *N Engl J Med* 350(17):1752–1762, 2004.
30. Koocher GP: Talking to children about death, *Am J Orthopsychiatry* 44:404–411, 1974.
31. Kenyon BL: Current research in children's conceptions of death: a critical review, *J Death and Dying* 43:69–91, 2001.
32. Furth GM: The secret world of drawings: a jungian approach to healing through art. Boston, 1988, Sigo Press.
33. Bertman SL: Grief and the healing arts: creativity as therapy. Amityville, NY, 1999, Baywood Publications.
34. Himebauch A, Arnold RM, May C: *Fast Fact and Concept #138, Grief in Children and Developmental Concepts of Death*, 2003. www.eperc.mcw.edu/fastFact/ff_138.htm. Accessed July 20, 2010.
35. Zeitlin SV: Grief and bereavement, *Prim Care* 2:415–425, 2001.
36. Dyregrov K: Bereaved parents' experience of research participation, *Soc Sci Med* 58(2):391–400, 2004.
37. Die Trill M, Kovalcik R: The child with cancer: influence of culture on truth-telling and patient care, *Ann NY Acad Sci* 809:197–210, 1997.
38. Martinson IM, Bi-Hui Z, Yi-Hua L: The reaction of chinese parents to a terminally ill child with cancer, *Cancer News* 17:72–76, 1994.
39. Papadatou D, Yfantopoulos J, Kosmides H: Child dying at home or in the hospital: experiences of Greek mothers, *Death Stud* 2:215–236, 1996.
40. Sagara M, Pickett M: Sociocultural influences and care of dying children in Japan and the United States, *Cancer Nurs* 274–281, 1998.
41. Linnard-Palmer L: *When parents say no: religious and cultural influences on pediatric healthcare treatment*, Indianapolis, 2006, Sigma Theta Tau International.
42. Noggle BJ: Identifying and meeting needs of ethnic minority patients, *Hosp J* 10:85–93, 1995.
43. Chan A, Woodruff RK: Comparison of palliative care needs of English and non-English-speaking Patients, *J Palliat Care* 15:26–30, 1999.
44. Gutheil TG, Gabbard GO: The concept of boundaries in clinical practice: theoretical and risk management dimensions, *Am J Psychiatry* 150:188–196, 1993.
45. Gobbard GO, Nadelson C: Professional boundaries in the physician-patient relationship, *JAMA* 273:1445–1449, 1995.
46. Farber NJ, Novack DH, O'Brien MK: Love, boundaries, and the patient-physician relationship, *Arch Intern Med* 157:2291–2294, 1997.
47. Spence S: Patients bearing gifts: are there strings attached? *Br Med J* 331:1527–1529, 2005.
48. Barnes LL, Plotnikoff GA, Fox K, Pendleton S: Spirituality, religion, and pediatrics: intersecting worlds of healing, *Pediatrics* 106 (4 Suppl):899–908, 2000.
49. American Academy of Pediatrics and Bioethics Co: Appropriate boundaires in the pediatrician-family-patient relationship, *Pediatrics* 104(2):334–336, 1999.
50. Barbour LT: *Fast Fact and Concept 3172. Professional-Patient boundaries in palliative care*, 2003. www.eperc.mcw.edu/fastFact/ff_172.htm. Accessed July 20, 2010.

51. Baverstock A, Finlay F: Specialist registrars' emotional responses to a patient's death, *Arch Dis Child* [0003-9888] Baverstock 91(9):774–776, 2006.
52. Jennings P: Should paediatric units have bereavement support posts? *Arch Dis Child* 87(1):40–42, 2002.
53. Valdimarsdottir U, Kreicbergs U, Hauksdottir A, Hunt H, Onelov E, Henter JI, et al: Parents' intellectual and emotional awareness of their child's impending death to cancer: a population-based long-term follow-up study, *Lancet Oncol* 8(8):706–714, 2007.
54. Surkan PJ, Dickman PW, Steineck G, Onelov E, Kreicbergs U: Home care of a child dying of a malignancy and parental awareness of a child's impending death, *Palliat Med* 20(3):161–169, 2006.
55. Wright LM, Leahey M: How to conclude or terminate with families, *J Fam Nurs* 10(3):379–401, 2004.
56. O'Donohue WT, Cuciarre M: *Terminating psychotherapy: a clinician's guide*, 2007, Routledge.

SUGGESTED READINGS

Aldred C, Green J, Adams C: A new social communication intervention for children with autism: pilot randomised controlled treatment study suggesting effectiveness, *J Child Psychol Psychiatry* 45(8):1420–1430, 2004.

Alderfer MA, Fiese BH, Gold JI, Cutuli JJ, Holmbeck GN, Goldbeck L, et al: Evidence-based assessment in pediatric psychology: family measures, *J Pediatr Psychol* 33(9):1046–1061; discussion 1062–1064, 2008.

Barrera M, D'Agostino NM, Schneiderman G, Tallett S, Spencer L, Jovcevska V: Patterns of parental bereavement following the loss of a child and related factors, *Omega (Westport)* 55(2):145–167, 2007.

Billings JA, Kolton E: Family satisfaction and bereavement care following death in the hospital, *J Palliat Med* 2(1):33–49, 1999.

Brown M: *When dinosaurs die: a guide to understanding death*, Boston, 1996, Little Brown.

Buchi S, Morgeli H, Schnyder U, Jenewein J, Glaser A, Fauchere JC, et al: Shared or discordant grief in couples 2–6 years after the death of their premature baby: effects on suffering and posttraumatic growth, *Psychosomatics* 50(2):123–130, 2009.

Burns CE: Diagnostic Reasoning: A complex issue for pediatric primary care. In Burns CE, Brady M, editors: *Pediatric primary care case studies*, Sudbury, 2009, Jones & Bartlett, p 450.

Chang PC, Yeh CH: Agreement between child self-report and parent proxy-report to evaluate quality of life in children with cancer, *Psychooncology* 14(2):125–134, 2005.

Chan K, Yeung K, Chu C, Tsang K, Leung Y: An evaluative study on the effectiveness of a parent-child parallel group model, *Research Social Work Pract* 12(4):546–557, 2002.

Clarke JN: Advocacy: essential work for mothers of children living with cancer, *J Psychosoc Oncol* 24(2):31–47, 2006.

Cohen MS: Families coping with childhood chronic illness: a research review, *Fam Sys & Health* 17:149–164, 1999.

Collins JJ, Byrnes ME, Dunkel IJ, Lapin J, Nadel T, Thaler HT, et al: The measurement of symptoms in children with cancer, *J Pain Symptom Manage* 19(5):363–377, 2000.

Collins JJ, Devine TD, Dick GS, Johnson EA, Kilham HA, Pinkerton CR, et al: The measurement of symptoms in young children with cancer: the validation of the Memorial Symptom Assessment Scale in children aged 7–12, *J Pain Symptom Manage* 23(1):10–16, 2002.

D'Agostino NM, Berlin-Romalis D, Jovcevska V, Barrera M: Bereaved parents' perspectives on their needs, *Palliat Support Care* 6(1):33–41, 2008.

De Cinque N, Monterosso L, Dadd G, Sidhu R, Macpherson R, Aoun S: Bereavement support for families following the death of a child from cancer: experience of bereaved parents, *J Psychosoc Oncol* 24(2):65–83, 2006.

Docherty SL, Miles MS, Brandon D: Searching for "the dying point:" providers' experiences with palliative care in pediatric acute care, *Pediatr Nurs* 33(4):335–341, 2007.

Duncan J, Spengler E, Wolfe J: Providing pediatric palliative care: PACT in action, *MCN Am J Matern Child Nurs* 32(5):279–287, 2007.

Eiser C, Morse R: The measurement of quality of life in children: past and future perspectives, *J Dev Behav Pediatr* 22(4):248–256, 2001.

Ellershaw JE, Peat SJ, Boys LC: Assessing the effectiveness of a hospital palliative care team, *Palliat Med* 9(2):145–152, 1995.

Fallat ME, Glover J: Professionalism in pediatrics: statement of principles, *Pediatrics* 120(4):895–897, 2007.

Gesundheit B, Greenberg ML, Or R, Koren G: Drug compliance by adolescent and young adult cancer patients: challenges for the physician. In Bleyer AW, Barr RD, editors: *Cancer in adolescents and young adults pediatric oncology*, 2007, Springer, NY, p 534.

Giannini A, Messeri A, Aprile A, Casalone C, Jankovic M, Scarani R, et al: End-of-life decisions in pediatric intensive care: recommendations of the Italian Society of Neonatal and Pediatric Anesthesia and Intensive Care (SARNePI), *Paediatr Anaesth* 18(11):1089–1095, 2008.

Glaser A, Bucher HU, Moergeli H, Fauchere JC, Buechi S: Loss of a pre-term infant: psychological aspects in parents, *Swiss Med Wkly* 137(27–28):392–401, 2007.

Grossoehme DH, Ragsdale JR, McHenry CL, Thurston C, DeWitt T, VandeCreek L: Pediatrician characteristics associated with attention to spirituality and religion in clinical practice, *Pediatrics* 119(1):e117–e123, 2007.

Hauksdottir A, Steineck G, Furst CJ, Valdimarsdottir U: Towards better measurements in bereavement research: order of questions and assessed psychological morbidity, *Palliat Med* 20(1):11–16, 2006.

Hechler T, Blankenburg M, Friedrichsdorf SJ, Garske D, Hubner B, Menke A, et al: Parents' perspective on symptoms, quality of life, characteristics of death and end-of-life decisions for children dying from cancer, *Klin Padiatr* 220(3):166–174, 2008.

Hellman J: Ethical issues in the neonatal intensive care unit. In Kirpalani H, Moore AM, Perlman M, editors. *Residents handbook of neonatology*, ed 3, Hamilton, Ontario: B.C., 2007, Decker, p 612.

Herr K, Coyne PJ, Key T, Manworren R, McCaffery M, Merkel S, et al: Pain assessment in the nonverbal patient: position statement with clinical practice recommendations, *Pain Manag Nurs* 7(2):44–52, 2006.

Hinds PS, Hockenberry-Eaton M, Gilger E, Kline N, Burleson C, Bottomley S, et al: Comparing patient, parent, and staff descriptions of fatigue in pediatric oncology patients, *Cancer Nurs* 22(4):277–288; quiz 288–289, 1999.

Hodges K: Depression and anxiety in children: a comparison of self-report questionnaires to clinical interview, *Psychol Assess: J Consult Clin Psychol* 2(4):376–381, 1990.

Hunt H, Valdimarsdottir U, Mucci L, Kreicbergs U, Steineck G: When death appears best for the child with severe malignancy: a nationwide parental follow-up, *Palliat Med* 20(6):567–577, 2006.

Hurwitz CA, Duncan J, Wolfe J: Caring for the child with cancer at the close of life: "There are people who make it, and I'm hoping I'm one of them," *JAMA* 292(17):2141–2149, 2004.

Hynson JL, Aroni R, Bauld C, Sawyer SM: Research with bereaved parents: a question of how not why, *Palliat Med* 20(8):805–811, 2006.

Jacobs HH: Ethics in pediatric end-of-life care: a nursing perspective, *J Pediatr Nurs* 20(5):360–369, 2005.

Jones BL: Companionship, control, and compassion: a social work perspective on the needs of children with cancer and their families at the end of life, *J Palliat Med* 9(3):774–788, 2006.

Jobe-Shields L, Alderfer MA, Barrera M, Vannatta K, Currier JM, Phipps S: Parental depression and family environment predict distress in children before stem cell transplantation, *J Dev Behav Pediatr* 30(2):140–146, 2009.

Jordan A, Eccleston C, McCracken LM, Connell H, Clinch J: The Bath Adolescent Pain—Parental Impact Questionnaire (BAP-PIQ): development and preliminary psychometric evaluation of an instrument to assess the impact of parenting an adolescent with chronic pain, *Pain* 73(3):478–487, 2008.

Joseph-Di Caprio J, Garwick AW, Kohrman C, Blum RW: Culture and the care of children with chronic conditions, *Arch Pediatr Adolesc Med* 153:1030–1035, 1999.

Kazak AE, Prusak A, McSherry M, Simms S, Beele D, Rourke M, et al: The Psychosocial Assessment Tool (PAT): Pilot data on a brief screening instrument for identifying high risk families in pediatric oncology, *Fam Syst Health* 19(3):303–317, 2001.

Keesee NJ, Currier JM, Neimeyer RA: Predictors of grief following the death of one's child: the contribution of finding meaning, *J Clin Psychol* 64(10):1145–1163, 2008.

Kirby D, Miller BC: Interventions designed to promote parent-teen communication about sexuality, *New Dir Child Adolesc Dev* 97:93–110, 2002.

Kreicbergs U, Valdimarsdottir U, Onelov E, Bjork O, Steineck G, Henter JI: Care-related distress: a nationwide study of parents who lost their child to cancer, *J Clin Oncol* 23(36):9162–9171, 2005.

Kreicbergs U, Valdimarsdottir U, Onelov E, Henter JI, Steineck G: Anxiety and depression in parents 4–9 years after the loss of a child owing to a malignancy: a population-based follow-up, *Psychol Med* 34(8):1431–1441, 2004.

Kreicbergs UC, Lannen P, Onelov E, Wolfe J: Parental grief after losing a child to cancer: impact of professional and social support on long-term outcomes, *J Clin Oncol* 25(22):3307–3312, 2007.

Lannen PK, Wolfe J, Prigerson HG, Onelov E, Kreicbergs UC: Unresolved grief in a national sample of bereaved parents: impaired mental and physical health 4 to 9 years later, *J Clin Oncol* 26(36):5870–5876, 2008.

Lynn-McHale DJ, Deatrick JA: Trust between family and health care provider, *J Fam Nurs* 6(3):210–230, 2000.

Mack JW, Evan EE, Duncan J, Wolfe J: Palliative care in pediatric oncology. In Orkin SH, Fisher DE, Nathan DG, Ginsburg D, editors: *Oncology of infancy and childhood: expert consult*, Philiadelphia, 2009, Elsevier, pp 1177–1202.

Mack JW, Hilden JM, Watterson J, Moore C, Turner B, Grier HE, et al: Parent and physician perspectives on quality of care at the end of life in children with cancer, *J Clin Oncol* 23(36):9155–9161, 2005.

Mack JW, Wolfe J: Early integration of pediatric palliative care: for some children, palliative care starts at diagnosis, *Curr Opin Pediatr* 18(1):10–14, 2006.

McCabe MA: Involving children and adolescents in medical decision making: developmental and clinical considerations, *J Pediatr Psychol* 21(4):505–516, 1996.

McCarthy MC, Clarke NE, Vance A, Ashley DM, Heath JA, Anderson VA: Measuring psychosocial risk in families caring for a child with cancer: the Psychosocial Assessment Tool (PAT2.0), *Pediatr Blood Cancer* 53(1):78–83, 2009.

Miller IW, Kabacoff RI, Epstein NB, Bishop DS, Keitner GI, Baldwin LM, et al: The development of a clinical rating scale for the McMaster model of family functioning, *Fam Process* 33(1):53–69, 1994.

Moon M, Taylor HA, McDonald EL, Hughes MT, Carrese JA: Everyday ethics issues in the outpatient clinical practice of pediatric residents, *Arch Pediatr Adolesc Med* 163(9):838–843, 2009.

Nitschke R, Meyer WH, Huszti HC: When the tumor is not the target, tell the children, *J Clin Oncol* 21(Suppl 9):40s, 2003.

Nitschke R, Meyer WH, Sexauer CL, Parkhurst JB, Foster P, Huszti H: Care of terminally ill children with cancer, *Med Pediatr Oncol* 34(4):268–270, 2000.

Parsons SK, Saiki-Craighill S, Mayer DK, Sullivan AM, Jeruss S, Terrin N, et al: Telling children and adolescents about their cancer diagnosis: Cross-cultural comparisons between pediatric oncologists in the US and Japan, *Psychooncology* 16(1):60–68, 2007.

Perce Hays RM, Valentine J, Haynes G, Geyer JR, Villareale N, McKinstry B, et al: The Seattle Pediatric Palliative Care Project: effects on family satisfaction and health-related quality of life, *J Palliat Med* 9(3):716–728, 2006.

Puchalski C, Romer AL: Taking a spiritual history allows clinicians to understand patients more fully, *J Palliat Med* 3(1):129–137, 2000.

Ruland CM, Hamilton GA, Schjodt-Osmo B: The complexity of symptoms and problems experienced in children with cancer: a review of the literature, *J Pain Symptom Manage* 37(3):403–418, 2009.

Seecharan GA, Andresen EM, Norris K, Toce SS: Parents' assessment of quality of care and grief following a child's death, *Arch Pediatr Adolesc Med* 158(6):515–520, 2004.

Sinal SH, Cabinum-Foeller E, Socolar R: Religion and medical neglect, *South Med J* 101(7):703–706, 2008.

Solomon M, Ono M, Timmer S, Goodlin-Jones B: The effectiveness of parent-child interaction therapy for families of children on the autism spectrum, *J Autism Dev Disord* 38(9):1767–1776, 2008.

Stephenson J: Palliative and hospice care needed for children with life-threatening conditions, *JAMA* 284(19):2437–2438, 2000.

Streisand R, Braniecki S, Tercyak KP, Kazak AE: Childhood illness-related parenting stress: the pediatric inventory for parents, *J Pediatr Psychol* 26(3):155–162, 2001.

Surkan PJ, Kreicbergs U, Valdimarsdottir U, Nyberg U, Onelov E, Dickman PW, et al: Perceptions of inadequate health care and feelings of guilt in parents after the death of a child to a malignancy: a population-based long-term follow-up, *J Palliat Med* 9(2):317–331, 2006.

Varni JW, Katz ER, Seid M, Quiggins DJ, Friedman-Bender A, Castro CM: The Pediatric Cancer Quality of Life Inventory (PCQL). I. Instrument development, descriptive statistics, and cross-informant variance, *J Behav Med* 21(2):179–204, 1998.

Wijngaards-de Meij L, Stroebe M, Schut H, Stroebe W, Van den Bout J, Van der Heijden PGM, et al: Parents grieving the loss of their child: Interdependence in coping, *Br J Clin Psychol* 47:31–42, 2008.

Wijngaards-de Meij L, Stroebe M, Schut H, Stroebe W, Van den Bout J, Van der Heijden PGM, et al: Patterns of attachment and parents' adjustment to the death of their child, *Pers Soc Psychol Bull* 33(4):537–548, 2007.

Wijngaards-de Meij L, Stroebe M, Stroebe W, Schut H, Van den Bout J, Van der Heijden PGM, et al: The impact of circumstances surrounding the death of a child on parents' grief, *Death Studies* 32(3):237–252, 2008.

Wilson E, Elkan R, Cox K: Closure for patients at the end of a cancer clinical trial: literature review, *J Adv Nurs* 59(5):445–453, 2007.

Woodgate RL: The 2002 Schering Lecture. Children's cancer symptom experiences: keeping the spirit alive in children and their families, *Can Oncol Nurs J* 13(3):142–150, 2003.

Woodgate RL: Living in the shadow of fear: adolescents' lived experience of depression, *J Adv Nurs* 56(3):261–269, 2006.

Woodgate RL: Feeling states: a new approach to understanding how children and adolescents with cancer experience symptoms, *Cancer Nurs* 31(3):229–238, 2008.

Woodgate RL, Degner LF: "Nothing is carved in stone!" uncertainty in children with cancer and their families, *Eur J Oncol Nurs* 6(4):191–202; discussion 203–204, 2002.

Woodgate RL, McClement S: Symptom distress in children with cancer: the need to adopt a meaning-centered approach, *J Pediatr Oncol Nurs* 15(1):3–12, 1998.

Woods M: Balancing rights and duties in "life and death" decision making involving children: a role for nurses? *Nurs Ethics* 8(5):397–408, 2001.

Yeates KO, Taylor HG, Drotar D, Wade SL, Klein S, Stancin T, et al: Preinjury family environment as a determinant of recovery from traumatic brain injuries in school-age children, *J Int Neuropsychol Soc* 3(6):617–630, 1997.

Zinner SE: The use of pediatric advance directives: a tool for palliative care physicians, *Am J Hosp Palliat Med* 25(6):427–430, 2009.

15 Parent and Sibling Relationships and the Family Experience

BARBARA L. JONES | MARY JO GILMER |
JESSICA PARKER-RALEY | DEBORAH L. DOKKEN |
DAVID R. FREYER | NANCY SYDNOR-GREENBERG

"I wish you knew ... how much difference your caring and support can make. We encountered so many people I view them as our comrades who were truly fighting for us and Ryan while our family was being bombarded. It is these relationships that gave me the strength to be brave, the strength to endure, and in some cases, the inspiration to be a better person."[1]
—Anne Willis

When a child is diagnosed with a life-threatening or life-limiting condition the entire family is also in a sense diagnosed as their lives are individually, collectively, and permanently altered. Relationships within the family and with the interdisciplinary healthcare team become crucially important. Understanding the unique meaning of the experiences for each family in their historical, cultural, spiritual, and environmental context is a key element of family-centered pediatric palliative care. Families caring for a child with a life-threatening condition have reported a wide range of experiences in the healthcare setting, from moments of insensitivity and hurt to profound compassion, support, and guidance.[2,3]

Contro and colleagues found:

"One of the most striking findings was how a single event could cause parents profound and lasting emotional distress. Parents recounted incidents that included insensitive delivery of bad news, feeling dismissed or patronized, perceived disregard for parents' judgment regarding the care of their child, and poor communication of important information. Such an event haunted them and complicated their grief even years later."[4]

The interdisciplinary pediatric palliative care team can play a critical role in facilitating the family's adaptation, wellness, and resilience. The key to this support is in the relationships formed with and between the family members. Pediatric palliative care is, by definition, about relationships: relationships with the child, the healthcare team, and the family. Ideally, interdisciplinary teams enhance the family's existing relationships and understand their experience while simultaneously forming a supportive relationship with the family. Relationship-building is a critical component of quality pediatric palliative care.[5]

The purpose of this chapter is to assist in understanding the meaning of experiences for each family faced with a life-threatening or life-limiting condition through appreciation of the historical, cultural, spiritual, and environmental context. An important key to this awareness lies in the relationships formed with and among family members.

Family-Centered Pediatric Palliative Care

After several decades, the philosophy of family-centered care has evolved in pediatrics and its principles are often cited in both literature and practice; indeed, family-centered care is now recognized as the standard of care for children, including those with life-threatening conditions.[6,7] Its principles provide a framework within which healthcare professionals can develop a broader understanding of all families, including those from many varied cultures. Box 15-1 summarizes five key components of care that are family-centered.

Central to family-centered care is the belief that a child is part of a family system and therefore both the child and his or her family are the unit of care. Perhaps no situation tests this belief more than the life-threatening illness or impending death of a child. Each child is part of a family; his or her illness impacts the family tremendously, in the present and in the unknown future. The family is the primary organizing structure for that child and it is the extended family that can be one of the main support structures for parents as they learn to cope and interact during a time of increased stress and heightened emotion. The entire family has a variety of needs, many of which can be addressed by healthcare professionals. In 2000, The Initiative for Pediatric Palliative Care conducted telephone interviews with parents or other adult family caregivers of deceased children who had been patients at three geographically dispersed pediatric teaching hospitals that served diverse patient populations in the United States. In the words of one mother from those interviews, "This was a whole family that was affected by this child..."[8] Recognizing and responding to those needs is the essence of family-centered practice.

While family-centered care does advocate respect for the family system, it also urges healthcare professionals to "recognize and build on the strengths of each child and family."[9] With a family-centered approach, professionals try to learn about the family's life, past and present, both inside and outside the healthcare system. Within that larger context, professionals can better understand and respond to each family's coping strategies. Practitioners, while remaining nonjudgmental and compassionate, attempt to assess the family's coping strategies in terms of how functional they are. While the approach is to honor the family as the expert in their own experience, there are still instances when the coping is not functional and potentially harmful, including situations such as family violence, substance abuse, and self-injurious behaviors. In these situations, healthcare professionals intervene to protect the child and, where possible, assist the family in maximizing safety, function, and wellness for each of its members.

BOX 15-1 Components of Family-Centered Care

- Recognizing and respecting the pivotal role of the family in the lives of children
- Striving to support families in their caregiving roles by building upon their unique strengths as individuals and as families
- Respecting and encouraging the choices families make for their children
- Promoting normal patterns of living in the hospital, at home, and in the community
- Promoting partnerships between families and professionals to ensure excellence at all levels of healthcare

In family-centered practice, family members are viewed as partners with healthcare professionals in caring for the child, providing information, and in making decisions about care and treatment. Families are recognized by the healthcare system for their essential role, as "nurturers, caregivers, and decision makers in their children's lives."[10] Professionals endeavor to understand the values and beliefs that are part of the family's world, and how those influence the family's understanding of situations they face and solutions they might find acceptable. "Family strengths and capabilities (not only problems and needs) are recognized and valued in the planning and provision of care."[11] While nothing can prepare a family for the challenges of caring for a child with a life-limiting condition, the guidance of an interdisciplinary team that can appreciate their needs is invaluable.[12]

In clinical care, we often refer to caring for and honoring the experience of the family. While it is true that each family will have a unique experience based upon its own psychosocial history, cultural and spiritual beliefs, and family composition, it is equally true that individual members of a family system will construct their own personal meaning out of the experience. Sometimes families are aligned in their approach to the experience, but just as often they are not. Family systems are affected by change in any one member, and certainly a child's life-threatening illness compels the entire system to renegotiate roles, rules, and experiences. The interdisciplinary pediatric palliative care team considers the entire family and provides support to each member. Pediatric palliative care is grounded in the principle of reducing suffering, both physical and psychological, for the child and the family. For healthcare professionals, the family is both an integral part in providing optimal care to the child and a part of the patient system that needs supportive services.

In providing care to the family of children with life-threatening or life-limiting conditions, the healthcare team should hold a broad definition of family to include parents, grandparents, siblings, cousins, and individuals who represent chosen family or are like family for the child. Family can be defined as "two or more people who are joined together by bonds of sharing and intimacy," which can include biological, adopted, step, multi-generational, transracial, same-sex, informal, and created families.[13,14] Additionally, given the mobility of today's modern family, members who are not living together should also be considered family for the child. Asking the child who his or her family is will likely elicit both the immediate family system as well as the extended and psychological family systems. The family system serves a foundational place in the life of a child and provides context for the experience of identity, meaning, and understanding of lived experiences. For many cultures, family almost always means a large and extended group of people who care about the child and may or may not be biologically related to the child. In a recent study of Latino adolescent cancer survivors, the participants indicated the importance of having their entire family, including distant aunts and uncles, present at many appointments and inpatient stays.[15]

While the philosophy of family-centered care is widely accepted in pediatric healthcare, including palliative care, its actual practice is not always consistent with the underlying philosophy. Indeed, "it is possible to affirm the philosophy, at least intellectually, without truly putting family-centered care into practice."[11] Another concern is that family-centered care can be misunderstood or not fully implemented. For example, in some institutions family-centered care consists merely of a visitation policy that allows more than two visitors to the bedside and a parent to stay overnight. That should be viewed as one facet, not the centerpiece, of family-centered care. Without an overarching commitment to fundamental principles of family-centered care and its comprehensive practice, families facing a life-threatening condition of a child frequently must endure confusion or even negative feelings about the healthcare system and their role within it, and second-guessing of their decisions. They also suffer an apparent lack of concern regarding aspects of their lives beyond the medical status of the ill child, such as siblings, work, marriage and other family relationships, and personal decisions.

The two vignettes that follow are from mothers of critically ill infants and powerfully illustrate these feelings and the discrepancy between theory and practice that can exist.

It was like a lost world. I felt totally removed from the "normal" world. I could spend a few hours there and experience the most amazing contradictions. Life and death; terrible anguish, and yet unbridled and sometimes senseless hope. A sense of urgent quiet, with the underlying whisper of nurses and the interruption of machine noise always warning of some impending disaster. I was expected, by both the staff and myself, to learn the medical minutiae of caring for a baby that was mine, and yet not quite mine. I tried my best to nurture, to behave like a mom; even to hold my baby close, while dressed like a surgeon ready to operate. The neonatologists and residents came in for rounds and discussed the babies at a normal volume; but we parents were asked to lower our voices when talking with each other. It often felt like our experience was not real, but some TV movie. Occasionally, a baby would burp loudly and I would laugh with relief, only to look up into the eyes of a mother who had just received some horrible news about the results of her child's last procedure. After a while I mastered walking a very thin behavioral and emotional line. Entering the subway to go home each day was such a rude transition that I often burst into tears.[16]

I think that in a high-tech environment, like a PICU, the feeling you get is that it's all here, it's available, we can just turn this on and add this and add that. As a parent you're given the feeling that if you say "no," you're making the wrong choice, and you're making a selfish choice, as opposed to a choice in the best interest of your child.... We were not in a situation that welcomed shared decision making. My main thought was, "Will they let us make the decision that we want for our daughter?" As empowered and resource-rich as we were, that situation was horrifying.[17]

As we are reminded by the following quote from a seasoned healthcare professional, the job of ensuring that family-centered pediatric palliative care moves from theory to practice falls to individual professionals, healthcare institutions, and a growing number of coalitions, it is hoped, in collaboration with family members themselves.

"In the NICU or other healthcare settings, confusion is not the 'fault' of parents. They are not confused because they lack intelligence or are troublesome. Rather, confusion is legitimate for the situation. It's the responsibility of professionals to adapt to different levels of confusion and understanding in parents."[18]

If family-centered care, including pediatric palliative care, is sometimes more theoretical than real, then healthcare professionals will need to move these principles into practice and support families of children with life-threatening conditions in two critical areas:

- Partnerships around the care of children and decision making
- Support to maintain family integrity and life, thus, providing a sense of control and normalcy

Maintaining integrity and some sense of normalcy for families also entails consideration and support of practical dimensions of life. The mother's following quote highlights the Herculean balancing act families are required to perform and the stresses and anxiety it causes:

"Being away from my other two kids (was difficult) because, I mean, they understood their brother was sick and I had to stay with him, but the only thing is that I was so far away from everybody and then my husband had to travel back and forth to work and I was already off from work, with my son being in the hospital."[8]

If family-centered care means that both the child and family are the units of care, then healthcare professionals and institutions must understand and address these practical needs in order to provide quality pediatric palliative care.

IMPACT ON FAMILY MEMBERS

Families of a child with a life-threatening condition find themselves on a roller coaster of uncertainty, anxiety, and anticipatory grief. From the time they realize something is wrong until they learn of the diagnosis, they are faced with stress of difficult decisions and feelings of failure as they struggle to find a cure or treatment. The family characteristics have an impact on both their specific needs and on the services that may be offered to them. Integral to the design of appropriate palliative care strategies is knowing the type of family, nuclear, single parent, blended, same gender parents, multigenerational and understanding the relationships among siblings, parents, and extended family members, and the roles members assume within the family. It becomes important to inquire about the members of the family and their respective roles in a child's care. Families may react in very different ways to the child's illness. If the family is a two-parent family, each of the parents may cope differently and therefore have difficulty supporting each other, resulting in a loss of intimacy and connection. Disease-directed treatment regimens typically necessitate that one parent takes a central role with the ill child, while the other continues to work outside the home. This may result in one parent feeling that he or she is taking all the responsibility for caregiving, or conversely, for holding the family together in a

financial sense. Through keeping the lines of communication open among family members, healthcare providers can provide needed opportunities for families to share their feelings.

Single parents may feel the burden of being alone in their decision making without support or a balanced perspective in providing care for a child with comprehensive needs. Healthcare providers may assist a single parent in identifying a support system. Unfortunately, families may dissolve as a response to a child's illness, magnifying the impact of a life-threatening condition.

Blended families have a unique situation where only one parent has decision-making authority, but both parents care deeply for the child and the non-custodial parent may feel marginalized. It becomes important for healthcare providers to assist with the identification of caregiving roles for the non-custodial parent, if he or she chooses to be involved.

Same-gender parents may be met with insensitivity to their individual needs and roles within the family. Some centers have support groups for mothers and different support groups for fathers. Helping same-gender parents respond to their needs for support without feeling ostracized is an important role of the healthcare team.

Multigenerational families may have the additional burden of caring for elderly family members. Often, these families experience not only the stress of caring for a child with a life-threatening condition, but they must also be concerned about aging parents. Managing the financial and emotional burdens takes a huge toll on these families, and social workers can be helpful in responding to their needs.

These diverse family structures require the healthcare team to make deliberate efforts to include parents meaningfully in communication and decision making. When illness is protracted, families often experience a loss of support over time, a loss of normalcy, ongoing financial stress, and an exaggeration of new and pre-existing stressors, such as financial strain or relationship difficulties.

Historically, family-focused research has emphasized needs of patients and parents. Siblings have received less attention but have been documented to be at risk for multiple psychological, social, and cognitive difficulties.[19] Healthy siblings may feel neglected, resentful, and confused as they struggle to find their own sources of support. Often a chronically ill child endures years of stressful treatments, and most of the family's attention is directed to the patient while the needs of siblings may be overlooked. Siblings of children with life-threatening conditions face unique challenges where their needs may have been neglected or deferred, leading them to wonder, "What about me?" They often report less quality time with parents, uncertainty about parents' ability to meet their needs, feelings of guilt, negative thoughts about their sibling-patient, and feelings of fear and anxiety due to changes in routine, and worry about the illness itself. Siblings often report feelings of isolation, withdrawal, sadness or depression, feeling not good enough, trouble with academic performance, and difficulty in relationships. As one sibling put it:

"The ache in my sister's side would begin a long journey for our family through distress, death, and love. We were all on the same road, but miles apart. As her illness became the focal point in our lives, jealousy, anger, and confusion jumbled in my mind. I wondered if our family would ever be the same....I became very tough on the outside, but I was dying on the inside."[20]

Beyond the sibling, only limited attention has been devoted to the needs or grief processes of grandparents.[21] In fact, grandparents have been called "forgotten grievers."[22] Not only are they forgotten, but also they may experience double pain.[23] Grandparents grieve for the dying grandchild, but they also grieve for their own child's loss and suffering. While extended families may be very close during a child's illness, grief may result in distancing and alienation. Clearly an appreciation of grandparents' grief, their roles in the family, and cultural sensitivities are integral to effective comprehensive family-centered care.

Comprehensive care for family members should involve including information they can understand, addressing emotional concerns, providing spiritual resources, and also helping with practical issues, such as managing health insurance forms, and having advanced directives at hand when needed. In order to consider the family, we use the following case to frame our discussion:

> *Michael was diagnosed with hypoplastic left heart syndrome while in utero. His mother had a routine ultrasound at five months' gestation and the defect was diagnosed at that time. Michael's mother and father decided to continue the pregnancy and make further decisions about treatment after delivery. At two days of age, Michael underwent open-heart surgery as the first stage of repair for the heart defect. He did well following the surgery in the pediatric intensive care unit, but developed complications and arrested while still in the PICU. Resuscitation was successful and his 5-year-old sister, Emily, was allowed to visit him briefly in the unit. Michael's parents took turns staying with him, alternating who was at the hospital and who tried to maintain normalcy for Emily at home. Unfortunately, Michael continued to have difficulties and arrested two more times. His parents decided to forego further CPR. Michael died in the hospital at two months of age, without ever having been home.*

INFORMATION NEEDS

When a child is diagnosed with a potentially life-threatening condition, families benefit from information about the probable progression of the condition, including what is known about life expectancy, physical and mental changes they might expect, and side effects of treatments. Clinicians need to provide all available information supplemented with their relevant clinical experience, while acknowledging an element of uncertainty. Parents and other family members often want to know how long the child has. While it may be certain that death will eventually ensue, forecasting its exact timing is impossible and may lead to confusion when reality does not correspond. Research has shown limitations of prognostic determinations for adults, and there is even less certainty with children, given the much lower numbers of deaths in children.[2,24] In general, it is preferable and usually possible to state an expected lifespan in general terms of months, weeks or days, and to revisit that timeframe as the child's changing conditions declares itself.

While the Internet can be a resource for general information and parent-to-parent support, it is important for families to be knowledgeable about credible sites, and avoid those intended for professionals as they may be highly technical and difficult to comprehend. Michael's parents accessed the American Heart Association website and found a link to an excellent description of their son's heart defect, specifically written for parents, which they could understand.

When there is very little chance of recovery, parents may choose to forego intensive treatments that may have questionable benefit for their child. Healthcare practitioners are challenged to provide honest, timely information while helping the family maintain hope that is appropriately tempered by realism. Unrealistic expectations for cure may deny parents the opportunities to build lasting memories crucial for negotiating the process of grief, such as taking one last trip, connecting with that special visitor, or saying good-bye. Michael's parents informed the palliative care team they wanted clear and timely information, even when there was uncertainty. But just as they want information, they told the team they wanted to impart information as well. They wanted to be listened to and recognized as the experts about Michael. They had spent much more time with him than any single healthcare provider. Even with a caring healthcare team and help from friends, much responsibility for implementing a child's care rests with parents. Many parents have asserted with good humor that they should receive honorary medical or nursing licenses.[25] In fact, in the case study; Michael's mother did go to nursing school a year after his death so she "could support other parents."

EMOTIONAL NEEDS

When a child is at risk of dying, the normal sequence of life events is disrupted. Initially, Michael's parents had to make a decision about whether or not to sustain the pregnancy. Then there was a decision after birth about whether to go through with a complex Norwood procedure, or provide comfort care. There was the relief that the first surgery went well and then the horrible realization that Michael would not survive. For Michael's family, there were ranges of emotion depending upon the content of the day and their son's medical and psychological status.

Healthcare providers should be mindful of the many dimensions and manifestations of emotional distress in parents. Parents may feel guilty that something they did resulted in their child's condition. Michael's mom was plagued by questions about prenatal care and early parenting decisions that caused her to need reassurance that she was not culpable in Michael's illness. Providing that support is more complicated if the actions of the parents contributed in any way to the child's health condition.

The emotional roller-coaster may impact the ability of parents to relate to siblings and extended family members. Support for parents may be provided best by family and friends, but parents may have difficulty accepting that support. They may also reach out to the healthcare team for that support. In addition, the team may help through referrals to other professionals for additional counseling.

SPIRITUAL NEEDS AND MAKING MEANING

Spirituality, broadly defined, encompasses all of the ways that we find understanding and make meaning out of our experiences.[26,27] Perhaps there are no circumstances where this definition is more important than in the life-threatening or life-limiting illness of a child. The essential question for these children and families is how they are to integrate the meaning of this experience into their lives. How does the illness, injury, loss, or death impact how they see themselves, their lives, their sense of family, and future? It is how meaning is derived from experience that determines the personal impact that experience will have.

Meaning is not a static state but instead the family and child are engaged in thousands of moments that create their understanding of the experience. We, as care providers, are charged with helping them integrate this experience and maintain connection to their loved ones and their sense of themselves. This may mean supporting the family in their religion or in any of the ways that they struggle to understand what is happening to them. One way to inquire about this without implying a religious connotation is to ask, "How are you and your family making sense out of what has been happening to you?" or, "What rituals are important to your family?" There are many rituals that can define a family's spiritual life and ability to make meaning out of their experiences.[27] These can include special family rituals, shared values, traditions, and a belief in the purpose of one's life. In all cases, care providers can offer loving support and opportunities for connection, healing, making meaning, and hope. Healthcare professionals do not necessarily have all of the answers about spirituality, and life and death, and cannot be expected to provide them to others. The most important roles for the healthcare provider are to be attentive to the child and family and to create opportunities for them to safely explore their own spiritual concerns. Michael's family decided to have his memorial service in the chapel at the children's hospital where he died. They were not religious but felt a spiritual bond with the staff they wanted to honor.

PRACTICAL NEEDS

Because families are so diverse, the needs for practical assistance vary enormously as do the challenges of meeting those needs. Opportunities to assist with the practical needs of families receiving palliative care range from finding housing to providing advice related to employment issues. Depending upon the socioeconomic status of the family, they may need significant support to provide for their family while struggling with their child's diagnosis. Families may need help with legal issues, financial assistance, housekeeping, lawn care, or some respite from the constant demands of care giving. For families who are recent immigrants or who have concerns about citizenship status, they may be concerned about seeking care in the medical system. Families that are separated by distance, families that have a member who is incarcerated, or those with significant members residing outside of the country all need specific support and intervention.

In addition to emotional support, siblings may need help with homework, babysitting, and transportation to activities that confer some normalcy in their lives. Contacting teachers to encourage creative ways for siblings of an ill child to complete assignments is helpful. In some cases, even visiting the classroom of a sick child or the sibling may improve peer support. In Michael's situation, a nurse and child-life specialist from the palliative care team visited his sister's classroom to help the kindergartners understand why Emily was missing so much school. The team members also suggested what the class might do to help her feel better, such as making a giant card telling her she was missed.

The Initiative for Pediatric Palliative Care (IPPC) developed Quality Domains, Standards, and Indicators of family-centered pediatric palliative care. The standards included the provision of "a range of practical (including financial assistance), emotional, and spiritual supports available to meet family-identified needs through the health institution and/or in the community in order to enable the family to maintain its usual life to the greatest degree possible."[28] A companion quality improvement tool developed by the IPPC, the Institutional Self Assessment Tool (ISAT), can be used as an assessment about resources for practical needs available within institutions and communities. Because of the uniqueness of each family, needs may vary widely and interventions must be tailored to each individual situation.

Developing and Changing Goals of Care

In family-centered care, the goals of care can be developed collaboratively with the family and may change repeatedly throughout the care trajectory. An important element of pediatric palliative care is balancing the desire to cure with the recognition that futile or burdensome medical intervention may not be in the child's best interest. There is never a situation when it can be said, "There is nothing more we can do." The goals of care may change, but there is always something an interdisciplinary team can do in providing palliative care. In today's world, the problem is that there is always more to do in terms of disease-directed treatment. Sometimes that treatment is inappropriate in the face of a life-limiting illness. The wisdom is in knowing when it is time to stop disease-directed treatments and focus on palliative interventions. Healthcare professionals can be companion to and guide the family as they navigate the challenges of making decisions, care giving, and providing support. A family systems approach involving the multidisciplinary team members may help those making decisions take into account all factors relevant to their situation. For example, a family having difficulty discontinuing futile disease-directed treatments may need to be supported and counseled about how their decisions affect the future of their family system. Continuation of futile therapy may not only threaten the well-being of their child, the patient, but also generate crushing debt and economic instability that jeopardizes the family's ability to provide a secure financial future for surviving siblings. Balancing such disparate considerations is not an easy task in the midst of a highly emotional situation. However, it is the multidisciplinary team's responsibility to provide both critical information and assist the family in synthesizing it and understanding its practical implications. A systematic evaluation of care goals may help families to change the focus from cure to comfort. Over time, parents may realize a cure is not possible and they are then better able to focus on goals of physical comfort, family functioning, and emotional support to enhance the quality of remaining time for both the child and family. Early introduction of parents and siblings to a palliative care team enables the development of relationships over the illness trajectory. Because goals of care fall into the realms of physical, emotional, spiritual, and mental needs, an interdisciplinary team consisting of nurses, physicians, social workers, child-life specialists, chaplains, and psychologists is needed to support a family undertaking these changes.

Some noteworthy tools have been developed to help interdisciplinary care teams work with families in developing and changing goals of care. Under the Robert Wood Johnson project, "Promoting Excellence in End-of-Life Care," The Pediatric Palliative Care Project of Seattle's Children's Hospital Regional Medical Center developed a decision-making tool to help families across the state of Washington plan care for children with progressive, potentially terminal illnesses. This tool allows family members and the healthcare team to view a complex case from four points of view: medical indications, quality of life, contextual issues, and patient and/or family preferences. The process of using the tool facilitates family-centered team communication and often leads to a collaborative plan of care.

SSM Cardinal Glennon Children's Medical Center in St. Louis collaborated with the Saint Louis University School of Medicine to build and maintain FOOTPRINTS, a statewide network of healthcare providers who care for terminally children and their families in their homes in Missouri. The FOOTPRINTS program also developed a care-planning tool to use with families of children with life-threatening conditions. The FOOTPRINTS program identifies difficult issues for families that may arise while caring for their children. Its care planning process acknowledges the family as the center of decision making and addresses not only the physical but also the psychosocial, spiritual, and emotional needs of the child and his or her family.

Considerations of Child Developmental Stages in Understanding and Discussing Death

Parents often ask care providers for advice on discussing with their child the topic of his or her impending death. Again, the multidisciplinary team, which should include a chaplain, psychologist, and child-life specialist, is positioned to assist parents in this difficult task. This requires understanding the child's cognitive, emotional, and spiritual development as these apply to acquiring a workable construct for the meaning of death. There are wide variations in this development, which is influenced by intellectual capacity, cognitive function, personal experiences, cultural and religious backgrounds, and emotional makeup.

A mature understanding of death as a biological event incorporates the constructs of irreversibility, finality or nonfunctionality, universality, and causality.[29] These can serve as a basis for evaluating a child's understanding of death. Irreversibility refers to awareness that when people die, their bodies do not become alive again. Universality refers to an understanding that all living things die. Nonfunctionality refers to lack of bodily functions such as breathing and eating. Finally, causality refers to being able to identify possible reasons why people die. In order to assess an understanding of this construct, healthcare providers might ask, "What makes people die?" Most children recognize a changed state and that something is dead (nonfunctionality) by 3 years. They realize all living things die at some time (universality) by 5 to 6 years, and that they will also die at some point by 8 to 9 years.[29,30] Healthcare providers may ask the child direct questions to begin to assess the child's understanding of their own health status and life expectancy. Especially for the younger child, more useful information may accrue from discerning answers through informal but directed conversation aimed at exploring a child's previous experience with death of family members, friends, or pets.

The point of conducting such an assessment is to provide parents and families with knowledge of their child's developmental understanding of death. The concerns that a child may have about dying stem from his or her understanding of death, and range from the concrete to the theological. Incomplete or wrong information can result in unnecessary anxiety. For most young children, their greatest fear is that they will be alone and/or in pain. Parents and the interdisciplinary team should be direct in reassuring them that this will not be the case. Older children should be offered access to spiritual support through the palliative care service or in conjunction with their own clergy. Parents should be supported to help them allow their children to discuss death as freely as they wish, without concern for upsetting their parents. It is not rare for parents to tell care providers that they do not want death to be discussed with their child for fear of upsetting him or her. While on some level this may reflect a genuine but misguided parental concern, far more often it is a symptom of parents who are experiencing difficulty coming to terms with the impending loss of their child. It can be useful to aid parents in gently gaining insight into the actual dynamic and to point out that even very young children are aware of their fate well before being told. Refusing to speak freely with children about death results in isolation and a loss of support at a critical time, and that isolation is from the most trusted individuals in their lives.

Family Conflict

Family variables such as conflict, cohesion, communication, and type of parenting are often used to describe a home environment and quality of a caregiving system. When parents are caring for a child with a life-threatening condition, it is likely there is an impact on parental functioning that may adversely affect the entire family through marital disruption, family conflict, lack of cohesion, and parenting. This may then lead to stress within the family that can spill over into relationships with extended family members, neighbors, teachers, and the healthcare team. Extended family members can pose their own challenges in the setting of life-threatening illness. Not uncommonly, relatives such as a child's grandparents, aunts, or uncles who have had little or no presence in the child's medical course will emerge at the child's demise. They will vociferously advocate for parents to continue all means of aggressive disease-directed treatment and not give up. Especially for families of a child with a prolonged course of treatment, as in cancer with multiple relapses, parents gain a unique perspective informed by firsthand experience with their child's suffering, which tends to moderate more extreme views of extended family. The extended family's views may be well-intentioned but are usually based on beliefs and theoretical values but not on medical experience. This places parents in the difficult position of considering a choice that best serves their child but directly opposes the strong opinions of extended family. Clinical experience suggests this type of conflict can often be resolved with help from the multidisciplinary team by:

- Affirming the parents are in a difficult position,
- Quietly supporting parents in their primary role of protecting their child's well-being,
- Offering to meet with extended family to remove suspicions and share essential medical information concerning prognosis and risks of continued treatment.

Few data are available regarding factors associated with illness and death to accurately predict the functional variability of families, especially siblings.[2] The evidence that does exist suggests that severe grief reactions among siblings and adults are more common when the deaths were recent, unexpected, in the hospital vs. at home, and associated with a lengthy illness or suffering.[2] Bereaved siblings may actually experience a two-fold loss when faced with not only the death of a sibling, but also the emotional unavailability of parents consumed by their own grief. As one mother stated, "I told (sibling) one day, I said, you know, you are a strong little boy.... I have cried and cried and you are just my little rock. And he said, 'Mom, he's right here' (mom stands up and puts her arm out like it's around shoulder of someone standing next to her)."[31] A death of a sibling is particularly challenging as it marks the end of what was expected to be a long and sometimes intimate relationship.[32,33] Common emotions expressed by siblings include anger, guilt, jealousy, fear, depression, and anticipatory grief.[34] Potential behavioral issues may be mitigated in families that are more cohesive and active in social and recreational activities and in those who put a greater emphasis on religion.[34]

However, there is also evidence that bereaved siblings exhibit positive attributes: increased maturity, self-esteem, empathy, and creativity.[35] Support from families' social, recreational, and religious activities may serve a protective function for bereaved siblings. Clinicians who show sensitivity to the amount of social support available to families can be especially beneficial in helping families when a child is ill or following the death of a child. Siblings can benefit from support groups, individual and group counseling, and from creative play activities, such as art and music therapy. Depending on their ages, they may not be able to verbalize their fears, but competent therapists can help them express themselves through alternative media. Child-life specialists and social workers are specially trained to assist siblings through this difficult time. Clinical experience suggests that siblings who play active roles in caring for the dying child, however simple those may be, adjust better to the future loss than those who are withdrawn or excluded. The extent to which these siblings are self-selected for better adjustment, possibly due to pre-existing family dynamics of greater openness and inclusion, is unclear.

Interdisciplinary Teamwork

In describing various roles related to palliative care, we frequently consider multidisciplinary, or a non-integrated mixture of disciplines, with a many-faceted team approach. Having experts work toward meeting the different needs of children and their families is often described as interdisciplinary, as team members combine their efforts and work together to address the needs. However, as team members become more adept at working together, they may even be called transdisciplinary. This transdisciplinary approach is a framework for facilitating healthcare team members to contribute knowledge and skills while collaborating with other members, and collectively determine the services that most would benefit a child and family. According to Bruder,[36] "This approach integrates a child's developmental needs across the major developmental domains" and "involves a greater degree of collaboration than other service delivery models" (p. 61).

Bruder describes this approach in more detail:

"A transdisciplinary approach requires the team members to share roles and systematically cross discipline boundaries. The primary purpose of this approach is to pool and integrate the expertise of team members so that more efficient and comprehensive assessment and intervention services may be provided. The communication style in this type of team involves continuous give-and-take between all members (especially with the parents) on a regular, planned basis. Professionals from different disciplines teach, learn, and work together to accomplish a common set of intervention goals for a child and her family. The role differentiation between disciplines is defined by the needs of the situation rather than by discipline-specific characteristics" (p. 61).

While it is important to consider discipline-specific roles, an interdisciplinary palliative care team, or even various members of a healthcare team, may experience overlapping roles without attempting to be discipline-specific. It may not really matter who does what as long as the family gets what it needs. Table 15-1 describes some of the roles of social workers, child-life specialists, chaplains, and nurses in caring for families needing palliative care, and dotted lines are important to note for delineation, to represent clearly overlapping functions. Sourkes and colleagues offer a complete picture of the multiple professionals who may also play a role in supporting children with life-limiting conditions and their families.[3]

TEAM CONFLICT

Given that by their very nature multidisciplinary teams involve several individuals representing various specialties, it is not surprising that occasionally differences of opinion may emerge on how certain palliative care issues should be addressed. In resolving these, it can be useful to incorporate several principles. First, not all conflict is bad and often it can serve a useful purpose. Through regular conferencing on children under their care, team members may find that what appears to be conflict is actually a misunderstanding of details concerning a child's prognosis or the risks and possible benefits of a proposed course of action. Related to this, addressing conflict through this type of dialogue first requires isolating the issue, reaching agreement on what the apparent conflict is about, and then seeking resolution if the conflict is real. Second, many palliative care decisions are objectively complex and nearly all are emotionally distressing. In such situations, decision-making is an iterative phenomenon in which the process is often critical to the outcome. Again, regular clinical conferences offer a forum where differences of opinion can be discussed openly and early before they create confusion among extended members of the clinical team and the family. Third, it is important to be both transparent to the family but to present, whenever possible, unambiguous care recommendations that represent a team consensus. Where differences of opinion remain, it may be the case that more than one option is reasonable for the family to choose. Rather than framing this for the family as a team conflict, care should be taken not to portray specific team members in opposition to each other, but to focus on the fact that the team recognizes more than one reasonable option exists and supports the parents in choosing as they think best. Finally, team member differences can sometimes be resolved by keeping the focus of recommendations on the well-being of

TABLE 15-1 Discipline-Specific Roles Related to Family Relationships

Role	Strategies
Social Work	• Provide individual counseling and brief psychotherapy with school-aged child and adolescent • Provide family counseling • Facilitate family-team conferencing • Provide initial crisis counseling • Offer referrals to support groups, bereavement groups, counseling • Collaborate with medical and case management team regarding discharge planning • Provide information and referrals for resources, including care-giving resources, financial and legal needs, advance directives • Assist with client advocacy and navigating the system
Child Life	• Facilite effective coping through play, preparation, education, and self-expression activities for child and siblings • Provide emotional support for families • Encourage optimum development of children facing a broad range of challenging experiences, particularly those related to healthcare and hospitalization • Provide information, support, and guidance to parents, siblings, and other family members, understanding that a child's well-being depends on the support of the family • Educate caregivers, administrators, and the general public about the needs of children under stress
Pastoral Care	• Assess spiritual needs of families • Coordinate notification of spiritual leaders of child's and family's choosing • Provide counseling for child and family • Assist with decision making
Nursing	• Pay attention to physical and emotional pain and symptom management needs of child and family • Coordinate care across settings, providing continuity of care • Facilitate integrative approaches to care, including complementary and alternative interventions • Assist family and team decision making and their understanding of the various treatment options • Offer referrals to other members of the interdisciplinary team, as needed • Assist with understanding symptoms of illness, provision of care, treatment options

the child and family in question. This may appear obvious, but it is not rare for conflict among team members to lose its proper context and appear intractable, but be resolved through refocusing the discussion on the patient. Unifying all the above is the need for excellent communication among team members, which is regular, frequent, and forthright.

Communication

When a child is facing a life-threatening condition, communication with the family is a critical tool that healthcare providers must use to ensure that the best decisions are being made for and with the child. Palliative care decisions such as limiting further aggressive treatments, signing. Do Not Resuscitate/Allow Natural Death (DNR/AND) orders, entering Phase I trials, providing palliative chemotherapy, or withdrawing life support represent just a few of the many choices that families are often required to make. Parents become the surrogate decision makers because pediatric patients are unable to legally make treatment decisions for themselves unless the child is an emancipated or mature minor. Ideally, the patient's preferences, hopes, desires, and goals should all be included as part of the decision-making process. However, this does not always occur in practice. Consequently, families are left to make palliative-care decisions for their child and they may feel unprepared to do so without the continued empathic support and communication from and with the interdisciplinary team.[37] Thus, a critical function of communication involving the child and the parent or responsible adult is to solicit the child's core values and preferences as they relate to end-of-life decision making. Ideally, these should be sought in advance through critical discernment and explicit discussion as the prognosis for recovery diminishes, well before death becomes imminent and difficult decisions must be implemented.

It is widely accepted that high-quality pediatric palliative care include effective and ongoing communication with the family that supports their wishes and engages them as partners in the decision-making process.[2,38] However, there are instances of families being asked to make care decisions before they completely understand the diagnosis or present condition of their loved one.[37] Studies of family members who have had a child die in the PICU all suggest that healthcare providers can continue to improve their communication with the families of dying patients.[39–42] Some institutions have begun to use family-centered language such as "allow natural death" when discussing end-of-life care decisions. PICU practitioners indicate that this terminology can sometimes be ambiguous but has the potential to ease difficult discussions for families.[43] Healthcare providers and families need to be allies in communication in pediatric palliative care to ensure that families have questions answered and understand all care options before making crucial decisions for their child. With that understanding, healthcare teams still need to keep the focus on well-being of the patient, not what makes parents feel better or less guilty.

COLLABORATIVE COMMUNICATION

The decision-making process can potentially be eased when family members are given the opportunity to engage in collaborative communication with healthcare providers. Collaborative communication is defined as the exchange of cooperative verbal and nonverbal messages between two or more parties that are committed to working toward a common goal.[44,45] Parties who engage in collaborative communication discuss shared interests and common goals while simultaneously exhibiting mutual respect and compassion for one another.[44] As a result, parties involved in the collaborative interaction are able to foster a supportive environment that encourages high levels of commitment,[46] satisfaction,[47] and coordination among all party participants.

A related but different aspect of collaborative communication and conflict involves how family members communicate with each other about the child's medical status. It is not altogether rare for parents to ask the physician not to disclose to the child the fact that he or she is not going to survive a worsening disease, such as multiply relapsed cancer. Almost always, this occurs in the context of pre-existing closed family communication patterns and where the parents are exhibiting other manifestations of difficulty accepting the child's coming death. A clinician's prior commitment to being honest with the child, in a developmentally appropriate way, must be respected. At the same time, handling such situations requires sensitivity, as well as candor. Especially in the case of school-aged children or older children dying of a chronic disease, it should be explained that most children already understand they are dying and that not speaking about it only isolates them and prevents discussion with those they need most for comfort. Support should be offered to the parents themselves for coming to terms with the impending reality they are finding so difficult to accept. Finally, there is no substitute for establishing healthy communication patterns throughout the trajectory of illness. Physicians, nurses, and other care providers can model good communication beginning at diagnosis of the life-threatening or life-limiting condition by speaking gently but openly of the possibility of death, and by always including the child in a developmentally appropriate way. Observing this approach may provide parents with the confidence and permission some need in being honest in this frightening and unfamiliar situation.

Collaborative Decision Making

Family members faced with difficult palliative care decisions welcome the opportunity to make shared decisions with healthcare providers by engaging in collaborative communication when treatment options are presented. Specifically, family members would rather take the time to walk through the different palliative care options with healthcare providers instead of being told that a particular course of treatment was the best way to proceed without further consideration.[37]

The following parental experience illustrates how important collaborative decision making is to family members faced with making palliative care decisions for their loved one.

> Author Deborah Dokken experienced collaborative decision making when she and her husband were presented with the option to transfer their daughter, Abby, to another hospital's PICU after a 5½ month stay in one NICU. Deborah said "Although the decision to move Abby was difficult, it was a shared decision made with healthcare providers who she and her husband trusted." Deborah also added that she and her husband were given enough time to think about the difficult decision and were encouraged to ask questions about the possible transfer without feeling rushed. Although Deborah and her husband experienced collaborative decision making when deciding to transfer their daughter to the PICU, Deborah also experienced how it felt for an intensivist to make a decision about Abby's care without her input. Deborah stated that the intensivist said, "The way I treat babies like your daughter is long-term ventilation." Deborah recalled that, "The intensivist announced the course of treatment instead of posing options or asking questions, or having a discussion of any sort."[17]

Contrasting the two different types of decision-making opportunities that the Dokken family experienced demonstrates how important it is to family members that they are given the opportunity to engage in collaborative decision making with healthcare providers. Families do not want to make such crucial decisions alone, nor do they want to be told what is best for their child. Instead family members are most satisfied when given the time to communicate collaboratively with healthcare providers about the best care options for their child. Thus, family members must not only be informed about the prognosis and treatment of their child but also given the opportunity to engage in detailed conversations with healthcare providers that explore treatment options to ensure families make the best decision for their loved one.

Collaborative decision-making also implies supporting medical decision-making by the child in the context of his or her family. As a child matures and gains decision-making capacity, he or she will become increasingly central in making important choices about end-of-life care. Especially for older children and adolescents, particularly those who have gained substantial medical experience through chronic illness, the child should be involved in a developmentally appropriate way in decisions concerning continuation of disease-directed treatment. The child should also be involved in what supportive care interventions may have adverse as well as beneficial effects and how remaining time will be spent. Again, depending on pre-existing family dynamics, parents may need to be guided in allowing their minor child to have a major, if not decisive, role in these choices. If their children have not been encouraged to develop personal autonomy through life decisions, it will be difficult for the family to embrace this approach at end of life. For this reason, it is useful for care providers to model good practice for the parents and promote decision-making experiences for the child beginning early in his or her care. Simple steps for this can include:

- Directing initial medical questions to the child during clinical encounters,
- Listening carefully to the child and acting on the information provided,
- Endeavoring to have the child's assent for interventions being considered,
- Providing graduated opportunities for the child to exercise choice over appropriate aspects of their care.

The goal is to reach the point where the family can embrace a decisional role for the child that maximizes his or her personal autonomy and dignity at end-of-life.

As is the case in communication, opportunities exist for conflict to develop within families over medical decision making by the child.

End-of-Life and Palliative Care Family Conferences

Family conferences enable families to make difficult decisions about palliative care options with the guidance and support of healthcare providers.[37] During these family meetings, healthcare providers and family members engage in collaborative communication that explores a variety of treatment options and considers all opinions, concerns, or worries in order to devise a medical plan that families and healthcare providers can support.[44] Reaching a consensus of care between family members and healthcare providers often takes time but ensures that all voices are heard and questions are raised before important decisions are made about end-of-life care for the patient.

Furthermore, family conferences have been shown to incorporate the strategies parents have recommended, such as clearer and more frequent communication with healthcare providers, to enhance communication and ultimately improve palliative and end-of-life care.[37] Additionally, studies have shown that family conferences help to reduce regret or guilt that family members feel after making crucial end-of-life decisions for their child.[37]

CONDUCTING PALLIATIVE AND END-OF-LIFE FAMILY CONFERENCE

Healthcare teams should consider the timing of palliative family conferences to provide the most benefit to the child. Ideally, this conference should occur in anticipation of the child's deterioration or impending death, not in a time of crisis. This is why it can be so helpful to introduce palliative care early in the treatment trajectory so that the team and family have a shared understanding of goals of care.

Before proceeding with family conferences it is helpful for healthcare providers to review the five steps that Feudtner[44] designed to ensure that family meetings are organized and successful: planning, beginning, dialogue, concluding, and actions and follow-up.

Planning

Healthcare providers should work with family members to arrange an appropriate date and time for the family meeting. At this time, family members need to be encouraged to brainstorm any questions, concerns, or ideas that they would like addressed in the meeting. Once the meeting date and time is set, an adequate location is required. It is important that the location be private with enough seating for all participants. Lastly, healthcare providers must make sure they have read all available information about the patient's case, are in agreement about treatment options, and have nominated one person to run the meeting.

Beginning

Open the meeting by first asking everyone to introduce themselves and highlight their roles in the child's care. Next, the healthcare provider running the meeting should present an agenda and ask the family to add to it. It is important that healthcare providers strive to capture all ideas, concerns, or input the family proposes and ensure they are addressed during the meeting. After collectively creating the agenda, briefly summarize the clinical status of the patient. When the summary is complete, ask the family members for feedback about the medical status of their loved one. Ensure that all family members understand the child's current condition.

Dialogue

Once healthcare providers are confident that all meeting participants are on the same page about the patient's clinical status, the meeting dialogue should be focused on establishing goals of care and exploring all treatment options available to the patient. To establish goals of care for the child it is important that healthcare providers attempt to balance interaction

patterns. For example, all parties should be voicing opinions and concerns rather than healthcare providers doing all the talking. Healthcare providers should gently help family members create goals of care for their loved one by asking questions and enabling the family to share their hopes, thoughts, fears, and emotions. The creation of care goals often fosters a supportive atmosphere that facilitates a collaborative exchange among the meeting's participants. After care goals have been collectively created, healthcare providers are ready to discuss the options available to the patient. When presenting the different courses of treatment, providers should help families visualize treatment options while discussing both the benefits and drawbacks of each course of action. It is helpful to keep referring to the established goals of care when families are attempting to make difficult decisions about treatment options. Once families have reviewed all treatment options, a consensus will likely emerge that reflects the most important goals of care and the treatment plan that family members agree is the best for their loved one.

Concluding

After meeting participants have reached a consensus of care the leader of the meeting should review the agenda, ensuring that all items were covered adequately and all questions, concerns, and ideas were addressed. Once the agenda has been revisited, the plan of care established at the meeting should be reviewed. It is important to confirm that all meeting participants can agree to support the palliative care plan.

Actions and Follow-Up

Following the family conference, it is important that the healthcare providers who participated ensure that the palliative care plan devised is followed. The palliative care plan must be shared with all healthcare providers that will be assisting the patient and family. In addition, healthcare providers should keep in mind that the condition of the patient could change, requiring a follow-up family meeting to alter the agreed-upon goals of care and palliative care plan.

Ultimately, end-of-life family conferences provide a forum for collaborative communication among the healthcare providers and families. Older, medically experienced children and adolescents need to be included in this decision-making process, either in real time during the conference with the family and practitioner, or in a co-occurring series of discussions. It is important for older children and adolescents that they not be kept in the dark about end-of-life conferences. They know when their parents are meeting with care providers and worry that information is being withheld from them. Involving them in the conference directly, or at least reassuring them that they will be told everything that was discussed, can prevent unnecessary anxiety. When healthcare providers, families, and children take the time to participate in end-of-life family conferences, a consensus of care can be reached. Family conferences empower family members to make the best care decisions for and with their children bolstered by the guidance and support of healthcare providers.

Providing Family Psychosocial Support and Enhancing Family Resilience

When a child is diagnosed with a life-threatening or life-limiting condition, the family is often overwhelmed, confused, and struggling to maintain or re-establish a sense of equilibrium.[2,3]

Simultaneously, most families are immediately calling in sources of support, mobilizing resources and using all of their pre-existing strengths to support the child and each other. Interdisciplinary pediatric palliative care teams can play a critical role in enhancing family resilience in this difficult time. One of the starting points for this is to assess both the strengths and challenges that the family has and to bring those to the awareness of the family and healthcare team. While providing empathic support to the distressing news of the child's diagnosis, the team can also begin to help the family identify their resources and resiliency.

In order to best support the family, the interdisciplinary team must truly work as a collaborative, coordinated, and compassionate team that is giving the same messages to the child and the family. Teamwork between various disciplines can be a struggle and communication is critical. Families feel frightened and less supported when they sense that the team is in disagreement or conflict. Ideally, an interdisciplinary pediatric palliative team will have many specialty disciplines that can include medicine, nursing, social work, psychology, psychiatry, child life, chaplaincy, rehabilitative services, educational support, art and music therapists, and supportive staff.[3] When the team is functioning well, the sense of support can enhance a family's functioning and increase their abilities to cope with their child's illness.

Siblings should be encouraged to be as involved in their brother's or sister's care as they want to be. They can also have opportunities to participate in their normal school and extra-curricular activities and peer groups. Siblings benefit from support groups and contact with other siblings who have been through similar experiences. Young children need to know that they are not responsible for their sibling's illness or their parent's distress. It can be very helpful to identify a safe adult who is designated specifically to support the sibling other than a parent. This person can be a teacher, family member, neighbor, friend, or healthcare professional. Child-life specialists and social workers can offer specific targeted support to siblings. Use local and national programs such as Supersibs (www.supersibs.org) to support siblings as well.

The interdisciplinary healthcare team can play a significant role in helping families by identifying family fears, challenges, loss and illness history as well as sources of strength and resilience. Pediatric palliative care teams can specifically listen to and support members of the family including grandparents and extended family. Healthcare professionals can empower the family to speak with children about their concerns and hopes and help the family identify the child's strengths, supports, and sources of resilience. Pediatric palliative care teams function as a witness to the trauma that families endure and can react with true compassion to their suffering and survival. As this family stated:

"We were made to feel as though we were part of a big family while we were there. Everyone cared for our son as though he were their own. In my opinion, that is what makes a good caregiver a great one."[48]

Family resilience can be fostered during times of stress, illness, trauma, and challenge.[49] Walsh identified three key domains of family functioning that relate to family resilience: some belief systems, organizational patterns, and communication processes. Belief systems that seem to foster resilience are those that include a positive outlook, a sense of making meaning out of struggle and a focus on transcendence or spirituality.[49] For families caring for a child who is ill, this may

imply that fostering realistic hopefulness and including discussions about spirituality and meaning making could be helpful tools to assist in the growth and wellness. Walsh indicated that a family's resilience can be enhanced by organizational patterns that display flexibility, connectedness and adequate social and economic resources. Interdisciplinary healthcare teams should continue to help families identify their natural sources of support, access critical financial resources, and maintain their attachments and sense of being a family facing struggle together. Finally, Walsh found that family communication that was categorized by clarity, open emotional expression, and collaborative problem solving fostered family resilience. Pediatric palliative care is ideally defined as providing clear, compassionate, collaborative information and decision making that encourages the expression and support of the child's and family's unique emotions and needs within their cultural and historical context. Knowing that this approach has the capacity to enhance the resilience of families should motivate all interdisciplinary pediatric palliative care providers.

Integration of Pediatric Palliative Care Principles into Practice

The following case demonstrates an interdisciplinary team working together to conduct a full assessment and respond to the patient and family facing end of life. Children and families may bring past traumas and histories into the current health care crisis and must have the opportunity to fully express their concerns in the context of the supportive palliative care team.

Future directions

Pediatric palliative care has always been dedicated to addressing the needs of the child and the family. The initial impetus for the field came largely out of the desire to design care that would be family-focused and offer alternatives to traditional medical models that do not include the family. As this young field moves forward, we gain a better understanding of what families truly experience and how we can best help them. In truth, we are learning that each family is as unique as the child they accompany, and that our best models of care involve listening, respect, collaborative decision making, partnerships, and fostering the existing strengths that families bring to the healthcare setting. Additional research that is under way to discover the key covariates and methods for palliative care and end-of-life decision making will help care providers understand and effectively address the most important needs of dying children and their families. There is no way to take away the pain of learning that a child has a life-threatening condition, but with compassion there are many ways to ease the suffering of families and to promote resilience, cohesion, and hope.

A 19-year-old with multiply relapsed acute lymphoblastic leukemia (ALL) (third relapse) who was receiving an investigational new drug on a phase II trial was admitted emergently with symptoms of spinal cord compression and paraparesis and neurogenic bowel/bladder. His medical status was quite complicated with many medical issues present, including pain, fevers, bleeding, and pancytopenia. He eventually developed hepatorenal syndrome. As it became more and more apparent that this young man was unable to survive his disease and was plagued by many symptoms, the need for an aggressive symptom-control regimen and adoption of "Allow Natural Death" (the institution's version of "Do Not Resuscitate") became urgent. Unfortunately, his family was initially quite opposed to the "AND" status because they felt it would be a sign of lack of religious faith that he would obtain a miracle. This was quite a difficult and challenging situation, as there was a strong, culturally-based value system at work that made it challenging to gain the family's trust and support for discontinuing disease-directed treatment while shifting to a focus on comfort-directed care. In contrast to the institution's general preference for home-based palliative care, it was decided that this young man and family would be best served by allowing him to stay in the hospital, both to reduce anxiety and also to address the extremely limited resources available to this family for home-based care. Finally, it became known to the inpatient clinical team that this young man had been plagued with guilt over a particularly traumatic event that occurred when he was barely 10 years old: A fire occurred in his house and he was unable to run back to save a small niece he knew was still in the house. He related that he could still remember how her badly burned body appeared when he watched first-responders remove it from the house. The patient was convinced that he was destined to go to hell as a result of failing to save her, and was thus afraid of dying. The team's multidisciplinary interventions focused on managing the physical concerns and also on supporting and re-educating the patient and his family in culturally-sensitive ways that would increase his likelihood of achieving inner peace and closure before passing. Ultimately, when the occasion of his death arrived a few days later, both he and his family were much more accepting of this outcome and able to focus on making his experience of death as comfortable and meaningful as possible.

REFERENCES

1. Wills AJ: I Wish you knew, *Pediatr Nurs* 35(5):318–321, 2009.
2. Field MJ, Behrman RE: *When children die: improving palliative and end-of-life care for children and their families*, Washington, DC, 2003, Institute of Medicine, National Academies Press.
3. Sourkes B, Frankel MD, Brown M, Contro N, Benitz W, Case C, Good J, Jones L, Komejan J, Modderman-Marshall J, Reichard W, Sentivany-Collins S, Sunde C: Food, toys, and love: pediatric palliative care, *Curr Probl Pediatr Adolesc Healthcare* 35:350–386, 2005.
4. Contro N, Larson J, Scofield S, Sourkes B, Cohen H: Family perspectives on the quality of pediatric palliative care, *Arch Pediatr Adolesc Med* 156(1):14–19, 2002.
5. Browning DM, Solomon MZ: Relational learning in pediatric palliative care: transformative education and the culture of medicine, *Child Adolesc Psychiatr Clin N Am* 15(3):795–815, 2006.
6. Dokken D, Ahmann E: The many roles of family members in "family-centered care"—Part I, *Pediatr Nurs* 32(6):562–565, 2006.
7. Johnson B, Jeppson E, Redburn L: *Caring for children and families: guidelines for hospitals*, Bethesda, Md, 1992, Association for the Care of Children's Health.
8. Initiative for Pediatric Palliative Care: *Unpublished interviews*, 2000.
9. American Academy of Pediatrics: Policy statement: family-centered care and the pediatrician's role, *Pediatrics* 112(3):691–696, 2003.
10. Ahmann E, Johnson BJ: Family-centered care: facing the new millennium, *Pediatr Nurs* 26(1):87–90, 2000.
11. Ahmann E: Examining assumptions underlying nursing practice with children and families, *Pediatr Nurs* 23(5):467–469, 1998.
12. Gilmer MJ: Pediatric palliative care: a family-centered model for critical care, *Crit Care Nurs Clin North Am* 14:207–214, 2002.
13. Hepworth DH, Rooney RH, Larsen JA, Strom-Gottfried K, Rooney GD: *Direct social work practice: theory and skills*, ed 8, Belmont, Calif, 2009, Brooks Cole Publishing.
14. Meyer C: *Can social work keep up with the changing family?* Monograph, The fifth annual Robert J. O'Leary Memorial Lecture, Columbus, Ohio, 1990, The Ohio State University College of Social Work, pp 1–24.
15. Jones B, Volker D, Vinajeras Y, Butros L, Fitchpatrick C, Rosetto K: The meaning of surviving cancer for Latino adolescents and emerging young adults, *Cancer Nurs* 33(1):74–81, 2010.
16. Sydnor-Greenburg N: *Personal communication*, May 10, 2005.
17. Dokken DL: In their own voices: families discuss end-of life decision making—Part I, *Pediatr Nurs* 32(2):173–175, 2006.
18. Dokken D, Simms R, Cole FS, Ahmann E: The many roles of family members in "family-centered care"—Part II, *Pediatr Nurs* 33(1):5151–5152, 5170, 2007.
19. Sharpe D, Rossiter L: Siblings of children with a chronic illness: a meta-analysis, *J Pediatric Psychol* 27(8):699–710, 2002.
20. Murray JS: The lived experience of childhood cancer: one sibling's perspective, *Issues Compr Pediatr Nurs* 21(4):217–227, 1998.
21. Dent AL, Stewart AJ: *Sudden death in childhood: support of bereaved family*, Butterworth, Heineman, 2004, Elsevier.
22. Ponzetti JJ, Johnson MA: The forgotten grievers: grandparents' reactions to the death of grandchildren, *Death Stud* 15:157–167, 1991.
23. Reed ML: *Grandparents cry twice*, Amityville, NY, 2000, Baywood Publications.
24. Thibault GE: Prognosis and clinical predictive models for critically ill patients. In Field MJ, Cassel CK, editors: *Approaching death: improving care at the end of life*, Washington, DC, 1997, National Academy Press, pp 358–362.
25. Hilden J, Himelstein BP, Reyer DR, Friebert S, Kane JR: End-of-life care: special issues in pediatric oncology. In Foley KM, Gelband H, editors: *improving palliative care for cancer*, Washington, DC, 2001, National Academy Press.
26. Canda E, Furman L: *Spirituality and social work practice: the heart of helping*, New York, 1999, Free Press.
27. Jones B, Weisenfluh S: Pediatric palliative and end-of-life care: spiritual and developmental issues for children, *Smith College Studies in Social Work: Special Edition on End of Life Care* 78(1):423–443, 2003.
28. Dokken DL, Heller KS, Levetown M, et al: *For The Initiative for Pediatric Palliative Care (IPPC). Quality domains, goals, and indicators of family-centered care of children living with life-threatening conditions*, Newton, Mass, 2002, Education Development Center, Inc.
29. Boyd-Webb N: *Helping bereaved children: a handbook for practitioners*, New York, 2002, Guilford Press.
30. Kenyon B: Current research in children's conceptions of death: a critical review, *Omega J Death Dying* 43:63–91, 2001.
31. Foster T: A mixed method study for exploring continuing bonds in children with cancer and their bereaved families, Unpublished dissertation.
32. Davies B: *Shadows in the sun: the experiences of sibling bereavement in childhood*, New York, 1998, Routledge.
33. Robinson L, Mahon M: Sibling bereavement: a concept analysis, *Death Stud* 21:477–499, 1997.
34. Davies B: The family environment in bereaved families and its relationship to surviving sibling behavior, *Children's Healthcare* 17:22–30, 1988.
35. Hogan NS, Schmidt LA: Testing the grief to personal growth model using structural equation modeling, *Death Stud* 26(8):615–634, 2002.
36. Bruder MB: Working with members of other disciplines: Collaboration for success. In Wolery M, Wilbers JS, editors: *Including children with special needs in early childhood programs*, Washington, DC, 1994, National Association for the Education of Young Children, pp 45–70.
37. Lautrette A, Ciroldi M, Ksibi H, Azoulay E: End-of-life family conferences: rooted in the evidence, *Crit Care Med* 34:364–372, 2006.
38. Meyer EC, Ritholz MD, Burns JP, Truog RD: Improving the quality of end-of-life care in the pediatric intensive care unit: parents' priorities and recommendations, *Pediatrics* 117:649–657, 2006.
39. Abbott KH, Sago JG, Breen CM: Families looking back: one year after discussion of withdrawal or withholding life-sustaining support, *Crit Care Med* 29:197–201, 2001.
40. Azoulay E, Sprung CL: Family-physician interactions in the intensive care unit, *Crit Care Med* 32:2323–2328, 2004.
41. Cuthbertson SJ, Margetts MA, Streat SJ: Bereavement follow-up after critical illness, *Crit Care Med* 28:1196–1201, 2000.

42. Hanson LC, Danis M, Garrett J: What is wrong with end-of-life care? Opinions of bereaved family members, *J Am Geriatr Soc* 45:1339–1344, 1997.

43. Jones B, Parker-Raley J, Higgerson R, Christie L, Legett S, Greathouse J: Finding the right words: the use of Allow Natural Death (AND) and DNR in pediatric palliative care, *J Healthc Qual* 30(5):55–63, 2008.

44. Feudtner C: Collaborative communication in pediatric palliative care: a foundation for problem-solving and decision-making, *Pediatr Clin North Am* 54:583–607, 2007.

45. Mohr JJ, Fisher RJ, Nevin JR: Collaborative communication in interfirm relationships: Moderating effects of integration and control, *Journal of Marketing* 60:103–115, 1996.

46. Morgan R, Hunt S: The commitment-trust theory of relationship marketing, *Journal of Marketing* 58:20–38, 1994.

47. Keith J, Jackson D, Crosby L: Effects of alternative types of influence strategies under different channel dependences structures, *Journal of Marketing* 54:30–41, 1990.

48. Meyer EC, Burns JP, Griffith JL, Truog RD: Parental perspectives on end-of-life care in the pediatric intensive care unit, *Crit Care Med* 30(1):226–231, 2002.

49. Walsh F: Family resilience: a framework for clinical practice, *Fam Process* 42:1–18, 2004.

16 Team Relationships

SARAH FRIEBERT | JODY CHRASTEK | MICHELLE R. BROWN

If they don't have scars, they haven't worked on a team.
Teams don't just happen. They slowly and painfully evolve.
The process is never complete. The work involved is usually
underestimated. —Balfour Mount

By its very nature, and in fact by legislative decree in the case of hospice, the discipline of palliative care is a team sport. The overall goal of teamwork is to enhance patient care through team performance, member satisfaction, and organizational commitment. Through a cyclic process of "forming, storming, norming, and performing,"[1] teams that are well-formed and well-maintained enhance the delivery of pediatric palliative care by far more than the sum of the individual disciplinary parts. Nevertheless, highly functional teams are not automatic—their creation and ongoing survival and growth require high-level, multimodal skills. This chapter will explore the basic types and dynamics of teams, their critical importance in pediatric palliative care, typical features of functional and dysfunctional teams, and practical strategies to prevent or remedy dysfunction to preserve and protect teams and their members.

Team Structures

Teams come in many flavors. Multidisciplinary teams are groups of individual practitioners who come together to report on what each is doing and work side by side but not necessarily together.[2] In multidisciplinary teams, professional identities are primary while team membership is a secondary priority. Leadership is generally hierarchical, and practitioners function as wedges in a pie.[3] Partly because these teams rarely meet face to face to discuss the needs of mutual clients, the multidisciplinary model is not a good fit for palliative care because the lack of regular communication increases burdens on families who become responsible for keeping their care professionals apprised of changing symptoms and treatments (Fig. 16-1).[4]

Most palliative care teams are self-described as interdisciplinary. In this model, different professionals combine resources and talents to deliver care in an interactive process by which collaboration reveals goals that cannot be delivered by one discipline alone,[5] and the synergy resulting from collaboration creates an "active, ongoing, productive process."[6] Team members engage in joint work from different orientations,[7] and the objective is to arrive at effective treatment decisions after considering input from all members. Leadership of interdisciplinary palliative care teams is often task-dependent

and decisions are usually made by consensus;[8] this process enables focus on medical concerns as well as wider issues of comfort and total patient-centered care—a founding principle of specialist palliative care practice.[9]

As mentioned above, the interdisciplinary team model of care is the standard of care in hospice, which is one of the only settings in the United States where interdisciplinary teamwork is regulated.[10,11] Functional interdisciplinary care can actually be measured through the Index of Interdisciplinary Collaboration. This instrument assesses teams based on a model of successful collaboration whose components are interdependence, newly created professional activities, flexibility, collective ownership of goals, and reflection on process.[12] Compared to multidisciplinary teams, interdisciplinary teams have been rated by members as higher in coherence, sense of responsibility, work climate, internal organization, and communication.[13] A true interdisciplinary team illustrates that the function of a hand is far more than the sum of each individual digit.[3,14] Most interdisciplinary teams are comprised of members who belong primarily to that team, service, program, or division.

Cross-functional teams are a subset of interdisciplinary teams with potential relevance in pediatric palliative care. Arising from the business world out of organizational theory, cross-functional teams are assembled to create sets of skills for a particular purpose. Members cover each other's weaknesses and maximize strengths as the team together takes responsibility for the well-being of a patient and family. In this way, resources are multiplied by the overlap of roles and a unique forum for problem-solving is developed.[14] A pediatric palliative care program in a large children's hospital discovered that families receiving care were being balance-billed when their insurance benefits did not cover palliative care services; worse yet, families were also receiving bills after their children had died. The program put together a cross-functional team, which included billing and finance personnel, a social worker, a parent liaison from the hospital's parent advisory committee, a department administrator, and leadership from the clinical palliative care program, to tackle the issue. Over an 18-month period, the team worked through the logistical confines of the hospital's accounting methods to create a system that satisfied everyone, especially the families. Some pediatric palliative care teams themselves can be described as cross-functional; in general, these are interdisciplinary teams at the core but also include members from other disciplines, departments, divisions, service lines, or the community, who have other job responsibilities and reporting structures but come together for a defined purpose or patient population.

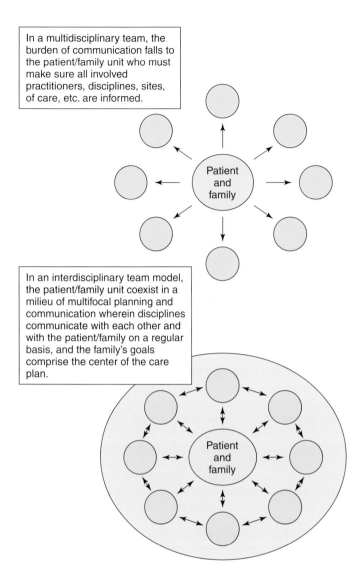

In a multidisciplinary team, the burden of communication falls to the patient/family unit who must make sure all involved practitioners, disciplines, sites, of care, etc. are informed.

In an interdisciplinary team model, the patient/family unit coexist in a milieu of multifocal planning and communication wherein disciplines communicate with each other and with the patient/family on a regular basis, and the family's goals comprise the center of the care plan.

Fig. 16-1 Communication burdens in different team types.

Benefits for pediatric palliative care teams are many:

- This model facilitates new ways of seeing and creating different frameworks, which can be helpful with both clinical and ethical dilemmas inherent in pediatric palliative care.
- Cross-functional team flexibility enables faster and more broad-based responses to patients and families in crisis.
- All members from diverse disciplines are fundamental to complex assessment, providing a much broader perspective than a straightforward medical or medicine or nursing approach.[3,14]
- Palliative care is a dynamic and uncertain environment.

From an organizational standpoint, cross-functional palliative care teams can enhance an organization's innovative capacities to match the organization to the environment by bundling a large range of discipline-based skills and competencies in different ways, using different team members.[15]

The last team type is transdisciplinary. This model is gaining in popularity, though not as commonly in healthcare. The fundamental concept is one of role release in which there exist few seams among member functions. Roles and responsibilities are shared and often blurred.[3,14] Members of transdisciplinary

teams have been heard to say, "Everyone on this team is a little bit nurse, a little bit social worker, a little bit physician. Whoever is in the clinical situation does what needs to be done since we all have a good basic knowledge of what our colleagues do." While this approach has its advantages, problems with role definition can lead to significant impairments in team functioning in palliative care; such potential downsides will be discussed later in this chapter.

The distinction between cross-functional and transdisciplinary is subtle but clinically relevant. A transdisciplinary team is composed of members of multiple disciplines who all function together with overlapping roles in the care of each family enrolled in the program. Team members do what is requested or required when they are present with a patient or family, which may include blending or blurring their roles. In contrast, a cross-disciplinary team would be made up of distinct disciplines that retain areas of practice and expertise but have a defined angle to approach in patient and family care. Though the team functions as a whole, each patient's plan of care is assessed through the lens of each discipline, so that each contributes specialized expertise to the overall plan of care. This approach enhances goal-directed or symptom-directed efficacy while preserving individual approach and minimizing blurring of boundaries.

Benefits and Challenges of Team-Based Palliative Care

While clear-cut advantages of high-functioning teams have not been demonstrated empirically in pediatric palliative care, the concept is central to the way in which most clinical work is performed, and its relevance cannot be overstated. Multiple potential and actual advantages of team-based care have been demonstrated for adults, particularly in palliative care, including:

- Higher quality of care due to improved goal setting and care delivery resulting from high-quality collaboration and the resultant synergy created by the collaborative relationship,[10,12]
- System and/or the organization benefits from more comprehensive care, reduction of overall health care costs, reduced medical services, fewer doctor visits, more complete attention to co-morbidities and complexities of care, and increased client satisfaction,[16–18]
- Team benefits from the development of joint initiatives not thought of individually, achievement of better care plans for holistic care, higher levels of productivity, and increased staff satisfaction,[19]
- Patient and family benefits from improved patient insight into illness,[20] self-reports of pain and non-pain symptoms,[21] quality of life, satisfaction with overall treatment, communication,[22,23] patient empowerment and education.[16]

Despite this lengthy list of benefits, some authors believe that the emphasis on the interdisciplinary team in palliative care is faulty. For example, Cott asserts that the value of team presupposes untested and perhaps unsustainable assumptions: that team members have shared understandings of norms, values, and roles; that the team functions in a cooperative, egalitarian, interdependent manner; and that the combined effects of shared, cooperative decision making are of greater benefit to the patient than the individual effects of the disciplines on their own.[24] At the very least, the as-yet untested benefits in pediatric palliative care necessitate that the team model be created, maintained, and sustained in the most productive and best way possible to maximize whatever potential benefits may be validated in actual practice.

Teams in palliative care have a number of specific challenges that are not faced as consistently by other healthcare teams. From the start members must form solid relationships with new colleagues to build an effective working group, acclimate to a field of work with a high emotional burden, and tolerate the significant uncertainty of practicing without defined standards compared to other medical fields.[4,13] The ever-increasing complexity of palliative medicine calls, in turn, for recognition of the increasing complexity and multiplicity of teams.[25] Teams must navigate more complex patient needs and work with more informed patients and families playing more significant roles in their own care—both a blessing and a challenge—in an environment in which ambiguity and uncertainty are the norms.

The context in which care is given is also increasing in complexity, requiring flexibility related to the diversity of location, culture, family structure, communities, privacy, and interconnectedness.[25] Practical conflicts exist as well. Team members must handle ever-changing communication patterns involving the use of alien technology and differences in terminology among disciplines.[26] Health-related priorities, targets, resources, and budgets are generally not set by palliative care teams, often resulting in scarcity of resources.[26] Increased access and equity, particularly as offered by community-based services, result in a larger service area with limited resources.[4] In fact, despite the continual change occurring for patients and families, the availability of resources for care is generally either constant or shrinking.[15]

In addition to the challenges inherent in clinical work, team functioning itself may be in conflict with the core values of palliative care. For instance, the philosophy of palliative care may be at odds with the clarification of team roles and procedures,[4] and the focus on team function may end up protecting team members rather than supporting patient and/or family needs.[26] Conflict may also occur between the democracy of palliative care teams and the traditional medical model.

Finally, the meteoric, successful rise of palliative care has created the potential that teams will fail to live up to unrealistic expectations. Often, palliative care teams are held up as the hallmark for interdisciplinary team functioning, creating more pressure under increased scrutiny.

Forming and Sustaining Teams: Recipes for Success and Failure

Despite these and other challenges, many pediatric palliative care teams are up and running, sustaining themselves and growing successfully. So how do functional, successful teams form? Many developmental models of team formation exist. One model includes five basic stages described by Lowe and Herranen, and it unites common themes:

1. Becoming acquainted, which represents a period of low group productivity but also minimal conflict,
2. Trial and error, during which team members test boundaries, seek allies, and engage in parallel play,

3. Collective indecision; without strong leadership and assumption of shared responsibility, the result is pseudo-consensus and unilateral action that leads to scapegoating,
4. If scapegoating occurs, generally an internal or external crisis happens, which forces teams to face their issues,
5. With strong leadership and committed team members, the final stage of resolution occurs, resulting in high individual and group productivity.[27]

The effectiveness of any team collaboration can be affected by structural characteristics, which are influenced by organizational processes contributing to the team's development and maintenance. Clearly, strong and visionary leadership is necessary for any team to succeed, and its importance cannot be emphasized enough. Box 16-1 describes some of the qualities of true team-centered leaders, which enhance the probability of developing and sustaining high-functioning teams. Further positive influences on team effectiveness comes from manageable caseloads, supportive and collaborative organizational culture, administrative support, professional autonomy, and time and/or space for collaboration.[6,7] The larger the team, and the more disciplines involved, the more time that team needs to achieve functionality and growth.[7]

In a survey of four nonprofit health care institutions, two of them pediatric, Proenca established that team empowerment is the mechanism through which team context and team atmosphere affect job satisfaction and organizational commitment.[28] This is helpful news for teams because it suggests that modifications of context and atmosphere that facilitate empowerment will lead to positive outcomes of improved satisfaction and organizational commitment. Said another way, direct strategies to empower team members can overcome a large number of variables that likely can't be modified or eliminated in daily life on a palliative care team.

Oliver et al used a modified Index of Interdisciplinary Collaboration and found that perceptions of interdisciplinary team collaboration can be measured, and that educational training in a specific discipline and clinical training do not create variance in perceptions of that collaboration. Instead, varied perceptions come from the interdisciplinary nature of the particular team.[10] In other words, it might be thought that collaboration is affected by the varied disciplines or training backgrounds or cultures of the individual team members. But it appears as though the team structure, leadership, empowerment, and functionality influence how members perceive how well the team collaborates. This again is heartening news for interdisciplinary and/or cross-functional teams because it suggests that effort directed at team functioning will overcome

---

BOX 16-1 Qualities of Team-Centered Leaders

Visionary, and able to share vision with team
Proactive in most relationships
Inspire teamwork and mutual support
Promote opportunities for teamwork
Build a team of individuals who can work constructively together
Consider problem solving a team responsibility
Communicate clearly and fully
Open to feedback and questions
Recognize that conflict is inevitable, and mediate conflict before it becomes destructive
Recognize both individual and team accomplishments appropriately
Honor commitments and expect the same in return

differences in individual background and training, which might seem to affect collaboration negatively.

TEAM COMPOSITION

The ideal makeup of a pediatric palliative care team will necessarily vary depending on site, goals, and scope of services, as well as on resources. Ideally, every team will be made up of medical; nursing; psychosocial, including social work, child life, and psychology; and spiritual and bereavement care; and will be able to access high-quality adjunct services such as pharmacology, nutrition, expressive therapy, rehabilitation, and education. When fully actualized, a pediatric palliative care team is like a tapestry in which different colors of threads are interwoven to produce a complete picture. At times one color—or one discipline—may be more prominent while others take a more background role. But the presence of each makes the tapestry complete when the weaving exists and comes together around a child and family's goals of care (Fig. 16-2).

Many programs, however, do not have a complete interdisciplinary team, especially when starting. Provision of high-quality pediatric palliative care can be challenging in this scenario, particularly for the solo provider with limited time and resources. Yet it is still possible for children and families to receive excellent interdisciplinary care through collaboration.

In the hospital setting, professionals who have a particular interest in palliative care can work together as an ad hoc team in the care of an individual child and family. More formally, a variety of departments may work together to provide parts of positions that together make up the needed team. For example, neurology may provide 10 hours of a social worker, NICU may provide 10 hours of nursing, hematology/oncology may provide 20 hours of both nursing and social work, and chaplaincy may provide hours from their department. Perhaps a specific physician in each specialty is willing to be the lead palliative care person for their patient population. Hospital-based volunteer services may have individuals who want to be part of a palliative care team as well. This kind of team is made up of individuals who together can provide excellent interdisciplinary care. Though true with any team, it is especially essential to have regular meetings to ensure good communication and foster the development of the team when members come from multiple departments.

One example of this was seen in a children's hospital in a small city with a new pediatric palliative care program. The program consisted of a part-time pediatric palliative care nurse, but no other disciplines were specifically designated to the team. The nurse knew that a few people in the hospital were very interested in palliative care and invited them to be on the pediatric palliative care advisory group. She looked for representation from chaplaincy, child life, social work, psychology, and physician groups. As she collaborated and built relationships, the group strategically planned the best way to fill the interdisciplinary needs of a palliative care team. They were able to negotiate parts of positions from a variety of departments. With program growth and demonstrated outcomes, more permanent positions were approved. Such a piecemeal approach can challenge cohesiveness, but with care, it can be done very successfully.

Creativity is essential when looking for palliative care team resources outside the hospital when a community-based team is not available. Certainly, area hospice and palliative care programs can be engaged in partnership with pediatric professionals to provide home-based care when available. Beyond existing community programs, providers can look for other professionals who are involved with the care of the child. These services may come from the county, school, religious community, or other private sources. Many children access county programs that provide social workers, physiotherapists, child development workers, counselors, and others involved in providing care for the child and family. Children on waiver or other support programs may have involved professionals who can be educated and trained in basic palliative care principles and practices. School-age children may be in close contact with the school nurse, counselor, social worker, and the teacher. With the permission of the parents, the palliative care provider or team can contact other caregivers, identified by the parents, and collaborate to enhance expert care within a palliative framework. County workers can help provide specific information from their disciplines, while teachers and counselors can assist adult hospice and palliative care providers to better understand the psychological needs of a child. School nurses can work with the team to ensure the child can attend school whenever possible. That may include working with the school to allow the school nurse to store the child's morphine in the office or facilitating discussion on how to handle Do Not Resuscitate orders. If the family belongs to a religious community, their spiritual care needs may be met; beyond this, it is essential to find out if the religious leaders should be part of the team. In some groups they may be instrumental in the healthcare decision-making process and should be included as part of the extended palliative care team. Throughout the process, care providers must be attuned to each aspect of the

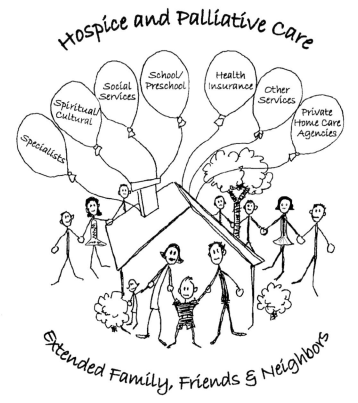

Fig. 16-2   A child's team.

child's and family's life so that this complex collaboration can be successful. It cannot be stressed enough that communication is essential to ensure everyone understands and supports the goals of care.

A basic understanding of palliative care concepts is essential for all team members. If this is not the case, then the plan of care can easily go wrong. Professionals who have always worked to cure or who are accustomed to practicing within a narrow discipline-based definition may need encouragement to focus on palliative care goals and the child's and parents' priorities. Consider the physiotherapist, whose goal for the child is to be in a stander for 1 hour three times a day; if the child is uncomfortable and progress is not the family's goal, then the therapist will need to adjust treatment goals to align with the family's goals for comfort. The child and family will benefit when every discipline understands the goals of care and works to align their plans to the overall palliative plan of care.

Palliative care staff can be instrumental in helping the extended team keep the focus on the family's stated goals of care. In one rural community where a child had very rapid disease progression and did not have any community services, the school played a major role in his care. The palliative home care nurse coordinated with the school nurse, teacher, and social worker who were eager to do what they could to help. The church community also stepped in to provide support. They worked with the rest of the child's expanded team to provide spiritual as well as practical support. The family practitioner provided medical oversight for symptom management, using the home-based expertise of the palliative care nurse in concert with phone support from the tertiary oncology center. The congregation provided help with yard work and extra attention for the siblings. This model of using community resources can work especially well for minority families who may not speak English or understand the dominant culture. Their cultural needs may be better served by collaborating with community members with whom the family most identifies.

Volunteers are an especially important part of the team for hospital- or community-based palliative care. They are an important link to the community and can extend the support that the team can provide. In addition to helping with office-based tasks, volunteers provide a number of services that others on the team cannot. This may include being the special friend for the sibling or reading a book to the child to provide a parent with time to take a nap. Careful screening, training, and follow-up are each key to ensure volunteers are prepared and supported in their work. There should be a professional contact person on the team as a point person for the volunteer to discuss questions and concerns. Clear guidelines of what their roles are in the home are essential for volunteers to maintain good boundaries.

Parents, as partners with the palliative care team, can play an important role. The child and family are the center of the unit of care, but are not truly members of the palliative care team (see Chapter 6). Nevertheless, parents and even patients themselves can and should play important roles. Mature patients, bereaved parents, or parents of chronically ill children, with appropriate training, can make excellent advisers to palliative care teams in terms of advocacy, clinical programming, and research initiatives. Parent and patient volunteers can take on team-based tasks such as assisting with bereavement outreach, memorial service planning, newsletter production and distribution, holiday or birthday and/or death day card writing. In addition, many hospitals and community agencies have mentor programs through which parents can be paired with others in similar circumstances to offer support and guidance. Resources such as the Institute for Family-Centered Care (www.familycenteredcare.org) provide excellent materials on training parent advocates to be effective members of the healthcare team.

Frameworks of Team Function and Dysfunction

The ways in which a palliative care team functions are influenced by a multitude of factors.

Based on purpose or mission, a team must have established goals or tasks and clearly defined objectives, and the strategies to achieve these, all of which need consensus and clarity.[5,25]

Interdisciplinary teams in particular need clearly defined internal and external role expectations. In practice, there is actually little congruence between the way a group of professionals defines its own roles and the way others define them.[27] Thus, because of the nature of the work, palliative care teams must delineate clear internal lines of responsibility and norms the unwritten rules governing the behavior of people in groups— before navigating the vague and changing environments in which they integrate.

Communication is perhaps the single most important factor in team success. Palliative care teams must establish defined communication patterns. At a minimum, this process should involve a clear definition of tasks and of responsibility and accountability for task completion.[25] Team members need accurate, common language for transmitting information and an agreed-upon philosophy of care, both of which incorporate mechanisms and capacity for team members to ascertain what others need to know to practice effectively.[4]

Other core concepts for functional teams include recognizing the specific personal contribution of every team member in their discipline, while respecting the same in others.[25] It is important to have a lack of hierarchy but a clear decision-making process. This allows for collaborative decision making while minimizing confusion about how things get decided. A culture that prioritizes autonomy, has realistic work expectations, and encourages high levels of personal feedback from colleagues as well as from patients and families[29] will strengthen the team. The successful team needs strong collaborative leadership that nurtures an atmosphere to cope with the specific challenges of palliative care. Factors particular to palliative care team success are procedures for evaluating effectiveness and quality of care, recognition of the contribution of patients in furthering professional understanding, and bereavement care of staff[25] (Box 16-2). Particularly in the challenging world of palliative care, team function and dysfunction come in many flavors and have been investigated by several authors. Some general observations about teams and categories of dysfunction in team based-care:

- Styles of decision making usually follow one of five patterns, in ascending order of functionality: default, unilateral, majority vote, consensus, or unanimity,[27]
- Types of intra-team conflict can generally be separated into conflicts around task or relationship,

BOX 16-2 Characteristics of Effective Palliative Care Teams

- The whole is greater than the sum of the individual component parts
- Interdependent—all members succeed or fail together
- Stimulating, and spurs individual members to greater achievement
- Fun—members enjoy a sense of belonging and camaraderie
- Civilized and structured: members blend individual aspirations into group objectives as they learn to share and interact. Roles are clearly defined.
- Demand a certain conformity, but not uniformity
- Members share their vulnerabilities as well as their strengths
- Difficult conversations are conducted face-to-face
- Deal with disagreement and anger in a constructive manner
- Work with existing healthcare teams without overstepping the advisory role
- Allow flexible professional roles
- Share difficult decisions
- Recognize that personal exchange can lead to professional growth
- Provide mechanisms for formal review to improve future performance

- Role stress is a frequent issue. New teams in particular face, three major role stressors: role ambiguity, role conflict, and role strain,[27,30]
- Poorly defined accountability is especially exemplified by poor performance feedback,[33]
- Lack of clear leadership designation,
- Poor or maladaptive communication, including underground communication or team secrets, which destroy trust and openness;[3,31] the gatekeeper phenomenon wherein a member who is not the team leader becomes the unofficial spokesperson for a subgroup of the team, withholding information or sharing information that may not reflect all opinions within the group,[32]
- Boundary violations may be rigid and/or blurred,
- Issues for long-standing or well-established teams in which there is resistance to change or new ideas,[3]
- A quasi-matrix system of authority, versus a traditional line model, where lines of authority are not clearly drawn and employees have more than one manager with specific areas of authority that are divided along professional or service lines,[33]
- Territoriality, usually stemming from lack of a common philosophy, language, and style among professions and services or from restricted contact among various busy professionals,[4]
- The formation of subgroups and alliances or other agendas distracting from the main mission, which may result in less connection to participation in what a service delivers or difficulty taking personal responsibility for the team's overall quality of care.[3]

EXAMINING TEAM HEALTH IN PEDIATRIC PALLIATIVE CARE

As is clear from the previous section, there are a multitude of frameworks in which to dissect the structure and function of interdisciplinary teams. In *The Five Dysfunctions of a Team*, Lencioni posits a helpful construct to discuss pediatric palliative care teams more specifically. Lencioni's five dysfunctions build on each other in pyramid fashion. An absence of trust, created from an unwillingness to be vulnerable, creates fear of conflict, which results in veiled discussions and guarded comments.

This environment generates lack of commitment, which progresses to avoidance of accountability resulting from lack of buy-in; and then to inattention to results, putting individual or divisional needs above those of the team. In contrast, truly cohesive teams trust one another, engage in unfiltered conflict, commit to decisions and action plans, hold each other accountable for delivering, and focus on the achievement of collective results.[34]

The costs of dysfunction in interdisciplinary teams can be extremely high. In addition to ineffectiveness and team member dissatisfaction, poorly functioning teams impact the patients and families we serve. Patient reactions to team dysfunction can lead to splitting or increased dependency on team members. For example, during the collective indecision phase of team development, patients and/or their families may ask multiple staff members the same questions and get different answers, leading to more anxiety. Even more significantly, patient or family lack of confidence in their care team may increase patient symptomatology.[27] Ultimately, of course, unnoticed or uncorrected dysfunction can lead to an implosion that results in the total dissolution of even the most well-intentioned group of like-minded people. Similar to what can be seen with individual patients and families, this so-called demoralization syndrome of teams stems initially from poor leadership and unreasonable burdens, and results in absenteeism, apathy, resistance to change, and deep sadness. Untreated, it progresses to a fatal loss of vision or loss of belief that objectives are worth striving for or even achievable.[25]

Viewed through the lens of Lencioni's model, the following sections of this chapter review five common pitfalls of team function in more detail that can deleteriously affect interdisciplinary pediatric palliative care teams.

Lack of Commitment

Although most, if not all, providers of palliative care likely maintain shared values and a common commitment to the cause, perceptions around appropriate goals and strategies for accomplishing such goals may vary widely. When team goals are undefined, care providers may be uncertain of their professional role or lack direction regarding their personal contribution to the team. Such ambiguity may thereby impair their sense of overall commitment to their team. Poorly defined goals are equally problematic. For example, a newly formed team in a pediatric hospital may identify the expansion of clinical services as a primary goal. Yet expansion can occur through various pathways. Should the team focus their limited resources on collaborating with a specific medical service such as neurology, which treats a large percentage of children with life-threatening conditions, or would resources be better spent working with the families of children admitted to the pediatric intensive care unit? Should financial resources be spent on a part-time nurse practitioner or a full-time clinical social worker? Without well-defined goals, individual members of the team may become frustrated with what they perceive as substandard care or limited progress of the program as a whole.

In contrast, clearly defined goals assist in orienting team members to the collective purpose. Similarly, the individual responsibilities of each care provider should be delineated in order to clarify personal role and obligation to the larger team. Sense of commitment is fostered when team members believe that duties have been appropriately distributed and that all members are working hard for the greater good. When roles are not adequately delineated, diffusion of responsibility becomes more likely. Team members may blame others for lack of progress, leading to hostility and ill will. Chronic unresolved conflict or dissatisfaction may lead to personal detachment or fractioning within the team.

In addition to clear, realistic, well-defined goals, commitment to supportive and collaborative relationships is equally important to healthy team functioning. As noted by Papadatou, "While team goals orient our actions, supportive and collaborative relationships help us to achieve them."[35] In fact, the two may be considered interdependent as the more supported we are by team members, the more likely we are to commit ourselves to work tasks and to the development of compassionate relationships. Thus committed care providers are dedicated to meaningful goals, rely upon each other in order to achieve them, and are mutually supported through the process. Four specific aspects of support that we seek and expect to receive from colleagues are informational support, instrumental support, emotional support, and support in meaning construction (Table 16-1). Each team values and encourages different aspects of support at different times. For mutual support to be effective, it must be timely and responsive to the specific needs and preferences of care providers, which vary from one team to another and at different times under different circumstances. Team functioning may be compromised when such support is unavailable or unresponsive to the needs of team members.

For example, care providers who are committed only to their own work tasks in their effort to demonstrate their own competency may fail to value or develop genuine interest in other team members. Relationships may even be experienced as competitive or conflicted. Although such care providers may offer sufficient informational support, they may be unable

to accept or supply emotional support to other team members when in need. If a mismatch exists between individual members and the team as a whole around areas of support that are highly regarded or considered essential, then team functioning may be negatively affected.

Other teams may be disrupted by limited instrumental support, such as when scarce financial resources require disparate allocation of job funding across individual team members. In such situations, team members may have similar task expectations yet are not equally compensated for the time provided to complete such tasks. Those individuals who receive less compensation for their time may be perceived as less committed to the team if they are less available to participate in activities or provide service to the team. Other times, disproportionate financial support may lead less-compensated team members to feel underappreciated or undervalued and, therefore, to feel less committed to the team as a whole.

Meaning-making support can be especially vital to palliative care teams and the absence of such support may degrade an individual's commitment to providing care. For example, while offering bereavement services to a parent whose child had recently died, the team nurse practitioner felt especially burdened by the mother's doubt around her decision to forgo a second stem cell transplant for her child. The mother had declined further curative efforts in order to allow the child more comfort yet, in the end, the child's last days were spent in an inordinate amount of pain and suffering. Upon reflection, the nurse practitioner worried that she had unwittingly influenced the mother to make the wrong decision. However, a later discussion with a fellow team member served to remind her that the mother's questioning was a normative feature of the grieving process. Without the opportunity to reframe her experience, the nurse practitioner may have been burdened by cognitive distortions that could negatively affect her commitment to working with other families.

Avoidance of Accountability and Conflict

Every PPC team needs to have a foundation of trust and openness among its members, wherein individuals can express their vulnerability with each other, disagree openly and remain respectful of one another. It is no surprise that team members who trust each other function effectively together to achieve their goals. This does not mean that they always agree with each other, but rather that there exists a basis of respect and openness that allows for expression of different views. Healthy discussion and effective resolution of conflict will enhance the level of trust and communication within the team.[34]

Although this sounds simple, it demands an ongoing commitment of time and energy by each team member and the team as a whole to ensure this process. Often people may not want to take the time to work on team building, given the intensity and the needs of the children and families we serve. Frustrated team members may think or actually say, "This work is hard enough without having to deal with my team members' dysfunction!" Unless individual team members deal directly with these issues and are open enough to accept responsibility for part of the dysfunction, they will be doing a disservice to the children and families they most want to help. If the team is not built on a solid foundation of trust and openness, it cannot serve those who need it most.

Few if any palliative care team members choose conflict over collaboration, yet conflict is a given part of the life of

TABLE 16-1 Types of Support

Informational support	Involves the exchange of information about the people served and the team's mode of operation; it comprises mutual feedback about and evaluation of individual or team performance with opportunities to expand one's knowledge and skills.
Instrumental support	Involves helping each other with practical issues such as sharing the workload, and the coordination of efforts toward the achievement of specific tasks. Shared goals, role clarity, and trust in each other's knowledge and skills enhance this form of support.
Emotional support	Involves opportunities for sharing personal feelings and thoughts in a safe environment in which one feels heard, understood, valued, and appreciated. Sometimes the presence of another colleague during stressful moments is all that is needed.
Support in meaning construction	Involves opportunities to reflect on and work through work-related experiences and invest individual and collective efforts with meaning. Care providers help each other understand their responses, correct distortions, and reframe situations in ways that make sense to them.

Adapted from Papadatou D. *In the face of death: professionals who care for the dying and bereaved.* New York, 2009, Springer Publishing.

any team. However, the way in which the conflict is handled between individuals and within the team can either strengthen or damage the whole group. Not uncommonly, in a misguided effort to be collaborative, the actual heart of the conflict may not be discussed and the source never identified or verbalized. When this occurs, people often become frustrated as they desperately try but fail to communicate without dealing with the conflict.[34] This is the proverbial elephant in the room that palliative care clinicians are so skilled at helping families face. Under the guidance of strong leadership, teams must draw upon their individual and collective skills in this area in order to address difficult issues in conflict resolution. Some helpful interventions are focusing on learning more about others' perspectives and using language that is open and less blaming. These strategies, explored in more detail later in this chapter, will go a long way in improving the functioning of team as a whole.[34]

As a practical example, one large team that did not have a strong foundation of trust addressed this issue by making a commitment to address every conflict within 24 hours of occurrence in a direct, private and personal way. This was a tough choice as it was a change from the norm, but the team as a whole agreed to it. The decision resulted in many private face-to-face meetings of team members as they worked to address issues head on. For most team members it was an uncomfortable and difficult task. Yet, it resulted in an overall reduction of underground discord and improved team functioning. Importantly, the team also needed to revisit this process periodically, as conflict resolution is not a one-time accomplishment but rather an ongoing process.

Practical applications of conflict resolution, encouragement of open and respectful debate, and using collaborative communication are important aspects in developing and maintaining an effective team.[36] A well-functioning team should be able to discuss disagreements openly and accept that there are often different ways to solve a problem. This environment allows individuals to be accountable for their mistakes, to avoid shame or punishment, and to use these situations as learning experiences for the team as a whole. An attitude of open discussion when things do not go well should be encouraged and supported both in word and deed. In one team interaction a clinician was offended by what was meant as an innocent action by another team member. She addressed this directly in the weekly interdisciplinary team meeting, and both clinicians shared their view of what had happened. Because this was not the way the team had operated previously, the process was somewhat uncomfortable for the individuals and the team as a whole. However, it was a growth experience for all. It did resolve the issue, and provided an example of how conflicts can be dealt with in a healthy way.

Boundary Issues and Role Blurring

A poorly functioning team without a strong foundation of trust can precipitate blurring of professional boundaries. Staff may overextend themselves to compensate for the perceived lack in other team members' abilities. People who provide palliative care for children and their families generally do this work because they find it fulfilling and enjoy working with children. They are personally interested in each child and family and strive to relieve suffering and provide support for families facing their child's death. This wonderful motivation can easily mutate to overextension of personnel, blurring of boundaries,

and eventual burnout when there is a lack of trust in the team. One clinician was working with a family much like her own; they shared interests and backgrounds, and had connected immediately. The family met with the clinician frequently and found the time extremely helpful. They told her they felt she was part of the family and they felt deeply connected to her. As the child's death came closer the family asked her to be personally available to them over a long weekend. Feeling appreciated and needed, she agreed and provided the family with her pager number, telling them to call any time. She believed this was the best solution, given her conviction that the weekend people were not as skilled in palliative care. Unfortunately, the child died suddenly on Saturday afternoon when the clinician was swimming and did not have her pager with her. The family tried desperately and unsuccessfully to reach her. Eventually they called the 24-hour emergency number, but the delay caused unnecessary distress for the family. This sad situation was the result of a team member trying to meet the perceived needs of the family by herself and demonstrating a fundamental lack of trust in her team. While this twofold problem is an easy trap to fall into, it is also one that can be avoided. The danger is greatly reduced by ensuring open communication and increasing the trust level among team members. Team members can help each other maintain good boundaries, as the fine line of professional boundaries can blur so easily. It is always essential to come back to the basic concept that palliative care is provided by a team, not just one individual.

Blurring of boundaries happens between clinical care providers and families, but also between providers. As mentioned earlier, the transdisciplinary model of palliative care is generating a growing interest and following. Although it has great benefits, it must be remembered that every discipline brings a unique dimension to the team, and specific roles must be respected. So when a social worker suggests a bowel medication to use, or a nurse starts to extend her role as a social worker beyond in-the-moment crisis management, other team members need to step in gently and rebalance the team roles as they should be.

Inattention to Results

Inattention to results is another potential risk for team dysfunction. Team members often rely upon subjective and unreliable means to assess the success of their program. As a result, various team members may have conflicting perceptions of the strengths of the program as well as areas in need of further development. For example, one team member who experiences a positive encounter with a family may perceive the program to be very successful, generalizing personal feelings about that one particular case to the effectiveness of the program as a whole. In contrast, another team member may conclude that the team is ineffective based upon opinions of others outside of the team, such as a comment made by a hospital staff member that "The palliative care team is never available when needed."

Conflict may also arise when team members have agreed to a broad goal such as "improving palliative care" without specifying the ways in which outcomes will be measured. Thus, despite the implementation of several initiatives and education of nursing and house staff, availability of various medical services and outreach to community providers, and enhancing clinical services already being provided, the effectiveness is equivocal without objective outcome measures. Such ambiguity can set the stage for burnout among team members when, despite significant time and energy, it is unclear whether their efforts have resulted in expected achievements. Furthermore, without evidence of positive outcomes, the team may fail to receive much deserved recognition from administrative figures who support the program financially and organizationally.

Team Identification with Patient Population

One potential consequence of the pitfalls is an observed but understudied phenomenon in healthcare teams of all types: the gradual, insidious shaping of a team to take on the issues or dysfunctions of the population it serves. This entity can be seen as an extreme example of role blurring, wherein the team's boundary as a whole becomes porous. Teams with a poor sense of group identity and cohesive organization around mission—lack of commitment stemming either from multidisciplinary practice on the one hand or too-amorphous interdisciplinary on the other—are more vulnerable to splitting behaviors that are usually unintentionally undertaken by patients and/or families who are searching for some type of stable mooring in an unsettling journey.

Consider a palliative care team caring for a child whose single parent has a long, untreated history of psychiatric impairment. Suppose this team has well-intentioned but unskilled leadership that creates gatekeepers and permits underground alliances. In this model, an individual accustomed to manipulating the environment is able to take advantage of team member alliances and vulnerabilities, such that communication and goal-directed treatment planning breaks down. It's not hard to see that over time, this dedicated team could come to resemble a dysfunctional family in which clients are unintentionally enabled and therapeutic outcomes are derailed.

As another example, consider a pediatric oncology team composed of multiple disciplines including child life, social work, pharmacy, chaplaincy, dietetics, and data management personnel. Here too, hierarchical and/or disorganized leadership that detracts from a team-based mission to improve comprehensive care can result, almost literally, in a cancerous team. Mistrust, lack of self-care in the ongoing practice of caring for children with a devastating illness, boundary issues, and a multitude of other problems can create situations in which passive-aggressive behavior spreads like a metastatic disease, wreaking havoc and eventually destruction among a group of professionals originally united around a common cause or enemy. The group may lose its therapeutic efficacy—a consequence that families are readily able to detect.

What is the relevance to pediatric palliative care? The very nature of our work necessitates a high level of attention to team dynamics and self-care of its members and the team as a whole. Every interdisciplinary pediatric palliative care team has, at some point, engaged with families or providers and/or referral sources who challenge the integrity of the team. Without careful housekeeping, pediatric palliative care teams can degenerate into ineffective multidisciplinary groups of individuals practicing from silos. The reason for the palliative care team becomes lost: care for children with life-threatening conditions and their families once again becomes fragmented, punctuated by crisis-driven interventions or decisions. The end result is that families shoulder the burdens of being in charge of navigating their child's journey through the healthcare system. Care returns to the very state from which the need for pediatric palliative care was born—only worse because of the lost promise of a better way.

SOLUTIONS AND TAKE-HOME MESSAGES

Fortunately, the picture is not one of inevitable failure. In fact, with attention to the issues, strong leadership, training, and a few key tactics, dysfunctional outcomes can be avoided relatively easily. Based on the discussions herein, a number of practical strategies can be outlined for team members and leaders to employ to create healthy and sustainable teams while avoiding the pitfalls that sink many well-meaning teams and organizations. Box 16-3 contains a list of some of the key points from this chapter to provide direction for pediatric palliative care teams.

Team Self-Care Plans

Pediatric palliative care team members work hard to develop and implement excellent, individualized, child-centered care plans. However, rarely if ever do they spend time working on care plans for themselves. Pediatric palliative care can exact a heavy toll on professionals.[37] Self-care plans are a formal way to examine how individuals can help themselves

---

BOX 16-3   Creating Healthy PPC Teams

- Keep staff meetings and interdisciplinary team meetings separate; staff meeting business should not interfere with the workings of the interdisciplinary team around patient and/or family care.
- Cultivate time, space, and patience: More disciplines and more people on a team both increase the need for role definition and mean more time and space will be needed for collaboration. Consider creating opportunities for team members to cross-train to understand each other's contributions.
- Establish clear policies and processes that value and support teamwork, including open discussion of contentious issues with reinforcement of boundaries.[33,38]
- Provide education on interpersonal team member communication, cultural norms, patterns of accountability, roles, processes and guidelines, and patterns of referral.[26]
- Undertake regular evaluation of psychological factors that impact team effectiveness, such as positive attitude toward interdisciplinary teamwork, including bringing in outside help for team rebuilding or re-examination of foundations.[26,39]
- Create a team covenant—a set of core principles agreed upon and signed by each team member that outlines shared ideals and procedures for resolution of disagreements—to facilitate development of trust, respect, understanding, and communication. Key message of the covenant: To be on this team requires the willingness to be vulnerable and transparent; personal agendas and turf issues must be replaced by openness, blending of roles, and nonjudgmental attitudes respecting the culture of each discipline on the team.[40]
- Establish and practice conflict resolution strategies within teams.
- Focus on creation of a team environment of optimistic approach, personal recognition, feedback, humor, informal exchange of ideas, subjective perceptions, anecdotes, openness, flexibility, empathy, egalitarianism, and mutual support.[13] Supportive behavior fosters sharing of information and group learning, which increases potency and impact perceived by members. It also empowers team members.[28]
- Perform repeated assessments and ongoing maintenance as teams are dynamic, including putting procedures in place for evaluating effectiveness and quality of team efforts.
- Design, enact, and revisit strategies for the care and feeding of the team with team self-care plans.

maintain healthy lives while working so closely with loss and sadness. The concept of the self-care plan is not new, yet its formal development and practical use are recent. When carefully developed, these documents can promote and sustain highly successful teams.

As a practical example, one large pediatric palliative care and hospice team asked members to develop their own self-care plans. These were detailed, private documents that served to remind members of how they were planning to care for themselves and how they would manage both distressing events and routine day-to-day events that increase stress. Although this was an informal and private exercise, it is important to address the issue holistically and to delineate some structure. Therefore the inclusion of physical, emotional, psychosocial, and spiritual domains is essential, as it is in all of palliative care.

For some staff members, the physical included very strenuous workouts such as running while for others it included a quiet walk in the woods. Emotional focus was addressed equally diversely, with some staff using journals to express emotions, and others identifying one or more team members who would provide support when needed. The psychosocial focus is especially important in this line of work; team members must be mindful to ensure that their social life either extends beyond or is separate from work. Team members identified activities such as bike rides, trips to an art museum, cooking, or roller coaster rides in their self-care plans. An important component is that team members enjoy themselves and have fun. However one describes it, fun is essential to maintaining balance in this work.

The fourth area of focus in the self-care plans was spirituality, which must be carefully distinguished from organized religion. For some people, this domain takes the shape of a particular faith, which can be a strong source of support and guidance. For others, enjoying quiet time or time to experience nature results in a sense of spiritual renewal. Team members need to recognize and care for their own spiritual needs in an individualized way.

As with the Team Covenant, team members who see others providing care in a difficult situation, or experiencing a particularly stressful period, can remind one another to revisit their own self-care plans.

Summary

As with many core concepts in pediatric palliative care, teamwork is not usually formally taught. Instead, most clinical teams learn these important skills by trial and error or by example, some good, some less than ideal. However, much more knowledge and training is available to guide the creation of unified, healthy, high-quality, effective and empowered interdisciplinary pediatric palliative care teams. "Providing team-based palliative care needs to be more than a set of assumptions about how teams can operate. … We need to move beyond the assumption that teams will operate effectively and toward a position that looks at their critical operation."[26] To place the primary focus of teamwork where it most belongs, team leaders and members would do well to remember that teams will form and reform "and change like the patterns in a kaleidoscope in the changing scenarios in healthcare systems—but what unifies the whole enterprise is the patient whose story is the common thread."[25]

Clinical Vignette

As like-minded individuals, palliative care team members often work together in a fluid, unencumbered process. However, in the pursuit of a so-called good death, disagreements can surface that lead to greater team conflict without open communication and respect for the personal and professional contributions of other team members.

Vanessa, 17, was a Hispanic female with a complicated medical history, including systemic lupus erythematosus and end-stage renal disease secondary to lupus nephritis; she had been dialysis-dependent for several years. Her illness had been well controlled over the past year, and she and her family were hopeful that she would receive a kidney transplant. After suffering new onset of chest pain, Vanessa was admitted to the hospital for pancreatitis. Approximately 2 weeks after her admission, she suffered a cardiac arrest due to severe retroperitoneal hemorrhage. She was temporarily stabilized but returned to the pediatric intensive care unit for closer monitoring after she developed fevers and lower blood pressures. A large pancreatic hematoma was identified. However, due to her hemodynamic instability, she was not considered a suitable surgical candidate. Surgical drains were placed in the hematoma but provided little fluid output. Lab results confirmed sepsis, which was unresponsive to broad-spectrum antibiotics.

Vanessa's family was devoutly religious and perceived this hospitalization as another test that they must endure. Vanessa had survived many near-death experiences in the past and her family strongly believed that with faith and prayer, she would pull through this episode as well. They asserted that they knew that miracles were possible and that only God could determine when her life would end. In the face of her family's wishes, the primary service continued to provide daily hemodialysis and life-sustaining medical interventions. However, as her condition continued to decline, the medical team and social worker requested the palliative care team review medical decision making with the family in the context of Vanessa's quality of life.

The palliative care team, which included a pediatric intensivist, a pain management specialist, and a psychologist, met with Vanessa and her family and separately with the medical team. Yet, at the conclusion of the initial consult, the team members had very disparate opinions regarding their goals in working with this family. The physicians, with the medical foresight to recognize that survival was extremely unlikely, believed that quality of life should be emphasized with the family and that comfort measures should be encouraged. Further, as treating clinicians, they felt burdened by the suffering caused by the treatments they were providing to prolong Vanessa's life. The psychologist believed that the family's wishes should be supported despite Vanessa's poor prognosis. Vanessa had deferred medical decisions to her parents, and the psychologist believed that the parents deserved to feel supported in their choices, as they would reflect upon them for years after her death.

Because they feared that the family would likely receive mixed messages, the palliative care team scheduled a meeting to discuss the case. Through their discussion, the intensivist was able to share that he believed he was doing harm in the process of providing care that was no longer beneficial. The pain and suffering caused by the medical interventions also challenged the pain specialist's sense of commitment and responsibility as a physician. The psychologist was also able to explain her own perspective: the family had only their experiences with Vanessa on which to base their decisions, in contrast to the physicians who had the experience of dozens of patients who had suffered a similar course of disease. As such, the physicians were able to interpret signs that were less obvious or meaningful to Vanessa's family. The psychologist also cautioned them against challenging a very strong faith upon which the family would continue to depend as they grieved the death of their daughter.

Although this meeting did not yield clear goals or unanimous opinions regarding the appropriate treatment course, the discussion allowed the members to more fully appreciate the others' perspectives and enabled each of them to have a bit more patience to allow the natural process to unfold. Despite their differing opinions, the members were mindful about presenting themselves to the family as a cohesive, unified team. They were also dedicated to interacting with the family in a way that would be experienced as supportive rather than confrontational. Through open-ended conversations, the team encouraged the family to share their thoughts, fears, and wishes, and in doing so, the family became more receptive to additional considerations presented by the team.

Within a few days, Vanessa's sepsis had progressed and her parents, although still hopeful for a miracle, acknowledged that God would not wish for their daughter to suffer. In her last days of life, she was made comfortable with opioids and benzodiazepines, and her epinephrine drip was gradually weaned off to allow for a natural death. The palliative care team remained involved with the family throughout this process and offered bereavement services to them following Vanessa's death.

REFERENCES

1. Tuckman B: Developmental sequence in small groups, *Psychol Bulletin* 63(6):384–399, 1965.
2. Lee S: Interdisciplinary teaming in primary care: a process of evolution and resolution, *Soc Work Health Care* 5(3):237–244, 1980.
3. Crawford GB, Price SD: Team working: palliative care as a model of interdisciplinary practice, *MJA* 179:S32–S34, 2003.
4. Street A, Blackford J: Communication issues for the interdisciplinary community palliative care team.
5. Rubin I, Beckhard R: Factors influencing the effectiveness of health teams, *Milbank Mem Fund Q Health Soc* 50(3):317–335, 1972.
6. Bronstein LR: A model for interdisciplinary collaboration, *Soc Work* 48(3):297–306, 2003.
7. Wittenberg-Lyles EM, Oliver DP, Demiris G, Courtney KL: Assessing the nature and process of hospice interdisciplinary team meetings, *J Hospice Palliat Nurs* 9(1):17–21, 2007.
8. Cummings I: The interdisciplinary team. In Doyle D, Hanks GW, MacDonald N, editors: *Oxford textbook of palliative medicine*, Oxford, 1998, Oxford University Press.
9. Arber A: Team meetings in specialist palliative care: asking questions as a strategy within interprofessional interaction, *Qual Health Res* 18(10):1323–1335, 2008.
10. Oliver DP, Wittenberg-Lyles EM, Day M: Variances in perceptions of interdisciplinary collaboration by hospice staff, *J Palliat Care* 22(4):275–280, 2006.
11. HCFA: *Medicare Program Hospice Care: Final Rule*, Health Care Financing Administration, Agency for Health Policy Research, 1983.
12. Bronstein LR: Index of interdisciplinary collaboration, *Soc Work Res* 26(2):113–126, 2002.
13. Junger S, Pestinger M, Elsner F, et al: Criteria for successful multiprofessional cooperation in palliative care teams, *Palliat Med* 21:347–354, 2007.
14. Parker GM: *Cross-functional teams: working with allies, enemies and other strangers*, San Francisco, 1994, Jossey-Bass Publishers.
15. Hyland P, Davison G, Sloan T: Linking team competencies to organizational capacities in health care, *J Health Organ Manag* 17(3):150–163, 2003.
16. Kemp KA: The use of interdisciplinary medical teams to improve quality and access to care, *J Interprof Care* 21(5):557–559, 2007.
17. Dyeson TB: The home health care team: what can we learn from the hospice experience? *Home Health Care Manage Pract* 17:125–127, 2005.
18. Reese DJ, Raymer TB: Relationships between social work involvement and hospice outcomes: results of the National Hospice Social Work Survey, *Soc Work* 49:415–422, 2004.
19. Opie A: Nobody's asked me for my view: users' empowerment by multidisciplinary health teams, *Qual Health Res* 8(2):188–206, 1998.
20. Jack B, Hillier V, Williams A, Oldham J: Hospital-based palliative care teams improve the symptoms of cancer patients, *J Palliat Med* 17(6):498–502, 2003.
21. Higginson IJ, Finlay IG, Goodwin DM, et al: Is there evidence that palliative care teams alter end-of-life experiences of patients and their caregivers? *J Pain Symptom Manage* 25(2):150–168, 2003.
22. Schrader SL, Horner A, Eidsness L, et al: A team approach in palliative care: enhancing outcomes, *S D J Med* 55(7):269–278, 2002.
23. Jack B, Hillier V, Williams A, Oldham J: Hospital-based palliative care teams improve the insight of cancer patients into their disease, *J Palliat Med* 18(1):46–52, 2004.
24. Cott C: Structure and meaning in multidisciplinary teamwork, *Sociol Health Illn* 20(6):848–873, 1998.
25. Lickiss JN, Turner KS, Pollock ML: The interdisciplinary team. In Doyle D, Hanks G, Cherny N, Calman K, editors: *Oxford textbook of palliative medicine*, ed 3, Oxford, 2004, Oxford University Press, pp 42–46.
26. O'Connor M, Fisher C, Guilfoyle A: Interdisciplinary teams in palliative care: a critical reflection, *Int J Palliat Nurs* 12(3):132–137, 2006.
27. Lowe JI, Herranen M: Conflict in teamwork: understanding roles and relationships, *Soc Work Health Care* 3(3):323–330, 1978.
28. Proenca EJ: Team dynamics and team empowerment in health care organizations, *Health Care Manage Rev* 32(4):370–378, 2007.
29. Graham J, Ramirez AJ, Cull A, et al: Job stress and satisfaction among palliative physicians, *Palliat Med* 10:185–194, 1996.
30. Vachon ML: Staff stress in hospice/palliative care: a review, *Palliat Med* 9(2):91–122, 1995.
31. Larson D: *The helper's journey: working with people facing grief, loss and life-threatening illness*, Champaign Ill, 2003, Research Press.
32. Bowen M: *Family therapy in clinical practice*, New York, 1978, Jason Aronson.
33. Butterill D, O'Hanlon J, Book H: When the system is the problem, don't blame the patient: problems inherent in the interdisciplinary inpatient team, *Can J Psychiatry* 37:168–172, 1992.
34. Lencioni PM: *The five dysfunctions of a team*, San Francisco, 2002, Jossey-Bass.
35. Papadatou D: *In the face of death: professionals who care for the dying and bereaved*, New York, 2009, Springer Publishing.
36. Feudtner C: Collaborative communication in pediatric palliative care: a foundation for problem-solving and decision-making, *Pediatr Clin North Am* 54:587–607, 2007.
37. Sourkes B, Frankel L, Brown M, et al: Food, toys and love: pediatric palliative care, *Curr Probl Pediatr Adolesc Health Care* 35(9):357, 2005.
38. Baggs JG, Norton SA, Schmitt MH, Seller CR: The dying patient in the ICU: role of the interdisciplinary team, *J Crit Care Clinics* 20:525–540, 2004.
39. Cohen L, O'Connor M, Blackmore AM: Nurses' attitudes towards palliative care in nursing homes in Western Australia, *Int J Palliat Nurs* 8(2):610–620, 2002.
40. Head B: The blessings and burdens of interdisciplinary teamwork, *Home Healthc Nurse* 20(5):337–338, 2002.

17 Relationships with the Community: Palliative Care and Beyond

DAVID M. STEINHORN | RICHARD GOLDSTEIN | STACY F. ORLOFF

This chapter is intended to provide the reader new to pediatric palliative care with an understanding of how to create an optimal environment for children and their families. For the experienced reader, this chapter provides an integrated, holistic perspective based upon the authors' experiences in several pediatric palliative care settings and, in doing so, offer new refinements and insights. The ultimate goal is to create the concept of seamless care, which assures that the child remains the central focus of continuous care independent of the setting in which it is provided.

Ben, 7, was in first grade when his general pediatrician determined that his knee pain was caused by leukemia. During his hospitalizations, he and his family developed relationships with hospital nurses, child life specialists, and social workers. Home nursing support became a regular part of their lives when he was discharged. The oncology team and his oncologist have been very involved, through induction chemotherapy, its failure, bone marrow transplant and its unfortunate failure. His teachers and schoolmates have stayed in touch throughout, wondering whether he would return to school. The general pediatrician has stayed involved and been an important resource for the family. Now the family is struggling with end of life and how it would best be for Ben. They are trying to understand hospice and what they will need to find it a secure option. Throughout it all, his family, his school, and his church community have grappled with his issues and how to support Ben, his brother, and his parents. While grateful, the family will sometimes lament how much energy it takes to keep it all straight.

Children don't live in a vacuum. Although children with life-threatening illnesses may feel isolated during the course of their treatment, they rarely live isolated lives. They have profound and defining relationships with family, friends, and community. They are connected to many different people and organizations such as schools, their community, pediatrician, pharmacies, durable medical equipment providers, hospice, the hospital, emergency responders, and service and faith-based groups. Their illness impacts all of these relationships. Excellent palliative care will include attention to them all, and perhaps some others.

For the pediatric palliative care team, finding effective means of incorporating the various relationships into a child's life is one of the greatest challenges. Failure to effectively do so creates the potential to increase the suffering and distress associated with the child's illness and death. As the World Health Organization emphasizes, a "broad multidisciplinary approach and one that includes the family and makes use of available community resources"[1] is central to the mission of pediatric palliative care. Palliative care providers must find ways to bridge the gap between the child's and family's needs for continuity and connection within their community of relationships and the larger context of multiple healthcare agencies and individuals providing palliative care. A fragmented approach to healthcare that does not connect the dots among the hospital, home, school, community healthcare providers, and other peer support groups can have a troubling negative impact on the lives of a child and his or her family.

Palliative and hospice medicine embodies a philosophy of care that is independent of the specific disease process or location of care delivery. It aims "to improve the quality of life of patients and their families facing life-threatening illness, through the prevention, assessment, and treatment of pain and other physical, psychosocial, and spiritual problems."[2] Providing palliative care for children who have life-limiting conditions is inseparable from all other aspects of their care and potentially impacts all of the relationships in their lives. Through its multidisciplinary composition, the palliative care team is ideally positioned to assist in optimizing the experience of patients and their families with the care provided in four domains (see Table 17-1). These domains broadly reflect the range of distinct care locations. The relationships in each must ideally be addressed from the perspective of the entirety of the child's care and life. This chapter will address the challenges of integrating palliative care into the various domains of a child's life and highlights its role in coordinating care across various domains.[3]

Palliative Care and the Community

One obstacle to the integration of palliative care into overall patient care stems from a limited understanding by many healthcare providers of its place and role. The field has come to be defined for children over the last 20 years through the efforts of leaders worldwide, culminating in important guidelines promulgated by the American Academy of Pediatrics and the Institute of Medicine regarding the importance of such care.[4,5] Such public statements have provided important guidance for the creation of palliative care services in many medical centers and some community-based hospice organizations and have spawned legislative efforts to improve reimbursement for palliative care separate from the existing hospice coverage. A set of best practice standards in pediatric palliative care promotes:

- Involving the PPC team as soon after determination of a disease with a grave prognosis is possible,
- Striving for meticulous symptom management,
- Addressing multiple sources of discomfort and suffering,
- Attempting curative therapy while focusing on optimal quality of life,

TABLE 17-1   Domains in Which Palliative Care May Be Provided

Location of care	Focus of pediatric palliative care team
Hospital-based medical care	Work collaboratively with primary medical team; assist, advise, advocate; help family explore options
Home-based care	Maintain contact with patient after discharge; liaison between hospital and home; sounding board for family, patient
Community-based medical care	Coordinate discharge to home; maintain contact to remain up to date on care needs at home and change in health status; support primary care provider
Community-based organizations	Liaison to school, religious organization, service organizations, clubs, sports teams

- Maintaining relationships and authority with primary care and subspecialty providers whenever possible,
- Providing care at home, school, and in the community,
- Providing family-supportive therapy to maintain integrity of family,
- Providing care as long as the child requires,
- Providing bereavement care.

The tasks associated with creating a palliative care plan for any child must be individualized and involve several interrelated areas.[6,7] They require identifying problems and obstacles, creating a set of interventions that improve quality of life, and solving logistical issues to permit care in the most appropriate setting. Using these points as a framework, a paradigm for integrating palliative care into overall patient care can be developed by the palliative care team working in close collaboration with the family and primary medical service.

The roles the palliative care team plays vary at different points throughout the illness.[8-11] It is important to remember that the disease process itself will ultimately determine which options are available at any point in the trajectory of an illness. As the disease progresses, certain options will no longer be possible yet the palliative care team can help the family in choosing from the remaining options, based upon their values and goals (Table 17-2).

The hospital-based palliative care team has an important role in creating a bridge to the community-based palliative care service. Frequently, the hospital-based team has the best feel for which community-based organizations in the child's home region have the proper resources such as a pediatric nurse or child life services to meet the patient's needs. Case management personnel and discharge planners can have a limited understanding of the needs of children being referred for home palliative care. Some discharge planners may be called upon infrequently to arrange a palliative care discharge. In contrast, the palliative care team may be involved in many more discharges each year to home care. Team members typically know the range of resources available in the child's community as well as how to expedite discharge or transfer closer to home when urgent situations arise.

This situation works well when the distances between a patient's home and the hospital is not too great and there is a well-defined collaborative relationship between the hospital- and home-based care providers. However, in many regions, the situation is very complex. For example, in metropolitan Chicago, there are more than eight hospitals providing tertiary pediatric care throughout the extended greater metropolitan area, covering eight counties and a population of 9.5 million. Hospice nurses may drive as much as 60 miles for one home visit. Within that large area, there are only six hospice organizations that have pediatric nurses who can provide home hospice and palliative care. No single community-based organization covers the entire area. Furthermore, the patients referred to any of the tertiary care centers may come from an equally long distance based upon the availability of special services or patterns of patient referral developed by each hospital's administrators. In other cities, such as Cleveland, Ohio, a single, well-established hospice

TABLE 17-2   Varying Roles of Palliative Care Team Throughout the Trajectory of Illness

Early	Middle	Late
Supportive and Anticipatory Care	Coordinating Interdisciplinary Care	Co-Management with First-Degree Caregivers
Early introduction of palliative care to family, optimizing child's life during an illness with an uncertain outcome	Longitudinal contact with family	Cure highly unlikely. Palliative care team takes more leading role in partnership with primary team
Consultation requested for in- or out-patient	Team visits in home or hospital	Support family decisions
Determine team's expectations	Frequent reassessment of goals in light of changing disease status	Complete end-of-life planning, including memory making, DNR status, desired location of death, funeral plans, and bereavement photography
Ascertain family's values and/or goals	Offers non-judgmental support	
Supportive role assuring attention to symptom management and quality of life	Offers ongoing family support	Immediate availability for difficult end-of-life symptom management
Consider referral to home palliative care agency	Discussion of options if disease progresses, the disease status determines the possible options	Attend death, when desired and/or needed
Anticipate needs for support of siblings and extended family	Optimize quality of life and symptom management	Consider autopsy follow-up
	Begin DNR and end-of-life planning	Provide bereavement service

Liben S, Papadatou D. et al. Paediatric palliative care: challenges and emerging ideas. *Lancet* 371(9615): 852-864, 2008.
Löfmark R, Nilstun T, et al. From cure to palliation: concept, decision and acceptance. *J Med Ethics* 33: 685-688, 2007.
Baker J N, Hinds PS, et al. Integration of palliative care practices into the ongoing care of children with cancer: individualized care planning and coordination. *Pediatr Clin North Am* 55(1): 223-250, xii. 2008.
Penson R, Partridge R, et al. Fear of death. *The Oncologist* 10: 160-169, 2005.
Heaston S, Beckstrand R, et al. Emergency nurses' perceptions of obstacles and supportive behaviors in end-of-life care. *J Emerg Nurs* 32: 477-485, 2006.
Levetown M, and Committee on Bioethics. Communicating with children and families: from everyday interactions to skill in conveying distressing information. *Pediatrics* 121(5): e1441-1460. 2008.

organization is able to provide pediatric care through satellite offices covering the entire metropolitan area. At the opposite end of the spectrum are areas where families live in very sparsely populated areas served only by adult hospice organizations (Table 17-3).

The care provided for the child and the support available to the family should ideally be the same regardless of where care is delivered. Because each palliative care family and child will inevitably face difficult and painful decisions, it is incumbent upon the healthcare system to provide an optimal environment for children on their palliative care journey. This care can only be provided by a cooperative, collaborative relationship between all care providers in a community. Because there is limited economic advantage to be gained in most medical markets by increasing market share in pediatric palliative care, a non-competitive relationship between providers in the community will ensure consistent standards of care and optimize the availability of resources for children. In addition, coalitions are beginning to develop in the United States that will create region-wide standards of care for pediatric palliative care and assure quality oversight in a non-competitive environment. The Greater Illinois Pediatric Palliative Care Coalition is one such evolving organization. It is highly likely that such region-wide coalitions will be able to more effectively leverage community philanthropy than individual organizations can, which will lead to greater ability of such coalitions to develop and expand shared services such as child life and music therapists.

At the other extreme are the rural families who depend upon adult hospices to help fill the gaps in care for their child at home. It has been a challenge at times to develop collaborative arrangements with the medical teams in adult hospices that are asked to care for children. A lack of nurses who have both pediatric assessment skills and comfort dealing with dying children makes it critically important for the palliative care team to maintain communication with the rural organization regarding symptom management, changes in the child's health status, and suggestions for psychosocial support for siblings and extended family. Attempts in Australia to employ videotelephony to remotely manage patients have met with mixed success, although the approach holds great promise.[12] In such situations, creative problem solving is required to achieve the palliative care goals.

In light of the rapid development of pediatric palliative care worldwide, there are multiple opportunities to provide education and in-service instruction at the community level. Palliative care team members should make themselves available for such community education and outreach activities. The goal of outreach in such circumstances is to engage the community providers in providing optimal care for the community's children. Blurring the message by highlighting the accomplishments of any individual institution or marketing will not serve those goals.

Clinical Vignette

A large, community-based palliative care organization supports two pediatric nurses to care for children requiring care at home. The organization cares for 18 children on average, without a full-time pediatric medical director, and relies upon a contract with a local teaching hospital that has pediatric palliative care specialists on staff. Every 2 weeks, the organization's entire interdisciplinary team (IDT) meets with one of the pediatric palliative care physicians and reviews all of the cases. Many of the pediatric patients were referred from other hospitals in the region, thus the pediatric palliative care physicians must oversee and clarify for the IDT medical orders from many other practitioners and institutions. Although the potential exists for institutional affiliations to become turf conflicts, the IDT recognizes that the patient's needs supersede all other considerations. Dispensing with institutional allegiances and keeping the patient's care foremost allows the palliative care pediatricians to optimize care, support the community-based nurses in their challenging practices, and to create goodwill and collegial dialog with referring physicians at other institutions. This process elevates the quality of care throughout the community and allows optimal continuity of care for patients.

Assurance at the Interface

Perhaps the most important goal in planning a discharge for a child with a life-threatening illness who requires palliative care services is the creation of a seamless transition to the out-of-hospital setting, which is typically the patient's home. Children thrive best in a predictable and consistent environment. The younger they are, then the more disruptive changes in caretakers and care settings may be. As children mature, they are able to deal intellectually with many of the demands of their illness and care but until mid- to late-adolescence, they remain children with the same needs for security, nurturing, and predictable caregivers. The optimal model of palliative care for children is one in which the palliative care team that visits them at home also provides supportive visits if they

TABLE 17-3 Relationships Between Institutions and Community-Based Care

Referring institution	Community-based care
Single children's hospital	Single palliative care organization
Pro: Single standard of care to adapt to	Pro: Concentrate resources, single standard
Con: Limited family choices for care	Con: Limited choices; no competition to excel; possibly limited geographic coverage
Multiple children's hospitals	Single, large palliative care organization
Pro: Greater choice, expertise	Pro: Concentrate expertise; set standard
Con: Multiple referring sources with varying expectations; variable expertise	Con: Single option for families; possibly limited geographic coverage
Multiple children's hospitals	Multiple palliative care organizations
Pro: Great choice in care; multiple specialists	Pro: Greater choice; competition promotes excellence
Con: Multiple referring sources with varying expectations; differing quality of care	Con: Lack of consistency; confusion in areas of coverage; logistical difficulties

are re-hospitalized. Similarly, the hospital-based palliative care team provides ongoing contact with the family at home via telephone and occasional home visits to assure that the philosophy and approach to care is consistent regardless of the location. As acknowledged by the American Academy of Pediatrics, care coordination is an area of critical importance for children with long-term, complex medical conditions[3] and requires both attention and unique skills.

The question becomes who is responsible for assuring the continuity of care among all the care providers so that truly seamless care is offered between hospital and home. There are also stops at school, visits to the community pediatrician, interaction with a faith community, and perhaps some assistance from emergency responders, and local support agencies such as pharmacies and durable medical equipment providers. It should quickly be apparent that one could not draw a straight line from one provider or institution to another. Children receiving palliative care often go back and forth among all of the named entities. How then do we ensure that these relationships are addressed and nurtured throughout the child's life and through the bereavement experience of the family? Some palliative care sites have done a reasonably good job in attempting to create seamless care transitions and management.

In order to best understand the consequences of not working well within this complex and interconnected web of relationships, we will consider the following important organizations or entities when designing seamless transitions within palliative care. Keep in mind that the connections among all of these entities is not linear. Diagramming this matrix relationship would be complex at best. The intent of this section is to provide thought-provoking scenarios. The reader, then, may wish to consider other ways in which a poor relationship between two or more of the following entities would decrease the potential for quality IDP care for the child and family, or conversely the many resultant benefits when consideration is made of and for this complex relational matrix.

- Tertiary care facilities
- Community pediatrician
- Community-based hospice programs
- Durable Medical Equipment providers
- Pharmacies
- Emergency responders
- Schools
- Peer, service, and/or faith groups

The impact of care fragmentation is great. Lack of communication or miscommunication may lead to unnecessary tests, treatments, or hospitalizations.[13] Community-based hospice providers may, unintentionally or not, neglect to inform hospital-based clinicians of changes in a child's condition thus impeding the hospital clinicians' ability to contact the family to offer support or say goodbye. In some cases clinicians involved in the child's prior care may not be notified of the child's death, which then prevents them from attending a funeral or wake. Lack of knowledge may also impede the family financially, creating barriers for further care.

Most children with a life-threatening illness have been treated for many years at a tertiary care facility. Over time many of these children and families have developed long lasting relationships with hospital clinicians. Many, if not most, of these clinicians want to maintain their connection to the child and family post discharge. The clinicians include: the referring physician within the hospital, the palliative care team, subspecialty physicians, child life specialists, nurses, social workers, and chaplains. It is not only the hospital-based staff members who express desire to be kept informed of the child's care management post hospital discharge. The child and family frequently want their hospital-based care team to be kept informed and involved, even if the likelihood of the child being readmitted to the hospital is slim. Keep in mind that the child may have developed a relationship with the hospital clinicians over many years and this emotional connection and relationship should be nurtured if requested by the child and family.

Sometimes this relationship makes it more difficult to refer a child and family to a community-based hospice provider, especially if there is a history of poor communication or care barriers between the two organizations. The referring hospital team may harbor ill feelings from a previous care relationship in which they believed the hospice team did not keep them informed about the child's care. The hospice team may have believed that the hospital team was over-reaching and did not allow the hospice team to do its job. Referrals may come late to a hospice with little resultant time to develop meaningful relationships with the child and family. This lack of time and meaningful relationship often makes it quite much more awkward and difficult for the hospice team to assist the child and family in talking about advance care planning and coordination. Hospital clinicians may believe that the hospice staff discourages a child and family from seeking the patient's readmission to the hospital, whereas it might be that no one is effectively communicating that the child and family have opted for no further hospitalization. This personal decision, and the decision-making process, is accurately reflected in care documentation and the plan of care but may not be effectively communicated to hospital staff.

This push-pull relationship is often related to miscommunication and lack of understanding of the goals of care. Frequently, too, all involved parties do not come to understanding the child's life expectancy at the same time. This leads to resentment and further barriers, or as we sometimes say, a lack of playing well together in the sandbox.

The inability of all care providers to acknowledge their own profound and important relationship with the child and family will potentially lead to inadvertent fragmentation of care and fewer options and opportunities for children and families to access quality palliative care. Effective and collaborative communication and problem solving must be a top priority. If poorly conducted, there will be a negative impact. The consequences are great when organizations don't acknowledge the relationships among one other and the child and family. Children suffer in pain. Parents feel isolated, siblings may feel abandoned. Additional patients who might be served by either institution don't get referred. Liben, Papadatou, Wolfe[1] describe cases in which Do Not Attempt Resuscitation (DNR) orders are instituted in hospitalized children close to the actual time of death. One can only wonder if these conversations had been undertaken sooner if more children would be discharged to home-based hospice or palliative care. Additionally, parents have described dissatisfaction with hospital clinicians who provided confusing and inadequate information regarding their child's treatment or prognosis. These confusing conversations may also lead to late hospice referrals programs, or no referral at all, as clinicians and parents don't mutually understand and communicate about the child's limited life expectancy. Perhaps a mediated conversation with the community-based hospice provider or child's community pediatrician would help in these circumstances.

The way out is a patient-centered approach in which important team relationships and contributions are valued and employed to support the child and family. It may not always be the same person in the lead, but there must always be the same commitment to working in concert, not in parallel or redundancy, to serve the needs of the patient. Hospice nurses and visiting nurses will have important insights to offer because of their closeness to the patient, but this also underscores an important coordination that should occur among palliative care, hospital-based programs, and community-based programs. The failsafe for this, given how central it is to its goals, is the pediatric palliative care team.

Relationships Within the Pediatric Palliative Care Team

The pediatric palliative care team has developed historically as a horizontally organized one in which the unique perspective and experience of each member is valued equally. This model contrasts with the hierarchical structure more typically seen in medical settings with each of the disciplines working under the physician's leadership. While there are frequently issues that require the physician to make decisions, the group must function as a cohesive team with mutual respect for what each member brings. Teams meet either weekly or biweekly to discuss the active patients and assess any change in status, function, or symptom management. In general, physicians make intermittent home visits on an as-needed basis with the majority of the work being carried out by the community-based team consisting of social worker, chaplain, nurse, and often a child life or music therapist. Thus the physician and the rest of the interdisciplinary team rely upon the home-care team to be effective eyes and ears, relaying necessary information for discussion at the weekly meetings.

The allocation of responsibilities within the team usually follows along the lines of each discipline's primary training. However, in pediatric palliative care, an interdisciplinary paradigm has emerged that represents an "approach that integrates the natural, social, and health sciences in a humanistic context, and in so doing transcends each of their traditional boundaries."[14,15] Organizing along such lines allows each discipline to extend beyond its traditional boundaries and take on other roles as needed, adapting in a dynamic fashion to the changing needs and realities of the patient and family.[16] Because the team is often spread over a large geographic area, an interdisciplinary approach allows members greater autonomy in problem solving, which permits the detection and resolution of problems more quickly and efficiently and contributes to better overall patient care (Box 17-1).

For an interdisciplinary team to function effectively and professionally, it is essential that each member be familiar with all of the various aspects of care that may be required. Open channels of communication are vitally important to avoid members working at cross-purposes. In addition, it is essential that each member of the team possess excellent interpersonal skills, maturity, and integrity. New members of the team must be carefully oriented to their roles and will develop their own style with ongoing experience and feedback from the group.

BOX 17-1 Advantages of Transdisciplinary Organization

- Improves quality of care
- Reduces errors in healthcare delivery
- Reduces duplication of services
- Provides cost-effective care
- Enhances efficiency of healthcare delivery
- Addresses medical and psychosocial aspects of care
- Is more convenient for the patient and family or caregiver
- Increases patient and family or caregiver satisfaction
- Promotes development of innovative approaches and solutions to complex problems
- Increases collaboration and networking among professionals
- Enhances individual professional development

Adapted from Patel D, Pratt H, et al. Team processes and team care for children with developmental disabilities, *Pediatr Clin North Am* 55:1375–1390, 2008.

Assuring Patient Privacy and Confidentiality

We must recognize that the protection of patient and family privacy is a central element in building the professional trust that families need. Members of the palliative care team will see families at their most vulnerable, when normal social checks and balances on behavior may have worn thin. Professionalism mandates that healthcare providers protect the intimate information pertaining to medical details, financial status, the family's functioning, and other private matters. Thus it is important that only information relevant to the care of the patient and family be provided to medical agencies that partner in caring for patients. The provision of various details to community organizations, including hospice organizations, schools, and churches, must be weighed against the rights of the family and patient to have their information kept private. Whenever possible, organizations should become familiar with the HIPAA guidelines and should use signed information release documents when these are available (see www.hhs.gov/ocr/privacy). Discussions of sensitive matters in interdisciplinary team meetings should remain professional with as little gossip as is humanly possible.

Palliative Care and the General Pediatrician

Successful collaboration between palliative care and primary care practitioners can contribute to improved care for children with life-threatening illnesses. These two areas of practice have great affinity in their emphasis on communication, the coordination of services, and the importance of family-centered solutions. There can, however, be great differences in the form as well as the success of the collaboration.

Parents often consider their primary care pediatrician their child's real doctor, while in fact that clinician may have a very limited role in medical decision making for children in palliative care. This confidence from the parents reflects strengths in a relationship that may pre-exist the circumstances prompting palliative care and the fact that the primary care doctor may have made the life-threatening diagnosis in the first place. The parents may believe that the primary care pediatrician is in a special position to understand the needs and values of the family. It is difficult to overestimate the importance of a relationship with a family and a child that may have begun at a prenatal visit and has been a part of every major health-related event in a child's life. It is not surprising that parents may desire the involvement of their primary care pediatrician in critical conversations and decisions. The palliative care team benefits when these strengths are incorporated into the overall care of the child.

One central challenge to effective, meaningful palliative care is to recognize and appreciate who the child is, separate from the ravages of disease and the sociologic stress of disease management. To the dismay of many parents, the healthcare team frequently understands and represents their child based upon their diagnosis and clinical course. However, the child under care has an identity and meaningful existence that, from a family-centered perspective, supersedes the identity of the patient the palliative care team may come to know in a specialized medical setting. The member of the child's healthcare team most likely to apprehend this fuller sense of the child is the primary care provider. Supporting the involvement of the primary care practitioner supports an emphasis on seeing decisions in the context of the children's undiseased lives, their families, and their communities, and can help assure that choices reflect deep-seated values and experiences.

The role of the primary care pediatrician in a child's care may be different depending on the kind of condition requiring pediatric palliative care. Broadly speaking, the more typically described patient categories of pediatric palliative care can be divided into four categories:

1. Conditions for which curative treatment is possible but may fail, such as advanced or progressive cancer with poor prognosis or severe or complex, congenital or acquired, heart disease
2. Conditions requiring intensive long-term treatment aimed at maintaining the quality of life, such as HIV, cystic fibrosis, severe immunodeficiency, or muscular dystrophy
3. Progressive conditions in which treatment is exclusively palliative after diagnosis, such as progressive metabolic disorders, severe chromosomal disorders, trisomy 13, trisomy 18, or severe osteogenesis imperfecta
4. Conditions involving severe, non-progressive disability, causing extreme vulnerability to health complications, such as severe cerebral palsy (CP) with recurrent infection or difficult to control symptoms, severe neurologic sequelae of infectious disease, anoxic or hypoxic brain injury

Realistically, primary care pediatricians have contributions to make in the care of children in all of these categories and, with the possible exception of the first category, most of the children's lives and their medical care are likely to occur in the community setting. While there may be differences in the willingness of primary care practitioners to become involved, practically speaking, in most communities he or she will be the central medical figure coordinating the child's medical care.

In addition, there are two other areas where the palliative care skill set is employed in pediatric primary care. The first is helping a family respond to the sudden, unexpected death of a child, generally from trauma such as motor vehicle accidents, falls, drownings, and Sudden Infant Death Syndrome. These constitute the leading causes of death in children. The primary care pediatrician may be involved at the time of death or may be involved in helping counsel the family on appropriate ways to assist the siblings. Secondly, primary care pediatricians are routinely consulted for advice about disclosure and planning related to children after a parent receives a life-threatening diagnosis. In both of these areas, there is great promise that the field of palliative care can support and potentially improve the care provided by pediatric primary care practitioners. Reciprocally, involvement of primary care practitioners can help improve the care delivered by practitioners of palliative care.

The needs of children and families in palliative care can be better addressed when their primary care pediatrician embraces the concept of the medical home.[17] The medical home can be characterized by a practice setting that incorporates commitments to access and care that is family centered, continuous, compassionate, culturally effective, comprehensive, and coordinated. This approach to child health is meant to offer an alternative to fragmented care lacking a sense of the whole child and family. While the approach is meant to improve the care delivered to children with a broad spectrum of chronic care needs, and not necessarily end-of-life care, the parallels and potential complements with palliative care are obvious. The medical home approach is based on confidence in the sympathetic perspective arising from a longstanding relationship to play an important role in the care of patients in palliative care. It meets the preferences of a family to have known, predictable sources of health care that understand the child, the family, and their community.

The primary care pediatrician with years of experience and trust with a family brings special expertise to the team of healthcare providers collaborating in the care of a child with life-threatening illness. One specific role is the potential to act as a two-way translator and communicator of medical information. Parents can sometimes have difficulty understanding medical facts and recommendations. They may not grasp the terminology used. The primary care pediatrician may have an accurate appreciation of how well a family understands things, and can help them bridge gaps in their understanding and knowledge. Conversely, a family may be more able to voice doubts and differences of opinion related to medical decision making with their primary care pediatrician. Once understood by the team, the family's concerns and how they might want them addressed can then be shared.

Another strength of the primary care pediatrician's role can be the fact that primary care is healthcare provided outside of the hospital and in the community. Families can feel overwhelmed with the logistical challenges of hospital-based care, and the child may have strong reactions to any return to the hospital setting. They may see healthcare delivered in the more normal setting of the primary care practice, when possible, as more tolerable.

Families and children place tremendous importance on maintaining normalcy. Primary care can be essential, in this sense, to maintaining quality of life. For the patient, this can mean routine visits, vaccinations, and developmental assessments. These visits may offer the only medical encounters where the rationale for involvement is not debilitating disease but the positive and ordinary characteristics of childhood. The primary care perspective also focuses on education and learning, social engagement, play, interests, and the child as part of a family and community. For parents and children interested in living a full life with the highest degree of quality, advice, and assistance in these areas can be extraordinarily meaningful.

A special case of this is the role of the primary care pediatrician for parents navigating palliative care. Matters of normal parenting can be challenging when children have life-threatening illnesses. Parents can come to see the impact of profound disease and its treatment as a kind of punishment, which they compensate for with lowered expectations of behavior, which can become its own burden. Consistent, sensible parenting in this alien terrain is important, even if it is tempered by a need for greater tenderness. Addressing basic parenting concerns such as sleep, diet, setting limits, and tolerating frustration and anxiety are important to parents and may have an important impact on the quality of a child's life. Indeed, these concerns may at times be more fundamental to parents' impressions of how well their child is doing than the actual physiologic markers of disease. Open discussions about parenting their child can be helpful.

The profoundly ill or dying child affects a whole family. The basic fabric of family life is at risk. Siblings have special needs and parents may need devoted settings where they can focus on how their other children are doing. The sibling's health needs and requirements of normal development demand their own attention. Parents also place great importance on discussions between the primary care pediatrician and siblings about how they are experiencing and coping with their sibling's illness. The appropriate topics and their depth of exploration may be affected by the age of the sibling, their relationship with the child requiring palliative care, the parental response, the sibling's perceived need to replace the positive characteristics of the ill sibling, and the sibling's capacity to grieve. The primary care setting is a place to begin to see that the sibling's needs are not being missed.

There is a further role for the primary care practitioner in the community. Schools and community programs may have good intentions to include the child with life-threatening illness for as long as possible but may need help understanding and managing potential risks to the child. They also may need help communicating to other children involved in these settings, generally to make contact with the ill child less worrisome to others.

Taken together, it should be seen that primary care has an important discipline-specific role in palliative care. Nonetheless, the reality of involvement in the care of a child with palliative care needs and complexities can be daunting to a primary care clinician. Primary care practitioners may be uncertain about performing at a level that reflects their commitment to the child and family. In a typical career, a primary care practitioner typically has two or three patients in his or her practice who will die, and may feel ill prepared to competently respond to the needs of a palliative care patient. There are considerable logistical challenges when a clinician needs to be available to the intense and dramatic needs of a palliative care patient while seeing patients in a typical day in primary care. Most practice settings involve groups and cross-coverage, requiring careful communication among all of the providers and agreement in attaining the goals of care. There is great variation in how much or how easily a primary care pediatrician wants to become involved in the palliative care of patients.

On the other hand, given the broad scope of children appropriately receiving palliative care, it cannot be expected that there will be a pediatric palliative care workforce sufficient to respond to all end of life and palliative care needs. Ideally, the primary care clinician would be a part of an interdisciplinary model where his or her contributions to the care of the child and family are valued and incorporated into the overall plan of care. A challenge for the nascent field of pediatric palliative care is thinking creatively about models of collaboration. In its policy statement on pediatric palliative care, the American Academy of Pediatrics (AAP) asserts that "minimum standards of pediatric palliative care must include a mechanism to ensure a seamless transition between settings."[4] Such a seamless transition relies on communication, mutual understanding, and mutual respect between the various parties involved in the child's care.

The successful collaboration and inclusion of primary care practitioners in palliative care is facilitated when certain conditions are met (Box 17-2). There must be a timely sharing of information, keeping primary care in the loop. Their contributions are only possible when the information necessary for relevant contribution is available. Obviously, more is needed than a discharge summary and efforts are best made to keep the contributing primary care practitioner updated on developments and involved in planning. As possible, the primary care practitioner should be invited to participate in discussions exploring goals of care and medical decision making. This not only has the promise of improving the planning itself but also helps ensure a more seamless transition for children between settings. Case coordination should explicitly include sharing responsibilities for outpatient management and acknowledge authority over turf. The care of children with life-threatening illnesses is undermined when the primary care pediatrician is unclear about whether certain decisions are out of their hands, just as it is undermining when plans carefully determined by the palliative care team are changed or ignored once the child has a change of setting. Social work and case management needs should be explored before discharge and reassignment of responsibility. Sensitivity to the different scale of available resources in the primary care setting will help assure a better quality of care for the child.

Finally, end-of-life care involving the primary care practitioner may also require backstopping on the technical matters of pain and symptom management where a potentially inexperienced or uncertain primary care clinician will be the first notified of changes and difficulties. Primary care pediatricians may also appreciate efforts to describe tasks necessary at the time of death.

Pediatric palliative care, working in coordination with the primary care pediatrician, can enhance and support community based models of care. Practical models will highlight the sharing of expertise with providers in the community and coordination at crucial times of decision making. Working together, the lives and the healthcare of children and families with life-threatening illnesses will be improved.

BOX 17-2 **Fundamentals of Successful Collaboration with Primary Care**

- Timely sharing of information
- Inclusion in clarifying goals of care and medical decision making
- Coordinated designation of responsibilities
- Explicit review of case management and social work needs
- Technical back-up for pain and symptom management

Clinical Vignette

A 5-year-old boy with progressive degenerative brain disease is being cared for by a community-based pediatric palliative care organization. The mother has been trying to contact the primary neurologist because her son is having increasingly painful muscle spasms. The office nurse has told her that no appointment would be available for five weeks. The home hospice nurse recognizes that such a delay would be harmful to the child and consults with the pediatric palliative care medical director. The medical director contacts the neurologist's office directly and finds that he is out of town, and the office nurse denies that the mother has been in contact with the office. The medical director obtains e-mail contact information for the primary neurologist and sends an e-mail indicating the steps planned to control the worsening spasms. The boy's medication is adjusted successfully in a timely manner and the primary neurologist is effectively kept in the loop on decisionmaking. This scenario demonstrates the palliative care team's advocacy role, use of the physician leader to overcome obstacles, and the focus on timely management of distressing symptoms. Primary caregivers can provide similar advocacy by contacting subspecialists directly or enlisting the palliative care physician in achieving timely resolution of difficulties.

Palliative Care and the Fabric of a Family's Life

The final domain of care involves the child in relation to the community organizations in which he or she has been involved. As is the case with adults, children are members of many communities. Beyond the nuclear and extended family units, the classroom situation is likely to be identified by most children as a strong point of reference. For pre-elementary children, the classroom provides fundamental lessons for social development. Elementary school provides opportunities to develop skills and competences in those things that our society values for achieving subsequent productive independence as adults. Middle school provides opportunities for individuation while high school provides the knowledge and skills to enter adulthood. The pursuit of developmentally appropriate learning is therefore critically important for the psychological well-being of children and adults in our society. When a child is confronted with a life-threatening illness, the attention will naturally be directed first at trying to combat and cure the condition. If it becomes clear that cure is not possible, a reappraisal of the goals of life is important to make plans in light of the new status. Throughout this process, keeping children engaged in the life activities that define normalcy for healthy children is psychologically beneficial and can serve to lift the spirits of an ill child. Simply getting to school for a few hours is often the most highly valued experience.

One's legacy is often manifested through the impact one has on others. This is true for adults as well as children no matter how long or short their lives may be. To impact another requires relationships between people and this is the very heart of much of the work done in end-of-life care. This area of palliative care work is one of the richest opportunities for personal growth and professional satisfaction. Many of the relationships exist in classrooms, with neighbors in the community, in faith-based organization, in youth groups, and in scouting and athletic organizations. The impact of a child's death reverberates through all of these communities and affects members who may not have directly known the child. In a society that has isolated the dying in institutions or hidden them at home, lay people have little exposure to terminal conditions except in the elderly in whom it is more to be expected. Palliative care organizations are routinely called upon to speak to school teachers and ministers to help them understand how to aid their constituencies in dealing with the death of a child in their midst. Other roles have included grief counseling for teachers when there are unexpected, tragic deaths in the student body such as from suicide or fatal motor vehicle accidents. These activities as community resources are vitally important to help members of the community process the death and grow from the experience to whatever extent possible. It is through such facilitation that the child's legacy is further developed and his or her impact on the community can be realized.

The impact of the death of a classmate can be a profound and life-changing experience for a young person. In a society that is focused on materialism and appearance, it is a call back to reality when a classmate dies. How many students have asked themselves if they really have such hard lives when they are confronted with the death of a fellow student? One of the tasks of the palliative care team is to seek opportunities to bring meaning and understanding to the surviving members of the community when asked to do so. Grief counselors and other support personnel associated with palliative care teams can serve as mentors for school and community officials in dealing with a childhood loss.

For the individual patient with a life-threatening condition in the community, the palliative care team can bring to bear its broad and deep perspective on life and how to live in preparation for a possible death. The goal of the child life therapists, chaplains, physicians, and nurses is to create the best experiences of life possible to whatever degree the child's condition permits. Through reinforcing relationships and finding creative ways for the child to remain involved with the community, the pediatric palliative care team can strive to give as much meaning to the child's life and to all whom he or she touches.

Other important community partners include community pharmacies that may have provided medications to the child for many years. Their role may change as the child becomes more ill and receives his or her medication through the hospice provider. It is the thoughtful hospice or hospital based team that, with parental permission, includes the community pharmacist in the communication loop. A simple phone call takes little time and does much to ensure that these important relationships are nurtured. The same may be true for the durable medical equipment (DME) company. DME companies may also have provided medical equipment and wheelchair adjustments to a child for many years. Informing them of the child's health status is more than a courtesy; doing so acknowledges the relationship between the child and family and the DME company.

By far the largest and one of the most important community partners is the child's school, and to a lesser extent the child's social, peer, and faith-based groups, religious youth groups, and scouting organizations (e.g., Boy and Girl Scouts). Child life specialists are often instrumental in assisting the ill child's return to school. The child life specialist may work with the school faculty, classroom peers, and other students closely associated with the ill child. Schools should be a safe haven for children and for the child with a life-threatening illness returning to school represents a return to normalcy. It is important to discuss with the parents how best to include key school personnel in ongoing discussions about the child's health status. This is in the best interest of the child. The ill child and his or her siblings may have attended the school for many years. The family may be well known and the teachers and office staff often have very warm and deep relationships with the child. It is important to determine from the parents how much information they would like the care program to share with school personnel.

Some school principals and other administrators become very concerned when a seriously ill child returns to school. Issues of DNR status are not uniformly acknowledged or followed.[18,19] This may create problems for the child and family as the school may call emergency responders even if the parents do not authorize such a call. Again, the care team might suggest a meeting with all involved clinicians and selected school personnel.

Service clubs and faith-based youth groups are also important social supports for the ill child and siblings. Knowing what information the family wants shared is important because these peers can be profoundly affected by the illness and death of their friend. Building relationships with these groups is important. Social workers and child life specialists have much to offer these often silent mourners. Their care needs are quite similar to the previous discussion of school classmates. Building rapport with these service and faith-based groups may also increase access for future care needs.

Summary

A hallmark of optimal pediatric palliative care is the seamless integration of the palliative care approach into total patient care. To achieve such integration requires the recognition of the complex relationships that create the safety net for children living with life-threatening and life-limiting conditions and their families. This chapter has provided many examples of such extended relationships and attempted to provide a context to permit practitioners to use the information in their own care settings. The reader is encouraged to consider this information and explore the myriad interactions, which directly affect the child's care whether as an in-patient or in the community setting. Following death, a part of each patient lives on through the consequences of the relationships he or she experienced.

REFERENCES

1. Liben S, Papadatou D, et al: Paediatric palliative care: challenges and emerging ideas, *Lancet* 371(9615):852–864, 2008.
2. Löfmark R, Nilstun T, et al: From cure to palliation: concept, decision and acceptance, *J Med Ethics* 33:685–688, 2007.
3. Ziring PR, Brazdziunas D, et al: American Academy of Pediatrics: Committee on Children with Disabilities. The treatment of neurologically impaired children using patterning, *Pediatrics* 104(5 Pt 1): 1149–1151, 1999.
4. Committee on Bioethics and Committee on Hospital Care: Palliative care for children, *Pediatrics* 106:351–357, 2000.
5. Field M, Behrman R: *When children die: improving palliative and end-of-life care for children and their families*, Washington, DC, 2003, National Academic Press.
6. Feudtner C: Collaborative communication in pediatric palliative care: a foundation for problem-solving and decision-making, *Pediatr Clin North Am* 54(5):583–607, ix, 2007.
7. Baker JN, Hinds PS, et al: Integration of palliative care practices into the ongoing care of children with cancer: individualized care planning and coordination, *Pediatr Clin North Am* 55(1):223–250, xii, 2008.
8. Penson R, Partridge R, et al: Fear of death, *Oncologist* 10:160–169, 2005.
9. Heaston S, Beckstrand R, et al: Emergency nurses' perceptions of obstacles and supportive behaviors in end-of-life care, *J Emerg Nurs* 32:477–485, 2006.
10. Levetown M, Committee on Bioethics: Communicating with children and families: from everyday interactions to skill in conveying distressing information, *Pediatrics* 121(5):e1441–e1460, 2008.
11. Davies B, Sehring SA, et al: Barriers to palliative care for children: perceptions of pediatric health care providers, *Pediatrics* 121(2):282–288, 2008.
12. Bensink ME, Armfield NR, et al: Using videotelephony to support pediatric oncology-related palliative care in the home: from abandoned RCT to acceptability study, *Palliat Med* 23(3):228–237, 2009.
13. Himelstein B: Palliative care for infants, children, adolescents, and their families, *J Palliat Med* 9:163–181, 2006.
14. Soskolne C: Transdisciplinary approaches for public health, *Epidemiology* 11:S122, 2000.
15. Batorowicz B, Shepherd T: Measuring the quality of transdisciplinary teams, *J Interprof Care* 22:612–620, 2008.
16. Patel D, Pratt H, et al: Team processes and team care for children with developmental disabilities, *Pediatr Clin North Am* 55:1375–1390, 2008.
17. American Academy of Pediatrics Medical Home Initiatives for Children With Special Needs Project Advisory Committee: The medical home, *Pediatrics* 110:184–186, 2002.
18. Kimberly MB, Forte AL, et al: Pediatric do-not-attempt-resuscitation orders and public schools: a national assessment of policies and laws, *Am J Bioeth* 5(1):59–65, 2005.
19. Ross ME, Hicks J, et al: Preschool as palliative care, *J Clin Oncol* 26(22):3797–3799, 2005.

SUGGESTED READING

Cassel C, Demel B: Palliative care and primary care. In Showstack J, editor: *The future of primary care*, San Francisco, 2004, Jossey-Bass, pp 223–242.

18 Self-Care: The Foundation of Care Giving

STEPHEN LIBEN | DANAI PAPADATOU

The best way to become a better "helper" is to become a better person. But one necessary aspect of becoming a better person is via helping other people. So one must and can do both simultaneously.[1]

From the basic principles of human physiology, such as the heart first pumps blood to itself, to airline instructions in case of emergency, put your oxygen mask on first and then assist those around you, emerges the underlying principle of self-care. Without caring for oneself there can be no caring for others.

As clinicians come face to face with the inevitable suffering of a child's dying and death, they have a choice, if not always consciously made, in how they approach their work. When they cope with suffering by seeing themselves as strong and giving to others who are perceived as weak, they are at high risk for burnout, becoming disillusioned and drained of energy. By contrast, if instead of helping the weak and vulnerable, they choose to offer themselves in service, then they assume a role of knowledgeable guide. As a knowledgeable guide they serve others with their whole selves that includes their particular strengths as well as vulnerabilities. Clinicians recognize the dark, the light, and the weak and strong aspects of their being and understand that are all needed in situations of intense suffering. They also recognize that despite their specialized knowledge in some areas, in most areas they share the sense of mystery experienced by those they serve. They can do only what they can, then they must let go of expectations that they can control outcomes that never were within our control. If they perceive their work as offering their whole selves in service, then the necessity to work on themselves becomes apparent. This self-work or self-care is both a requirement of their roles as well as a privilege they are being offered: to be allowed to become more themselves and to move toward their own potential as part of their daily jobs. As Robert Coles said, "I had begun to see how complicated this notion of service is, how it is a function of not only what we do but who we are (which of course, gives shape to what we do)."[2]

What do care givers have to offer families of children who live with a life-threatening illness? What more can they possibly do or say when all has been done in terms of pain and symptom control? How can each of the care givers be enough in the face of such suffering? They know that what children and parents value during these times is the abiding presence of a trusted person who listens and bears witness to their suffering, even better if that person has experience in being present in similar life-threatening situations, and has walked that path with others.[3,4] "All I want is what is in your mind and in your heart," said dying patient David Tasma to Cicely Saunders, founder of the modern hospice movement. Tasma shared and supported her dream to develop a hospice. The quality of care is not limited to professional expertise but is greatly affected by what each clinician, as individuals and as members of a professional team, brings into relationships with children, adolescents, and parents. While bringing their imperfect selves to the service of others is necessary, it is not, however, sufficient. What is also required is that clinicians care for themselves in an ongoing reflective and systematic way.

The term self-care has been used in a variety of activities and in its most reductive sense is understood superficially as taking time for ourselves or taking a vacation. While it is important to balance work-life with other activities, the kind of self-care that leads to enduring personal resilience and growth requires more than time away because clinicians can never get away from themselves. In the words of Jon Kabat Zinn, "Wherever you go, there you are."[5] Self-care, when stripped of self-reflection, meaning making and paying attention in the present moment, becomes a self-centered exercise that is about I, Me, and Mine. Self-care activities based solely on distractions, such as vacations and other means to get away from work, can become selfish. If distractions and running away, including reliance on drugs and alcohol, are exclusively what self-care consists of, then inevitably there is never going to be enough time away. When the habit of running away from what is in the present moment becomes an established practice, then caregivers find that each distraction is good for a while but inevitably tolerance develops and no time away or distraction is ever enough. It is important to clarify that distraction, in and of itself, is not bad or unhealthy; and when entered into mindfully it is one of many strategies that can be helpful. Rather than being harmful, distraction, in the correct balance, is necessary but not enough to encompass the self-care needed in pediatric palliative care. While eating well, getting adequate sleep, regular medical care, physical exercise, having interests outside work, and making time for oneself are all important and necessary aspects of self-care, they are not sufficient. What follows in this chapter is a focus on the deep work of caring for the caregivers, which is essential when attending to the suffering of others.

The first part of this chapter outlines the relationship to self for professionals in the care of the seriously ill, caregivers' suffering within the work and the possibilities of personal growth that comes with accepting things as they are. The second part of this chapter introduces self-reflective practice with specific exercises in awareness that clinicians may choose to experience.

Relationship to Self

"How can you do this job?" "How can you bear the pain of children who are seriously ill… children who die… parents who grieve?" "Isn't your life deeply affected, or are you used to death?" Such questions, often asked by colleagues, friends, patients, and their families, have no easy answer. These questions invite caregivers to turn their gazes inward and reflect both upon the process by which they cope with the life-threatening illness or death of a child, as well as with their own mortality. In reality, they never get used to or become immune to the suffering of children, adolescents, and families that dream of a future yet live with uncertainty and in the shadow of loss. Nevertheless, caregivers often do get used to the sight, the touch, the sounds, or smells of the child's frail body that may or may not survive the ravages of a life-threatening illness. With growing experience, caregivers learn to anticipate the disease trajectory and recognize the symptoms of remission or deterioration identify signs of anticipatory grief, facilitate its unfolding, and help families accept and eventually temper their suffering or transform it into opportunities for development and growth. Over time caregivers gain specialized knowledge that can be of use to those they accompany down a path many have never been down before, while at the same time caregivers recognize that they never know all there is to know about the inevitably unknowable journey of each particular child and family.

All of that is possible in the context of relationships that are personal. Personal relationships both make the job highly stressful but also deeply fulfilling, and determine the degree of satisfaction that families experience with regard to the care being offered to them. We have come to understand that the relationships developed with the parents of seriously ill children are often problematic, and professionals who are insensitive, unavailable, or impersonal in their approaches elicit parental dissatisfaction and increased distress.[3,6–13] Parental satisfaction with care is directly related to the nature of the relationships held with the care providers. These relationships have a positive or negative impact upon how families experience the dying process and death of a child, and seem to affect their long-term adjustment to loss. These findings make self-reflective practice a necessary part of the job, and encourage caregivers to review the relationships developed as well as challenge some of the mistaken beliefs according to which specialized knowledge, refined skills, and clinical experience are thought to be enough to ensure quality of care. While knowledge, skills, and experience are undoubtedly critical, families of seriously ill children demand more than that and expect a personal, human, and caring relationship. The following example illustrates how quality of care extends beyond the provision of expert care, and encompasses the development of nurturing and meaningful relationships with children and parents.

Mrs. Lauver gave birth to Maria, and 2 years later to Stella. Both of her daughters were born with a rare, undiagnosed syndrome that resulted in serious retardation, neurological and motor problems, frequent seizures, and pulmonary infections. Each of them lived until age 9 and died in an intensive care unit as a result of their health complications. When the mother was asked to describe her experiences with the care her daughters had received, she chose to focus on their last hospitalization in two different intensive care units. With regard to Maria's hospitalization in the first ICU she shared the following account:

"Her hospitalization lasted 10 days, and during those days, staff members did their duty.…The care she received, from the first physician to the last nurse, was very professional but what was missing was personal warmth and humanity. It was a physician who informed me that Maria's condition was critical and that it was uncertain whether she would survive. The way he imparted this information was so cold, so distant.… Some doctors avoid giving time to parents and I fully understand it because they have to attend to several children besides our own. But, we, the parents who have children with major problems, have the right to clear explanations, to some compassion, to be treated as if we are their own people.

"The night Maria died, they told us that it would be a difficult night.… But we, the parents, always hope for a miracle.…What I remember is that when I squeezed her hand, she bit the breathing tube. When I saw the machines react, I hurt. I realized that she was aware I was there. I then left the ICU, and 10 minutes later she left [died]. The following day when her grandfather came to take her body from the morgue, he realized that the she had been removed from the ICU unwashed, uncombed, and with blood on her cheek that they did not even bother to wipe off after taking out the respirator. This infuriated me as well as her grandfather. They ought to take greater care of such things."

In contrast to Maria's death, Stella's hospitalization in another ICU was experienced by Mrs. Lauver quite differently:

"Stella was admitted to another ICU and was hospitalized for 40 days due to her apneas. From the moment we were admitted to the moment she left [died], we experienced a tremendous difference in our relationships with the staff compared with our other daughter. The doctors outdid themselves; they were very human, warm, and made us feel as if we were their family. Yes, we were indeed their family. My child was also their child. There are no words to describe it. We just felt it. And to tell you the truth, Stella felt it too.… Although she was on a respirator, she felt the care, the concern, and the love that staff members expressed to her. I could see it in her face. She was content, happy.… In this unit, professionals had a place for her and for us. They were interested in my concerns, and discussed Stella's condition and what would be in her best interest. We did not want her to suffer. They gave us some choices.… And they respected our decisions, and I am deeply grateful for that.

"I remember it was Sunday when the physician on call informed us that she presented arrhythmias and that, sadly, the end was close. Again, I did not want to believe it.… I sat next to her until the moment she died. I expressed the desire to hug her one last time, which was difficult because she was on the respirator. The staff removed the respirator to help me take her in my arms for one last hug (cries).

"The following morning when her grandfather went to pick her up [from the morgue], he saw a totally different child from the one he had encountered in the case of her sister Maria. It was obvious that they had treated Stella with total respect. She was clean and combed.… they had honored my child."

In her account, Mrs. Lauver acknowledged that professionals in both intensive care units dealt with the physical aspects of her daughters' care with great competence and also had informed her and her husband about the imminence of death. Of note, however, is that Mrs. Lauver's satisfaction with regard to the care that each of her children and family received was directly related to the nature of the relationships with the care providers. The impact of what had transpired in those relationships was so profound that Maria's death was experienced as highly traumatic, while Stella's death was comforting, affecting the family's bereavement in distinct ways.

This example illustrates how quality of care is not limited to professional expertise but is greatly affected by what each caregiver, as individuals and as members of a professional team, bring into the relationships with children, adolescents, and parents. It is critical to better understand how caregivers' values, attitudes, and beliefs affect those served, and also to understand that they themselves are also affected by the challenges, uncertainties, hopes, and losses they experience.

A Relationship-Centered Approach to Care

Papadatou[14] suggests that it is necessary to expand our view of the care of seriously ill children beyond the family-centered approach that limits focus to the needs, concerns, and preferences of young patients and their families. This broader outlook is possible if a relationship-centered approach is adopted. Such an approach illuminates the dynamics that develop in life-and-death situations among patients, family members, professionals, and teams, and considers the larger organizational and sociocultural contexts in which care is offered and received. It explores the reciprocal influence of patients, families, and professionals and sheds light upon their subjective experiences and interactions in the context of healthcare.[15] In essence, the relationship-centered approach focuses on whatever transpires when the private and social worlds of a sick child or family interacts with the private and social worlds of care providers in a given work and social environment. To better understand the outcomes of such encounters, it is important to consider its basic components (Fig. 18-1):

1. The subjective world of the child, adolescent, or parent understood in light of his or her personal and family history and sociocultural background.
2. The subjective world of the clinician understood in light of his or her personal, family and professional history and sociocultural background.
3. The culture of the team, organization, or service that offers services to children with a life-threatening illness and to their families.
4. The larger social, economic, and cultural context in which care is offered and received.
5. The intersubjective space that is formed when the child, adolescent, or parent meets and interacts with a clinician or team in a given work and sociocultural context; this space belongs to their unique relationship.

According to Stern,[16] the intersubjective space is "the domain of feelings, thoughts, and knowledge that two (or more) people share about the nature of their current relationship" (p. 243). When the clinician and the patient or parent are open to each other, and to their respective worlds, then the intersubjective space is enlarged to include a rich partnership, a fruitful collaboration, and the co-creation of new narratives. It also includes opportunities for increased self-awareness, new learning, positive changes, and personal growth in the midst of uncertainty and hope. Such experiences render the process of care human, meaningful, and rewarding. By contrast, when both clinicians and family members enact prescribed roles and focus solely on what needs to be done, which is often accomplished in a ritualistic or detached manner—then the intersubjective space becomes limited in its capacity to offer opportunities for genuine connection. It is also limited for viewing reality in a new way, and for containing, tempering, and transforming suffering in meaningful ways while developing resilience in the midst of adversity and loss.

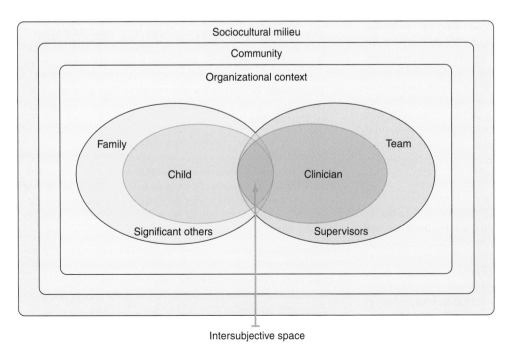

Fig. 18-1 Sociocultural milieu, community, organizational context.

The relationship-centered approach does not limit its focus solely upon the identification of specific goals that aim to meet the physical, psychosocial, and spiritual needs of seriously ill children and of their families. It emphasizes the importance of developing a partnership in caring relationships that allow for needs to be met and goals accomplished. One of the challenges posed by the relationship-centered approach is the development of an increased awareness and understanding of the clinician's private worlds in the context of relationships that aim to be truly and genuinely caring and enriching.

The Private Worlds of Professionals

To engage in a process of self-exploration and self-understanding, caregivers must first recognize such commonly held mistaken beliefs as:

- Suffering affects only seriously ill children, adolescents, and the people who are significant in their life; professionals do not and should not experience suffering.
- Effective care is ensured through specialized skills, rational thinking, and objectivity; emotions are subjective and lead to biases and mistaken clinical judgments.
- Clinicians must adopt an attitude of detached concern that involves an intellectual interest, and concern and understanding of others, along with emotional detachment that aims to protect them from occupational hazards such as burnout and compassion fatigue.

These beliefs prevent clinicians from developing caring relationships in which they are fully present and aware of what unfolds in the intersubjective space that is shared between themselves and others. As caregivers, knowing oneself is equally important as knowing the child, the adolescent, or the family to whom services are provided. Such 'self-knowledge' should not be limited to cognitive understanding, but also includes the integration of information gathered from emotional responses, physical senses, and bodily reactions, all of which contribute to self-understanding. When caregivers accompany families through illness, dying, and bereavement they cannot promise a cure, a perfect death, or recovery from bereavement. All they can assure is a committed and authentic relationship in which they will strive to remain fully present and open to the child's and family's experiences, no matter how painful or distressing these may be. According to Papadatou[14] such openness "permits us to meet the unknown in life, in others, or in ourselves without preconceived ideas or rigid theories and planned interventions. It allows us to welcome the unexpected without always trying to provide a logical explanation, and to work through the paradoxes that are inherent in life and death situations.… This process demands time, energy, and commitment. When we are consumed by the everyday and rush from one activity, task, or crisis to the next, we do not engage in a deep examination of our experiences and we restrict our capacity to provide effective care and to reap the rewards."

Openness toward self, others, and life is the antithesis of detachment and goes against any attempt to identify a precise distance that is believed to be correct in clinician's relationships with children and their families. Such clinical detachment is touted as protecting us from the suffering, the unexpected, the unfamiliar, or the surprise that occurs in intimate relationships.

Openness is associated with vulnerability. Contrary to the view that vulnerability is a weakness in situations that are perceived as harmful to well-being, it is the ability to be vulnerable enough that enables caregivers to remain open and permeable to others, and to their shared relationships.

What does the experience of being vulnerable enough entail and how does it differ from the experience of being highly vulnerable or invulnerable? Differences are of a qualitative nature. When caregivers cannot differentiate which aspects of an experience belong to them and which to another person with whom they totally identify and develop an enmeshed relationship, they tend to experience self as being highly vulnerable and overwhelmed by care giving. By contrast, when caregivers are threatened or terrified by their increased vulnerability, they tend to hide fears and instead project an image of over-competence, power, and control over situations and relations that evoke anxiety or suffering in themselves. In striving to appear unaffected and invulnerable, caregivers build rigid boundaries and remain oblivious to the private worlds of children and parents, as well as to their own experiences. They limit their attention to a prescribed role and to defined functions that are performed with great efficacy in the pursuit of specific goals.

The experience of being vulnerable enough involves an openness and permeability that enables caregivers to develop a deeper understanding of others, contain suffering without being threatened by it, assist with the challenges of illness, and gives the flexibility to adjust to emerging needs. This same openness and permeability is also experienced in the relationship to self. Caregivers take the time to process experiences, attend to distress or pain, cope with personal issues that have remained unaddressed, and develop a deeper understanding of how caregivers affect and are being affected by encounters with children and their families. When caregivers acknowledge and befriend a suffering that is unavoidable in the face of death, they are more likely to maintain relationships that are authentic, personal, and meaningful to those whom they accompany as well as to themselves.

When caregivers remain open and vulnerable enough, they acknowledge the presence of death in all relationships and cope with its effects upon patients, families, teams, and themselves. Only then may they recognize its violent impact upon relationships which are threatened, broken, or severed forever, as well as its vitalizing force that motivates families to live more fully and confronts us with life's value and meaning.[14,17]

When caregivers perceive their relationships to children and their families as emerging solely in pain and suffering, they tend to neglect the potential of deriving rewards from care giving, and of growing to value life and their existence into the world.

WHAT ARE SOME ASPECTS OF CAREGIVERS SUFFERING?

In the healthcare professions, it is often believed that clinicians do not and should not suffer. However, at the same time, it is often recognized that caring for children who are going to die is filled with stressors or occupational hazards. Previous work has focused on the stressors clinicians encounter, such as exposure to childhood death, communication difficulties, team conflicts, lack of support, and work overload. Some of the responses have been associated to concepts such as burnout, while others to vicarious trauma and compassion fatigue. These conceptualizations describe aspects of professionals' suffering when their ability to care is impaired. However, suffering does not always lead to impairment. The challenge is to distinguish when suffering is a normal, necessary, healthy, unavoidable aspect of the work that can lead to enrichment, and when suffering is unnecessary and indicative of increased anxiety, depression, or disillusionment that requires the help of a senior colleague, mentor, counselor, or psychotherapist. Distinctions between normal and necessary and unnecessary suffering are not always evident, and require both an in-depth knowledge and ongoing awareness of how they are affected by the nature of their work.

Suffering That Leads to Impairment

Suffering that leads to impairment may develop progressively, as in the case of burnout, while at other times may appear to occur suddenly when caregivers are exposed to highly traumatic situations, as in the case of compassion stress or compassion fatigue. Overwhelmed by care giving, clinicians remain limited in their capacities to care for children and families, and concurrently tend to needs for self care. Following is a brief description of some aspects of suffering that lead to impairment, including burnout, compassion stress, and compassion fatigue, which have been studied to great extent among healthcare professionals.

Burnout is a "state of physical, emotional, and mental exhaustion caused by long-term involvement in emotionally demanding situations."[18] Although described as a static state, burnout is more of a process that develops gradually, when:

- Workload is increased or highly stressful, such as the constant exposure to death,
- When caregivers feel powerless or unable to achieve goals,
- When required to display or suppress certain emotions on the job.

Burnout is worsened by not coping adequately with these emotional responses or taking the necessary time to process experiences, review goals, and recharge batteries by addressing the need for self care. Sometimes burnout stems from the long-term effects of caring for others, called caring burnout. At other times it is from becoming disillusioned and losing a sense of purpose and meaning in the care provided, called meaning burnout, either because the job becomes routine, boring or insignificant, or because caregivers doubt the value or effectiveness of the work.[19] The key dimensions of burnout involve emotional exhaustion, a depersonalized approach toward patients and detachment from the job, and a sense of incompetence and lack of achievement.[20] Although the term burnout is used quite casually in the workplace, it is important to recognize that it is a severe psychological condition that is often associated with depressive symptoms, anxiety, and demoralization.

Other times, however, caregivers' suffering occurs suddenly in situations that we experience as highly traumatic. Faced with the trauma of others, we experience compassion stress, which is defined as "the natural consequent behaviours and emotions… resulting from helping or wanting to help a traumatized or suffering person."[21] Figley argues that when caregivers are not satisfied with the help provided, and fail to reduce the suffering of traumatized people, caregivers experience secondary traumatic stress, compassion stress, which can develop

into a secondary traumatic stress disorder that he named compassion fatigue. Symptoms of compassion fatigue are similar to symptoms of a post-traumatic stress disorder (PTSD) and can be grouped in three categories:

- Re-experiencing, that is having intrusive thoughts, feelings, nightmares, re-experiencing symptoms or physiological and psychological distress when exposed to reminders of work with the dying child or bereaved parents,
- Avoidance, that is avoiding thoughts, feelings, rooms, or circumstances that have been experienced as traumatic in our work with the family,
- Hyperarousal, that is irritability, hypervigilance, sleep problems, outbursts of anger or crying.

In reality, compassion fatigue is a disorder that requires professional help.

When caregivers are burned out or seriously traumatized by their involvement with families of seriously ill children and the exposure to dying and death, they experience disruptions in our world view, thinking the world is unjust, They also experience disruptions in the view of self, thinking "I'm powerless" or "I'm incompetent" and in the meaning they attribute to life and existence. These inner transformations negatively affect caregivers' well-being, as well as the nature of relationships with those they serve. Such pervasive suffering requires the help of a mental health professional.

Suffering That Is Unavoidable

Not all suffering is hazardous to caregivers' well-being and to the quality of their work. Some of their distress to the pain and suffering of seriously ill or dying children, and grieving parents, is unavoidable (Fig. 18-2). Not infrequently it reflects a grieving process over losses that are experienced in acute

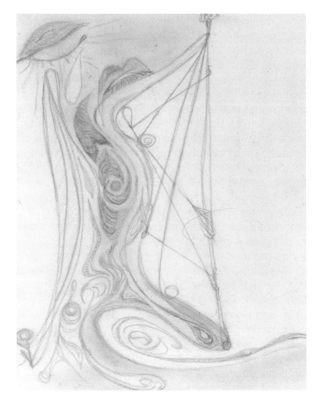

Fig. 18-2 Grief. Illustration by Danai Papadatou.

or chronic life-and-death situations.[22–26] Papadatou[14] offers a model that describes the healthy, unavoidable grieving process triggered by an event or situations that are perceived as losses. For example, some clinicians experience as loss the death of a child and grieve over a special bond that has been severed forever; others experience as loss the non-realization of professional goals to cure a child; still others grieve over personal loss that surfaces with exposure to a child's death. Most often such losses trigger a grieving process that presents unique characteristics. It involves an ongoing fluctuation between experiencing grief responses, and avoiding or repressing them. This fluctuation enables clinicians to acknowledge their losses but also set them aside in order to function appropriately without being overwhelmed. Moving in and out from grief helps to attribute meaning to their experiences with regard to the dying process and death of a patient, as well as to their roles and contributions in the care of families of seriously ill children.

By contrast, the lack of fluctuation between experiencing and avoiding loss and grief may lead to manifestations of grief overload and complications that compromise the quality of services caregivers provide and may leave them to feel overwhelmed.

There are times when caregivers' suffering seems more intense or pervasive; such intense feelings may be particularly invoked when work experiences resonate with unresolved personal issues. It is not uncommon to feel overwhelmed by the care of an adolescent patient who reminds a caregiver of an adolescent at home, or to avoid a family who is faced with decisions regarding end-of-life care, when the caregivers are confronted with similar dilemmas and decisions in the care of a dying parent. When work experiences invade personal lives or when personal experiences invade work lives, caregivers need to seek supervision or mentoring that can help set boundaries, explore suffering and seek helpful ways to mitigate it by addressing their own needs.

The progressive understanding of caregivers' private worlds has several benefits. First, it makes them aware that they are not immune to suffering; expertise in this field of work does not guarantee immunity to pain, uncertainty, loss, and death. Second, it normalizes several of their responses and sensitizes them to some aspects of suffering that impair the provision of care and negatively affect their mental health. Third, it motivates caregivers to develop coping patterns that can help them accept their suffering, ease its distressing effects, transform it in creative ways, and seek help when suffering is unbearable. Fourth, it uncovers vulnerability in the face of death and confronts caregivers with their limitations, as a result of which they may become more humble in their approach. Fifth, it offers opportunities to examine expressed or latent motives for assisting families in life-and-death situations and to address caregivers' anxieties and review their coping patterns in the face of loss and suffering. Finally, it incites caregivers to develop resources that enhance their resilience in adversity. Wisdom and growth can stem from accepting both their strengths and limitations and from acknowledging the rewarding aspects of care giving in life-and-death situations.

What Are Some of the Rewards?

Rewarding experiences have several sources (Fig. 18-3). Sometimes they are associated with the outcomes of caregivers' interventions, the achievement of a desired goal, the

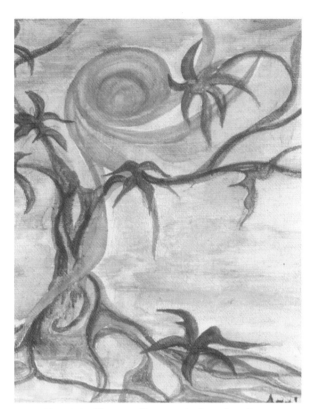

Fig. 18-3   Nurturing. Illustration by Danai Papadatou.

accomplishment a specific task, or the effective management of a challenging situation. While the ultimate goal in pediatric palliative care is to enhance the quality of life of seriously ill children and of their family members by attending to their physical, psychosocial, and spiritual needs, the criteria that define quality of life are often vague and subjective because they vary among patients and families. At times the goals that, according to one set of values enhance quality of life do not coincide with the priorities of families who strive for a cure, the prolongation of life even when its quality is seriously compromised, or hope for a miracle. Unfortunately, in pediatric palliative care, what families desire most, the cure of their child, cannot be provided. This explains why the rewards caregivers derive are most often associated with the process by which services are provided. They involve, for example, the establishment of caring relationships or bonds; an availability, presence, and compassion through the diagnosis, illness, or dying trajectory; the creativity and resourcefulness by which caregivers respond to needs; or the fruitful collaboration with co-workers in the pursuit of shared goals.

Rewards are profound when caregivers find value and attribute meaning to a job that is well done and contributes to the fulfillment and growth of others, whose lives are positively affected. Caregivers derive meaning from assisting families in coping with major challenges and, despite their suffering, sometimes live peak experiences that function as a source of comfort after the child's death. Such peak experiences are uncommon experiences that are experienced as intensely meaningful or highly significant and unforgettable and are usually associated with feelings of awe, wonder, connection, and love.[27]

When caregivers value their services, they pass their knowledge and seek to affect others by sharing their experiences and wisdom. Caregivers experience what Yalom[28] describes as "rippling." Through actions that are not aimed at fame, prestige, or self-elevation, but rather toward a social good, caregivers create multiple concentric circles of influence that effect, oftentimes without their conscious knowledge, the lives of others for years and generations.

Rewards in Palliative Care

Finally, rewards in palliative care are associated with a sense of personal growth that may be experienced at various levels[14]:

Growth Associated with Perception of Self Caregivers develop an altered and expanded view of self that results from an increased awareness of who they are. They perceive self as more able to cope with stress and suffering, and more appreciative of the many common joys of life. Caregivers feel more competent to deal with adversities, remain humble about their achievements, and acknowledge their strengths, vulnerabilities, and limitations.

Growth Associated with Perception of and Connection to Others Caregivers relate to others with greater compassion and understanding and remain open to their experiences, both in suffering and in joy. They are authentic, genuine, and expressive, and connect with greater warmth, caring, and respect.

Growth Associated with Life Perspective Life is not perceived superficially, but valued and lived with increased awareness. Caregivers reflect upon their personal goals and priorities and actively strive to live a life that is enriching to them and their loved ones. Frequent reminders of their own mortality encourage them to review their own lives, imagine their ultimate end, and contemplate the finality of valued relationships. Despite the anxiety that such a process engenders, it usually becomes an awakening experience through which caregivers can change unfulfilling lives, or cope with regrets over missed opportunities and any sense that life has slipped away. Through this process caregivers develop new perceptions of who they are, make new choices over what is important to strive for, and feel free to live differently.[28]

To experience the rewards of care giving in pediatric palliative care, caregivers must first be willing to illuminate what Jellinek[29] described as the "dark side" of caring for seriously ill children. That involves an acceptance of a suffering that is inevitable when life is threatened and caring bonds are severed by death. This demands a willingness to create the space and time to reflect over caregivers' work experiences in order to better understand how they affect and are being affected by the children and parents served. It also requires that caregivers explore the meaning they attribute to their experiences, to personal issues that compromise the care provided, and to identify those resources that help them do a good enough job.

However, caregivers must keep in mind that this process is not solely an individual affair. Their suffering and rewarding experiences in pediatric palliative care are also affected by professional, social, and cultural variables. As long as the education of physicians and nurses reinforces a biomedical approach to care and socializes future clinicians to maintain a stoic and detached approach toward the suffering of others, then self-awareness and self-care will continue to be discarded as unimportant and remain exclusively a private affair. Moreover, sociocultural values and norms determine how clinicians are expected to cope

with death, how they express and manage their grief, what meaning they attribute to patient loss, and what types of support, if any, are available to them. When Greek and Hong Kong pediatric nurses were compared with regard to their responses to the dying process and death of a child, it was found that all experienced a grieving process that remained largely disenfranchised because, in their social contexts, they were expected to be strong and brave in the face of death. However, nurses in these cultures had distinct ways of expressing and coping with their grief.[30] Greek nurses displayed their grief openly, cried more frequently, and supported each other within the confines of their unit, which valued and enhanced mutual support. By contrast, Hong Kong nurses were more private and tended to suppress their grief by resorting to practical duties and work responsibilities. Differences were also found when Greek nurses were compared to Greek physicians.[31] The latter were more likely to perceive the death of a child as a failure to achieve their professional goals to cure the disease and to prevent death, and reported more avoidant strategies with regard to their grief.

Clinician Suffering and Self-Care

While some clinician suffering may seem inevitable, much unnecessary suffering is caused by specific maladaptive attitudes of the caregiver themselves. Fortunately, once recognized these maladaptive attitudes can be corrected and suffering lessened by practical actions such as mindful practice (Box 18-1). The second part of this chapter offers step-by-step examples of mindful practice skills;[32,33] a set of practical, learnable life skills for self-care that serves to reduce or transform suffering in meaningful ways.

Awareness itself is not a thought, but is more a state of being fully in the present non-judgmentally. Rather than a thought, awareness is a lived experience. The difficulty in conveying mindful awareness lies in the limits of words and their ability to convey concepts better than ideas. Concepts need only words to be understood and communicated while ideas include a component that needs to be experienced if they are to be fully communicated.[34] For example while the concept of the physiology of taste can be communicated via words, that is the pathway from taste receptors in the tongue and the neurophysiology of neurotransmitters leading to the sensory cortex, the idea of what a piece of chocolate actually tastes like cannot be effectively communicated by words alone.

BOX 18-1 Suffering in Clinicians

By bearing witness to the suffering of others, clinicians involved in relationships with ill children and their families will themselves experience suffering.

Some aspects of living with grief and loss are unavoidable, and are healthy and adaptive, leading to an enriched relationship with children and their families. However, unnecessary and avoidable suffering occurs when there is either prolonged attachment to, or non-acceptance of, grief, loss, and other emotions that may contribute to clinicians becoming overwhelmed or depressed.

Clinicians can learn to reduce or transform the suffering caused by attachment or the non-acceptance of grief and loss. Moving from suffering toward acceptance is a process that leads to wholeness and healing.[38,39]

Reducing clinicians' suffering may be achieved by cultivating specific practical actions, including finding a healthy balance between work-life and outside interests, seeking medical and psychological support when needed, and integrating mindfulness and mindful practice into daily life.

Awareness, while an individual experience, is cultivated through relating to others and to the world around us. Sometimes it occurs on its own, spontaneously, even if it is not necessarily recognized as awareness at the time it is happening. Such moments are often described as being out of time when, in the space that exists between thoughts and feelings, we exist within a field of pure awareness of moment to moment lived experience. In sports or while being fully engaged in any activity, this has been described as being in the flow. Being completely aware of the moment to moment experience that develops in the flow is an example of active awareness. Such a feeling is to be fully awake, receptive to what is. It is devoid of thought or judgment about how good, bad, or special the experience is.

Awareness is important because it increases insight into the personal feelings, biases, and experiences that each person brings into relationships including those with seriously ill children and their family members. It renders caregivers open to the experiences of others and to becoming attuned to their responses and needs in the present moment. Being aware means accepting that while clinicians may experience many things, including sorrow, loss, and anger, they are aware that these responses are happening and do not mistake these feelings as being either necessarily true or self-defining. When caregivers feel sorrow over the impending death of a child they cared for, they can meet the sadness with an awareness of feelings and an awareness of the need to let go of unrealistic goals. There is also understanding of the healing role yet to be played in the remaining, perhaps brief, life of the child, as well as the lives of family members. In recognizing personal sadness, we acknowledge that these are simply thoughts and feelings and that they will come and go like all thoughts and feelings eventually to dissipate and be replaced by others. Thus being aware moment to moment means being less attached to our thoughts and feelings and more ready to observe them in the moment as they flow one to another. While feeling sadness, caregivers are aware they are having feelings of sadness rather than seeing the sadness as who they are. Caregivers themselves are not sad, but rather are aware that they are experiencing sadness. Sadness is not them.

So if mindful practice depends on cultivating awareness, and awareness cannot be understood until it is experienced then tasting awareness is needed to know awareness. While there are different ways to be aware, and to be mindful, there are also specific practices or exercises that facilitate the experience of active awareness.

The following exercise relates to the awareness of the breath as an example of how to cultivate awareness. What you need for this five-minute exercise is a physical place where you will not be disturbed during the exercise. Read through the instructions in Box 18-2, then simply put the book down for a few minutes and try the exercise for yourself.

REACTING VERSUS RESPONDING

Paying attention purposefully, moment to moment, is a simple concept to understand but for most is not easy in practice. Focusing attention on the breath is very challenging as it is difficult (at first) to not be carried away by a stream of thoughts that lead away from focusing on the sensations of breathing. Being mindful, even for a brief period of time such as during

---

BOX 18-2 Five-Minute Seated Awareness Exercise

You might consider doing this exercise as an experiment in self-care. The following questions will help set the tone to enter into this exercise:

What do you have to lose in trying this exercise? What barriers, such as negative thoughts and pre-judgments, are you experiencing as you consider trying this exercise?

Can you give yourself permission to have nothing to do and nowhere to go for 5 minutes in your life to try this exercise? Are you able to dismiss any thoughts that come up during the 5-minute period that might stop you from completing it?

What are your expectations as you enter into this exercise? Can you enter into the exercise with as few expectations as possible?

1. In your seated position, in a chair or on a pillow on the floor, place yourself comfortably upright. Your back should be a few inches forward from the backrest so that you are supporting yourself. Your arms can be relaxed and supported on armrests, in front of you on your knees, or overlapping in front of you. Your eyes can be directed forward and slightly downward so that your gaze falls softly on a point two or three feet in front of you. If you feel comfortable you may allow your eyes to close at any point during this exercise.

2. Rock very gently back and forth in your seat a few times. Feel your body, feel your arms, your hands. Feel your weight being supported by the chair and the floor and the earth beneath you.

3. Sitting in this posture, awake and alert, take three deliberate deep, slow breaths. Allow your belly to expand fully on the inhale and relax completely on the exhale.

4. Allow your natural rhythm of breathing to unfold. When thoughts arise, just notice the thought. There is no need to control your thoughts, no need to judge them, just become aware of them as they come and go.

5. Settle your awareness into the breath. Focus your awareness on the different components of breathing, such as the feeling of the air going in and out of your nostrils and mouth; the feeling of your belly rising and falling. Notice the rhythm of breathing, that sometimes comes in short bursts and other times in slower waves. Avoid judging or trying to control the breath; just notice its character from moment to moment.

6. Become aware of the still point between inhalation and exhalation.

7. Allow your awareness to ride the waves of breathing as you inhale and exhale. If thoughts or emotions arise, then note them and let them go. Give yourself permission to not chase after thoughts of "I should," "I need to," and so on. No matter what the thought or emotion or feeling is, notice it and let it be. Notice how one thought is always followed by another.

8. If sensations arise such as an itch or a pain, notice them and experiment with not reaching out with your hand to alleviate them by scratching or rubbing. What happens to the sensation if you focus your awareness on the sensation rather than seeking to alleviate it? If you do scratch or shift position notice how another sensation often takes its place and continues the cycle of sensation-action. What happens if you choose to observe the sensation rather than seek to alleviate it? What thoughts arise during these sensations? Do you label them as good or bad, tolerable or intolerable?

9. If you get lost in thought, then notice that has occurred, let go of the thought and bring your awareness back to your breath. You may need to do this again and again even during only a 5-minute period. This process of beginning again and again and coming back to the breath is part of the process of awareness.

10. Sit like this for about 5 minutes. Many find it easier to focus on the breath with eyes closed but if you feel more comfortable with your eyes open, then do so.

When you are ready, gently open your eyes. Notice how you are feeling, right now, in this moment.

If you managed, even once in the 5-minute period, to feel the difference between you and your thoughts, then you were experiencing active awareness, even if it was frustrating and if many thoughts kept intruding one after the other. It is your attention to whatever is going on inside and outside you that matters.

the previous exercise, is practice in breaking the old habit of mindless reactivity that fills most of our lives. When caregivers are immersed in the stream of their own thoughts and associated emotions, they experience the opposite of mindful attention. Such a state of inattention, of mindless immersion, does not allow for an examination of the quality of our inner experiences, such as physical sensations, thoughts, and emotions.

However, as in the example of the seated awareness exercise, caregivers can develop personal habits that help create a space between the unconscious automatic reactions, such as thoughts and feelings, and create a possibility of transforming them into conscious responses. Strengthening this new habit of being aware requires a commitment to change old habits of thinking and being, which have usually been the default mode. The reactive, mindless, automatic pilot mode of believing each thought, feeling, and reaction as true is not an easy one to break. Sustained practice encourages moment to moment non-judgmental awareness and acceptance of what is rather than how one wishes things were. Bringing an open awareness and attitude of acceptance to the bedside of ill people is not only good for clinicians, but also for their patients and colleagues. Such an attitude of acceptance of the way things actually are evolves over time as the byproduct of such a mindful awareness practice.

One common question that arises when beginning an awareness practice is how to differentiate acceptance of the way things are from passive acceptance and inaction. True acceptance of the way things are does not mean that everything is OK. Nevertheless, accepting the way things are is the first step to clearly identifying what needs to be done without resorting to automatic reacting. Reacting is an autopilot response to both the external and internal world. For example, when faced with a distressing situation, caregivers' bodies may react with flushing, sweating, tachycardia, or a minor irritation may be fueled into anger with thoughts of past grievances. Becoming aware of these reactions, through regular awareness practice, gives caregivers the ability to re-examine their responses and decide whether they are helpful or not. If they are aware of their reactions, in the moment, they can choose to decide whether the reaction is based on limited information or triggered by past hurts or sleights, then open up the possibility for transforming the automatic reaction into a conscious response. Reactions that are evaluated upon then become responses that have been chosen.

While a regular practice of between 5 and 30 minutes a day is the mainstay of a regular mindful practice,[33] it is also possible to practice mini deliberate moments of active awareness throughout the day. Kearney and colleagues[35] have outlined awareness practices that can be incorporated into the caregivers' workplace, some of which are included in the following list:

- Each day set aside a few moments at the very beginning of the day, while brushing your teeth or after parking your car, to remind yourself what your goal or desire is for your day and why you are doing the work. For example, you might say to yourself that you are entering into your day with the intention to do work that reduces the suffering of others and with attention to being aware of your thoughts, bodily sensations, and feelings as they emerge. Give yourself permission to fail many times during the day, indeed expect to forget your intention and attention several times, and then come back to your intention and attention whenever you can with warmth and gentleness toward yourself.

- As you walk from one place to the next during your day, pay attention to the sensation of contact between your feet and the ground. If you find yourself rushing while walking, see if you can give yourself permission to slow your pace and feel each step. When sitting, become aware of the feeling of the chair holding you up.

- When it comes to mind, pay attention to how you are breathing. If you are aware of physical tension take a deep slow breath letting your belly expand fully on the in breath. This can be particularly helpful during meetings when you are sitting for long periods of time.

- At set points during the day, such as before lunch or between patient visits, take three deliberate slow breaths and bring yourself back to the moment and whatever you are feeling and thinking at the time.

- When you complete a task, take a moment to reward yourself with a deep breath, a stretch, or a brief walk.

- After very emotional events, take some time, even just a few minutes, to re-center yourself before heading into the next task. This is best accomplished by physically removing yourself from the place the event occurred and finding some time and space to take a few breaths and come back to your sense of self in your body.

- Focus your attention on a visual or written cue that you find peaceful, such as a treasured oasis photograph, a brief poem or prayer that you find especially meaningful, or something in nature that you can see out the window. If you can see a tree or a bird, focus your vision and full attention on the nature object and rest in awareness of that object for a few moments.

- Before a meeting with colleagues, take a moment to center yourself with a breath and remind yourself of your intention to serve to reduce suffering and your attention to being aware of the flow of thoughts and feelings as they occur. Should you feel angry or bored, be aware of that feeling or thought, and instead of reacting you can decide how to respond. When taking the time to respond, you may find that no action is needed.

- How is your effectiveness changed when you fail to listen to your body? Becoming aware of your body more often opens the possibility for you to take better physical care of yourself. If hungry, then have a snack; when the need occurs go to the washroom.

- When washing your hands, use the time to be more aware of what you are doing, with active awareness. Can you feel the sensation of the water on your hands, the soap on your skin, the temperature of the water? Take a slow centering breath while drying your hands.

- See how often you can make connections with others throughout the day and observe how you feel when you do so. Make eye contact with colleagues and see if you can listen without thinking of the next thing you will say. When you greet other workers in the hospital, experiment with making eye contact and asking them something about themselves or their work. How does this affect the quality of your day?

- Try writing down your thoughts, feelings, and experiences in a notepad by your desk or at home at the end of the day (a narrative writing exercise). You may choose to share some of this writing with colleagues when the time feels right, perhaps during a debriefing session after a patient's death (Box 18-3).

- If you have a long drive to work, try listening to a book on CD or tape instead of the radio. At another time, experiment with not listening to anything at all for the drive and observe the stream of thoughts as they come and go. Where does the need for distraction come from? What are you distracting yourself from?
- When appropriate, find a way to make physical contact with the patient in some appropriate way during the encounter. If while performing a physical exam you are listening to the heart, place your hand gently on the patient's shoulder or arm at the same time.
- Be gentle with yourself. Expect to make many mistakes over and over. Simply restate your intention and attention, and begin again.

BOX 18-3 Narrative Writing Exercise

A 13-year-old girl with end-stage advanced leukemia is the type of palliative care consult that is among the hardest for me and I do not need a psychotherapist to help me figure out why. She is the same age as my own daughter. I have been following her and her family for 7 months and have found myself pulled along as they rode the ups and downs of remission and relapse. Now I am about to ring the doorbell for what will be the last or near to last home visit, because she has slipped to the point of being unresponsive now for two days. I stand outside the door of their home and I feel both the urge to run away and the desire to enter into their situation; somehow co-existing despite the lack of sense that makes. I need to, I need to think, or perhaps instead I need to just be. Before I ring the bell and enter the home I pause and take a few moments: three slow deep breaths. I return my attention to my breath each time my mind wanders from one anxious thought to the next. I recognize that I am making my own suffering worse because I'm imagining that this is my own daughter. But she is not my daughter and it is not helpful to me or to them for me to imagine that it is. I ask myself to focus on my intention to be with the way things are and not to get lost in imaginary thoughts of what if this was my own precious girl. Can I stay with the energy of the moment and drop the storyline that imagines this as my own daughter? I bring attention to what I am thinking and feeling; I focus on my breathing and the task ahead. My intention is clear: to be as present for this family and ill child as I can, and to be with them and attend to what they tell me they need. I ring the bell and enter.

Team Care

While the individual clinician needs to establish his or her own self-care practice, working within teams of colleagues presents its own opportunities and challenges. Team dynamics and implicit or explicit rules can promote or negate individual efforts to reduce suffering. In some teams, admissions of individual suffering is perceived as unacceptable, upsetting, and threatening to team functioning. In this environment, clinicians learn to repress and hide their own suffering; they display an outwardly stoic approach to loss and death, and support each other in the suppression of their suffering. This group dynamic of mutual suppression leads to dysfunctional team patterns. By contrast, functional patterns occur when the team's culture acknowledges individual and collective suffering, and sets as a priority the establishment of a holding environment for its members.[14] A holding environment:

- Contains the clinicians' suffering without dismissing, repressing, masking, or distorting it,
- Facilitates the elaboration of painful experiences by inviting sharing, reflection, and the circulation of information among team members,
- Tempers suffering by reframing painful events by planning activities and rituals that acknowledge the clinicians' grief, and by using resources to build upon a collective sense of resilience,
- Cultivates interconnectedness and mutual support among team members.

Establishing a holding environment is not a responsibility assumed solely by the team's leader, but rather is shared by all team members who display genuine acts of compassion and support among each other. However, the team leader has the responsibility of embodying self-care as well as establishing a safe environment in which clinicians communicate openly and freely and share personal feelings, thoughts, and experiences. Team leaders adopt different approaches in their work with professionals and teams. One common approach focuses on the analysis and management of specific cases or events. Emphasis is placed on understanding the specifics of a work situation and alternative coping patterns and solutions to problems are considered. Clinicians become more aware of their actions and develop an increased sense of control and self-efficacy. Another approach focuses on individual and team functioning in the face of crisis, loss, and death. Conflicts, tensions and dynamics are exposed, reviewed, and analyzed, while emphasis is placed on strengthening relationships among professionals and building personal and team resources in order to cope with the challenges of a child's death and family bereavement. Team leaders may implicitly bring self-care awareness practices to team meetings by the leader's ability to be aware of his or her own thoughts, feelings, judgments, and reactions; that is, to be a mindful team leader. A team leader who is mindful of his or herself, others, and the environment will be less reactive and more responsive, and will embody the practice of mindful awareness through their own behaviors. Mindful practice may also be explicitly introduced to the team by the introduction of half- or full-day workshops, outside of patient care demands, that offer different kinds of mindfulness-awareness practices, such as group-guided sitting meditation, walking meditation, silent meal, and mindful yoga .

Summary

This chapter was conceived as one that would provide background to better understand the need for self-care and its entwined relationship with care giving to those who suffer. Understanding the underlying dynamics in relationships in which patients, family members, and care providers are mutually and reciprocally influenced is not enough to bring about increased awareness, and to that end, the chapter outlines specific awareness self-care practices that infuse conceptual understanding with experiential learning. There are many resources available for developing mindfulness self-care practice in books; on Internet sites such as www.umassmed.edu/Content.aspx?id=41252, in seminars, and workshops.[5,36,37] It is also important to be reminded that self awareness and self-care, although inherently individual processes, are developed and enriched through relationships with others. Being open to new understandings and experiences is itself rewarding as we mindfully walk along the path this work offers us.

REFERENCES

1. Maslow AH: *Religions, values, and peak experiences*, Harmondsworth, Engl. Markham, Ont: 1976, Penguin Books.
2. Coles R: *The call of service: a witness to idealism*, Boston, 1993, Houghton Mifflin.
3. Meyer EC, et al: Improving the quality of end-of-life care in the pediatric intensive care unit: parents' priorities and recommendations, *Pediatrics* 117(3):649–657, 2006.
4. Macdonald ME, et al: Parental perspectives on hospital staff members' acts of kindness and commemoration after a child's death, *Pediatrics* 116(4):884–890, 2005.
5. Kabat-Zinn J: *Wherever you go, there you are*, London, 2005, Piatkus.
6. Contro N, et al: Family perspectives on the quality of pediatric palliative care, *Arch Pediatr Adolesc Med* 156(1):14–19, 2002.
7. Contro NA, et al: Hospital staff and family perspectives regarding quality of pediatric palliative care, *Pediatrics* 114(5):1248–1252, 2004.
8. Heller KS, Solomon MZ: For the Initiative for Pediatric Palliative Care Investigator: Continuity of care and caring: what matters to parents of children with life-threatening conditions, *J Pediatr Nurs* 20(5):335–346, 2005.
9. Kreicbergs U, et al: Care-related distress: a nationwide study of parents who lost their child to cancer, *J Clin Oncol* 23(36):9162–9171, 2005.
10. Mack JW, et al: Parent and physician perspectives on quality of care at the end of life in children with cancer, *J Clin Oncol* 23(36):9155–9161, 2005.
11. Steinhauser KE, et al: Factors considered important at the end of life by patients, family, physicians, and other care providers, *JAMA* 284(19):2476–2482, 2000.
12. Steinhauser KE, et al: In search of a good death: observations of patients, families, and providers, *Ann Intern Med* 132(10):825–832, 2000.
13. Solomon MZ, Browning D: Pediatric palliative care: relationships matter and so does pain control, *J Clin Oncol* 23(36):9055–9057, 2005.
14. Papadatou D: *In the face of death: professionals who care for the dying and the bereaved*, New York, 2009, Springer, pp 330.
15. Beach MC, Inui T, Relationship-Centered Care Research: Relationship-centered care: a constructive reframing, *J Gen Intern Med* 21(Suppl 1):S3–S8, 2006.
16. Stern D: *The present moment in psychotherapy and everyday life*, New York, 2004, WW Norton.
17. Hennezel M: *La mort intime*, París, 1995, Editions Robert Laffont SA.
18. Pines A, Aronson E: *Career burnout: Causes and cures*, New York, 1988, Free Press.
19. Skovholt T: *The resilient practitioner: burnout prevention and self-care strategies for counselors, therapists, teachers, and health professionals*, Boston, 2001, Allyn and Bacon.
20. Maslach C: Job burnout: new directions in research and intervention, *Curr Dir Psychol Sci* 12(5):189–192, 2003.
21. Figley C: Compassion fatigue: psychotherapists' chronic lack of self care, *J Clin Psychol* 58(11):2002.
22. Davies B, et al: Caring for dying children: nurses' experiences, *Pediatr Nurs* 22(6):500–507, 1996.
23. Hinds PS, et al: The impact of a grief workshop for pediatric oncology nurses on their grief and perceived stress, *J Pediatr Nurs* 9(6):388–397, 1994.
24. Kaplan LJ: Toward a model of caregiver grief: nurses' experiences of treating dying children, *Omega: J Death Dying* 41(3):187–206, 2000.
25. Rashotte J, Fothergill-Bourbonnais F, Chamberlain M: Pediatric intensive care nurses and their grief experiences: a phenomenological study, *Heart Lung* 26(5):372–386, 1997.
26. Shanfield SB: The mourning of the health care professional: an important element in education about death and loss, *Death Educ* 4(4):385–395, 1981.
27. Clarke-Steffen L: The meaning of peak and nadir experiences of pediatric oncology nurses: secondary analysis, *J Pediatr Oncol Nurs* 15(1):25–33, 1998.
28. Yalom ID: *Staring at the sun: overcoming the terror of death*, San Francisco, 2008, Jossey-Bass.
29. Jellinek MS, et al: Pediatric intensive care training: confronting the dark side, *Crit Care Med* 21(5):775–779, 1993.
30. Papadatou D, Martinson IM, Chung PM: Caring for dying children: a comparative study of nurses' experiences in Greece and Hong Kong, *Cancer Nurs* 24(5):402–412, 2001.
31. Papadatou D, et al: Greek nurse and physician grief as a result of caring for children dying of cancer, *Pediatr Nurs* 28(4):345–353, 2002.
32. Epstein RM: Mindful practice, *JAMA* 282(9):833–839, 1999.
33. Kabat-Zinn J, C.W. University of Massachusetts Medical: *Full catastrophe living: using the wisdom of your body and mind to face stress, pain, and illness*, New York, 2005, Delta Trade Paperbacks.
34. Hutchinson TA, Dobkin PL: Mindful medical practice: just another fad? *Can Fam Physician* 55(8):778–779, 2009.
35. Kearney MK, et al: Self-care of physicians caring for patients at the end of life: "Being connected… a key to my survival," *JAMA* 301(11):1155–1164, E1, 2009.
36. Tedeschi R, Calhoun L: *Trauma and transformation: growing in the aftermath of suffering*, Thousand Oaks, Calif, 1995, Sage Publications.
37. Halifax J, Byock I: *Being with dying: cultivating compassion and fearlessness in the presence of death*, Boston, 2008, Shambhala Publications.
38. Kearney M: *A place of healing: working with suffering in living and dying*, Oxford; New York, 2000, Oxford University Press.
39. Mount BM, Boston PH, Cohen SR: Healing connections: on moving from suffering to a sense of well-being, *J Pain Symptom Manage* 33(4):372–388, 2007.

19 Practical Aspects of Communication

JENNIFER W. MACK | PAMELA S. HINDS

People are disturbed not by things but by the view they take of them. They may forget what you said, but they will never forget how you made them feel. —Carl W. Buechner

Perhaps the most important thing we bring to another person is the silence in us. Not the sort of silence that is filled with unspoken criticism or hard withdrawal. The sort of silence that is a place of refuge, of rest, of acceptance of someone as they are. We are all hungry for this other silence. It is hard to find. In its presence we can remember something beyond the moment, a strength on which to build a life. Silence is a place of great power and healing.

—Rachel Naomi Remen, M.D., in *My Grandfather's Blessing*

When our daughter was dying in the intensive care unit, our physician was in the room with us and he did not say anything, but he put his hand on my shoulder and joined us in prayer. And that is what I remember still six months after my child died and that quiet touch is what comforts me.

—Mother of a deceased child

Juan was a 10-year-old boy with refractory leukemia. He was a boy full of love for his family and friends. As Juan's cancer progressed, it became clear to his clinicians and parents that the end of his life was near. His parents wanted to make sure he was aware that he was dying and that he had the opportunity to talk about it, but they felt unable to initiate this conversation themselves because of their intense sadness. They asked his physician, Dr. K., to speak with Juan privately.

After a conversation about how Juan was feeling, Dr. K. asked Juan what else he would like to talk about during their time together. Juan's eyes widened, he sat up in bed, and said, "Am I going to die?" When Dr. K. responded by asking Juan what he thought about that, Juan said, "I think I am." "Yes, Juan," Dr. K. replied quietly, "I think you will die, too." Dr. K. paused, then asked, "How do you feel about that?" Juan described worries about his parents and brother and sister, wondering how he could help everyone if he was no longer alive. Dr. K. asked Juan what he believed would happen to him when he died. Juan replied, "Heaven." "What does Heaven mean to you?" Dr. K. asked. Juan replied,

"It means that my family will be OK, and that they will know I love them." Dr. K. affirmed the beauty of this Heaven. Juan spoke at length about his thoughts of Heaven while Dr. K. quietly listened. As the conversation drew to a close, Dr. K. spoke about the special things she would always remember about him. Dr. K. asked Juan's permission to talk about their conversation with his family.

Being able to effectively talk to children honestly about their physical status and illness, their treatment, and their prognosis in ways that are matched with their age, maturation and clinical situation is expected of clinicians.[1-5] This expectation spans all clinical settings from primary care to emergency care[6,7] unless there are extreme circumstances such as a parent or legal guardian forbidding that kind of talk[8,9] or the treating culture is opposed.[10] The American Academy of Pediatrics (AAP) has produced a technical report, which states communication competency that includes cultural effectiveness is part of the ideal standards of behavior and professional practice for pediatricians.[11] The AAP also issued a policy statement indicating that primary care pediatric clinicians need to be able to elicit concerns from children within their cultural context.[7] Even more specifically, professional specialty associations have issued position papers making explicit the expectations that clinicians will be willing and able to effectively and compassionately share information with a child regarding the nature of the child's illness, the type, duration and likely experience and outcomes of its treatment, and to be readily available to revisit the discussion as the child signals need.

For most child patients, life is centered within a family and communication occurs within that context. Although communication with children is a crucial skill, communication with the entire family is no less vital to care for the child with a life-threatening illness. Thus the guidance offered below considers communication in the setting of a relationship among the clinician, child, and family, with respect for the highly individualized nature of family relationships.

What Is Effective Communication?

Effective communication is the making of a human connection with a child and family. The transmission of information, while essential, is by no means the only role of effective communication. In addition, the communication encounter serves as the foundation for a relationship that unfolds over time. Communication provides the clinician with the opportunity to learn about the child and family: who they are as people, their beliefs and sources of support, the meaning of the illness in their lives, their needs, their goals, their hopes, and their fears. As such, vital roles by the clinician include listening and eliciting information in the encounter. Resulting knowledge allows the clinician to communicate in a way that is helpful for this child and family, to provide care specifically tailored to them, and to consider who they are as people along the illness trajectory. This knowledge serves as a foundation for effective decision making and as a foundation for a meaningful therapeutic alliance, which in itself can support end-of-life decision making.[12] Much of this can be achieved not through the use of particular words, but through caring interaction among the child, family, and clinician. Although the language used matters,[13] the emerging clinician-child-parent relationship matters more. Therefore, although specific words and phrases may be considered as possible tools for these conversations, clinicians who approach these encounters with a sincere desire to listen and get to know the child and family, and to be trusted by them, are likely to be the most successful.

Although the clinician may come into the communication with an agenda for transmitting information about the child's illness or plans for care, quiet presence and a willingness to allow the encounter to unfold cannot be overemphasized as a foundation for the interactions that form a relationship. This conversation is part of a relationship, and not a single interaction; the outcome of any one conversation is less important than the family's and child's experience of the relationship over time. Even when medical information must be discussed or decisions about medical care are critical, parents and children need the opportunity to raise the issues most important to them. Often the issues important to the team and family are similar, but when they are not, forgoing the family's and child's interests to address the medical issues is rarely productive; instead, a joint agenda should be developed. As with other aspects of communication, this allows the clinician to understand what is most important to the child and family, and also reminds the family that what is important to them is also important to the clinician.

WHY IS EFFECTIVE COMMUNICATION IMPORTANT IN PEDIATRIC PALLIATIVE AND END-OF-LIFE CARE?

The attention given to communicating with a seriously ill child and his or her family is attributed to the belief that effective communication helps the child and family to:

- Anticipate what they will likely experience secondary to the illness or its treatment, including adversities,[4]
- Make effective decisions about care,[14]
- Cope with the clinical and life situations,[5]
- Have less confusion and anxiety or depression related to both the illness and the treatment,[15]
- Feel respected by the clinicians,[8]
- Establish a trusting relationship with the healthcare team,[16]
- Establish a forum and process for ongoing support, transmission of information, and making decisions.

Additionally, providing children with information about their diseases and treatments meets legal regulations and ethical considerations[8,17] in terms of assent and consent. Finally,

carefully communicated information about illness and treatment can also promote self-care behaviors in the ill child, such as learning to recognize and avoid high-risk situations,[18] and promote child participation in treatment decision making.[16,19,20] On the other hand, insensitive or incomplete communication is reported to be distressing to the pediatric patient and his or her family, including the siblings.[21]

WHAT ARE THE GUIDING PRINCIPLES OF COMMUNICATING EFFECTIVELY WITH THE SERIOUSLY ILL CHILD AND FAMILY?

The complexity of communicating with seriously ill children is well recognized by clinicians and is underscored in their reported anxiety about discussions with these children and their families.[4,22] Perhaps as a direct result of the complexity and importance of communicating with children and families, clinicians have created guides and principles intended to assist in their efforts to communicate with children (Table 19-1). The first principle of communication between a child and a clinician is that the communication needs to always take place within a family context.[23] Families enter into an illness experience with a style of communication already in place. Effective communicators recognize that parents and guardians are the most knowledgeable about their child and are thus the experts about the child[24] (Box 19-1).

Just as every family is different, children and families experience illness in their cultural context, and medical communication should be sensitive to the differences in information needs and decision-making styles. Although many clinicians in the United States prefer to provide information about diagnosis or prognosis, internationally this is not always the case, and in part these clinician traditions reflect the pervading beliefs and preferences of the families in those areas.[10,25] Whenever possible, clinicians should accept the standards within a family. Some knowledge of the family's culture of origin may be helpful; cultural brokers, for example, may be able to offer insight into general standards of communication and areas that are particularly different or sensitive.[26] However, assumptions about the meaning of culture in a particular family should be avoided.[26,27] The clinician's best tool for learning about communication within a family is often humility; a willingness to ask about the way the family likes to communicate and make decisions should be accompanied by an openness to respect that family's style.

Parents can vary in their preferences for who shares serious information with their child. Some may prefer that a trusted clinician have these discussions alone with the child or in the presence of the parents; while other parents may not want the clinician to be the one to initiate certain discussions with their child. They may prefer to initiate the discussion themselves. In the latter case, there remain important roles for the clinicians, including preparing parents for the discussions with their child and being well informed or even present when the parents share information with their ill child. There may be a natural parent reluctance to share serious information with their child.[28] Reluctance could include fear of the child's emotional reaction, loss of hope about the situation, or diminished willingness on the child's part to interact with the parents and others. Clinicians can help prepare parents for these discussions by exploring underlying reasons for concerns, offering suggestions for possible ways to share the information or even

TABLE 19-1 Guideline Examples Based on Principles of Communication

7-step communication tool[*]	Guidelines for communication of the diagnosis[†]	Six E's of communication[‡]	SEGUE[§]	PACE[‖]	SPIKES[¶]
1. Prepare for the discussion 2. Establish what the patient and family already knows 3. Determine how the information is to be handled 4. Deliver the information 5. Respond to emotions 6. Establish goals for care and treatment priorities 7. Establish a plan	1. Establish a protocol for communication 2. Communicate immediately at diagnosis and follow up later 3. Communicate in a private and comfortable space 4. Communicate with both parents, and other family members if desired 5. Hold a separate session with the child 6. Solicit questions from the child and parents 7. Communicate in ways that are sensitive to cultural differences 8. Share information about the diagnosis and the plan for cure 9. Share information on lifestyle and psychosocial issues 10. Encourage the entire family to talk together	1. Establish an agreement about communication 2. Engage child at opportune time 3. Explore what child already knows 4. Explain medical information according to child's developmental status and needs 5. Empathize with child's emotions 6. Encourage child that you will be there when needed	1. Set the Stage 2. Elicit the information 3. Give information 4. Understand the recipient's perspective 5. End the encounter	1. Plan the setting 2. Assess the recipient's knowledge/needs 3. Choose appropriate strategies 4. Evaluate their understanding	1. Setting up the interview 2. Assessing the patient's perceptions 3. Obtaining the patient's invitation 4. Giving knowledge and information to the patient 5. Addressing the patient's emotions with empathic responses 6. Strategy and summary

[*]Von Gunten CF, Ferris FD, Emanuel LL: Ensuring competency in end-of-life care, *JAMA* 284(23):3051-3057, 2000.
[†]Masera G, Chesler MA, Jankovic M, et.al: SIOP Working Committee on Psychosocial Issues in Pediatric Oncology: Guidelines for communication of the diagnosis, *Med Pediatr Oncol* 28:382-385, 1997.
[‡]Beale EA, Baile WF, Aaron J: Silence is not golden: communicating with children dying from cancer, *J Clin Oncol* 20(15):3629-3631, 2005.
[§]Makoul G: The SEGUE Framework for teaching and assessing communication skills, *Patient Educ Couns* 45(1):23-34, 2001.
[‖]Garwick AW, Patterson J, Bennett FC, Blum RW: Breaking the news: how families first learn about their child's chronic condition, *Arch Pediatr Adolesc Med* 149(9):991-997, 1995.
[¶]Baile WF, Buckman R, Lenzi R, Glober G, Beale EA, Kudelka AP: SPIKES: A six-step protocol for delivering bad news: application to the patient with cancer, *Oncologist* 5(4):302-311, 2000.

role-playing with the parents in advance of the discussion. Parents have indicated that after they or the clinicians have serious conversations with their child, they want clinicians to treat their child the very same as before the child's condition became more serious.[29]

The second guiding principle is that communication is making a human connection. Literature offers instructions on how to deliver bad news.[30,31] These are helpful tools but the most central point to effective communication between a clinician and a child is the intention to make a human connection in which honest information and feelings are shared. Clinicians are first providing care for a person, and then for the person's condition.[6]

BOX 19-1 Principles of Communication with a Seriously Ill Child and the Child's Family

1. The context for communication is the family.
2. Communication is intended to make a human connection with the seriously ill child and family.
3. Each serious discussion requires careful preparation regarding timing, place, who needs to be included in the discussion from the team and family, and adequate time to remain to address lingering questions.
4. Communication is never a one-time interaction, but is ongoing.
5. Clinicians need to be invited to communicate by the ill child.
6. A single mode of communication is most commonly insufficient in pediatric palliative and end-of-life care.
7. All members of the interdisciplinary pediatric palliative care or end-of-life team are integral to communicating effectively with the child and family.

The third guiding principle is to thoughtfully prepare for sharing information and feelings. As noted in Table 19-1, the guidelines for communication include steps to assure that all relevant individuals are included in the discussion. It is also important that a quiet setting is available for an uninterrupted discussion and that to the fullest extent possible no anticipated interruptions occur, instead ask a team member to handle the pagers for those who will be in the discussion. Openness to conversation is particularly important. With children, an open invitation to talk should be accompanied by careful listening for cues that the time is right. A clinician who is too busy when such glimpses into a child's thoughts occur may miss important opportunities. In addition, clinicians may wish to create opportunities for interaction including quiet presence on a regular basis, not just when there is medical news to be delivered. The spaces between the news may be rich with meaning that informs all other interactions. Presence also sends a powerful message about the consistent caring the clinician provides and the value of the child and family.

The fourth guiding principle is that communication is never a one-time event but is instead ongoing,[32] with the clinician being attuned to clues from the child about information needs. In addition to being sensitive to clues from the child, it is helpful when the clinician directly offers to revisit a topic or conversation or specifically solicits questions about any aspect of care. Communication is not limited to when a change in the child's condition or treatment is occurring, but it is especially critical for such times. Children find it helpful when clinicians address how the clinical change occurred, if this can be determined, and particularly for the younger child, when clinicians clearly state that the child is not to blame for the change.[3]

The fifth guiding communication principle is for the clinician to get invited by the child to engage in sharing information, thoughts, and feelings. Clinicians will seek the invitation through their unique styles that develop over time; some may do it directly, others using a metaphor or vehicle such as sports, play items, or books. The likelihood of being invited is increased from the point of diagnosis forward when the clinicians tell the child about their willingness to keep the child informed and to answer questions. Being invited signals respect for the child, as it allows the child to decide the timing for the exchange of information, ideas, and feelings. This is taking time to establish a relationship and a rapport and seeking to build a partnership between the clinician and the child.[16]

A sixth guiding principle is there are times when a single mode of communication will be insufficient with a child or the family. Helpful examples of verbiage have been published.[3,33] Other forms of media can also be very helpful in sharing information and feelings between clinicians and children include drawings.[34] Perhaps one of the most powerful of communication tools that a clinician can use is silence. Clinicians must be able to quiet their own thoughts and not try to plan their next comment but instead listen with the intention of discovering an insight about this child, family, situation, or about self.[35] Listening without interruptions is a very sophisticated skill and one that is least-frequently practiced by clinicians. Communication is sharing information and feelings that is intended to be understood in the same way by the child and the clinician and most typically requires more than one method. Whatever mode is selected for communication, the endpoint goal is the same: The child and parents will feel listened to and respected.[36]

The seventh principle is to recognize that communication, as with all other skills in pediatric palliative care, involves a team of clinicians. Before the meeting with the family, team members may wish to meet together to plan and designate a team member to lead the discussion. In certain discussions, particularly those involving a change in the child's condition, the physician may take the lead in initiating the conversation. However, when a team approach is used, non-physician team members may be effective leaders of the conversation, with the physician present for input when necessary. In addition, certain team members may wish to address specific issues without leading the entire meeting. For example, a psychologist may wish to address the child's emotional needs as an important component of the meeting, or a physician may wish to clarify recent medical events. The team's pre-meeting discussion can help to plan which roles individual team members will take and the best ways for the team to collaborate during the meeting itself.

What transpires during the discussion is important, and what transpires after the discussion is as well. Commonly, some members of the interdisciplinary team are present during the discussion without leading the conversation. These team members may insert comments meant to clarify content and confirm the child's understanding.[37] Following the discussion, individual team members may linger with the patient and family or return subsequently to encourage the child and family to ask questions.[38] Careful documentation of all of these exchanges is needed so that all clinicians can be well informed and not need to ask the family to repeat to them what transpired. One professional organization, the SIOP Working Committee on Psychosocial Issues in Pediatric Oncology, recommends that a communication protocol be created for each healthcare setting that contains the expected behaviors of each member on the clinical team for communication including that related to diagnosis.[4] In addition to providing the family with the opportunity to reflect on the conversation afterward, interdisciplinary team members may actively participate by observing interactions carefully, recognizing and attending to emotional content, and being alert to miscommunications. These roles may be difficult for the clinician who is leading the conversation to fully take on. The team can also serve as a source of support to one another, working together to reflect on these encounters and helping one another feel sustained in this difficult work. Finally, team members have a role in simply witnessing these profound discussions. Even if some members of a team don't say a word in a family meeting, simply by being present they convey a message that the conversation is important and meaningful and that the child and family are as well.

WHEN COMMUNICATION EFFORTS DO NOT GO WELL

Even seasoned clinicians at times find that, despite their best efforts, a communication interaction has not gone well. There are many reasons why these interactions sometimes feel difficult, not the least of which is the overpowering emotions that families often feel in these encounters. It is natural that at times their anger or sense of powerlessness at a difficult situation sometimes emerges through displacement of emotion onto the team. In addition, even the most caring clinicians will at times say or do something that causes distress to the family or child.

When this happens, it can be helpful to process the experience with the help of the interdisciplinary team, to reflect honestly on one's role in the difficult encounter and the emotions that such an encounter produced in the child and family, as well as in the clinician. The team can then develop a plan for how best to move forward with the child and family.

Sometimes families are simply unable to move forward with a particular clinician or even the entire team, and when this happens, the family's needs should be respected whenever possible. Most of the time, however, children and their families are able to recognize that every encounter will not be as difficult, particularly when a caring relationship has already been established among the child, family, and clinician. The clinician may wish to meet with the family to discuss the encounter, to express regret over the family's distress, and to express caring for them and a desire to work toward a better relationship in the future. When the family is willing to discuss the difficult encounter, a discussion about the process can be helpful. For example, the clinician may wish to ask the family for guidance about how best to discuss some of these issues in the future. The clinician should listen openly to concerns and respond honestly with hopes for things to go better with time. Impossible promises, such as promising to avoid ever making mistakes in the future, should be avoided, but honest statements about a desire to always listen and work toward meeting the needs of the family may be appreciated.

Clinicians should remember to be forgiving of themselves in such encounters as well. Much of the time, difficult encounters are not a result of a thoughtless or unskilled clinician, but rather the result of a situation that is painful for the clinician. Clinicians who have difficulty talking with the child about diagnosis, treatment, and prognosis are likely struggling themselves with the sad clinical situation.[39,40] All clinicians need support during these difficult times but clinicians who avoid communicating honestly with children need immediate support from other members of the healthcare team and particularly from a senior clinician who has recognized abilities to communicate well with seriously ill children, a willingness to demonstrate those abilities and who has respect for fellow clinicians who do not yet have such skills.

Specific Palliative Care Communication Topics

SHARING INFORMATION ABOUT PROGNOSIS

Much of the literature on communicating about advanced illness comes from studies of adults with metastatic cancer, in which the disease course is often relatively predictable and typically involves a progressive decline from diagnosis to death. For children with life-threatening illnesses, however, the trajectory can be unpredictable, often lasting over many years, and marked by exacerbations and reprieves from symptoms.[28] For families and children who experience these long, complex illnesses, the ups and downs of illness can make the larger picture difficult to fathom. It is particularly important, then, for clinicians caring for the child to help the child and family understand what the future may hold, so that appropriate decisions can be made all along the trajectory.

One aspect of this is communicating about the child's prognosis, including the possibility of death and when that may occur. Previous literature suggests that physicians are often reluctant to discuss prognosis with patients, in part because they worry about causing distress and taking away hope.[41–45] Yet parents tend to have less distress when they have received the information they want about prognosis,[46,47] perhaps because such information gives them a sense of some control over the situation and alleviates uncertainty, which itself can be extremely upsetting. In addition, parents often want prognostic information, reporting that accurate prognostic information helps them to make the best possible decisions for their children.[47]

Evidence from the adult cancer setting suggests that prognosis communication does affect end-of-life decision-making. For example, adult patients with metastatic cancer who have unrealistic expectations about a long lifespan are more likely to choose life-prolonging therapy over comfort-directed care.[48] Similarly, adult patients with advanced cancer who report having discussed their wishes for end-of-life care with a physician are less likely to use mechanical ventilation, resuscitation, or care in the intensive care unit at the end of life, and are more likely to enroll in hospice care.[49] Although it is possible that some patients will continue to desire life-prolonging care at the end of life, communication about the expectation that death is likely to occur allows patients to make decisions based on their own values, and not on unrealistic expectations.[50,51]

In addition to the importance of having discussions about the possibility of death, the timing of such discussions is also important. There are reports that bereaved parents' understanding that their children with cancer had no realistic chance for cure tended to lag behind physicians' knowledge of the child's incurability by several months.[14] Earlier parental recognition of the child's limited chance of cure was associated with earlier discussions about hospice care, earlier institution of do-not-resuscitate orders, and decreased use of cancer-directed therapy at the end of life.[14]

Similarly, in a study of 318 bereaved family members of adults who had died of cancer, half believed that palliative care services were provided later than they would have wanted, while less than 5 % believed that referrals for palliative care were provided too early. Families were more likely to say palliative care was instituted too late when they also reported feeling inadequately prepared for changes in the patient's medical condition and when they believed that discussion about end-of-life care preferences with physicians was insufficient, suggesting that communication about a poor prognosis and institution of palliative care often jointly occur late in the disease course.[52]

Despite the potential benefits of early conversations about a child's life-limiting condition, the diversity of life-limiting illnesses in pediatrics means that the perceived optimal timing of referrals to palliative care varies widely among pediatricians.[53] Pediatric clinicians report feeling inexperienced with communication about end-of-life issues, including transitions to palliative care and resuscitation status,[40] and this inexperience may also lead to delays in such communication.

Clinicians may also be faced with uncertain clinical situations, in which the timing of death or even whether death is expected cannot be determined with certainty. Communication is particularly challenging in this setting, but even so an honest conversation about possible outcomes can be important to families. Previous work has suggested that clinicians tend to give no information or overly optimistic information to patients and families in uncertain times.[54,55] However, just as in situations where the prognosis is known with greater certainty, an honest estimate may best allow families to prepare for possible outcomes. The clinician may also wish to discuss a range of possible outcomes but, again, with honesty and not with undue optimism.

Throughout this discussion, we have described prognostic disclosure as an important aspect of clinical care. This strategy supports ethical principles of patient autonomy and informed decision making. The evidence suggests that for most families, disclosure also supports principles of beneficence rather than undermining them, that is, disclosure may promote hope and well-being rather than taking those feelings away. However, for individual patients and families, clinician disclosure of prognostic information may be difficult and associated with real harm. At times the clinician may feel that disclosure of prognostic information is ethically necessary even if the family does not wish for such information. But when the act, nature, or timing of disclosure is open to consideration, clinicians would do well to strongly consider the wishes of the family.

APPLYING A FRAMEWORK FOR COMMUNICATING EFFECTIVELY ABOUT PROGNOSIS

Clinician inexperience or anxiety can lead to delays in communication about prognosis. Offered here is a framework for talking about prognosis and plans for care in the end-of-life period with a child and family. This framework is presented in the context of the SPIKES format described in Table 19-1. However, there is no single way of holding this discussion, and as always the most important element is the caring child-parent-clinician relationship that forms the context for this discussion. A second vitally important aspect of the discussion is tailoring the information and its presentation to the needs of the child and family, a strategy that can best be enacted by eliciting their preferences and needs and by listening carefully. There are six steps to this process:

1. Setting up the interview. A meeting with the child and/or family should be scheduled in advance in a quiet setting. Ideally such a meeting occurs when the child is doing relatively well, so that the decision making does not have urgency. However, this should not preclude the clinician from holding a meeting when there is medical need. The interdisciplinary team may wish to prepare the child and family for the importance of the discussion, perhaps by mentioning that this is an opportunity to review our expectations for the next months and years of the child's life, and to think about the child's and family's goals for that time.

2. Assessing the patient's perceptions. The clinician may wish to start by assessing the child's or parents' understanding of the child's illness and its implications for his or her life and lifespan. A question could be, "As you think about your child's illness, what do you think is likely to be ahead?" A general question like this one may be useful initially, but for some families and children, more specific questions are helpful. For example, the clinician may wish to specify a timeframe by asking about what may be ahead for the next months or years, or what can be expected as the child's illness progresses.

3. Obtaining the patient's invitation. The invitation to discuss these topics is particularly important. The clinician might ask the child or parent, "Would it be helpful to talk about what may be ahead for you and/or your child?" A clinician who asks this question, however, should be prepared for refusal. As described by The and colleagues,[41] "awareness cannot be forced, it can only be supported." A child or family who is not ready for such a conversation should not be pushed unless the interdisciplinary team believes that the conversation is critically important. If the team chooses not to address the topic at the request of the family, the team may wish to tell the family that they can have this conversation at another time, if and when the time is right.

4. Giving knowledge and information to the patient. As the clinician prepares to provide information, he or she may wish to ask the child and family about how they like to receive information, and what kind of information would be most helpful. For example, some patients prefer to hear quantitative estimates of the likelihood of cure or expected lifespan, while others prefer to hear a general idea without numbers. For some families, detailed information about timing is less important than information about what the child's life will be like during that period of time. First making an assessment of information needs and preferences can allow the clinician to tailor the information given to the needs of the child and family. Some clinicians are worried about providing estimates because of their inherent inaccuracy—no course is predictable, and any estimate may be wrong.[43,54] Some clinicians therefore provide no estimate, or even an overly optimistic estimate.[54] Because this practice can contribute to inaccurate parental expectations about prognosis, which could in turn alter end-of-life decision making, we recommend providing the most accurate possible estimate when one is requested. Uncertainty can be addressed using a statement such as, "We never know how long any one patient will live, but children in this circumstance usually don't live more than about six months." A range of possible outcomes can be discussed if a more precise estimate is not possible, for example, the possibility of living from days to weeks.

5. Addressing the patient's emotions with empathic responses. Prognostic information can be very difficult for parents and children to hear, and clinicians are often acutely aware of the pain such conversations can cause.[42] Yet literature also suggests that empathic opportunities are often missed.[56] Clinicians can support parents and children by listening carefully for affect and acknowledging and/or exploring it when it surfaces. For example, the clinician may wish to name the emotion that the child or parent is expressing, such as "you seem sad," and then follow up with a request to "tell me more about that." In addition, a willingness to listen and be quietly present can help parents and children to feel most comfortable expressing their feelings. When needed, the clinician may wish to ask directly how the parent or child is feeling. For example, a clinician might follow a conversation about prognosis by saying, "This kind of information can be difficult to hear. Can you tell me how you are feeling now?" Alternatively, the clinician may be able to open up the discussion to the emotional response by simply asking, "How did this information differ from what you were expecting?"

6. Strategy and summary. As this difficult conversation draws to a close, the clinician can provide some reassurance to the parent or child whose worlds may have changed. Perhaps most important is an offer of ongoing presence, including plans for the next visit or discussion if appropriate. A review of the information may accompany an offer to continue this conversation. In addition, the clinician may wish to offer some information about what can be achieved in this difficult situation. At times, discussion about goals of care is a natural next step; for some families, however, the promise that such a conversation will occur is enough for the moment. As always, the interdisciplinary team will want to be sensitive to the child's and parents' experiences in the conversation, leaving them neither completely overwhelmed with information, nor lost after difficult news with no understanding of the next steps. Asking the child and parents how they are doing and what they hope for is useful.[57] In addition, it is sometimes helpful to let the family know that not every conversation has to touch on these difficult topics. Rather, the team will try to let the family know in advance when this kind of hard conversation must take place.

APPLYING A FRAMEWORK FOR COMMUNICATING EFFECTIVELY ABOUT PALLIATIVE AND END-OF-LIFE CARE GOAL-SETTING

The child's and parents' goals of care form the foundation of the care plan. Once goals are defined, all decisions about care can be considered in light of these goals, with the clinician and family jointly considering the extent to which specific interventions meet the desired goals or not. Involving the child and family in care goal-setting from the point of diagnosis or injury forward provides opportunities for them to become accustomed to this aspect of care. This can also avoid only using goal-setting at the end of life, when such a shift in language could be disconcerting for the child and family.

Goal-setting has also been associated with facilitating patient-family-clinician general communication and trust[58] as well as future decision making.[59]

Goal-setting is influenced by the child and parents' and clinical team's understanding of the child's prognosis, suffering and care preferences.[60–61] Because goals can change over time, reassessment is important.[33] In addition to changing goals, children and their parents may change their preferences for involvement in goal setting and related decision making. This change can range from having been somewhat involved at one point in care to becoming directive or passive in other points in care. Differences in preference for involvement may also differ in geographically distinct parts of the world thus making it important for clinicians to be responsive to the child's and parent's preferences for involvement.[62–64]

Goal-setting discussions include two major foci: goals for the life plan and for the treatment plan.[65] The life-plan goals are related to personal values, priorities, and commitments whereas treatment goals are related to medical-care priorities. Together, the goals from these directly influence the child's quality of life (see Fig. 19-1). The life-plan goals and the treatment goals, though both of primary concern, are not necessarily in equal balance with each other as at times one or the other may carry more weight. However, consideration of both concurrently throughout palliative care will help achieve quality of life considerations for the seriously ill child. Certain categories of factors influence goal-setting discussions about the life plan and the treatment plan, including characteristics of the child and the parents such as family culture and communication style; the child's injury or acute or chronic illness; treatment options; and characteristics and values of the clinical care team members. When discussing life plans and treatment plans, it is important to have the primary physician present, because the majority of parents report that physicians are the primary source of information for them about their child's clinical status and prognosis. No single member of a team can be expected to lead all goal-setting discussions as a different team member may be more informed or familiar with a patient's or parents' unique style of communication and thus would more expertly facilitate the discussion for that family. Another reason to have multiple team members skilled at facilitating goal-setting discussions is that a member of a team may be unable to serve in that way at certain times and for a number of reasons, not the least of which is a deep sadness about the child's cir-

cumstances. It is important for each clinical team to be able to examine their abilities and strengths in communicating with patients, parents, and each other about care goals.

The discussion about prognosis and goals of care may take place in a single conversation. Certainly the topics tend to be inextricably linked; the goals of care almost always take into account expectations for the future and the extent to which goals can be achieved. In addition, a discussion about a poor prognosis may feel incomplete without some discussion about what is possible in the child's life. Here is a format for goal-setting and translation of goals into care plans, based on the SPIKES format.

1. Setting up the interview. When conversation about goal-setting includes prognosis, the conversation about both issues can allow parents an opportunity to focus on what is possible for the child, not simply on the difficult course ahead. However, some parents may need time to process the prognostic information, and may wish for a separate opportunity to discuss their goals of care. In either case, the conversation should best be set up in advance, so that parents can have any needed supports present and are aware of the important topic.

2. Assessing the patient's perceptions. A conversation about goals of care should begin with assessment of the child's and parents' understanding of what is ahead. The perception about the child's prognosis and expected course of illness forms the foundation for their goals of care, and if the child or parents have significant misperceptions, then these should be addressed before goals are discussed in detail. Once this foundation has been established, then the clinician can ask the child and parents about their goals for care. Often, several questions are helpful to elicit this information. Examples include: "As you think about what is ahead for your child and/or yourself, what is most important to you?" "As you think about what is ahead, what are you most worried about?" "What do you think has caused your child to suffer the most?" "What does good quality of life look like for your child?" "What makes your child feel most joyful?" "What makes your child feel most at peace and comfortable?" Exploratory questions about the meaning of goals can be very helpful in eliciting a vision for the best and worst possible situations.

3. Obtaining the patient's invitation. Once the child's and parents' goals are established, the clinician can talk about the translation of these goals into plans for care. First, though, the clinician should ask if this is wanted. Possible phrases include: "You have told me about what is most important to you as you look ahead to a time when your child's illness gets worse. I am wondering if I could make some suggestions, based on what you have told me is important to you, about how we should think about his or her care when that time comes."

4. Giving knowledge and information to the patient. We would particularly emphasize the importance of making a recommendation rather than asking the child or parents to decide on the course of care. Although shared decision making is widely used, physicians typically make recommendations for most aspects of medical care in other phases of life. Clinicians would not routinely ask the parents of a healthy child to decide on

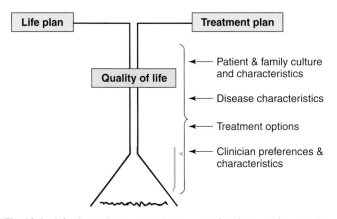

Fig. 19-1 Life plan and treatment plan aspects of goal setting that together influence the quality of life of the patient.

which antibiotic for an infection. The desire to defer to parents about end-of-life decisions often emanates from compassion; clinicians may wish to be sensitive to the fact that multiple courses of action may be appropriate at the end of life and that a clinician should not dictate care. However, parents may find that holding substantial responsibility for decision making in the end-of-life setting is burdensome.[66,67] As an example, when specific issues such as resuscitation are considered, a clinician who is aware of the parents' goals for care can often recommend a course of action that is most consistent with those goals. If parents wish to limit the child's suffering and maximize quality of life as death approaches, then a clinician may be able to honestly recommend that efforts at resuscitation not be provided, because such efforts are likely to cause suffering when death is near. Even when a parent wishes to prolong life, the clinician may be able to provide realistic recommendations about whether resuscitation is expected to meet that goal. In doing so, the clinician can take the parent's goals into account but also enter into shared responsibility with the parent for what may be a painful and difficult decision.

5. Addressing the patient's emotions with empathic responses. As described above, attentive listening and openness to affect should be part of such a difficult discussion. When discussions involve challenging and potentially burdensome care decisions, the clinician may also wish to affirm the love that went into these decisions.

6. Strategy and summary. A summary of the child's and parents' goals of care affirms that they have been heard and that their wishes are known and understood. Once again, the clinician should make plans for the next visit or discussion, signifying the ongoing nature of the relationship.

HOPE AND REALITY AS FRAMEWORKS FOR PARENTING AT THE END OF LIFE

Clinicians who care for children at the end of life may look for evidence that parents have accepted their child's impending death. Parents and children, however, may not consider the child's condition in such black-and-white terms, with a clear separation between curable and incurable disease. Instead, parents may hold hopes for their child that are inconsistent with what they believe is likely to happen. This state of cognitive dissonance may allow them to preserve some hope and ambiguity about the future as they also try to live in a difficult present. Importantly, the expression of hope does not necessarily indicate that the child or parents have not accepted the likelihood of death.

As an example, researchers found that parents of children who have died of cancer tend to express dual goals of using cancer-directed therapy to extend life and symptom-directed therapy to address the child's suffering or symptoms.[14,68] Instead of seeing these goals as conflicting, parents may find care that addresses both sets of goals to be most comfortable. The clinician may wish to allow for a range of goals when communicating with the parents, and may wish to explore hopes and perceived reality as separate but complementary aspects of the parents' present. Some have recommended allowing for hopes by talking about end-of-life care in a hypothetical manner with

patients who have a great deal of difficulty accepting death as a likely reality.[69] This strategy, termed "hope for the best, prepare for the worst," can allow for end-of-life care planning concurrent with the hope that such plans will not be necessary.[69]

In addition, hope may not always be focused on cure or a long life.[57] A previous study evaluated the extent to which discussion about a child's prognosis affected the parents' sense of hope for their children with cancer. Strikingly, parents who had received more extensive prognostic information were also more likely to report that communication had made them feel hopeful, even when the child's prognosis was poor.[55]

This study raises the possibility that knowledge of a poor prognosis can actually increase hope. Although this relationship seems counterintuitive, recent literature affirms the possibility that clinician honesty, even about difficult news, can help patients to feel more hopeful. For example, 126 patients with metastatic cancer were surveyed about physician behaviors they considered to be hope-giving. Realistic communication about prognosis was considered by the majority of patients to be hope-giving; communicating in euphemistic terms or avoiding honest disclosure of bad news, on the other hand, engendered more hopelessness.[70] Along similar lines, a study of surrogate decision makers for patients receiving mechanical ventilation revealed that 93% of surrogates considered avoidance of discussion about prognosis to be an unacceptable way to maintain hope.[71]

The reasons that hope may be enhanced by honest communication of difficult issues are not understood, though there are some possible explanations. First, knowledge of a poor prognosis could relieve the anxiety of uncertainty about the future. Others have reported that the experience of uncertainty about one's medical situation can result in a diminished sense of hope.[72] In contrast, clear communication about the illness and its expected trajectory may positively impact adjustment to illness and the individual's sense of hope. Among adult patients with end-stage renal disease on hemodialysis, receipt of information, including prognostic information, allowed for a sense of empowerment about medical care and decision making, which was in turn an important component of hope. Because many patients relied on physicians to initiate discussions about advance care planning, however, fears for the worst possible outcomes sometimes threatened hope when discussions did not take place.[73]

A second possible explanation is that direct acknowledgement of a life-limiting condition allows patients to formulate alternative hopes not focused on the disease.[57] Because most previous studies have assessed the general experience of hope without examining what hope means, an assumption that hope equals hope for a cure has persisted in the medical literature and in the minds of many clinicians. However, if prognosis communication can support hope, then hope must be broader than hope for a cure. Hope may encompass life-prolongation or palliation, or broader hopes that are focused on meaningful relationships, beliefs, and experiences. The formulation of hopes not focused on the disease could be a component of finding meaning in the end-of-life experience. Among adolescents with cancer, for example, hope has been defined as a belief in a "personal tomorrow" with highly individual meanings.[74]

Finally, it is possible that hope can be derived from the communication interaction itself. It may not be the discussion of difficult issues itself that provides hope, but the fact that the discussion occurs in the context of a caring parent-child-clinician relationship. A 2008 editorial speaks to this issue by describing hope as an experience related to caring, consolation, relief from disquiet, and meaning in relationships. This definition suggests that the clinician may have a meaningful role to play in the development and maintenance of hope, and that this role emanates from a caring, human connection between caregiver and patient.[75]

For clinicians working with children with life-threatening illnesses and their parents, recognition of these many possible meanings of hope may be important. Because the meaning of hope may be so individualized, the clinician may wish to explore what hope means for the child and family, so that these can be considered in plans for care and the team can support these hopes when possible and return to them over time. Listening and engaging in a caring relationship with the child and parents serve as a foundation for this exploration rather than using any specific words. However, the clinician could consider asking parents questions such as, "What are you hoping for most as you look at your child's life and illness and your lives?" In addition, the clinician may consider following this question with "What else are you hoping for?" so that a range of hopes can be elicited. Drawing out the child's and parents' hopes does not necessarily need to be followed with an immediate assessment of how realistic such hopes are, particularly if the clinician has already communicated an honest assessment of the child's prognosis. Instead, the clinician may wish to acknowledge the profound importance of such hopes by commenting on the beauty of these hopes, or perhaps by noting that he or she will hope for the same thing. A clinician who allows space for hopes, fears, and worries may be best able to support children and parents in the face of those feelings.

Children, like their parents, may develop deeply meaningful hopes near the end of life, such as hoping that their family will be OK after their death, or hoping to be remembered. A clinician who explores these issues with the child may be able to offer support and reassurance. For example, for children who hope to be remembered after death, the clinician may honestly be able to say that he or she will always remember the child. Specific examples of what will be remembered about the child can serve the child as a review of the relationship, a model of one way to reflect with a loved one and say goodbye, and a reminder of how very special the child is. In addition, simply by taking the time to talk about these important issues, the clinician sends the implicit message that the child is valued.

Communicating Effectively About What to Expect When Death Is Near

While medical caregivers ensure detailed communication with parents and children about side effects and expected symptoms during self-limiting illnesses, clinicians may find that conversations about the child's experience when death is imminent may be too difficult to broach. This sympathy with the pain parents may experience at such conversations can lead clinicians to avoid providing detailed information about how the death may unfold. For parents, however, receipt of information about what to expect at the end of life is a component of high-quality care.[76,77] The deep pain parents experience

in such conversations may be outweighed by the need to know what is ahead, and in knowing this, to gain some sense of control over an uncontrollable situation.

Children should also be offered the opportunity to talk about what happens as death nears. While parents may need to know specific information about the dying process and the care of the body after death, children's questions often focus on existential concerns about what will happen to them and to their family after the death. The clinician may best be able to respond to these concerns by serving as a willing and open listener. For children who wish to protect their parents from topics that their parents may find distressing, this can be a particularly important role for the clinician.

APPLYING A FRAMEWORK FOR COMMUNICATING EFFECTIVELY ABOUT WHAT TO EXPECT AT END OF LIFE

The following is guidance for the conversation with parents about what to expect at their child's end of life, again using the SPIKES format.

1. Setting up the interview. As with any important conversation, offer parents the opportunity to plan for this conversation, so that they can have the important people in their lives and on their care team present. This conversation is usually most helpful in the days or weeks before the child's death, although some parents may wish to learn about these issues earlier.

2. Assessing the patient's perceptions. As with other important conversations about the end-of-life period, the clinician also needs to know what the parents understand about the child's prognosis; if a parent does not know that death is likely to occur, then a discussion about the dying process is inappropriate, and the physician should first focus communication on prognostic information.

   For parents who recognize that death is likely, begin by asking the child and parents what is most important to them as they look to the child's time ahead before providing information about what may be ahead for the child. Understanding their goals helps to frame the conversation about the future, because caregivers are able to directly address the ways that symptoms and care can be managed to meet those goals. A family who wants to allow the child to remain in school for as long as possible, for instance, may find a discussion about the expected trajectory of symptoms to be helpful, as well as information about how clinicians can work with the school to maximize the quality of the child's time there. Even when parents do not state control of suffering explicitly as a goal, clinicians also always discuss how to work to alleviate any suffering associated with symptoms. It may also be helpful to ask if the parents have experience with another loved one who has died.

3. Obtaining the patient's invitation. Parents may be asked if it would be helpful to talk about what to expect as the child's illness progresses. When parents decline, caregivers can let them know that they are available to discuss this if there is ever a time when talking about this would be helpful.

4. Giving knowledge and information to the patient. A range of topics may be appropriate in this conversation,

according to the expected course for the child and to the needs of the child and parents. Clinicians often discuss specific symptoms and their management. For each symptom, talk about what the symptom will look and/or feel like, whether the symptom is likely to cause suffering, and how suffering will be managed. Along with the discussion about symptoms, discuss how caregivers will assess distress, particularly if the child is not able to communicate. For example, many children develop stridor or other noisy breathing due to upper airway secretions and obstruction as the end of life nears. Preparation for this symptom may help parents to feel less distressed when the symptom appears.[76] Clinicians let them know that, as the child's consciousness wanes, the muscles of the upper airway often relax and cause the stridor. However, also tell them that this symptom often appears without other signs of distress, which could include increased respiratory effort and a distressed facial expression. If the stridor is associated with signs that the child is distressed, then clinicians can work to manage discomfort, such as using opioids. However, if the child appears comfortable, no additional management may be needed.

Clinicians can also offer information about natural changes to the body as death nears. For example, the wane of consciousness, decreased urine output, and changes in perfusion may all be particularly distressing to parents if they are not prepared for such changes. Parents also often want to consider the location of death as part of this discussion. Finally, parents may find it helpful to learn about the moment of death and the practicalities of what they can and should do after the child dies. A conversation about washing the body, spending time with the child's body for a period of time, and also about autopsy and preparation of the body for services or burial, may help the parent to prepare for this period.

5. Addressing the patient's emotions with empathic responses. It is impossible to have a conversation about what to expect at the end of life without laying bare some of the anguish parents experience in this terrible situation. A careful assessment and ongoing reassessment of how the parents are feeling and what they want to know is essential.

6. Strategy and summary. At the close of this conversation, the clinician may wish to reiterate some important points. For example, the clinician might restate the goals of care, the ways that as death approaches caregivers will continue to work to meet those goals, and the ways that the team will work to help the child feel as good as possible. In addition, reassurance about the presence of the team during this time, and ongoing availability, may be helpful.

Using Communication to Affirm Core Values

Caring for children with life-limiting illnesses is not easy, but those who do it know this work comes with great gifts. Among them is the opportunity to build unique and meaningful relationships with patients and families and to witness the beautiful work they do together all along the course of the child's illness, to the death and beyond. While communication allows the clinician to convey information that can help the family and child with this process, communication can also allow the clinician to engage fully with the family in this work.

We have described a number of roles for communication: the development of a relationship with the child and parents, the transmission of information that will allow the child and parents to make decisions for care based on their personal goals, the provision of emotional support, and the creation of a forum for ongoing support and communication. A final role for communication should be noted. At its best, communication affirms the core values of palliative care: that the child has value as a person, that the child-parent relationship is meaningful, that clinicians' relationships with these children and their families have meaning to us personally, and that these relationships will endure.

REFERENCES

1. Goldie J, Schwartz L, Morrison J: Whose information is it anyway and informing a 12-year-old patient of her terminal prognosis, *J Med Ethics* 31:427–434, 2005.
2. Levetown M: Ensuring that difficult decisions are honored—even in school settings, *Am J Bioeth* 5(11):78–81, 2005.
3. Hurwitz CA, Duncan J, Wolfe J, et al: Caring for the child with cancer at the close of life: "There are people who make it, and I'm hoping I'm one of them," *JAMA* 292(17):2141–2149, 2004 doi:10.1001/jama.292.17.2141.
4. Masera G, Chesler MA, Jankovic M, et al: SIOP Working Committee on psychosocial issues in pediatric oncology: guidelines for communication of the diagnosis, *Med Pediatr Oncol* 28:382–385, 1997.
5. Ranmal R, Prictor M, Scott JT, et al: Interventions for improving communication with children and adolescents about their cancer, *Cochrane Database Syst Rev* (1):2009 DOI: 10.1002/14651858. CD002969.pub2.
6. O'Malley PJ, Brown K, Krug SE, et al: Patient- and family-centered care of children in the emergency department, *Pediatrics* 122(2):2008.
7. Garwick AW, Patterson J, Bennett FC, Blum RW: Breaking the news: how families first learn about their child's chronic condition, *Arch Pediatr Adolescent Med* 149(9):991–1107, 1995.
8. Freyer DR: Care of the dying adolescent: special considerations, *Pediatrics* 113:381–388, 2004 DOI: 10.1542/peds. 113.2.381.
9. Gupta VB, Willert J, Pian M, Stein MT: When disclosing a serious diagnosis to a minor conflicts with family values, *J Dev Behav Pediatr* 29(3):231, 2008.
10. Parsons SK, Saiki-Craighill S, et al: Telling children and adolescents about their cancer diagnosis: cross-cultural comparisons between pediatric oncologists in the US and Japan, *Psychooncology* 16(1):60–80, 2007.
11. Fallat ME, Glover J: Professionalism in pediatrics, *Pediatrics* 120(4):e1123–e1133, 2007.
12. Mack JW, Block SD, Nilsson M, et al: Measuring therapeutic alliance between oncologists and patients with advanced cancer: the Human Connection Scale, *Cancer* 115(14):3302–3311, 2009.
13. Pantilat SZ: Communicating with seriously ill patients: better words to say, *JAMA* 301(12):1279–1281, 2009.
14. Wolfe J, Klar N, Grier HE, et al: Understanding of prognosis among parents of children who died of cancer: impact on treatment goals and integration of palliative care, *JAMA* 284(19):2469–2475, 2000.
15. Last BF, van Veldhuizen AM: Information about diagnosis and prognosis related to anxiety and depression in children with cancer aged 8–16 years, *Eur J Cancer* 32A(2):290–294, 1996.
16. Levetown M: Communicating with children and families: from everyday interactions to skill in conveying distressing information, *Pediatrics* 121:e1441–e1460, 2008 DOI: 10.1542/peds.2008-0565.
17. Bradlyn AS, Kato PM, Beale IL, Cole SW: Pediatric oncology professionals' perceptions of information needs of adolescent patients with cancer, *J Pediatr Oncol Nurs* 21(6):335–342, 2004.
18. Hinds PS, Gattuso JS, Mandrell BN: Nursing care. In Pui CH, editor: *Childhood leukemias*, ed 2, New York, 2006, Cambridge University Press, pp 882–893.
19. Knafl K, Deatrick JA, Gallo AM, et al: The interplay of concepts, data, and methods in the development of the family management style framework, *J Fam Nurs* 14(4):412–428, 2008.

20. Snethen JA, Broome ME, Knafl K, Deatrick J, Angst D: Family patterns of decision making in pediatric clinical trails, *Res Nurs Health* 29(3):223–232, 2006.

21. Contro N, Larson J, Scofield S, et al: Family perspectives on the quality of pediatric palliative care, *Arch Pediatr Adolesc Med* 156:14–19, 2002.

22. Feudtner C, Santucci G, Feinstein JA, Snyder CR, Rourke MT, Kang T: Hopeful thinking and level of comfort regarding providing pediatric palliative care: a survey of hospital nurses, *Pediatrics* 119(1):e186–e192, 2007.

23. Clarke SA, Davies H, Jenny M, Glaser A, Eiser C: Parental communication and children's behaviour following diagnosis of childhood leukaemia, *Psychooncology* 14(4):274–281, 2005.

24. Young B, Dixon-Woods M, Windridge K, Heney D: Managing communication with children who have a potentially life threatening chronic illness: children's and parents' accounts, *BMJ* 326:305–308, 2003.

25. Mystakidou K, Parpa E, Tsilila E, Katsouda E, Vlahos L: Cancer information disclosure in different cultural contexts, *Support Care Cancer* 12(3):147–154, 2004.

26. Surbone A: Cultural aspects of communication in cancer care, *Support Care Cancer* 16(3):235–240, 2008.

27. De Trill M, Kovalcik R: The child with cancer. influence of culture on truth-telling and patient care, *Ann NY Acad Sci* 809:197–210, 1997.

28. Mack JW, Wolfe J: Early integration of pediatric palliative care: for some children, palliative care starts at diagnosis, *Curr Opin Pediatr* 18(1):10–14, 2006.

29. Barrera M, D'Agostino N, Gammon J, Spencer L, Baruchel S, et al: Health-related quality of life and enrollment in phase 1 trials in children with incurable cancer, *Palliat Support Care* 3(3):191–196, 2005.

30. Himelstein BP, Jackson NL, Pegram L: The power of silence, *JCO* 19(19):3996, 2001.

31. Mack JW, Grier HE: The day one talk, *J Clin Oncol* 22(3):2004.

32. Ishibashi A: The needs of children and adolescents with cancer for information and social support, *Cancer Nurs* 24(1):61–67, 2001.

33. Baker JN, Hinds PS, Spunt SL, Barfield RC, Allen C, Powell BC, Anderson LH, Kane JR: Integration of palliative care practices into the ongoing care of children with cancer: individualized care planning and coordination, *Pediatr Clin North Am* 55(1):23–50, 2008.

34. Rollins JA: Tell me about it: drawing as a communication tool for children with cancer, *J Pediatr Oncol Nurs* 22(4):203–221, 2005.

35. Rushton CH: A framework for integrated pediatric palliative care: being with dying, *J Pediatr Nurs* 20(5):311–325, 2005.

36. Clark JN, Fletcher P: Communication issues faced by parents who have a child diagnosed with cancer, *J Pediatr Oncol Nurs* (4):175–191, 2003, 2000.

37. Ahmann E: Reviews and commentary: two studies regarding giving "bad news," *Pediatr Nurs* 24(6):554–556, 1998.

38. Mahany B: Working with kids who have cancer, *Nursing* 20(8):44–49, 1990.

39. Chanock S: Reflections on events surrounding the time of diagnosis in pediatric oncology, *J Pediatr Hematol Oncol* 23(4):211–212, 2001.

40. Contro NA, Larson J, Scofield S, Sourkes B, Cohen HJ: Hospital staff and family perspectives regarding quality of pediatric palliative care, *Pediatrics* 114(5):1248–1252, 2004.

41. The AM, Hak T, Koeter G, van Der Wal G: Collusion in doctor-patient communication about imminent death: an ethnographic study, *BMJ* 321(7273):1376–1381, 2000.

42. Gordon EJ: Daugherty CK. "Hitting you over the head": oncologists' disclosure of prognosis to advanced cancer patients, *Bioethics* 17(2):142–168, 2003.

43. Miyaji NT: The power of compassion: truth-telling among American doctors in the care of dying patients, *Soc Sci Med* 36(3):249–264, 1993.

44. Ruddick W: Hope and deception, *Bioethics* 13(3–4):343–357, 1999.

45. Kodish E, Post SG: Oncology and hope, *J Clin Oncol* 13(7):1817, 1995.

46. Mack JW, Cook EF, Wolfe J, Grier HE, Cleary PD, Weeks JC: Understanding of prognosis among parents of children with cancer: parental optimism and the parent-physician interaction, *J Clin Oncol* 25(11):1357–1362, 2007.

47. Mack JW, Wolfe J, Grier HE, Cleary PD, Weeks JC: Communication about prognosis between parents and physicians of children with cancer: parent preferences and the impact of prognostic information, *J Clin Oncol* 24(33):5265–5270, 2006.

48. Weeks JC, Cook EF, O'Day SJ, et al: Relationship between cancer patients' predictions of prognosis and their treatment preferences, *JAMA* 279(21):1709–1714, 1998.

49. Wright AA, Zhang B, Ray A, et al: Associations between end-of-life discussions, patient mental health, medical care near death, and caregiver bereavement adjustment, *JAMA* 300(14):1665–1673, 2008.

50. Block S: Psychological considerations, growth, and transcendence at the end of life, *JAMA* 285:2898–2905, 2001.

51. Lamont EB, Christakis NA: Complexities in prognostication in advanced cancer: "to help them live their lives the way they want to," *JAMA* 290(1):98–104, 2003.

52. Morita T, Akechi T, Ikenaga M, et al: Late referrals to specialized palliative care service in Japan, *J Clin Oncol* 23(12):2637–2644, 2005.

53. Thompson LA, Knapp C, Madden V, Shenkman E: Pediatricians' perceptions of and preferred timing for pediatric palliative care, *Pediatrics* 123(5):e777–e782, 2009.

54. Christakis NA, Iwashyna TJ: Attitude and self-reported practice regarding prognostication in a national sample of internists, *Arch Intern Med* 158(21):2389–2395, 1998.

55. Mack JW, Wolfe J, Cook EF, Grier HE, Cleary PD, Weeks JC: Hope and prognostic disclosure, *J Clin Oncol* 25(35):5636–5642, 2007.

56. Pollak KI, Arnold RM, Jeffreys AS, et al: Oncologist communication about emotion during visits with patients with advanced cancer, *J Clin Oncol* 25(36):5748–5752, 2007.

57. Hinds PS: The hopes and wishes of adolescents with cancer and the nursing care that helps, *Oncol Nurs Forum* 31(5):927–934, 2004.

58. Eiser C, Jenney M: Measuring quality of life, *Arch Dis Child* 92:348–350, 2007.

59. Varni JW, Burwinkle TM, Lane MM: Health-related quality of life measurement in pediatric clinical practice: an appraisal and precept for future research and application, *Health Qual Life Outcomes* 3:34, 2005.

60. Hays RM, Valentine J, Haynes G, et al: The Seattle Pediatric Palliative Care Project: effect on family satisfaction and health-related quality of life, *J Palliat Med* 9(3):716–728, 2006.

61. Klopfenstein KJ, Hutchinson C, Clark C, et al: Variables influencing end-of-life care in children and adolescents with cancer, *J Pediatr Hematol Oncol* 23(8):481–486, 2001.

62. Hinds P, Birenbaum L, Clarke-Steffen L, et al: Coming to terms: parents response to a first cancer recurrence, *Nurs Res* 45(3):148–153, 1996.

63. Hinds PS, Oakes L, Quargnenti A, et al: An international feasibility study of parental decision making in pediatric oncology, *Oncol Nurs Forum* 27(8):1233–1243, 2000.

64. Hinds P, Birenbaum L, Pedrosa A: Guidelines for the recurrence of pediatric cancer, *Semin Oncol Nurs* 18(1):50–59, 2002.

65. Policy Statement—The Future of Pediatrics: Mental Health Competencies for Pediatric Primary Care, *Amer Acad Pediatr* 124(1), 2009.

66. Carnevale FA, Canoui P, Hubert P, et al: The moral experience of parents regarding life-support decisions for their critically-ill children: a preliminary study in France, *J Child Health Care* 10(1):69–82, 2006.

67. Sharman M, Meert KL, Sarnaik AP: What influences parents' decisions to limit or withdraw life support? *Pediatr Crit Care Med* 6(5):513–518, 2005.

68. Bluebond-Langner M, Belasco JB, Goldman A, Belasco C: Understanding parents' approaches to care and treatment of children with cancer when standard therapy has failed, *JCO* 2414–2419, 2007.

69. Back AL, Arnold RM, Quill TE: Hope for the best, and prepare for the worst, *Ann Intern Med* 138(5):439–443, 2003.

70. Hagerty RG, Butow PN, Ellis PM, et al: Communicating with realism and hope: incurable cancer patients' views on the disclosure of prognosis, *J Clin Oncol* 23(6):1278–1288, 2005.

71. Apatira L, Boyd EA, Malvar G, et al: Hope, truth, and preparing for death: perspectives of surrogate decision makers, *Ann Intern Med* 149(12):861–868, 2008.

72. Hsu TH, Lu MS, Tsou TS, Lin CC: The relationship of pain, uncertainty, and hope in Taiwanese lung cancer patients, *J Pain Symptom Manage* 26(3):835–842, 2003.

73. Davison SN, Simpson C: Hope and advance care planning in patients with end stage renal disease: qualitative interview study, *BMJ* 333(7574):886, 2006.

74. Hinds PS: Inducing a definition of 'hope' through the use of grounded theory methodology. *J Adv Nurs* 9(4):357–362, 1984.

75. Harris JC, DeAngelis CD: The power of hope, *JAMA* 300(24):2919–2920, 2008.

76. Pritchard M, Burghen E, Srivastava DK, Okuma J, Anderson L, Powell B, Furman WL, Hinds PS: Cancer-related symptoms most concerning to parents during the last week and last day of their child's life, *Pediatrics* 121(5):e1301–e1309, 2008.

77. Mack JW, Hilden JM, Watterson J, et al: Parent and physician perspectives on quality of care at the end of life in children with cancer, *J Clin Oncol* 23(36):9155–9161, 2005.

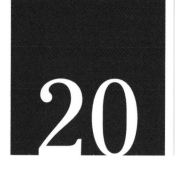

20 Introducing Palliative Care

JOETTA DESWARTE WALLACE | LINDA MURO-GARCIA

Hope is the thing with feathers that perches on the soul and sings the tune, without the words, and never stops at all.

—Emily Dickinson

The introduction of palliative care into the plan of care for a pediatric patient can be challenging. It is important to understand that palliative care is not synonymous with end-of-life care. The World Health Organization (WHO) defines palliative care as:

- The active total care of the child's body, mind and spirit, and also involves giving support to the family,
- Beginning when illness is diagnosed, and continues regardless of whether or not a child receives treatment directed at the disease,
- Requiring healthcare providers to evaluate and alleviate a child's physical, psychological, and social distress,
- Incorporating a broad interdisciplinary approach that includes the family and makes use of available community resources; it can be successfully implemented even if resources are limited,
- Being provided in tertiary care facilities, in community health and hospice centers, and in children's homes.

End-of-life care refers to the care delivered when death is almost certain and close in time. Care at end of life can be incorporated into palliative care as the approaches to cure become less of a focus and symptom control becomes the goal. At this stage, the primary team may change its approach, leaving the life-limiting diagnosis aside, and focus on symptom control, quality time with loved ones and assurances of dignity and respect for the child and family.

Care at end of life can be synonymous with hospice care, but in the United States hospice is a Medicare benefit and is defined as a special way of caring for people who are terminally ill. As in palliative care and end-of-life care, hospice care involves a team-oriented approach that addresses the medical, physical, social, emotional, and spiritual needs of the patient and support to the patient's family or caregiver. Hospice care, however, is usually given by a public agency or private company approved by Medicare and is different from the original primary care team. The goal of hospice is to care for a terminally ill patient and family, not to treat the illness (http://www.medicare.gov/publications/pubs/pdf/hosplg.pdf). Several basic differences between palliative care and hospice are listed in Table 20-1.

Incorporating palliative care at diagnosis can be challenging, even though approaches to control symptoms of discomfort and care for the psychosocial needs of the family are usually incorporated into excellent pediatric care specialties. Tertiary care centers, complete with specialists in most conditions, provide state-of-the-art treatment aimed at the cure of most life-threatening conditions. The hope for success is expected by the healthcare professionals as well as the families, and usually accomplished. Technological brinkmanship is described as pursuing aggressive treatment as far as it can go in the hope it can be stopped at just the right moment it turns out to be futile. As medical care accelerates in its technical and scientific sophistication, the fine line between prolonging life and prolonging suffering may become blurred.[1] Acknowledging that not all children will be cured and that approaches to cure can cause discomfort or even harm can be difficult. Physicians may find it difficult to acknowledge to a child or family that cure is not likely and may feel that they have failed professionally when curative options have been depleted. Families may suspect that they are not receiving all possible information about treatment options from their healthcare team, or that potentially curative therapies are being withheld because the center where they are receiving care is not as capable as another center, or for financial reasons. The family and the healthcare team may struggle with the feeling of giving up on the child and not continuing to fight for the child's life. When palliative and curative approaches are offered in tandem throughout the illness, there is less of a sense of transitioning to a different plan of care.[2]

The realization that a child will not be cured may be clear at the time of diagnosis or it may become apparent only later in the course of treatment. Reports from the Institute of Medicine (IOM)[2] and the American Academy of Pediatrics (AAP)[3] include recommendations that discussions of palliative care begin at diagnosis for some conditions. This allows for curative therapies to include measures to assure comfort and enhance quality of life throughout the disease process. The AAP policy includes statements that indicate inclusion of palliative care early in diagnosis could be of tremendous benefit to the children who eventually lose their lives to their diseases as well as to those who recover. Because the term palliative is frequently perceived as meaning a step away from curative approaches, it can be difficult to introduce the concept early in the plan of care.[4] Identified obstacles include an uncertain prognosis, parents not being ready, and time and staff limitations.

When dealing with a diagnosis for which the outcome is uncertain, healthcare providers may be reluctant to introduce the perceived opposites of curative vs. comfort-focused approaches. This dichotomous model can be challenging for families and healthcare providers.[5] A diagnosis with an uncertain outcome can instead be the signal to offer palliative care, even if end-of-life care discussions are not yet appropriate.

TABLE 20-1   Hospice vs. Palliative Care

Hospice	Palliative care
No further curative approaches	Concurrent with therapies against underlying disease
<6 months' life expectancy	Incorporated at diagnosis and not time limited
MediCare benefit with daily reimbursement (approximately $125/day)	Charges reimbursed as a component of care for the underlying disease
Hospice team becomes the sole provider of services	Primary care provider directs care and services

Pediatric oncologists surveyed by American Society of Clinical Oncology report a key factor in their decisions to shift from curative to palliative care is the absence of effective therapy.[6] This reluctance can subject the child to multiple treatment regimens in desperate attempts to find the elusive cure and can result in increased toxicities and potentially hampered quality of life. Healthcare professionals may find it challenging to confront the truth of a poor prognosis without removing hope and the decision to involve palliative care may be feared to constitute an abandonment of hope for a cure, regardless how remote. Allowing the family to hear possible outcomes of a diagnosis may offer them the opportunity to better collaborate with healthcare professionals and prepare for what may lie ahead for them.

The idea that a parent will ever be ready to hear that their child will probably not survive is inconceivable. Parents may intellectually understand that the prognosis is very poor but remain reluctant to accept the likelihood of their child's death while waiting for a cure. Denial can be an important coping mechanism, but it can also function as a barrier to providing comfort and quality-of-life choices to a child during intensive treatments and at end of life. Denial can be damaging to relationships within the family and can result in moral distress for healthcare providers as further curative attempts become perceived as prolonging suffering.[7] Research findings indicate that parents want to know as soon as the healthcare team knows that their child may not survive and what assurances they have that their child's comfort needs and quality-of-life issues will be addressed. It has also been shown that families are more satisfied with their relationships with the healthcare providers when they are better informed of possible outcomes, even if discomforting.[8] In a study looking at parents' priorities for quality end-of-life care in an intensive care setting, honesty and access to complete information were the key recommendations from families.[9] Rather than parents' perceived readiness, the healthcare professional's comfort with discussing the topic that can be expected to be difficult and time consuming may be a more important issue.

The time and expertise required to discuss issues of symptom control and quality of life can easily exceed a healthcare team's resources. At the same time, social workers, chaplains, nurses, and physicians may believe that comfort and supportive care are included in their existing plan of care without the need to add a palliative care specialist specifically. However, a retrospective study looking at healthcare record documentation did not reflect the use of these services for supportive care for children at end of life.[10] The need for more education and mentorship in palliative care to improve staff members' knowledge and experience in this area is well recognized.

Reimbursement for specific palliative care services remains limited, but can usually be included as routine services charged along with treatment support.

Introducing Palliative Care

The introduction of palliative care can be done using three different approaches.

AN ADDED DIMENSION TO CARE

Many disciplines are involved in the treatment of a child with challenging conditions. These may include medical subspecialists, surgeons, nurses, social workers, pharmacists, dieticians, child life specialists, and many others. As with any of these disciplines, palliative care can be introduced as a component of the care team whose focus will be to provide comfort from disturbing physical, social, or spiritual challenges. Palliative care specialists participate in developing a plan of care that is collaboratively established along with the patient's and family's goals of care. A palliative care model has been proposed for children with cancer in which components of quality of life care are integrated into family care along the illness trajectory. This model demonstrated how palliative care was essential regardless of the child's prognosis, because even children with an essentially good prognosis could eventually require end-of-life care.[11] Including palliative care at the time of diagnosis allows palliative care to become the foundation upon which additional treatment modalities are built. If all involved can assure that comfort and quality of life are key components of care, then additional interventions such as surgery and medical treatments can be evaluated by their contribution to or deterrence from that base. This modality allows for palliative care to be incorporated at the earliest time and can be accomplished by adding skills and experiences to the basic healthcare team or can include the incorporation of new members specializing in palliative care to the primary team.

By allowing the palliative care team to join at diagnosis, the family does not feel that strangers are being added when the family needs support and consistency from those who have cared for them along the course of the illness. An example of this approach to timing could be the extreme premature infant. A child born at 25 weeks' gestation is considered viable, but will remain in the neonatal intensive care unit for several months and will likely require extended community support for developmental delays, supplemental oxygen requirements, and specialized feeding requirements for years. Although the child may ultimately survive, the child's and family's needs for information support and coordination of complex care needs can be facilitated with the early involvement of palliative care professionals. In this case, a palliative care consult may be included in the order set for premature infants less than 28 weeks' gestation. The primary physician or the palliative care professional can introduce the concept by saying, "In our NICU, we include professionals who will help us address your and your baby's physical, social, and spiritual needs. Working with our doctors, nurses, and social workers will be a palliative care team. You will be introduced to that team sometime this first week, and they may remain involved with your child's care even after discharge."

MOVEMENT FROM CURE TO PALLIATION

When conditions have a high likelihood of cure, it is not uncommon for healthcare practitioners to exclude the topic of palliative care until it becomes obvious that a cure will not be accomplished. At this time, specialists are usually added to the primary team to introduce a change in treatment approach from curative to palliative. This approach allows for continued therapy toward the possible cure, but the goal of comfort and quality time with loved ones becomes a priority. With the primary team still managing care, new treatment and outcome goals may be established collaboratively with the patient and family, using concepts of palliative care. An example of this approach to palliative care can be seen with a child diagnosed with a relapsed medulloblastoma. While the concepts of palliative care may have been incorporated into the primary team's approach to the condition at original diagnosis, treatment of this recurrence is unlikely to result in a cure. While additional chemotherapy, radiation therapy, and alternative approaches may be considered, the palliative care perspective would assure that approaches to treat the underlying cancer did not deter unacceptably from the child's comfort, quality time with those who love him or her and assurance of dignity and respect. The toll upon the child and family can be weighed against the potential prolongation of life.

Palliative care could be introduced at this time by the primary physician saying, "As we consider treatment options for your child, I am asking another specialty to join us. The palliative care service will work with us to assure that while we continue to consider perhaps aggressive treatment options, we are equally aggressive in addressing any signs of discomfort or worries that could arise. These professionals are part of the excellent care we want to continue to provide to you and your child."

TRANSITION TO HOSPICE

The hospice approach is employed when all attempts toward a cure are abandoned and all efforts are placed on comfort and quality time with loved ones. At this time, specialists in hospice may enter the care team, and as a result of restrictions imposed by third-party payers, the primary team may become less involved. Care is provided by the hospice service, which will include physicians, nurses, social workers, chaplains, and child life specialists who are not necessarily the same people as those on the primary treatment team. This transition can be very difficult for families who have come to rely upon the collaborative care provided by their primary team. Families have been known to express feelings of abandonment and desertion at this time. Healthcare professionals may be concerned about their lack of involvement at a very vulnerable time with families with whom they may have had several years of involvement. It would be ideal if the primary team could continue to be involved and coordinate this aspect of care, which would include bereavement support.[12]

An example of this approach could be the child with a severe cardiac defect which is not surgically correctable. The child would be given medications to alleviate fluid retention, control pain and dyspnea, and oxygen supplementation, but could be followed by a hospice team that visits him or her in the home and provides support at end of life and through bereavement. Again, the primary physician is best to introduce this transition in care. A typical introduction could be, "We have exhausted

TABLE 20-2 Examples of End-of-Life and Palliative Care Language

End-of-life language	
Helpful phrases	**Avoid**
May I just sit here with you?	It was a blessing…
Is there anyone I can call for you?	You have other children and your family to think about.
I can't imagine how difficult this must be.	I know how you feel.
Would you like me to talk with your other family members, or be there with you when you talk with them?	You must be strong for your family and other children.

Palliative care language	
Helpful phrases	**Avoid**
Let's talk about the lab tests and treatments that are not providing benefit for your child and talk about discontinuing these.	It's time to pull back in her treatment and not order expensive tests.
Let's review what we have done so far in care, what has been the outcome, and what our goals of care are now.	There is nothing more we can do.
In my experience, I have not seen a child in this situation survive. We will continue to hope for his comfort and quality time with those who love him.	A miracle may turn things around.

all approaches that could be expected to cure your child. It is now time to change our care plan away from her underlying heart problem and instead challenge anything that is making her uncomfortable, or that decreases the quality time she has with you or others who love her or that in any way impact her dignity. I would like to ask our hospice team to meet with you to offer their services." It is important to remember that hospice service could be provided by existing, and possibly already involved, palliative care professionals, without a change in service providers or loss of primary care provider.

The timing and wording used for introducing the concept of palliative care can be as varied as the conditions that warrant it. If not incorporated at the time of diagnosis, establishment of clear guidelines for when it should be introduced need to be established in areas where concerns for the child's and family's comfort and relief from distressing symptoms would be helpful. Early inclusion, prior to discussions about preparations for death, are particularly helpful to foster the inclusion of the patient and family in the multidisciplinary care plan. Examples of language that may be used by clinicians when discussing palliative care and end-of-life issues are included in Table 20-2.

Clinical Vignette

Sarah Kohn, 6, was recently diagnosed with recurrent acute myelogenous leukemia after previously being treated with chemotherapy and hematopoietic stem cell transplant from a sibling donor. Her parents are meeting with the pediatric oncologist, social worker, and primary nurse. The palliative care nurse practitioner has been asked to join the multidisciplinary conference, and will be meeting the family for the first time.

MD: Mr. and Mrs. Kohn, we have the results of Sarah's bone marrow aspiration biopsy. As you probably suspected by us asking to meet with you as a team, our concerns have been confirmed and her AML has returned.

Mother: I just knew it! She hasn't been herself for the last two weeks and her counts were dropping.

Father: Now what do we do? More chemo? Another transplant?

MD: We have some options that we would like to discuss with you, but I must be honest with you. Our chances to cure Sarah are very remote. We have other chemotherapy regimens to try, but her leukemia has proven to be stronger than our best therapy. Other therapies are less likely to be more effective at eradicating her cancer.

Mother: So what happens if you can't get rid of the cancer? Is she going to die? Please don't tell us that!

SW: I know this is very difficult for you. Let's hear what therapies the doctor has to offer, then make a plan to do the very best we can do for Sarah.

MD: I have asked the nurse practitioner in charge of supportive and palliative care to join us. I believe that her services can add much to what we are going to offer.

PCNP: I'm so sorry that you have received such devastating news. My role on her treatment team is to assure that regardless of the treatment options that we decide upon for her cancer, we will always strive to make sure that she is comfortable, that she has the best quality time with those who love her, and that we treat her with respect and dignity for the fabulous person that she is. We promise to do the same for you. I suggest that we use these three goals as our base upon which any treatment options are built. I will explain further as we discuss her treatment options.

MD: There are basically three different approaches open to us at this time. The first is to give Sarah another very strong chemotherapy regimen; even stronger than her previous therapy. This will probably result in her being in the hospital for four to six weeks, possibly in the PICU, and with a serious risk of multiple infections and toxicities; any of which could take her life, even if we are successful in getting her back into another remission. If she does go into remission, we could consider another bone marrow transplant (BMT), but the toxicities would be greater yet.

The second choice would be to give Sarah an experimental therapy that has not been proved to be effective against AML in children, but has shown some promise in the laboratory and with adult studies. The purpose of giving her this therapy would primarily be to learn more about that specific drug and how a child who has been heavily pre-treated would tolerate it. The toxicities to this therapy would be expected to be less than the first option, and Sarah could benefit from the therapy.

The third option is for us to use just enough chemotherapy to minimize her symptoms, while allowing her to be at home with the fewest side effects. Again, none of these three options have the potential to cure her disease. We don't have a therapy that can offer that to Sarah at this time. I have already checked with colleagues specializing in AML therapies nationwide and no one has any other options that they would recommend.

SW: Please understand that you are not making the decision of which therapy to give her by yourself. We will be making this decision together as a team. No parent should be expected to make the decision alone, and the medical team can't make the decision without taking into consideration what is important to you and Sarah.

PCNP: As we think about these options, why don't we talk about what is really important to Sarah. Because I don't know her yet, what can you tell me about her? What is she like when she isn't in the hospital?

Mother (sobbing): She is the most energetic, happy, positive little girl that I have ever known. She always has a smile for everyone. She loves to play with her dog, and her friends and her little sister.

RN: Sarah is loved by all the nurses for exactly those attributes, even though she never likes to be in the hospital! She is always showing us pictures of her dog, and places and people she likes to visit. She is an avid artist and we have lots of her creations posted in the nurse's station.

Father: I don't want to give her any therapy that will take Sarah away from us again. I thought I would die when she was hospitalized for so long for her transplant. And she was so sick. I don't want to do that again, but I also don't want to give up! You can't ask us to do that!

MD: No one is suggesting that we give up. We have treatment options, and we will continue to hope for the best outcome for Sarah. If we can get her into another remission, we may be able to give her some more time, possibly even another BMT.

SW: Would you be interested in talking about an aggressive approach, including another BMT?

Mother: I'm not sure I could handle that again, and I don't think Sarah is strong enough for it. I would want to offer her the best chance she has for a cure so that she can live and grow up.

PCNP: Again, regardless of the treatment option that we all decide upon, we all agree that we will build upon our promise to assure her comfort and quality time with you. Some of these options may make that goal easier than others.

Father: If we choose to give her the experimental chemotherapy, there might be a chance for a cure, and it doesn't sound as hard as the stronger chemo and BMT. Is that right?

MD: It would be possible, but not expected, for the experimental chemo regimen to place her into a remission and again, it is not expected to cure her. Our hope would be that we learn more about this medication, a child's tolerance of it, and any effect that it may have on her disease.

SW: Hope is a very important part of any choice that we make at this time. We will all work together to foster that hope that Sarah can live along with her cancer, comfortably, for as long as possible.

PCNP: Would you like to talk about some of the symptoms that bothered Sarah the most during her previous therapies? This could help us anticipate and prevent their occurrence in whichever subsequent therapy we decide upon.

The meeting continued with discussions about pain, mouth sores, septic shock episodes, nausea and vomiting, anorexia, fear, and loneliness. The PCNP, SW, MD, and RN all provided suggestions that may prevent or minimize each symptom in the future, while the parents offered specifics as to what had worked in the past. Upon completion of this conference, the parents asked for a day to discuss it with their family and rabbi. They returned to further discuss their options, and eventually, along with the healthcare team, chose the experimental regimen. A plan of care was developed with palliative care and symptom control as the base and additional approaches to assure comfort and as much quality time with loved ones outside the hospital as possible. All hoped for and worked toward minimizing Sarah's hospital stays, and eventually she experienced a peaceful, dignified death at home, surrounded by loved ones, including her dog.

Summary

When a child is diagnosed with a life-threatening or life-limiting condition, the lives of their entire family is changed forever. Their physical and affective world is immediately changed, regardless of the outcome of treatment. A multidisciplinary healthcare team is required to offer hope to children and families regardless of the possibility of a cure. This approach focuses not only on cure, but also incorporates the understanding that quality of life must be assured regardless of length of life and that compassionate care can be provided in all stages of treatment. Palliative care adds much to the plan of care for children and their families regardless of the underlying prognosis.[13] It allows the patient and family to partner with the healthcare team to assure that along the disease trajectory, comfort and quality of life remain the base upon which therapeutic interventions are offered and assures a partnership among the patient, family, and healthcare team.

REFERENCES

1. Callahan D: *The troubled dream of life: in search of a peaceful death*, Washington, DC, 2000, Georgetown University Press.
2. Field M, Behrman R: *When children die: improving palliative and end-of-life care for children and their families*, Washington, DC, 2003, National Academies Press.
3. American Academy of Pediatrics, Committee on Bioethics and Committee on Hospital Care: Palliative care for children, *Pediatrics* 106(2):351–357, 2000.
4. Davies B, Sehring SA, Partridge JC, Cooper BA, Hughes A, Philp JC, Amidi-Nouri A, Kramer RF: *Pediatrics* 121(2):282–288, 2008.
5. Selwyn PA, Forsetin M: Overcoming the false dichotomy of curative vs palliative care for late-stage HIV/AIDS: "Let me live the way I want to live, until I can't." *JAMA* 290(6):806–814, 2003.
6. Hilden JM, Emanuel EJK, Fairclough DL, Link MP, Foley KM, Clarridge BC, et al: Attitudes and practices among pediatric oncologists regarding end-of-life care: results of the 1998 American Society of Clinical Oncology Survey, *J Clin Oncol* 19:205–212, 2001.
7. Davies B, Clark D, Connaughty S: Caring for dying children: nurses' experiences, *Pediatr Nurs* 22(6):500–507, 1996.
8. Wolfe J, Grier HE, Klar N, Levin SB, Ellenbogen JM, Salem-Schatz S, et al: Symptoms and suffering at the end of life in children with cancer, *N Engl J Med* 342(5):326–333, 2000.
9. Meyer EC, Ritholz MD, Burns JP, Truog RD: Improving the quality of end-of-life care in the pediatric intensive care unit: parents' priorities and recommendations, *Pediatrics* 117(3):649–657, 2006.
10. Carter BS, Howenstien M, Gilmer MJ, Throop P, France D, Whitlock JA: Circumstances surrounding the deaths of hospitalized children: opportunities for pediatric palliative care, *Pediatrics* 114(3):361–366, 2004.
11. Harris MB: Palliative care in children with cancer: which child and when? *J Natl Cancer Inst Monogr* 32:144–149, 2004.
12. Docherty SL, Miles MS, Brandon D: Searching for 'the dying point': providers' experiences with palliative care in pediatric acute care, *Pediatr Nurs* 33(4):335–341, 2007.
13. Hutton N, Jones B, Hilden JM: From cure to palliation: managing the transition, *Child Adolesc Psychiatr Clin North Am* 15(3):575–584, 2006.

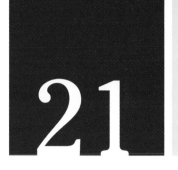

Introducing Home-Based Palliative Care and Hospice

ROSS M. HAYS | LESLIE ADAMS | MICHELLE FROST

Only connect. That was the whole of her sermon. Only connect the prose and the passion, and both will be exalted, and human love will be seen at its height. Live in fragments no longer. —E. M. Forster, in *Howards End*

The majority of children who die in the United States do not die at home. Nearly three-fourths of pediatric deaths occur in the hospital, mostly in intensive care units (ICUs) where aggressive, life-sustaining medical therapy is typically provided.[1] Home-based palliative care and hospice programs serve less than a third of the children who die, and the majority of those hospice agencies do not have specially trained pediatric teams. Even when this specialized service is available in the community, it is often underused.

The number of children who die at home as a result of complex chronic conditions has been steadily increasing during the last twenty years. The growing number of these children has been cited as a justification to expand the capacity for home-based hospice and home-nursing care in order to meet the increasing palliative care needs of these complicated pediatric patients.[2]

In 2008, the availability of home-based hospice care was demonstrated to have an indirect positive effect on the quality of end-of-life experience and bereavement. The study showed that families of children with severe life-limiting illnesses who have home care available are five times more likely to participate in the planning of their child's location of death. The opportunity to plan was associated with better experiences at the end of life and less prolonged grief afterward.[3]

Home-based palliative care and hospice is one dimension of care for children with severe life-limiting diseases, yet the introduction of home-based palliative care and hospice is often difficult and fraught with anxiety for both the family and the medical team. Clinicians may be more successful in providing home-based palliative care and hospice if we understand its component parts, including recognizing the barriers to palliative care, forgoing the search for the dying point, avoiding abandonment, and maintaining hope. Based on our combined experiences in home-based palliative care and hospice and gleanings from the literature, we describe these components and the clinical practices that help the goals of each component.

Recognizing the Barriers to Palliative Care

The barriers to the introduction of palliative care and hospice for children are often different than those identified for adult hospice referrals. Fear of addiction to pain medication, fear of hastening death through use of opioids and concerns about legal action are common problems in the recommendation of hospice care for adults, but are rarely encountered in pediatrics. The barriers to referral for children can be roughly divided into two groups: those that are associated with constraints within our national medical culture and those that are related to clinical practice.

Constraints within our medical culture include limited financial resources for specialized pediatric palliative care, limited access in rural regions, lack of research and evidence-based guidelines, and lack of provider training and expertise. These barriers are best addressed at the level of resource allocation, policy, local and governmental advocacy, and curriculum development.[4] There has been a gratifying, if small, increase in the awareness of these issues in the last decade but clearly the gains accomplished so far have only advanced the frequency of referrals by a small amount.

Historically, palliative care has been confused with a subset of palliative care: hospice. Hospice in the United States traditionally has been reserved for children whose doctors were willing to predict that they had 6 months or less to live and whose families were willing to forgo curative treatment. This confusion over palliative care and hospice often led to an awkward introduction of palliative care to the family late in the child's illness, preventing children and their families from receiving comfort care at home. The criteria for enrollment into hospice, especially agreeing to forgo curative treatment, have been stumbling blocks that have interfered with the opportunity for children to receive home-based hospice care at the end of their lives. The most encouraging models now include home-based palliative care programs that provide community-based care without the strict eligibility requirement for hospice but also allow patients to transition into hospice when it is appropriate.

The barriers to palliative care and hospice referral that are related to clinical practice are more subtle. In 2008, Davies and colleagues identified 26 barriers to palliative care referral within a large pediatric teaching hospital. The five most frequently cited barriers from the providers' perspective were uncertainty of prognosis, families not being ready to acknowledge the incurable condition, language barriers, time constraints, and families' preferences for life-sustaining care.[1]

Uncertainty of prognosis is much more common in pediatric patients than in adults. In most pediatric palliative care programs, cancer represents less than half of all diagnostic groups. Children with chronic and complex life-limiting conditions now represent a wide variety of illnesses, including those caused by prematurity, congenital disorders of every organ system, neurodegenerative abnormalities, and malignancies. All of these disorders are relatively rare and often do not lend themselves to accurate predictions about either the response to treatment or the likelihood of survival. This uncertainty can lead to confusion

195

that undermines the goals of care and leads to a "dichotomous cure vs. palliative care" approach.[1] In this framework neither parents nor medical teams are willing to pursue palliative care or hospice until all are sure that no curative option exists. Thus referral occurs inevitably late when the opportunity to plan and arrange for quality care at the end of life may no longer be possible. Uncertainty also has the ability to undermine the medical team's credibility with families who expect expert medical personnel to be able to predict the natural history of their child's disease. Uncertainty over prognosis in this situation can erode the family's trust, it can impede the development of consensus for care, and delay spiritual and psychosocial support, all of which may contribute to increased suffering.

The death of a child is never within the natural order of things and is therefore "always out of season."[5] It is not surprising then that the second- and fifth-most common barriers to referral are the families' lack of readiness to acknowledge an incurable condition and families' preference for life-sustaining treatment. There is considerable overlap among these barriers. Families are often confronted with unexpected reversals, idiosyncratic responses to therapy and plateaus of relative stability that inspire them to hope for a positive resolution of their child's disease. Their best hopes for recovery are often supported by the promises of the latest treatment and the newest technology or by the recounting of miraculous recoveries promoted by the media and the hospital's own marketing department. At times, some members of the clinical care team are unable to stop aggressive medical treatment, even while they are discussing end-of-life options, because they cannot know with absolute certainty that a child will die. This mixed message adds to the family's uncertainty. The medical team often recognizes a terminal prognosis before families do.[6] Bridging the gap between the team's and the family's understanding of the child's terminal diagnosis is difficult. If done too abruptly it can create tension between the staff and family; if it is delayed and aggressive curative care is continued beyond the limits of perceived benefit, then both the staff and the family can suffer acute moral distress.[7] There is growing evidence that the introduction of skilled communicators at this point may facilitate clearer understanding of the prognosis and promote a unified approach to goals of care.

The increasingly technological sophistication of diagnostic and treatment procedures and the sensitive nature of end-of-life communication challenges the assurance that the family's understanding is adequate to meet the minimum requirements of informed consent. This challenge is increased when families have limited proficiency in English. U.S. federal antidiscrimination laws require that healthcare facilities receiving federal funds provide professional interpreter services for families with limited English proficiency, but the mandate is seldom enforced. The cultural barriers extend beyond language. For example, many Latino families view the physician as a figure of authority and consider it impolite to question, correct, or disagree. Some promising innovations include states that have adopted Medicaid codes that include compensation for medical translation and health organizations that have diversity centers which employ cultural navigators for families.[8]

Forgoing the Search for the Dying Point

The majority of medical providers view home-based palliative care and hospice as a changed dimension of care instituted once it is agreed that death is the likely outcome for the patient.[9]

Conflict from many sources occurs when the provision of palliative care or hospice is viewed as a new approach to care distinct from aggressive medical management. Because providers view palliative care as a distinctly different model of care, they are tempted to search for the point along the illness trajectory when they are sure death is inevitable, the dying point, and then transition to palliative care or hospice. This approach is not helpful because there is rarely agreement about the timing of the dying point.[6] Empirical attempts to predict which children will need palliative care when it is tied to the timing of death have been unproductive.[10,11]

Home-based palliative care and hospice should be considered in terms of the patient's and family's needs rather than as a wholesale change in approach that occurs at a single point along the disease trajectory. To search for the dying point only delays the provision of services and leads to missed opportunities for better managed care at the end of life. When palliative care and hospice are conceptualized as models of care that seek to prevent, relieve, reduce, or soothe the symptoms produced by serious medical conditions to maintain the quality of life for seriously ill children and their families, they can be integrated with curative or life-prolonging care. This model may begin at diagnosis in many cases where the disease is known to be potentially life limiting and be continued throughout the disease trajectory regardless of the outcome.

Adopting such a model of palliative care and hospice as timely and coincident treatment requires a shift in the attitudes of many of the acute care services. New educational programs are helping to promote this model of palliative care. Recently some programs have reported success with prospective agreements on referral criteria that automatically trigger referrals to palliative care and hospice. By doing so, these agreements obviate the search for the dying point and ensure that, at a minimum, the hospice and palliative care services have the chance to assess families' needs in a timely manner.[12] More progress will likely come by sharing the emerging evidence about the benefits of palliative care and hospice as early intervention with acute care providers. Eventually these interventions may help to create an environment where the introduction of home-based palliative care and hospice is less abrupt, more readily accepted by families and associated with better quality of life outcomes at the end of life.[12]

Avoiding Abandonment

Perhaps the area where adult and pediatric care differ the most is the transition process. Adults with severe life-limiting illnesses are frequently transferred to a new caregiver team for home-based hospice, with progressively limited contact from the acute service. A 2000 study suggests that adults tolerate this transfer from one team to another fairly well.[13] The nature of pediatrics, the special place that the ill child occupies in the clinical milieu, and the needs of young families make the traditional model of transfer ineffective for children.

Although continuity of care has been a focus on neonatal and pediatric units for more than a decade, it is easy to see how this critical attribute is degraded when an acute care team terminates their relationship with the family and the home based palliative care team or hospice assumes a management role. Patients and their families form strong, healthy relationships with their acute providers. Nurses particularly form very strong attachments to their patients and have intimate knowledge of families' needs and strengths.[9] An abrupt transfer to a new team, regardless of the skills of its members and the best intentions of all those involved, has a profound and usually negative impact on the continuity of care that the child and the family need.[14] At its worst, the transition takes on the quality of abandonment.

A model of home-based palliative care and hospice that integrates curative care would most effectively be implemented by the acute team. It is most successful when both teams work cooperatively to introduce the transition and continue to stay in contact through the duration of the child's illness up to, and including, death.

One example of introducing home-based palliative care includes tasks that are shared by the acute and the palliative care teams. The earlier in the trajectory of illness that the discussion occurs, the more likely it is to be helpful to the patient, the family, and to all care providers. Although the acute and the palliative care teams may take turns taking the lead on different aspects of the conversation, it is imperative that the discussions occur with both teams with the family at the same time. The advantages of this approach are many; it reduces the risk of miscommunication and misunderstanding of the goals of care, but most importantly it demonstrates the partnership in continuity of care that both teams are committed to provide.

The acute team is best equipped to provide the most accurate understanding of the diagnosis and prognosis. With the palliative care team present, the acute team can introduce the patient and family to members of the home-based team. Then it is best to review the patient's medical status. This should include a sensitive recounting of the testing and treatments provided thus far, and include unambiguous explanations of the negative outcomes. For medically fragile children with complex care needs or children with degenerative disorders whose course is somewhat predictable, this description may occur quite early in the trajectory of illness and contain a review of what is known about the natural history of the disease. For children who have life-threatening illnesses, the discussion should begin as soon as possible. An example might be, "We had hoped that the pathology report would suggest a benign tumor, but unfortunately this is a malignant tumor that is presenting in a very aggressive way. We will do everything we can to treat this successfully and restore your child to health but we may come to the place where we cannot cure this disease." This can be followed by a discussion of the family's questions and concerns. Within this discussion it is important to be realistic about treatment options and to provide accurate information free from speculation about options that are truly not available, For example, statements such as "if this were a less-aggressive cancer we would be considering x or y treatment" creates needless ambiguity in the minds of patients and families and may undermine the goals of care.

This honest accumulation of negative medical evidence must be balanced with a holistic approach to continued care, with assurances that the child's needs will still be aggressively assessed and treated. It also must be communicated that the team will continue to work toward the highest degree of comfort and quality of life possible throughout the child's illness and even at the end of life. Both teams can then move ahead with the discussion by assessing the patient's and family's understanding of the prognosis. This part of the discussion is often the most sensitive and should be led by the family with open, cooperative responses from both teams. The next step is to encourage the family to articulate their goals of care. Both teams may then assist the family in reviewing their goals, and in the cases where it is necessary, reframing their goals. The palliative care team may then lead with a discussion of the family's needs and proceed with dialogue that links the needs to the goals of care. When the link between needs and goals is established, at least temporarily, the home-based team can then proceed with more detailed descriptions of the services available and the methods by which they can be accessed by the patient and the family. The most appropriate conclusion to this introductory discussion is a clear reinforcement of the commitment from both the acute care team and the home-based team to continue to work together to provide the highest level of care for the patient and the family.

The approach described above may be a best case scenario and may not be possible in every patient setting. However, if the best intentions, honoring the family's perspective, maintaining honest communication, and creating an atmosphere of genuine cooperation are honored then the risk of abandonment will be reduced.

Maintaining Hope

Hope is not a singular entity that can be created or destroyed by circumstances or conversations. It is an essential component of the human spirit and a way of living in the world. Truthful disclosure about life-limiting pediatric disease, even when the prognosis is poor or uncertain, does not have the power to diminish hope.[15] Truth telling and compassionate listening build rapport that enables hope to flourish, regardless of the circumstances. Realistic perceptions of prognosis, sensitively communicated, have the potential to transform hope into meaningful goals for children and their families, even at the end of life. An experienced clinician might explain that there are no more curative options by first reviewing all the treatment that has taken place thus far and then following with a statement such as: "If we could find another treatment that would cure this disease, we would offer it to your child, but we have tried everything and have exhausted all of our options. At this point a cure would be a miracle. We want you to know that we will continue to care for your child, and work to meet her needs, regardless of the outcome. And as we do, we will join you in hoping for a miracle."

Compassionate relationships are the vehicles that impart hope, regardless of the trajectory of illness.[15] Eliciting and establishing goals of care is essential throughout the course of treatment and has the ability to promote and transform hope. Evaluating where the family may be on the continuum of hope at any moment is a necessary starting point for conversations that build relationships. These conversations should include the sharing of specific recommendations that invite further conversation, the introduction of the possibility of death when appropriate, and the elicitation of goals of care as they continue to change. Continuity of care is central in the promotion of hope. Families and providers both benefit from maintaining the relationship with their acute care providers, even after the majority of the curative treatment has concluded.

Families value honest and complete information. The relationships that foster their hope require ready access to trusted staff. Relieving some of the burdens of care with the provision of care coordination can provide relief that allows families the emotional space to grow in hope. Hope can be supported by appropriate and honest emotional expression on the part of staff members. Parents' hopes are supported by continuing efforts that maintain the integrity of the parent-child relationship. Religious faith can be very meaningful to families as they approach their child's life-limiting illness. Creating a culture of acceptance and integration of spiritual belief may be crucial for some families in the promotion of hope throughout the course of the illness.[16]

Families' beliefs and experiences inform their hopes. It can sometimes be helpful to families if clinicians help them to locate their hope when it appears to be elusive. An example of this might include asking the family what they hope for. When the answer they provide is "We are hoping for a cure," then a helpful response might be "I am hoping for a cure, too. And I hope we get one, but if we are not able to have a complete remission, what else do you hope for?" Frequently families will respond with a more proximate hope, such as "I hope she will live until Thanksgiving." By locating the nature of their deepest hopes, families can direct the goals of care in a constructive direction. The child's care can proceed with realistic hopes without sacrificing hope at a higher level.[17,18]

Hope can extend into bereavement by affirming a lifelong bond with the child that continues after death. Bereaved parents strive to find ways of sustaining that lifelong bond.[19] Hope can continue by sustaining belief in the possibility of making meaning out of their child's death. Home-based programs that include bereavement, sibling programs, and ongoing support groups can assist families as they search for meaning in their child's death and grow in the relationship with their child after death.[20] Families hope to sustain life and the physical and emotional union of relationship throughout their child's illness. That same hope can continue into bereavement as parents nurture and create lifelong bonds with their deceased children.

REFERENCES

1. Davies B, Sehring SA, Partridge JC, Cooper BA, Hughes A, Philip JC, Amidid-Nouri A, Kramer RF: Barriers to palliative care for children: perceptions of pediatric health care providers, *Pediatrics* 121(2): 282–288, 2008.
2. Feudtner C, Fienstein J, Satchell M, Zhao H, Kang T: Shifting place of death among children with complex chronic conditions in the United States, 1989–2003, *JAMA* 297(24):2725–2732, 2007.
3. Dussel V, Kreicsbergs U, Hilden J, Watterston J, Moore C, Turner BG, Weeks J, Wolfe J: Looking beyond where children die: determinants and effects of planning a child's location of death, *J Pain Symptom Manage* 37(1):33–43, 2008.
4. Himelstein B, Hilden JM, Boldt AM, Weissman D: Pediatric palliative care, *N Engl J Med* 350(7):1752–1762, 2004.
5. Hinds PS, Schum L, Baker JN, Wolfe J: Key factors affecting dying children and their families, *J Palliat Med* 8(Suppl 1):S70–S78, 2005.
6. Wolfe J, Klar N, Grier H, Duncan J, Salem-Schatz S, Emanuel E, Weeks JC: Understanding of prognosis among parents of children who died of cancer: impact on treatment goals and integration of palliative care, *JAMA* 284(19):2469–2475, 2000.
7. Elpern EH, Covert B, Kleinpell R: Moral distress of staff nurses in a medical intensive care unit, *Am J Crit Care* 14(6):523–530, 2005.
8. Hunt LM, de Voogd KB: Are good intentions good enough? Informed consent without trained interpreters, *J Gen Intern Med* 22(5):598–605, 2006.
9. Docherty DL, Miles MS, Brandon D: Searching for the "dying point:" providers' experiences with palliative care and acute care, *Pediatr Nurs* 33(4):335–341, 2007.
10. Feudtner C, Connor SR: Epidemiology and health services research. In Carter BS, Levetown M, editors: *Palliative care for infants, children and adolescents*, Baltimore, 2002, Johns Hopkins Press, pp 3–22.
11. Sahler OJ, Frager G, Levetown M, Cohn F, Lipson M: Medical education about end of life care in the pediatric setting: principles, challenges and opportunities, *Pediatrics* 105(4):575–584, 2000.
12. Hays RM, Valentine J, Haynes G, et al: The Seattle pediatric palliative care project: effects on family satisfaction and health-related quality of life, *J Palliat Med* 9(3):716–728, 2006.
13. Steinhauser KE, Christakis NA, Clipp EC, McNeilly M, McIntyre L, Tulsky J: Factors considered important at the end of life by patients, family and physicians, and other care providers, *JAMA* 284(10):2476–2482, 2000.
14. Bak AL, Young JP, McCown E, Engelberg RA, Vig EK, Reinke LF, Wenrich MD, McGrath BB, Curtis JR: Abandonment at the end of life from patient, caregiver, nurse and physician perspectives, *Arch Intern Med* 169(5): 474–479, 2009.
15. Mack J, Wolf J, et al: Hope and prognostic disclosure, *J Clin Oncol* 25(35):5636–5642, 2007.
16. Meyer E, Ritholz M, Burns J, Truog R: Improving the quality of end-of-life care in the pediatric intensive care unit: parents' priorities and recommendations, *Pediatrics* 117(3):649–657, 2006.
17. Feudtner C: Hope and the prospects of healing at the end of life, *J Altern Complement Med* 11(1):S23–S30, 2005.
18. Feudtner C, et al: Hopeful thinking and level of comfort regarding providing pediatric palliative care: a survey of hospital nurses, *Pediatrics* 119(1):186–192, 2007.
19. Finkbeiner A: *After the death of a child: living with loss through the years*, Baltimore, 1996, Johns Hopkins.
20. Murphy S, Johnson C: Finding meaning in a child's violent death: a five-year prospective analysis of parents' personal narratives and empirical data, *Death Stud* 27(5):381, 2003.

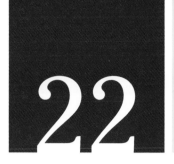

Resuscitation

JUSTIN N. BAKER

The kid is a full code. We can't get the parents to sign a Do Not Resuscitate (DNR) order. They just don't get it. ...

The expression "the parents signed the DNR" is erroneous because, in most instances, they are not required to do so. It is more acceptable to state that the parents "agreed to the recommendations of the healthcare team regarding resuscitation status."

Open discussions between clinicians and the patient and family about the goals of care and recommendations regarding resuscitation status are encouraged. Taking a "hope for the best, but plan for everything" approach may help parents during this difficult time of decision making.

Although technological and medical advances have led to an increase in pediatric patients' survival rates, the number of children living with life-threatening conditions is on the rise.[1] Many of these children are medically fragile and face uncertain prognoses with regard to cure, life expectancy, and functional outcome.[2] End-of-life decisions such as forgoing life-sustaining medical treatments or placing a DNR or similar order in the medical record are extremely complex, and parents report that decisions such as these are most difficult for them to make for their child with a life-threatening illness.[3] Frequently, these decisions have to be made at a time when the patient has experienced clinical deterioration, causing great duress for family members as they witness the significant suffering associated with their child's advancing illness. Communication and decision making with patients and parents regarding resuscitation and forgoing artificial life-sustaining medical treatments (ALSMT) must therefore be based on a framework that is both humanistic and ethical.[4] Although attempting to predict outcomes in this group of highly complex patients may be difficult, performing cardiopulmonary resuscitation (CPR) or other medical and procedural interventions may seriously impair the quality of life of patients. It may also negatively impact the ability of children and parents to achieve important life goals. In an effort to minimize this risk, clinicians, parents, and pediatric patients frequently struggle to decide if or when to place a DNR or similar order in the medical record.

A patient's resuscitation status is usually determined by the clinician through discussions with the patient and family on the potential use of certain medical interventions, such as CPR or endotracheal intubation and mechanical ventilation in the care of a patient with life-threatening illness. In the context of clinical care, these discussions are frequently summarized by the simple phrases code or no code. These discussions, however, have to be individualized and based on the overall goals of care for the patient and family.[5] Specific interventions such as non-invasive respiratory support or other ALSMT may be appropriate early in the disease trajectory, but as death becomes imminent, goals as well as interventions to support them may likely change. The primary purpose of such resuscitation discussions is to attempt to secure for the incurable child a death filled with dignity and free from excessive suffering and treatment-related morbidity.[6]

The American Academy of Pediatrics (AAP) has adopted the definition of ALSMT as "all interventions that may prolong the life of patients."[7] This includes such technologically advanced measures as solid organ and bone marrow transplantation, but also includes less technically demanding measures such as antibiotics, support from blood products, artificial hydration or nutrition, and CPR. There has been a general consensus in pediatric medical literature that decisions regarding starting or forgoing ALSMT should be based primarily on the relative benefits and burdens to the patient and family.[8,9] Therefore, the goals of the patient and family need to be elucidated and the potential benefits and burdens of CPR and other ALSMT clearly explained. Clinicians must understand the goals and needs of patients and their families for making suitable recommendations to forgo an attempt at resuscitation or withhold or withdraw ALSMT (Table 22-1). CPR is unique in that an order is required to forgo it, and it is presumed that resuscitation is desired unless explicitly refused through a DNR or other similar order.[10] Most healthcare facilities have a specific form, such as a DNR order, that is used to denote the patient's resuscitation status. The specific contents of a DNR order vary widely, depending on legal jurisdiction and individual facility interpretation.[10] Terms such as "Do Not Attempt Resuscitation" (DNAR) and "Allow Natural Death" (AND) have been proposed as alternatives to DNR in order to emphasize differing qualities of such orders. DNAR, for example, attempts to negate the underlying assumption that CPR will be successful if it is employed; AND has been recommended as a more acceptable term from a patient's perspective, although this has not been explicitly studied among families of children with life-threatening illness.[11] Physician Orders for Life Sustaining Therapies (POLST) and Physician Orders for Scope of Therapy (POST) forms are goal-oriented documents that incorporate specific decisions regarding resuscitation status. The forms function more as a means for advance care planning and may be used earlier in the disease trajectory.[11,12] Medical institutions should examine their order forms, policies and procedures in order to ensure they are goal-based and meet state and federal guidelines. Clinicians need to be familiar with specific state and institutional requirements in order to best educate patients and families on this

TABLE 22-1   Resuscitation Scenarios and Probing Questions

Clinical Scenario and Example	Probing Question	Potential Response Regarding Resuscitation
Very poor long-term prognosis Child completing radiation therapy for diffuse intrinsic pontine glioma	Given your understanding of your child's illness, what are your goals for you, your child, and your family? Would you like to talk about what to expect if the tumor grows in size despite treatment?	We will continue to readdress our goals of care for Jack throughout the time we have together. We are going to continue to hope for the best, but it is important to begin to think about what happens if the tumor grows. Would you like to discuss this more? If the tumor grows we will need to make sure we are meeting your and Jack's goals. This will include looking at issues such as further cancer-directed therapy, home-based care versus coming to the hospital and attempting CPR.
Chronic disease with slow progression Child with hypoxic ischemic encephalopathy and seizure disorder	How has being sick been for Emma? What about for you? What makes her happy? What seems to bother her or make her sad? It seems that you have a good understanding of your child's illness. Given this understanding, can you tell me what is most important for you right now? Having a better understanding of Emma and of your goals for her care will allow me to better make recommendations to support these goals.	Some families with a goal of prolonging a life of good quality for their child recognize the hospital and ICU as a source of distress. Since this is how Emma seems to view the hospital, we need to discuss ways to accomplish the overall goal trying our best to stay away from the hospital. It may be that using oxygen and other breathing support interventions from home are able to keep her comfortable and help prolong her life. We need to discuss what to do if Emma's breathing does not get better, though. One question to consider is, "Is it more important to stay at home and focus on comfort or to come to the hospital and consider using machines to support the breathing?" We can always change our decision; it will be an ongoing conversation as Emma feels better and worse.
Incurable genetic disorder with no disease-directed therapy available Baby with spinal muscular atrophy type I	Lisa seems comfortable right now. I am so happy for her. One of the purposes of my meeting with you today is to help you better understand her illness and what you might expect as the illness advances. I also want to learn more about your goals for Lisa. Do you have any questions for me before we begin this conversation?	At some point, most children with Lisa's illness begin to have trouble breathing. There are specific interventions we can do to help Lisa breath better and to ensure she is comfortable, but there is no intervention to make Lisa's breathing ability return or to make Lisa breathe better on her own. It is important for the medical team to understand your goals of care for Lisa so we can best know how to respond when this happens. We want to make sure that all of our responses are done for Lisa and not simply to her.
Death is imminent Progressive respiratory failure in child with widely metastatic cancer	Do you sense that Mike is suffering from his difficulty breathing? Do you see him as comfortable overall? What is your greatest concern right now?	As we have established a goal of helping Mike be comfortable as the first priority, breathing machines and CPR do not accomplish this goal and may actually do more harm than good. I, as a physician, would like to write an order to allow the medical community to focus on comfort and not need to attempt CPR if Mike stopped breathing. We will also be escalating interventions aimed at ensuring Mike's comfort.

topic as well as become more effective at leading conversations and making recommendations on resuscitation status and forgoing ALSMT.

Patients and parents may be hesitant to agree to forgo some ALSMT or an attempt at resuscitation because they believe that other care interventions not otherwise specified in their decision may change once an order has been placed in the medical record. Early published guidelines for DNR orders urge that "nothing in the entire procedure should indicate to the patient and family any intention to diminish the appropriate medical and nursing attention to be received by the patient."[13] A DNR order simply indicates that no resuscitation should be attempted in the event of cardiopulmonary arrest. In the absence of cardiopulmonary arrest a DNR order should not alter a patient's care, and medically appropriate treatment options that help facilitate the goals of care for the patient and family should be provided.[14,15] In end-of-life care for adults, however, a DNR order is in practice often one of a series of measures to limit aggressive life-prolonging interventions for severely or terminally ill patients.[16] Studies have also shown that treatments other than CPR may be withheld from critically ill adults with a DNR.[17,18] There are few data on this topic with regard to children and adolescents, but an early report suggests that at a tertiary pediatric oncology referral center, clinical care interventions other than CPR and mechanical ventilation did not seem to be limited by a DNR order.[19] Because it remains unclear whether a DNR or other similar orders affect the provision of interventions other than CPR in children, it is important to discuss with the patient and family all the aspects of care that will be continued or added. This discussion can facilitate accomplishing the goals of care instead of focusing on the recommendation to forgo ALSMT or an attempt at resuscitation. Clinicians need to avoid phrases such as "withholding or withdrawing care." In fact, the difficult nature of end-of-life care requires that care be actually increased during this trying time. Families need to be assured that clinicians are dedicated to upholding the standard of care and support end-of-life goals of care for patients.

Another difficulty with discussing resuscitation status with families is the misinformation that has been propagated through media sources.[20] CPR has been shown to be almost always successful on television shows. However, the literature reports that only approximately 25 percent of hospitalized, critically ill pediatric patients who undergo CPR survive until hospital discharge, and this number is even lower for patients with underlying medical conditions and co-morbidities. There is a plethora of information available about CPR in children, but much of this is in the acute setting, the ICU and emergency department, where the medical team likely believed that CPR was clinically appropriate and the goals of care may not have primarily focused on comfort. A recent report has shown that hospitalized pediatric patients with advanced cancer have poorer outcomes after receiving CPR than other hospitalized pediatric patients when undergoing in-hospital resuscitation.[21] The same is likely true for many patients with advancing life-threatening illnesses. A meta-analysis of studies on adults with metastatic cancer who undergo in-hospital CPR shows that these patients have a rate of survival to discharge of only 5.6%.[22] These statistics can be shared with patients and families while providing recommendations and making decisions.

Another difficult aspect of discussing resuscitation status is to determine how and when to incorporate children into the decision making. Children and adolescents are likely capable of understanding complex decision-making processes and of using the information for end-of-life issues and other related topics to make a decision.[23] Also, speaking to their children about dying seems to be beneficial for bereaved parents: parents who reported speaking to their children about dying and death did not regret discussing these issues. However, a significant proportion of those who did not speak to their children about these issues reported regretting not doing so, especially if they believed that their child wanted to discuss death-related issues.[24] However, many children do not desire to participate in end-of-life decision making and are comfortable with their clinicians and parents discussing and deciding on these issues. Therefore, clinicians are advised to encourage the inclusion of children in resuscitation discussions, but at the same time also be very sensitive to the potential harm that can come from doing so. Clearly, the approach to such a sensitive topic must be individualized and the benefits and burdens of involving the patient in decision making discussed with the family.

Even though resuscitation is difficult to talk about, there has been a trend over the past decade to discuss end-of-life issues early on and integrate palliative care principles into the continuum of care of children suffering from life-threatening illnesses. Care interventions in the treatment of children with life-threatening illnesses seem to be inclined toward decreasing attempts at resuscitation and increasing use of DNR orders, hospice, and home-based care.[25–27] This likely represents a systematic shift toward a more family-centered approach to end-of-life care that is goal-based and aimed at maximizing comfort. Earlier agreement between families and clinicians that cure is an unrealistic goal increases the likelihood of the use of hospice, earlier institution of a DNR order, and an earlier focus on issues related to comfort and quality of life.[28] Children with life-threatening illnesses and their families need to be informed that early integration of palliative care principles and increased emphasis on end-of-life care discussions has also helped bereaved parents to be better prepared during the child's last month of life and at the time of death.[25] Introducing the concept of palliative care in the context of options, planning for now or the future, or decision making for your child and family during this most difficult chapter of the illness, may be helpful.[29]

Discussions regarding forgoing ALSMT or resuscitation status can be best accomplished through an interdisciplinary approach of a team familiar with the hopes, values, needs, and goals of patients and families. The use of psychosocial resources during these difficult conversations can enable more effective communication.[28,30] Families must be reassured that they are not alone, and the team needs to encourage a family-oriented approach that fosters open communication, psychosocial and spiritual support, and timely access to care, with the primary purpose of ensuring that goals of care are supported. Use of a multidisciplinary approach while discussing end-of-life decisions can facilitate achieving the goals of care, as many of these goals may not be treatment-related and may be best addressed by members of the team other than the physician.

In an increasingly diverse cultural society, it is also likely that clinicians need to discuss end-of-life issues with patients and families with diverse backgrounds and cultural needs. An interdisciplinary team can facilitate conversations in such situations by developing greater sensitivity and awareness as to how cultural factors influence end-of-life decisions and finding solutions to overcome barriers. Teams are encouraged to use professional interpreters when there are language barriers in order to assure accurate communication and understanding.[31] A multidisciplinary approach may also allow the family to feel an increase in the level of care rather than a pulling back of the team as forgoing ALSMT and resuscitation issues are discussed. This is critical as abandonment, or a sense of abandonment, during the end-of-life period can cause significant distress to the primary care team and to families.[32]

As stated earlier, there has been a shift toward more children with life-threatening illness dying at home and having a DNR or other such order in place. It needs to be ensured that these documents do not influence interventions other than those described in the order. Children with out-of-hospital DNR or other similar orders deserve to have their wishes honored to forego CPR and have their goals of care supported even if they call 911 or activate the emergency response system. In-hospital and out-of-hospital advance care planning documents such as the POST and the POLST are becoming common, but a consistent DNR form and documentation is not yet universal. Outpatient orders to forego resuscitation efforts for adults can be honored with the assurance of protection against liability,[33] and arguments have been made that this right to self-determination should be given to children as well.[34] Clear documentation of advance directives and desired resuscitation status has been demonstrated to lead to effective responses to emergency management issues, even if a parent is not present, without performing unwanted CPR.[35] Clinicians are encouraged to work with first responders in the community and the emergency medical system (EMS) to clarify the goals and plan for patients in the community setting. To facilitate the plan of care, families can also be encouraged to use alternative services such as hospice rather than activating the EMS.[10]

One specific example of how out-of-hospital orders to forego CPR can be used is the school setting. Many children with a DNR order want to attend school, in fact, this is a primary palliative care intervention for some patients.[36] Schools are unlikely to have specific policies in place for children who have decided to forego CPR or other ALSMT. The majority state that they do not know how they would handle a patient with such an order or that they would not honor the DNR.[37] School officials may also be uncomfortable with the considerable uncertainty surrounding the care of a child with a life-threatening illness and the impact that child's care may have on other students. Communication with school officials, teachers, and other students' families is recommended in order to provide the best care for the child while also ensuring the well-being of other children. Furthermore, clinicians should regularly update the school authorities about changes in the overall plan of care and be available to assist teachers, administrators, and other children and their families when the child dies.[38] Clinicians can also help guide decision making regarding the child attending school during times of clinical deterioration or when acute deterioration is anticipated.[39]

Clinical Vignette

Autumn is a 6-year-old girl whose family includes her mother, Sarah, her father, Nick, and her 1-year-old brother, Sammy. Autumn recently developed left-sided weakness, swallowing difficulties and a left outward gaze deficit. She went to her pediatrician, who referred her for an urgent MRI. The MRI revealed a large non-enhancing lesion in the region of the pons that essentially replaced the pons. Her pediatrician called Sarah with the horrible diagnosis: a diffuse intrinsic pontine glioma (DIPG). She was referred to the local oncologist for further evaluation and management.

While waiting for the appointment, Sarah and Nick went on the Internet and began to learn of the horror that is DIPG. They read that it was essentially incurable; this was later confirmed by Dr. Peete, Autumn's oncologist. The family met with him, their social worker and nurse who went on to describe the proposed treatment plan of six weeks of radiation therapy plus an oral chemotherapy agent. Dr. Peete stated this would be provided with a goal of prolonging a life of good quality, but that it would not cure Autumn's disease. He also brought up the options of experimental trials and pursuing comfort measures exclusively by aggressively treating Autumn's symptoms, but not using medical interventions to treat her cancer. Within the context of this discussion, Dr. Peete brought up hospice enrollment and how this could fit into the overall care plan for Autumn. He also brought up other very difficult decisions Sarah and Nick would likely need to make in the future, including withholding and withdrawing medical interventions and resuscitation decisions including the provision of CPR if Autumn were to stop breathing. These conversations happened over the span of many days with the support of an interdisciplinary team and were always brought up with an approach of hope for the best, but plan for everything. Sarah and Nick were very appreciative of Dr. Peete's bedside manner and his ability to empathically listen, as well as the involvement of the truly interdisciplinary team caring for Autumn and the family. They decided to pursue local radiation therapy and oral chemotherapy.

Dr. Peete and his team saw them weekly during the radiation therapy and monthly thereafter. Autumn's symptoms vastly improved and she was even able to return to school. When the time came for her first follow-up MRI, Dr. Peete asked the family about their hopes for the therapy and about their expectations for the MRI. He listened intently and stated that he hoped the same, but that he needed to hope for the best, but plan for everything. He then brought up some of the issues he had mentioned earlier, including hospice and resuscitation. He stated that at some point, CPR and other medical interventions were unlikely to fit into the goals of care for Autumn. He stated that he would help them make these

difficult decisions. The next day Autumn underwent an MRI that demonstrated tumor regression, but the tumor continued to infiltrate throughout the pons. This MRI was shared with the family and with Autumn. It was celebrated as great news that the tumor was smaller, but that things were going very much as expected and that the tumor was still present.

Autumn returned to her normal routine and the family focused on living every day to its fullest. Approximately 10 months later, after three other MRIs and similar discussions, Autumn began to exhibit the same symptoms as when she was first diagnosed and an MRI revealed rapid progression of the pontine tumor. Dr. Peete and his team sat with the family and began to discuss the overall goals of care for Autumn. Sarah and Nick felt strongly that comfort needed to be the primary goal of care at this point. Dr. Peete recommended against further cancer-directed therapy. He also recommended hospice enrollment with primarily home-based care provision. He brought up the issue of resuscitation by saying, "Breathing machines and CPR do not accomplish our goal of focusing on comfort for Autumn. In fact, they may actually do more harm than good. I would like to write an order to allow the medical community to focus on comfort and not need to attempt CPR if Autumn stops breathing." Sarah and Nick agreed with each of Dr. Peete's recommendations. A DNAR order was placed in the medical record and provided to the family. Autumn was enrolled in hospice where her symptoms were aggressively treated and the family was supported with a strong interdisciplinary team. The excellent anticipatory guidance provided by Dr. Peete and his team and the hospice team allowed for recognition of Autumn's symptoms and needs and allowed for the family to provide her care in the home setting. She died comfortably at home 3 weeks later surrounded by her family and friends.

Summary

Discussions and decision-making regarding resuscitation status for children with life-threatening illness are difficult for patients, families, and clinicians. It is crucial to continue to advance the science of pediatric resuscitation, but clinicians must also realize that some patients are unlikely to benefit from this potentially burdensome intervention. It is vital that discussions about resuscitation status be based on mutually acceptable goals of care for the patient and family, and the child's participation is encouraged. Decisions should be made on the basis of recommendations of clinicians on whether or not CPR or specific ALSMT fit into the goal-based plan of care. Furthermore, clinicians should ensure that if families agree to the recommendations of clinicians regarding resuscitation status, patients continue to receive all treatments that help achieve the goal of care, including potentially life-sustaining medical treatments. Each intervention needs to be discussed with respect to how it will integrate into the overall plan of care and how it may help achieve the goals of the patient and family. It is essential that the medical team display a sense of increasing care rather than of withdrawing care to the patient and family during these times of difficult decision making.

REFERENCES

1. Martin JA, Kung HC, Mathews TJ, et al: Annual summary of vital statistics: 2006, *Pediatrics* 121(4):788–801, 2008.
2. Feudtner C, Hays RM, Haynes G, Geyer JR, Neff JM, Koepsell TD: Deaths attributed to pediatric complex chronic conditions: national trends and implications for supportive care services, *Pediatrics* 107(6):E99, 2001.
3. Hinds PS, Oakes L, Furman W, et al: Decision making by parents and healthcare professionals when considering continued care for pediatric patients with cancer, *Oncol Nurs Forum* 24(9):1523–1528, 1997.
4. Baker JN, Barfield R, Hinds PS, Kane JRA: Process to facilitate decision making in pediatric stem cell transplantation: the individualized care planning and coordination model, *Biol Blood Marrow Transplant* 13(3):245–254, 2007.
5. Baker JN, Hinds PS, Spunt SL, et al: Integration of palliative care practices into the ongoing care of children with cancer: individualized care planning and coordination, *Pediatr Clin North Am* 55(1): 223–250, xii, 2008.
6. Freyer DR: Children with cancer: special considerations in the discontinuation of life-sustaining treatment, *Med Pediatr Oncol* 20(2): 136–142, 1992.
7. American Academy of Pediatrics Committee on Bioethics: Guidelines on foregoing life-sustaining medical treatment, *Pediatrics* 93(3): 532–536, 1994.
8. Wanzer SH, Adelstein SJ, Cranford RE, et al: The physician's responsibility toward hopelessly ill patients, *N Engl J Med* 310(15):955–959, 1984.
9. Wanzer SH, Federman DD, Adelstein SJ, et al: The physician's responsibility toward hopelessly ill patients: a second look, *N Engl J Med* 320(13):844–849, 1989.
10. Morrison W, Berkowitz I: Do not attempt resuscitation orders in pediatrics, *Pediatr Clin North Am* 54(5):757–xii, 2007.
11. Jones BL, Parker-Raley J, Higgerson R, Christie LM, Legett S, Greathouse J: Finding the right words: using the terms allow natural death (AND) and do not resuscitate (DNR) in pediatric palliative care, *J Healthc Qual* 30(5):55–63, 2008.
12. Baumrucker SJ: Physician orders for scope of treatment: an idea whose time has come, *Am J Hosp Palliat Care* 21(4):247–248, 2004.
13. Rabkin MT, Gillerman G, Rice NR: Orders not to resuscitate, *N Engl J Med* 295(7):364–366, 1976.
14. Burns JP, Edwards J, Johnson J, Cassem NH, Truog RD: Do-not-resuscitate order after 25 years, *Crit Care Med* 31(5):1543–1550, 2003.
15. Smith CB, Bunch OL: Do not resuscitate does not mean do not treat: how palliative care and other modalities can help facilitate communication about goals of care in advanced illness, *Mt Sinai J Med* 75(5):460–465, 2008.
16. Beach MC, Morrison RS: The effect of do-not-resuscitate orders on physician decision-making, *J Am Geriatr Soc* 50(12):2057–2061, 2002.
17. La PJ, Silverstein MD, Stocking CB, Roland D, Siegler M: Life-sustaining treatment: a prospective study of patients with DNR orders in a teaching hospital, *Arch Intern Med* 148(10):2193–2198, 1988.
18. Uhlmann RF, Cassel CK, McDonald WJ: Some treatment-withholding implications of no-code orders in an academic hospital, *Crit Care Med* 12(10):879–881, 1984.
19. Baker JN, Kane JR, Hinds PS: Clinical care interventions are not limited by a "do not resuscitate" order at a tertiary pediatric oncology referral center. In *Annual Assembly of the American Academy of Hospice and Palliative Medicine,* January 30, 2008.
20. Diem SJ, Lantos JD, Tulsky JA: Cardiopulmonary resuscitation on television: miracles and misinformation, *N Engl J Med* 334(24):1578–1582, 1996.
21. Wu ET, Li MJ, Huang SC, et al: Survey of outcome of CPR in pediatric in-hospital cardiac arrest in a medical center in Taiwan, *Resuscitation* 80(4):443–448, 2009.
22. Reisfield GM, Wallace SK, Munsell MF, et al: Survival in cancer patients undergoing in-hospital cardiopulmonary resuscitation: a meta-analysis, *Resuscitation* 71(2):152–160, 2006.
23. Hinds PS, Drew D, Oakes LL, et al: End-of-life care preferences of pediatric patients with cancer, *J Clin Oncol* 23(36):9146–9154, 2005.
24. Kreicbergs U, Valdimarsdottir U, Onelov E, Henter JI, Steineck G: Talking about death with children who have severe malignant disease, *N Engl J Med* 351(12):1175–1186, 2004.
25. Wolfe J, Hammel JF, Edwards KE, et al: Easing of suffering in children with cancer at the end of life: is care changing? *J Clin Oncol* 26(10): 1717–1723, 2008.
26. Baker JN, Rai S, Liu W, et al: Race does not influence do-not-resuscitate status or the number or timing of end-of-life care discussions at a pediatric oncology referral center, *J Palliat Med* 12(1):71–76, 2009.
27. Feudtner C, Feinstein JA, Satchell M, Zhao H, Kang TI: Shifting place of death among children with complex chronic conditions in the United States, 1989–2003, *JAMA* 297(24):2725–2732, 2007.
28. Wolfe J, Klar N, Grier HE, et al: Understanding of prognosis among parents of children who died of cancer: impact on treatment goals and integration of palliative care, *JAMA* 284(19):2469–2475, 2000.
29. Wolfe J, Sourkes B: Palliative care for the child with advanced cancer. In Pizzo PA, Poplack DG, editors: *Principles & practice of pediatric oncology,* ed 5, 2009, Lippincott Williams & Wilkins, pp 1531–1534.
30. Tan GH, Totapally BR, Torbati D, Wolfsdorf J: End-of-life decisions and palliative care in a children's hospital, *J Palliat Med* 9(2):332–342, 2006.
31. Smith AK, Sudore RL, Perez-Stable EJ: Palliative care for Latino patients and their families: whenever we prayed, she wept, *JAMA* 301(10): 1047–1057, E1, 2009.
32. Back AL, Young JP, McCown E, et al: Abandonment at the end of life from patient, caregiver, nurse, and physician perspectives: loss of continuity and lack of closure, *Arch Intern Med* 169(5):474–479, 2009.
33. Iserson KV: Foregoing prehospital care: should ambulance staff always resuscitate? *J Med Ethics* 17(1):19–24, 1991.
34. Sahler OJ, Greenlaw J: Pediatrics and the Patient Self-Determination Act, *Pediatrics* 90(6):999–1001, 1992.
35. Walsh-Kelly CM, Lang KR, Chevako J, et al: Advance directives in a pediatric emergency department, *Pediatrics* 103(4 Pt 1):826–830, 1999.
36. Ross ME, Hicks J, Furman WL: Preschool as palliative care, *J Clin Oncol* 26(22):3797–3799, 2008.
37. Kimberly MB, Forte AL, Carroll JM, Feudtner C: Pediatric do-not-attempt-resuscitation orders and public schools: a national assessment of policies and laws, *Am J Bioeth* 5(1):59–65, 2005.
38. American Academy of Pediatrics Committee on School Health and Committee on Bioethics: Do not resuscitate orders in schools, *Pediatrics* 105:878–879, 2000.
39. Weise KL: The spectrum of our obligations: DNR in public schools, *Am J Bioeth* 5(1):81–83, 2005.

Palliative Sedation

AMRITA D. NAIPAUL | CHRISTINA ULLRICH

The world is full of suffering, it is also full of overcoming it.

—Helen Keller

Relief of suffering is fundamental to the practice of palliative care. On occasion, children with life-threatening illness may suffer from severe or escalating symptoms that are not ameliorated by the usual palliative interventions. When the overriding goal is comfort for the child, palliative sedation therapy (PST) provides a means to relieve extreme suffering in such critical situations. Even in such challenging circumstances, patients and families may find opportunities for choices, to maintain self-actualization and to preserve their dignity and integrity through the possibility of PST.

Open, honest, and clear communication among the care team and patients and their families is paramount before, during, and after the implementation of palliative sedation therapy. It is central to everyone's ability to consider the complexities of PST and to feel as comfortable as possible with decisions rendered along the way. This chapter will provide foundational information related to PST to enhance a clinician's ability to communicate with patients, families and other healthcare providers in such a manner.

Terminology

Terminal sedation was described in the literature in 1991 as "as the intention of deliberately inducing and maintaining deep sleep, but not deliberately causing death in very specific circumstances."[1] However, a lack of consensus over the definition of terminal sedation exists amongst palliative care experts. In addition, it does not convey or emphasize the aim of sedation, to palliate symptoms, or the possibility that the patient may awaken or recover. In fact, terminal could be interpreted to mean the intentional ending of life. In one survey of 61 palliative care experts (59 physicians and two nurses, response rate of 87 percent) only 21 (40 percent) agreed that terminal sedation was "the intention of deliberately inducing and maintaining deep sleep, but not deliberately causing death in very specific circumstances."[2] In response to this continued lack of consensus, other terms such as *sedation for intractable distress in the dying* or *sedation in the imminently dying* arose as alternatives in the literature,[3] and have evolved into the most commonly used term, *palliative sedation*.[4] While there is not complete agreement on the optimal terminology or definition, most would agree that PST is "the use of sedative medications to relieve intolerable suffering from refractory symptoms by a reduction in patient consciousness."[5] PST is usually administered for intractable symptoms at the end of life. Because the addition of "therapy" to the term emphasizes that it is an accepted palliative treatment for symptoms rather than an end in and of itself, palliative sedation therapy is used in this chapter.

PST may be further described in terms of the level of sedation achieved, that is from mild to deep, as well as the intended duration, such as continuous versus intermittent or respite sedation. In general, the goal of PST is for the child to be in a state of conscious sedation, with relief from symptoms but still able to communicate. In rare situations requiring urgent relief of suffering, deep sedation may instead be the goal. If there is no intention of waking the patient, then continuous sedation is used. Both deep and continuous sedation can be recommended only for patients with an expected prognosis of hours to days without a treatable condition.[6] *Respite sedation* is a subtype of palliative sedation therapy intended to be time-limited and temporary in nature. Such temporary respite from suffering may allow continued or future therapy to provide relief,[7,8] or may provide relief and rest for a patient when their perception of intolerability is impacted by factors that create severe physical and emotional fatigue.[6,7]

A clear definition for *refractory symptom* is central to the discourse regarding palliative sedation. Cherny and Portenoy's definition of refractory symptoms is widely accepted: "symptom[s] for which all possible treatment has failed, or it is estimated that no methods are available for palliation within the time frame and the risk-benefit ratio that the patient can tolerate."[7] Refractory symptoms can be categorized by the clinician using the diagnostic criteria as those symptoms in which further interventions are:

- Incapable of providing further relief
- Efforts are incapable of providing relief with acceptable toxicity and/or morbidity
- Efforts are incapable of providing relief in an acceptable time frame
- Or intensive efforts to relieve the symptom have been exhausted[7]

Despite controversy surrounding nomenclature as well as some of the specific indications for PST, this treatment modality is by and large accepted worldwide as an intervention for patients with refractory suffering at the end of life. In 2007, international guidelines and recommendations for standards were developed with representation from the United Kingdom, the Netherlands, Belgium, France, Germany, Switzerland, Finland, Canada, the United States, Argentina, South Africa, Israel, Japan, Australia and New Zealand.[5] The European Association for Palliative Care developed a recommended 10-point framework for the use of palliative sedation based on existing guidelines, literature, and extensive peer review. This framework supports the use of palliative sedation as important and necessary, when used appropriately and ethically, in patients with otherwise refractory distress.[6] However, literature regarding the provision of PST in the pediatric population is scant, and outside of one review,[9] largely consists of case reports. Except where specified in this chapter, evidence presented reflects PST in adults. Issues regarding PST in children that require special consideration are discussed later in this chapter.

Setting the Stage

A variety of factors may influence the decision to initiate PST (Box 23-1). While PST is an effective palliative intervention for relief of suffering, the risks and potential controversy surrounding it require careful consideration of the situation from a variety of perspectives. This section describes some key issues that must be taken into account before this therapeutic option is employed. Communication with the family and entire care team around these issues is essential.

INTOLERABLE SUFFERING

If refractory symptoms escalate to the point of intolerability, the predominant goal of care may shift from extension of life or preservation of function to that of alleviating of suffering. Suffering and distress are subjective phenomena (Fig. 23-1). As such, only the individual experiencing such suffering can truly deem his or her condition intolerable.[10] However, many patients at the very end of life are unable to express whether their degree of suffering warrants sedation. In studies of adult palliative care patients, 22 percent to 49 percent of adult patients were not involved with the decision to undertake sedation for intolerable suffering.[2,11,12] In these instances, proxies, in conjunction with the medical team, decided whether PST should be implemented. In pediatrics, parents most commonly serve as the surrogate decision makers for children. Skillful discussions with families regarding the distinction between the child's suffering and their own are needed when PST is under consideration.

Developmental limitations or neurocognitive impairment are frequent conditions in children with life-threatening illnesses. In situations involving a pediatric patient, it is even more likely that a parent or guardian will make the decision about PST on behalf of the patient (Fig. 23-2). That is not to say that children should be routinely excluded from such discussions. Many children are able to consider significant decisions such as resuscitation status.[13] The extent to which a particular

BOX 23-1 Factors Influencing the Decision to Initiate Palliative Sedation Therapy

Child and Family-Specific Factors
- Prognosis, or estimate of the patient's proximity to death
- Severity of distress
- Tolerability of suffering
- Availability of alternative interventions to relieve suffering
- Whether PST is consistent with the patient's wishes, if the child's wishes are known
- Values and preferences of the family
- Emotional well-being of the family and how PST may influence bereavement

Care Team-Specific Factors
- Personal, moral or religious beliefs*
- Experience and/or confidence with psychological care†
- Palliative care experience
- Emotional burnout†

Setting-Specific Factors
- Availability of PST in the desired location of care, such as a hospital ward vs an ICU
- Prevalence of PST, and thus familiarity of PST, in the culture in which care is provided

*Curlin FA, Lawrence RE, Chin MH, Lantos JD. Religion, conscience, and controversial clinical practices. *N Engl J Med* 356:593–600, 2007.
†Morita T, Akechi T, Sugawara Y, Chihara S, Uchitomi Y. Practices and attitudes of japanese oncologists and palliative care physicians concerning terminal sedation: a nationwide survey. *J Clin Oncol* 20:758–764, 2002.

child participates in a decision about PST depends greatly on the child as well as his or her family. Whether and how a child is involved in the determination of whether his or her suffering justifies PST should be decided by the family and care team on an individual basis, and include consideration of the extent to which the child can express his or her own will, understand the relevant information, and understand and acknowledge the implications of the choice.[6]

DISTINGUISHING REFRACTORY SYMPTOMS FROM DIFFICULT SYMPTOMS

Before embarking on a consideration of PST, it is essential to distinguish symptoms that are challenging to manage from those that are not relieved by available measures within an

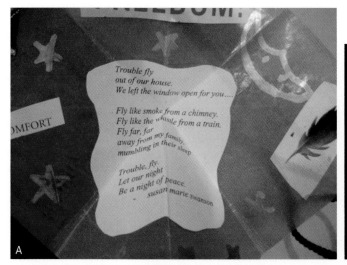

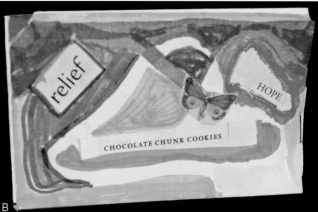

Fig. 23-1   A, A child's response to the question "What is comfort to you?" **B,** An adolescent's response to the same question.

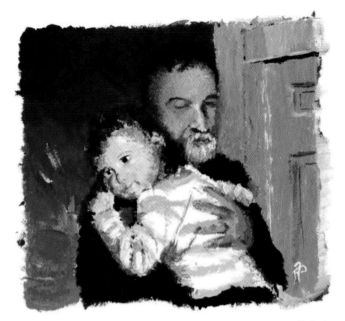

Fig. 23-2 In situations involving a pediatric patient, it is even more likely that a parent or guardian will make the decision about palliative sedation therapy on behalf of the patient. (Artwork by Brett Rogers, www.beatcanvas.com)

acceptable timeframe and with acceptable toxicity. Further consideration of a symptom's refractoriness should also include whether the patient's medical team has enough expertise and experience to truly judge the symptom as refractory.[5] Palliative care consultation, if available, should be a requisite condition whenever PST is considered. A palliative care team can help establish that all acceptable interventions to relieve suffering have been considered. In addition, a palliative care team can also ensure that the circumstances are considered from an interdisciplinary perspective, and that the physical, emotional, existential, and social dimensions of suffering have been thoroughly explored and addressed. If palliative care consultation is not an option, input from clinicians from different disciplines and with expertise in symptom control, ethics or the care of seriously ill children should be sought.

Symptoms Prompting Consideration of PST

Refractory physical symptoms such as pain, delirium and/or agitation, dyspnea, and nausea and/or vomiting may prompt consideration of PST. The published relative frequencies of physical symptoms invoking PST vary across settings and populations, and with the type of sedation studied.[14,15] Large studies to determine the prevalence of indications for PST in children have not been conducted.

While the relative frequencies of refractory physical symptoms prompting PST may vary, refractory physical symptoms are generally accepted as potential indications for PST. This is largely due to the presence of well-established therapeutic strategies to be considered before the symptom is deemed refractory. Such physical symptoms also tend to occur late in the illness trajectory, when the proximity of death is incontrovertible.[16]

In contrast, distress from non-physical symptoms is less clear. In adults, such distress may involve feelings of meaninglessness and worthlessness; being a burden on others; dependency and/or the inability to take care of oneself; death

anxiety, fear, and/or panic; a wish to control the time of death by oneself; and isolation or lack of social support.[17] Therapeutic strategies are often less established and symptoms may fluctuate, complicating evaluation. These issues may all influence whether a nonphysical symptom is considered refractory, and whether the use of PST is proportionate to the suffering inflicted by the symptom. Finally, the beliefs of the members of the care team are likely to shape the determination of whether PST is acceptable treatment for refractory psychological and existential distress.[18,19]

Because nonphysical symptoms may not correlate with proximity to death, adults who receive PST for this indication may be sedated for a longer time before death. Some opponents of PST for psychological and existential distress argue that establishment of such suffering as refractory is difficult, and that it may be implemented earlier in the illness trajectory, with a concomitant increase in risk from PST and blurring of the distinction between PST and euthanasia.[16,20,21] On the other hand, proponents of PST for psychological or existential suffering maintain that such suffering may cause more suffering than physical symptoms, with fewer therapeutic options. To facilitate decision making regarding PST and psychological and/or existential distress, there is a set of proposed clinical rules for consideration.[16] This issue clearly requires further investigation prior to recommendation of it as a standard indication for PST in pediatrics.

Location of Care

The location of the child's care should also be determined before initiating discussion of PST, because this is likely to affect PST option. In a multicenter study in Italy, wide variations in whether and how PST was implemented among centers was more reflective of differences in institutional policies and provider behavior rather than the patients' preferences or needs.[22] The availability of continuous palliative sedation or sedation to unconsciousness may be particularly uneven or unpredictable. Offering to relieve a child's suffering through sedation when this is not a realistic option can leave a family feeling abandoned and the care team demoralized and guilty.[23] Therefore, determining the range of options before presenting them to the family is recommended.

PST in adults is more commonly provided in inpatient settings, such as palliative care units. Institutional policies may restrict the availability of particular sedatives, such as propofol or dexmedetomidine, to the operating room, intensive care unit, or other specific clinical settings. Policies that permit the use of particular agents, such as midazolam or propofol, for the express purpose of PST in other settings do exist.[24] Even with such policies, barriers such as logistical or clinical constraints and the healthcare team's ethical or legal concerns may also determine whether PST is a viable option in certain settings.[25]

PST may also be implemented in the home setting; however, a high degree of cooperation and commitment from both staff and family is needed. Additionally, home-care staff are likely to be increasingly needed as the intensity of treatment increases.[26] PST at home may present greater demands on home-care staff, with these individuals providing more emotional support for the family and experiencing more stress from the decision making.[26]

Artificial Hydration and Nutrition

Although provision of artificial hydration and nutrition (AHN) is not contraindicated during PST, it is unlikely to contribute to the patient's comfort. It may actually detract from the goal of maximizing comfort by contributing to fluid overload or gastrointestinal discomfort.[27] Discontinuation of AHN when PST is implemented has not been associated with shorter survival times,[12] perhaps because patients with severely distressing and uncontrolled symptoms are unlikely to sustain themselves with oral intake for extended periods of time. In some cases where respite sedation is intended, ongoing provision of AHN may be consistent with the family's primary goals. The interdisciplinary team approach is key in exploring the family's personal or religious beliefs with regard to AHN. Some strongly believe that AHN be continued; in this case, AHN may be continued.

Resuscitation Status

Given the premises of PST, that the child has a life-threatening illness with a very limited prognosis and the primary goal of care is comfort, an order should be in place indicating that no resuscitation attempts should be made if the child has a life-ending event. Implementation of a DNR order is required if there are no intentions to lift sedation. Even if sedation is intended to be temporary, or respite sedation, it is possible that the child will not regain consciousness. To prevent undue suffering, it is recommended that a DNR order be in place for respite sedation in patients with advanced illness and a limited prognosis.

Respite Sedation

Respite sedation may be initiated with the intention of maintaining unconsciousness for a limited period, such as while waiting for treatment benefit or until preplanned family interactions. Before beginning respite sedation, it is important to establish an endpoint and plan to re-awaken the patient. It is equally as important to discuss with the family beforehand the fact that the patient may not regain consciousness.

Emergency Sedation

In rare instances, such as catastrophic and distressing bleeding, urgent sedation may be initiated without the same forethought or discussion that normally occurs. In ideal situations, the potential for emergency sedation is recognized by the care team and discussed with the family, with plans for such sedation ready to implement. If there has not been an opportunity for proactive planning, the care team must rapidly evaluate the child's prognosis, goals of care, resuscitation status, and the benefits and burdens of sedation.

Communication with the Family Before and During PST

Frequent, open and honest communication with the family both before and during the provision of PST is crucial. Knowledge of end-of-life treatment options is highly variable in adult patients,[28] and care teams should be aware of such variability when broaching the topic of PST with families. Decisions of great import, such as forgoing life-sustaining therapy, frequently require multiple conversations to reach consensus with families.[29] Once initiated, PST is also associated with families expressing more concerns, so the importance of ongoing communication to readdress goals, plans, and the family's needs persists, and may increase as duration of sedation increases.[30]

Bereaved family members of patients who received PST report having concerns about the patient's distress, whether maximum efforts to control symptoms had been made before initiating PST, having opportunities to say important things to the patients before sedation, to understand their suffering, and for professionals to treat patients with dignity.[31] Families also report feeling guilt, helplessness, and exhaustion during the process.

Opportunities, both initially and during follow-up conversations, are needed to address these concerns and feelings, which may compound the suffering that families endure during their loved one's last days. Families report that information reduced their anxiety and confusion and gave them confidence that the staff was in control and would be able to help the patient.[32] If care teams do not proactively create opportunities for ongoing communication to clarify the care plan, provide relevant information, and address questions during the provision of PST, then families may experience frustration and disappointment[32] (Box 23-2).

Morita and colleagues have demonstrated that feeling the responsibility for the decision is an independent predictor of high distress in bereaved family members.[33] It is therefore particularly important for the healthcare team to share the responsibility for the decision to administer PST, alleviating some of the burden that the family may feel. Frequent communication not only allows the transmission or clarification of information, but also allows for the development of rapport and the sense of a joint endeavor between the care team and family.

Concern that sedation may shorten life is common among family members,[33] although several empirical studies have shown no differences in survival when patients who received PST are compared with those who did not.[14,15,34-36] It is therefore important to discuss with families that PST, as with other forms of sedation, is generally very safe although rarely patients experience complications that may shorten life. The degree of focus on risks should also be influenced by the clinical context. For example, presentation of the risks and plans to reduce them, such as monitoring vital signs, may be different depending on whether there is a plan to reverse sedation and awaken the patient after a certain period of time. In any event, discussion of the risks should never leave families feeling as though they must choose between their child's life and comfort.

Families should have the opportunity to meet with the care team every 24 to 48 hours, to revisit the plan of care and

---

BOX 23-2 Communication-Related Factors as Sources of Family Dissatisfaction or Distress During Provision of Palliative Sedation Therapy

- Inadequate opportunities for sharing of information and clarification of questions
- Family perceives inadequate relief of symptoms
- Family members doubtful that PST was indicated, perhaps wondering if suffering could have been relieved in some other way
- Family's concern that PST may shorten life
- Family feeling the burden of responsibility for the decision
- Family members feeling unprepared for changes in the patient's condition
- Family's observation that the patient is not cared for in a sensitive or respectful manner
- Lack of opportunities for the family to say important things to the patient before sedation

Brajtrnan S: The impact on the family of terminal restlessness and its management, *Palliat Med* 17:454–460, 2003.
Monta T, Ikenaga M, Adach I. et al: Concerns of family members of patients receiving palliative sedaion therapy, *Support Care Cancer* 12:885–889, 2004.

discuss concerns that may have arisen. All discussions should be documented in the medical record as they occur to maximize clear and consistent communication between staff members and the family (Box 23-3). Such documentation should be readily accessible by all members of the child's care team, particularly if those administering PST are not directly part of ongoing discussions with the family regarding it. Special attention to regular interdisciplinary communication with families may be needed if PST is administered in the home. Such communication is important not only for the family, but also for staff providing direct care in the home. PST places higher demands on home-care staff.[26] Routine interdisciplinary team meetings may lessen the burden that individual staff members in the home may feel.

Communication with the Child

Although conscious sedation may sometimes be the targeted level, the ability to communicate is diminished in the majority of patients who receive PST.[37,38] The ability to communicate without hindrance with a loved one who is seriously ill is precisely why PST is not routinely used in patients facing the end of life.[7] Most families deeply miss the ability to communicate with their loved one, and once the patient is comfortable and sedated, they often wish for opportunities to reawaken and communicate with their loved one.[8,32] Such longing may lead to feelings of anger, frustration, and disappointment. Families should be encouraged to continue to talk to their child and to participate in their care if desired. Some family members may be hesitant to touch their child. To the extent that they are comfortable doing so, family members should be encouraged to do certain things for their child, such as washing and dressing, or holding or massaging the child (Fig. 23-3). The use of respite sedation may be another strategy for permitting meaningful

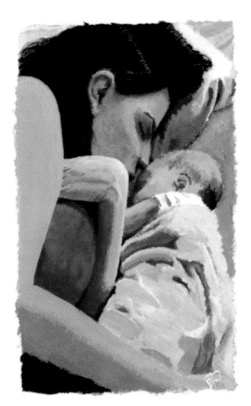

Fig. 23-3 Families should be encouraged to continue to talk to their child and to participate in the child's care if they wish. (Artwork by Brett Rogers, www.beatcanvas.com)

interactions with their loved one, if interrupted sedation does not evoke a crisis of uncontrolled suffering.

During PST, families are also acutely aware of the manner in which the care team interacts with their loved one. Even small gestures, such as talking to the child and attending to the environment, conveys compassion for the child as well as the message that the child will continue to receive the same attentive care received before sedation. A respectful manner that preserves the individual's dignity and individuality is needed from all members of the care team. When respectful interactions that preserve the child's dignity and individuality are not provided by all members of the care team, it may deeply impact families and their subsequent bereavement.[31,32]

Team Communication

Caring for a patient with intractable suffering can strain every member of a care team physically, emotionally, and morally. Although PST is a widely accepted therapy for otherwise intractable suffering at the end of life in many countries,[2,5,19,39] including Japan, Europe, Canada, and the United States, support for PST may not necessarily be unanimous, particularly so when PST is administered for non-physical suffering. Serious disagreement among team members can jeopardize a team's ability to function as a cohesive unit in effectively caring for a patient who is suffering at the end of life. It is imperative that all members have the freedom to share their views with others on the team in a non-judgmental and respectful environment. Those who object or who are significantly distressed by providing palliative sedation should be given the opportunity to change patient assignments without concern

---

BOX 23-3   Communication Documentation

When beginning palliative sedation therapy, the physician should be responsible for documenting the following, which will enhance communication among members of the care team:

- Elements of documentation include the nature of the child's life-threatening illness and their limited prognosis, death anticipated in hours to days
- The patient's and/or family's goals of care. For PST to be considered, the overriding goal must be comfort as opposed to function or preservation of consciousness
- The nature of the distressing and intolerable symptom
- Refractoriness of symptom
- Outcomes of interdisciplinary assessment
- Findings of relevant consultants
- Limitations of the available techniques
- The option of PST
- Intended outcome of sedation, the degree and duration of sedation, its goals, and expected outcomes
- Risks, aspiration, paradoxical agitation, respiratory suppression, and treatment alternatives should be discussed.
- Indications for titrating the sedative upward or downward
- Plans for monitoring the child with vital signs, laboratory tests
- Location of care
- Provision of artificial nutrition and hydration
- Resuscitation status and life-sustaining treatments, such as dialysis
- If the child is involved in the decision, the child's ability to make decisions about their ongoing care should be specified.
- Any specific goals that the patient or family may have, such as a visit from a family member before initiating sedation

for repercussions. For those who continue to provide care for the child, frequent opportunities to debrief are essential.

Even when support for PST is unanimous, evidence exists that caring for patients who are receiving it may place a significant strain on care team members. For example, nurses report a significant burden providing PST for patients.[40,41] Among a study of 3187 nurses in Japan, 30 percent reported wanting to leave their current work situation at least occasionally due to sedation-related burden.[40] In qualitative work with nurses in the Netherlands, others found that a significant number of nurses believed that PST shortened life or was equivalent to euthanasia.[41] Similarly, concern that sedation may shorten life is not infrequent among physicians.[2,39] The Japan study also demonstrated that physicians who report higher levels of emotional exhaustion and depersonalization, indicators of professional burnout, were more likely to choose deep, continuous sedation for patients with refractory physical and psychological distress.[39] Strategies to prevent occupational overload, including provision of PST by an interdisciplinary team and opportunities for staff to debrief in a supportive, nonjudgmental environment, are clearly needed and should be considered routine whenever PST is used.

Documentation

The importance of documentation whenever PST is considered cannot be underestimated. Outcomes of interdisciplinary assessments in determination of a symptom's refractoriness, discussions with families regarding the PST option, and ongoing assessments of clinicians caring for a child receiving PST must all be thoroughly and routinely documented (see Box 23-3). Such documentation should be readily accessible by all members of the child's care team. Documentation is particularly important for caregivers who may not have had participated in discussions, but are involved in providing sedation.

Physician Considerations

DEPTH OF SEDATION

In general, the targeted level of sedation should be the lowest that relieves distress. Conscious sedation, where the patient is calm and able to respond to verbal commands, is often considered the ideal level of sedation for PST. This mild degree of sedation should be attempted first because it preserves interactive function. If the patient experiences persistent distress, deeper sedation should be pursued. Once symptoms are controlled, the sedative dose may be titrated downward in an attempt to re-establish consciousness after a specified interval in order to allow for planned family interactions and to re-evaluate the child's condition and the family's preferences for sedation. In other instances, such as intense distress, severely refractory symptoms, anticipated death within hours to a few days, or emergency sedation, continuous deep sedation may be indicated.

CHOICE OF SEDATIVE

In the absence of controlled trials evaluating sedatives for PST, the drug choice is largely empirical. The choice of sedative is often driven by the particular clinical scenario, including the nature of the refractory symptoms, location of care, and whether continuous or respite sedation is desired. A rapid onset and short duration of action are properties that are frequently desirable for medications used to deliver PST (Table 23-1 and Box 23-4). The sedatives used in PST are usually benzodiazepines, neuroleptics, or barbiturates, although in recent years successful use of other anesthetic agents such as propofol has been reported.[42,43]

While opioids are sometimes used expressly for their sedating properties, they are not effective in producing reliable, prolonged sedation. Furthermore, escalating opioids may have neuroexcitatory side effects such as delirium, hyperalgesia, or myoclonus. Therefore, opioids should not be delivered expressly for the purpose of achieving palliative sedation. However, for children already receiving opioids, they should be continued to provide ongoing analgesia and to prevent symptoms of withdrawal. The use of dexmedetomidine may permit discontinuation of opioids and benzodiazepines, as discussed later. Although ketamine has sedative and analgesic properties, it may cause unpleasant dysphoric or dissociative reactions, particularly in older children, and is not recommended as monotherapy for PST. Neuroleptics such as chlorpromazine, haloperidol, and methotrimeprazine are often cited in the PST literature,[14,15] but do not by themselves reliably induce unconsciousness. However, for agitated delirium, a neuroleptic in conjunction with another agent, such as a benzodiazepine, may be a reasonable choice.

Midazolam and barbituates such as pentobarbital were some of the first agents reported to be used for PST.[44,45] In the absence of delerium, midazolam is the agent of choice and is the most commonly used agent for PST.[46] It has a rapid onset and short duration of action, facilitating titration. Pentobarbital also has a short onset of action and may alternatively be used, but it has a long half-life and is not readily reversed. Because of these properties, pentobarbital is not ideal for respite sedation.

Propofol and dexmedetomidine may be used for PST but are often not available outside the operating room or intensive care unit. If available, propofol is frequently an excellent choice because its rapid onset and duration of action allow for close control of sedation in response to symptoms and for variable depths of sedation.[43] In fact, its onset and duration of action is 5 to 10 minutes, shorter than that of midazolam. A recent case series reported that propofol was able to provide relief of symptoms and conscious sedation by careful titration of the dose in nine of 22 patients.[42] The remaining patients had symptoms that necessitated doses that kept them asleep. Propofol also has many other beneficial properties, including anxiolytic, antiemetic, antipruritic, anticonvulsant, and anti-myoclonic effects.

Dexmedetomidine acts in the descending pain modulating system on post-synaptic alpha-2 receptors.[47] It is associated with less delirium than midazolam in intubated ICU patients,[48] has analgesic effects, and frequently allows patients to be sedated but communicative and cooperative.[47] Dexmedetomidine is used for sedation during withdrawal of ventilatory support[49] and may hold promise as a new agent for PST. If dexmedetomidine is used for sedation, opioids and benzodiazepines may be discontinued. Because this approach is novel, use of dexmedetomidine and discontinuation of opioids and benzodiazepines should be considered only in consultation with an anesthesiologist or a clinician with expertise in pain medicine.

TABLE 23-1   Medications Commonly Used for Palliative Sedation Therapy

	Dose	Titration	Symptom control	Comments
Benzodiazepines			Anxiolytic, amnestic, and anticonvulsant properties. Synergistic sedative effect with opioids and neuroleptics	Monotherapy with benzodiazepines occasionally fails to provide adequate sedation. May cause paradoxical agitation, especially in those with impaired liver function.
Midazolam	Loading dose 0.03-0.05 mg/kg slow push IV/SC; may repeat loading dose every 5 min to achieve desired effect (to maximum of 2 mg). Continuous infusion: hourly dose 25%-33% of the cumulative loading dose.	Additional bolus doses equal to the hourly infusion dose may be given up to every 5-15 min. If >3 boluses are required within an hour, the continuous infusion may be increased by 30%. Tolerance may develop.		One of the most commonly used drugs for PST. Short-acting benzodiazepine; because of rapid redistribution, administer by continuous infusion. Maintain continuous infusion because of short duration of action. Compatible with many other IV medications, including opioids. Midazolam infusions are stable for 24 hrs after preparation by pharmacy.
Lorazepam	0.05 mg/kg every 2-4 hrs as intermittent bolus			Peak effect 30 min after IV administration. Because of slower pharmacokinetics, less amenable to titration than midazolam.
Other anesthetics				
Pentobarbital	Loading dose 2-3 mg/kg IV over 30 min (no faster than 50 mg/min). If inadequate sedation after 30 min, a second loading dose of 1-2 mg/kg should be administered over 30 min. At the time of initial loading dose, begin continuous infusion at 1-2 mg/kg/hr	For escalating symptoms, a bolus dose of 1 mg/kg IV over 30 min may be given. Tolerance may develop quickly, prompting increases in infusion rate. Titrate continuous infusion every 30-60 min.	Anticonvulsant, antipruritic, antiemetic properties; No analgesic properties	Pentobarbital infusions are stable for 7 days after preparation by pharmacy.
Dexmedetomidine	Initial loading infusion of 1 mcg/kg IV over 10 min; continuous infusion of 0.1-1 mcg/kg/hr). Dosing guidelines are undetermined in pediatrics and warrant further investigation	Titrate infusion up to 1 mcg/kg/hr every 10 min to reach desired effect. Maximum dosing in pediatrics requires further investigation	Analgesic, sympatholytic, and anxiolytic effects	Alpha-2 agonist; May cause sedation without respiratory depression; may cause bradycardia and hypotension; has a rapid distribution phase with a distribution half-life (t1/2) of approximately 6 minutes. Consider close monitoring of heart rate and blood pressure during initiation and with increases in dose. However, gradual changes in blood pressure and heart rate unrelated to dose changes should not be attributed to dexmedetomidine and are more likely to be a reflection of the dying process.
Propofol	Start at 1 mg/kg/hr IV	Titrate dose in steps of 0.5 mg/kg/hr every 30 min. For acute management of severe symptoms, may give bolus dose every 10 min. With prolonged use tolerance may develop-dose range usually 1-4 mg/kg/hr Most respond to 1-2 mg/kg/hr. Avoid exceeding 3 mg/kg/hr long-term.	Anxiolytic, antiemetic, antipruritic, anticonvulsant, antimyoclonic bronchodilation. No analgesic effects	Widely used for general anesthesia and sedation of ICU patients. Can NOT be given SC. May be used for PST if midazolam fails.[42] Incompatible with other IV meds commonly given at end of life, therefore requiring a dedicated line. Onset of action 30 sec, allowing for rapid titration Change tubing every 12 hrs and discard vial and any unused drug if not infused after 12 hrs. Duration of action 5-10 min, do not interrupt infusion for >60 sec when changing tubing. Useful for renal or hepatic insufficiency; metabolites not thought to have biologic activity. Mechanism of action includes inhibition of GABA uptake Negative inotrope; high doses may cause hypotension, bradycardia, respiratory depression May cause pain on infusion into small peripheral veins Risk of infection due to high lipid content; change tubing every 12 hrs and discard any unused drug not infused after 12 hrs Synergistic with midazolam in causing sedation

BOX 23-4 Guidelines for Administration of Palliative Sedation Therapy

- After an initial steady dose is found that maintains the desired level of sedation, dose adjustments require documentation for the adjustments and the level of comfort before and after the adjustments.
- Once the desired level of symptom control is achieved, the infusion should be maintained at the lowest rate that supports this desired level of symptom control.
- Continuous infusions must be administerd via an infusion pump and should be interrupted or discontinued only upon a physician's order.
- To ensure that a continuous supply of medication is readily available for the patient, the pharmacy should be notified well in advance of the anticipated need for additional supply of medication.
- The patient's nurse and prescribing physician should remain with the patient during the initiation and initial titration of sedative to achieve relief from suffering.
- Drug solutions should be inspected visually for evidence of precipitaion prior to administration. If precipitaion is present, the solution should not be used.
- The physician should administer the loading dose.
- An initial bolus (loading) dose should be accompanied by the start of a continuous infusion.
- Additional boluses may be delivered to capture uncontrolled symptoms. A nurse or physician should remain at the bedside to observe the effect, about 5 minutes for propofol, 10 minutes for midazolam, and 15 minutes for pentobarbital.
- The infusion rate may also be increased until sedation is achieved or should the patient exhibit evidence of distress or other target symptoms.
- The infusion should be titrated to achieve the desired level of sedation and comfort and not in response to vital signs, if monitored. Lowered blood pressure, and gradual changes in respiratory rate or oxygen saturation, are expected in a dying patient and should not, by themselves, lead to reduction of the infusion rate.
- However, abrupt onset of apnea or snoring may indicate oversedation, and should prompt consideration of decreasing sedative infusion rate.

OTHER PHYSICIAN CONSIDERATIONS

The physician should document the outcome of the discussion with the family in the medical record (see Box 23-3), including the indication for PST, desired outcomes, and the family's agreement with the plan. The physician should also ensure that a DNR order is in the chart. Once sedation has been titrated to relieve symptoms, the physician should ensure that clear parameters for sedative titration and notifying the physician are documented and discussed with the care team. The parameters are the initial infusion rate, rate of continuous infusion, time interval for infusion increases, dose and time interval for bolus doses, indications for infusion rate increases or bolus dose administration. The physician should also discontinue all orders not contributing to the patient's comfort or goals of care. During ongoing PST, the physician should evaluate the child, and document efficacy of PST and occurrence and outcomes of ongoing discussions with the family and staff. Finally, even after PST has been initiated, the physician should continue to ensure ongoing interdisciplinary assessment of the patient for new and ongoing sources of distress.

Nursing Considerations

During the planning and implementation phases of PST, the nurse has crucial roles in monitoring the patient and participating in the ongoing communication with the patient, family, and healthcare team. During the initiation of PST, continuous nursing care will be required with a nurse/patient ratio of 1:1 preferred until the desired treatment effects are reached.

Once the titration of medications is completed, then nurse and patient ratios may be reconsidered. As a member of the healthcare team, the nurse caring for the patient needs to be actively involved in the family and team decision-making processes. Every setting environment will offer different challenges and both ethical and practical considerations should be discussed, anticipated, and addressed. The nurse will be the consistent presence at the patient bedside and will provide ongoing guidance to the patient and family in relation to PST. Depending upon the goal of PST in each patient situation, the nurse may also be actively assisting the family with anticipatory guidance for the child's death. The nurse's presence at the bedside is an important source of information for the other members of the team and thus the role includes timely sharing of relevant information with the team.

Monitoring

Patient monitoring must consider goals of treatment, effectiveness of the intervention in relieving symptoms, and the degree of sedation achieved. For continuous sedation when there is no intent to awaken the patient, and a DNR order is in place, cardiopulmonary monitoring is usually not necessary, and the key monitored parameters are those that reflect the patient's comfort.[6] For example, respiratory rate may be monitored as a measure of respiratory distress. However, for respite sedation when death may not be imminent, monitoring of routine physiologic parameters such as heart rate, blood pressure, respiratory rate, and oxygen saturation may be in order. Observational assessments and physical exam can be used to make adjustments to therapy and the desired effects.

MONITORING COMFORT

Optimal tools to quantitatively measure comfort are not yet established. Monitoring comfort level will vary among each patient and family's perspective. Because of the individualized approach, when communicating with the family, the nurse should avoid ambiguous terms such as comfort care. The nurse has an important role in establishing with the patient and family what comfort means to them and what the individual's goal is to be comfortable throughout the initiation and treatment of PST. The nurse will continually re-evaluate these measures of comfort with, when possible, the patient and family's input.

MONITORING SEDATION

To minimize the risk of treatment failure during PST, the degree of sedation should be regularly assessed.[50] Awareness in patients undergoing surgery or conscious sedation is a rare event, but when it occurs it may be intensely distressing for patients. A large, multicenter study of adults undergoing PST in Japan found that 49 percent of patients awoke after falling into a deeply sedated state. Although awakening in this instance was defined as eye-opening, any movement of the extremities, or speech, it usually did not indicate distress.[38]

During the initiation and titration of therapy, the level of sedation is monitored frequently. Once sedation has been achieved, the level of sedation should be evaluated and documented at least every 4 hours. The level of sedation may be documented as mild, intermediate or deep or using a tool such as the Ramsay Scale.[51] Consistent use of a sedation scale may be useful in monitoring the degree of sedation because comfort as well as degree may guide subsequent dosing of the sedative (Box 23-5).

OTHER NURSING CONSIDERATIONS

The level of sedation will impact the intensity of nursing care. A patient may experience diminished or loss of protective reflexes such as blinking, gagging, and coughing. Routine eye and mouth care, as well as skin protection to prevent breakdown, will be necessary and important to maximize comfort. Families can be provided with the opportunity to participate in the patient's hygiene.

Considerations for the Interdisciplinary Team

Interdisciplinary care should continue unaltered once PST has been initiated. For example, the presence of a chaplain may facilitate exploration of religious, spiritual, or cultural beliefs that could impact a family's decision regarding PST. Ongoing visits from chaplaincy are often a source of great support for family and staff alike. Psychosocial clinicians can support the family's coping styles and identify ways in which ongoing communication with their loved one is possible. The clinicians' involvement with the child's care before and during PST provision will position them especially well to provide bereavement support. Child life therapists can support involvement of siblings and facilitate communication with them in a developmentally appropriate manner. Together, interdisciplinary team members can support opportunities for the family to participate in meaningful activities regardless of whether a decision is made for palliative sedation.

Interdisciplinary care is also a crucial element of bereavement follow-up after PST. Issues around PST and the circumstances

leading up to PST may impact bereavement. For example, uncontrolled symptom distress, a prerequisite for PST, may place surviving loved ones at increased risk for complicated grief. As a complex and multifaceted palliative care intervention for proportionally serious distress, bereavement necessitates skilled interdisciplinary follow-up, preferably from the same team that followed the patient and family during PST.

Ethical Considerations

PST has been criticized as a slow form of euthanasia. Euthanasia is the deliberate termination of a patient's life by active intervention, at the request of the patient in otherwise uncontrollable suffering. The aim of PST is the relief of suffering, and not the shortening of life.[5] The major distinguishing factor between slow euthanasia and palliative sedation is the intent of the clinician and care providers. The intent of the clinician, patient, and family receiving PST is to relieve suffering, not to cause death. Another distinguishing factor is the use of the lowest dose of medication in PST to relieve suffering, versus the use of lethal doses in euthanasia. The amount of medication, dose, and route for PST needs to be slowly titrated and the patient frequently monitored to establish the minimal level of sedation required to relieve the amount of intolerable suffering. The doctrine of double effect is often used to justify PST, but invocation of the doctrine is often unnecessary and overemphasizes an association between PST and hastening death.

Controversy with PST will continue to exist, which makes it imperative to have guidelines and frameworks to assist with the implementation of PST. As stated by Cherny for the European Association of Palliative Care, "inattention to potential risks and problematic practices can lead to harmful and unethical practice."[6] Each patient situation will vary and questions related to the ethics of PST will need to be evaluated. Ethics consultation is highly advisable in instances where disagreement exists, or consultation would support the patient, family, and healthcare team members in the decision-making process.

BOX 23-5 **Monitoring Recommendations**

Patient monitoring recommendations during the initiation and titration of palliative sedation therapy in the hospital or home environment:

Degree of comfort, level of consciousness (using scale below), and potential adverse effects of sedation (e.g., agitation) should be evaluated regularly:
- Every 15 minutes × 1 hour
- Then, every 30 minutes × 1 hour
- Then every 2 hours × 6 hours
- Then may increase interval to every 4 hours

Note: Cardiac monitors, oxygen monitors and other monitors are generally not used, or discontinued, except in the case of respite sedation

A scale such as the modified Ramsay Scale should be used to consistently rate degree of sedation*
1 Patient is anxious and agitated or restless, or both
2 Patient is cooperative, oriented, and tranquil
3 Patient responds to commands only
4 Patient exhibits brisk response to light glabellar tap, or equivalent, or auditory stimulus
5 Patient exhibits a sluggish response to light glabellar tap, or equivalent, or auditory stimulus
6 Patient exhibits no response

*Ramsay MA. Savege TM. Simpson BR. Goodwin R: Controlled sedation with alphaxalone-alphadolone, *Br Med J* 2:656–659, 1974.

Summary

Rather than being a concession that routine palliative care interventions have failed, PST is better viewed as an extension of many of the basic tenets of palliative care. While some aspects of PST may challenge the care team, successful implementation of PST rests on some of the core principles of palliative care. Such principles include providing expert interdisciplinary care and clear, open and honest communication, in order to provide optimal compassionate care for a suffering patient and his or her family. In this light, PST may be viewed as one of the ultimate interventions offered by palliative care today.

In pediatrics, palliative sedation is rarely needed. However, knowing that their child's care team will remain with them and that they are prepared to offer this modality can be a great comfort to families. When the rare need does arise, it can provide a rare opportunity for trainees and staff to grow personally and professionally, stimulating rich discussions and opportunities for exceptional interdisciplinary collaboration.

During the past decade, inroads in understanding the end-of-life experiences of children have been made. However, the presumed rarity of sedation in pediatric palliative care may pose a particular challenge for investigators aiming to further elucidate this treatment for children. While numerous retrospective and a few prospective studies in adults have been published,[52] the pediatric palliative sedation literature is remarkably sparse. Practice is largely based on extrapolation from adult studies and anecdotal knowledge. Further study of this area is needed in order to understand the prevalence, practices, and needs of children with refractory suffering for whom PST might bring relief.

REFERENCES

1. Enck RE: Drug-induced terminal sedation for symptom control, *Am J Hosp Palliat Care* 8:3–5, 1991.
2. Chater S, Viola R, Paterson J, Jarvis V: Sedation for intractable distress in the dying: a survey of experts, *Palliat Med* 12:255–269, 1998.
3. Krakauer EL, Penson RT, Truog RD, King LA, Chabner BA, Lynch TJ Jr: Sedation for intractable distress of a dying patient: acute palliative care and the principle of double effect, *Oncologist* 5:53–62, 2000.
4. Jackson WC: Palliative sedation vs. terminal sedation: what's in a name? *Am J Hosp Palliat Care* 19:81–82, 2002.
5. de Graeff A, Dean M: Palliative sedation therapy in the last weeks of life: a literature review and recommendations for standards, *J Palliat Med* 10:67–85, 2007.
6. Cherny NI, Radbruch L: European Association for Palliative Care (EAPC) recommended framework for the use of sedation in palliative care, *Palliat Med* 23:581–593, 2009.
7. Cherny NI, Portenoy RK: Sedation in the management of refractory symptoms: guidelines for evaluation and treatment, *J Palliat Care* 10:31–38, 1994.
8. Morita T, Inoue S, Chihara S: Sedation for symptom control in Japan: the importance of intermittent use and communication with family members, *J Pain Symptom Manage* 12:32–38, 1996.
9. Kenny NP, Frager G: Refractory symptoms and terminal sedation of children: ethical issues and practical management, *J Palliat Care* 12:40–45, 1996.
10. Cassell EJ: Diagnosing suffering: a perspective, *Ann Intern Med* 131:531–534, 1999.
11. Rietjens JA, van Delden JJ, van der Heide A, et al: Terminal sedation and euthanasia: a comparison of clinical practices, *Arch Intern Med* 166:749–753, 2006.
12. Hasselaar JG, Reuzel RP, van den Muijsenbergh ME, et al: Dealing with delicate issues in continuous deep sedation: varying practices among Dutch medical specialists, general practitioners, and nursing home physicians, *Arch Intern Med* 168:537–543, 2008.
13. Hinds PS, Drew D, Oakes LL, et al: End-of-life care preferences of pediatric patients with cancer, *J Clin Oncol* 23:9146–9154, 2005.
14. Chiu TY, Hu WY, Lue BH, Cheng SY, Chen CY: Sedation for refractory symptoms of terminal cancer patients in Taiwan, *J Pain Symptom Manage* 21:467–472, 2001.
15. Ventafridda V, Ripamonti C, De Conno F, Tamburini M, Cassileth BR: Symptom prevalence and control during cancer patients' last days of life, *J Palliat Care* 6:7–11, 1990.
16. Cherny NI: Commentary: sedation in response to refractory existential distress: walking the fine line, *J Pain Symptom Manage* 16:404–406, 1998.
17. Morita T: Palliative sedation to relieve psycho-existential suffering of terminally ill cancer patients, *J Pain Symptom Manage* 28:445–450, 2004.
18. Rietjens JA, Buiting HM, Pasman HR, van der Maas PJ, van Delden JJ, van der Heide A: Deciding about continuous deep sedation: physicians' perspectives: a focus group study, *Palliat Med* 23:410–417, 2009.
19. Curlin FA, Lawrence RE, Chin MH, Lantos JD: Religion, conscience, and controversial clinical practices, *N Engl J Med* 356:593–600, 2007.
20. Sanft T, Hauser J, Rosielle D, et al: Physical pain and emotional suffering: the case for palliative sedation, *J Pain* 10:238–242, 2009.
21. Rousseau PC: Palliative sedation and the fear of legal ramifications, *J Palliat Med* 9:246–247, 2006.
22. Peruselli C, Di Giulio P, Toscani F, et al: Home palliative care for terminal cancer patients: a survey on the final week of life, *Palliat Med* 13:233–241, 1999.
23. Quill TE, Lo B, Brock DW, Meisel A: Last-resort options for palliative sedation, *Ann Intern Med* 151:421–424, 2009.
24. Elsayem A, Curry Iii E, Boohene J, et al: Use of palliative sedation for intractable symptoms in the palliative care unit of a comprehensive cancer center, *Support Care Cancer* 17:53–59, 2009.
25. Braun TC, Hagen NA, Clark T: Development of a clinical practice guideline for palliative sedation, *J Palliat Med* 6:345–350, 2003.
26. Rosengarten OS, Lamed Y, Zisling T, Feigin A, Jacobs JM: Palliative sedation at home, *J Palliat Care* 25:5–11, 2009.
27. Siden H, Tucker T, Derman S, Cox K, Soon GS, Hartnett S, Straatman L: Pediatric enteral feeding intolerance: a new prognosticator for children with life-limiting illness? *J Palliat Care* 25(3):213–217, 2009.
28. Silveira MJ, DiPiero A, Gerrity MS, Feudtner C: Patients' knowledge of options at the end of life: ignorance in the face of death, *JAMA* 284:2483–2488, 2000.
29. Garros D, Rosychuk RJ, Cox PN: Circumstances surrounding end of life in a pediatric intensive care unit, *Pediatrics* 112:e371, 2003.
30. van Dooren S, van Veluw HT, van Zuylen L, Rietjens JA, Passchier J, van der Rijt CC: Exploration of concerns of relatives during continuous palliative sedation of their family members with cancer, *J Pain Symptom Manage* 38:452–459, 2009.
31. Morita T, Ikenaga M, Adachi I, et al: Concerns of family members of patients receiving palliative sedation therapy, *Support Care Cancer* 12:885–889, 2004.
32. Brajtman S: The impact on the family of terminal restlessness and its management, *Palliat Med* 17:454–460, 2003.
33. Morita T, Ikenaga M, Adachi I, et al: Family experience with palliative sedation therapy for terminally ill cancer patients, *J Pain Symptom Manage* 28:557–565, 2004.
34. Stone P, Phillips C, Spruyt O, Waight C: A comparison of the use of sedatives in a hospital support team and in a hospice, *Palliat Med* 11:140–144, 1997.
35. Morita T, Tsunoda J, Inoue S, Chihara S: Effects of high dose opioids and sedatives on survival in terminally ill cancer patients, *J Pain Symptom Manage* 21:282–289, 2001.
36. Maltoni M, Pittureri C, Scarpi E, et al: Palliative sedation therapy does not hasten death: results from a prospective multicenter study, *Ann Oncol* 20:1163–1169, 2009.
37. Mercadante S, Intravaia G, Villari P, Ferrera P, David F, Casuccio A: Controlled sedation for refractory symptoms in dying patients, *J Pain Symptom Manage* 37:771–779, 2009.
38. Morita T, Chinone Y, Ikenaga M, et al: Efficacy and safety of palliative sedation therapy: a multicenter, prospective, observational study conducted on specialized palliative care units in Japan, *J Pain Symptom Manage* 30:320–328, 2005.
39. Morita T, Akechi T, Sugawara Y, Chihara S, Uchitomi Y: Practices and attitudes of Japanese oncologists and palliative care physicians concerning terminal sedation: a nationwide survey, *J Clin Oncol* 20:758–764, 2002.
40. Morita T, Miyashita M, Kimura R, Adachi I, Shima Y: Emotional burden of nurses in palliative sedation therapy, *Palliat Med* 18:550–557, 2004.
41. Rietjens JA, Hauser J, van der Heide A, Emanuel L: Having a difficult time leaving: experiences and attitudes of nurses with palliative sedation, *Palliat Med* 21:643–649, 2007.
42. Lundstrom S, Zachrisson U, Furst CJ: When nothing helps: propofol as sedative and antiemetic in palliative cancer care, *J Pain Symptom Manage* 30:570–577, 2005.
43. McWilliams K, Keeley PW, Waterhouse ET: Propofol for terminal sedation in palliative care: a systematic review, *J Palliat Med* 13:73–76, 2010.
44. Truog RD, Berde CB, Mitchell C, Grier HE: Barbiturates in the care of the terminally ill, *N Engl J Med* 327:1678–1682, 1992.
45. Burke AL, Diamond PL, Hulbert J, Yeatman J, Farr EA: Terminal restlessness: its management and the role of midazolam, *Med J Aust* 155:485–487, 1991.
46. Cowan JD, Walsh D: Terminal sedation in palliative medicine: definition and review of the literature, *Support Care Cancer* 9:403–407, 2001.
47. Soares LG, Naylor C, Martins MA, Peixoto G: Dexmedetomidine: a new option for intractable distress in the dying, *J Pain Symptom Manage* 24:6–8, 2002.
48. Riker RR, Shehabi Y, Bokesch PM, et al: Dexmedetomidine vs midazolam for sedation of critically ill patients: a randomized trial, *JAMA* 301:489–499, 2009.

49. Kent CD, Kaufman BS, Lowy J: Dexmedetomidine facilitates the withdrawal of ventilatory support in palliative care, *Anesthesiology* 103:439–441, 2005.

50. Davis MP: Does palliative sedation always relieve symptoms? *J Palliat Med* 12:875–877, 2009.

51. Ramsay MA, Savege TM, Simpson BR, Goodwin R: Controlled sedation with alphaxalone-alphadolone, *Br Med J* 2:656–659, 1974.

52. Hasselaar JG, Verhagen SC, Vissers KC: When cancer symptoms cannot be controlled: the role of palliative sedation, *Curr Opin Support Palliat Care* 3:14–23, 2009.

24 Organ Donation

AMY DURALL

The world is round and the place which may seem like the end may also be the beginning. —Ivy Baker Priest[1]

Organ transplantation is a potentially life-saving treatment option for those with end-stage organ failure. When organ transplantation began in the 1950s, kidneys were procured from either living related donors or from patients who suffered cardiopulmonary arrest after illness or injury. Legislation, passed in 1968 in the Uniform Anatomical Gift Act, authorized individuals to donate all or a part of their or a family member's body after death for education, research, therapy or transplantation. The Act was revised in 1987 to reflect changes in practice. Subsequent revisions in 2006 emphasized an individual's donation rights as described in the previous versions of the Act. In addition, language prohibiting others from overruling a person's decision regarding organ donation after his or her death was reinforced.[1]

In 1984, The National Organ Transplant Act was approved, establishing the Organ Procurement and Transplantation Network (OPTN). The OPTN is responsible for the nationwide, equitable distribution of organs for transplantation using specific allocation policies.[2] Due to advances in surgical technique and immunosuppression therapy, the number of organ transplantations has grown, with both early and late outcomes improving.[3] Since 1998 there have been more than 460,000 transplantations in the United States: 78 percent were from deceased donors and 22 percent were from living donors. Patients less than 18 years of age comprised nearly 8 percent of the total number of transplants. Furthermore, approximately 7 percent of organ recipients from deceased donors and 9 percent of organ recipients from living donors were children.[2] However, the demand for organs continues to exceed the supply, and patients die awaiting transplant.[3] As of August 2009, there were approximately 103,000 people awaiting transplantation, of which 1,800 were pediatric patients.[2]

In this part of the chapter, we will discuss the complexity that surrounds organ donation, including: religion, race and ethnicity, the perspectives of individuals involved in the process, and the role of interdisciplinary communication.

Factors Influencing Willingness to Donate

Multiple studies have evaluated factors that influence a person's willingness to donate his or her own or a family member's organs.[4–10] There are specific patient and family characteristics, beliefs, attitudes, and experiences that have been identified as positively correlated with consent to organ donation[4,6,8,11,12] (Box 24-1).

A principal limiting factor to organ donation is the low percentage of families who agree to organ donation. Several factors have been associated with refusal to donate[5,6,8,12] (Box 24-2).

Overall, there are many complex, interactive variables involved in a person's willingness to donate. It is important for the medical team to understand how these factors may influence the organ-donation request process.

Religiosity

Religion encompasses principles and traditions that are related to God or a higher power.[13] Most major religions support organ donation,[11,13,14] but a significant number of people cite their religious beliefs as a reason not to donate.[8,11,13,15] In particular, persons who are concerned about maintaining the body's integrity after death and/or believe that organ transplantation is against God's will have more negative attitudes toward organ donation.[11,13,15] Many religions consider organ donation to be an act of compassion and altruism; one that is permissible because of the life-saving potential. Although many religions encourage their members to be donors, the decision is ultimately left up to the individual.[13,14] The role of religiosity as a positive or negative influence in the organ-donation process has been explored, with many conflicting conclusions.[8,11,13,15,16] This may be due to an incomplete understanding of the complex interactions among religion, societal norms, family dynamics, and personal organ-donation beliefs.[13] Despite conflicting data, religion is a part of many peoples' lives and religiosity may indeed influence perspectives on organ donation. It is essential for the medical team to understand and respect the religious beliefs of patients and families in order to provide unconditional support during the decision-making process. When appropriate, it may be helpful to encourage the involvement of a religious adviser to dispel any misconceptions.

Race and Ethnicity

Studies have shown differences in attitudes toward organ donation as well as the process itself in persons of different racial and ethnic backgrounds.[8,11,12,15,17–19] Differences include knowing the patient's organ-donation preferences, communication with the healthcare team, and trust in the healthcare system. Studies have shown that individuals from minority racial and/or ethnic backgrounds are less willing to donate their organs, are less likely to discuss organ donation with family members, and are less likely to carry a donor card compared with whites.[8,11,12,17,19] In addition, minority individuals tend to have less trust in the healthcare system. For example, more minorities than whites believe that doctors will not try as hard to save a person's life if doctors know that person is willing

BOX 24-1 Factors Associated with Consent to Organ Donation

- Sense of altruism
- Perceived good quality patient care
- Understanding the concept of brain death
- Families given enough information and time to make an informed decision
- Separation in the timing of discussions relating to brain death and organ donation
- High level of interpersonal skill of the person making the donation request
- High level of trust in the physician and healthcare system
- Communication with others about organ donation preferences
- Younger patient
- Private location to hold organ donation discussions
- Families being informed of the potential to help others
- Death resulting from trauma
- Increased knowledge about organ donation and transplantation

Alden DL, Cheung AH: Organ donation and culture: a comparison of Asian American and European American beliefs, attitudes, and behaviors, *J Appl Soc Psychol* 30(2):293–314, 2000.

Jeffres LW, Carroll JA, Rubenking BE, Amschlinger J: Communication as a predictor of willingness to donate one's organs: an addition to the Theory of Reasoned Action, *Prog Transplant* 18(4):257–262, 2008.

Siminoff LA, Lawrence RH, Arnold RM: Comparison of black and white families' experiences and *perceptions* regarding organ donation requests, *Crit Care Med* 31(1):146–151, 2003.

Simpkin AL, Robertson LC, Barber VS, Young JD: Modifiable factors influencing relatives' decision to offer organ donation: systematic review, *BMJ* 338:b991, 2009.

Thornton JD, Wong KA, Cardenas V, Curtis JR, Spigner C, Allen MD: Ethnic and gender differences in willingness among high school students to donate organs, *J Adolesc Health* 39(2):266–274, 2006.

to be an organ donor.[12,15] Furthermore, blacks are less likely than whites to agree that doctors can be trusted to pronounce death correctly when a patient is eligible to be an organ donor.[17]

One study evaluating the experiences of black and white families found discrepancies in the communication process at the organ donation request. White families initiated donation discussions more often than black families. In addition, black

BOX 24-2 Factors Associated with Refusal to Donate Organs

- Poor communication between healthcare providers and family members
- Emotional exhaustion
- Religious beliefs
- Family's belief that a patient would not have wanted to be an organ donor
- Family's perception of uncaring healthcare providers
- Feeling pressured to make a decision
- Families being told that healthcare providers are required to ask about donation
- Potential for disfigurement
- Poor timing of the request

Siminoff LA, Gordon N, Hewlett J, Arnold RM: Factors influencing families' consent for donation of soid organs for transplantation, *JAMA* 286(1):71–77, 2001.

Siminoff LA, Lawrence RH, Arnold RM: Comparison of black and white familes, experiences and perceptions regarding organ donation requests, *Crit Care Med* 31(1):146–11, 2003.

Simpkin AL, Robertson LC, Barber VS, Young JD: Modifiable factors influencing relatives' decision to offer organ donation: systematic review, *BMJ* 338:b991, 2009.

Thornton JD, Wong KA, Cardenas V, Curus JR, Spigner C, Allen MD: Ethnic and gender differences in wilingness among high school students to donate organs, *J Adolesc Health* 39(2):266–274, 2006.

families felt more pressure to make a decision. Although the number of total discussions was the same for black and white families, fewer donation-related topics were discussed with black families. For example, black families were less likely to have spoken with a chaplain or an organ procurement organization (OPO) representative.[12] This could have a significant impact upon the donation process because speaking to and spending more time with an OPO representative is strongly associated with families' willingness to donate.[5] In addition, black families were less likely to have discussed two specific issues: families are not responsible for the costs of donation, and the impact of organ donation on funeral arrangements. These discussions may help dispel misconceptions about the donation process and could affect a family's willingness to donate.

Inconsistencies are present in the organ donation request process for individuals of different ethnic and racial backgrounds. Compared with whites, minorities may have different beliefs about organ donation based on their experiences and lack of trust in the medical system. Consequently, medical professionals need to understand these issues in order to eliminate barriers in the organ donation process for all individuals, regardless of race and ethnicity.

Parent and Adolescent Perspectives

In 2006, children under the age of 18 years made up 12% of the donor organ pool, and more than half of those were aged 11 to 17 years.[3] As such, it is important for healthcare providers to appreciate the perspectives of children and their parents regarding organ donation. Studies from various countries have shown that many adolescents believe that transplantation is an acceptable practice that could provide benefit to others.[20,21]

Many students are willing to donate their own organs to help others.[21–23] Students who either oppose organ donation or express discomfort with the issue do so because of distrust, lack of information, uneasiness with a body being cut up, fear of being disrespectful to the deceased, discomfort of having one's organs in another body, and fear of not being dead.[22,23] Despite some knowledge about organ donation and transplantation, students would like to be better informed on the topic and many believe that it should be included in the school curriculum.[21–23] Consequently, many schools have established organ donation educational programs for their adolescent students, which have been met with a favorable response.[20,22–26] Furthermore, teenagers who were involved in these programs were more inclined to register as organ donors, had greater knowledge of the topic and had more positive opinions regarding organ donation than students who did not participate.[24,25]

One study examined a number of domains concerning organ donation and transplantation such as knowledge, personal experience, and attitudes.[8] Differences in ethnicity, gender, religious views, and other factors were assessed. Approximately one-fourth of students who had driver's licenses or learner's permits had designated themselves as organ donors. Girls were more likely than boys and white students were more likely than minority students to have signed an organ donor card. Among those who intended to be donors, only slightly more than half shared this with their family. All students had a low level of knowledge regarding organ donation, allocation, and the transplantation process. For instance, more than half of all students believed that organs are bought and sold in the United States. Nevertheless, several positive predictors of willingness to donate were identified: female gender, white ethnicity, not religious, previous organ donation discussions with family and friends, increased knowledge of organ donation and a wish to receive a transplant, if necessary.[8]

The decision to donate a family member's organs is influenced, in part, by whether or not the decision maker is aware of the wishes of the potential organ donor.[5,7,12] Families with knowledge of the patient's wishes are more likely to agree to donation.[5,7] However, many people do not discuss their preferences with their family and this may make the decision difficult.[7] Although many adolescents are willing to discuss the subject with their parents,[21,22] anxiety and discomfort about death and organ donation could be a barrier to adolescent-parent communication. To address this issue, a study examined the impact of a school-based program to assist students aged 11 to 18 years in initiating organ donation discussions with their families.[26] Approximately one-third of students thought that the discussion went "OK" and over half believed that it "went very well." Initiating the conversation was the most difficult aspect of the discussion for many of the students, and feelings of anxiety, discomfort, and unease were expressed. Talking about death, either one's own or another's was also difficult. Interestingly, a small number of parents became angry or refused to discuss the topic. Positively, the students and their parents were able to talk about things that they had never discussed before. This study illustrates barriers to communication about death and organ donation between adolescents and their parents. Despite some difficulties with these conversations, there were positive aspects, such as overall enhanced communication within the family.[26] Encouraging adolescents and their parents to engage in such conversations may assist families if they are ever in the position of making a decision regarding organ donation.

While there has been progress in understanding the perspectives of adolescents, there is a paucity of data regarding the meaning of organ donation in younger children. This is an important understudied area of investigation that could benefit from formal research.

In addition to children, it is important to understand the perspectives of parents. A research team conducted interviews with 74 parents who had previously been approached about donating their child's organs.[27] Parental characteristics that were associated with a higher likelihood of consent included no college education, interest in organ donation for themselves, and a complete understanding of brain death. Having rapport with the person requesting the donation was also associated with a favorable decision. With regard to communication, parents were more likely to consent to organ donation when they perceived the timing of the request to be appropriate, when they had enough time to discuss their decision with others and when there was no conflict within the family about the decision. The majority of parents were satisfied with their decision but, interestingly, 10% of those who consented to organ donation would not make the same decision again; 16 percent of those who had declined now wished that they had agreed. Thus, a parent's decision to donate their child's organs is influenced by a number of factors, including satisfaction with the healthcare team, requestor characteristics, and the communication process.[27]

Pastoral Care Perspectives

Hospital chaplains are valuable members of the healthcare team and their involvement in the organ donation process can be extremely beneficial to a patient's family. Chaplains are especially skilled in communication, providing support to bereaved families, and being sensitive to ethnic, cultural, and religious values.[28]

To better understand the perspectives of clergy toward organ donation, researchers surveyed 110 hospital chaplains to assess their level of participation in organ donation.[29] The likelihood of chaplain participation in the organ donation process of a brain-dead patient was approximately 50%. Interestingly, the level of participation was slightly less in the chaplains who served in university-based hospitals rather than in other settings, such as private or community hospitals. The reasons for this difference were not evident but it was speculated that brain death was an infrequent event in non-university hospitals and chaplain participation was desired more often. Many chaplains believed that they should take a purely supportive position and should not be primarily involved in approaching the family to request organ donation. However, several university-based chaplains believed that they could take a more active role in the organ donation process.[29]

In addition to participation, attitudes and religious issues were explored. Respect of the donor and not viewing the donor as a means to an end were very important to chaplains. Most chaplains viewed organ donation as consistent with their religious values. Some believed their role was to protect a family's decision to decline organ donation on religious grounds. Apart from their religious views, chaplains were concerned about families being coerced during the decision-making process, and considered themselves advocates for the patient and family. Another important concern among chaplains regarded the timing of organ donation discussions. Many chaplains believed that families were approached about organ donation too soon after their loved one's death. In some cases, the families were not given enough time to come to terms with the patient's death. Overwhelmingly, chaplains believed that they could be extremely valuable because of their training in grief and crisis counseling.[29]

Social Work Perspectives

Social workers play a key role in the transplantation process by evaluating the psychosocial profile of potential transplant recipients and then helping recipients and their families cope with the implications of transplantation. Furthermore, social workers meet with family members of potential organ donors to assist them in the decision-making process and to support them in their grief.[30] Social workers can also assist the medical team by educating clinicians about ethnic and cultural issues pertaining to organ donation. In addition, social workers can assist the medical team as they deal with their own emotions surrounding dying patients and grieving families. Social workers are an essential part of the clinical team.[30,31]

Nursing Perspectives

The organ-donation process involves a complex set of interactions among the medical team, patients, and their families. Nurses are an integral part of the healthcare team and are directly involved in this process. They may have a significant impact upon end-of-life care and, more specifically, organ donation. Because of the large amount of time that the bedside nurse spends interacting with the patient and family, nurses are in a strong position to provide support to families considering organ donation.[7,32] Nurses focus on respect and dignity of the potential organ donor and their family. In fact, they view protection of these individuals as one of their major responsibilities.[33] However, nurses may not be comfortable in this role due to lack of experience in this area, deficient education about the topic, and their own personal views of organ donation. Strategies to assist nurses in this role include educational programs related to organ donation, programs to improve communication skills, and ensuring a work environment that promotes excellent end-of-life care. Intensive care unit leadership must promote a culture that recognizes nurses as valued members of the team. As such, the bedside nurse should be present at family conferences, nurse performance evaluations should include end-of-life care skills, patient assignments must promote continuity of care, and unit policies and guidelines regarding the care of potential organ donors must be readily accessible.[32]

Physician Perspectives

Physicians are responsible for coordinating patient care within the interdisciplinary medical team. As part of that responsibility, physicians must assure accurate and consistent transmission of information among members of the medical team, the patient, and the family. Initiating the request for organ donation has typically been the responsibility of the attending physician. In 1998, changes in federal regulations concerning organ and tissue donation stipulated that individuals initiating the organ donation request process must be properly trained.[34] This was misinterpreted by some to mean that only OPO staff members could approach families, excluding physicians from the process.[9] However, there now appears to be more of an understanding that request for donation is a collaborative process between OPOs and the medical team. The physician's relationship with the family is invaluable, but so is the training and skill of the OPO representatives. An important physician responsibility is to incorporate OPO staff members into the medical team and coordinate efforts in the organ request process.[9]

Organ Procurement Organizations' Perspectives

There are 58 OPOs in the United States and Puerto Rico.[35] These organizations serve a specific geographic area and coordinate organ procurement efforts. Specifically, OPOs evaluate potential organ donors, discuss donation with families, facilitate surgical removal and preservation of donated organs, and coordinate their distribution according to national organ sharing policies.[36] Factors that are important for success of OPOs include experienced leadership, adequate staffing, allocation of responsibilities, strong relationships with donor hospitals and transplant centers, and support of donor families. Highly efficient and successful OPOs have a management team that is focused on the donation process, systems for monitoring activity and tracking outcomes, and efficient mechanisms for resolving conflict with hospitals and within the organization itself.[37]

The United States Health Care Financing Administration changed the federal Conditions of Participation for tissue and organ donation such that hospitals must notify their OPO of any patients who are potential donors. The intention was to increase OPO referral rates so that all families would have the option of tissue and/or organ donation. Furthermore, the person making the donation request must be adequately trained to do so. This stipulation was based on evidence that suggested healthcare providers lack sufficient knowledge and training to effectively approach families about organ donation.[9] Involvement of the local OPO is imperative to the process, and families have reported that discussing organ donation with an OPO representative is crucial to their decision-making process. In fact, talking with an OPO staff member prior to the request for organ donation and spending more time with an OPO representative have been positively correlated with the decision to donate.[5]

Ethical Considerations

Many complicated ethical issues surround organ donation and transplantation. Laws and regulations have been put forth to increase organ donation in light of the shortage of organs. It is imperative to identify the correct outcome measure. For instance, ethical quandaries may arise if the desired outcome is increased consent rate. Focusing on consent rate is problematic because the decision to decline organ donation is seen as negative. Conflicts of interest may occur because efforts to increase consent rate may divert attention away from the best interests of the patient and family. When the primary outcome is improving the process itself, however, then the decision to decline donation is no longer seen as negative.[9] Another issue is the timing of organ donation discussions. Discussions informing families of brain death testing and death should be independent of organ donation requests. The concern is that if the subjects are discussed concurrently then questions arise as to whose interests, the potential donor's or the potential recipients', take precedence. The medical team should have an understanding of the pertinent ethical issues so that the best interests of the potential organ donor and their family are maintained.

Discussing Organ Donation with the Family

Joey was a bright and energetic 7-year-old. One Saturday morning he was riding in a car to baseball practice with his dad. It started to rain and Joey's dad lost control of the car when the road became slippery. The car rolled over several times and, unfortunately, neither Joey nor his dad was wearing a seatbelt. When rescuers arrived at the scene Joey was in cardiopulmonary arrest. He was resuscitated and then transported to a pediatric trauma center while his dad was transported to a nearby hospital with serious injuries that were not life-threatening. Joey's initial assessment demonstrated a severe traumatic brain injury, and it was a distinct possibility that he might progress to brain death. The attending physician, Dr. Smith, Joey's nurse, and the unit social worker met with Joey's mom, updating her on Joey's clinical status and poor prognosis. As the day progressed, Joey showed no neurologic response, and his exam was consistent with brain death. The clinical team contacted the local OPO and a member of its team came to the hospital to offer expertise. Dr. Smith met again with Joey's mom and gently explained the results of the test and the fact that a second brain death exam would be conducted after a number of hours. Joey's mom was devastated and quietly acknowledged her son's condition. At this time, Dr. Smith told Joey's mom that she would like to tell her about an opportunity to help others through organ donation. Dr. Smith explained the process and assured Joey's mom that no matter what decision she chose, the clinical team would respect and fully support her decision. In addition, Dr. Smith encouraged Joey's mom to take as long as she needed to think about the situation and that the team was always available to answer any questions. Joey's mom was receptive to the idea and agreed that she needed time to think about it. After a short period, Joey's mom told Dr. Smith that she was interested in Joey being an organ donor but that she wanted to speak with Joey's dad about it. Dr. Smith offered to walk with Joey's mom over to the hospital where Joey's dad was admitted. On the way, Joey's mom spoke very little. The silence made Dr. Smith uncomfortable but she followed the cues from Joey's mom and allowed her to guide the amount of discussion. At the hospital Dr. Smith discussed Joey's condition and the results of the brain death exam with his dad. Joey's dad was heartbroken and agreed that Joey should be an organ donor. Dr. Smith accompanied Joey's mom back to the children's hospital, respecting the silence as they walked.

Approaching a family about organ donation is never an easy process and no two conversations are the same. Every patient, family, and set of circumstances is unique and this requires the clinical team to adjust its approach to the discussion based on the situation. Several approaches have been put forth, including the standard approach, the presumptive approach, and dual advocacy.[38-40] The standard approach may be described as value-neutral and unbiased. The organ donation discussion is balanced and the goal is to help the family reach the choice that is best for them.[39,40] On the other hand, the goal of the presumptive approach is to increase the number of organs available for transplantation. Requestors view themselves as advocates for both donors and recipients. There is a shift from value-neutral language to value-positive language, and the discussion is biased toward supporting organ donation.[39,40] Dual advocacy considers the interests of both donors and recipients and promotes the family's right to make a decision based on complete information, including the positive impact that organ donation can have. Dual advocacy recognizes that requestors must also consider the needs of the family.[38] Currently, there is controversy concerning the best way to approach families.[38-40] Some believe that in order to respect the rights of patients and families, clinicians must be fully transparent, fair and evenhanded in discussions with families regarding organ donation.[39] This philosophy most closely aligns with the standard approach[40] (Box 24-3).

BOX 24-3 Standard Approch-Specific Language

- This is Mary. She works with families like yours who have lost a loved one. Would it be possible for her to speak with you for a moment?
- I am very sorry for the loss of your loved one. You now have the option of organ donation. Have you ever had a discussion about organ donation?
- Some families choose the option of donating their loved one's organs. I am here to help you make the decision that is best for you and your family.
- Would you like me to give you some time before you make final decision?
- If you decide to donate, I can provide you with a letter that will tell you about the who receive your loved one's organs.

Models for Interdisciplinary Communication

Excellent communication between the clinical team and families is essential for a collaborative relationship. Professional competence and clear delineation of roles and responsibilities among the medical team are important for building trust with families.[28,31,33] Some institutions have addressed these issues by creating programs to enhance communication both within the medical team as well as between clinicians and families.

In 1997, the Medical College of Virginia Hospitals (MCVH) convened the MCVH Organ Donation Task Force to improve the organ donation process by emphasizing family care and communication. A multidimensional approach was taken and, among other things, a standard organ donation protocol and a hospital-based support team were created. The *Family Communication for Potential Organ Donation Protocol* was developed to ensure reliable identification of all potential brain-dead organ donors, optimize family communication, and to maximize the organ donation request process. The protocol clearly defined roles and responsibilities for individuals involved. The hospital-based support team was staffed 24 hours per day by the Department of Pastoral Care chaplains, who were named the Family Communication Coordinators (FCCs). Chaplains were chosen to staff the support team due to their expertise in family counseling and crisis intervention. In addition to providing spiritual and emotional support to families, the FCCs managed communication with the family by coordinating a communication plan between the family and the medical team. In addition, the FCCs were present at family conferences when there was discussion of a grave prognosis and/or brain death. The FCCs introduced the family members to the OPO representative and remained with the family throughout the donation request process. Organ donation consent rates increased nearly 40% after implementation of this program. The protocol's authors concluded that increased support and communication with families contributed to this increase. Several benefits were observed by the medical staff:

- Improved relationship with the local OPO,
- Standardization of care due to guideline development,
- Increased emotional support of the medical staff,
- Increased focus on bedside care of the patient due to shared emotional care of the family,
- Improved timeliness and consistency of information given to families.[28]

Similarly, a teaching hospital in Iowa developed a family support person (FSP) team that was composed of social workers. The responsibility of the FSP team was to oversee the organ donation process. Specifically, the team promoted effective communication between medical staff and families by creating a communication plan to ensure clear, consistent transmission of information. A key responsibility of the team was to prohibit the family from being approached for organ donation until it was clear that the family understood the meaning of brain death. The program was supported by the medical staff, who felt increased confidence that the needs of the family were met. Strengths of the program were consistent communication between the family and the medical team and family support regardless of organ donation decision.[41]

Overall, these programs serve as models for interdisciplinary communication and enhanced family support during the organ donation process. A collaborative approach between physicians and OPO staff members has resulted in higher consent rates.[6]

Summary

The organ donation process is very complex and may be influenced by a variety of factors. Systems must be in place to optimize the process so that all families who are interested in participating are able to do so. However, it is equally important to respect and support families who decline organ donation so that patient and family interests are preserved. Fundamental to this approach is clear, efficient communication, understanding of divergent belief systems, and respect for all individuals.

REFERENCES

1. Uniform Anatomical Gift Act website: www.anatomicalgiftact.org Accessed August 31, 2009.
2. Organ Procurement and Transplantation Network website: http://optn.transplant.hrsa.gov/. Accessed August 31, 2009.
3. Scientific Registry of Transplant Recipients website: http://www.ustransplant.org/. Accessed August 10, 2009.
4. Jeffres LW, Carroll JA, Rubenking BE, Amschlinger J: Communication as a predictor of willingness to donate one's organs: an addition to the Theory of Reasoned Action, *Prog Transplant* 18(4):257–262, 2008.
5. Siminoff LA, Gordon N, Hewlett J, Arnold RM: Factors influencing families' consent for donation of solid organs for transplantation, *JAMA* 286(1):71–77, 2001.
6. Simpkin AL, Robertson LC, Barber VS, Young JD: Modifiable factors influencing relatives' decision to offer organ donation: systematic review, *BMJ* 338:b991, 2009.
7. Thomas SL, Milnes S, Komesaroff PA: Understanding organ donation in the collaborative era: a qualitative study of staff and family experiences, *Intern Med J* 2008.
8. Thornton JD, Wong KA, Cardenas V, Curtis JR, Spigner C, Allen MD: Ethnic and gender differences in willingness among high school students to donate organs, *J Adolesc Health* 39(2):266–274, 2006.
9. Williams MA, Lipsett PA, Rushton CH, et al: The physician's role in discussing organ donation with families, *Crit Care Med* 31(5):1568–1573, 2003.
10. Siminoff LA, Marshall HM, Dumenci L, Bowen G, Swaminathan A, Gordon N: Communicating effectively about donation: an educational intervention to increase consent to donation, *Prog Transplant* 19(1):35–43, 2009.
11. Alden DL, Cheung AH: Organ donation and culture: a comparison of Asian American and European American beliefs, attitudes, and behaviors, *J Appl Soc Psychol* 30(2):293–314, 2000.
12. Siminoff LA, Lawrence RH, Arnold RM: Comparison of black and white families' experiences and perceptions regarding organ donation requests, *Crit Care Med* 31(1):146–151, 2003.
13. Stephenson MT, Morgan SE, Roberts-Perez SD, Harrison T, Afifi W, Long SD: The role of religiosity, religious norms, subjective norms, and bodily integrity in signing an organ donor card, *Health Commun* 23(5):436–447, 2008.
14. al-Mousawi M, Hamed T, al-Matouk H: Views of Muslim scholars on organ donation and brain death, *Transplant Proc* 29(8):3217, 1997.
15. Alvaro EM, Jones SP, Robles AS, Siegel J: Hispanic organ donation: impact of a Spanish-language organ donation campaign, *J Natl Med Assoc* 98(1):28–35, 2006.
16. Morse CR, Afifi WA, Morgan SE, et al: Religiosity, anxiety, and discussions about organ donation: understanding a complex system of associations, *Health Commun* 24(2):156–164, 2009.
17. Siminoff LA, Burant CJ, Ibrahim SA: Racial disparities in preferences and perceptions regarding organ donation, *J Gen Intern Med* 21(9):995–1000, 2006.
18. Pietz CA, Mayes T, Naclerio A, Taylor R: Pediatric organ transplantation and the Hispanic population: approaching families and obtaining their consent, *Transplant Proc* 36(5):1237–1240, 2004.
19. Manninen DL, Evans RW: Public attitudes and behavior regarding organ donation, *JAMA* 253(21):3111–3115, 1985.
20. Jafri T, Tellis V: Attitudes of high school students regarding organ donation, *Transplant Proc* 33(1–2):968–969, 2001.
21. Lopez-Navidad A, Vilardell J, Aguayo MT, et al: Introducing an informative program on donation and transplantation into secondary education, *Transplant Proc* 34(1):25–28, 2002.
22. Pierini L, Valdez P, Pennone P, et al: Teenager donation: investigation of 848 high school students, *Transplant Proc* 41(8):3457–3459, 2009.
23. Sanner MA: A Swedish survey of young people's views on organ donation and transplantation, *Transpl Int* 15(12):641–648, 2002.
24. Piccoli GB, Soragna G, Putaggio S, et al: Efficacy of an educational program on dialysis, renal transplantation, and organ donation on the opinions of high school students: a randomized controlled trial, *Transplant Proc* 36(3):431–432, 2004.
25. Reubsaet A, Brug J, Nijkamp MD, Candel MJ, van Hooff JP, van den Borne HW: The impact of an organ donation registration information program for high school students in the Netherlands, *Soc Sci Med* 60(7):1479–1486, 2005.
26. Waldrop DP, Tamburlin JA, Thompson SJ, Simon M: Life and death decisions: using school-based health education to facilitate family discussion about organ and tissue donation, *Death Stud* 28(7):643–657, 2004.
27. Rodrigue JR, Cornell DL, Howard RJ: Pediatric organ donation: what factors most influence parents' donation decisions? *Pediatr Crit Care Med* 9(2):180–185, 2008.
28. Tartaglia A, Linyear AS: Organ donation: a pastoral care model, *J Pastoral Care* Autumn, 54(3):277–286, 2000.
29. DeLong WR: Organ donation and hospital chaplains. Attitudes, beliefs, and concerns, *Transplantation* 50(1):25–29, 1990.
30. Geva J, Weinman ML: Social work perspectives in organ procurement, *Health Soc Work* 20(4):287–293, 1995.
31. Truog RD, Christ G, Browning DM, Meyer EC: Sudden traumatic death in children: "We did everything, but your child didn't survive." *JAMA* 295(22):2646–2654, 2006.
32. Daly BJ: End-of-life decision making, organ donation, and critical care nurses, *Crit Care Nurse* 26(2):78–86, 2006.
33. Meyer K, Bjork IT: Change of focus: from intensive care towards organ donation, *Transpl Int* 21(2):133–139, 2008.
34. Medicare and Medicaid programs; hospital conditions of participation; identification of potential organ, tissue, and eye donors and transplant hospitals' provision of transplant-related data—HCFA. Final rule, *Fed Regist* 63(119):33856–33875, 1998.
35. Association of Organ Procurement Organizations: www.aopo.org/aopo/. Accessed August 14, 2009.
36. OrganDonor.gov: http://organdonor.gov/ Accessed August 14, 2009.
37. Bollinger RR, Heinrichs DR, Seem DL, Rosendale JD, Johnson KS: Organ procurement organization (OPO), best practices, *Clin Transplant* 15(Suppl 6):16–21, 2001.
38. Luskin R: Glazier, Alexandra, Delmonico, Francis: organ donation and dual advocacy, *N Engl J Med* 358(12):1297–1298, 2008.
39. Truog RD: Consent for organ donation: balancing conflicting ethical obligations, *N Engl J Med* 358(12):1209–1211, 2008.
40. Zink S, Wertlieb S: A study of the presumptive approach to consent for organ donation: a new solution to an old problem, *Crit Care Nurse* 26(2):129–136, 2006.
41. Thall CR, Jensen G, Wright C, Baker S, Meade R: The role of hospital-based family support teams in improving the quality of the organ donation process, *Transplant Proc* 29(8):3252–3253, 1997.

25 Autopsy

ALBERTO BRONISCER

Something can come out of the child's death that will help others.

I feel good knowing that it (autopsy) could help to prevent this from happening to another child or family.

—Quotes from parents whose children died of
a rare brain cancer, and whose tumors were collected
at autopsy

Post-mortem examination or autopsy, meaning to see for oneself, has been an important foundation of medicine since ancient times. Descriptions of autopsies have been found as early as the third century BC.[1] However, it was not until the middle of the nineteenth century that pathologists started to follow strict scientific methods to perform autopsies.[1] Although autopsies had been considered standard practice until the middle of the twentieth century, most recently the hospital autopsy rates for adults have been steadily declining, particularly in Western countries.[2,3] The decline in autopsy rates has been attributed to multiple causes, including:

- The belief that the procedure is less relevant in face of technological advances,
- The procedure's cost,
- Lack of time and expertise among pathologists,
- Lack of experience and interest among clinicians to pursue consent from families,
- Concern that autopsy could upset bereaved families or create litigation.[3]

Unlike adults, the decline in autopsy rates has been less pronounced in the pediatric age group.[4,5] Although autopsies in adults and children share some common goals, this procedure has particular characteristics and may serve specific objectives when performed in children, particularly for the grieving family.

Unique Characteristics of Autopsies in the Pediatric Age Group

The description of the characteristics of autopsy in the pediatric age group, including consent process, objectives, and perspective of families and physicians about the procedure, is more complex than that for adults. Whereas the attributes of this procedure in adolescents and young adults may be very reminiscent of those in older adults, there are unique characteristics associated with this procedure in younger children, especially in neonates and infants. A competent review of some of the issues surrounding autopsies in children is

available.[6] Unlike past times when childhood mortality accounted for most deaths within the community, the advances of modern medicine have transformed the death of a child into an uncommon event, at least in developed countries. The unexpected death of a child commonly brings upon parents or relatives the feeling of guilt or blame, which is generally unjustified. After all, the rearing of children in modern societies is so dependent on parents or guardians that the death of a child is commonly attributed to direct or indirect fault of an adult. The death of a child, particularly at an early age, can commonly raise concerns among families about genetic disorders and/or predispositions, which may have caused or contributed to the child's demise. The latter issue is of particular importance for parents who are still of their reproductive age and information obtained during autopsy may help their decision making about having additional children. In all the situations previously described, the results of the autopsy may be helpful for families, whether or not the procedure is able to confirm the cause and contributing factors of the child's death. Finally, sometimes the death of a child is unexpected and cannot be attributed with certainty to any specific cause. In that case, an autopsy may be required for forensic reasons to ascertain the cause of death, such as in cases of sudden infant death syndrome (SIDS).

FACTORS THAT INFLUENCE CONSENT TO AUTOPSY IN CHILDREN

The success in obtaining consent for autopsy in children is influenced by the interaction of multiple factors within society, the families of the deceased children, and the team of healthcare providers. It is also dependent on the context and characteristics surrounding the death of the child. It is essential to emphasize the variability in public attitude toward autopsy in different countries and sometimes within the same country, which are based on secular and religious characteristics.[3] Different religions have more or less permissive attitudes toward autopsies.[3] Whereas some religions place limitations on autopsy because of the need to bury all body parts within a short interval, several other religions pose no obstacles toward this procedure.[3] Culture consists of a set of shared values, beliefs, attitudes, goals, and behaviors that characterize a human group. Cultural influences, which are very difficult to quantify, are presumed to affect the acceptance of autopsies by families. Although very little has been described about how culture influences the consent for autopsy, two studies addressed some of the subtle cultural differences between Hispanics and non-Hispanics, which affected the rates of consent to autopsy.[7,8] In my own practice, I have not been able to clearly determine the influence of cultural background on the rate of consent to autopsy. Anecdotal reports from physicians in several developed countries or regions in Europe and South America describe their difficulties in obtaining consent to autopsies, which were attributed to cultural influences. Further study is required to address the influence of cultural factors in pediatric autopsy.

The success or failure to obtain consent to autopsy is also dependent on the setting in which it takes place and who is asking for consent. Unfortunately, the responsibility for initiation of the process for consent to autopsy commonly relies on a junior physician, who is unfamiliar with the deceased child and inexperienced in addressing issues associated with autopsy. Success in obtaining consent to autopsy is more likely to occur when this task is undertaken by a healthcare provider who was directly involved in the care of the deceased child and/or acquainted with the family. That may be the primary physician, a nurse, a social worker, or a bereavement counselor. Several studies have also demonstrated that more experienced physicians have more positive and accepting views of the procedure than junior colleagues, which may have an an impact on their success rate of persuading families about the importance of autopsy.[9,10] However, no study to date has shown a better success rate in obtaining consent to autopsy among more experienced compared to junior physicians.[9] The involvement of the pathologist who will perform the autopsy may benefit bereaved parents in their decision to consent.[11] Pathologists do not directly participate in the care of children, nor are they acquainted with the child's family. However, their abilities to provide accurate details about the autopsy, including the procedure, aspects related to removal and retention of tissue and organs, and planned tests, add transparency to the process and help in the family's decision.

One study analyzed maternal and infant factors that could be determinants of parental autopsy consent after neonatal death in a large tertiary center.[9] Whereas history of previous perinatal loss or abortion was significantly associated with an increased consent rate to autopsy, low gestational age, extreme prematurity and/or low birth weight, and death due to extreme prematurity were significantly associated with failure to obtain consent to autopsy. On the other hand, none of the socioeconomic characteristics analyzed, including occupation and employment, had any influence on the success of obtaining consent to autopsy. In this study, blacks were associated with a marginally significant increase in failure to obtain consent to neonatal autopsy.[9]

The Consent to Autopsy

There is extreme variability in the logistical issues associated with the consent to autopsy, which are dependent on the following factors:

- Nature of death, including sudden vs. following a chronic disorder, expected vs. unexpected,
- Place where child dies, home vs. hospital,
- Laws at the place of death.

The consent to autopsy generally starts after the child's death. However, it is not uncommon for an autopsy to be discussed before death along with other end-of-life issues in chronically ill children or when death is expected. In fact, physicians or parents may raise this issue long before the child's death. Although the issue of autopsy may be discussed beforehand, the formal consent to autopsy is invariably signed after death, except in states or regions that permit signing the consent before death. Because there are regulations regarding the body's disposal, the consent to autopsy in fact allows for the release of the body for the procedure.

The consent to autopsy usually takes place in face-to-face meetings between families and healthcare providers when children die in the hospital or at home. However, the consent to autopsy may occasionally need to be obtained via telephone conversations, particularly for children who die at home. In a 2009 report, researchers prospectively contacted by telephone the parents of children who died unexpectedly in order to obtain consent for research imaging studies during autopsy.[12] Parents were approached by a senior family liaison experienced in dealing with bereaved families. Thirty-one of 32 families contacted by telephone consented for the procedure. It is common now for families to pursue specialized care for their children far from home. In this setting, face-to-face meetings with the primary care team may not be feasible. Consent to autopsy may need to be obtained over the telephone in such circumstances. However, it is important to emphasize that regulations within the jurisdiction where the child died will dictate if telephone consent is permissible; and requirements for autopsy consent obtained over the telephone may vary. In my institution, we recommend that a witness listen to the consent on an interconnected line or confirm permission for the procedure by communicating directly with the person who provided the consent. The person obtaining the consent should go over all the information contained in the autopsy consent form and fill out the information about the person providing the consent including name, address, relationship to the deceased child, and telephone number called. In my experience, the consent to autopsy obtained over the telephone worked well when death was expected and a good support system, such as hospice, was already in place. In particular, a local healthcare team member such as the hospice nurse may provide essential guidance so that consent is done at the appropriate time and in the least intrusive way to grieving families.

Most commonly the consent process and the topic of autopsy is led by a physician whose practice is hospital-based. However, the consent to autopsy can certainly be raised by other healthcare providers who are knowledgeable about autopsy process and can adequately address the questions and concerns raised by families.

The individual who is legally allowed to give autopsy consent is generally the person assuming custody of the child's body for burial. Next of kin and the person authorized to consent to autopsy are dictated by the law in the jurisdiction where the child died. In the absence of any of those options, the consent to autopsy may need to be obtained from a representative of governmental agencies charged by law with the responsibility for burial. However, I have witnessed situations where the determination of the person who should be able to provide consent to autopsy was not straightforward. For example, a deceased child had been under state custody. The state's representative relinquished the consent decision to the child's biological parent. I have also raised the issue of autopsy with parents who were separated, divorced, or never married. In these cases, unless both parents had already reached an agreement, the decision to consent to autopsy should rely on the child's primary caregiver. Irrespective of the legal status of their relationship, I have not pursued consent to autopsy for my patients when there was a disagreement among parents about the procedure. Guidelines for introducing the topic of autopsy are shown in Box 25-1.

BOX 25-1 Guidelines on How to Introduce the Topic of Autopsy to Parents or Guardians of Children

1. Anticipate that the opportunities to discuss autopsy with parents and/or legal guardians can take place at different times during the child's illness, but most commonly at the end of life.
2. Anticipate that parents and/or legal guardians are most responsive to this discussion when they have a good understanding of the child's illness and the inevitability of the child's death, and when they trust the healthcare provider.
3. A particularly productive way to introduce the issue of autopsy is to first have a global discussion about the challenges faced by parents, families, and clinicians in relation to the child's specific medical problem. Suggested discussion points include:
   1. Describe how common or rare the illness or specific medical problem is
   2. Discuss why more effective therapies are not available and the shortcoming of current therapies
   3. Depict aspects of the problem and/or illness to which parents can envision a more humane relationship, such as other affected children, families, or social groups
4. Offer a description of the goals of autopsy, including tissue collection for research purposes, and clarification or elucidation of cause of death, and link these to this child's clinical circumstances.
5. Discuss with parents all aspects of autopsy, including details about the procedure, potential to interfere with grieving process or planned rituals, retention of tissues if applicable, costs, and particularly potential limitations and shortcomings, including the possibility that no cause of death may be found, tissue and fluids collected may not be suitable for analysis.

Legal Aspects of Autopsy

Healthcare providers need to be knowledgeable and prepared to address multiple legal issues when consenting or performing autopsies in children. Because the legal requirements for autopsy consent vary among different countries, regions, or states, it is important to know the laws applicable both where the death occurs and where the autopsy takes place. Some countries, for example, allow autopsies to be done without consent for medical, scientific, or educational reasons.[3] The legislation associated with autopsy may also vary over time. A 2002 survey provided examples of inconsistencies over time of legislation pertaining to tissue retention at autopsy in different countries.[13]

It is critical that a proper consent process be followed, which must include:

- Transparent and thorough discussion of the proposed procedure with families,
- The use of the appropriate consent forms that provides details about the scope of the procedure,
- Intent to retain tissue or organs and for what purposes,
- Plans to return body parts.

Practical issues associated with the consent process have been previously addressed.

The form used to obtain autopsy consent needs to provide details about the type of autopsy to be done, such as complete or limited to particular areas or organs, and whether tissue retention is requested. The examiner can be liable for failure to obtain consent to autopsy or failure to comply with the scope of the consent to autopsy.[14]

Two incidents in the United Kingdom, one at the Bristol Infirmary Hospital and the other at the Alder Hey Hospital, highlight the importance of clear disclosure of tissue retention to families.[15] Both incidents, which resulted from inappropriate retention of body parts of deceased children without parental consent, generated enormous controversy and resulted in a large public backlash against pediatric autopsies in the United Kingdom. Therefore, it is imperative that autopsy consent forms contain a request for tissue retention for additional studies, and for research and educational purposes. The consent form also must include contingency plans to return body parts to families, if necessary.

As a result of the incidents described, the law for tissue retention after autopsy has been changed in the United Kingdom by the approval of the Human Tissue Act of 2003.[16] The Act declared lawful only the post-mortem retention of body parts done with appropriate consent. Failure to obtain appropriate consent to retain body parts is considered a criminal offense with specified penalties. However, this law is not applicable to coronial cases, which constitute the majority of autopsies in the United Kingdom. A similar law, the Human Tissue and Anatomy Legislation Amendment Act of 2003, was also approved in New South Wales, Australia.[16] The Australian law dictated that retention of human tissue after post-mortem examination of a child could be done only upon consent from a senior available next of kin. Human tissue was defined as organs or body parts and excluded small samples, such as slides and blood smears, which are routinely retained as part of the standard goals of the autopsy. Identical to the law in the United Kingdom, this new legislation applied only to non-coronial cases.

Unlike the United Kingdom, organ retention is regulated under state, not federal, law in the United States.[16] No uniform national legislation has been instituted to regulate organ retention after autopsy, and the judicial authorities in the different states have not reached a consensus about this issue. With few exceptions, most of the state statutes do not address the retention of body remains whether the autopsy is performed after consent from next of kin or if it is mandated by the state.[16] Organ retention in the United States is regulated under the common law, which as a general rule considers that the survivors of the deceased have no property rights over the human body or its parts. Therefore, the courts have generally not imposed liability over unauthorized tissue and/or organ retention after autopsy in the United States, except in cases where there was no consent to a general autopsy at all.

It is also critical for the pathologist performing the autopsy that the body be identified by someone familiar with the child, or by appropriate means of identification, such as a wristband with the child's name.

Finally, most jurisdictions authorize autopsies when the death of a child younger than 18 years is traumatic, unexpected, obscure, suspicious, or otherwise unexplained. The American Academy of Pediatrics (AAP) has set recommendations to perform a complete autopsy in such cases, including cases suspicious for SIDS.[17] Complete autopsy consists of external and internal examination, microscopic examination, removal and examination of the eyes, and toxicologic, microbiologic, and other pertinent studies. The AAP recommendations for unexplained deaths apply even to children with chronic conditions. As described before, it is imperative that the examiner be familiar with the law because some states in the United States allow exceptions for autopsies in unexplained deaths when this procedure is believed to be contrary to the religious beliefs of the decedent.[14]

Logistics of Autopsy

The description of a standard autopsy is outside the scope of this review. A 2007 study reviewed alternative methods of performing an autopsy, including minimally invasive procedures and verbal autopsy.[3]

There are preparations that need to take place in order to have an autopsy done. In my experience, parents or legal guardians greatly appreciate if they do not have any involvement in preparing the autopsy at a time of tremendous grief. Not having someone outside the family to coordinate preparation for autopsy by itself could represent an obstacle to this procedure.

Another major concern among parents is the feasibility of autopsy if the child dies at home. Two main problems are the ability to transport the child's body to the site where autopsy will take place and the possible delay in starting autopsy when death occurs outside the hospital. I have been conducting a prospective study to obtain brain-only autopsies in children with diffuse intrinsic pontine glioma (DIPG), a rare and lethal type of brain cancer in children.[18] More than 80% of the children who underwent autopsy in our study died at home. The median interval from death to autopsy was 7.5 hours. We were able to arrange transport of the body with funeral homes for all children who died at home. The delay in the start of autopsy is particularly concerning when metabolic disorders are suspected. A recent review described the importance of tissue and fluid collection as soon as possible after death and the procedures that need to be followed in these special autopsies, also called metabolic autopsy, to rule out metabolic disorders.[19] In the latter cases, further arrangements need to be in place to assure a very short interval between death and autopsy and the expeditious collection of tissue samples.

Lastly, in the majority of cases there may be financial costs associated with the transportation of the child's body and autopsy that may not be covered by the insurance plan or by the hospital where the autopsy takes place. In my experience, the potential financial burden of the procedure may also influence the decision of families to consent or not to this procedure.

Perspective of Families about Autopsy

Among the main reasons raised by physicians not to initiate the discussion about autopsy are the perception of futility of this procedure in view of what was already known before death, and the assumption that such discussion could further upset bereaved families. Only a few studies to date have investigated the pros and cons of having an autopsy done from the perspective of parents who had lost a child.[5,20-22] The perception of bereaved parents varied from one study to another depending on several factors, including the medical problem, the design of the study, the overall context of death such as the child's age, type of illness, and expected vs. unexpected death, and how the process was handled by medical personnel.

In a report published in the 1980s, researchers reported the opinion about autopsy among family members who had recently lost a child or adult relative in a large tertiary center.[5] One-fifth of the study subjects were parents who had lost a child. The authors contacted not only family members who had consented but also those who had not consented to an autopsy. Strikingly, family members who consented to autopsy for deceased children reported significantly more comfort in knowing the cause of death than relatives of adult patients who had also provided consent to the procedure. Family members of deceased children also expressed their concern significantly more often about body disfigurement with autopsy and the stress associated with autopsy consent than

relatives of deceased adults. Overall, the role of autopsy was seen as beneficial in 91% and 83% of relatives who consented or did not consent to autopsy, respectively.

A survey was conducted among 59 sets of parents whose children had died in three neonatal units in Scotland between 1996 and 1998.[20] Autopsy consent had been initiated for all but one set of parents, and two-thirds had consented to the procedure. The main reasons for parents to consent to autopsy were to obtain answers to their questions, to help others, and to obtain information that could influence future pregnancies. The main reasons parents declined consent to autopsy were dread of mutilation to the child's body and the absence of questions to be answered about the child's death. When reached 13 months after death, none of the parents regretted the decision either way.

A 2002 study interviewed, via questionnaire, mothers who had lost a child during pregnancy or infancy over a 4-year period.[21] Of the 148 respondents, 120 had consented to autopsy. Almost half of mothers consented to autopsy because they wanted to learn more about what happened to their child and 25% believed that it would improve medical knowledge and research. On the other hand, 7% of those who consented to autopsy regretted the decision because no clear reason for the death was identified, the procedure produced more questions than answers, or they believed that their children had suffered too much. Four of the 28 mothers who declined autopsy regretted their decision. Almost half of mothers who declined autopsy believed that their children had already suffered too much, 26% did not believe the procedure would help them, and 10% were concerned about the effects of autopsy on the child's appearance.

A 2006 follow-up survey of 373 parents who lost a child to SIDS,[22] was conducted by questionnaire 4 to 7 years after death, and all children underwent autopsy. Response was obtained from 141 (38%) of parents. There were no differences between respondents and no-respondents in regards to sex of the deceased child and whether the diagnosis of SIDS was confirmed. However, parents who responded to the survey had a higher socioeconomic level. Two-thirds of parents believed that the autopsy was helpful in the bereavement period, 17% thought autopsy was wrong at the time of death but now believed that it was the right decision, and 3% thought autopsy was the right decision at the time of death but now regretted their decision. Thirteen percent of parents believed that autopsy was wrong at the time of death and at follow-up. The authors concluded that the high approval rate of autopsy in the context of infants who were suspected to have died of SIDS was because the procedure generated helpful information for parents, families, and the surrounding community. In the latter situation, the authors emphasized the importance of autopsy to show that the parents were not responsible for their child's death.

In our own study conducting autopsies in children who died of DIPG, a survey of 25% who consented to autopsy has been conducted to obtain their feedback about the procedure. Within this context, we have not witnessed any regrets about the autopsy among parents. So far, the most common reasons reported by parents to consent to autopsy have been to help with research to find a cure for this lethal cancer, to help physicians advance knowledge, and to protect future patients and families.

Several of the previously described studies emphasized the importance for parents of obtaining the results of the autopsy in a timely manner, and also that the results be reported in clear terms.[5,20] It also needs to be emphasized to parents that there is always a risk that autopsy may not contribute to better understanding of the child's death, so that further frustration is avoided.[21]

One major limitation common to all the studies is the difficulty or complete inability in obtaining feedback from parents who declined or were never asked about autopsy because of logistical and ethical reasons. The lack of knowledge about the perception of a larger share of parents about autopsy creates a bias in the results and limits our ability to transform this entire process to one more acceptable to families.

Perspective of Physicians about Autopsy

Despite all technological advances in diagnosing and treating acute and chronically ill children, autopsy remains the gold standard to assure appropriateness of care. Autopsy is an important tool to confirm primary or concomitant conditions, and even to detect conditions that may have been unknown before death. Several prospective and retrospective studies have reported the impact of autopsy in providing a standard for the quality of care of children in different contexts, be it in general pediatrics or specialty services, including neonatology, pediatric cardiology, hematology-oncology, critical care, and emergency medicine.[23–25] Autopsy produced new major diagnoses, which would have been relevant for the care of these children in 20% to 50% of the cases.[23–25]

Two surveys conducted in the 1990s evaluated the knowledge and opinion of pediatric residents and/or pediatricians about autopsy.[10,26] In the first study, 98% of responding physicians believed that autopsy provided valuable information. However, less experienced physicians and those who had not witnessed an autopsy were less cognizant of the importance of this procedure.[10] A significant share of physicians reported discomfort in informing parents of the death of a child who they were treating or raising the issue of autopsy; these feelings were less relevant for more experienced physicians. The most common reasons described for physicians not to make efforts to get consent to autopsy were fear of upsetting families and the belief that the results of autopsy would not be valuable. The physicians believed that the most common reasons for failure to get consent to autopsy were concern about desecration of the body among families and that family members were too upset to consider the procedure. The second study demonstrated lack of knowledge about autopsies among senior pediatric residents.[26] Senior residents were shown to be unfamiliar with the procedures involved in autopsy and therefore unable to correctly pass this information to families. More alarming, two-thirds of senior pediatric residents had not had any training about procedures associated with autopsy, and half of senior pediatric residents had not had any training on how to obtain consent to autopsy.

A survey of residents, fellows, and faculty neonatologists at a tertiary neonatal unit in the 1980s also showed that the most experienced physicians considered neonatal autopsy important more often than their junior colleagues.[9]

Future of Pediatric Autopsy

As discussed previously, I believe that autopsy continues to provide a relevant service to the families of deceased children, physicians and trainees, and society as a whole. The availability of new technologies, particularly in the diagnosis of pediatric illnesses, may have supplanted the need for autopsy in several situations where the cause of death has been well established. However, autopsy will continue to be useful in multiple other situations in children.

Significant research has been conducted in tissue obtained at autopsy in several debilitating and catastrophic disorders in childhood such as autism, SIDS, and cancer.[18,27–29] One study reported the importance of basic research done in tissue specimens collected at autopsy in children who died of SIDS, to investigate the mechanisms of death.[27] In this study, researchers described the key collaboration between bereaved parents of children who died of SIDS and investigators to push legislation in California to assist in the creation of protocols for scene investigation and postmortem examination.[27] The authors also emphasized the opportunity for families and investigators elsewhere to follow this same paradigm to help enhance the acceptance of pediatric autopsies.

Although the cause of SIDS in most children remains unknown, previously undiagnosed inborn errors of metabolism account for a significant percentage of these deaths.[30] Since the first description of metabolic causes of SIDS in 1976,[31] major progress has been accomplished in the biochemical, molecular, histochemical, and genetic analysis of tissue and fluids obtained at autopsy. A 2004 review of the most common metabolic disorders associated with SIDS and the new techniques that are available for their diagnosis[19] emphasized the importance of multidisciplinary discussion in metabolic autopsy, if possible with direct involvement of the metabolism specialist. This is crucial to guarantee the proper collection of samples and the timing of collection. For example, some organs, such as the liver, undergo rapid proteolysis and tissue collection needs to occur as soon as possible after death. Collection of cerebropsinal fluid, when clinically indicated, needs to occur before death. The metabolic autopsy has provided crucial information not only in deaths suspicious for SIDS but also in other cases in which inborn errors of metabolism are suspected to play an important role.

Another study described the efforts to collect and bank brain tissue collected at autopsy from children and adults with autism.[29] Because little is known about the pathophysiology of autism, researchers hope to better understand the neurobiology of this disorder by studying the brains of affected individuals.

We have been conducting a clinical trial to prospectively collect tumor tissue in children with DIPG.[18] Radical surgical resection of DIPGs is impossible due to the critical location and the infiltrative nature of this tumor. Biopsy of the tumor for histological confirmation is only recommended in cases with atypical imaging characteristics.[32] Because tissue samples from DIPG are hardly ever available for research purposes, very little is known about the biology of this cancer. We have successfully collected a large number of tissue samples from children with DIPG at autopsy. Of note, we have obtained DNA of excellent quality from these tumor samples obtained at autopsy even several hours after death. Extensive molecular studies of these precious tissue samples are ongoing.

As described before, appropriate legislation that regulates autopsy and tissue retention makes the process of consent particularly transparent for families, which may ultimately increase society's support for this procedure. However, there is significant concern among physicians and researchers about some aspects of these new regulations. For example, the requirement for full description of the tests planned to be done in retained tissue samples after autopsy, as mandated by the Human Act of 2003, is not believed feasible by many scientists.[33] Therefore, there has been concern that some of the new legislation may serve as a deterrent for future research based on tissue samples obtained at autopsy.

We also described how legislation in California was modified to foster the acquisition of tissue at autopsy from infants who died of SIDS. This change was possible only because of cooperation among families, investigators, and the government. Likewise, the success of our own study in acquiring tumor tissue samples from children with DIPG is a result of cooperation between investigators and affected families. In fact, several organizations formed by parents and families have created networks to support some of this research based on tissue obtained at autopsy.[34-36] Therefore, this paradigm of cooperation among affected families, healthcare providers, and government may be paramount in establishing an important role for research based on tissue obtained at autopsy in other settings of pediatric disease.

For this cooperation to take place, it is crucial that physicians continue to learn from affected families the pros and cons associated with this procedure. For example, it is clear that a significant proportion of parents are concerned about disfigurement and/or desecration of the child's body at autopsy. In such cases, minimally invasive autopsies may provide enough information after the death without creating significant objection from parents.[3]

Summary

It is clear that continued education of medical students and physicians about autopsy is required. It is obvious that the curriculum of medical schools and residency programs needs to be changed to emphasize the importance and potential gains when autopsy is performed. Medical students and physicians in training will only feel comfortable in raising the issue of death and the possibility of autopsy to families if they undergo appropriate training and exposure to these issues.

Pediatricians need to continue to teach and learn about the pros and cons of autopsy. Pediatricians are well positioned to influence other healthcare providers and bereaved families, and hopefully to lead to a change in attitude within society about the importance of this procedure.

REFERENCES

1. King LS, Meehan MC: A history of the autopsy: a review, *Am J Pathol* 73:514–544, 1973.
2. Kircher TL: Autopsy and mortality statistics: making a difference, *JAMA* 267:1264–1268, 1992.
3. Burton JL, Underwood J: Clinical, educational, and epidemiological value of autopsy, *Lancet* 369:1471–1480, 2007.
4. Ahronheim JC, Bernholc AS, Clark WD: Age trends in autopsy rates: striking decline in late life, *JAMA* 250:1182–1186, 1983.
5. McPhee SJ, Bottles K, Lo B, et al: To redeem them from death: reactions of family members to autopsy, *Am J Med* 80:665–671, 1986.
6. Beckwith JB: The value of the pediatric postmortem examination, *Pediatr Clin North Am* 36:29–36, 1989.
7. Perkins HS, Supik JD, Hazuda HP: Autopsy decisions: the possibility of conflicting cultural attitudes, *J Clin Ethics* 4:145–154, 1993.
8. González-Villalpando C: The influence of culture in the authorization of an autopsy, *J Clin Ethics* 4:145–154, 1993.
9. VanMarter LJ, Taylor F, Epstein MF: Parental and physician-related determinants of consent for neonatal autopsy, *Am J Dis Child* 141:149–153, 1987.
10. Stolman CJ, Castello F, Yorio M, et al: Attitudes of pediatricians and pediatric residents toward obtaining permission for autopsy, *Arch Pediatr Adolesc Med* 148:843–847, 1994.
11. McDermott MB: Obtaining consent for autopsy, *BMJ* 327:804–806, 2003.
12. Thayyil S, Robertson NJ, Scales A, et al: Prospective parental consent for autopsy research following sudden unexpected childhood deaths: a successful model, *Arch Dis Child* 94:354–358, 2009.
13. Skene L: Ownership of human tissue and the law, *Nat Rev Genet* 3:145–148, 2002.
14. Bierig JR: A potpourri of legal issues relating to the autopsy, *Arch Path Lab Med* 120:759–762, 1996.
15. Hall D: Reflecting on Redfern: What can we learn from the Alder Hey story? *Arch Dis Child* 84:455–456, 2001.
16. Klaiman MH: Whose brain is it anyway? The comparative law of postmortem organ retention, *J Leg Med* 26:475–490, 2005.
17. Kairys SW, Alexander RC, Block RW, et al: American Academy of Pediatrics. Committee on Child Abuse and Neglect and Committee on Community Health Services. Investigation and review of unexpected infant and child deaths, *Pediatrics* 104:1158–1160, 1999.
18. Broniscer A, Baker JN, Baker SJ, et al: Prospective collection of tissue samples at autopsy in children with diffuse intrinsic pontine glioma, *Cancer* 116(19):4632–4637.
19. Olpin SE: The metabolic investigation of sudden infant death, *Ann Clin Biochem* 41:282–293, 2004.
20. McHaffie HE, Fowlie PW, Hume R, et al: Consent to autopsy for neonates, *Arch Dis Child Fetal Neonatal Ed* 85:F4–F7, 2001.
21. Rankin J, Wright C, Lind T: Cross sectional survey of parents' experience and views of the postmortem examination, *BMJ* 324:816–818, 2002.
22. Vennemann MM, Rentsch C, Bajanowski T, et al: Are autopsies of help to the parents of SIDS victims? A follow-up on SIDS families, *Int J Legal Med* 120:352–354, 2006.
23. Kumar P, Taxy J, Angst DB, et al: Autopsies in children: are they still useful? *Arch Pediatr Adolesc Med* 152:558–563, 1998.
24. Buckner T, Blatt J, Smith SV: The autopsy in pediatrics and pediatric oncology: a single institution experience, *Pediatr Dev Pathol* 9:374–380, 2006.
25. Feinstein JA, Ernst LM, Ganesh J, et al: What new information pediatric autopsies can provide: a retrospective evaluation of 100 consecutive autopsies using family-centered criteria, *Arch Pediatr Adolesc Med* 161:1190–1196, 2007.
26. Rosenbaum GE, Burns J, Johnson J, et al: Autopsy consent practice at US teaching hospitals: results of a national survey, *Arch Intern Med* 160:374–380, 2000.
27. Krous HF, Byard RW, Rognum TO: Pathology research into sudden infant death syndrome: where do we go from here? *Pediatrics* 114:492–494, 2004.
28. Kinney HC: Neuropathology provides new insight in the pathogenesis of the sudden infant death syndrome, *Acta Neuropathol* 117:247–255, 2009.
29. Haroutunian V, Pickett J: Autism brain tissue banking, *Brain Pathol* 17:412–421, 2007.
30. Boles RG, Buck EA, Blitzer MG, et al: Retrospective biochemical screening of fatty acid oxidation disorders in postmortem livers of 418 cases of sudden death in the first year of life, *J Pediatr* 132:924–933, 1998.
31. Sinclair-Smith C, Dinsdale F, Emery J: Evidence of duration and type of illness in children found unexpectedly dead, *Arch Dis Child* 51:424–429, 1976.
32. Albright AL, Packer RJ, Zimmerman R, et al: Magnetic resonance scans should replace biopsies for the diagnosis of diffuse brain stem gliomas: a report from the Children's Cancer Group, *Neurosurgery* 33:1026–1030, 1993.
33. Mavroforou A, Giannoukas A, Michalodimitrakis E: Consent for organ and tissue retention in British law in the light of the Human Tissue Act 2004, *Med Law* 25:427–434, 2006.
34. www.brainbankforautism.org.uk/documentation_library/support-leaflet.pdf.
35. www.brainbank.org/advocates.php.
36. www.justonemoreday.org/Research/TumorTissueAnalysis.html.

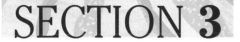

SECTION 3 Easing Suffering

Pain has an element of blank;
It cannot recollect
When it began, or if there were
A day when it was not.

It has no future but itself,
Its infinite realms contain
Its past, enlightened to perceive
New periods of pain.
  —Emily Dickinson

Pain is the symptom most commonly associated with suffering, and studies from across the globe over the past decade suggest that suffering from pain remains highly prevalent in children at the end of life. The chapters in this section will show that children with life-threatening illness face a myriad of symptoms including pain, and they experience suffering throughout their illness trajectory.

According to Dr. Eric Cassell, suffering is a specific state of distress that occurs when the intactness or integrity of the person is threatened or disrupted. It lasts until the threat is gone or integrity is restored.[1] The meanings and fears related to suffering are personal and individual, so that even if two patients have the same symptoms, their suffering would be different. This far-reaching definition of suffering can be applied to the child with life-threatening illness and family. Importantly, when the integrity of a child is threatened and disrupted, so too is the integrity of the entire family; and when there is child suffering, there is family suffering. The "threats" as described by Cassell can be *visible*, such as the underlying illness and observable symptoms, and they can be *invisible*, such as disruptions to everyday life, social needs, and psychological and existential concerns.

It is the primary responsibility of the interdisciplinary pediatric palliative care team to ease suffering of the child and family with the goal of rebuilding child and family integrity. Though the family's pre-illness integrity can never be fully restored, a reintegration can be achieved that incorporates the experience of the family living with an ill child. Strategies to re-establish family integrity include *global approaches* such as team work, and *targeted strategies* such as symptom management. The preceding section and chapters focused on broad approaches to ease suffering in children with life-threatening illness and their families, through relationships, structure and communication. The chapters that follow focus primarily on specific symptom experiences of the child and comprehensive strategies to evaluate and treat such symptoms. We chose to order these chapters from broad symptoms experiences to more specific, closing the section with distress in the child and family when death is near. And as is the case throughout this textbook, the interdisciplinary team emerges as the common thread to achieve comfort for the child and family.

REFERENCE

1. Cassell EJ: *The nature of suffering and the goals of medicine*, ed 2, New York, 2004, Oxford University Press.

26 Psychological Symptoms

MARYLAND PAO | LORI WIENER

As I stand in the night the fear approaches

I stand strong and face it with all I have

It tears and beats down on me

I stand my ground and face whatever it comes at me with

It reaches to the darkest part of my soul

It flows through me and never seems to go away

It comes right back

But I stand my ground

For the hopes of the end and of something better

I stand strong for the things that help me fight it

In the end it does not end but I still stand strong

Into the night I stand bold till the end

But then there is another journey ahead

Another challenge to face

I will face sadness, humiliation, opinion, pain, disgrace, and choice as they tear me apart.

The medicine from friendship, family, love, and life experiences heal me.

—Derick Mount, whose osteosarcoma was diagnosed at age 12. (12/3/1986–8/17/2005)

When a child faces a chronic or life-threatening illness, families immediately inherit myriad challenges. First and foremost, the family is thrust into living with uncertainty. Concerns about the child's health status are accompanied by additional stresses, including parental ability to maintain employment with associated financial implications; the child's ability to negotiate school and maintain relationships; and the ongoing negotiation of other difficult events or traumas that occur in everyday life. Worry and sadness are natural psychological reactions in this context. However, when should clinicians be concerned that these responses, secondary to the illness or treatment, are becoming pathologic in and of themselves? When do worry and sadness translate into anxiety and depression?

Symptoms such as anxiety and depressed mood are evaluated on a continuum (Fig. 26-1). In general, increasing frequency of a symptom, lasting longer than two continuous weeks, and the presence of significant impairment in functioning or the expressed desire for death should alert clinicians to pursue an

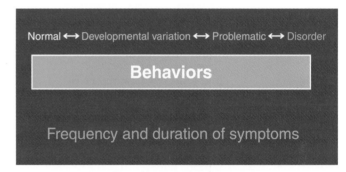

Fig. 26-1 Spectrum of clinical concerns.

in-depth mental health assessment to explore the need for specific psychological intervention. Such assessments must take into account the cultural background of the family, because psychological symptoms may be either minimized or emphasized in certain cultural contexts.[1]

There are particular junctures in the illness where strong psychological reactions may be expected. The diagnosis of a life-threatening illness such as cancer and the subsequent aggressive treatment may be disruptive, frightening, and potentially traumatic for children and their families. Anxiety or depression may emerge at multiple stages of illness: during and immediately after diagnosis and treatment from the uncertainty of outcome, as well as during survivorship, treatment for relapses and end-of-life care, and when worries appear about how death might affect the family. Hospitalization may create more anxiety in children under the age of 5 years or in those who already had difficulty separating from caregivers. Just thinking about chemotherapy or hospital smells may trigger feelings of anxiety. Youth, particularly adolescents, are concerned about the effects the illness and treatment may have on their appearance. Additionally, the further a child gets from a normal routine, the more anxiety-inducing it may be to try to re-enter his or her previous life with school, family, and friends. Anxiety, depression, post-traumatic stress, disordered sleep, and adequate pain control must all be addressed for optimal care to be provided.

Anxiety in Pediatric Patients

Anxiety emerges in response to perceived or real threats to our physical integrity or our sense of self, that is, our identity or self-esteem. It is a universal but subjective experience often based on a person's knowledge, judgment, expectations, and previous experiences. Anxiety can range from transient mild discomfort or uneasiness to pervasive and paralyzing fear. It

TABLE 26-1 Anxiety Disorders Seen in Medically Ill Children

Diagnosis	Key symptoms and/or considerations
Generalized anxiety disorder	Excessive worry with associated restlessness, fatigue, difficulty concentrating, irritability, muscle tension, sleep disturbance
Obsessive-compulsive disorder	Obsessive preoccupation or fears about physical illness
Acute Stress/ post-traumatic stress disorder	Numbness, intrusiveness and hyperarousal; diagnosis depends on duration greater than one month; can occur as a reaction to hearing diagnosis, aspects of medical treatment, or memories of treatment; common in chronic physical illness
Separation anxiety disorder	Inappropriate and/or excessive worry about separation from home and/or the family; common in children younger than age 6, resurgence around age 12
Phobias	Specific fear of blood and/or needle, claustrophobia, agoraphobia, white coat syndrome; may lead to difficulty with MRI scans, confinement in isolation, treatment compliance, etc.
Panic disorder	Severe palpitations, diaphoresis, and nausea; feeling of impending doom; resulting panic attacks lasting at least several minutes
Anxiety disorder caused by general medical condition	Should be considered if history is not consistent with symptoms of primary anxiety disorder/is resistant to treatment; more likely if physical symptoms such as shortness of breath, tachycardia, or tremor are pronounced
Substance-induced anxiety disorder	May result from direct effect of substance or withdrawal; particular awareness to medication history, start of new medication, change in dosage

Adapted and reprinted with permission from the *Diagnostic and Statistical Manual of Mental Disorders*, Text Revision, Fourth Edition (DSM-IV-TR). ©2000, American Psychiatric Association.

BOX 26-1 Possible Medical Conditions Precipitating Anxiety in Medically Ill Patients

Metabolic
- Electrolyte disturbances
- Uremia
- Vitamin B_{12} and/or folate deficiency

Pulmonary
- Hypoxia
- Pneumothorax
- Pulmonary edema and/or embolism
- Asthma
- Anaphylaxis

Neurologic
- Encephalopathy
- Mass/lesion
- Post stroke
- Post concussion
- Seizure
- Vertigo

Endocrinologic
- Cushing syndrome
- Adrenal insufficiency
- Hypopituitarism
- Pheochromocytoma
- Thyroid dysfunction

Cardiovascular
- Ischemic heart disease
- Arrhythmias
- Congestive heart failure
- Hematologic, such as anemia

Neoplasms
- Brain tumors
- Insulinoma
- Lymphoma
- Small cell carcinoma
- Pancreatic cancer
- Leukemia

Other
- Transplantation
- Pain (uncontrolled)
- Caffeine
- Substance abuse or withdrawal

Adapted and reprinted with permission from the *Clinical Manual of Pediatric Psychosomatic Medicine*. © 2006, American Psychiatric Association.

is accompanied by psychological, cognitive, and behavioral symptoms. Psychological symptoms of anxiety include dread and anticipation of negative outcomes, an inability to turn off one's thoughts, and feeling helpless. Physical symptoms include feeling tense, palpitations, chest tightness or shortness of breath, nausea, tremors, crying spells, and difficulty sleeping. Behaviorally, people may become jumpy, irritable, avoidant, talk too fast, and have trouble concentrating.

Anxiety is thought to be problematic when its intensity and duration begin to affect functioning and quality of life, especially in the context of childhood cancer or other life-threatening illness. It can develop as a primary disorder, as a psychological reaction to illness, as a secondary disorder, or may be comorbid with other psychiatric disorders such as depression (Table 26-1). Anxiety may be acute or chronic. It is important to identify any underlying treatable medical etiologies for new onset anxiety (Box 26-1). For example, akathesia, a common side effect of medications, may be misdiagnosed as anxiety.

Anxiety disorders are common in the general population in the United States, with the prevalence of any lifetime anxiety disorder estimated to be 28.8%, with 11 years as the median age of onset.[2] Age of onset varies for particular anxiety disorders, with a median onset at 7 years for separation anxiety and phobia disorders, at 13 years for social phobias, and at 19 to 31 years for other disorders. Anxiety is common in children, with

a lifetime prevalence of any anxiety disorder at 15% to 20%.[3] In children with chronic illness, an estimated 20% to 35 % have an anxiety disorder. In a study assessing anxiety in pediatric oncology patients, 14.3% of 63 children met diagnostic criteria for an anxiety disorder.[4] The prevalence of anxiety in other disorders, such as asthma, ranges from 9%[5] to 37%,[6] while in diabetes anxiety symptoms range from 0.8%[7] to almost 20%. One study found anxiety symptoms persisting 10 years after diagnosis of diabetes.[8] High rates of anxiety, up to 63%, have been reported in children with epilepsy.[9] Clearly, age at onset, sample selection, method and timing of ascertainment of anxiety disorders need to be considered when interpreting the literature on anxiety disorders in chronically ill children.

Recognition of severe anxiety is important because it may affect symptom management, treatment adherence, medical outcome, or the ability of the patient to cope with the illness. Severe anxiety may even exacerbate pre-existing physical conditions such as nausea, pain, and irritable bowel syndrome. Procedural anxiety related to the anticipation or performance of specific medical procedures could interfere with treatment. Anxiety is also common in parents, so it is critical to monitor their anxiety when discussing treatment options and decisions, communicating with them throughout the course of treatment, and coordinating post treatment care. Parental anxiety can exacerbate the child's anxiety. It is important to document if there is a family history of anxiety.

Post-traumatic stress has emerged as a possible model for understanding cancer-related distress across family members during the illness and beyond.[10] Pediatric medical traumatic stress is a set of psychological and physiological responses of children and their families to pain, injury, serious illness, medical procedures, and invasive or frightening treatment experiences. Traumatic stress responses include symptoms of arousal, re-experiencing, and avoidance or a constellation of these symptoms consistent with post-traumatic stress disorder (PTSD) or acute stress disorder.[11] Traumatic stress responses are more related to one's subjective experience of the medical event than its objective severity and are seen in children as well as in parents across the course of treatment and into survivorship.[12] Anticipatory anxiety can develop initially or during the course of treatment and clinicians need to monitor vigilantly for increased irritability, resistance, and outright refusal to cooperate with procedures. Many clinicians have found providing anticipatory guidance about normative psychological symptoms, including anxiety and worry about tests, procedures, and hospitalizations, to children and their parents is helpful in decreasing the stress of uncertainty.

EVALUATION OF ANXIETY IN A PEDIATRIC SETTING

Assessment by a palliative care team member for anxiety begins with a careful medical history including the current subjective symptoms to rule out possible medical conditions precipitating anxiety, such as the use of drugs or alcohol (see Box 26-1). It is critical to evaluate for pain because pain can affect mood and anxiety (see Chapter 22). It is also imperative to ask if the child has a history of anxiety disorders, current or previous use of prescribed medications, or a family history of psychiatric disorders, especially anxiety or mood disorders. It is important to learn about previous anxiety and coping around the initial diagnosis; anxiety surrounding hospitalizations; fear of needles and/or procedures; anticipatory anxiety; or the physical effects of illness. Be specific as to whether there are rooms, people, sights, times during the day, days of the week, sounds or smells that the child finds aversive in order to better understand how to modify these factors. The clinician should be alert to previous difficulties with separation from home and/or other familiar settings or people. Worries about death or dying need to be explicitly questioned, using developmentally appropriate language. Assessment of sources of anxiety such as academic and social impact and financial burden of illness may add important information.

A thorough assessment for an anxiety disorder includes a review of:
- Heart rate, respiratory rate, and temperature,
- Complete blood count,
- Glucose,
- Electrolytes,
- Blood urea nitrogen,
- Creatinine,
- Liver enzymes,
- Thyroid function tests,
- Urinalysis with toxicology screening,
- Arterial blood gas and/or oxygen saturation measurements to rule out respiratory causes,
- Central nervous system scans.

Depression in Pediatric Patients

Depression describes transient sad feelings in combination with a sustained low mood leading to impairment in overall functioning and may present with both psychological and physical symptoms. In general, the most prominent symptoms of depression are sadness, dysphoria, and anhedonia (inability to experience pleasure). Depression may exist as a primary disorder, as a psychological reaction to illness, as a secondary disorder to an organic etiology, or may be comorbid with other psychiatric disorders such as anxiety (Table 26-2). Even if patients do not meet diagnostic criteria for a depressive disorder, they should still receive appropriate clinical follow-up and continued monitoring.

Childhood depression does not look identical to adult depression and may be more difficult to diagnose, particularly with a concurrent medical illness. Children are more likely than adults to present with irritability, guilt, and somatic complaints. Physical symptoms include joint, limb, back, and abdominal pain; headaches, gastrointestinal problems, fatigue, weakness, and changes in appetite. It may be expressed in apathetic mood, non-adherence and changes in behavior, including regression. Depression affects school performance and peer relationships and can be associated with substance use and suicidal thoughts and behaviors. When diagnosing depression in a child with a medical illness, consideration must be given to the fact that the medical symptoms and/or side effects of serious illness can be confused with, or co-exist with, symptoms of depression. Depressive responses may be a normal response to the diagnosis and treatment of cancer and to medical events that occur during the course of treatment. Physicians and nurses are less accurate at assessment of depression than of physical distress and sometimes overestimate psychological distress. However, persistent depressed mood or irritability associated with anhedonia and withdrawn behavior that lasts for 2 or more week, should signal the need for additional monitoring and intervention.

The lifetime prevalence of a major depressive disorder in the general population in the United States is 16.6%. Approximately 2% of school age children and 4% to 8% of adolescents meet criteria for major depressive disorder (MDD) with gender differences becoming more apparent with age (females greater than males).[2] A meta-analysis estimates a 9% prevalence of depression in chronically ill children and some studies show a lower-than-normal rate of depression in pediatric cancer.[13] Generally, studies using clinical interview methodologies, rather than self report, tend to report higher levels of depression. Some large samples have shown no difference in the prevalence of depression in children with other conditions such as asthma,[6] while others[14] found that 16.3% of youths with asthma compared with 8.6% of youths without asthma met DSM-IV criteria for one or more anxiety or depressive disorders. The prevalence of depression in youth with diabetes is believed to be two to three times greater than in those without diabetes.[15] A study[8] found that in the

TABLE 26-2 Depressive Disorders Seen in Medically Ill Children

Diagnosis	Key symptoms and/or considerations
Major depressive episode	Primary mood disorder most often associated with previous psychiatric history. Must exhibit at least 5 symptoms for at least 2 weeks of: persistent depressed mood, anhedonia, irritability, change of weight, change of appetite, sleep disturbance, fatigue, feelings of worthlessness and/or guilt, diminished ability to concentrate, recurrent thoughts of death.
Dysthymia	Chronically depressed or irritable mood for at least 1 year that is less disabling than MDD. At least 2 symptoms of: sleep disturbance, fatigue, diminished ability to concentrate, feelings of hopelessness.
Adjustment disorder (that is, the adjustment to diagnosis, course, and treatment of illness)	Depressed mood in reaction to medical illness; the most common mood disorder in cancer patients. Symptoms of depression do not meet criteria for major depression but are associated with mildly impaired functioning or shorter duration.
Mood disorder caused by general medical condition	Depressed mood, elevated mood, or irritability caused by underlying medical condition; may be one of first symptoms of medical illness. Relationship to significant physical examination and study findings; particular attention to any central nervous system (CNS) lesions in frontal, limbic, and temporal lobes as possible cause.
Substance-induced mood disorder	Depression induced by medication, drugs, or alcohol. Usually resolves within 2 weeks of abstinence. Important to note the course of depression in initiation and/or dosage of a medicine (for example, high-dose α interferon).
Primary or secondary mania	Manic symptoms as a primary disorder, secondary to medical condition, induced by medication (such as corticosteroids) or toxicity. Symptoms include abnormally elevated, expansive, or irritable mood, rapid speech. Patients with brain atrophy or sleep deprivation are more prone.
Behavioral considerations	Regression: When stress of illness leads to behavioral regression and manifests as clinginess, social withdrawal, tearfulness, depressed mood. Very common in children and adolescents. Generally resolves after illness and/or hospitalization.
Bereavement	Fleeting thoughts of sadness or suicide that are part of normal mourning process. Complicated bereavement, prolonged and more persistent symptoms of mourning, needs to be distinguished from depression.

Adapted and reprinted with permission from the *Diagnostic and Statistical Manual of Mental Disorders*, Text Revision, Fourth Edition (DSM-IV-TR). ©2000, American Psychiatric Association.

10 years of post-diabetes diagnosis, 27% of the children and adolescents developed depression. Children with complex partial seizures and absence epilepsy are five times more likely to have a mood or anxiety disorder than healthy children.[9] Depression, although common, is often unrecognized and untreated in children and adolescents with epilepsy.[16] These data taken across chronic illnesses suggest that screening at regular intervals for depression and anxiety should be considered in chronically ill children, but rates may vary with the particular disease group.

Depression affects quality of life and psychological well-being. In the medically ill, depression may affect symptom management, treatment adherence, and medical outcomes. Depression is associated with higher morbidity, increased length of hospital stay, increased complaint of somatic symptoms, and is a risk factor for nonadherence with medical care. As with anxiety, patients may feel depressed at multiple points throughout the illness. The diagnosis and subsequent arduous treatment for many serious conditions may trigger feelings of overwhelming helplessness and depression.

At terminal stages of an illness, clinicians can help the child and family work through feelings of loss and should recognize symptoms of depression as part of the grieving process. Whenever possible, it is important to find ways to help children communicate their worries to family or the clinical team, so that the diagnosis of depression or anxiety can be properly made or ruled out. For example, emotional withdrawal should not be confused with depression. Emotional distancing provides the opportunity to conserve energy to focus on a few significant relationships rather than dealing with multiple painful separations.[17] In addition, chronic and severe pain is exhausting, and once under control, the child's distress may improve. Therefore, it is essential that the palliative care team assess for the role that pain and withdrawal

might have in depressive symptoms. Yet, as psychiatric symptoms can be reactive to the stresses and disruptions being experienced, a good history that includes knowledge of these conditions can help the palliative care team anticipate problems and provide them with the time to engage additional resources as needed.

One of the most frequent reasons for a psychiatric consult in a pediatric hospital setting is depression, especially within one year of a cancer diagnosis. Pediatric oncologists in the United States commonly prescribe antidepressants. A survey of 40 pediatric oncologists found that half had prescribed a selective serotonin reuptake inhibitor (SSRI)[18] while a review of a children's hospital reported that 10% of pediatric oncology patients received an antidepressant medication within one year of diagnosis.[19] On admission to the NIH Clinical Center, 14% of pediatric oncology patients had been prescribed a psychotropic medication.[20] These clinicians appear to be responding to significant distress associated with medical illness and its treatments.

EVALUATION OF DEPRESSION IN A PEDIATRIC SETTING

A detailed patient history is needed to determine the etiology of psychological and physical symptoms consistent with depression. Symptoms of depression can be difficult for clinicians to differentiate from medical and treatment side effects of cancer, which often include fatigue, decreased appetite, and sleep disturbances. Careful attention is needed to discern whether physical symptoms can be attributed to the illness process and/or treatment, or to a depressive disorder. Often, the diagnosis of depression is based on psychological symptoms such as anhedonia, feelings of worthlessness, and feeling like a burden to others.

Determining whether depressive symptoms are related to an expected course of grief or to a clinical depression is another important consideration, particularly in patients at the end of life. Consideration must be given to the patient's and family's psychiatric history, which may reveal genetic vulnerability for mood disorders. Evaluation for depression includes the assessment: symptom severity, duration, and impact on quality of life. Both the patient and primary caregivers should be interviewed to obtain information most comprehensively.

Assessment for depression in a child begins with a careful medical history including the current subjective symptoms to rule out possible medical conditions precipitating depression, such as use of drugs or alcohol (Box 26-2; see also Box 26-1). It is critical to evaluate for pain, as significant pain can affect mood and anxiety (see Chapter 22). It is also imperative to ask if the child has a history of mood disorders, previous suicide attempts, current or previous use of prescribed medications, or a family history of psychiatric disorders, especially suicidal behavior. It is useful to elicit a history of prior losses, including serious illness and/or death of family members, parental divorce, loss of pet, disappointments in school or social relationships, and how the child has, until this point, coped with his or her illness.

A thorough assessment for major depression may include:

- A review of vital signs and laboratory tests and/or procedures, including heart rate, respiratory rate and temperature,
- Complete blood count,
- Glucose,
- Electrolytes,
- Blood urea nitrogen,
- Creatinine,
- Liver enzymes,
- Thyroid function tests,
- Urinalysis with toxicology screening,
- Central nervous system scans,
- Possibly an electroencephalogram (EEG).

BOX 26-2 **Additional Considerations for Medical Conditions Precipitating Depression in Medically Ill Patients**

Medications
- Corticosteroids (may cause depressive or mania symptoms)
- Opioid analgesics
- Benzodiazepines
- Barbituates
- Narcotics
- Interferon
- Interleukin-2
- Chemotherapy agent (e.g., prednisone, vincristine, vinblastin, procarbazine, L-asparginase)

Metabolic Abnormalities
- Electrolytes
- Calcium
- B$_{12}$
- Folic acid
- Parathyroid function
- Thyriod function

Tumor
- Primary brain tumors
- Central nervous system lymphomas or metastases
- Carcinoma of pancreas

Pain
- Severe, uncontrolled pain
- Fear of unrelieved pain

Adapted and reprinted with permission from Abraham J, Gulley JL, Allegra CJ, editors: *The Bethesda Handbook of Clinical Oncology*, Lippincott, Williams and Wilkins, Philadelphia, 2005.

Assessment and Management of Suicide in Children and Adolescents

Completed suicide is rare in children. The prevalence is unknown in children with chronic illness because few healthcare professionals assess for suicide risk in pediatric patients presenting with medical complaints.[21] Suicide risk increases with age in the general population. Increased rates of suicidal ideation are found in pediatric epilepsy,[9] adult survivors of childhood cancer,[22] and in adults with medical diagnoses that are also common in childhood such as asthma[23] and pulmonary disease.[24] Previous studies indicate that chronic physical illness is a risk factor for suicide in adults[25,26] and adolescents[27] with variability by particular underlying medical diagnoses. There are no pediatric suicide-screening tools that have been validated on a general medical population. Therefore, assessing risk specific to suicide is critical. To provide a comprehensive evaluation, clinicians should inquire about suicidal ideation and history of previous suicide attempts and/or ideation, along with the stated intent and belief of lethality of attempt of suicide with or without a plan. Other risk factors include comorbid psychiatric disorders; symptoms of helplessness, hopelessness, impulsivity; social isolation; uncontrolled pain; advanced disease; male gender; history of abuse or violence; and family history of suicidal behavior or psychopathology.[28]

Ongoing assessment of suicide risk begins with the first report of suicidal ideation including passive thoughts such as being tired of fighting, or feeling it would be OK not to wake up from sleep. Other specific times for assessment should occur with any change in mental status, during worsening of illness-related symptoms and pain, and at times of management transition such as a change of healthcare provider. Immediate interventions should include environmental restrictions particularly removal of any firearms from the home, appropriate support, observation, and monitoring at home or in the hospital if actively suicidal, with available care providers to be contacted in an emergency. Passive suicidal thoughts should be taken seriously for the distress and possible depression they indicate but may not always require immediate one-to-one monitoring. Specific mental health consultation is essential to further assess suicidal comments even in the medically ill. Treatment must simultaneously address underlying psychopathology, disease-related factors, and pain, and may include psychopharmacology and/or psychotherapy.[29]

INTERVENTIONS FOR ANXIETY AND DEPRESSION

One of the challenges in evaluating anxiety or depression in children is the differentiation of symptoms that are secondary to the cancer or treatment. Somatic symptoms of depression, such as difficulty sleeping or fatigue, are also common symptoms of both depression and cancer. It is also important to differentiate symptoms that might be interpreted as depression as they may be more accurately an expression of grief. Such symptoms, regardless of whether they are normal rather than pathological require intervention. Therapeutic interventions are designed to reduce distress and to help the child integrate the facets of his or her illness and life into expression.[30] For some, talk therapy can provide a vehicle for communication of profound grief. For others, different forms of self-expression are equally powerful and effective including behavioral and cognitive techniques, play, bibliotherapy, storytelling, writing, art, music, and animal-assisted therapy. Most often, a combination of approaches is used.

Behavioral and cognitive behavioral approaches for reducing procedural distress are well established.[31] These should be tailored developmentally and include distraction, guided imagery, hypnosis, and relaxation.[32] Parents and staff members can be trained in the use of these approaches. Other treatments for anxiety and depression include cognitive behavioral therapy and family therapy to reduce anxiety and provide patients and families with adaptive strategies.

Effective treatment of a depressive disorder is best accomplished in collaboration with a mental health professional. Clinical social workers, psychologists, and/or child psychiatrists familiar with children with serious illness should be consulted in this process. There are few reports of interventions for depression that are specific and exclusive to pediatric cancer or other life-threatening illnesses. Fortunately, literature in this area is growing and the results of more general literatures are relevant. For example, individual psychotherapy for depression, especially cognitive behavioral therapy, is effective for youth in general, both alone and in combination with medication.[33] There is less empirically driven data to support other interventions known to be effective in caring for psychological distress in end-of-life care.

Bibliotherapy is an interactive therapeutic intervention that uses literature and storytelling as a means to reduce anxiety, gain insight into behavioral or psychological symptoms, enhance self-understanding, and promote coping skills and personal growth. Stories can shape one's response to later events, make connections between seemingly random events, address unfair suffering, and provide meaning. After an assessment and the identification of clear therapy goals, the basic technique begins with a therapist choosing a story to read to a child that includes characters the child may relate to and whose struggles and triumphs the child can identify with. The therapist reads the story, followed by a discussion of the themes by the child and the therapist.[34,35] The child may be asked to suggest additions or changes in the story, or he or she may share stories that are similar but have different outcomes. Together, the child and therapist might write a book or story that exemplifies the individual child's struggles, strengths, and gives meaning to his or her life. By externalizing a problem and re-creating endings, children can begin to experience a sense of mastery over their circumstances. An example of a book that addresses cancer, hair loss, courage, and resiliency is *Kathy's Hats*, by T. Krisher.

Bibliotherapy is effective in groups as well as in individual sessions. For children able to address end-of-life concerns, reading books, such as *The Fall of Freddie the Leaf* by L. Buscaglia, *The Dream Tree* by S. Cosgrove, or *Waterbugs and Dragonflies* by D. Stickney, allows group participants to talk about their personal thoughts about death, transitions, spiritual concerns, the afterlife, or even to make a book together that has a different ending.[36] Viewing films can also be used to impart therapeutic messages and to help the child obtain greater insight into his or her own life circumstances.[37,38] The goal of each of these techniques is to foster emotional expressiveness, which in turn, reduces psychic distress.

While most adults use words to express emotions as well as to address conflicts, play is the language and vehicle for a child's expression and the mechanism for therapists to promote healing. There are a variety of play therapy approaches to reduce the anxiety and depression that critically ill children may experience at the end of life. To create a therapeutic relationship based on trust, safety, and acceptance, a non-directive or child-centered approach during the first few sessions with the child is useful.[39] The therapist provides several games,

objects, and therapeutic toys the child can choose from. These may be medical play materials such as oxygen masks, alcohol pads, syringes, blood pressure cuff, or stethoscope. Objects that the child can control and can be used to facilitate mastery include play dough, bubbles, finger paints, and sand. Creating an environment of safety and trust that fosters freedom and acceptance is particularly significant for children who often experience a loss of control, privacy, and freedom of choice.

Depending on the child's health, more directive sessions are useful, particularly when a specific issue needs to be addressed quickly. Children should be told that sometimes he or she gets to choose the therapy activity, and sometimes the therapist will choose. Medical play can be valuable when the child is struggling with specific procedures that can be frightening such as the need for oxygen. Board games created to allow the child to share end-of-life worries, concerns, and fears in a non-threatening and fun way can also be informative and effective in identifying major stressors.[40] Because an important goal is to create open communication and closeness between the child and parents, it may be useful to have the parents join the child in playing such games. For the child who may be too ill or weak to play, vicarious enjoyment and expression may be accomplished by playing for the child. Through a nod or by pointing a finger, the child can direct the therapist to roll a die, choose paint colors, or create images that express his or her inner emotional state.[36]

Writing is another useful medium for working with medically ill children. Anxiety about the unknown is common and therefore, at the end of each session, providing validation of one's existence and a sense of continuity from one session to the next is useful. Completing a page of a personalized workbook for children living with a life-threatening illness[41] or a list of feelings or statements written by both the therapist and child about what activities and feelings were evident that day, can be helpful. A narrative therapy approach of letter writing, postal or e-mail, between sessions can also be used to maintain open communication. A relatively new technique, computer-assisted art therapy,[42] can enable online interactive communication between the child and the therapist in real time.

Children often fear that they will be forgotten after death. The workbook and letters written during sessions may be material that the children wish their parents to keep and cherish following their death. "My Mock Will," a page in the workbook, *This Is My World*, has been especially instructive for parents who were not able to communicate with their child about his or her last wishes or who the child would like to have some of his or her most meaningful belongings. As death approaches, feelings of loneliness and the need for expression often intensify. Adolescents particularly appreciate the opportunity to use writing techniques to counteract their anxiety, sadness, and grief. This can take the form of a personal narrative, song, poem, or combination of all. Many find that addressing issues such as funeral arrangements, giving away belongings, and discussion of how they wish to be remembered[43] less threatening through writing than verbal communication. Offering children the opportunity to use creative writing to document what they would want to happen after they are gone and to leave something of themselves behind can lessen anxiety as it affirms that an important part of their existence is still under their control.

Art therapy is another creative technique to enable children to express their conscious and unconscious concerns and to externalize their fears and anxieties. The use of art media can be used as memory-making or legacy-building activities for the child to do alone or with family members. Treasure boxes, pillow cases, outlining and then painting of a parent and child's hands touching, and family quilts, especially those that includes photographs, can also be a potent form of self-expression and healing. Photography can be used as a powerful avenue to reduce distress, increase a sense of control, and promote family interactions and communication. Following instructions pertaining to confidentiality, providing a child with a camera and asking him or her to take pictures that will show others what it is like to be sick can provide the family and providers insight into the child's perspective. Self-portraits are perhaps the most powerful and valuable photos to work with therapeutically. Asking the child to choose where they would like their portrait taken or what they would like to be doing or wearing when their portrait is created allows others to bear witness to what is most important to that child. Using phototherapy techniques, children can connect the past with the present,[44] critical steps in integrating their life experience.

Animal-assisted therapy has been gaining popularity. In this form of therapy, children are able to interact with trained animals. Volunteers whose family pets have been trained to work in a hospital setting often provide animal-assisted therapy programs. Some hospitals and long-term care facilities have also reported placing an animal on a unit with patients and staff sharing responsibilities for the animal's care. Dogs are most commonly involved, although therapeutic activities with cats, fish, guinea pigs, dolphins, and horses have also been described. Interaction between the patient and animal may simply be an informal, unstructured visit that includes play, petting, and talking with the animal and its owner. The presence of an animal seems to lessen the threat of the hospital setting, reminding many children and families of their own pet. Time with the animal may also be integrated into the goals of a therapeutic intervention. For example, a child who is resistant to leaving the hospital room or having social interaction may be willing to take a dog for a walk around the unit. Similarly, for a child who is feeling alone, snuggling with an assist animal can provide a sense of unconditional love, acceptance, and a connection to the world outside of the hospital environment.

The contact comfort of tactile stimulation and the gentle presence of the animal has both physical and psychosocial effects on children.[45] Animal-assisted therapy tends to reduce heart rate, blood pressure, and respiration rate, inducing a physiologic relaxation response. Reduction in anxiety and improvement in confidence, self-image and self-esteem has been found.[46] Children participating in animal-assisted therapy may also experience a significant reduction in pain, perhaps due to the release of endorphins that occurs during interaction with a friendly animal.[47] Additionally, the animal provides a distraction from pain and the hospital experience as well as direct enjoyment. According to a review of articles addressing the healing power of the human-animal connection, the affection shared between the child and animal promotes healing, and provides motivation. Patients also enjoy having a sense of control and a sense of calm when they are able to help care for the animal.[45]

When anxiety or depression is so severe that the child cannot participate or make use of the psychotherapeutic techniques offered, pharmacologic interventions may need to be considered. Combining pharmacological and psychological interventions is often effective. Before prescribing anxiolytic or antidepressant agents, considerations include knowing the body weight, Tanner staging, and clinical status. Drug-drug interactions should also be factored into medication and dose selection. Benzodiazepines can cause sedation, confusion, and behavioral inhibition, especially in children. Antihistamines are not helpful for persistent anxiety and their anticholinergic properties can precipitate or worsen delirium (Table 26-3). For pharmacologic treatment of depression, both citalopram and fluvoxamine have been shown to be well tolerated in empirical trials in pediatric oncology patients.[4,48] Case reports for use of tricyclic antidepressants,[49,50] low-dose atypical antipsychotics (e.g., risperidone)[51] and low-dose stimulants[52] in medically ill children are in the literature. Similarly, there is evidence for family interventions in childhood disorders, including depression.[53] Many families may be reluctant to try psychotropic medications for a variety of cultural and personal beliefs. However, they are often more willing to consider them when it is explained, for example, how the symptoms of cancer and cancer treatment may be due to a shared biologic mechanism of cytokine-induced mood changes.[54,55]

The need for intervention may continue after the end of treatment or throughout critical periods of development in a child with a chronic illness. For adolescent survivors of childhood cancer and their families, participation in a combined cognitive behavioral therapy (CBT) and family therapy intervention reduced symptoms of traumatic stress in all members of the family.[56,57] Resources for multiinterdisciplinary members of pediatric oncology teams to promote trauma informed practice are in the Medical Traumatic Stress Toolkit[58] produced by the National Child Traumatic Stress Network and available by download at: www.nctsnet.org/nccts/nav.do?pid=typ_mt_ptlkt.

Parents often question for years to come whether they made the right treatment decisions for their child, about their decision to pursue palliative or aggressive treatment, or even about having conceived or given birth to a child who developed a terminal illness.[59] The need to review events over and over, until acceptance or peace comes is common. Some are able to eloquently express these deep emotions and find gratitude for the time they did have, albeit too brief, as the following poem illustrates:

To my precious son,

If before you were born, I could have gone to heaven and saw all the beautiful souls, I still would have chosen you…

If God had told me "this soul will one day need extra care and needs," I still would have chosen you…

If he had told me "that one day this soul may make my heart bleed," I still would have chosen you…

If he had told me "this soul would make me question the depth of my faith," I still would have chosen you…

If he had told me "this soul would make tears flow from my eyes that would overflow a river," I still would have chosen you…

If he had told me, "our time spent together here on earth could be short," I still would have chosen you…

If he had told me, this soul may one day make me witness overbearing suffering," I still would have chosen you…

If he had told me, "all that you know to be normal would drastically change," I still would have chosen you…

Of course, even though I would have chosen you, I know it was God who chose me for you….

Thank You God For Letting Me Be Your Mommy.

—TERRI BANISH

TABLE 26-3 Preparations and Dosages of Anxiolytics and Antidepressants in Children

Formulation/tradename	Prescribing information ‡ (dose ranges)	Clinical information
Benzodiazepines		Chronic use will lead to tolerance and dependence.
Clonazepam/Klonopin	0.25-3 mg/day 0.01 mg/kg/24 hr ÷ every 8 hr PO	Longer coverage of persistent, pervasive anxiety, may decrease anxiety rebound symptoms. Drowsiness, sedation, may lead to behavioral disinhibition.
Diazepam/Valium	0.5-10 mg/day 0.04-0.2 mg/kg/dose IV 0.12-0.8 mg/kg/24 hr ÷ every 6-8 hr PO	Longer coverage of persistent, pervasive anxiety, may decrease anxiety rebound symptoms, but long-half-life may interfere with other medications. Less likely to need taper. Drowsiness, sedation, may lead to behavioral disinhibition.
Lorazepam/Ativan	0.25-6 mg/day 0.05 mg/kg/dose every 4-8 hours PO/IV, max dose 2 mg/dose	Quick onset, useful for acute anxiety and procedures. Drowsiness, sedation, may lead to behavioral disinhibition. Should be tapered.
Midazolam/Versed	0.025-0.05 mg/kg IV Max 0.4 mg/kg 0.25-1.0 mg/kg PO Max 20 mg	Drowsiness, sedation, may lead to behavioral disinhibition. Should be tapered; be especially careful of transitions from intensive care settings (using high doses) to the floors (using none) can lead to withdrawal.
Selective serotonin reuptake inhibitors (SSRIs)		Have a black box warning for suicidal ideation in children under 18 years. Risk of serotonin syndrome with toxicity.
Citalopram/Celexa	5-20 mg/day Max 40 mg	Dry mouth, somnolence, insomnia, GI symptoms. Has fewer drug-drug interactions.
Fluoxetine/Prozac*	5-60 mg/day Max 60 mg	Dry mouth, somnolence, insomnia, GI symptoms. Long-half-life may interfere with other medications.
Fluvoxamine/Luvox*	25-200 mg/day Max 300 mg	Dry mouth, somnolence, insomnia, GI symptoms. Some drug-drug interactions.
Paroxetine/Paxil	5-20 mg/day Max 50 mg	Dry mouth, somnolence, insomnia, GI symptoms. Withdrawal effects with abrupt cessation.
Sertraline/Zoloft*	12.5-150 mg/day Max 200 mg	Dry mouth, somnolence, insomnia, GI symptoms. Has fewer drug-drug interactions.
Serotonin norepinephrine reuptake inhibitors (SNRIs)		Have a black box warning for suicidal ideation in children under 18 years.
Venlafaxine/Effexor	75-225 mg/day	Dry mouth, somnolence, insomnia, GI symptoms.
Duloxetine/Cymbalta	20-60 mg/day	Dry mouth, somnolence, insomnia, GI symptoms.
Tricyclic antidepressants (TCAs)		Have a black box warning for suicidal ideation in children under 18 years.
Amitriptyline/Elavil*	5-50 mg/day Max 300 mg	Dry mouth, constipation, weight gain, hypotension. Greater sedation than other TCAs.
Desipramine/Norpramin	10 mg/day Max 30 mg	Sedation, dry mouth, constipation, weight gain, hypotension.
Nortriptyline/Pamelor	10 mg/day Max 150 mg	Sedation, dry mouth, constipation, weight gain, hypotension. TCA blood levels more easily monitored.
Other antidepressants		Have a black box warning for suicidal ideation in children under 18 years.
Bupropion/Wellbutrin	37.5-300mg/day Max 450 mg	Activation, agitation, anxiety, headaches, GI symptoms. Fewer sexual side effects. Increased risk of seizures.
Alternative anxiolytics		
Buspirone/Buspar	15-60 mg/day	Tachycardia, headache, GI symptoms, dizziness, insomnia.
Stimulants		
Methylphenidate†	2.5 mg-40 mg/day	Useful for fatigue, depressed, sedated person at end-of-life, rapid on and off. Insomnia, appetite suppression.

*Has an FDA indication in children or adolescents.
†Has multiple formulations.
‡Prescribing information adapted from Johns Hopkins Hospital, Custer, Rau, and Lee (eds.). The Harriet Lane Handbook, 18th Edition, Mosby: An Imprint of Elsevier Science, 2008.
mg, milligram; *kg*, kilogram; *hr*, hour; *po*, per os or by mouth; IV, intravenous; *Max*, maximum dose/day; *GI*, gastrointestinal.

Clinical Vignette

Sandra was a 16-year-old high school sophomore when she was diagnosed with osteosarcoma. As a cross-country runner and an avid dancer, she was devastated not only by the diagnosis itself but also by the recommendation that she undergo an above the knee amputation. For weeks, she refused to listen to any discussion by her oncologists of surgery. She was
referred to a psychosocial clinician for counseling. During the first session, Sandra tearfully reflected on all the losses she had already experienced and anticipated experiencing in her life. She was concerned about how poorly her mother was handling the thought of her daughter losing her leg, not being able to run with her cross country team or dance in competitions, as well as how much more difficult it would be to fulfill her dream of becoming a doctor. Taking

risks was something Sandra had always avoided and the surgery represented such an enormous "unknown" that just the thought of it initiated mild panic attacks. During the following two weeks, Sandra met with the psychosocial clinician several times a week and explored the range of intense emotions associated with her diagnosis and future surgery. The team social worker also worked closely with the family on how best to support and prepare Sandra for surgery and on how to help her to maintain healthy self-esteem afterward. In addition, the whole psychosocial team identified several goals with Sandra that were mutually agreed upon and carried out:

1. Sandra *identified two activities that previously had frightened her. Together with the recreational therapist, she participated in both of these activities.*
2. *Sandra loved to sing. Together with a music therapist, they searched for and recorded songs that best described the anxiety that she was experiencing and how she would like to ultimately conquer her fears.*
3. *Sandra read short stories by peers who had also lost a limb and learned how they had adapted to their life since the amputation. A librarian worked closely with Sandra to help identify these stories.*
4. *Sandra was introduced by her nurse practitioner to another teenager who recently had an amputation. It took a little time before she was ready to look at the stump.*
5. *Sandra wrote a letter to her leg during an individual psychotherapy session.*
6. *Sandra met with a psychologist and together they identified soothing images. A relaxation CD was created that included a guided imagery of all that Sandra could and would do with one leg.*
7. *Sandra met with a child psychiatrist who agreed with the multimodal therapies and recommended in addition the limited use of short-acting benzodiazepines for acute procedures such as scans, but did not recommend additional psychotropic medication during this time.*
8. *Sandra met with a chaplain to discuss her spiritual concerns.*
9. *Sandra met with the surgeon and expressed her thoughts, wishes, questions, and fears about the amputation.*

The interventions listed above took place over a month. At the meeting with the surgeon, Sandra said she had two remaining questions to ask. The first question was whether she would be able to obtain a prosthetic leg that would allow her to wear high heels. The second was whether he would keep the leg, so that when she became a doctor, she could study the tumor and "eradicate this disease once and for all."

Sandra and her family coped well with her surgery. No one provider could have helped Sandra grieve, prepare for her surgery, or prepare for her life without a limb. Each specialist brought an approach that complemented the others and allowed her physical, psychological, social, and spiritual concerns to be integrated into her care. Each discipline also provided a web of support to Sandra and her family. With each person, Sandra developed a strong relationship—each of which brought unique meaning to her experience.

Within a year of Sandra's surgery, she joined a Special Olympics cross-country team. As a result of significant neurotoxicity, she was not able to pursue a medical degree. A vocational therapist helped Sandra identify other skills and areas of strength. She currently works with children and hopes to run her own day care center one day.

Summary

Anxiety and depression are common symptoms in the seriously medically ill child. This chapter has reviewed clinical presentations of anxiety and depression along with means for assessing and treating these symptoms. As the child's well-being is intrinsically linked to parents' overall coping and functioning,[60] of great importance, regardless of the specific intervention used, is the establishment and maintenance of a developmentally appropriate and supportive therapeutic relationship that involves the family in a meaningful way. These children and their families are eager for help and support. By understanding their worries, concerns, and grief and by building on their strengths throughout the unpredictable course of the illness, tremendous growth, and resilience can shine through the pain of loss and grief.

REFERENCES

1. Field MJ, Behrman RE, editors: *When children die: improving palliative and end-of-life care for children and their families, Board on Health Sciences Policy (HSP)*, Washington, DC, 2003, Institute of Medicine (IOM), The National Academies Press.
2. Kessler RC, Berglund P, Demler O, et al: Lifetime prevalence and age of onset distributions of DSM-IV disorders in the national comorbidity survey replication, *Arch Gen Psychiatry* 62:593–602, 2005.
3. Beesdo K, Knappe S, Pine DS: Anxiety and anxiety disorders in children and adolescents: developmental issues and implications for DSM-V, *Psychiatr Clin North Am* 32:483–524, 2006.
4. Gothelf D, Rubinstein M, Shemesh E, et al: Pilot study: fluvoxamine treatment for depression and anxiety disorders in children and adolescents with cancer, *J Am Acad Child Adolesc Psychiatry* 44:1258–1262, 2005.
5. Richardson LP, Lozano P, Russo J, et al: Asthma symptom burden: relationship to asthma severity and anxiety and depression symptoms, *Pediatrics* 118:1042–1051, 2006.
6. Ortega AN, Huertas SE, Canino G, et al: Childhood asthma, chronic illness, and psychiatric disorders, *J Nerv Ment Dis* 190(5):275–281, 2002.
7. Chavira DA, Garland AF, Daley S, et al: The impact of medical comorbidity on mental health and functional health outcomes among children with anxiety disorders, *J Dev Behav Pediatr* 29(5):394–402, 2008.
8. Kovacs M, Goldston D, Obrosky DS, et al: Psychiatric disorders in youths with IDDM: rates and risk factors, *Diabetes Care* 20(1):36–44, 1997.
9. Caplan R, Siddarth P, Gurbani S, et al: Depression and anxiety disorders in pediatric epilepsy, *Epilepsia* 46:720–730, 2005.
10. Kazak A, Simms S, Barakat L, et al: Surviving Cancer Competently Intervention Program (SCCIP): a cognitive-behavioral and family therapy intervention for adolescent survivors of childhood cancer and their families, *Fam Process* 38:175–191, 1999.
11. *Diagnostic and statistical manual of mental disorders, fourth edition,* Washington, DC, 1994, American Psychiatric Association.
12. Stuber ML, Shemesh E: Post-traumatic stress response to life-threatening illnesses in children and their parents, *Child Adolesc Psychiatric Clin North Am* 15:597–609, 2006.
13. Bennett DS: Depression among children with chronic medical problems: a meta-analysis, *J Pediatr Psychol* 19:149–169, 1994.

14. Katon W, Lozano P, Russo J, et al: The prevalence of DSM-IV anxiety and depressive disorders in youth with asthma compared with controls, *J Adolesc Health* 41:455–463, 2007.

15. Kokkonen J, Taabuka A, Kokkonen ER: Diabetes in adolescence: the effect of family and psychologic factors on metabolic control, *Nord J Psychiatry* 51:165–172, 1997.

16. Plioplys S, Dunn DW, Caplan R: 10-year research update review: psychiatric problems in children with epilepsy, *J Am Acad Child Adol Psychiatry* 46(11):1389–1402, 2007.

17. Kubler-Ross E: *On death and dying*, New York, 1969, Macmillan.

18. Kersun LS, Kazak AE: Prescribing practices of selective serotonin reuptake inhibitors (SSRIs) among pediatric oncologists: a single institution experience, *Pediatr Blood Cancer* 47:339–342, 2006.

19. Portteus A, Ahamd N, Tobey D, et al: The prevalence and use of antidepressant medication in pediatric cancer patients, *J Child Adolesc Psychopharmacol* 16:467–473, 2006.

20. Pao M, Ballard ED, Rosenstein DL, et al: Psychotropic medication use in pediatric patients with cancer, *Arch Pediatr Adolesc Med* 160:818–822, 2006.

21. Habis A, Tall L, Smith J, et al: Pediatric emergency physicians' current practices and beliefs regarding mental health screening, *Pediatr Emerg Care* 23(6):387–393, 2007.

22. Recklitis CJ, Lockwood RA, Rothwell MA, et al: Suicidal ideation and attempts in adult survivors of childhood cancer, *J Clin Oncol* 24:3852–3857, 2006.

23. Goodwin RD, Eaton WW: Asthma, suicidal ideation, and suicide attempts: findings from the Baltimore Catchment Area follow-up, *Am J Public Health* 95:717–722, 2005.

24. Goodwin RD, Kroenke K, Hoven CW, et al: Major depression, physical illness, and suicidal ideation in primary care, *Psychosom Med* 65:501–505, 2003.

25. Ratcliffe GE, Enns MW, Belik SL, et al: Chronic pain conditions and suicidal ideation and suicide attempts: an epidemiologic perspective, *Clin J Pain* 24:204–210, 2008.

26. Hughes D, Kleespies P: Suicide in the medically ill, *Suicide Life Threat Behav* 31(Suppl):48–59, 2001.

27. Blumenthal SJ: Youth suicide: risk factors, assessment, and treatment of adolescent and young adult suicidal patients, *Psychiatr Clin North Am* 13:511–556, 1990.

28. Simon RI, Hales RE: *The American psychiatric publishing textbook of suicide assessment and management*, Washington, DC, 2006, American Psychiatric Press.

29. Berman A, Jobes D, Silverman M: *Adolescent suicide: assessment and intervention*, Washington, DC, 2006, American Psychological Association.

30. Sourkes B, Frankel L, Brown M, et al: Food, toys, and love: pediatric palliative care, *Curr Probl Pediatr Adolesc Health Care* 35:350–386, 2005.

31. Spirito A, Kazak AE: *Effective and emerging treatments in pediatric psychology*, Oxford, 2006, Oxford University Press.

32. Power SW: Empirically supported treatments in pediatric psychology: procedure-related pain, *J Pediatr Psychol* 24:131–145, 1999.

33. TADS Team: The treatment for adolescents with depression study (TADS), *Arch Gen Psychiatry* 64:1132–1144, 2007.

34. Kreitler S, Oppenheim D, Segev-Shoham E: Fantasy, art therapies, humor and pets as psychosocial means of intervention. In Kreitler S, editor: *Psychosocial aspects of pediatric oncology*, Bognor, England, 2004, John Wiley & Sons, pp 351–388.

35. Rokke K: A place for children's literature in dealing with cancer, *J Pediatr Oncol Nurs* 10:57, 1993.

36. Brown CD: Therapeutic play and creative arts. In Armstrong-Daily A, editor: *Hospice care for children*, New York, 2009, Oxford University Press, pp 305–338.

37. Kalm MA: *The healing movie book—precious images: the healing use of cinema in psychotherapy*, 2004, Lulu Press.

38. Wolz B: *E-motion picture magic: a movie lover's guide to healing and transformation*, Centennial, Colo, 2005, Glenbridge.

39. Landreth GL: *Innovatizons in play therapy: issues, process, and special populations*, New York, 2001, Brunner-Routledge.

40. Wiener L: Shop talk: a new therapeutic game for youth living with cancer and other life-threatening illnesses, *Psychooncology* 18(Suppl 2):S240–S241, 2009.

41. Wiener L: *This is my world*, Washington, DC, 1998, CWLA Press.

42. Malchiodi CA: *Art therapy and computer technology: a virtual studio of possibilities*, London, 2000, Jessical Kingsley.

43. Wiener L, Ballard E, Brennan T, et al: How I wish to be remembered: the use of an advance care planning document in adolescent and young adult populations, *J Palliat Med* 11:1309–1313, 2008.

44. Weiser J: Phototherapy techniques: using clients' personal snapshots and family photos as counseling and therapy tools; in memory of Arnold Gassan photographer, poet and phototherapy pioneer—feature, findarticles.com. Available at: http://findarticles.com/p/articles/mi_m2479/is_3_29/ai_80757504/ 2009, Accessed August 10.

45. Halm MA: The healing power of the human-animal connection, *Am J Crit Care* 17:373–376, 2008.

46. Willis DA: Animal therapy, *Rehabil Nurs* 22:78–81, 1997.

47. Braun C, Stangler T, Narveson J, et al: Animal-assisted therapy as a pain relief intervention for children, *Complement Ther Clin Pract* 15:105–109, 2009.

48. DeJong M, Fombonne E: Citalopram to treat depression in pediatric oncology, *J Child Adolesc Psychopharmacol* 17:371–437, 2007.

49. Maisami M, Sohmer BH, Coyle JT: Combined use of tricyclic antidepressants and neuroleptics in the management of terminally ill children: a report on three cases, *J Am Acad Child Psychiatry* 24:487–489, 1985.

50. Pfefferbaum-Levine B, Kumor K, Cangir A, et al: Tricyclic antidepressants for children with cancer, *Am J Psychiatry* 140:1074–1076, 1986.

51. Bealke JM, Meighen KG: Risperidone treatment of three seriously medically ill children with secondary mood disorders, *Psychosomatics* 46:254–258, 2005.

52. Walling VR, Pfefferbaum B: The use of methylphenidate in a depressed adolescent with AIDS, *J Dev Behav Pediatr* 11(4):195–197, 1990.

53. Diamond G, Josephson A: Family-based treatment research: a 10-year update, *J Am Acad Child Adolesc Psychiatry* 44:872–887, 2005.

54. Cleeland CS, Bennett GJ, Dantzer R, et al: Are the symptoms of cancer and cancer treatment due to a shared biological mechanism? A cytokine-immunologic model of cancer symptoms, *Cancer* 97:2919–2925, 2003.

55. Miller AH, Maletic V, Raison CL: Inflammation and discontents: the role of cytokines in the pathophysiology of major depression, *Biol Psychiatry* 65(9):732–741, 2009.

56. Kazak AE, Alderfer MA, Streisand R, et al: Treatment of posttraumatic stress symptoms in adolescent survivors of childhood cancer and their families: a randomized clinical trial, *J Fam Psychol* 18:493–504, 2004.

57. Stuber ML, Shemesh E: Post-traumatic stress response to life-threatening illnesses in children and their parents, *Child Adolesc Psychiatr Clin North Am* 15:597–609, 2006.

58. Stuber ML, Schneider S, Kassam-Adams N, et al: The medical traumatic stress toolkit, *CNS Spectr* 11:137–142, 2006.

59. Worden JW, Monahan JR: Caring for Bereaved Parents. In Arnstrong-Daily A, editor: *Hospice care for children*, ed 2, New York, 2001, Oxford University Press, pp 137–156.

60. American Academy of Pediatrics: Family pediatrics: report of the Task Force on the Family, *Pediatrics* 111:1541–1571, 2003.

27 Neurological Symptoms

RICHARD HAIN | HELEN DOUGLAS

We have scotch'd the snake, not kill'd it.
She'll close and be herself, whilst our poor malice Remains in
danger of her former tooth.
— William Shakespeare, in *Macbeth*, Act II, Scene I

The purpose of this chapter is to address symptoms etiologies that are an abnormality or dysfunction of the nervous system, and are not covered elsewhere in the book.

Neurological symptoms present particular difficulties for those working in pediatric palliative medicine. The evidence base for most symptom interventions derives largely from work done in adults. Historically, adult palliative medicine has largely addressed the needs of patients with cancer, while it is in the large group of children with non-cancer conditions that neurological symptoms occur most commonly.[1] Typically, they are neurodegenerative conditions in which deterioration to death occurs over years or decades, and are characterized by severe neurological symptoms that may be difficult to treat.

The management of neurological symptoms in childhood is complicated both by the inherent intractability of many, and by the lack of a robust evidence base to support effective management. Nevertheless, the broad principles of good palliative care can and should be applied.

General Principles

The most important preparations for providing palliative care to children who may experience neurological symptoms are anticipation, education, and discussion. Informing the child, family, and caretakers about the potential symptoms at an appropriate time can help to reduce anxiety, stress, and unwanted admissions. Ensuring that families have strategies for managing symptoms in a way acceptable to them, even if it is only having the telephone number of someone who can help, will help meet the aims of palliative care. Many families report that honesty and unlimited support are critical elements of the palliative care process. Palliative care approaches should be multidimensional, in the best interest of the child, and rational.

MULTIDIMENSIONAL

In considering the impact of neurological symptoms, professionals need to consider not only their physical effects, but also their influence on psychosocial, emotional, and spiritual issues. In focusing on reducing the frequency of seizures, for example, professionals should not lose sight of the need to allow a child to engage meaningfully with his or her family. This can lead to the involvement of a potentially large and extended team with varying but, at times, over-lapping roles (Box 27-1).

ALWAYS IN THE BEST INTERESTS OF THE CHILD

Palliative care is, at its heart, a logical and rational specialty. Professionals should always carefully consider whether a proposed intervention is likely to do more good than harm; whether, on balance, it is in the child's best interest. To be consistent with the principle of multidimensionality above, this clearly means that sometimes professionals will be called on to balance physical benefits with, for example, psychosocial or emotional burdens. In considering the relative weight that should be given to these, it is essential that professionals engage in ongoing dialogue with the family and, where possible the patient. It is rarely possible to make objective judgments about dimensions of experience other than the physical.

RATIONAL

In establishing that a given intervention is in the child's best interest, it is clearly necessary to be aware of the existing evidence. In an age where evidence-based medicine is a professional requirement,[2] it is important that practice is not just based on anecdotes and experience, but also is justified with research. Critical appraisal and clinical reasoning must underpin practice. Systematic reviews or meta-analyses, where they exist, are authoritative sources of such evidence. Individual carefully designed double-blind trials are also powerful evidence. Anecdote and case history, however, are not indicators of effectiveness. They are important signposts to studies that should take place, but should not result in an uncritical change of practice by themselves.

The literature pertaining to non-pharmacological approaches to the management of neurological symptoms is particularly sparse. A rational and logical approach does not, however, mean that practice should be limited only to that rather narrow range of therapeutic options that have been subjected to study in children. It is often necessary to extrapolate from evidence in the adult specialty, or from related disciplines such as acute pain management. Sometimes, professionals working in pediatric palliative care need to be therapeutically creative, using a sound knowledge of pharmacology and therapeutics to develop an approach that, while it may not be fully supported by evidence, is nevertheless rational.

Complementary and alternative medicine (CAM) approaches should be used in conjunction with conventional medicine to aim to provide better symptom control and meet the cultural, spiritual, and psychosocial needs of the child and family.[3] Many neurological symptoms are exacerbated by

BOX 27-1 The Interdisciplinary Team

- Doctors: from acute, community, and palliative care settings. Those already involved in the management of the child's long-term symptoms and those with the specialist knowledge of management of symptoms experienced toward the end of life.
- Nursing staff: again they can be involved in each setting; acute hospital, hospice, and in the home and will offer more than physical care but should be specialists in advocating for the child and family when working with the wider team.
- Therapists and allied health professionals: of varying different specialties; movement and handling, equipment, diet and feeding, communication, learning and education, complementary and alternative medicine treatments.
- Psychologists: from neuro-psychology and child specialties. They can provide assessment and advice on the child's ability to understand and manage the situation and psychological support to the child, family, and staff involved in the palliative care process.
- Social workers, bereavement counselors, chaplin, etc.: to offer practical, emotional, and spiritual support to the child and family during the palliative care process and ongoing after the child has died.
- Key worker: this role helps to access and coordinate appropriate care and is a key point of contact and support for the child and family. Each situation must be assessed when deciding which professional will take on this role. It often falls to nursing staff but in some circumstances another health professional, such as a physiohtherapist, may know the child and family and their needs better.

depression, anxiety, and/or fatigue. There is evidence to suggest these are ameliorated by some CAM approaches, including massage,[4–12] acupuncture,[8,10,13–16] and transcutaneous electrical stimulation (TENS)[8,17] can offer some assistance with this. The effectiveness of TENS is unclear[18,19] but it is well tolerated by most patients. Music therapy and hydrotherapy are naturally enjoyable interventions for children (Fig. 27-1).

Symptoms

For a summary of doses and indications of medications in this chapter, see Table 27-1.

SEIZURES

Management of seizures outside the terminal phase is beyond the scope of this chapter. The palliative care professional should continue to liaise carefully with colleagues in neurology,

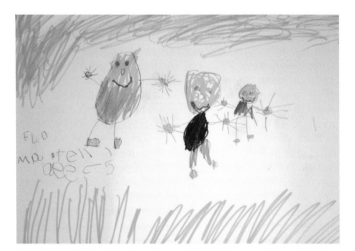

Fig. 27-1 Child's depiction of successful family-centered interdisciplinary care of child with neurological symptoms.

even as death approaches. Potentially, this can achieve several important objectives:

- Rationalization of anticonvulsant medications

Children with life-limiting conditions in ACT categories III and IV (Table 27-2), which are often chronic neurological conditions, are likely to have seizures that have been difficult to control for some time. The result is typically that, at the time it is clear a palliative phase has been entered, children are on a large number of different anticonvulsants.

The long-term management of seizures requires a neurologist to balance carefully immediate benefit with long-term side effects. In the palliative phase, such a balance may no longer be necessary. Discussion with neurology colleagues may allow:

- Discontinuation of some anticonvulsants,
- Reduction in the number of anticonvulsants,
- Substitution of specific anticonvulsants with broader range ones with additional desirable benefits such as anxiolysis or activity against neuropathic pain.

Management of breakthrough seizures usually requires a parenteral approach. This presents a conflict with one of the aims of palliative care, which is to offer the family the choice of locations, typically home, hospital, or hospice, for death to occur. The intravenous and subcutaneous routes may not be appropriate, because they are not usually available except to professionals who may not be immediately on hand.

The solution to this is to use the buccal route. Small volumes of water soluble drugs such as midazolam and diamorphine can be administered between the cheek and the gum. They are absorbed rapidly through the oral mucosa, effectively providing an alternative parenteral route without needles. This is increasingly used for management of breakthrough seizures in neurology[20] and is ideally suited to their management in the terminal phase.

- Management of terminal seizures

The two mainstays of seizure management in the terminal stages are phenobarbital and midazolam. Both may be given as continuous subcutaneous infusion, though phenobarbital must be given separately from other medications. The decision as to which of these should be first-line use is largely up to the clinician; there is little evidence to suggest which is likely to be more effective, and it may depend on the individual circumstances and patient.

- Phenobarbital

Phenobarbital is rarely used in seizure disorders because of the risk of adverse effect in long-term use. In the palliative phase, however, where these are unlikely to be a significant consideration, it has a number of potential advantages over many other anticonvulsants, though not all are proved. It is anxiolytic, rather than simply sedative,[21] effective against cerebral irritation; is sedating it may have some activity against neuropathic pain.[22] It can also be given orally or through a gastrostomy tube.

It does, however, also have some disadvantages:

It induces its own metabolism, so the dose may need to be kept under review; and its long half-life means it cannot easily be titrated against its effect, particularly if given orally.

- Midazolam

Midazolam is a short-acting benzodiazepine. It is often used by neurologists for breakthrough seizures, but rarely for background control because of its short half-life. In the

TABLE 27-1   Doses and Indications for Medications Mentioned in This Chapter

Medication	Indication	Dosage
Midazolam	Status epilepticus and terminal seizure control. Breakthrough anxiety, such as panic attacks. Adjuvant for pain of cerebral irritation. Dyspnea	For status epilepticus: By buccal administration, Neonate 300 micrograms/kg as a single dose Child 1-6 mo, 300 micrograms/kg (max. 2.5 mg), repeated once if necessary Child 6 mo-1 yr, 2.5 mg, repeated once if necessary Child 1-5 yrs, 5 mg, repeated once if necessary Child 5-10 yrs, 7.5 mg, repeated once if necessary Child 10-18 yrs, 10 mg, repeated once if necessary For terminal seizure control: By subcutaneous or intravenous infusion over 24 hrs, 50-300 mcg/kg/hour up to maxi. 160 mg For anxiety or dyspnea: Approximately 50% above doses
Diamorphine	As for morphine. Useful where large doses need to be dissolved in small volume	Relative potency parenteral preparations 3x that of oral morphine.
Phenobarbital	Adjuvant in pain of cerebral irritation. Control of terminal seizures. Sedation	By mouth: Neonates, loading dose by slow intravenous injection, then 2.5-5 mg/kg by mouth once a day Child 1 mo-12 yrs, 1-1.5 mg/kg twice a day, increased by 2 mg/kg daily as required (usual maintenance dose 2.5-4 mg/kg once or twice a day) Child 12-18 yrs, 60-180 mg once a day.
Diazepam	Short-term anxiety relief. Relief of muscle spasm. Treatment of status epilepticus	Short-term anxiety relief: By mouth: Child 2-12 yrs, 2-3 mg three times a day Child 12-18 yrs, 2-10 mg three times a day Relief of muscle spasm: By mouth: Child 1-12 mo, initially 250 mcg/kg twice a day Child 1-5 yrs, initially 2.5 mg twice a day Child 5-12 yrs, initially 5 mg twice a day Child 12-18 yrs, initially 10 mg twice a day, maxi. Total daily dose 40 mg Status epilepticus: By intravenous injection over 3-5 min: Neonate, 300-400 mcg/kg repeated after 10 min if necessary Child 1 mo-12 yrs, 300-400 mcg/kg repeated after 10 min if necessary Child 12-18 yrs, 10-20 mg repeated after 10 min if necessary By rectum: Neonate, 1.25-2.5 mg repeated after 10 min if necessary Child 1 mo-2 yrs, 5 mg repeated after 10 min if necessary Child 2-12 yrs, 5-10 mg repeated after 10 min if necessary Child 12-18 yrs, 10 mg repeated after 10 min if necessary
Levomepromazine	Antiemetic where cause is unclear, or where probably multifactorial. Secondary effects include sedation and analgesia	Antiemetic: By mouth: Child 2-12 yrs, starting dose 0.1-1 mg/kg, max 25 mg Child greater than 12 yrs, 6.25-25 mg by mouth once or twice daily By continuous intravenous or subcutaneous infusion over 24 hrs: Child 1 mo-12 yrs, 100-400 mcg/kg over 24 hrs Child greater than 12-18 yrs, 5-25 mg over 24 hrs For sedation: By subcutaneous infusion over 24 hrs: Child 1 yr-12 yrs, 0.35-3 mg/kg over 24 hrs Child over 12-18 yrs, 12.5-200 mg over 24 hrs Analgesic: May be of benefit in a very distressed patient with severe pain unresponsive to other measures Stat dose 0.5 mg/kg by mouth or subcutaneously. Titrate dose according to response; usual maximum daily dose in adult 100 mg subcutaneous or 200 mg by mouth
Fentanyl	Severe pain (synthetic opioid analgesic), particularly as rotation from morphine or if patch formulation desirable	By transmucosal application (lozenge with oromucosal applicator): Child 2-18 yrs, 15-20 mcg/kg as a single dose, max. dose 400 mcg By transdermal patch: Based on oral morphine dose-equivalent Product monogram, Oral morphine 60-134 mg = 25 mcg/h patch of fentanyl Oral morphine 180-224 mg = 50 mcg/h patch of fentanyl Oral morphine 27-314 mg = 75 mcg/h patch of fentanyl
Hydromorphone	Severe pain (opioid analgesic) especially if diamorphine unavailable and solubility is an issue	By mouth: Child 12-18 yrs, initially 1.3 mg every 4 hrs, increasing as required

Continued

TABLE 27-1 Doses and Indications for Medications Mentioned in This Chapter—cont'd

Medication	Indication	Dosage
Tizanidine	Muscle spasm	By mouth: Adult dose, initially 2 mg increasing in increments of 2 mg at intervals of 3 to 4 days. Give total daily dose in divided doses up to 3-4 times daily. Usual total daily dose 24 mg. Maximum total daily dose 36 mg
Baclofen	Chronic severe spasticity of voluntary muscle	By mouth: Initially, Child 1-10 yrs 0.75-2 mg/kg daily or 2.5 mg 4 times daily. Increased gradually to maintenance: Child 1-2 yrs, 10-20 mg daily in divided doses Child 2-6 yrs, 20-30 mg daily in divided doses Child 6-10 yrs, 30-60 mg in divided doses
Melatonin	Sleep disturbance caused by disruption of circadian rhythm (not anxiolytic)	By mouth: Dose unknown, initially 2-3 mg, increasing every 1-2 wk dependent on effectiveness up to maximum 10 mg (higher doses have been used)

palliative phase, Midazolam is usually given by continuous subcutaneous infusion although there is no reason in principle why it should not also be given intravenously. It can be mixed with other medications in the same syringe driver, including diamorphine, morphine, levomepromazine, and other medications commonly used in the final days of life. It is easy to titrate against symptoms due to its short half-life;[23] powerfully anxiolytic, amnestic and sedating; and has a broad range of anticonvulsant activity. Midazolam is widely used in pediatric palliative care, so it has reasonable clinical experience and evidence base. Also, it is highly soluble so can be given by buccal route.

Midazolam's disadvantages are that paradoxical agitation can occur in some children[24] and its short half-life makes it inappropriate for background control of seizures except by parenteral infusion. The drug can cause confusion; and in cognitively aware children, loss of memory may be a disadvantage, particularly if it impairs family relationships.

The decision as to which is the better first-line approach will depend largely on individual circumstances. For a child who has otherwise no need for parenteral access, phenobarbital given orally may be preferable. For a child needing benzodiazepines for other reasons, midazolam may be the logical choice. For many children, adequate control of seizures in the terminal phase will in practice require both drugs to be given parenterally as the swallowing reflex becomes lost.

BREAKTHROUGH SEIZURES

Before embarking on management of breakthrough seizures, it is important to discuss with the child's family what their expectations are. Most families have lived with a child with complex seizure disorder for many years and will be able to fully engage in a discussion about what can and cannot be achieved in the way of control in the final days and weeks of life.

It is important to acknowledge that seizures are more unpleasant and frightening for those observing them than they are for the child who experiences them. If seizures do not appear to distress the child, then vigorous attempts to abolish them may result in replacing acceptable seizures with unacceptable adverse effects. For families used to a child who has many seizures a day, reducing them to only one or two seizures a day may be an acceptable outcome.

It is also important to acknowledge that complete control of seizures may simply not be possible. If complete absence of seizures can only be achieved by means of anesthesia and ventilation, from which there is no realistic prospect of the child's recovering, it is a price too high for the child to pay.

TABLE 27-2 Life-Limiting Conditions

The original ACT/RCPCH categories[25]

Category	Definition	Example conditions	Characteristic
I	Life-threatening conditions for which curative treatment may be feasible but can fail. Palliative care may be necessary during phases of prognostic uncertainty and when treatment fails.	Cancer, cardiac anomalies	Possible cure
II	Conditions in which there may be long phases of intensive treatment aimed at prolonging life and allowing participation in normal childhood activities, but premature death is still possible	Cystic fibrosis, Muscular dystrophy, HIV/AIDS with antiretroviral treatment	Normal phase
III	Progressive conditions without curative treatment options, in which treatment is exclusively palliative and may commonly extend over many years	Batten's disease, Mucopolysaccharidosis, HIV/AIDS without antiretroviral treatment	Relentless progression
IV	Conditions with severe neurological disability, which may cause weakness and susceptibility to health complications, and may deteriorate unpredictably, but are not considered progressive	Severe cerebral palsy	Unpredictable

Adapted from *Categories of life-timing and life-threatening conditions.* Available from www.act.org.uk.

This needs to be explored with the family at the time management of terminal seizures is initiated.

It is usual for children with complex seizure disorders to have a detailed seizure protocol that has been agreed between neurologist and family. It is important that the palliative care pediatrician be aware of this protocol, and that he or she work carefully with the neurology team and the family themselves before suggesting any modification. This protocol should be accessible to all those involved with the child and identify what is normal for that child, when a seizure has become prolonged and requires medication, and at what stage and to what level further help should be sought if seizure activity continues.

One common medication used for treatment of breakthrough seizures, when indicated, is diazepam, which may be given by the rectal route. The metabolites of diazepam are active and long-lasting, but this is rarely a problem in children. Children prefer to avoid the rectal route where possible, as it is uncomfortable and undignified. Nevertheless, it is certainly preferred to a needle by most and may be the most accessible in the midst of a seizure. The rectal route is contraindicated in neutropenia or marked thrombocytopenia.

NON-PHARMACOLOGICAL MANAGEMENT

Even in the terminal phase, immediate nursing interventions aimed at making the child comfortable are important. These would include correct positioning of the child, and oxygen if indicated. The timing of anti-seizure medications should be carefully defined ahead of time in a clear seizure protocol, that takes account of the needs and priorities of the individual child and family. Short, self-limiting seizures will commonly need no such intervention.

The mainstay of non-pharmacological management of seizures is to avoid over-handling. Intractable seizures are likely to be exacerbated by stimulation and, as most therapeutic interventions entail touch and some stimulation of the senses, involvement of therapists is likely to be in managing co-existing symptoms such as pain and muscle spasms. If triggering seizures is perceived by the child, family, and care team to be a small burden whilst the benefit gained from a pleasurable intervention such as music therapy or massage is more significant, then such therapies should be offered. The therapist should, however, be cautiously aware and constantly re-evaluate.

Because many children who experience seizures near the end of life have chronic neurological conditions, it is likely that they will also have other symptoms that may benefit from therapeutic involvement. Although not directly treating the seizures, effective tone-reducing positioning may ensure that the child is more comfortable and functional between seizures. Positioning aids such as sleep systems and soft splinting should not forcibly restrain abnormal movement patterns but should encourage comfort positions and allow function by supporting where required. For example, a child with trunk and lower limb hypertonia, when positioned in supine is likely to extend. By positioning the child on his or her side in flexion or in supine but with appropriate soft positioning aids to encourage trunk, hip, and knee flexion, even if a tonic-clonic seizure occurs, the child is not going to injure himself or herself but once resolved they will recover back into a tone-minimizing and, by the same token, comfortable position.

Non-Seizure Movements

It is not always possible to distinguish definitively between seizures and non-seizure abnormal movements. The purpose of making such a distinction is to establish the most appropriate therapeutic intervention. Where there is diagnostic uncertainty, it may sometimes be necessary to institute a trial of therapy.

Again, it is important to discuss with family and the child when possible in order to establish their expectations, and to negotiate reasonable and attainable goals. It is rarely possible to abolish abnormal movements completely, and attempts to do so may risk jeopardizing a child's quality of life through overmedication.

Many children with abnormal movement patterns due to any neurological condition, palliative or not, have developed ways in which to use the fluctuations in muscle tone to enable them to carry out functional activities, such as walking. The aim, particularly in the palliative phase when these movements are likely to be increasing in amount and severity, should be to minimize the negative effects but optimize function to enable the child to manage desired activities (Box 27-2).

DYSTONIA

Dystonia is characterized by repetitive and sustained contraction of the muscles, leading to abnormal posture. It can result from the underlying condition, or from medications used in its treatment. Prolonged dystonia is referred to as status dystonicus.[26]

Drug-induced dystonias are associated with drugs that block dopamine receptors. These particularly include pure dopamine antagonists such as haloperidol and dopamine. The actual incidence of dystonic reactions with these medications is small, but more likely in pediatric than in adult practice.[27] The medications are relatively frequently used in the palliative phase, however, and are important causes. Dystonic reactions caused by medication can be reduced or even avoided by the use of anticholinergics such as procyclidine or antihistamines such as diphenhydramine.

Phenothiazines such as levomepromazine, chlorpromazine, or prochlorperazine are also dopamine antagonists, but the incidence of dystonia is rather rare. This may be because they are also anticholinergic and are antihistamines.

BOX 27-2   Movement Disorders

Explore impact of symptoms on family, and negotiate achievable goals, particularly distinguishing between painful and painless movements.

Review existing medications, particularly identifying combinations that multiply the risk of adverse effects without significantly increasing the likelihood of effectiveness, such as anti-dopamined domperidone in a patient already receiving phenothiazine nozinan.

Remove medications that are unnecessary because of duplication or because their effect is no longer necessary in the palliative phase.

Reconsider medications in discussion with neurologist. Medications that are contraindicated because of adverse effects in long-term use, such as phenobarbital, may have valuable effects in the shorter term of palliative care.

Introduce any new interventions in proportion to the severity of the symptom, its importance to the child and family, the relative balance of good and harm that are likely, and the stage of illness.

Drug-induced dystonias, while frightening, are not usually painful or dangerous. It is important to warn patients and families of the possibility that they may occur before prescribing haloperidol or metoclopramide. The usefulness of these medications in managing nausea and vomiting associated with metabolic causes, haloperidol, or with gastric outflow obstruction, metoclopramide, is such that they are valuable medications in palliative medicine and should not be unreasonably withheld.

Conditions causing dystonia in the absence of medication include many of the metabolic disorders, particularly metachromatic leukodystrophy, the gangliosidoses and mitochondrial disorders. Deep brain stimulation,[28] in which electrodes are placed in the globus pallidus area of the brain, is effective in such primary dystonias in children. This should be combined[26] with attention to hypertonia.

MYOCLONUS

Myoclonus describes jerking interactions of a muscle or muscle group. They are typically brief, abrupt, and involuntary.[29]

In contrast with dystonia, myoclonus characteristically occurs in children who are cognitively aware. Although not usually painful, it can be disproportionately distressing.

The most common single cause of myoclonus in palliative care is as a consequence of opioid therapy. The risk is minimized by careful titration in strict accordance with the World Health Organization (WHO) guidelines. The appearance of myoclonus generally indicates that opioid dose is too high, either because titration has been too rapid, such as when it has been escalated with insufficient regard to pain intensity, or because the pain is partially or completely opioid unresponsive. This is usually due to significant emotional and spiritual components to the pain that are not amenable to analgesics alone. It can also result from physical pain that is inherently less opioid-responsive, such as when neuropathic in origin.

In the presence of opioid induced myoclonus, two approaches should be considered simultaneously. The first is the immediate prescription of a benzodiazepine. The first-line choice, if it is available, would be midazolam by continuous infusion. If this is not available, or it is important to avoid parenteral medications, long- or medium-acting benzodiazepines such as lorazepam or diazepam can be considered instead. In either event, a breakthrough dose of midazolam buccally should be made available should the problem recur.

At the same time, an opioid substitution should be carried out. As always, the effectiveness of this relies on incomplete cross-tolerance; that is, the fact that tolerance to adverse effects may occur later than tolerance to analgesia. In this instance, the hope is that it is possible to obtain at least the same analgesia with a lower dose of opioid by substituting an opioid of a different class, to which tolerance has not yet occurred.

To be effective, substitution should be to an opioid of a structure as different as possible from the original. There would, for example, be little point in substituting diamorphine for morphine, because the two medications are almost identical. If myoclonus occurs on morphine, substitution should be to a synthetic opioid such as fentanyl. If this is not available, a semi-synthetic opioid such as hydromorphone may be sufficiently different.

It should be noted that myoclonus can also be associated with normal phenomena such as anxiety, exercise or as one falls asleep.

CHOREA

Chorea can be seen as intermediate in duration between myoclonus and dystonia.[29] Like them, it is brief and purposeless and can seem to flow from limb to limb, called choreoathetosis.

Again, it is associated with neurodegenerative diseases in children's palliative care, as well as with cerebral palsy. The choreoathetotic type of cerebral palsy is thought to be due to anoxic damage at the basal ganglia.

Again, chorea can be associated with complications of some of the important medications used in pediatric palliative care such as haloperidol, metoclopramide, or phenothiazines. Withdrawal of these medications, if responsible, is clearly a first important step.

Non-Pharmacological Treatment

Dystonic and choreoathetotic movements are usually not painful but can cause distress, discomfort, and frustration. Positioning, soft splinting, and proprioceptive feedback may help to reduce and control the movements and enable a child to function or rest. For example, a therapist may improve the repetitive, writhing choreoathetotic movements of an upper limb by placing a firm, but not restrictive, hand cupping the shoulder of the child and applying firm but gentle pressure diagonally over the child's chest toward the opposite hip with the therapist's forearm. The movement is not restricted but the proprioceptive feedback provided around the key point of the shoulder and across the core of the trunk may normalize the fluctuating tone and reduce more distal involuntary movement. If effective, this technique should be taught to the family and caretakers to enable them to assist the child. Often, the ability to soothe through touch benefits not only the child but the family as well by enabling physical contact and the feeling of doing something practical to help settle the child, a nurturing instinct frequently limited in palliative care. This dynamic form of splinting can be replicated by applying stocking bandage to the key points to provide similar feedback. It is important that movement is not restricted, preventing any potential injury to the child.

HYPER- AND HYPOTONIA

Alongside dystonia, chorea, athetosis and spasms, abnormalities in the underlying tone in children with chronic neurological conditions often changes toward the end of life. Hypertonia is almost universal among children with conditions in ACT/RCPCH groups III and IV, particularly those with cerebral palsy.

Pharmacological Interventions

A number of interventions can reduce muscle tone.[30]

Benzodiazepines and baclofen are enhancers of activity of the neurotransmitter GABA, while tizanidine is a centrally acting α_2-adrenergic agonist.

Midazolam infusion can relieve hypertonia in the short term, but is not suitable for long-term management. Longer-acting benzodiazepines such as diazepam or clobazam are more appropriate. Tizanidine has to be titrated carefully against its adverse effects, which include hypotension. It is a relatively novel drug, and should probably be used only in discussion with neurologists.

Baclofen can be given orally, but in some children its effect on truncal muscle tone is more marked than in the limbs, impairing posture so that the net impact can be adverse. The effectiveness of intrathecal baclofen in generalized hypertonia of cerebral palsy,[31] particularly using a surgically implanted pump, is such that it is a useful modality despite its complications.[32] A risk of accelerating the progression of scoliosis has been suggested,[33,34] but remains unproved.[35] Baclofen may have an additional effect as an adjuvant in neuropathic pain.[36,37]

Botulinum toxin[38] binds irreversibly to the motor endplate, causing paralysis of a muscle unit until the endplate is re-synthesised. The safety profile is good.[39]

Non-Pharmacological Approaches

The same principles apply as in treating movement disorders. Normalizing tone through proprioceptive feedback and appropriate positioning to promote comfort and function is key. Encouraging weight-bearing exercise may also help with control. For example, supported sitting may enable a child to participate more in activities than being positioned in bed. Side-lying may encourage an increase in tone around the shoulder enabling better hand function in a child who previously has had little control. In addition, hypertonic postural patterns can be released with passive range of movement and stretching exercises and then positioning with the tight muscle group at its longest to maintain a more comfortable position. In addition, minimizing stimulation to overactive muscle groups will help to prevent hypertonic postural patterns that are difficult to release.

Again, anxiety, pain, and distress compound non-seizure movements and tonal abnormalities and ensuring that these are minimized will help with control. CAM therapies can play a valuable part.

CEREBRAL IRRITATION

One of the basic principles of palliative care in children is that it should flow from the child's own subjective experience of their symptoms. This is difficult when the child is pre- or non-verbal. Children in ACT/RCPCH group IV includes those with cerebral palsy as a result of perinatal events. Typically, a long period of chronic disability is preceded by many weeks or months of acute symptoms arising out of the brain injury itself. This is the most common form of cerebral irritation.

It is likely that the neonate with acute brain injury experiences at least three elements of total pain:

1. Acute pain arising from physical injury.
2. Fear and anxiety as a result of trauma and changed environment.
3. Amplification of both fear and pain as a result of failure of processing by damaged neurones and psyche.

The neonate is, in effect, experiencing at the same time severe acute pain and an inability to begin to make sense of it.

The clinical causes and features of cerebral irritation should be distinguished from those of central thalamic pain (Table 27-3), a specific example of neuropathic pain (see Chapter 31) caused by damage to the pain-perceiving part of the brain.

TABLE 27-3 Distinction Between Central, or Thalamic, Pain and Cerebral Irritation

The distinction may not always be possible in clinical practice, and both may need to be treated in a single patient.

	Central Pain	Cerebral Irritation
Pathophysiology	Thalamic damage	Meningeal inflammation/infiltration/stretch
Causes	Cerebral vascular accident, tumor, probably metabolic conditions	Hypoxic ischemic encephalopathy, post-infection, post-trauma, leptomeningeal spread of malignancy
Type of pain	Neuropathic	Nociceptive
Chronicity	Often chronic, may be permanent	Follow acute injury, usually self-limiting over months
Characteristics	Difficult to pinpoint, all over body, often dysaesthesia	Abnormal processing, exaggerated startle, amplification of pain by unfocused anxiety, difficult to pinpoint
Pharmacological treatments	Antineuropathic agents (amitriptyline, anticonvulsants)	Aimed at reducing neuronal firing, anxiety and pain (phenobarbitone, benzos and opioids)

However, in practice the two may co-exist in a child unable to communicate his or her experience. It is often necessary to treat both simultaneously.

Pharmacological Management

Management of cerebral irritation in the neonate requires a three-pronged attack:

1. Phenobarbital. The evidence base for phenobarbital in cerebral irritation is largely from metastatic disease in adults.[40] It is a powerful anxiolytic sedative with probable anti-neuropathic properties.[22] It has the additional benefit in neonates of a long track record as an effective anticonvulsant for seizures occurring in the early neonatal period.
2. Benzodiazepines. Prompt intervention with effective doses of benzodiazepines can be dramatically effective. Midazolam by subcutaneous or intravenous continuous infusion is rapidly effective and easily titrated against the child's symptoms. Once an infusion is no longer appropriate, this should be converted to a longer-acting benzodiazepine such as lorazepam or diazepam. Breakthrough episodes of anxiety can be treated with midazolam buccally[22] because midazolam's short half-life[23] makes it ideal for this purpose. Frequent requirements for breakthrough midazolam are an indication that the background benzodiazepine dose should be reviewed.
3. Major opioids. Major opioids should always be commenced if there is significant hypoxic brain injury. The dose and interval are not always straightforward. The painful stimulus is potentially intense, but it is hard to quantify in the absence of subjective reporting. There is animal evidence to suggest[41] that the blood-brain barrier of the neonate, particularly in the presence of inflammation, may be more permeable to opioids than in older children. Furthermore, elimination of opioids is influenced strongly by renal function.[42] A reasonable starting dose

in the absence of hypoxic renal damage would be 0.5 mg/kg oral morphine equivalent given 8 hourly regularly, with the same dose for breakthrough as needed. Titration should then progress in the usual way, that is, by reviewing every 48 hours and increasing the average 24 hourly breakthrough requirements, being careful to ensure that regular and breakthrough doses remain in proportion.

These medications should be reviewed after six months. At that time, most neonatologists would wish to substitute an alternative anticonvulsant for phenobarbital. It is usually clear at that time whether a child has required escalation of benzodiazepine and opioid doses to account for growth, or whether these are in effect sub-therapeutic and can and should be actively weaned and discontinued.

Although cerebral irritation is most commonly associated with hypoxic ischemic encephalopathy in the neonatal period, it can of course complicate brain injury at any age and a similar approach should be considered.

Non-Pharmacological Approaches

As with controlling seizures, minimizing stimulation is important for managing the neonate suffering with cerebral irritation. This time period is often one of trauma for a family. The birth and immediate post-natal period is likely to have involved unexpected complications and interventions, leaving a family feeling confused and distressed. After the initial acute stage, further neurological symptoms may evolve and must be managed effectively by the whole interdisciplinary team, as described in the other sections of this chapter.

The most important aspect of managing the care of a child with cerebral irritation is supportive care to the family. A new baby who cries or screams for hours on end and is unable to be settled, compounded by lack of sleep and grieving for the loss of the child that they had expected, can leave parents feeling anxious and struggling to cope. Respite care and support must be provided, especially when the child is cared for at home.

The use of craniosacral therapy for children who have experienced birth trauma has become more popular in recent years, although there is little clinical evidence for this, supportive or otherwise.[16]

SLEEP-WAKE CYCLE

Diurnal sleep-wake cycle is coordinated centrally in the region of the hypothalamus. Even in the normally functioning brain, it can be disrupted easily by physical, emotional, and spiritual factors. Lying awake at night with worry is a common human experience.

In ACT groups III and IV particularly, disruption of normal brain function is the rule. It is perhaps unsurprising that in this group disruption of the sleep-wake cycle is common.[43,44] Its impact on the family can be profound. Endless nights of broken sleep inevitably accumulate and contribute to the global exhaustion reported by many families.[45]

One chemical mediator of the normal diurnal rhythm is melatonin, synthesized in the pineal gland and in T-lymphocytes.[46] Exogenous melatonin is now available for oral use, and this can be a helpful intervention.[44] The fact that it is not universally effective underlines the fact that disruption of the sleep-wake cycle is a complex and multidimensional phenomenon rather than simply a function of melatonin deficiency.

A therapeutic approach to disruption of the sleep-wake cycle can consist in three simultaneous and parallel approaches:

1. Prescription of melatonin at night. The usual starting dose is 3 mg. It is not clear what the maximum dose should be, but doses several times this have been used.[47] Other medications that can facilitate sleep include those that reduce anxiety, such as benzodiazepines, and those that are soporific but not anxiolytic, for example chloral hydrate. In the presence of probable or possible neuropathic pain, amitriptyline may be preferable to these. Larger doses of antidepressants may also be effective if the cause for poor sleep is depression itself.

2. Exaggeration of the distinction between day and night (see following). For example, ensure that lights are extinguished and noises kept to a minimum during the night. Conversely, it is important to avoid being over quiet during the day.

3. Review of prescriptions. Many of the medications required by children in ACT Groups III and IV can potentially cause drowsiness. It is often possible to review the timings of these, so that drugs with sedative or soporific effects are given at night.

Non-Pharmacological Management

The sleep-wake pattern of any ill child is often disturbed. For those children nearing the end of their lives, sleep can become further disturbed by troublesome symptoms and the effects of medication. Maintaining a routine may benefit the rest of the family and help in the palliative process.

In addition to pharmacological management, maintaining the pattern of night and day is of paramount importance. This should involve allowing the child to access natural light, if possible, and dark at the appropriate times and increasing stimulation during daytime hours and reducing it overnight. Ensuring the child is kept as physically active as possible, with regular rests, during the day is important even in the non-ambulant child. Continuing with previously enjoyed physical activities, such as hydrotherapy, may enable a child to relax more afterward. Position changes, to show the child a difference between day and night, may promote sleep and wakefulness at appropriate times. Even when a child is bed-bound, his or her positioning can be directed to restful or activity. Using high sitting or head-up side-lying in bed during the day can promote more interaction in a neurologically impaired child, while more reclined positions can be saved for sleep.

Sleep is often disturbed by anxiety, pain, depression, and other symptoms.[48] It is important to ensure that these have been addressed as much as possible, even in the pre- or non-verbal child. There is evidence from the adult palliative care research that aromatherapy and massage can help to promote better sleep patterns.[11] It is feasible that this may also be the case within the pediatric population.

FATIGUE

Fatigue is one of the most common symptoms experienced by children with cancer.[49] (See Chapter 29.) Furthermore, it is an obvious complication of many of the conditions in ACT/RCPCH Group II, such as Duchenne muscular dystrophy. Despite this, the symptom of fatigue has received little attention in the pediatric literature. Even in adult palliative medicine, there is no single agreed-upon therapeutic approach.

It is a multifactorial phenomenon, caused not only by the disease and the body's defenses against it, but also therapeutic interventions themselves.

Fatigue is described as one of the symptoms that causes most distress[49–54] and has received some attention in the adult cancer literature.[55] Despite its apparent high prevalence in children with life-threatening conditions,[49,51,52] it is relatively under-recognized in children,[56] perhaps because it is difficult to diagnose and assess, and there are few effective interventions.

Fatigue, like all symptoms, is multidimensional,[56] including symptoms directly arising from the underlying condition, and those arising from its treatment. These include:

- Anemia. Although anemia seems an obvious cause for fatigue, in practice the two are not always closely associated, suggesting other factors may also contribute.
- Muscle abnormalities. Some of the more common non-malignant life-limiting conditions in childhood, such as Duchenne muscular dystrophy, are primary causes of muscle weakness. The cachexia associated with cancer is an immune-mediated inflammatory phenomenon rather than simply a nutritional one. Even where the underlying condition does not directly cause muscle weakness, it can cause immobility, which itself impairs muscle strength and stamina. Medications, particularly steroids,[57] can cause muscle weakness.
- Endocrine abnormalities, particularly involving endogenous steroids, thyroid or hypothalamo-pituitary axis, can lead to a sense of fatigue. Such abnormalities may be common where there is central neurological damage, such as children in ACT/RCPCH Groups III and IV, or those with brain tumors.
- Depression and anxiety can both manifest as a sensation of tiredness. Both are difficult to diagnose in children, particularly those who are cognitively impaired or non-verbal. A high index of suspicion, together with a willingness to collaborate with child mental health services in actively treating psychological illness in children with life-limiting conditions, will minimize this.
- Sleep disturbance. Many children with non-malignant life-limiting conditions in Groups II, III, and IV will also have disruption of their circadian rhythm.

Management of fatigue should, in the first instance, be directed at the underlying cause if possible. Correction of anemia may relieve symptoms of fatigue, though the benefit of this should be weighed against the difficulty of the child having to be admitted to the hospital and establish intravenous access. A review and rationalization of medication, particularly aiming to reduce co-prescription of duplicative and/or centrally acting medications, can often result in significant improvement.

Activity should be maintained at an appropriate level. The golden rule for the patient is to do as much as you can, but no more. This avoids the extremes complete bed rest and too vigorous physical demands on the principle of no pain, no gain. Neither extreme is helpful.

Diagnosis and appropriate treatment of depression or anxiety is important. Guidelines[58] suggest that management of depression in children should be undertaken in collaboration with child mental health services if possible. Correction of an altered sleep pattern should be attempted as much as possible.

There is some literature in adults suggesting that pharmacological stimulants can improve fatigue.[59–61] In young people, this evidence is limited to reduction of opioid-induced drowsiness.[62] Although the evidence base is weak, methylphenidate is familiar to most pediatricians and its safe use in children has been established, albeit in a different therapeutic context. In the absence of approaches supported by better evidence, it seems a reasonable therapeutic trial where fatigue is identified as a significant problem.

Other pharmacological treatments such as steroids, adenosine triphosphate, megestrol acetate, and carnitine have been proposed, but though all are plausible none has shown unequivocal effectiveness.

Non-Pharmacological Management

The main approach for rehabilitating a patient suffering fatigue uses paced exercise programs.[63] For those children and families who are still able and wanting to participate in active rehabilitation, a graded, functional exercise program should be designed and implemented. For those unable or not wanting to take part in this, physical activity should be encouraged in a way and to a level that is appropriate and acceptable to the child and family. Again, this should be functionally aimed, enabling the child to participate in activities that he or she enjoys. A fine balance in the amount and frequency of activity should be found to ensure that the fatigue-reducing physiological benefits of physical activity are experienced without the child overdoing it and becoming exhausted. "Little and often" is a useful adage to follow.

During the palliative phase, fatigue may become more and more a limiting factor in a child's ability to take part in everyday activities. Some families may require guidance as to prioritizing tasks to ensure that the child is using his or her small amounts of energy on meaningful activities. Many families in this situation will be in a routine of care and treatment provided to their child. In the latter stages it may be more desirable to enable the child to take part in his or her own chosen, pleasurable activities even if that means a more mundane, non-essential task has to be sacrificed, such as a wash or stretching regime. At this point an occupational therapist may be able to offer energy preservation advice and aids to maintain as much independence as possible for the child whilst minimizing the energy expended on activities of daily living.

Studies of CAM approaches in the treatment of palliative adult cancer patients with fatigue[4,7,17,64,65] suggest that massage, homeopathy, TENS, acupuncture, and even Reiki had a positive effect on participants' perception of fatigue. There are far fewer studies in children, and all are in cancer.[9,66] These suggest that massage measurably reduced anxiety, though it did not improve the patient's perception of fatigue. The lack of evidence for these approaches in treating children with fatigue in palliative care should not prevent their use, however, as with all treatment, the clinician, child, and family must be able to balance the potential good and harmful effects to establish what is in the child's best interest before deciding on the course of action.

Summary

Management of neurological symptoms in palliative care is complicated by a number of factors. Those caring for children nevertheless need to feel confident enough to address effectively a range of symptoms that cause distress to a large number of children needing palliative care.

Children at risk of neurological symptoms are often pre- or non-verbal and find it difficult to express their discomfort. A key for physicians and nurses is to have a high index of suspicion and to respond appropriately when caretakers bring signs of distress to their attention.

Neurological symptoms are often intractable in that they do not completely resolve with treatment. Nevertheless, with good palliative care, improvement is usually possible and often considerable. Discussion with the family and, where possible, the child, is important, both to identify which symptoms are most distressing and to establish realistic treatment goals.

The evidence base is small. Nevertheless, there is such an evidence base, both for pharmacological and non-pharmacological approaches in neurological symptoms. Clinicians should derive their practice from published experience in children where possible and in adults where necessary. An overly cautious insistence on robust evidence must inevitably lead to underusing approaches that are intuitively harmless and valuable such as music therapy and hydrotherapy.

Pharmacological approaches demand a higher level of evidence, but even with these a pragmatic approach is sometimes necessary, adopting as a trial therapeutic interventions that are plausible and rational, but not yet proved.

Management of neurological symptoms is therefore a perfect exemplar for palliative care in children. It combines an analytical approach with a holistic one, rational considerations with pragmatic ones, and the application of research to the care of a group of vulnerable patients.

Clinical Vignette

Anna was offered palliative care at thirteen years old. Born by forceps delivery for fetal distress, she presented at birth with respiratory distress and seizures. A diagnosis of hypoxic ischemic encephalopathy (HIE) was made.

Anna had total-body involvement cerebral palsy with hypertonic presentation and frequent muscle spasms, epilepsy, cortical blindness, and developmental delay. She required regular hospital admissions throughout her life for recurrent chest infections, always effectively treated with a short course of intravenous antibiotics, and various elective procedures including gastrostomy and intrathecal baclofen. The health professionals involved in Anna's care at this point included a neurologist and epilepsy nurse specialist, neurosurgeon and baclofen pump nurse specialist, community pediatrician, dietician, physiotherapist, nurse and occupational therapist, general practitioner, acute hospital pediatrician, nursing staff and physiotherapist, and school care team.

Between acute illnesses, Anna attended school and enjoyed teenage life. She was a fan of pop music, Disney films and spending time with her family, friends, and regular caretakers. Although unable to speak or use communication aids, Anna was able to communicate pleasure and discomfort to those around her.

At thirteen, Anna became unwell with another chest infection requiring an episode of invasive ventilation recovering with a course of intravenous antibiotics and chest physiotherapy. Because her episodes of acute respiratory illness had become increasingly frequent and severe, on this occasion she was reviewed by the respiratory physician and an interdisciplinary team meeting was called to plan her future care. The meeting involved the intensivist, neurology consultant, respiratory consultant, community pediatrician, Anna's parents, and her school care worker. Following the discussion, Anna's parents decided that, should she become unwell in the same way again, they wished for her to have an active treatment or antibiotics, chest physiotherapy and non-invasive ventilation, but not to be admitted to the intensive care unit for invasive ventilation, or to be given cardiopulmonary resuscitation in the event of arrest. This decision was supported by the team involved and a specific care plan was drawn up and made easily available in all accessed medical, school, and care plan notes. Anna was also referred to the local children's hospice.

Anna's main symptom was muscle spasms, and her baclofen dose was reviewed with good effect. Her epilepsy was well-controlled at this point with anti-convulsants and she appeared to have no other symptoms. Over the next year Anna visited the hospice for regular planned respite care and support to her and her family. She required three admissions for chest infection, all requiring non-invasive ventilation, chest physiotherapy, and intravenous therapies. At the request of her parents, Anna always had a step-down discharge via respite admission in the hospice.

Anna's fourth admission was with unexplained pain and an increase in her seizures and muscle spasms. Her symptoms were treated with further anti-convulsant medication and opioids. Her previous splinting was reviewed and changed for soft splints to one hand only, where she was experiencing discomfort from spasms into thumb opposition. Anna's parents were also taught a limb massage technique as she appeared to settle and enjoy this. Anna returned home and was reviewed regularly by hospice medical and nursing staff and her established community health care team.

Two months later Anna died in her sleep, at home with her family. She was taken to the hospice where she and her family were cared for until her funeral. Her family still receives support from the hospice team who have worked particularly closely with Anna's younger sister. Anna's family and care team were not imminently expecting her death but, because it had been anticipated and her care planned, the last few months of her life were managed in the way that her family had wished. It was important to them that, during her final illness, Anna was cared for by a team that they already knew well and who had got to know Anna well.

REFERENCES

1. Hain RD: Palliative care in children in Wales: a study of provision and need, *Palliat Med* 19(2):137–142, 2005.
2. Health Professions Council: Standard 2b. Standards of Proficiency - Physiotherapists 2007.
3. CAM basics Internet database: Available from: http://nccam.nih.gov/health/whatiscam/D347.pdf, 2007. (Accessed August 2, 2009.)

4. Cassileth BR, Vickers AJ: Massage therapy for symptom control: outcome study at a major cancer center, *J Pain Symptom Manage* 28(3):244–249, 2004.
5. Gray RA: The use of massage therapy in palliative care, *Complement Ther Nurs Midwifery* 6(2):77–82, 2000.
6. Kutner JS, Smith MC, Corbin L, Hemphill L, Benton K, Mellis BK, et al: Massage therapy versus simple touch to improve pain and mood in patients with advanced cancer: a randomized trial, *Ann Intern Med* 149(6):369–379, 2008.
7. Lafferty WE, Downey L, McCarty RL, Standish LJ, Patrick DL: Evaluating CAM treatment at the end of life: a review of clinical trials for massage and meditation, *Complement Ther Med* 14(2):100–112, 2006.
8. Pan CX, Morrison RS, Ness J, Fugh-Berman A, Leipzig RM: Complementary and alternative medicine in the management of pain, dyspnea, and nausea and vomiting near the end of life: a systematic review, *J Pain Symptom Manage* 20(5):374–387, 2000.
9. Post-White J, Fitzgerald M, Savik K, Hooke MC, Hannahan AB, Sencer SF: Massage therapy for children with cancer, *J Pediatr Oncol Nurs* 26(1):16–28, 2009.
10. Sellick SM, Zaza C: Critical review of 5 nonpharmacologic strategies for managing cancer pain, *Cancer Prev Control* 2(1):7–14, 1998.
11. Soden K, Vincent K, Craske S, Lucas C, Ashley S: A randomized controlled trial of aromatherapy massage in a hospice setting, *Palliat Med* 18(2):87–92, 2004.
12. Wilkie D, Kampbell J, Cutshall S, Halbisky H, Harmon H, Johnson L: Effects of massage on pain intensity, analgesics and quality of life in patients with cancer pain: a pilot study of a randomized clinical trial conducted within hospice care delivery, *Hosp J* 15:31–53, 2000.
13. Dillon M, Lucas C: Auricular stud acupuncture in palliative care patients, *Palliat Med* 13(3):253–254, 1999.
14. Filshie J: Acupuncture in palliative care, *Eur J Palliat Care* 7(2):41–44, 2000.
15. Leng G: A year of acupuncture in palliative care, *Palliat Med* 13(2):163–164, 1999.
16. Liptak GS: Complementary and alternative therapies for cerebral palsy, *Ment Retard Dev Disabil Res Rev* 11(2):156–163, 2005.
17. Gadsby J, Franks A, Jarvis P, Dewhurst F: Acupuncture-like transcutaneous nerve stimulation within palliative care: a pilot study, *Complement Ther Med* 5:13–18, 1997.
18. Robb K, Oxberry SG, Bennett MI, Johnson MI, Simpson KH, Searle RD: A cochrane systematic review of transcutaneous electrical nerve stimulation for cancer pain, *J Pain Symptom Manage* 37(4):746–753, 2009.
19. Robb KA, Newham DJ, Williams JE: Transcutaneous electrical nerve stimulation vs. transcutaneous spinal electroanalgesia for chronic pain associated with breast cancer treatments, *J Pain Symptom Manage* 33(4):410–419, 2007.
20. Klimach VJ: The community use of rescue medication for prolonged epileptic seizures in children, *Seizure* 18(5):343–346, 2009.
21. Uhlig T, Huppe M, Nidermaier B, Pestel G: Mood effects of zolpidem versus phenobarbital combined with promethazine in an anesthesiological setting, *Neuropsychobiology* 34(2):90–97, 1996.
22. Tremont-Lukats IW, Megeff C, Backonja MM: Anticonvulsants for neuropathic pain syndromes: mechanisms of action and place in therapy, *Drugs* 60(5):1029–1052, 2000.
23. Nahara MC, McMorrow J, Jones PR, Anglin D, Rosenberg R: Pharmacokinetics of midazolam in critically ill pediatric patients, *Eur J Drug Metab Pharmacokinet* 25(3–4):219–221, 2000.
24. Kanegaye JT, Favela JL, Acosta M, Bank DE: High-dose rectal midazolam for pediatric procedures: a randomized trial of sedative efficacy and agitation, *Pediatr Emerg Care* 19(5):329–336, 2003.
25. Categories of life-limiting and life-threatening conditions: Available from www.act.org.uk/page.asp?section=164&sectionTitle=Categories+and+life%2Dlimiting+and+life%2Dthreatening+conditions. Accessed January 10, 2010.
26. Mariotti P, Fasano A, Contarino MF, Della Marca G, Piastra M, Genovese O, et al: Management of status dystonicus: our experience and review of the literature, *Mov Disord* 22(7):963–968, 2007.
27. Bateman DN, Rawlins MD, Simpson JM: Extrapyramidal reactions to prochlorperazine and haloperidol in the United Kingdom, *Q J Med* 59(230):549–556, 1986.
28. Starr PA, Turner RS, Rau G, Lindsey N, Heath S, Volz M, et al: Microelectrode-guided implantation of deep brain stimulators into the globus pallidus internus for dystonia: techniques, electrode locations, and outcomes, *Neurosurg Focus* 17(1):E4, 2004.
29. Schlaggar BL, Mink JW: Movement disorders in children, *Pediatr Rev* 24(2):39–51, 2003.
30. Tilton A: Management of spasticity in children with cerebral palsy, *Semin Pediatr Neurol* 16(2):82–89, 2009.
31. Albright AL, Ferson SS: Intrathecal baclofen therapy in children, *Neurosurg Focus* 21(2):e3, 2006.
32. Kolaski K, Logan LR: A review of the complications of intrathecal baclofen in patients with cerebral palsy, *NeuroRehabilitation* 22(5):383–395, 2007.
33. Sansone JM, Mann D, Noonan K, McLeish D, Ward M, Iskandar BJ: Rapid progression of scoliosis following insertion of intrathecal baclofen pump, *J Pediatr Orthop* 26(1):125–128, 2006.
34. Senaran H, Shah SA, Presedo A, Dabney KW, Glutting JW, Miller F: The risk of progression of scoliosis in cerebral palsy patients after intrathecal baclofen therapy, *Spine* (Phila, Pa 1976) 32(21):2348–2354, 2007.
35. Ginsburg GM, Lauder AJ: Progression of scoliosis in patients with spastic quadriplegia after the insertion of an intrathecal baclofen pump, *Spine* (Phila, Pa 1976) 32(24):2745–2750, 2007.
36. Vissers KC, Geenen F, Biermans R, Meert TF: Pharmacological correlation between the formalin test and the neuropathic pain behavior in different species with chronic constriction injury, *Pharmacol Biochem Behav* 84(3):479–486, 2006.
37. Yomiya K, Matsuo N, Tomiyasu S, Yoshimoto T, Tamaki T, Suzuki T, et al: Baclofen as an adjuvant analgesic for cancer pain, *Am J Hosp Palliat Care* 26(2):112–118, 2009.
38. Simpson DM, Gracies JM, Graham HK, Miyasaki JM, Naumann M, Russman B, et al: Assessment: Botulinum neurotoxin for the treatment of spasticity (an evidence-based review): report of the Therapeutics and Technology Assessment Subcommittee of the American Academy of Neurology, *Neurology* 70(19):1691–1698, 2008.
39. Albavera-Hernandez C, Rodriguez JM, Idrovo AJ: Safety of botulinum toxin type A among children with spasticity secondary to cerebral palsy: a systematic review of randomized clinical trials, *Clin Rehabil* 23(5):394–407, 2009.
40. Stirling LC, Kurowska A, Tookman A: The use of phenobarbitone in the management of agitation and seizures at the end of life, *J Pain Symptom Manage* 17(5):363–368, 1999.
41. Lynn AM, McRorie TI, Slattery JT, Calkins DF, Opheim KE: Age-dependent morphine partitioning between plasma and cerebrospinal fluid in monkeys, *Dev Pharmacol Ther* 17(3–4):200–204, 1991.
42. Mercadante S, Arcuri E: Opioids and renal function, *J Pain* 5(1):2–19, 2004.
43. Adlington K, Liu AJ, Nanan R: Sleep disturbances in the disabled child: a case report and literature review, *Aust Fam Physician* 35(9):711–715, 2006.
44. Zucconi M, Bruni O: Sleep disorders in children with neurologic diseases, *Semin Pediatr Neurol* 8(4):258–275, 2001.
45. Wood F, Simpson S, Barnes E, Hain R: Disease trajectories in paediatric palliative care: towards validation of the ACT/RCPH categories, *Palliat Med*, 2010. In press.
46. Lardone PJ, Carrillo-Vico A, Naranjo MC, De Felipe B, Vallejo A, Karasek M, et al: Melatonin synthesized by Jurkat human leukemic T cell line is implicated in IL-2 production, *J Cell Physiol* 206(1):273–279, 2006.
47. Hancock E, O'Callaghan F, Osborne JP: Effect of melatonin dosage on sleep disorder in tuberous sclerosis complex, *J Child Neurol* 20(1):78–80, 2005.
48. Sateia M, Santulli R: Sleep in palliative care. In Doyle D, Hanks G, Cherny NI, Calman K, editors: *Oxford textbook of palliative medicine*, ed 3, Oxford, 2004, Oxford University Press.
49. Goldman A, Hewitt M, Collins GS, Childs M, Hain R: Symptoms in children/young people with progressive malignant disease: United Kingdom Children's Cancer Study Group/Paediatric Oncology Nurses Forum survey, *Pediatrics* 117(6):e1179–e1186, 2006.
50. Hechler T, Blankenburg M, Friedrichsdorf SJ, Garske D, Hubner B, Menke A, et al: Parents' perspective on symptoms, quality of life, characteristics of death and end-of-life decisions for children dying from cancer, *Klin Padiatr* 220(3):166–174, 2008.
51. Jalmsell L, Kreicbergs U, Onelov E, Steineck G, Henter JI: Symptoms affecting children with malignancies during the last month of life: a nationwide follow-up, *Pediatrics* 117(4):1314–1320, 2006.
52. Pritchard M, Burghen E, Srivastava DK, Okuma J, Anderson L, Powell B, et al: Cancer-related symptoms most concerning to parents during the last week and last day of their child's life, *Pediatrics* 121(5):e1301–e1309, 2008.

53. Theunissen JM, Hoogerbrugge PM, van Achterberg T, Prins JB, Vernooij-Dassen MJ, van den Ende CH: Symptoms in the palliative phase of children with cancer, *Pediatr Blood Cancer* 49(2):160–165, 2007.

54. Wolfe J, Grier HE, Klar N, Levin SB, Ellenbogen JM, Salem-Schatz S, et al: Symptoms and suffering at the end of life in children with cancer, *N Engl J Med* 342(5):326–333, 2000.

55. Stone PC, Minton O: Cancer-related fatigue, *Eur J Cancer* 44(8):1097–1104, 2008.

56. Ullrich CK, Mayer OH: Assessment and management of fatigue and dyspnea in pediatric palliative care, *Pediatr Clin North Am* 54(5):735–756, xi, 2007.

57. Batchelor TT, Taylor LP, Thaler HT, Posner JB, DeAngelis LM: Steroid myopathy in cancer patients, *Nuerology* 48:1234–1238, 1997.

58. National Institute for Clinical Excellence: *Depression in Children and Young People Identification and management in primary, community and secondary care*, London, 2005, The British Psychological Society.

59. Breitbart W, Rosenfeld B, Kaim M, Funesti-Esch J: A randomized, double-blind, placebo-controlled trial of psychostimulants for the treatment of fatigue in ambulatory patients with human immunodeficiency virus disease, *Arch Intern Med* 161(3):411–420, 2001.

60. Bruera E, Miller MJ, Macmillan K, Kuehn N: Neuropsychological effects of methylphenidate in patients receiving a continuous infusion of narcotics for cancer pain, *Pain* 48(2):163–166, 1992.

61. Bruera E, Valero V, Driver L, Shen L, Willey J, Zhang T, et al: Patient-controlled methylphenidate for cancer fatigue: a double-blind, randomized, placebo-controlled trial, *J Clin Oncol* 24(13):2073–2078, 2006.

62. Yee JD, Berde CB: Dextroamphetamine or methylphenidate as adjuvants to opioid analgesia for adolescents with cancer, *J Pain Symptom Manage* 9(2):122–125, 1994.

63. Cramp F, Daniel J: Exercise for the management of cancer-related fatigue in adults, *Cochrane Database Syst Rev* (2):CD006145, 2008.

64. Frenkel M, Shah V: Complementary medicine can benefit palliative care, Part 1, *Eur J Palliat Care* 15(5):238–243, 2008.

65. Thompson EA, Reillly D: The homeopathic approach to symptom control in the cancer patient: a prospective observational study, *Palliat Med* 16(3):227–233, 2002.

66. Williams PD, Schmideskamp J, Ridder EL, Williams AR: Symptom monitoring and dependent care during cancer treatment in children: pilot study, *Cancer Nurs* 29(3):188–197, 2006.

28 Delirium

MICHELLE GOLDSMITH | PAULINA ORTIZ-RUBIO |
SANDRA STAVESKI | MELANIE CHAN | RICHARD J. SHAW

*When a man lacks mental balance in pneumonia he is said
to be delirious. When he lacks mental balance without the
pneumonia, he is pronounced insane by all smart doctors.*
  —Martin Henry Fischer

Pediatric delirium is an under-recognized and often reversible complication of critical illness that is considered a medical emergency demanding immediate management.[1] New research on the clinical presentation of pediatric delirium and age-appropriate assessment tools for prompt identification have highlighted some of the differences between the adult and pediatric populations.[2–6] In the context of palliative care, delirium is one of many crises, including pain, anxiety, and dyspnea, which require a thorough and collaboratively developed plan of care.[7]

In the adult palliative care setting, delirium has been carefully studied and identified as a sign of impending death.[8,9] Among adult patients who are terminally ill, delirium is the most common neuropsychiatric disorder with a prevalence estimated as high as 85%.[10] In a palliative care setting, researchers[11] identified 42% of the patients with a diagnosis of delirium at the time of hospital admission, and an additional 45% who developed delirium during their hospital stay. These data suggest that delirium occurs in the majority of patients nearing the end of life and that improved methods of diagnosis and management are warranted for this highly distressing and often reversible condition. Therefore, in all critically ill patients of every age, mental status should be carefully evaluated in addition to conventional monitoring of pulse, temperature, respiratory rate, blood pressure, and pain.[12]

The study of delirium is at the confluence of a number of clinical disciplines including anesthesiology, critical care medicine, pediatrics, geriatrics, oncology, pain medicine, palliative medicine, neurology, psychiatry, psychology, nursing, pharmacy, and bioethics. Across these domains, there has been a recent groundswell of interest in delirium,[13] and specifically pediatric delirium, after a long period of neglect between 1980 and 2003.[2,3] Advances in medical care that prolong life place critically ill patients at greater risk for delirium. In addition, awareness of potential cognitive and psychological sequelae of delirium has led to efforts directed at early recognition and treatment. Goals of palliative and general clinical care target delirium as a symptom that necessitates immediate care.[14]

The aim of this chapter is to provide an overview of pediatric delirium and its clinical relevance in the palliative care setting. An additional goal includes underscoring the interdisciplinary nature of delirium. Any clinician or caregiver, including respiratory therapist, nurse, doctor, pharmacist, and parent, has the opportunity to screen patients for delirium. Delirium has many causes, occurs in both simple and complex clinical situations and should be suspected in all circumstances when mental status is altered. One long-term study has shown that nurse-directed delirium prevention and management programs, involving multidisciplinary education and collaboration, have led to a decrease in delirium and clinician workload.[15] Every member of the treatment team serves as a resource in the prevention, recognition, and management of delirium.

Topics addressed in this chapter include definitions, phenomenology, prevalence and epidemiology, etiology and risk factors, pathogenesis, assessment, and treatment. Finally, there is a review of the relationship between delirium and posttraumatic stress symptoms, including its effects on caregivers.

Definition

According to the *Diagnostic and Statistical Manual*[16] the core features of delirium include a disturbance of consciousness, change in cognition, and perceptual disturbance that develops over a short period, usually hours to days, and fluctuates over time (Box 28-1). Delirium has been associated with rates of morbidity and mortality that surpass those of all other psychiatric diagnoses.[17] Across clinical disciplines and countries, there are many ambiguities in the terminology used to describe delirium.[18] Such terms as acute brain failure, encephalopathy, acute confusional state, and intensive care unit (ICU) psychosis have been widely employed, and the critical care literature has now conformed to the recommendations of the American Psychiatric Association, and other experts, that the term delirium be used uniformly to describe this syndrome of brain dysfunction.[19] The need for shared terminology reflects the challenges clinicians face in diagnosing delirium across clinical settings and age groups.

CLINICAL PRESENTATION

Although the clinical presentation of delirium in children and adolescents is considered to be similar to that of adults, there are observed differences in the type and frequency of symptoms across various age groups.[4,5,6] Clinician-observed features of pediatric delirium varied across several studies. Pediatric patients are described as having more frequent fluctuation in symptoms, greater affective lability, impaired attention, and disturbances in their sleep-wake cycle.[4] By contrast[6] a study described pediatric patients as having lower rates of sleep disturbance, fewer cognitive deficits, and lower levels of symptom fluctuation.

BOX 28-1 DSM-IV-TR Diagnostic Criteria for Delirium

Disturbance of consciousness
- Reduced clarity in awareness of the environment, that is a reduced ability to focus, sustain, or shift attention

Change in cognition
- Memory deficit, disorientation, language disturbance, or development of a perceptual disturbance not better accounted for by a pre-existing cognitive disorder

Temporal character
- Develops over a short period, usually hours to days, and fluctuates during the course of the day

Etiology
- There is evidence from the history, physical examination, or laboratory findings of a general medical condition, including possible substance intoxication or substance withdrawal, that is deemed etiologically related to the disturbance

Adapted from the American Psychiatric Association: *Diagnostic and Statistical Manual of Mental Disorders*, 4th edition revised, (DSM-IV-TR).Washington, DC, American Psychiatric Press, 2000.

With regard to psychotic symptoms, authors have described both lower and higher prevalence of perceptual disturbances and delusions among children compared to adults.[4,6] Some[4] have suggested that delusions and hallucinations may not be core symptoms of pediatric delirium. Alternatively, a study of pediatric patients emerging from anesthesia reported that younger children had higher rates of hallucinations and other perceptual disturbances, compared with older children.[20] These differences may reflect variations in brain function across the age span, developmental immaturity in children, functional decline in old age, and differences in the expression of distress during hospitalization.[21] The variance in observed clinical features is wide and may result from the fluctuating nature of the illness, the subjective nature of clinical assessment, lack of age-appropriate screening tools, and the various causes of delirium.

Subtypes of Delirium

Three motoric subtypes of delirium–hypoactive, hyperactive, and mixed–have been well described in the adult literature.[22] Delirium is also categorized on the basis of symptom severity, with terms such as pre-delirium, sub-syndromal, veiled,

and full-blown used to designate differences in presentation.[23] These additional terms reflect growing research into the phenomenology of delirium. Although few studies have focused on categorizing delirium temporally or by severity, the practical finding from this work is that delirium may be detectable earlier in its course with vigilant screening. In this chapter, a discussion of motoric subtypes is reviewed with vignettes (Table 28-1).

Anna was a 14-year-old previously healthy girl who presented with the sudden onset of dizziness, shortness of breath, lethargy, and chest pain. Chest x-ray showed signs of cardiomegaly which prompted cardiology consultation. Following a cardiology workup, including an echocardiogram, Anna was diagnosed with idiopathic dilated cardiomyopathy, and hospitalized in the ICU. By hospital day 4, Anna's cardiac function had declined rapidly, and she was placed on the cardiac transplant waiting list. Despite intensive pharmacologic treatment, her worsening cardiac status necessitated Anna being placed on a ventricular assist device. Anna's course was further complicated by a small cerebral vascular accident on hospital day 17. The night following her stroke, Anna was unable to sleep and became acutely agitated, and needed soft physical restraints to prevent her from pulling out her lines and catheters. She was clearly confused and disoriented, and unable to reason with the medical staff. By the following morning, Anna said she was hearing the voice of her deceased grandfather, and believed that he had visited her the previous night. She also reported seeing blood coming out of the faucet in her room, and the feeling of spiders walking over her face.

Anna received a psychiatric consultation and was diagnosed as having a hyperactive delirium with a score of 22/32 on the Delirium Rating Scale-Revised-98 (DRS-R-98). Recommendations were made for treatment with intravenous (IV) haloperidol 0.5 mg q6h, pending review of her ECG. Although Anna's ECG showed evidence of a prolonged QTc interval (410 mseconds), it was considered safe to

TABLE 28-1 Characteristics of Delirium Subtypes

Subtype	Hyperactive	Hypoactive	Mixed
Clinical features	• Psychomotor agitation • Increased verbal fluency and volume • Restlessness • Hyperarousal • Hallucinations	• Psychomotor retardation • Diminished speech production and volume • Apathy • Withdrawal	• Presence of hyperactive and hypoactive symptoms
Notes	• More easily identified • May demand a higher level of care • May need restraint for safety of self and others • Often more distressing to family, staff, and patient	• Often overlooked • Often misdiagnosed as depression or oversedation from medication	• Diagnosis confounded by mixed clinical picture
Likely etiologies	• Drug withdrawal • Anti-cholinergic induced	• Hepatic • Metabolic encephalopathies • Acute sedative or analgesic intoxication • Hypoxia	• Multiple etiologies
Common EEG findings and pathophysiology	• EEG: fast or normal • Increased cerebral metabolism • Reduced activity in the GABA system	• EEG: diffuse slowing • Decreased cerebral metabolism • Increased activity in the GABA system	• Multiple pathways
Treatment options[17]	• Haloperidol	• Second-generation antipsychotic	• Second-generation antipsychotic

prescribe the haloperidol with close cardiac monitoring. This was very helpful in reducing her level of agitation, and re-establishing her normal sleep-wake cycle. By hospital day 20, Anna's symptoms of delirium had resolved and her DRS-R-98 score was 5/32. The following day, an organ became available, and Anna underwent cardiac transplant surgery.

The term *hyperactive* refers to patients who present with symptoms of confusion, psychosis, disorientation, agitation, hypervigilance, hyperalertness, fast or loud speech, combativeness, and behavioral problems such as pulling out catheters and lines. These patients quickly come to the attention of the medical staff and are less likely to be overlooked.

By contrast, patients with hypoactive or silent delirium present with somnolence, decreased activity, slow or decreased speech, psychomotor slowing, withdrawal, apathy, and confusion. These patients may also be perceived as calm and somnolent by the medical and nursing staff. Patients with this latter presentation who demand less care are less likely to be diagnosed with delirium, or may be misdiagnosed with depression.

In these cases, parental opinion comparing current presentation and baseline functioning can be very useful. Often it is a parent's observation, such as *this is not my child* that alerts clinicians to assess mental status more carefully and frequently.

Barry was a 16-year-old male with a history of acute lymphoblastic leukemia with central nervous system involvement. Although he initially responded well to chemotherapy, his treatment was complicated by both herpes simplex virus as well as hemorrhagic stroke requiring intensive rehabilitation. Although Barry made a good recovery, residual damage to his frontal lobes was evident on MRI scan. After 3 years in remission, Barry relapsed and was restarted on a re-induction regimen of methotrexate, vincristine, daunorubicin, and asparaginase. After his second dose of chemotherapy, Barry developed fever and signs of neutropenia, and was admitted for intravenous antibiotics. By hospital day 3, although Barry's fever had resolved and his white blood count was recovering, he was noted to be increasingly withdrawn, spending much of the day in silence, avoiding eye contact, and appearing internally distracted. He started to refuse food, was sleeping excessively during the day, and became almost mute. On hospital day 5, Barry was referred for psychiatric consultation due to concerns about possible depression related to his relapse. Barry was quite uncommunicative during the assessment and either unable or unwilling to cooperate with simple tests of attention and cognition. However, he did appear quite profoundly impaired even with respect to simple questions about orientation and memory. Due to concerns about a possible hypoactive delirium, recommendations were made for a comprehensive medical workup, including an MRI scan, as well as a trial of treatment with risperidone at a dose of 0.5 mg bid. By the following day, although still slowed motorally, Barry had made a quite remarkable improvement. He was more talkative, expressive, and able to answer questions. He was

noted to have difficulty with several items on his mental status examination, in particular questions about his level of orientation, tests of attention and memory, and pen and paper tests of his visual-spatial abilities. He also endorsed vague but strongly held beliefs that "men in black were outside his room, waiting for him to die." His score on the DRS-R-98 was 18/32, and he was thought to meet criteria for hypoactive delirium. Barry was continued on risperidone for a further 5 days. His medical workup was unremarkable, and no etiology was ever established to explain his symptoms. His psychotic symptoms resolved quite rapidly, and by hospital day 9, he was fully oriented, with a score of 3/32 on the DRS-R-98. One week after discharge Barry was titrated down to risperidone 0.5 mg qhs, and after 5 days it was discontinued. Both he and his mother reported that his mood and affect remained appropriate, and he did not exhibit any further evidence of symptoms of delirium.

Adapted from Karnik NS, Joshi SV, Paterno C, Shaw R: Subtypes of pediatric delirium: a treatment algorithm. Psychosomatics. *2007;48:254. Copyright 2007 American Psychiatric Publishing, Inc. Used with permission.*

Mixed delirium describes patients who fluctuate between hyperactive and hypoactive states.[22,25] These critically ill patients present with an array of symptoms, in the context of possible pain, anxiety, and nausea, making it difficult to recognize delirium and identify the cause.

Jackie is a 9-year-old girl with a glioblastoma who, during hospitalization for chemotherapy, developed pressured speech, periods of confusion, and occasional disorientation.

She was noticed to be sleeping as little as 4 hours a night. Her level of activity was also increased, and nursing staff reported that she would spend significant periods of time cleaning and ordering items in her hospital room. She expressed less interested in toys and games, or participating in care. She had a score of 18/32 on the DRS-98, and was diagnosed with acute delirium. Jackie was initially treated with risperidone 0.5 mg qhs. She seemed to improve on this regimen, with better sleep and less pressured activity, but continued to have episodes of increased confusion, disorientation, apathy and talking to herself during the day. Her risperidone dose was increased to 0.5 mg bid, with the addition of zolpidem 5 mg for insomnia. She showed improvement on this regimen and gradually returned to her baseline over several days, at which time she had a score of 4/32 on the DRS-R-98.

Prevalence and Epidemiology

Among adult studies, delirium has been reported in 15% to 18% of patients on acute medical and surgical wards, with higher rates in specific populations.[17] One of the largest retrospective pediatric studies on delirium,[3] reported a 9% prevalence of delirium in a sample of 1027 patients referred for psychiatric consultation (Table 28-2). Another

TABLE 28-2   Studies Examining Clinical Aspects of Pediatric Delirium

Study	Objectives	Population	Clinical symptoms	Etiology	Findings	Comments
Prugh et al,[2] 1980	• To compare hospitalized children with acute central nervous system (CNS) disorder to matched controls • To investigate potential recovery from associated CNS impairments	• 33 hospitalized children and adolescents • 19 controls • Average age 11-13 yrs • Age range 6-17 yrs • Test categories were mental status exam, neurological exam, EEG testing, neuropsychological, and psychodynamic testing • 22 variables measured and remeasured	• Severe delirium • Subclinical delirium • Developmental implications General features: • Patients with delirium may be perceived as acting out • Regressive behaviors are observed • Perceptual-motor abnormalities are common	Not studied	• 17 test items were found clinically useful distinguishing delirium, including EEG slowing, memory impairment, disorientation, severity of illness • Many clinical tools did not discriminate between the two groups and revealed soft neurological signs • Important developmental differences compared with adults • Children with delirium improved on re-testing except with some perceptual motor tests and EEG organization	• This is the first study to closely observe and compare children with and without delirium • It provides well-described cases of various types • This study closely examined variables affected by impairments in brain functioning and showed both persistent negative outcomes from delirium and also recovery in other areas • Etiology and treatment are not examined
Turkel et al,[3] 2003	• Describe the phenomenology, and outcome of delirium	• Retrospective study reviewing 1027 consecutive psychiatric consultations over 4 yrs • 84 patients diagnosed with delirium • Age range 6 mo-18 yrs	• Impaired attention in every patient • Hypoactive subtype, 68% • Hyperactive subtype, 69% • Anxiety noted in 61% of patients • Impaired consciousness more often seen in younger children • Delusions were rare • Hallucinations, 43% • Memory impairment is more common in older patients	• 33% infection • 19% drug-induced • 10% trauma • 8% autoimmune • 8% transplant • 7% postoperative • 7% neoplasm • 7% organ failure	• Incidence of delirium 9% • Mortality 20% • No deaths in group following surgery or trauma • Prolonged hospital stay associated with delirium • First-generation antipsychotics with no reported adverse effects • Second-generation antipsychotics not available at the time of the study	• Pediatric delirium and adult delirium present similarly • The DSM criteria field tested in adults were applicable to children in this cohort • Similar rates of mortality in children and adults • Anti-dopaminergic agents are beneficial in the treatment of delirium in adults and children
Turkel et al,[4] 2006	• Literature review and comparison of adult and pediatric delirium symptoms and their frequency	• 10 adult studies (n=968) • Ages 30-100 yrs • Mean age over 60 yrs • 1 pediatric study (n=84) • Ages 1-18 yrs • Mean age 10.4 yrs	• Frequent symptoms among children: • Psychomotor changes • Mood and affect changes • Sleep-wake disturbance • Fluctuating symptoms • Impaired attention • Irritability • Agitation • Affective liability Frequent symptoms among adults: • Impaired memory • Depressed mood • Speech disturbance • Delusions and paranoia Frequent symptoms in both groups: • Apathy • Impaired alertness • Anxiety • Disorientation • Hallucinations	• Same cohort as Turkel et al, 2003[3]	• Hypoactive delirium occurred in similar rates in the pediatric (68%) and adult groups (combined rate 59%) • Hyperactive delirium occurred more frequently in the pediatric group (69%) than in adults (combined rate 44%) • Mortality rates were not compared in this study • Response to treatment was not studied here	• Inconsistent use of terminology to describe symptoms • Across adult studies there were no consistently used validated instruments to assess delirium • Although impaired attention is a core symptom in the DSM-IV, it was not present 100% in the adult group • Hallucinations and delusions were reported less often than other symptoms and thought not to be a core feature of pediatric delirium

Study					
Schieveld et al,[5] 2007	• Analysis of demographic data, clinical presentation and response to treatment	• Descriptive cohort study of 877 admissions to an 8-bed tertiary PICU over 3 yrs • 61 assessments for delirium • 40 patients diagnosed • Age range 3 mo-17 yrs	• Orientation was difficult to assess in children • Subtypes observed: 43% veiled 35% hyperactive 23% hypoactive Pediatric delirium has distinct neuropsychiatric signs: • Decreased awareness of caregivers and/or environment • Purposeless actions • Restlessness • Inconsolability • Signs of autonomic dysregulation • Subtle higher cortical dysfunctions	• Often multifactorial 55% drug-induced 53% neurological 50% infection 30% respiratory	• Incidence of delirium 4.6% • Mortality data on those not diagnosed with delirium not provided • Mortality rate of those with delirium 12.5% • Data provided on age and gender • Greatest incidence of delirium occurred in the 15-18 yr-old group at 19.4%, but they were the least represented age group in the PICU (only 31 of 877 patients) • 38 of the 40 patients' delirium resolved with antipsychotic medication • 2 out of 27 children had dystonic reactions with haloperidol • Differential diagnosis includes other psychiatric disorders such as acute stress, anxiety, adjustment disorder, child onset psychosis, dissociative disorder
					• Unusually low incidence of delirium compared with adults • Delirium not reliably identified by caregivers and clinicians • Evaluation for delirium may have been requested more often in cases of hyperactive or mixed delirium as opposed to hypoactive cases • Adult DSM criteria do not apply equally to all age groups or settings, such as the PICU • Parents are particularly good at discriminating subtle changes in their children • Risperidone is preferred to haloperidol because of more favorable side effect profile
Leentjens et al,[6] 2008	• Compare the phenomenology of delirium in children, adults, and geriatric patients using the Delirium Rating Scale (DRS) as the assessment tool	• Two separate study groups from two different facilities • The adults and seniors were from the same palliative care setting • The children were the same cohort as Schieveld et al,[5] 2007 • Children n = 46 Mean age 8.3 yrs Age range 0-17 yrs • Adults n = 49 Mean age 55.4 yrs Age range 18-65 yrs • Seniors n = 70 Mean age 76.2 yrs Age range 66-91 yrs	• The range of symptoms by type among all three populations was similar. • Symptoms reported among children were: • More acute onset • More severe perceptual disturbances • More frequent visual hallucinations • More severe delusions • More severe mood lability • Greater agitation • Less severe cognitive deficits • Less severe sleep-wake cycle disturbance • Less variability of symptoms over time	• Reason for pediatric admissions (not the proposed etiology of the delirium): • 39% neurological • 26% respiratory • 17% circulatory • 13% other • 4% trauma	• 4.6% incidence of delirium • Items 2, 3, 4, and 6 on the Delirium Rating Scale (DRS) could not be reliably scored in younger children, i.e., perceptual disturbances, hallucination type, delusions, and cognitive deficits • To allow for statistical analysis, the average score on each individual DRS was substituted for missing items • This accommodation in scoring occurred 57 times across four items in the pediatric population • 16.8% of the adult and seniors had dementia • 37% of adults and 50% of the geriatric patients were already on antipsychotics at the time of the rating
					• The range of symptoms was similar across all groups • The symptom profile on every item of the DRS differed in children and adults • Possible confounding factors include: sedated children in the PICU setting are too impaired to participate, the DRS is not applicable to young children, missing items on the DRS were substituted with the average score • Symptoms of delirium used for screening were limited to the phenomenology described by the DRS • Etiology for delirium in the pediatric group was not described • Outcomes were not studied

study[5] reported a lower prevalence of 4.6% in a pediatric sample of 877 critical care patients.

Among pediatric patients, age as a risk factor for delirium is not well known. The study of 1027 patients[3] identified 84 patients with delirium ages 6 months to 18 years and there was no significant difference in mean and median age based on the cause of delirium. The study did not assess whether age itself was risk factor for delirium. According to the study[5] that presented data stratified by age, the greatest incidence of delirium occurred among the oldest children (15 to 18 years), but these data were not analyzed for statistical significance. Conversely, another study[26] found a negative correlation between age and delirium among post-anesthesia patients suffering with emergence delirium.

Although studies to assess the prevalence of delirium in children receiving end-of-life care have not yet been undertaken, data from adult studies suggest potentially much higher rates in this population. For example, immediately before death, delirium rates of 68% to 88% have been reported in adult oncology patients.[11,27] More specifically, according to a review[8] hypoactive delirium, which is easily overlooked, has been reported as high as 40% to 78% in adult palliative care patients.[11,28,29]

Attempts to quantify the prevalence of delirium by subtype among adults have resulted in a range of findings. For example, a study[30] reported hypoactive delirium (43.5%) occurring considerably more often than "purely" hyperactive delirium (1.6%), and mixed delirium was the most frequently observed subtype (54.1%). The low number of cases with hyperactive delirium in this cohort is unusual when compared with other studies that report rates of hyperactive delirium ranging from 15% to 80%.[22,31] On the other hand, the high number of cases in the cohort[30] of 375 elderly diagnosed with hypoactive delirium suggests that careful screening may accurately identify more subtle presentations of delirium. The only comparison[4] of the prevalence of hyperactive and hypoactive states in adults to children found across three adult studies there was an average of 59% hypoactive delirium, similar to a pediatric prevalence of 69%. Agitation was noted in the adult studies at a combined rate of 44%, which was significantly lower than the pediatric rate of hyperactive delirium of 68%.

In adult palliative care literature, the rates of hypoactive delirium are as high as 86%, mean prevalence 48% in one meta-analysis, while rates of hyperactive delirium vary between 13% to 46% of patients.[29,32] Figures for the prevalence of delirium by subtype in the pediatric palliative care setting are not known.

Despite the varied estimates on prevalence, numerous studies suggest that the motoric subtypes of delirium differ beyond the degree of psychomotor activity. Studies show variation between hypoactive, hyperactive, and mixed delirium with regard to other non-motoric features of delirium,[33] etiology and pathophysiology,[34] ease of detection and assessment, response to treatment,[24] and outcome.[35] Notably, clinician observations of patient psychomotor disturbance were less reliable when compared with data from electronic motion detectors.[36] Because recognition of delirium continues to be challenging and machine-assisted assessment is helpful, there is the potential that future technological innovations may enhance clinician assessment. For example, similar to the use of heart monitors in the ICU, motion

detection may be used to help alert clinicians to the presence of delirium among high-risk groups (see Table 28-2).

Etiology

Causes and risk factors for delirium are often multifaceted and include vascular, infectious, neoplastic, degenerative, organ failure, toxic, deficiencies including vitamin, congenital, central nervous system pathologic, traumatic, endocrinological, metabolic, dehydration, heavy metal, and anoxic phenomena.[17] Medication-related etiologies, as a result of toxic effects or withdrawal reactions, are also common. As with adults, certain classes of medications such as steroids, opiates, benzodiazepines, and anticholinergic agents are frequent precipitants.

Tristan, a 16-year-old boy with chronic myelogenous leukemia (CML), was scheduled to receive a blood transfusion. He was pretreated with IV diphenhydramine to prevent allergic reactions. He had previously received three doses of diphenhydramine in the prior 36-hour period for itching and insomnia. After transfusion, he complained of blurry vision, appeared flushed and became agitated. He also reported that there were cameras in his room and snakes coming out of his arm. On examination, he had dilated pupils, dry mucous membranes, and flushed skin. He was assessed as having classic signs of an anticholinergic delirium related to his treatment with diphenhydramine.

In the palliative care setting, delirium often results from aggressive treatment of pain and suffering, which can lead to drug-induced change in mental status.[9] A study of 40 critically ill children[5] found that the most frequent causes of delirium in decreasing order included a change in analgosedative medication, neurological disorders, infections, and respiratory disorders. Often there were multiple causes for delirium. Infection was twice as often the precipitating factor compared with drug induced-delirium in one report.[4] A thorough diagnostic workup to identify the cause is the standard of care[37]; however, in the palliative care setting where the goal of care is to decrease pain and suffering, this approach is often modified.

Pathogenesis

Delirium is a neuropsychiatric disorder involving global encephalopathy dysfunction caused by multiple impaired neural pathways and physiologic compromises. The neurotransmitters that have been implicated in the pathophysiology of delirium include acetylcholine, dopamine, glutamine, gamma aminobutyric acid (GABA), and serotonin.[34] Dopamine is thought to modulate mood and cognitive function, and in excess can lead to psychotic disorders. Similarly, acute alterations in dopamine levels may contribute to the characteristic symptoms of delirium. Antipsychotic medications that inhibit the dopamine pathway are effective in treating delirium.[38] Alteration of GABA, an inhibitory neurotransmitter, may also cause changes in cerebral functioning, possibly by affecting sleep patterns. In the critical and palliative care setting medications such as benzodiazepines and propofol, which directly affect

GABA receptors, are frequently used and have been found to contribute to the development of delirium in the ICU setting.[39] Likewise, acetylcholine deficiency is associated with delirium and the use of anticholinergic drugs has been found to precipitate and worsen symptoms of delirium.[40] These neurotransmitter perturbations are thought to cause neuronal membrane hyperpolarization, thus spreading neuronal depression, which is seen on EEG as a diffuse slowing.[41]

Other insults to cerebral functioning such as inflammation, hypoxia, metabolic encephalopathies, and drugs or toxins, are implicated in the development of delirium. Inflammation, caused by infection, surgery or other tissue injury, heightens blood-brain barrier permeability leading to translocation of inflammatory mediators, such as cytokines and chemokines, into the CNS, causing encephalopathy dysfunction.[42] Cytokines such as interleukin (IL)-1, IL-2, interferon (IFN) and tumor necrosis factor (TNF) can affect neuronal pathways by inhibiting acetylcholine, leading to agitation, perceptual disturbances, seizures, and delirium.[43] There are reports of chemokine elevations in patients with delirium, and one study found IL-6 increase in children with influenza that developed delirium.[44] Inability to meet oxygen needs, either because of increased demand or decreased delivery, contributes to development of delirium because of disruption of ionic gradients, neurotransmitter homeostasis, and neurotoxic byproduct elimination. The compromise of oxygen metabolism can be due to hypoglycemia, hyper- or hypothermia, and vitamin or amino acid deficiencies. Impaired oxygen metabolism leads to reduced neurotransmitter synthesis, causing a deregulation of sleep-wake cycle, behavior and mood, and psychomotor activity, all of which are clinical manifestations of delirium.[38,45]

Assessment

The diagnosis of delirium is primarily made on clinical examination, which should always include an interview with parents and primary caregivers. There should also be a review of the medical chart, including laboratory and imaging test results. Nursing staff and parents' observations are particularly important to evaluate fluctuations in levels of consciousness and sleep disturbance. The Nursing Staff Delirium Screening Scale (NDSS) provides a quick and consistent measure for the clinicians who have the most frequent clinical contact with patients.[46] Although not generally standard of care, EEG findings may offer diagnostic support of delirium and perhaps subtype.[41] Additionally, family members serve as a valuable clinical resource regarding the patient's state of arousal, activity, and orientation, especially in the pediatric population. In palliative care, the education of patients and family members in recognizing signs of delirium can aid in assessment and early intervention, minimize distress to the patient and family, and support clinical decision making in end-of-life care.

To supplement and help guide the direct clinical evaluation, there are a number of structured assessments and rating scales to diagnose and track symptoms related to delirium (Table 28-3). These tools include assessment for cognitive impairment, such as Mini Mental Status Exam[47]; screening for delirium using DSM-IV-TR diagnostic criterias including the Confusion Assessment Measure[48,49]; and delirium-specific numeric scales to rate severity, that is, Delirium Rating Scale-Revised-98 (DRS-R-98).[50] The DRS-R-98 is widely used to assess delirium in adults

using a 16-item scale with items that include disturbances of cognition, perception, thought, language, sleep, affect, and psychomotor function. Items are rated based on direct observation, data from the medical record, and accounts from caregivers. The DRS-R-98 has been proved reliable for both the diagnosis and the serial assessment of delirium, and has been used and validated for pediatric patients.[51] The Pediatric Anesthesia Emergence Delirium Scale (PAEDS) is a measure designed to rate post-surgical emergence delirium and has been validated for use in children.[26] Unlike other scales, the PAEDS is a clinician report of observed behaviors and responses to stimuli, which differentiate it from the DRS-R-98. The pediatric Confusion Assessment Measure (p-CAM) is a two-part assessment tool that screens for overall cognitive impairment using the Richmond Agitation Sedation Scale (RASS) and then distinguishes delirium from other causes of cognitive impairment.[52,53] Unlike the DRS-R-98, the p-CAM is designed to diagnose delirium rather than to rate symptom severity. The Pediatric Index of Mortality (PIM)[54] and the Pediatric Risk of Mortality (PRISM II)[55] are scales used in the pediatric intensive care setting to predict outcome. Using PIM and PRISM, one study[56] found the positive predictive value was low mostly due to few identified cases of delirium, 40 out of 877 patients, the negative predictive value was very high at 99%, suggesting that these scales can be used to rule out non-occurrence of delirium.[56] A 2009 study suggested an algorithm for diagnosing and managing pediatric delirium using the RASS and PAEDS.[23] As the authors point out, further research is required to validate any proposed methods. Likewise, the overview (see Fig. 28-1, p. 262) included in this chapter highlights important aspects of identifying and treating pediatric delirium. Further research will be needed to establish best evidenced-based practices (see Table 28-3).

Treatment

An interdisciplinary approach for the clinical management of delirium combines the identification of risk factors, patient and family education, environmental modification, treatment of underlying etiologies, and use of appropriate medications. In the setting of comfort care, the management of delirium is further complicated by the goal of providing relief from suffering while avoiding medication-induced delirium when treating pain and other discomforts. For example, patients with terminal illness often receive, or are withdrawn from, high doses of opiates and benzodiazepines, which may cause delirium. Another challenge in the pediatric population is differentiating between agitation, delirium, fear, anxiety, and pain. Few age-appropriate validated assessments tools are available that easily make the distinction in young patients.[57,58] Parents often are the best indicators of the nature and intensity of their child's distress. Parent opinion regarding symptoms of discomfort should be sought by clinical staff. The interdisciplinary treatment team, the patient, and the family should create repeated opportunities to discuss goals of care regarding treatment and comfort. When illness cure is no longer the goal, symptomatic control remains the sole aim; refractory symptoms of discomfort may necessitate deeper or palliative sedation.[8]

The first step in the management of delirium should be to treat the underlying cause. In the palliative population this approach requires prudence and collaboration. More simple, less invasive interventions may include restoring electrolyte

TABLE 28-3 Scales to Assess Pediatric Delirium

Scale	Objective and intended use	Development	Areas assessed and items rated	Validity and strengths	Questions and possible limitations
Pediatric Anesthesia Emergence Delirium Scale (PAEDS)[26]	Assessment of emergence delirium post sedation	Sikich and Lerman[26] (2004) 5 of 27 proposed items were validated for the measurement of delirium emerging from anesthesia	Assesses: • Disturbance of consciousness • Change in cognition Items rated: • Eye contact with caregiver • Purposeful actions • Awareness of surroundings • Restlessness • Inconsolability	• Deemed valid and reliable in children in its intended clinical context • Used with children 2 yrs and older	• Based on the subjective rating by clinician • Lacks validation against DSM-IV criteria for diagnosis of delirium • Most easily identifies hyperactive delirium and may fail to detect cases of hypoactive delirium
Pediatric-Confusion Assessment Measure (p-CAM)[52]	Diagnosis and screening of delirium in PICU patients Ratings may be completed by clinicians without psychiatric specialty training	Vanderbilt Pediatric Delirium Group Adaptation of the adult CAM-ICU[48,49] The Richmond Agitation Sedation Scale (RASS)[53] is used in conjunction with the p-CAM	Assesses: • Level of consciousness via the RASS • Content of consciousness Items rated: • Acute change in mental status or fluctuating course • Inattention • Altered level of consciousness • Disorganized thinking	• Piloted in children 5 yrs and older in a small clinical group • Adapted from the CAM-ICU to be age appropriate • Validations studies currently in progress	• Suitable for use in non-sedated patients • Low scores on the RASS may lead to failure to recognize cases of hypoactive delirium • May not be suitable for use in children under 5 yrs old
Delirium Rating Scale-Revised-98 (DRS-R-98)[50]	Initial assessments of delirium and sequential ratings over time to track clinical progress and response to treatment	Trzepacz et al[50] (1998) Turkel et al[51] (2003)	Assesses: • DSM criteria for delirium Items rated: • Two items to assess onset and temporality • Eight items to assess symptoms	• Deemed valid and reliable in children • Used widely with adults and available in multiple languages • Used for diagnosis and ongoing assessment of illness course	• Turkel et al[4] (2006) report that hallucinations and delusions occur less frequently in children than adults and may not be required symptoms in the diagnosis of pediatric delirium • Total scores did not predict mortality or length of hospital stay in pediatric patients in contrast to studies of adult patients
Pediatric Risk of Mortality (PRISM II)[55] Pediatric Index of Mortality (PIM)[54]	Originally designed to predict mortality in critically ill patients	Schieveld et al[56] Four-year prospective study in an ICU setting following 877 consecutive admissions	Assesses: • Medical stability • Severity of illness Items rated: • Vital signs • Acid/base status • Ventilation status • Pupillary dilatation • Coagulation • Electrolytes	Ability of scale to predict pediatric delirium: PRISM • Sensitivity, 76% • Specificity, 62% PIM • Sensitivity 82% • Specificity, 62%	• Low number of children with delirium in the study (40/877; 4.6%) • Low positive predictive value • High negative predictive value • Useful in predicting the likely non-occurrence of delirium

imbalances, ensuring adequate hydration and oxygenation, judicious tapering of medications, controlling pain, and treating infections.[1] Clinicians should conduct a diagnostic workup taking into account the treatment goals of the specific patient and weighing such factors as distress related to invasive procedures as well as the potential efficacy of the intervention.[37] In an effort to minimize suffering, it should be noted that in one prospective adult study[59] the cause of delirium was identified in less than 50% of terminally ill patients. Advanced care planning involving the family, and the patient when age appropriate, is essential in managing palliative care crises such as delirium. Anticipating delirium, which can occur in 85% of adult palliative care patients,[10] should be an essential step in end-of-life treatment planning. Children as young as 10 years old have demonstrated the ability to express preferences regarding end-of-life treatment, an understanding of possible consequences to their decisions, and the capacity to weigh complex issues.[60] Education about delirium before onset is an opportunity for pediatric patients and their families to participate in care, especially those with chronic illness, and thereby minimize distress and promote a sense of agency.

PREVENTION

Awareness of the major risk factors for delirium is critical for prevention and early recognition. Although current research focuses on risk factors in adults, there is overlap with the pediatric population. Risk factors can be divided into three categories: predisposing, precipitating, and environmental factors (Table 28-4).

Delirium prevention involves clinical staff and family education, recognition of high-risk populations, correction of underlying illness, appropriate medication management, and environmental interventions. Education of family members can be an investment in comprehensive clinical care. Education of medical staff, both physicians and nurses, is also important because they have control over such issues as rate of medication tapering and maintenance of an appropriate environment. High-risk populations, such as post-surgical patients, those being weaned from intubation and those with underlying neurological and psychiatric conditions, should be closely monitored. Environmental interventions include orientation to date and time, social interactions and activities during the day, sleep hygiene at night, such as light and noise reduction, relaxation including calming music, massage and reassurance, and avoidance of immobility with ambulation or bedside exercises.

TABLE 28-4   Risk Factors for Delirium

Predisposing factors	Precipitating factors	Environmental factors
Age	Electrolyte imbalance	Immobility
Genetic predisposition	Hypoxia	Light
	Acidosis	Noise
Neurological disease	Hypoalbuminemia	Reduced social interactions
	Fever	
Psychiatric illness	Hypotension	Pain
Visual impairment	Sepsis	Use of IV lines
Hearing impairment	Infection	Physical restraints
	Polypharmacy	
Surgery	Oversedation	
	Medication withdrawal	
	Sleep deprivation	

Medications, which are often major contributors to the development of delirium, should be chosen with care and with appropriate evaluation of possible unwanted drug-drug interactions. In the palliative care setting, careful attention to the dosing and scheduling of sedatives, analgesics, anticholinergics, including some low-potency antipsychotics, corticosteroids, and anticonvulsants, is essential in reducing the incidence of delirium. In particular, tapering medications should be carefully managed because withdrawal from drugs such as opioids and benzodiazepines can trigger or worsen symptoms of delirium. Pain should also be frequently assessed and appropriately managed. In the palliative care setting, avoiding medications that may exacerbate delirium is often the first and only step taken to treat delirium, particularly when it is not possible to treat the primary immediate cause, such as cancer.[61]

NONPHARMACOLOGIC TREATMENT

Nonpharmacologic treatment of delirium should focus on correction of underlying causes, reorientation, and patient safety. Interventions such as restoring electrolyte imbalances, ensuring adequate hydration and oxygenation, improving bowel and bladder function, slow taper of medications, controlling pain, and treating infections have been shown to improve the rate of delirium recovery.[1,62]

Environmental modifications are also beneficial. An effort should be made to orient the patient using calendars, clocks, and familiar objects such as toys and pictures.[5] There should be a clear distinction between night and day to help restore disturbances in the sleep-wake cycle. Some options include the minimization of noise and light at night, organizing vital sign checks, procedures, and medications at a time that does not interrupt sleep, and massage and music for relaxation. During the day, social interactions that are soothing and familiar should be encouraged. Every effort should be made to minimize the use of catheters, intravenous lines, and other items that limit physical mobility. Family, visitors, and clinical staff should attempt to speak in short simple sentences, avoiding confrontation and provide reassurance whenever possible. Patients should ideally be placed in a single-patient room with either one-on-one nursing or a family member present. This direct observation is important to ensure patients do not harm themselves or others. If the patient is highly agitated, physical restraints may be necessary to prevent dislodgement of lines or catheters. However, physical restraints have been reported as an independent risk factor for delirium and should be used only with careful monitoring and a clear, time-limited plan.[62] The appropriate use of the nonpharmacologic measures should include a thoughtful and supportive discussion with family members (Table 28-5).

PHARMACOLOGIC INTERVENTIONS

While a diagnostic workup of potential causes is being conducted, pharmacologic interventions may still be required to manage symptoms in patients with delirium (Table 28-6). Antipsychotic and sedative agents can be used to diminish levels of agitation, correct disturbances in the sleep-cycle, and minimize perceptual disturbances. Haloperidol, second-generation antipsychotics, and benzodiazepines have all been used in the treatment of delirium with varying degrees of success. The side effect profile of each agent should be

TABLE 28-5 Nonpharmacologic Management
Guideline for Pediatrics

Intervention type	Potential activities
Sensory and environmental modification	Favorite or soothing music Gentle touch and massage Minimize immobilizing lines, catheters, and restraints Minimize noise Calming and clear speech Lighting Familiar objects in the room and with patient when leaving the room
Caregiver measures	Proper body alignment • Assist with passive range of motion • Avoid immobility Time and place re-orientation • Boards to communicate with pictures or words • Clocks • Photos • Daily schedules to promote sleep-wake cycles Sleep protocols Play favorite movies and/or shows Parental participation in care Parental and significant other presence Parents holding child in bed or chair Scheduling medications and treatments to accommodate child's routine and minimize intrusion

considered and individualized to each patient. Moreover, treatments should always be accompanied by adequate pain management and monitoring of potential medication withdrawal reactions.

Haloperidol, one of the first-generation antipsychotics, is the most frequently used pharmacologic treatment of delirium.[63] Although not approved by the Federal Drug Administration (FDA) for treatment of delirium, reasons for its use include considerations of efficacy, cost, and intravenous route of administration. Intravenous use results in more reliable absorption, decreased incidence of extrapyramidal reactions, and minimal effects on blood pressure, respiration, and heart rate.[64,65] The intravenous dose is twice as potent as oral administration. This high-potency agent is preferred to low-potency antipsychotics because of the decreased likelihood of hypotensive and anticholinergic effects, and has been found to be safe and effective in managing cases of pediatric delirium.[66] In the palliative care population, subcutaneous and intramuscular injection are also convenient options. The primary mechanism of haloperidol's action is inhibition of dopaminergic pathways that may be overstimulated in states of hyperactive delirium, thus helping restore normal thought patterns and sensorium. The cautious use of haloperidol is recommended in patients with hypoactive delirium, who may already have dopaminergic suppression and consequently its use may exacerbate symptoms of delirium.[39] A double-blinded, randomized control trial compared haloperidol, chlorpromazine, and lorazepam for the treatment of delirium reports both haloperidol and chlorpromazine as effective in improving symptoms of delirium and cognitive function, while lorazepam was not only ineffective but also worsened symptoms in some patients.

All antipsychotics have side effects and patients must be closely monitored. Serious adverse reactions requiring immediate medical attention include malignant hyperthermia. Also, extrapyramidal movement disorders including laryngeal spasm, hypotension, and glucose and lipid dysregulation; anticholinergic effects, such as constipation, urinary retention, and dry mouth; and cardiac effects such as QTc prolongation and torsades de pointes, need to be monitored. Electrocardiogram monitoring is strongly recommended for those on intravenous haloperidol. Significant complications such as dystonia, hypotension, and hyperpyrexia in more than 20% of pediatric burn patients treated with haloperidol were reported.[68]

Second-generation antipsychotics, such as risperidone, olanzapine, and quetiapine, is another option for the treatment of delirium. Most second-generation antipsychotics act on both dopaminergic and serotonergic receptors. Their side effect profile is commonly reported as more favorable than that of the first-generation antipsychotics. Although there have been few efficacy studies directly comparing the second-generation antipsychotic agents and haloperidol, there may be some benefits in terms of the second-generation antipsychotic side effect profile.[62,69] A review on the topic concluded that second-generation antipsychotics are effective in treating delirium and have fewer side effects compared with high-dose haloperidol. In addition, in the case of hypoactive delirium, second-generation antipsychotics may be indicated because their mechanisms of action extend beyond dopamine blockade and affect other pathways likely implicated in the pathophysiology of delirium.[24] Disadvantages of second-generation antipsychotic agents include the lack of an intravenous formulation. Although most of these agents must be given orally, some, such as risperidone and olanzapine, have intramuscular and sublingual formulations (see Table 28-6).

Like haloperidol, second-generation antipsychotics also carry an FDA warning of increased risk of death, mostly cardiovascular related, in elderly patients. Controlled studies for delirium in the pediatric population, comparing both classes of antipsychotics for efficacy and safety, have yet to be undertaken. Of note, all of the antipsychotics are employed off-label when used to treat delirium. The second-generation antipsychotics have been tested in children with approval for other indications. For example, risperidone has been approved for use in children ages 5 to 16 for management of aggressive behavior related to autism. Olanzapine is indicated for the treatment of schizophrenia and manic or mixed episodes of bipolar disorder in 13- to 17-year-olds. These medications can be safely used at low doses in young children with appropriate monitoring when treating delirium.[70]

Benzodiazepines, such as lorazepam and diazepam, are GABA agonists that treat distress related to anxiety and sleep-wake cycle disturbance in delirious patients. They have amnesic properties and consequently can worsen cognitive impairment. There are also reports of paradoxical effects, such as aggression, violence, and irritability in pediatric patients.[71] In general, there appears to be some consensus that benzodiazepines should not be used as first-line agents in the treatment of pediatric delirium. In addition, a longer duration of benzodiazepines and opiate use in critically ill children was associated with increased reports of delusional memory, which is associated with greater risk for post-traumatic stress disorder.[72] In some cases when a benzodiazepine is required, lorazepam combined with haloperidol for severe agitation in older adolescent and adult patients has been beneficial.[62]

Figure 28-1 describes an algorithm that depicts the key factors and decision points salient to education, assessment, and treatment of delirium in the pediatric palliative care setting. Although

TABLE 28-6 Pharmacologic Management Guidelines for Pediatrics

Clinical Scenario: Agitated or NPO

Medication: Haloperidol IV

Dosing: 0.01-0.02 mg/kg q1h prn agitation or psychotic symptoms x 3 days then reassess

Age	Weight	Low end of range (per dose)	High end of range (per dose)	Max daily dose
1-3 yrs	10-20 kg	0.1 mg	0.4 mg	1 mg/day
>3-6 yrs	20-30 kg	0.2 mg	0.6 mg	2 mg/day
>6-10 yrs	30-40 kg	0.3 mg	0.8 mg	4 mg/day
>10-18 yrs	>40 kg	0.4 mg	1 mg	7 mg/day

Clinical Scenario: Not Agitated and Taking PO

Medication: Risperidone

Dosing: 0.0125-0.025mg/kg q6h prn psychotic symptoms x 3 days then reassess

Age	Weight	Low end of range (per dose)	High end of range (per dose)	Max daily dose
1-3 yrs	10-20 kg	0.125 mg	0.5 mg	1 mg
>3-6 yrs	20-30 kg	0.25 mg	0.75 mg	2 mg
>6-10 yrs	30-40 kg	0.375 mg	1 mg	3 mg
>10-18 yrs	>40 kg	0.5 mg	1 mg	4 mg

Clinical Scenario: Agitated with insomnia and taking PO,

Medication: Olanzapine

Dosing: QHS for delirium with insomnia x 3 days then reassess

Age	Weight	Low end of range (per dose)	High end of range (per dose)	Max daily dose
7-10 yrs	30-40 kg	1.25 mg	2.5 mg	2.5 mg
>10-18 yrs	>40 kg	2.5 mg	5 mg	5 mg

this algorithm is not an evidenced-based protocol, it does suggest a paradigm for understanding delirium and its management.

Palliative care, as an interdisciplinary field, lends itself to the management of delirium with its fluctuating course and multiple causes. All members of the care team should play a role in the education, prevention, detection, and treatment of delirium. Roles can be divided into educator, detector, screener, and treater. Anyone with patient contact should be warned about the potential for delirium and become an educator. For example, the evening shift nurse can educate the mother about delirium. The mother then teaches the sibling, who will be with the patient during the day about the possibility of confusion, agitation, and other associated signs. The ultimate goal is to educate the patient and all caregivers about the phenomenon of delirium for the purpose of preventing and identifying signs and symptoms if they occur. Anyone with patient contact should be trained as a detector. This includes primary and consulting physicians, nurses, social workers, psychologists, chaplains, dieticians, and therapists (respiratory, physical, occupational, and child-life specialists).

A smaller subset of the care team, which manages daily patient care responsibilities, will be systematic screeners and treaters. If delirium is suspected as a result of systematic screening, and the primary team has evaluated for poly-pharmacy intoxication or withdrawal, and has made the appropriate intervention without improvement, a pediatric psychiatry con-

sult should be requested. At that time, further information from detectors and screeners should be collected to develop a longitudinal picture of the patient's mental status. Once delirium is diagnosed, every member of the care team should be instructed in the appropriate nonpharmacologic interventions. Screeners and treaters, that is, nurses and doctors, will administer pharmacologic treatment and track progress. This team approach also suits the goals of comfort care for monitoring pain, anxiety, and nausea.

Sequelae of Delirium

The psychological and cognitive impact of delirium on patients, families, and caregivers of critically ill adults at the end of life has been well explored and reviewed.[8] Delirium is related to longer hospital stay, higher rates of morbidity and mortality, and negative outcome post recovery.[73,74] Post-traumatic stress disorder (PTSD) in adults following the experience of delirium has also been reported.[75,76,77]

POST-TRAUMATIC STRESS DISORDER

The recognition of post-traumatic stress disorder in medically ill patients, including those receiving treatment in ICUs, is now well recognized. These symptoms include flashbacks, nightmares, avoidance of reminders, anger, and hypervigilance.[16] More recently, there have also been a number of studies examining the relationship between PTSD and the experience of delirium. This is particularly relevant because there is evidence that a great number of patients with mild to moderate delirium (43% of those with hypoactive delirium and 66 % of patients with hyperactive features), recall their experience.[75] This vignette describes the traumatic experience of delirium and its impact.

> *Cassie, a 14-year-old girl with a history of asthma, was admitted for treatment of acute respiratory distress syndrome. After initial continuous nebulized albuterol treatments, she went into respiratory failure and was intubated and transferred to the ICU. She remained on the ventilator for 3 days before being extubated. Although Cassie improved medically, she became increasingly anxious, particularly when approached by nursing staff. She also had increased difficulty sleeping at night. At one point, she became combative, and hit her nurse while she was attempting to administer an IV medication with a syringe.*
>
> *Cassie received a psychiatry consultation, and was noted to be confused and disoriented during her evaluation. Careful questioning elicited the history that Cassie believed that her nurse was attempting to kill her by injecting poison into her IV line. She also reported being afraid to fall asleep at night, believing that someone might come into her room at night to turn off her oxygen supply. Cassie was diagnosed with acute delirium and started on risperidone 0.5 mg bid. She made a rapid recovery, and was soon transferred to a general pediatric unit, and then home.*
>
> *Cassie was seen in follow-up a month after her discharge. A psychiatric consultation was requested again after her mother reported that Cassie was still having difficulties sleeping at night and had missed 13 of her last 17 regular school*

days. Cassie reported persistent distressing dreams as well as intrusive memories of her hospitalization, prompted by events such as watching television episodes of "ER" or visiting the hospital. She described conscious efforts to avoid things that reminded her of her experience. She tried to be outside as much as possible because being indoors gave her a boxed-in feeling that reminded her of the ICU. She was also reluctant to take her asthma medications, and stated that she worried that they might be contaminated, even though she knew this to be impossible. In addition, she described a feeling of a foreshortened future and fear that she was likely to die at an early age because of asthma. Cassie was assessed as having symptoms of post-traumatic stress disorder related to the traumatic medical experience during her inpatient hospitalization. Her symptoms persisted despite vigorous attempts by her parents to reassure her, and were clearly interfering with her ability to function at school. She was referred to the local university child psychiatry clinic for further evaluation and treatment.

Adult and pediatric studies have explored the association between delirium and PTSD in intensive care patients and have found that those with delusional memories have increased risk of developing PTSD symptoms compared with those with factual memories.[72,78] Because alterations in memory and perception are common presentations of delirium, children with delirium may be at greater risk of developing PTSD. Such sequelae should not be taken lightly because it can cause significant social impairment and can negatively impact academic performance.[79]

If pediatric patients experience delirium, when they recover it is appropriate to ask what they remember. Some children do not recall the experience or report positive associations.[72] The specifics of delusions should not be over-interpreted (e.g., intravenous lines being perceived as snakes) rather, themes of fear, anxiety, loss, and mortality can be considered and explored. Further psychological support is recommended both for patient and the family if delirium has been distressing whether for themselves or for anyone else, including caregivers and staff.

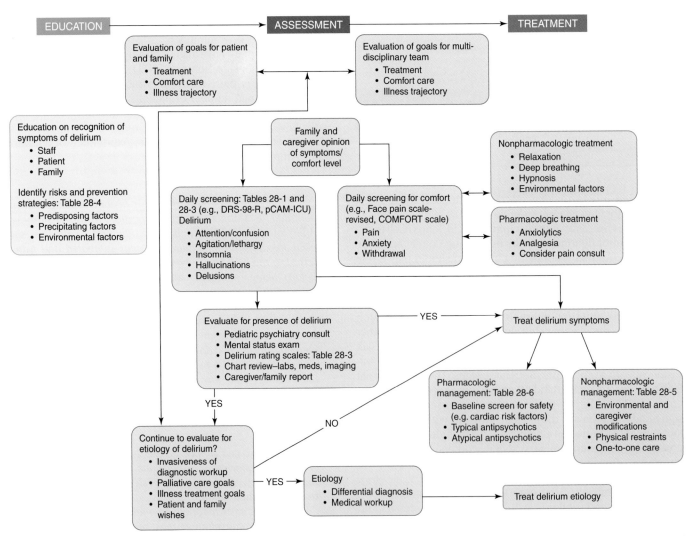

Fig. 28–1 Algorithm for education, assessment, and treatment of delirium. (Redrawn from Niranjan S. Karnik, Shashank V. Joshi, Caroline Paterno, and Richard Shaw. Subtypes of Pediatric Delirium: A Treatment Algorithm Psychosomatics, May-June:48:253–257 in Pediatric Delirium in Palliative Care. *Reprinted with permission from Psychosomatics, [copyright 2007]. American Psychiatric Publishing, Inc.*)

IMPACT ON CAREGIVERS

Delirium affects not only patients but also family members and medical staff. Mean distress levels regarding delirium on a 4.0 scale were highest among spouses (3.75), nurses (3.09), and then patients (3.02).[77] For families, hyperactive delirium and severe physical debilitation were the strongest predictors of distress in contrast to nurses who rated the severity of the delirium and perceptual disturbances more highly.[77] Interviews conducted of bereaved family members who witnessed delirium revealed they were often troubled by feelings of guilt and helplessness, struggled with making proxy decisions, and worried about the burden of care.[80] Families often equate signs of delirium with pain or discomfort, going crazy, and death anxiety.[80] In addition, family members of patients with delirium reported both concerns about inadequate medical care as well as a desire for more information about the condition.[81]

These accounts by families likely reflect the challenge that medical staff face when caring for patients with delirium. Nurses commonly reported stress from increased workload, safety concerns for themselves and their patients, and difficulty finding a balance between connecting with the patient and being on guard.[82] Long-term consequences for caregivers are yet to be fully investigated. Similarly, parents who have children hospitalized in intensive care are at increased risk of developing PTSD.[83] All caregivers, including parents, siblings, nurses, doctors, other clinicians, social workers, and clergy are at risk of psychological sequelae from traumatic experiences with critically ill patients.

Summary

Pediatric patients experiencing delirium constitute a high-risk population because of developmental vulnerabilities associated with their neurophysiology, challenges in assessment, and advancements in life-prolonging medical therapies. Delirium is associated with a number of indices of medical morbidity that include increased length of hospital stay and elevated rates of both morbidity and mortality.[84,85] In addition, research has shown associations with poor functional outcome, cognitive decline, and patient and family emotional distress in patients with delirium.[77,86,87] Research in adult intensive care patients has shown a threefold increase in mortality in patients diagnosed with delirium independent of other risk factors.[88] Similarly, studies in pediatric patients have reported mortality rates as high as 20%.[3] Because pediatric delirium is an often under-diagnosed and reversible complication of serious illness with significant negative impact, further research has the potential to improve patient care and outcome across all disciplines.

Many challenges await additional study. The diagnosis of delirium in children is based on DSM-IV-TR criteria described for adult patients and may not be applicable to the pediatric population. Efforts to improve the prospective assessment of pediatric delirium may benefit from incorporating advancements in medical technology, including motion detectors, as well as expanded knowledge of motoric subtypes. Valid and reliable assessment tools that are age appropriate and based on interdisciplinary agreed-upon diagnostic criteria are few. There are no evidence-based treatment guidelines existing for the management of pediatric delirium or for pediatric delirium in the palliative care setting. In addition, variations in the treatment of delirium based on differences in genetic predisposition, etiology, and pathophysiological disturbance demands further exploration. Finally, educational materials for clinicians and families about the risk factors and signs of delirium as well as the potential for cognitive impairment and PTSD are limited. Delirium should be recognized as a medical complication that spans many clinical domains and all age groups. In managing delirium, clinicians can capitalize on interdisciplinary collaboration and research with the goal of enhancing patient care, family support, and clinical outcomes.

REFERENCES

1. Smith HA, Fuchs DC, Pandharipande PP, et al: Delirium: an emerging frontier in the management of critically ill children, *Crit Care Clin* 25(3):593–614, 2009.
2. Prugh DC, Wagonfield S, Metcalf D, et al: A clinical study of delirium in children and adolescents, *Psychosom Med* 42:177–195, 1980.
3. Turkel SB, Tavaré CJ: Delirium in children and adolescents, *J Neuropsychiatry Clin Neurosci* 15:431–435, 2003.
4. Turkel SB, Trzepacz PT, Tavare CJ: Comparison of delirium in adults and children, *Psychosomatics* 47:320–324, 2006.
5. Schieveld JN, Leroy PL, van OSJ, et al: Pediatric delirium in critical illness: phenomenology, clinical correlates and treatment response in 40 cases in the pediatric intensive care unit, *Intensive Care Med* 33:1033–1040, 2007.
6. Leentjens AF, Schieveld JN, Leonard M, et al: A comparison of the phenomenology of pediatric, adult, and geriatric delirium, *Psychosomatics* 64:219–223, 2008.
7. Nauck F, Alt-Epping B: Crises in palliative care: a comprehensive approach, *Lancet Oncol* 9:1086–1091, 2008.
8. Leonard M, Agar M, Mason C, et al: Delirium issues in palliative care settings, *J Psychosom Res* 65:289–298, 2008.
9. Breitbart W, Lawlor P: Delirium in the terminally ill. In Chochinov M, editor: *Oxford handbook of psychiatry in palliative care medicine*, ed 2, Oxford, 2009, Oxford University Press, pp 81–100.
10. Massie MJ, Holland J, Glass E: Delirium in terminally ill cancer patients, *Am J Psychiatry* 140:1048–1050, 1983.
11. Lawlor PG, Gagnon B, Mancini IL, et al: Occurrence, causes, and outcome of delirium in patients with advanced cancer: a prospective study, *Arch Intern Med* 160:786–794, 2000.
12. Flaherty JH, Rudolph J, Shay K, et al: Delirium is a serious and under-recognized problem: why assessment of mental status should be the sixth vital sign, *J Am Med Dir Assoc* 8(5):273–275, 2007.
13. Leentjens AFG, MacLullich AF, Meagher DJ: Delirium, Cinderella no more . . . ? *J Psychosom Res* 65:205, 2008. Epub 2008 Jul 24.
14. Institute of Medicine of the National Academies: *When children die: improving palliative and end of life care for children and their families*, New York, 2003, The National Academies Press.
15. Manuela Pretto M, Spirig R, Milisen K, et al: Effects of an interdisciplinary nurse-led Delirium Prevention and Management Program (DPMP) on nursing workload: a pilot study, *Int J Nurs Stud* 46(6):804–812, 2009. Epub 2009 Feb 27.
16. American Psychiatric Association, *Diagnostic and statistical manual of mental disorders*, ed 4 revised, (DSM-IV-TR), Washington, DC, 2000, American Psychiatric Press.
17. Wise MG, Trzepacz PT: Delirium (Confusional States). In Rundell JR, Wise MG, editors: *Textbook of consultation-liaison psychiatry*, Washington, DC, 1996, American Psychiatric Press, pp 258–275.
18. Morandi P, Pandharipande M, Trabucchi, et al: Understanding international differences in terminology for delirium and other types of acute brain dysfunction in critically ill patients, *Intensive Care Med* 34:1907–1915, 2008.
19. Girard TD, Pandharipande PP, Ely EW: Delirium in the intensive care unit, *Crit Care* 12(Suppl 3):S3, 2008.
20. Przybylo HJ, Martini DR, Mazurek AJ, et al: Assessing behaviour in children emerging from anaesthesia: can we apply psychiatric diagnostic techniques? *Paediatr Anaesth* 13:609–616, 2003.
21. Gupta N, de Jongheb J, Schieveld J, et al: Delirium phenomenology: what can we learn from the symptoms of delirium? *J Psychosom Res* 65:215–222, 2008.
22. Liptzin B, Levkoff SE: An empirical study of delirium subtypes, *Br J Psychiatry* 161:843–845, 1992.

23. Schieveld JNM, van der Valk JA, Smeets I, et al: Diagnostic considerations regarding pediatric delirium: a review and a proposal for an algorithm for pediatric intensive care units, *Intensive Care Med* 35:1843–1849, 2009.

24. Karnik NS, Joshi SV, Paterno C, Shaw R: Subtypes of pediatric delirium: a treatment algorithm, *Psychosomatics* 48(3):253–257, 2007.

25. Gupta AK, Saravay SM, Trzepacz PT, et al: Delirium motoric subtypes, *Psychosomatics* 46:158, 2005.

26. Sikich N, Lerman J: Development and psychometric evaluation of the pediatric anesthesia emergence delirium scale, *Anesthesiology* 100(5):1138–1145, 2004.

27. Morita T, Tei Y, Tsunoda J, et al: Underlying pathologies and their associations with clinical features in terminal delirium of cancer patients, *J Pain Symptom Manage* 22:997–1006, 2001.

28. Lam PT, Tse CY, Lee CH: Delirium in a palliative care unit, *Prog Palliat Care* 11:126–133, 2003.

29. Spiller JA, Keen JC: Hypoactive delirium: assessing the extent of the problem for inpatient specialist palliative care, *Palliat Med* 20:17–23, 2006.

30. Peterson JF, Pun BT, Dittus RS, et al: Delirium and its motoric subtypes: A study of 614 critically ill patients, *J Am Geriatr Soc* 54:479–484, 2006.

31. Kobayashi K, Takeuchi O, Suzuki M, et al: A retrospective study on delirium type, *Jpn J Psychiatry Neurol* 46:911–917, 1992.

32. Ross CA, Peyser CE, Shapiro I, et al: Delirium: phenomenologic and etiologic subtypes, *Int Psychogeriatr* 3(2):135–147, 1991.

33. Meagher DJ, O'Hanlon D, O'Mahony E, et al: Relationship between symptoms and motoric subtype of delirium, *J Neuropsychiatry Clin Neurosci* 12:51–56, 2000.

34. Maldonado J: Pathoetiological model of delirium: a comprehensive understanding of the neurobiology of delirium and an evidence-based approach to prevention and treatment, *Crit Care Clin* 24:789–856, 2008.

35. O'Malley G, Leonard M, Meagher D, et al: The delirium experience: a review, *Psychosom Res* 65(3):223–228, 2008.

36. Godfrey A, Conway R, Leonard M, et al: A classification system for delirium subtyping with the use of a commercial mobility monitor, *Gait Posture* 30(2):245–252, 2009.

37. Trzepacz PT, Breitbart W, Franklin J, et al: Practice guideline for the treatment of patients with delirium, *Am J Psychiatry* 156:11, 1999.

38. Van der Mast RC: Pathophysiology of delirium, *Geriatr Psychiatr Neurol* 11:138–145, 1998.

39. Maldonado JR: Delirium in the acute care setting: characteristics, diagnosis and treatment, *Crit Care Clin* 24(4):657–722, vii, 2008.

40. Rummans TA, Evans JM, Krahn LE, et al: Delirium in elderly patients: evaluation and management, *Mayo Clin Proc* 70(10):989–998, 1995.

41. Jacobson S, Jerrier H: EEG in delirium, *Semin Clin Neuropsychiatry* 5:86–92, 2000.

42. Rudolph JL: Chemokines are associated with delirium after cardiac surgery, *J Gerontol Med Sci* 63A:184–189, 2008.

43. Dunlop RJ, Campbell CW: Cytokines and advanced cancer, *J Pain Symptom Management* 20:214–232, 2000.

44. Fukumoto Y, Okumura A, Hayakawa F, et al: Serum levels of cytokines and EEG findings in children with influenza associated with mild neurological complications, *Brain Dev* 29(7):425–430, 2007. Epub 2007 Feb 6.

45. Eikelenboom P, Hoogendijk WJG, Jonker C, et al: Immunologic mechanisms and the spectrum of psychiatric syndromes in Alzheimer's disease, *J Psychiatric Res* 36:269–280, 2002.

46. Gaudreau JD, Gagnon P, Harel F, et al: Fast, systematic, and continuous delirium assessment in hospitalized patients: the nursing delirium screening scale, *J Pain Symptom Manage* 29:368–375, 2005.

47. Folstein MF, Folstein SE, McHugh PR: "Mini-mental state": a practical method for grading the cognitive state of patients for the clinician, *J Psychiatr Res* 12:189–198, 1975.

48. Inouye SK, Vandyck C, Alessi C, et al: Clarifying confusion: the confusion assessment method: a new method for the detection of delirium, *Ann Intern Med* 113(12):941–948, 1990.

49. Ely EW, Margolin R, Francis J, et al: Evaluation of delirium in critically ill patients: validation of the Confusion Assessment Method for the Intensive Care Unit (CAM-ICU), *Crit Care Med* 29(7):1370–1379, 2001.

50. Trzepacz PT, Mittal D, Torres R, et al: Validation of the Delirium Rating Scale-Revised-98 (DRS-R-98), *J Neuropsychiatry Clin Neurosci* 12:156, 2001.

51. Turkel SB, Braslow K, Tavare CJ, et al: The Delirium Rating Scale in children and adolescents, *Psychosomatics* 44:126–129, 2003.

52. Smith H, Ely W: *A multi-site validation study for the Pediatric Confusion Assessment Measure: Vanderbilt delirium group*, Nashville, Tenn, in process via personal communication with Dr. Heidi Smith.

53. Sessler CN, Gosnell MS, Grap MJ: The Richmond Agitation-Sedation Scale: validity and reliability in adult intensive care unit patients, *Am J Respir Crit Care Med* 166(10):1338–1344, 2002.

54. Shann F, Pearson G, Slater A, et al: Pediatric index of mortality (PIM): a mortality prediction model for children in intensive care, *Intensive Care Med* 23:201–207, 1997.

55. Pollack MM, Ruttimann UE, Getson PR: The Pediatric Risk of Mortality (PRISM) score, *Crit Care Med* 16:1110–1116, 1988.

56. Schieveld JNM, Lousberg R, Berghmans E, et al: Pediatric illness severity measures predict delirium in a pediatric intensive care unit, *Crit Care Med* 36(6):1933–1936, 2008.

57. Hicks CL, von Baeyer CL, Spafford P, et al: The *Faces Pain Scale—Revised*: Toward a common metric in pediatric pain measurement, *Pain* 93:173–183, 2001.

58. Ambuel B, et al: Assessing distress in pediatric intensive care environments: The COMFORT Scale, *J Pediatr Psychol* 17:95–109, 1992.

59. Breura E, Miller L, McCallion J: Cognitive failure in patients with cancer: a prospective study, *J Pain Symptom Manage* 7(4):192–195, 1992.

60. Hinds PS, Drew D, Oakes LL, et al: End-of-life care preferences of pediatric patients with cancer, *J Clin Oncol* 23(36):9146–9154, 2005.

61. Gagon R: Treatment of delirium in supportive and palliative care, *Curr Opin Support Palliative Care* 2:60–66, 2008.

62. Breitbart W, Alici Y: Agitation and delirium at the end of life, *JAMA* 300(24):2898–2910, 2008.

63. Ely EW, Stephens RK, Jackson JC, et al: Current opinions regarding the importance, diagnosis, and management of delirium in the intensive care unit: a survey of 912 healthcare professionals, *Crit Care Med* 32(1):106–112, 2004.

64. Beliles KE: Alternative routes of administration of psychotropic medications. In Stoudemire A, editor: *Psychiatric care of the medical patient*, ed 2, Oxford, 2000, Oxford University Press, pp 395–405.

65. Menza MA, Murray GB, Holmes VF, et al: Decreased extrapyramidal symptoms with intravenous haloperidol, *J Clin Psychiatry* 48:278–280, 1987.

66. Brown RL, Henke A, Greenhalgh, et al: The use of haloperidol in the agitated, critically ill pediatric patient with burns, *J Burn Care Rehabil* 17:34–38, 1996.

67. Breitbart W, Marotta R, Platt M, et al: A double-blind trial of haloperidol, chlorpromazine, and lorazepam in the treatment of delirium in hospitalized AIDS patients, *Am J Psychiatry* 153(2):231–237, 1996.

68. Ratcliff SL, Meyer WJ, Cuervo LJ, et al: The use of haloperidol and associated complications in the agitated, acutely ill pediatric burn patient, *J Burn Care Rehabil* 25(6):472–478, 2004.

69. Liu CY, Juang YY, Liang HY, et al: Efficacy of risperidone in treating the hyperactive symptoms of delirium, *Int Clin Psychopharmacol* 19(3):165–168, 2004.

70. Turkel SB: Delirium. In Shaw RJ, DeMaso DR editors: *Textbook of pediatric psychosomatic medicine*, Washington, DC, 2010, American Psychiatric Publishing, Inc, pp 63–75.

71. Saïas T, Gallarda T: Paradoxical aggressive reactions to benzodiazepine use: a review, *Encephale* 34(4):330–336, 2008. Epub 2007 Dec 26.

72. Colville G, Kerry S, Pierce C: Children's factual and delusional memories of intensive care, *Am J Respir Crit Care Med* 177(9):976–982, 2008. Epub 2008 Jan 31.

73. Levkoff SE, Evans DA, Liptzin B, et al: Delirium: the occurrence and persistence of symptoms among elderly hospitalized patients, *Arch Intern Med* 152(2):334–340, 1992.

74. Newman MF, et al: Report of the sub-study assessing the impact of neurocognitive function on quality of life 5 years after cardiac surgery, *Stroke* 32(12):2874–2881, 2001.

75. DiMartini A, Dew MA, Kormos R, et al: Posttraumatic stress disorder caused by hallucinations and delusions experienced in delirium, *Psychosomatics* 48(5):436–439, 2007.

76. Dew MA, Kormos RL, DiMartini AF, et al: Prevalence and risk of depression and anxiety-related disorders during the first three years after heart transplantation, *Psychosomatics* 42(4):300–313, 2001.

77. Breitbart W, Gibson C, Tremblay A: The delirium experience: delirium recall and delirium-related distress in hospitalized patients with cancer, their spouses/caregivers, and their nurses, *Psychosomatics* 43:183–194, 2002.

78. Jones C, Griffiths RD, Humphris G, et al: Memory, delusions, and the development of acute posttraumatic stress disorder-related symptoms after intensive care, *Crit Care Med* 29(3):573–580, 2001.

79. Yasik AE, Saigh PA, Oberfield RA, et al: Posttraumatic stress disorder: memory and learning performance in children and adolescents, *Psychiatry* 61(3):382–388, 2007. Epub 2006 Aug 22.

80. Morita T, Akechi T, Ikenaga M, et al: Terminal delirium: recommendations from bereaved families' experiences, *J Pain Symptom Manage* 34(6):579–589, 2007. Epub 2007 Jul 26.

81. Namba M, Morita T, Imura C, et al: Terminal delirium: families' experience, *Palliat Med* 21(7):587–594, 2007.

82. Lou MF, Dai YT: Nurses' experience of caring for delirious patients, *J Nurs Res* 10(4):279–290, 2002.

83. Balluffi A, Kassam-Adams N, Kazak A, et al: Traumatic stress in parents of children admitted to the pediatric intensive care unit, *Pediatr Crit Care Med* 5(6):547–553, 2004.

84. Inouye SK, Rushing JT, Foreman MD, et al: Does delirium contribute to poor hospital outcome? *J Gen Intern Med* 13:234–242, 1998.

85. McCusker J, Cole M, Abrahamowicz M, et al: Delirium predicts 12-month mortality, *Arch Intern Med* 162:457–463, 2002.

86. Trzepacz PT, Meagher DJ: Delirium. In Levenson JL, editor: *Textbook of psychosomatic medicine*. Washington, DC, 2005, American Psychiatric Publishing, pp 91–130.

87. Morita T, Akechi T, Ikenaga M, et al: Terminal delirium: recommendations from bereaved families' experiences, *J Pain Symptom Manage* 34:579–589, 2007.

88. Ely EW, Shintani A, Truman B, et al: Delirium as a predictor of mortality in mechanically ventilated patients in the intensive care unit, *JAMA* 291(14):1753–1762, 2004.

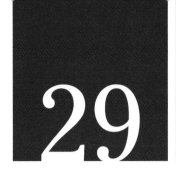

29 Fatigue

JOY HESSELGRAVE | MARILYN HOCKENBERRY

It's like my legs weigh 100 pounds…[1]
You think about it, dwell on it and it makes it worse. So, part of it is mental and part of it is physical fatigue. You are not your normal self and you are just tired of everything that has happened.[1]
It's like being wiped out … my body is just too tired for me to care.[2]

Fatigue, physical, mental, and emotional, is an under-studied symptom in children living with a life-threatening illness. Despite its prevalence throughout the trajectory of many conditions, clinicians tend to focus on the more obvious side effects of illness and treatment. This chapter reviews the research in management of fatigue in children with implications for clinical assessment and intervention.

The direct effects of disease, side effects of treatment[3] and medications prescribed to manage these contribute to fatigue in children with life-threatening illnesses. Infection, electrolyte imbalance, anemia, dehydration, malnutrition, endocrine dysfunction, and organ impairment are all factors. Psychological states including anxiety, fear, depression, and feelings of isolation and loneliness also influence the frequency and intensity of fatigue.[4] Sleep disruption and poor sleep quality contribute to fatigue in children, particularly at the end of life. Sleep deprivation may worsen pain that exacerbates their tiredness. Children with cancer identify the hospital environment as a major contributing factor to fatigue because of the frequent disruptions in their sleep[5] (Tables 29-1 and 29-2).

Children's Descriptions of Fatigue

Children are able to use expressive descriptors of physical fatigue such as "not being able to 'run or play with friends'" or looking in a mirror and seeing themselves as a "dull face." They also describe aspects of emotional fatigue in terms of withdrawing from others, being irritable and feeling "mad" or "sad."

Researchers exploring fatigue in seriously ill children confirm that perceptions of fatigue differ by developmental age.[6–8] Younger children tend to emphasize the physical sensation of fatigue more than emotional aspects, and describe, for example, how watching television or reading comprise their main activities.

Adolescents tend to be more cognitively aware of the impact of fatigue on their lives, and often describe the symptom in terms of its effect on their lifestyle. They also highlight mental tiredness that alternates and at times merges with the physical sensation of fatigue.[3,7–10] Teens describe activities that they can no longer perform and their inability to be with peers as significant changes brought on by fatigue. They are more aware of the relationship of the symptom to their overall illness or treatment. For example, adolescents can define when fatigue occurs in relation to their chemotherapy cycle.

Research on Fatigue in Children

Research on fatigue in children has focused primarily on children with rheumatologic disorders and cancer. Fatigue is characterized as a distressing, pervasive symptom with physical, mental, and emotional components characterized by a lack of energy.[9,10]

Children with juvenile rheumatoid arthritis and systemic lupus erythematous (SLE) describe fatigue as a common symptom.[11,12] In a study of 51 children with juvenile polyarticular arthritis, researchers found fatigue present along with pain and joint stiffness on more than 70% of days with significant variability in symptom levels.[13] Researchers found a positive relationship between stress and mood and same-day variations in fatigue. A study of 15 children with SLE found fatigue to be a significant symptom in 67% of the children.[14] These children also had reduced aerobic fitness compared to age and sex-matched reference norms. Fatigue was a significant symptom in a group of 52 children with Crohn's disease.[15] They had lower quality of life scores and significantly more fatigue compared with healthy controls.

Fatigue is the most frequent symptom experienced by children with cancer.[9,10,16–20] In a survey of parents of children with cancer and their treating clinicians, 57% in each group reported fatigue as a frequent symptom.[19] In a qualitative study of children receiving treatment for cancer, researchers generated a detailed description of fatigue: a core concept or energy, a core process or managing dwindling energy, and a typology of three types of fatigue: typical tiredness, treatment fatigue, and shutdown fatigue.[18] Children with leukemia described fatigue, both disease and treatment-related, as having the greatest impact on their quality of life by altering participation in school, sports, and family activities. In a pilot study of nine school-age children with leukemia, diaries revealed evening fatigue and sleep disturbances[21] during the maintenance phase of treatment. Fatigue was also the most frequently reported symptom in a group of 161 acute lymphocytic leukemia survivors,[22] even many years after treatment.

Studies have specifically addressed fatigue at the end of life within the childhood cancer population.[23] A landmark study of symptoms and suffering at the end of life found that all 103 families surveyed report that their child had experienced fatigue during the last month of life.[4] In a Swedish nationwide survey of 449 parents of children with cancer, 86% reported physical fatigue as the most frequently reported symptom that had moderate or high impact on their child's well-being.[24]

TABLE 29-1 Fatigue: Contributing Factors in Children with a Life-Threatening Illness

Factor	Possible causes
Physical	Infection
	Electrolyte problems
	Metabolic abnormalities
	Dehydration
	Malnutrition
	Organ dysfunction
	Inactivity
	Anemia
	Hormone imbalance
	Sleep deprivation
	Medications, such as opioids, antiemetics, antidepressants, antihistamines
	Pain
Psychological	Anxiety
	Fear
	Loneliness
	Isolation
	Decreased enjoyment
	Depression

A study of 65 parents of children who had died of cancer within the previous 6 to 10 months revealed that fatigue was one of the most frequently reported symptoms, along with pain, and changes in behavior, appearance, and breathing.[25] Similar findings were found in 32 parents whose child had died within the past 3 years. They reported that the symptom burden was high during the palliative phase, with pain, poor appetite, and fatigue as the most frequently reported physical symptoms. Emotional symptoms included sadness, difficulty talking about feelings, and fear of being alone.[26] Fatigue was a prevalent symptom in a group of 28 Japanese children at the end of life.[27] In interviews with 30 parents whose children had received pediatric home hospice services, fatigue was one of the most frequently identified symptoms during the last week of their child's life[28] (Fig. 29-1).

A qualitative study exploring factors that influence quality of life in 49 children and adolescents with epilepsy found excessive fatigue as a barrier to academic and social pursuits. Participants described how intermittent or continuous fatigue made it difficult to think clearly and to fully participate in classroom learning.[29]

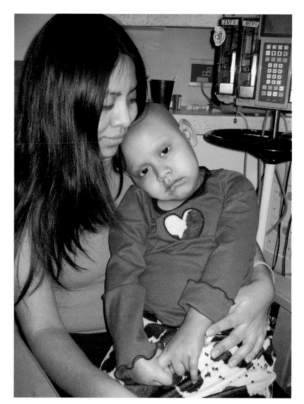

Fig. 29-1 Parents need help with understanding the significant effects fatigue can have on their child.

Fatigue may provide protection, as a shield from suffering, during the final stages of life; and treatment of fatigue at this stage of palliative care may be detrimental.[30] When the death of a child is imminent, fatigue often intensifies and withdrawal from family and friends occurs as a result of diminished energy. Preparing the family for this eventuality may prevent their misinterpretation of tiredness as depression, or, even more painful, as a rejection of them (Fig. 29-2).

Assessment of Fatigue

Many patients and families assume that fatigue is an inevitable and untreatable side effect of disease or treatment and thus often do not report it as a symptom. Furthermore, until recently, standardized assessment of fatigue by clinicians has been oversimplified, as a yes or no checklist,[6] or entirely absent.

Guidelines from the National Comprehensive Cancer Network recommend routine screening for fatigue as the sixth vital sign. Those older than 12 years of age should be screened using a simple numeric rating scale such as 0, no fatigue, to 10, worst fatigue. For children 7 to 12 years of age, a 1 to 5 point scale is recommended. For children aged 5 and 6 years the words tired or not tired should be used to determine fatigue. Once screened, patients should be evaluated for the seven treatable contributing factors to fatigue, which is informally referred to as the gang of seven: anemia, pain, sleep difficulties, nutrition issues, changes in activity patterns, emotional distress, and presence of co-morbidities.[31–33] The health care team should assess for the onset and type of fatigue, aggravating or alleviating factors, and degree of interference with the child's functioning.

TABLE 29-2 Signs and Symptoms of Fatigue in Children

Domain	Clinical findings
Cognitive	Inability to concentrate
	Not able to think
	Forgetfulness
	Lack of focus
Physical	Weakness
	Difficulty walking or running
	No energy
	Tiredness
	Heaviness throughout body
	Lethargy
	Desire to rest and lie down
Emotional	Irritability
	Depressed
	Non-communicative
	Sad or mad

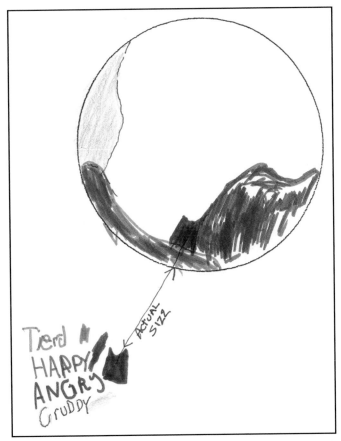

Fig. 29-2 "Tired." Katie, age 10, did her last drawing days before her death from neuroblastoma. She was calm and deliberate, although very weak as she chose these feeling and color matches: tired is medium blue; happy is deep blue; angry is dark green; cruddy is pale blue. Her one comment, spoken quietly with a smile, was: "I wanted to make 'happy' bigger, but I am too tired to draw anymore....I am happy with my family." (Reprinted with permission from Sourkes, B. Pediatric Palliative Care: An Overview. In *INSIGHTS*, A Publication of the National Hospice and Palliative Care Organization. Alexandria: 2004).

Several research instruments are available to assess symptom clusters in children, including fatigue, although none was designed specifically for end of life. Once fatigue has been identified as a specific symptom it may be useful to use one of the validated and reliable pediatric fatigue scales, such as the Memorial Symptom Assessment Scale (MSAS), Edmonton Symptom Assessment Scale (ESAS), or the Pediatric Quality of Life (PedsQL) scale.[34]

The Childhood Fatigue Scale (CFS) is a 14-item (four-point Likert scale) questionnaire that asks children (ages 7 to 12 years) about their tiredness during the previous week. The three subscales are: lack of energy, inability to function, and altered mood.[8,35] Parent Fatigue Scale (PFS) is a 17-item inventory of parents' perception of their child's fatigue in the previous week. In addition to the three subscales on the children's version, it also included a scale of altered sleep. The Fatigue Scale-Adolescent (FS-A) is a 14-item questionnaire that asks adolescents (ages 13 to 18 years), to evaluate their fatigue experience during the previous week. The child and parent scales are available in English and Spanish; the adolescent form in English only. The CFS, PFS, and FS-A are validated research instruments, easy to administer, and require limited time to complete in the clinical setting.[8,35,36]

The PedQL Multidimensional Fatigue Scale is an 18-item research instrument (ages 2 to 18) with three subscales: general fatigue, sleep-rest fatigue, and cognitive fatigue. The scale is self-administered for 8 to 18 year olds, interview-administered in 5 to 7 year olds and done by parent proxy for the youngest children. It is available in 22 languages.[37,38] The Pediatric Functional Assessment of Chronic Illness Therapy-Fatigue (Peds FACIT-F) is an 11-item scale for children with cancer that measures fatigue in the past 7 days. It is correlated with the Peds QL Multidimensional Fatigue Scale and is available in English and Spanish.[35,39]

Interventions for Fatigue

Research on interventions for fatigue in children is at an early stage of development. The following two studies describe selected variables in exploring the management of fatigue.

Sixty Turkish children, ages 7 to 12 years, with leukemia or lymphoma, who were receiving their first 7- to 10-day course of chemotherapy, were randomized to an experimental group who received fatigue education or a control group who received standard care. The experimental group received a handbook on fatigue and nutritional counseling. Children and their mothers identified strategies that could decrease fatigue, such as minimizing interruptions at night during hospitalization. Developmentally appropriate activities included reading, art, music, and walking in the hallway for 10 to 15 minutes. After a 7-day period, the children were evaluated using the Child Fatigue Scale (CFS) and Parent Fatigue Scale (PFS). Mean scores for the experimental group was significantly lower than the control group. Methods that helped alleviate fatigue were taking naps, walking, eating well-balanced meals, increasing visitor interaction, and having fun activities to distract from the sense of being tired.[40]

In another study, 13 children ages 5 to 15 years with leukemia and lymphoma and their parents were interviewed regarding quality of life during therapy.[18] One area dealt with ways to replenish, conserve, and preserve energy to alleviate physical, mental, and emotional fatigue. Strategies to replenish energy or promote relaxation included taking hot baths and naps, receiving massage, or engaging in quiet activities. Distractions such as watching television, playing with animals, and doing puzzles were also helpful. Conserving strategies included activities that required minimal energy expenditure such as watching television without the sound, resting the mind, having only familiar people around, sleeping, being read to, and having alone time. Children's preserving strategies to minimize further energy loss were more inward: withdrawing, ignoring people, and creating a quiet environment. Teenagers reported that the loss of control over their environment and a lack of age-appropriate activities contributed to their fatigue.[18]

The management of fatigue is most effective when an interdisciplinary team contributes to the plan for an individual child[33] (Table 29-3). Strategies to alleviate fatigue should be an intrinsic part of dealing with a complex of associated symptoms, such as anemia, pain, sleep disturbances, and depression (Table 29-4). Children and families should be taught that while fatigue is a normal and expected symptom, there are strategies to mitigate its effects. Suggestions include setting priorities for activities and scheduling them during peak energy times, maintaining a consistent daily routine, limiting naps to

TABLE 29-3 Interdisciplinary Approach to Fatigue Interventions

Discipline	Interventions
Nursing	• Develop plan to minimize energy expenditure • Develop a schedule and routine for each day • Encourage short rest periods during the day • Stress importance of self pacing to prevent tiredness • Encourage development of specific bedtimes and wake times • Prevent sleep interruptions at night
Medicine	• Provide information on the impact cancer treatment can have on energy level and performance • Participate in the development of interventions that minimize energy expenditure
Psychology and/or social work	• Provide opportunities for child and family to express concerns regarding decreased energy capacity
Child life	• Encourage activities that minimize energy expenditure • Teach child and/or family stress reduction techniques such as relaxation, guided imagery, and distraction to facilitate rest
Nutrition	• Encourage good nutrition to promote energy
Physical and/or occupational therapy	• Discuss important of exercise to promote energy • Encourage activities that involved rhythmic or repetitive movement of large muscle groups • Emphasize importance of a developmentally appropriate exercise program

20 to 30 minutes so as not to interfere with nighttime sleep, and using play and distractions.[32,33,41]

Johnny, an 8-year-old boy with a progressive neurologic illness, was hospitalized frequently because of an increase in his uncontrolled seizures. During one of these admissions, his mother commented that he had less energy than before and would often fall asleep during the day, something he had not done since he was 3. The interdisciplinary team worked with Johnny's mother to establish a schedule and routine for each day. Specific bedtime and wake times were established and a rest period was encouraged each afternoon. The child life specialist identified Johnny's favorite activities and encouraged play that minimized energy expenditure. The nutritionist worked with the mother to identify Johnny's favorite foods and emphasized the importance of choosing those that promote energy. The social worker spent time with the parents, allowing them to express their concerns about the changes that they were observing in Johnny. A physical therapy consult was set to develop an age-appropriate exercise plan for Johnny. In a follow-up outpatient appointment, the mother reported that she had implemented all the strategies and that Johnny was showing renewed strength and energy.

SLEEP

Inquiry and guidance regarding sleep hygiene should be integrated into regular clinic and hospital visits. The need for regular and adequate sleep is particularly important to emphasize when counseling adolescents. Considerations in the hospital include clustering care and creating a restful environment in the room.[18] Limiting caffeinated drinks and foods as well as vigorous exercise within 4 hours of bedtime can promote better rest. Maintaining a consistent bedtime routine, quiet environment, and the presence of a security object are effective in promoting sleep.[33] Pharmacologic interventions may be used[3] and are further discussed in Chapter 30.

EXERCISE

Randomized controlled trials have demonstrated that exercise decreases fatigue in adults.[3] Recommendations for both adults and children include starting with a low-intensity exercise regimen and adjusting as needed based on the patient's clinical condition.[32] Before initiating an exercise program, a referral to physical therapy, occupational therapy, or physical medicine should be considered.

TABLE 29-4 Possible Interventions for Fatigue and Contributing Symptoms

Correct potential factors associated with fatigue	Medical/pharmacologic interventions	Nonpharmacolgic interventions
Anemia	Transfusion Erythropoeitin Supplemental iron	Educate regarding foods high in iron
Pain	Provide adequate pain management, including adjuvants	Cognitive behavioral therapies Complementary and alternative medicine (CAM)
Sleep disturbances*	Careful consideration of hypnotics	Modify activity and rest Sleep hygiene Minimize nighttime interruptions while hospitalized CAM
Inactivity		Incorporate activity, exercise regimen as tolerated
Depression	Antidepressants	Cognitive behavioral therapies CAM
Symptomatic fatigue	Consider pscho-stimulants such as methylphenidate, detroamphetamine Low-dose steroids	Patient education Exercise Adequate nutrition and hydration Stress management Cognitive and behavioral therapies CAM

*Increasing periods of sleep are normal at the end of life

NUTRITION

Children with chronic illnesses or debilitating conditions may be at particular risk for nutritional deficits that exacerbate fatigue. Interventions are guided by the assessment of caloric intake, fluid and electrolyte imbalances, and any barriers to intake. Megestrol acetate has been used to increase appetite but there is limited research in children.[42] Correcting sodium, potassium, calcium, or magnesium electrolyte imbalances may improve fatigue symptoms as well as providing nutritional supplements. It is well recognized that decreased appetite and oral intake are common at the end of life and that the interventions at this phase of life will be different[33] (Chapter 33).

ANEMIA

Some adult studies indicate correcting anemia with erythropoietin for cancer patients has improved their quality of life.[3,33] However, in children with cancer, erythropoietin improved the anemia but it did not significantly improve their quality of life. Correcting anemia alone does not address the multidimensional factors associated with fatigue.[43] If anemia is identified as the significant factor in the child's fatigue, red cell transfusions and erythropoietin may be considered.

PHARMACOLOGIC AGENTS

Psycho-stimulants may be considered after careful evaluation of fatigue. Improvement in fatigue in adults has been documented with the use of methylphenidate and modafinil. While there is extensive evidence that methylphenidate is useful in the treatment of attention deficit hyperactivity disorder in children, there are no studies evaluating its use for fatigue.[42] Only one case series supports the use of methylphenidate to decrease fatigue in adolescents who were receiving opioids.[44] Corticosteroids and adenosine triphosphate infusions are described as pharmacologic therapies for fatigue but there are no data for their use in children.[3,33]

Complementary and Alternative Medicine

Complementary and alternative medicine (CAM) is a growing field and data suggest that many parents pursue these therapies for their children. Estimates of pediatric CAM use range from 2% to 70%.[45] A 2007 National Health Interview survey evaluated CAM use in 9000 children under 17 years and found that 12% had used some form of CAM during the previous 12 months.[46] A recent survey of 281 families reported that 52.3% of children had used one or more types of CAM therapies in the previous year. Children with epilepsy and cancer used CAM most frequently.[47] In a review of 482 pediatric and adolescent charts, 34.6% were taking 1 to 10 CAM products. A significant predictor of this use was a presenting symptom of poor energy or fatigue.[45]

When faced with life-threatening illnesses, parents often pursue CAM therapies to ensure that they have left no stone unturned.[48] Patients and families tend to seek CAM when symptoms are not adequately treated with conventional approaches.[49] The National Center for Complementary and Alternative Medicine has identified four major domains of CAM therapies: mind-body medicine, manipulative body-based practices, energy, and biologic therapies.[48] Massage is the CAM most frequently cited for fatigue management. Incorporating cognitive behavior therapy (CBT), stress management, guided imagery, and relaxation also may reduce fatigue.[33]

Over a 1-year period, 17 parent-child dyads were randomized to receive massage therapy or quiet time and then crossed over to the other treatment option. Pain, nausea, anxiety, fatigue, vital signs, and cortisol levels were assessed. There were no significant changes in fatigue with either the massage or the quiet time. Children reported feeling relaxed but some had a difficult time conceptualizing the difference between fatigue and relaxation.[50] A study of 68 mothers who received massage while their children were hospitalized had decreased fatigue and increased vigor. Researchers suggested that decreasing fatigue in mothers caring for their sick children may lead to improved support to their children.[51] Healing touch and acupuncture in adults have demonstrated effectiveness in reducing cancer-related fatigue but no studies are available in children.[48]

L-Carnitine deficiency is observed in pediatric AIDS patients and both adult and pediatric cancer patients presenting with fatigue.[48,52] Earlier studies suggest that a week of carnitine supplementation reduced fatigue and improved functioning in adult hospice patients without adverse events. However, a recent double-blind, placebo-controlled study in adults did not support the reversal of cancer-related fatigue even though serum levels improved with L-carnitine supplementation.[48,52] In a double-blind randomized controlled trial with 15 adult hospice patients who received transcutaneous electrical nerve stimulation (TENS) for 6 days found that fatigue improved significantly over the sham TENS.[53]

Summary

Children with life-threatening illnesses frequently experience fatigue. Repeated assessment is essential, because this symptom can wax and wane greatly over time and is influenced by numerous factors. Interventions provided by an interdisciplinary health care team allow for strategies that focus on minimizing energy expenditure and promoting quality of life.

REFERENCES

1. Hockenberry-Eaton M, Hinds PS, Alcoser P: Fatigue in children and adolescents with cancer, *J Pediatr Oncol Nurs* 15(3):172–182, 1998.
2. Hicks J, Bartholomew J, Ward-Smith P, et al: Quality of life among childhood leukemia patients, *J Pediatr Oncol Nurs* 20(4):192–200, 2003.
3. Ullrich CK, Mayer OH: Assessment and management of fatigue and dyspnea in pediatric palliative care, *Pediatr Clin North Am* 54:735–756, 2007.
4. Wolfe J, Grier HE, Klar N, et al: Symptoms and suffering at the end of life in children with cancer, *N Engl J Med* 342:326–333, 2000.
5. Hinds PS, Hockenberry M, Rai SN, et al: Nocturnal awakenings, sleep environment interruptions, and fatigue in hospitalized children with cancer, *Oncol Nurs Forum* 34:393–402, 2007.
6. Eddy L, Cruz M: The relationship between fatigue and quality of life in children with chronic health problems: a systematic review, *J Spec Pediatr Nurs* 12:105–114, 2007.
7. Hockenberry-Eaton M, Hinds PS: Fatigue in children and adolescents with cancer. In Winningham ML, Barton-Burke M, editors: *Fatigue in cancer*, Boston, 2000, Jones and Bartlett Publishers, pp 71–85.
8. Hockenberry MJ, Hinds PS, et al: Three instruments to assess fatigue in children with cancer: the child, parent and staff perspectives, *J Pain Symptom Manage* 25(4):319–328, 2003.
9. Hockenberry-Eaton M, Hinds PS, Alcoser P: Fatigue in children and adolescents with cancer, *J Pediatr Oncol Nurs* 15(3):172–182, 1998.

10. Hockenberry-Eaton M, Hinds P, O'Neill JB, et al: Developing a conceptual model for fatigue in children, *Eur J Oncol Nurses* 3(1):5–11, 1999.

11. Ward TM, Brandt P, Archbold K, et al: Polysomnography and self-reported sleep, pain, fatigue, and anxiety in children with active and inactive juvenile rheumatoid arthritis, *J Pediatr Psychol* 33:232–241, 2008.

12. Sällfors C, Hallberg LR, Fasth A: Well-being in children with juvenile chronic arthritis, *Clin Exp Rheumatol* 22:125–130, 2004.

13. Schanberg LE, Gil KM, Anthony KK, et al: Pain, stiffness, and fatigue in juvenile polyarticular arthritis: contemporary stressful events and mood as predictors, *Arthritis Rheum* 52:1196–1204, 2005.

14. Houghton KM, Tucker LB, Potts JE, et al: Fitness, fatigue, disease activity, and quality of life in pediatric lupus, *Arthritis Rheum* 59:537–545, 2008.

15. Marcus SB, Strople JA, Neighbors K, et al: Fatigue and health-related quality of life in pediatric inflammatory bowel disease, *Clin Gastroenterol Hepatol* 7:554–561, 2009.

16. Perdikaris P, Merkouris A, Patiraki E, et al: Changes in children's fatigue during the course of treatment for pediatric cancer, *Int Nurs Rev* 55:412–419, 2008.

17. Whitsett SF, Gudmundsdottir M, Davies B, et al: Chemotherapy-related fatigue in childhood cancer: correlates, consequences, and coping strategies, *J Pediatr Oncol Nurs* 25:86–96, 2008.

18. Davies B, Whitsee S, Bruce A, et al: A typology of fatigue in children with cancer, *J Pediatr Oncol Nurs* 19(1):12–21, 2002.

19. Gibson F, Barnett M, Richardson A, et al: Heavy to carry, a survey of parents' and healthcare professionals perceptions of cancer-related fatigue in children and young people, *Cancer Nurs* 28(1):27–35, 2005.

20. Erickson JM: Fatigue in adolescents with cancer: a review of the literature, *Clin J Oncol Nurs* 8:139–145, 2004.

21. Gedaly-Duff V, Lee KA, Nail LM, et al: Pain, sleep disturbance, and fatigue in children with leukemia and their parents: a pilot study, *Oncol Nurs Forum* 33(3):641–646, 2006.

22. Meeske KA, Hicks J, Bartholomew J, Ward-Smith P, et al: Quality of life among childhood leukemia patients, *J Pediatr Oncol Nurs* 20(4):192–200, 2003.

23. Mooney-Doyle K: An examination of fatigue in advanced childhood cancer, *J Pediatr Oncol Nurs* 23:305–310, 2006.

24. Jalmsell L, Kreicbergs U, Onelov E, et al: Symptoms affecting children with malignancies during the last month of life: a nationwide follow-up, *Pediatrics* 117:1314–1320, 2006.

25. Pritchard M, Burghen E, Srivastava DK, et al: Cancer-related symptoms most concerning to parents during the last week and last day of their child's life, *Pediatrics* 121:e1301–e1309, 2008.

26. Theunissen JM, Hoogerbrugge PM, van Achterberg T, et al: Symptoms in the palliative phase of children with cancer, *Pediatr Blood Cancer* 49(2):160–165, 2007.

27. Hongo T, Watanabe C, Okada S, et al: Analysis of the circumstances at the end of life in children with cancer: symptoms, suffering and acceptance, *Pediatr Int* 45:60–64, 2003.

28. Hendricks-Ferguson V: Physical symptoms of children receiving pediatric hospice care at home during the last week of life, *Oncol Nurs Forum* 35(6):E108–115, 2008.

29. Elliott IM, Lach L, Smith ML: I just want to be normal: a qualitative study exploring how children and adolescents view the impact of intractable epilepsy on their quality of life, *Epilepsy Behav* 7:664–678, 2005.

30. Radbruch L, Strasser F, Eisner F, et al: Fatigue in palliative care patients-an EAPC approach, *Palliat Med* 22:13–32, 2008.

31. Piper BF, Borneman T, Sun VC, et al: Cancer-related fatigue: role of oncology nurses in translating national comprehensive cancer network assessment guidelines into practice, *Clin J Oncol Nurs* 12:37–47, 2008.

32. Mock V, Atkinson A, Barsevick AM, et al: Cancer-related fatigue: clinical practice guidelines in oncology, *J Natl Compr Canc Netw* 5:1054–1078, 2007.

33. National Comprehensive Cancer Network (NCCN). Available at www.ncc.org/professionals/physician_gls/f_guidelines.asp. Originally accessed July 25, 2009.

34. Paice JA: Assessment of symptom clusters in people with cancer, *J Natl Cancer Inst Monogr* 32:98–102, 2004.

35. Hockenberry M: Nausea, vomiting, anorexia and fatigue. In Wiener LS, Pau M, editors: *Quick Reference for Pediatric Oncology Clinicians: The Psychiatric and Psychological Dimensions of Pediatric Cancer Symptom Management*, Charlottesville, Va, 2009, IPOS Press, pp 104–107.

36. Hinds PS, Hockenberry M, Tong X, et al: Validity and reliability of a new instrument to measure cancer-related fatigue in adolescents, *J Pain Symptom Manage* 34:607–618, 2007.

37. Varni JW, Burwinkle TM, Szer IS: The PedsQL multidimensional fatigue scale in pediatric rheumatology: reliability and validity, *J Rheumatol* 31:2494–2500, 2004.

38. Varni JW, Burwinkle TM, Katz ER, et al: The PedsQL in pediatric cancer: reliability and validity of the pediatric quality of life inventory generic core scales, multidimensional fatigue scale, and cancer module, *Cancer* 94:2090–2106, 2002.

39. Lai JS, Cella D, Kupst MJ, et al: Measuring fatigue for children with cancer: development and validation of the pediatric functional assessment of chronic illness therapy-fatigue (peds FACIT-F), *J Pediatr Hematol Oncol* 29:471–479, 2007.

40. Genc RE, Conk Z: Impact of effective nursing interventions to the fatigue syndrome in children who receive chemotherapy, *Cancer Nurs* 31:312–317, 2008.

41. Radbruch L, Strasser F, Eisner F, et al: Fatigue in palliative care patients-an EAPC approach, *Palliat Med* 22:13–32, 2008.

42. McCullough R, Comac M, Craig F: Paediatric palliative care: coming of age in oncology? *Eur J Cancer* 44:1139–1145, 2008.

43. Razzouk BI, Hord JD, Hockenberry M, et al: Double-blind, placebo-controlled study of quality of life, hematologic end points, and safety of weekly epoietin alfa in children with cancer receiving myelosuppressive chemotherapy, *J Clin Oncol* 27:3583–3589, 2006.

44. Yee JD, Berde CB: Dextroamphetamine or methylphenidate as adjuvants to opioid analgesia for adolescents with cancer, *J Pain Symptom Manage* 9:122–125, 1994.

45. Wilson K, Busse J, Gilchrist A, et al: Characteristics of pediatric and adolescent patients attending a naturopathic college clinic in Canada, *Pediatrics* 115:e338–343, 2005.

46. National Center for Complementary and Alternative Medicine. Complementary and Alternative Medicine use in children. Available at http://nccam.nih.gov/health/children/ (Originally accessed July 25, 2009.)

47. Post-White J, Fitzgerald M, Hageness S, et al: Complementary and alternative medicine use in children with cancer and general and specialty pediatrics, *J Pediatr Oncol Nurs* 26:7–15, 2009.

48. Ladas E, Post-White J, Hawks R, et al: Evidence for symptom management in the child with cancer, *J Pediatr Hematol Oncol* 28:601–615, 2006.

49. Steinhorn DM, Rogers M: Complementary and alternative medicine. In Goldman A, Hain R, Liben S, editors: *Oxford textbook of palliative care for children*, Oxford, 2006, Oxford University Press, pp 484–496.

50. Post-White J, Fitzgerald M, Savik K, et al: Massage therapy for children with cancer, *J Pediatr Oncol Nurs* 26:16–28, 2009.

51. Iwasaki M: Interventional study on fatigue relief in mothers caring for hospitalized children-effect of massage incorporating techniques from oriental medicine, *Kurume Med J* 52:19–27, 2005.

52. Cruciani RA, Dvorkin E, Homel P, et al: L-carnitine supplementation in patients with advanced cancer and carnitine deficiency: a double-blind, placebo-controlled study, *J Pain Symptom Manage* 37:622–631, 2009.

53. Pan C, Morrison S, Ness J, et al: Complementary and alternative medicine in the management of pain, dyspnea, and nausea and vomiting near the end of life: a systematic review, *J Pain Symptom Manage* 20:374–387, 2000.

Sleep and Insomnia

ANTHONY HERBERT | CHRIS SETON | AMANDA GAMBLE

Disease exists, if either sleep or watchfulness be
excessive. —Hippocrates

Since antiquity, sleep has been considered a time of healing, mending, and restoration.[1] Sleeping difficulties are a significant issue for many healthy children and adolescents and are further increased in children suffering from life-threatening conditions. This can have a significant impact on both the child and his or her family. Lack of restful sleep can lead to impaired daytime functioning, increased pain, mood disturbances, altered immune function, and school or work problems for both children and parents.[2-3] Sleep also provides an important respite for children with life-threatening conditions and their parents from the daily burden associated with managing their conditions.[4]

Classification of Sleeping Problems in Childhood

Sleep problems for children and adolescents can include:

1. Disorders of initiating and maintaining sleep include difficulties at sleep onset and problems occurring during sleep that may disrupt sleep or lead to awakenings. The period of wakefulness in bed that is of concern is generally longer than 30 minutes.[5] Insomnia has been defined as an almost nightly complaint of an insufficient amount of sleep, or not feeling rested after sleep. In adults, its severity is judged by evidence of impairment of social or occupational functioning.[6] A primary form of insomnia often arising in childhood exists. In the palliative care context, the most common form of insomnia is "Sleep Disorder Due to General Medical Condition" as per the American Psychiatric Association [DSM-IV, 780.52],[7] or "Sleep Disorders Associated with Mental, Neurologic and Other Medical Disorders."[6]
2. Inability to awaken from sleep at the desired time and daytime sleepiness.[8]
3. Sleep-related behaviors in children, which include rhythmic movement disorders such as head banging and body rocking, and parasomnias. Parasomnias are abnormal behaviors during partial arousals from non-REM (rapid eye movement) sleep. They include sleep talking, sleep walking, teeth grinding or bruxism, enuresis, and night terrors. Night terrors are the most dramatic of these and occur in approximately 6% of children. Night terrors differ from a nightmare; in that there is no memory of the sleep behavior the following morning.[9]
4. Sleep disordered breathing is the general term used to describe obstructive sleep apnea (OSA), central sleep apnea (CSA), and hyperventilation or hypoventilation occurring in patients suffering from chronic respiratory diseases.

Growth and Development

An understanding of normal developmental changes in children's sleep patterns is helpful for both practitioners and families. Regular sleeping patterns generally become established by 12 months of age. Total sleep duration decreases from an average of 14.2 hours at 6 months of age to an average of 8.1 hours at 16 years of age[10] (Fig. 30-1). There is a decreasing trend for daytime napping beyond the age of 12 months, with the most prominent decline in napping habits occurring between 18 months and 4 years of age.[10] There is also a trend for children, particularly adolescents, to go to sleep at a later time compared with earlier eras, and this can be attributed to academic demands and entertainment, such as the Internet and television.[10-12]

Sleeping Difficulties in Healthy Children

Sleeping problems occur in healthy children. It has been found that 24% of children between 1 and 2 years still wake regularly at night.[13] The frequency of disrupted sleep at night continues to decrease with age, with 10% of children waking at age 8.[14] Sleeping problems are also important for adolescents, with 10% to 15% having difficulties falling asleep.[14] Erratic sleeping patterns, partly associated with hormone secretion related to puberty, can make it difficult for some adolescents to fall asleep at bedtime. While nearly all teenagers show this tendency toward delayed sleep onset, approximately 7% will be diagnosed with delayed sleep phase syndrome in which the adolescent is typically unable to fall asleep before midnight and has extreme difficulty waking up in the morning.[15] A national survey of 70,000 healthy children in the United States aged between 6 and 18 years showed 31.9% experienced more than one night of inadequate sleep in the week before the survey.[16]

Children with Life-Threatening Conditions

Sleep problems are magnified in children with respiratory, metabolic, neurologic, and malignant conditions. Insomnia can be considered a symptom in this group of children rather than a diagnosis. The cause may be peripheral in origin, such as gastroesophageal reflux causing pain or adenoidal hypertrophy with nasal obstruction causing respiratory difficulty. Alternatively, the causes of poor sleep may be central in origin, related to medications, brain tumors, seizures, and syndrome

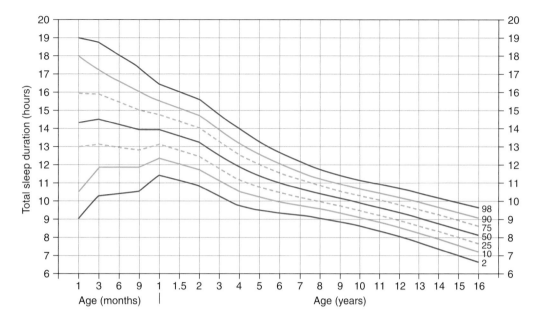

Fig. 30-1   Percentiles for total sleep duration per 24 hours from infancy to adolescence. *(Redrawn from Iglowstein I, Jenni O, Molinari L, and Largo R. Sleep Duration from Infancy to Adolescence: Reference Values and Generational Trends. Pediatrics 2003; 111: 302–307. Copyright 2003 by the AAP.)*

abnormalities with dysfunction of central sleep systems.[17] In particular, pain and sleep-disordered breathing are prevalent problems in this patient population. Sleeping difficulties have also been noted to be present in children receiving end-of-life care.

Sleep complaints are common in children and adolescents diagnosed with cystic fibrosis (CF) with approximately 40% of children reporting difficulty falling asleep and a similar proportion having difficulty staying asleep.[18] Hypoxemia and nocturnal cough account for some of these difficulties.[19,20] Various metabolic and genetic syndromes are also associated with sleep disturbance, including Rett syndrome and Angelmann syndrome.[21,22] Approximately 90% of children diagnosed with Sanfilippo syndrome have sleep disturbance.[23]

Structural brain lesions in infants and children are also often associated with difficulty falling asleep at night and nocturnal awakenings.[24] States of wakefulness are regulated by brainstem nuclei, while the establishment of circadian rhythms is dependent upon the hypothalamus and its connections. Children with midline brain pathology and blindness are at high risk for sleep disorders resulting from desynchronization of the 24-hour sleep-wake rhythm. Children with hydranencephaly, in particular, can suffer from severe sleep disturbance, demonstrating the importance that intact cerebral hemispheres have in maintaining sleep-wake cycles.

Sleep-disordered breathing can occur in patients with chronic respiratory illnesses such as chest wall, neuromuscular, primary lung diseases and heart failure. Obstructive sleep apnea in children can be caused by enlarged tonsils or adenoids. Obesity, severe scoliosis, and craniofacial deformities may also contribute to sleep-related breathing problems.[19] All of these risk factors for sleep-disordered breathing occur in children with life-threatening conditions.

Central and obstructive apneas are common and problematic for children with myopathies and other neuromuscular disease. Respiratory disorders during sleep, including apnea and hypoventilation, have been described in Duchenne muscular

dystrophy and spinal muscular atrophy.[19,24] Such children can experience ventilatory muscle fatigue, particularly in the latter hours of the night, resulting in disrupted sleep, daytime sleepiness, and headaches. Excessive daytime sleepiness was also a common sleep disturbance in children with brain tumors.[25] Problems included resumption of daytime naps, difficulty waking in the morning, and inability to remain awake during daytime activities such as school.

Approximately 31% of children with cancer treated as outpatients experienced sleeping difficulties.[26,27] This symptom was particularly distressing to 39% of 7- to 12-year-old children while 59% of 10- to 18-year-old children found this symptom to be particularly distressing. Children with cancer who are admitted to hospital for chemotherapy sleep for a longer duration and have more frequently disrupted sleep.[28] One study revealed that 80% of children with cancer experienced significant pain at the time of their diagnosis. Almost 75% of children reported that this pain led to sleep disruption.[29] The disruption of the sleep-wake pattern is a common issue adding to the fatigue that often accompanies cancer and its treatments.[30]

A survey of children attending a chronic pain clinic found that 71% had sleep disruptions.[31] Pain has been found to contribute to children waking from sleep and affecting the overall quality of sleep in a number of studies.[32,33] Pain may interfere with the ability to sleep because it can fragment sleep with frequent awakening, activate threat-related arousal to more pain, and increase vigilance that something worse may happen.[34,35] Pain and discomfort affect sleep, while poor sleep predisposes a patient to increased, pain experiences.[35,36] A study of healthy young adults found that reduced sleep led to increased sensitivity to pain.[37] A bidirectional relationship between pain and sleep may ensue such that children enter a negative downward spiral in which worsening pain disrupts sleep, which then further heightens their pain experience.

Retrospective studies of children who died found insomnia to occur in 20% to 25% of children in the terminal stage of their disease.[38,39] Fatigue is the most common symptom experienced at the end of life.[39,40] Fatigue in children with cancer has been found to negatively correlate with sleep quality.[28] Although anemia and metabolic changes may contribute to fatigue, sleeping poorly at night may be another important factor.[34] Further, medications used to treat symptoms, such as opioid analgesics, antiepileptic drugs, and benzodiazapines, and keep children comfortable can also disrupt normal sleep patterns.[41,42] Assessment can be difficult in the palliative care context where fatigue and sleepiness can arise from the disease state as well as sleep disturbance.

Effect of Hospitalization on Sleep

One survey of children ages 3 to 8 years who were admitted to a general pediatric unit found that they lost 20% to 25% of their usual sleep time.[43,44] Children admitted to intensive care lost up to 50% of their sleeping time. These changes in sleep, such as reversal of the sleep-wake cycle, can persist for up to 7 weeks after discharge from the intensive care unit.[45] A survey of children and adolescents admitted to The Children's Hospital at Westmead, Sydney, Australia, found that the overall prevalence of poor sleep in children admitted to hospital was 52%.[32] This survey included children with malignant and non-malignant life-threatening conditions, 19 and 11% of sample, respectively. The causes that woke children, in this survey, are presented in Fig. 30-2.

Sleep loss in the hospital is due to the underlying disease as well as environmental and psychosocial aspects associated with hospital admission.[35] Many factors contribute to disturbed sleep, including noise, lights, lack of control, separation from parents, unfamiliar environment, loss of normal routine, anxiety, depression, and pain.[28,44,46] Children may also have negative associations with their hospital bed if it is linked with stressors such as pain or procedures.

These studies highlight the benefits of home care in the palliative care context, given the numerous hospital related factors that disrupt sleep in children. Nevertheless, some children receiving palliative care will still require admission to the hospital at times for symptom management, respite, and end-of-life care.[47] It is therefore important for hospital environments to be conducive to sleep for children, siblings, and parents in this context.

Psychosocial Factors

Although sleep is a physiologic process, it occurs in a psychosocial context. Psychological stressors that hinder sleep onset, such as anxiety, are common in pediatric palliative care. Other psychosocial factors known to impact sleep include parental education, family stress, and cultural factors.[14,48] Children themselves may have worries about their clinical status, their situation, and fears of the dark compounded by legitimate fears of death. Fear, anxiety, depression, and anger at bedtime may make it difficult for the child to transition smoothly to sleep both at bedtime and at subsequent awakenings throughout the night. For the transition to sleep to be smooth, a child must feel safe.

Both research and clinical experience supports a relationship between childhood sleep problems and anxiety and other alterations in mood. Even modest amounts of sleep restriction result in difficulties regulating emotion and subsequent elevations in anxiety and depression.[49] Sleep problems are commonly associated with anxiety with as much as 83% of anxious children experiencing significant sleep disturbance.[50] Difficulty falling asleep, refusing to sleep alone, and nightmares are common, along with reduced total sleep time on school nights, frequent nighttime waking, and decreased deep sleep.[50-52]

The link between anxiety and sleep disturbance is both biological and behavioral. From a biological perspective, anxiety is characterized by dysregulation in the Hypothalamic Pituitary Adrenal (HPA) axis, resulting in increased secretion of cortisol which may negatively impact the timing and patterns of children's sleep. Anxious children have been found to secrete higher levels of cortisol during the pre-sleep period than depressed and healthy controls.[53] Children with anxiety may also elicit parenting responses that inadvertently maintain their sleep problems. Parents of anxious children frequently respond to their child's anxiety by over-protecting and enabling avoidance, which inadvertently maintains anxiety by limiting opportunities for children to test their fearful predictions and develop coping skills.[54,55] Parent-child interactions are similarly important in maintaining childhood sleep problems. Studies show that children who require or receive a high level of parental involvement at bedtime are more likely

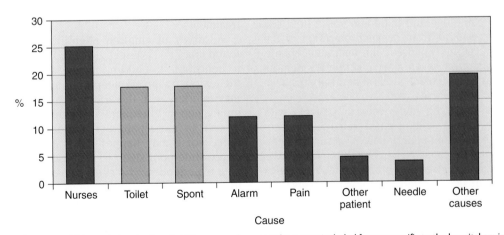

Fig. 30-2 Cause of awakenings in children admitted to hospital. The causes shown on the x-axes included factors specific to the hospital environment (e.g., nurses, alarms, pain, other patients, procedures, and others) as well as unprompted awakenings (e.g., toileting and spontaneous). The percentage of children awakened by each cause is represented on the y-axes. *(Data from Herbert A, De Lima J, Seton C, et al. A survey of sleeping patterns in children admitted to the hospital. Sleep Biologic Rhythms 6(Suppl 1); A49:2008.)*

to have night-waking problems and vice versa.[56] Thus, the interaction between anxiety, sleep problems and parent-child bedtime interactions may be particularly complex in the palliative care context.

Sleep problems are similarly associated with depression in young people. Sleep disturbances are reported in up to 90% of adolescents with major depression.[57] Depression in young people tends to be associated with symptoms of insomnia, with polysomnogram (PSG) studies revealing reduced total sleep time, longer sleep onset latencies and shorter latency to REM sleep.[58] Poor sleep quality and daytime sleepiness are also frequently reported.[59] At times it can be unclear whether the sleep or the emotional disturbance is the primary problem. Traditionally, disturbed sleep has been viewed as a manifestation or symptom of psychological disorder. Increasingly, however, there is evidence of a bidirectional relationship between sleep and emotional and behavioral functioning. It also has a huge impact on the emotional status of the family who looks after the child. Parents and caretakers at night need rest and sleep to continue the taxing nature of caring for children on a daily basis.

Adolescents with a life-threatening illness will also have concerns related to growing up and planning for the future combined with a grief relating to multiple losses, including changes in friendships, physical appearance, and modification of future aspirations. Supportive communication with their parents may be lacking, and as a consequence they may stay in bed, awake, trying to deal with poorly understood anxieties.[60] As the cartoon (Fig. 30-3) "3 AM Wakeup" illustrates, it can be difficult for health professionals to fully appreciate the impact of a disturbed night's sleep, particularly when we observe and assess patients in the light of day. Worries may occur at night when in a dark room and defenses are least able to cope. Sometimes as health professionals we may minimize sleeping difficulties and see it like a "sardine on toast," while our patients see it as a "great whale of doom." There is also a spiritual dimension to this distress (Fig. 30-4).

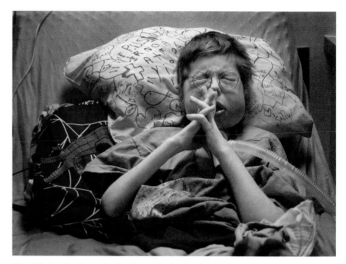

Fig. 30-4 At the end of a day in the hospital, this patient prays for his family and friends, and for his own healing from the cancer that has invaded his body and subjected him to a long series of painful treatments. *(Photograph by Monica Lopossay. Courtesy the Baltimore Sun Company, Inc., All rights reserved.)*

Assessment

It is important to undertake a thorough history and examination when assessing a child with sleeping difficulties. If children are fully awake for long periods at night and miserable despite being held, walked or fed, offered playtime, or brought into the parents' bed, medical causes such as pain and cerebral irritability should be considered.[17] Older children and adolescents are able to recall whether their sleep was restful and refreshing or restless and disturbed. In younger children, the parent acts as proxy. A simple and effective subjective method of rating sleep is that of a visual analogue scale —a 100-mm horizontal line with opposing statements such as "best sleep ever" and "worst night ever" at each end. The subject being assessed is asked to place a mark on the line in a position corresponding to their perception of the previous night's sleep. The distance of

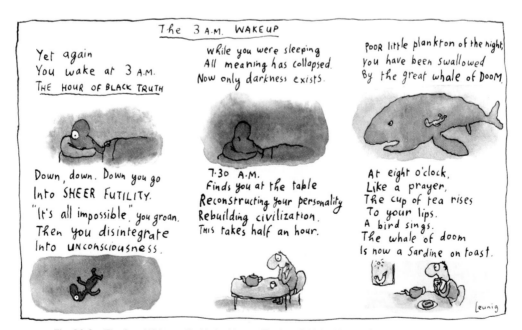

Fig. 30-3 The **3 AM Wakeup.** *(By Michael Leunig, The Age. ©Michael Leunig. Reproduced by permission.)*

TABLE 30-1 Sleep Assessment Using BEARS Proforma

Domain	Toddlers / preschool (2-5 years)	School age (6-12 years)	Adolescents (13-18 years)
Bedtime issues	Does your child have problems going to bed and/or falling asleep? (p)	Does your child have problems at bedtime? (p) Do you have problems going to bed? (c)	Do you have problems going to bed? (c) Do you have problems going to sleep? (c)
Excessive daytime sleepiness	Does your child exhibit tired and sleepy behavior during the day? (p)	Does your child have problems waking in the morning? (p) Do you often feel tired? (c)	Do you feel sleepy during the day? (c)
Night awakenings	Does your child wake frequently during the night? (p)	Does your child wake frequently during the night, sleepwalk, or suffer nightmares? (p) Do you wake frequently in the night and have trouble getting back to sleep? (c)	Do you wake and have difficulty re-sleeping at night? (c)
Regularity and duration of sleep	Does your child have a regular bedtime and waketime? What are they? (p)	What time does your child go to bed and get up on school days and on weekends? Is he or she getting enough sleep? (p)	What time do you go to bed and get up on weekdays, and on weekends? How much sleep do you get? (c)
Snoring	Does your child regularly snore or have breathing difficulty at night?	Does your child snore regularly or loudly, or have breathing difficulty at night? (p)	Does your teenager snore loudly and regularly at night? (p)

P, Question for parent; *C*, Question for child.

that mark along the line may then be measured in millimeters, providing a numerical value for satisfaction with the previous night's sleep. Each subject creates his or her own scale, which is extremely sensitive to change and therefore particularly useful for serial assessments.[61]

BEARS (**Bedtime** issues, **Excessive** daytime sleepiness, night **Awakenings**, **Regularity** and duration of sleep, **Snoring**) is a five-item pediatric sleep screening instrument that is useful in obtaining sleep-related information and identifying sleep problems and can be incorporated into taking a sleep history from a child or parent[62] (Table 30-1). A sleep diary is another assessment tool that allows parents or older children to record periods of being asleep and being awake over a 24-hour period. There are also provisions to record the times, duration, and causes of awakenings throughout the night. Sleep diaries completed by parents are an accurate way of measuring sleep-schedule measures, that is sleep duration and sleep onset time, and can be completed over a number of days. It is often necessary for parents to complete sleep diaries on their child's behalf, particularly

where the child may still be developing an accurate sense of time. Children older than 12 years can accurately and reliably complete a sleep diary themselves[63] (Fig. 30-5). Online sleep diaries are also available.[51]

An actigraph monitor is a small, lightweight, and watch-like device attached to the wrist and is capable of collecting time-based activity data over extended intervals. It is the gold standard to which sleep diaries are compared. Parents can overestimate the time their children spend in actual sleep and underestimate the number of their night-time awakenings.[64] Actigraphy provides a non-invasive objective measure of sleep per week parameters in the child's home environment. Nevertheless, sleep diaries remain an accessible and inexpensive way of assessing sleep in the clinical setting.

A number of outcomes can be measured when analyzing sleep diaries or actigraph recordings. These include:
- Sleep period or duration: the time from sleep onset to morning awakening.
- Sleep efficiency: percentage of time in bed that is spent asleep. Greater than 85% is considered normal.

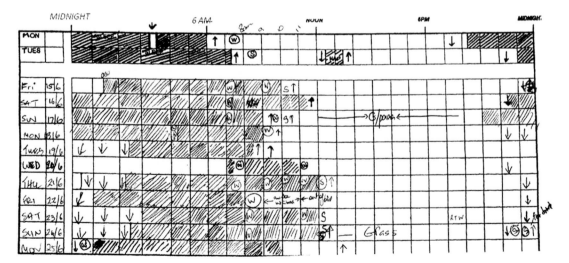

Fig. 30-5 Sleep diary from a 17-year-old boy with an undiagnosed neuromuscular condition demonstrating a delayed sleep phase. Co-morbidities included depression, need for nocturnal non-invasive ventilation, severe scoliosis causing chronic pain, and grief over the death of his grandmother.

- Sleep Onset Latency: defined as the time it takes to fall asleep at night, normally less than 30 minutes.
- Number and length of night awakenings.

On occasion, it may be appropriate to use more advanced technology, such as a polysomnograph study. A polysomnograph is a laboratory-based test to diagnose and evaluate sleep disorders. It measures sleep, respiratory and other parameters (Table 30-2). It is not helpful in assessing insomnia because patients may sleep better than they normally do, or alternatively not sleep at all, due to the artificial environment of a sleep laboratory. It is particularly helpful for evaluating sleep-disordered breathing, or the assessment of upper airway obstruction and central sleep apnea. It also has a role in the pre-surgery assessment of patients at increased risk of anesthetic complications, such as spinal fusion for muscular dystrophy patients, and evaluation of patients after a brain tumor removal or spinal decompression. It can assist in the assessment of when to start non-invasive ventilatory support for at risk children, including those with neuromuscular conditions, and monitoring children receiving respiratory support during sleep such as supplemental oxygen, continuous positive airway pressure, and non-invasive ventilation.[65] Collaboration and guidance from an experienced sleep pediatrician in relation to the appropriateness and use of these investigations is important.

Management

Health professionals caring for a child with a life-threatening condition should screen for insomnia as a potential symptom, given its potential to cause distress for both the child and his or her family. The above assessment tools are important to guide accurate initial assessment of sleep problems. Where possible, these should be repeated at various times to monitor the progress of sleeping difficulties and assess for changes following interventions. Where possible, these should be repeated at various times to monitor the progress of sleeping difficulties and assess for changes following interventions. This is particularly the case if other causes, such as gastro-esophageal reflux, seizures or anxiety, and symptoms such as pain, itch, nausea, and dyspnea can be better managed.

The management of sleeping problems in children requires an interdisciplinary approach, not dissimilar to the management of chronic pain (Table 30-3). When symptoms are persistent and severe, there is a role for pharmacologic management. However, these must be used in conjunction with other nonpharmacologic strategies. This includes the management of psychologic distress, such as depression and anxiety, with input from a psychologist or psychiatrist. Because of the frequent coexistence and bidirectional effects of sleep disturbances and mood disorders, the most-effective treatment strategy generally involves an integrated approach that addresses both concerns simultaneously.

The approach to healthy children with sleeping problems has been either to avoid the use of medications or use medications only for a short duration.[66] This is due to concerns over addiction to medications and lack of evidence for their long-term effectiveness in clinical studies. There is more evidence for developing nonpharmacologic strategies to manage sleep problems and many parents would also prefer this. Nonpharmacologic interventions may also be appealing for patients who are already taking a number of medications, such as in oncology.[28,67]

However, the symptom burden of insomnia may be quite high in a patient requiring end-of-life care, and in this context it may be more appropriate to use medications to assist with sleep. This is particularly the case in a child who has a progressive condition and whose physical symptoms will worsen with time. Assessment of life expectancy may assist in determining the balance between pharmacologic and nonpharmacologic methods of managing insomnia. Further, some patients with life-threatening conditions will have sleep disturbances and associated behavior, which is so severe or refractory that there is no other option except to use medications.

Provision of supplemental oxygen at night to patients with severe lung disease, such as CF and neuromuscular conditions, can improve daytime function and quality of life.[68,69] The use of other respiratory support therapies should be evaluated in reference to the value in maintaining or improving quality of life. Children may benefit from non-invasive ventilation (NIV) during sleep for symptom management. NIV is readily available in most pediatric teaching hospitals and is increasingly available in the home and hospice settings. NIV can be seen as a treatment alternative to enotracheal ventilation for patients with end-stage terminal illness with a respiratory deterioration and in whom intensive care is electively declined or deemed inappropriate.[69]

The use of NIV in the pediatric palliative setting is limited by lack of experience, cost, access because therapy was being previously restricted to teaching hospitals, and lack of published trials to assess its efficacy.[69] Symptoms related to upper airway obstruction, dyspnea associated with severe restrictive lung disease and problems of clearing secretion in children with suppurative lung disease and neuromuscular conditions might warrant consideration of a trial of NIV. Pediatric data are limited to case reports and small series of patients with neuromuscular conditions such as spinal muscular atrophy, particularly type II and III, Duchenne muscular dystrophy, and children with brain tumors.[25,70]

Pharmacologic Management

The American Academy of Pediatrics (AAP) and the National Sleep Foundation in America recognize that there are inadequate data to guide pharmacologic treatment of insomnia

TABLE 30-2 Components of Polysomnograph

Category	Parameter and what it measures	Abbreviation
Sleep	Electroencephalogrampm - electrical activity of brain and seizures	EEG
	Electro-oculogram-eye movements	EOG
	Electromyography-chin diaphragmatic or intercostal muscles	EMG
Respiratory	Blood O_2 and CO_2 levels	
	Respiratory movements of abdominal and chest wall	
	Oronasal airflow	
	Diaphragmatic or intercostals EMG	
	Oximetry - blood oxygen saturation	
	Capnography - CO_2 levels	
Other	Electrocardiogram	ECG
	Body position	
	Leg movements	
	Microphone-snoring, noisy breathing	
	Esophageal pH	

TABLE 30-3 Discipline-Specific Contributions to the Management of the Child with Insomnia

Discipline	Discipline specific contributions	Overlapping contributions
Medical	Assessment for underlying medical conditions. Prescription of medications to assist sleep and manage other symptoms. Collaboration and/or referral to another specialist such as a psychiatrist or sleep physician, for complex cases. Collaboration with family physician, for management of sleeping problems of parents or siblings. Advanced practice nurses may assume some of these roles dependent on scope of practice	Being polite, gentle, respectful, and quiet in providing care for children at night. Be aware of sleeping difficulties and screen for this when assessing patients. Monitor poor sleep as a symptom and provide empathetic support during ongoing assessment. Avoid painful and fearful procedures around bedtime and in the room that the child will be sleeping as much as possible. Ensure observations taken on patient maximize comfort and sleep. Being mindful of minimizing noise at night in hospital, such as door closing and alarms. Avoid prescription of medications at nighttime, which will disrupt sleep because of their effects or administration, where possible. Provide emotional and spiritual support, including active listening and focusing on the patient, and family's strengths. Provide information and brochures on sleep hygiene. Provide practical assistance and equipment, such as hospital bed, mattress, pillows. Wake patients at night only when it is essential and explain the reason to the parents if the child is to be woken. Referral to community agencies and supports. Collaborate with respiratory and sleep practitioners in relation to educating healthcare teams about how to assess for and management sleep problems. Undertake research to better define epidemiology and evaluation of efficacy of management options. Flexibility to allow co-sleeping during end-of-life care. Encourage parents to show affection with touch
Nursing	Work collaboratively with other team members to implement and evaluate holistic treatment in home, hospice or hospital settings, including provision of durable medical equipment. Provide after-hours care in a hospital or hospice setting or at home including after hours support by telephone. Offer the patient measures designed to assist sleep, including provision of a place to sleep which is safe • Environment: lighting, temperature • Diet: snack, glass of milk, or herbal tea • Quiet activities such as relaxation tapes, music, reading a story, talking about worries. Administering as required, rescue, pro re nata (PRN) medications as ordered	
Psychosocial specialist	Psycho-education about sleeping difficulties. Supportive counseling for the patient and family, including cognitive-behavioral management of insomnia. This also includes management of pain, and anxiety and/or depression, resulting from, or co-morbid with, the illness. Adjustment to physical deterioration and psychological distress associated with end-of-life phase of illness. Bereavement care to the family and siblings, including anticipatory care before the death of the child	
Other allied health	Physiotherapy: assist with mobility and activity, including exercise, during day time. Occupational therapy: Equipment, relaxation techniques, therapeutic play. Speech pathology: Communication	
Child life specialist, other expressive therapies (such as music, art, play)	Provide developmentally appropriate media for expression of emotions such as fear and anxiety (such as use of a worry doll). Instructional play and tools to assist children with sleep, such as provision of relaxing music at bedtime and the use of a "dreamcatcher". Physiologically enhancing play, daytime activity, or play away from bed to facilitate sleep at night	
Teacher and/or school	Provide mental and physical stimulation during day	
Pastoral care	Address patient's and family's spiritual needs and distress through prayer, meditation	
Integrative therapies	Massage, acupuncture, hypnosis	

in children. There is no sleep medication for children that is approved by the Food and Drug Administration.[66,67] There is an absence of safety and efficacy data for the use of benzodiazepines or newer non-benzodiazapine hypnotics for children with insomnia. This chapter summarizes the authors' opinions regarding the pharmacologic management of sleeping problems in the pediatric palliative care context and acknowledges the need for more research in this area (Table 30-4). Surveys of hospital patients have shown that just 3% of patients are prescribed medications for sleep, with antihistamines being commonly prescribed at 37% followed by benzodiazapines at 19%.[71] One randomized controlled trial found that antihistamines were no more effective than placebo.[72] Other research has suggested that sedating antihistamines should be used only as a short-term adjunct to a behavioral therapy program in healthy children and are unlikely to be of benefit to children with severe neurologic dysfunction.[73,74]

Sleep disruption caused by dysfunction of the central nervous system will often require a trial of medication. Benzodiazapines target the GABA receptor and have been shown to increase total sleep duration. However, a recent meta-analysis of 45 randomized controlled trials have documented daytime drowsiness and other adverse effects in adults.[75] Agents that have short half-lives, such as temazepam and oxazepam, may be advantageous in minimizing residual

TABLE 30-4 Summary of Various Medications That Can Promote Sleep in Children

Medication	Indications and notes
Analgesia (including opioids)	Consider slow-release preparation or infusion and/or patient-controlled analgesia (PCA) at night time May also assist cough and dyspnea

Benzodiazapines
  Lorazepam
  Clonazepam
  Diazepam
	Relieve anxiety, sedation, dyspnea, and cerebral irritability
	Lorazepam can also relieve nausea
	Clonazepam can treat seizures and parasomnia
	Diazepam can treat seizures and muscle spasm

Adjuvant analgesics
  Amitriptyline
  Gabapentin
  Pregabalin
	Neuropathic pain

Alpha-agonist-clonidine	Cerebral irritability

Sedating antihistamines
  Trimeprazine
  Promethazine
  Diphenhydramine
	Itch, irritability

Chloral hydrate	Severe cerebral irritability, especially at night Dosing ranges between 10-50 mg/kg/dose up to a maximum of 1 g per dose orally or rectally Higher doses, 80 to 100 mg / kg have been given to children younger than 5 years with good effect and minimal toxicity.[41]

Antidepressants
Tetracyclic antidepressants
  Mirtazapine
  Trazodone
Selective serotonin reuptake inhibitors
  Fluoxetine
  Sertraline
Serotonin and norepinephrine reuptake inhibitors
  Venlafaxine
  Duloxetine
	Major Depression or Anxiety.
	Recommend consultation with psychiatrist.
	Tetracyclic antidepressants have a sedative effect which can assist sleep.
	SSRIs can exacerbate insomnia.
	SNRIs can assist neuropathic pain.

Atypical antipsychotics
  Quetiapine
  Olanzapine
  Risperidone
	At low doses are extremely useful in treating severe agitation in combination with insomnia.
	Recommend consultation with psychiatrist.
	Risperidone can worsen insomnia.

daytime drowsiness. Common adverse effects from over-sedation are respiratory depression and the rapid development of tolerance, which limits their usefulness. The newer non-benzodiazapine hypnotics including zolpidem or zopiclone, have the advantage of a short half-life and are therefore useful in the treatment of sleep onset insomnia while causing minimal morning hangover. These medications have less effect on sleep architecture and do not have the insomnia rebound effect experienced when benzodiazepine hypnotics are stopped abruptly. However, there is lack of experience or research in the effectiveness, dosing, and side effects of these medications in pediatrics.[41,76]

At times, nocturnal irritability may be so severe that sedation is required to provide comfort to the child and rest to the caretakers. Clonidine and chloral hydrate are described in the literature as being particularly effective for children with cerebral irritability.[17] Factors such as the child's overall level of function, both baseline and sleep loss–related, the degree of nighttime disturbance, and the desires of the parents or other caretakers should be carefully considered.[17] If used, one should be sure that daytime function is improved, that the lowest effective dose is chosen, and that periodic drug withdrawals are trialed to ensure the drug's continued necessity.[60]

Endogenous melatonin is a hormone produced by the pineal gland at night and also plays a major role in the synchronization of circadian rhythms. There are a number of randomized controlled studies on the use of melatonin in children published in the literature, but more research is required.[77] These studies are generally small in number and vary in the dosage of melatonin given from 0.3-10 mg. Melatonin usage appears safe in the short term with minimal side effects; however, there are concerns that melatonin can lower the seizure threshold. There has been one randomized, placebo-controlled trial of controlled release melatonin in children with neurodevelopmental disability showing benefit in terms of sleep latency, clinician and patient rated variables, sleep efficiency and reduced family stress.[78] In a survey of children with Sanfilippo syndrome, parents found melatonin used in conjunction with benzodiazepines was the most effective pharmacologic treatments of sleeping difficulties.[23]

Some medications, such as diuretics and steroids, which the child is on may also be contributing to sleep disturbance and these should be reviewed.[19] Switching drugs, dosage regimens, or routes of administration may assist sleep. A combination of medications, each at lower doses, from two or three classes is sometimes more effective and preferred over increasing the dose of a single agent. Opioid analgesics can cause a delirium, and sometimes vivid dreams, and, in this context, a switch to an alternative opioid may be appropriate.[79] Lamotrigine is an anti-seizure medication that can cause irritability and sleep disturbance. Consideration of switching to another anti-epileptic that also sedates, such as clobazam or phenobarbitone, could be considered.

Nonpharmacologic Management

Providing children and parents with nonpharmacologic methods of sleep management can assist children to sleep and empower the family. Simple measures may go a long way to increasing restful sleep for the whole family. This includes both environmental modifications and behavioral therapies.[23] Behavioral approaches can be rapidly successful for treating sleep problems, even where the sleep problems are long-standing, severe and associated with physical, psychologic, or intellectual problems.[80]

Feedback from children and parents shows a number of small practical steps that can be undertaken to improve children's sleep when they are hospitalized.[32] Examples include avoiding oral medications at times when children would be expected to be asleep, turning off monitor alarms as soon as possible and keeping other night time interventions to a minimum. Ward routines that are flexible in allowing children to fulfill their own sleep requirements are important to consider, including allowing children to go to sleep at a similar time as they would at home, and use of activities such as bedtime reading or having a glass of milk or small snack just before bedtime.

Sleep hygiene relates to creating a sleep-friendly bedtime routine. It can be challenging to implement such a routine when children have a medical illness or neuro-developmental disability.[81] The hour before bedtime should be a quiet time for shared pleasures, with television, computer games, and other stimulating activities restricted. A cool, quiet, comfortable bedroom will also promote sleep. Special overlays may be used to manage temperature-regulation difficulties. A variety of specialized positioning equipment can be used to provide postural support during sleep, for management of deformity, comfort, breathing, digestion, and safety. Specialized beds, mattresses and pillows can also be beneficial. Children are also often comforted by a dim nightlight, and a familiar transitional object such as a stuffed animal.

Thirty minutes of bright light exposure in the early morning will lead to better modulation of melatonin in the child's body between daytime and nighttime. This also improves daytime functioning. Restful sleep is promoted by trying to aim for a regular waking time, both on school days and weekends. Where possible it is helpful to keep a child busy and active during the day, and limit naps to mid-afternoon. Children that are forced by illness or incapacitation to spend long amounts of time in bed run greater risk of associating their bed with wakefulness rather than sleep, which can further compound sleep difficulties. Thus, even very sick children might benefit from having different places to spend during the day. There is some evidence that daytime activities, such as a short time of exercise, will enhance sleep at night in children undergoing chemotherapy.[28] Ongoing involvement at school, visits by friends, or the use of expressive therapies, such as play and music, can also help to keep children occupied during the day.

While it can be difficult for parents to set firm limits around a bedtime routine in the palliative care context, sometimes this is required to allow both the child and family to have adequate sleep and maintain quality of life during the day.[60] Some balance needs to be maintained when negotiating this with children and families, because some parents may be happy to stay up late at night with their child if that is the time that they are most interactive with their family. Such interaction is only sustainable for a short period of time and may not be appropriate to facilitate if the child is not at an end-of-life phase of their illness. Some children during the end stages of their disease, and for various reasons, will develop a delayed sleep phase of going to bed later and waking late in the morning. Some parents are happy to accommodate this change in sleeping pattern and acknowledgement of this is all that may be required.

Commonly used intervention techniques in adults include training in relaxation strategies and mind meditation techniques.[30] A recent study of adult patients with persistent insomnia, showed the addition of medication, Zolpidem, to cognitive behavioral therapy (CBT) produced added benefits during acute therapy, but long-term outcome was optimized when medication was discontinued during maintenance CBT.[82] A recent study demonstrated that trained and supervised nurses can effectively deliver cognitive behavioral therapy for insomnia in general practice.[83] This included education about sleep hygiene and establishing a bedtime routine.

Research into the effectiveness of CBT has also focused on children with anxiety and insomnia.[84] CBT focuses on helping children to learn the connections among thoughts, feelings and behaviors, and learn specific skills to begin to think, feel, and behave in more positive and helpful ways. There is also a role for resources that provide children psycho-education and give them autonomy in managing their sleep problems, such as books and group work.[60,85] An integrated approach is beneficial in that cognitive restructuring strategies can be highly effective for both sleep disturbance and psychiatric issues.[54] Cognitive restructuring involves an active process of challenging negative, unhelpful or unrealistic thoughts and generating more accurate or helpful interpretations of situations in order to facilitate coping. Aside from changes to bedtime routines and behavior, behavioral components of CBT can involve gradual exposure to situations that are feared or avoided. Facing feared situations provides opportunities to test fearful predictions, while also providing self-mastery experiences and an opportunity for children to develop coping skills. More significant and chronic fears cannot be dealt with by such behavioral methods alone and counseling must be considered. It is important that both children and parents are given close follow-up and support.[60]

Co-sleeping or bed sharing is another strategy that parents adopt to assist their children to sleep. In some studies, bed sharing of at least once per week was noted in 44% of the children between age 2 and 7 years old.[86] There are also significant cultural variations in this practice. In cultures where children share their parents' bed, night waking is not such a problem.[60] An increased prevalence of bed and room sharing has been found amongst Asian, African American, and indigenous children.[87–90] Factors associated with this practice in China included younger age, large family, children without their own bedrooms, and parents' approval of a co-sleeping arrangement.[87] Swedish children also often co-sleep with both their parents until school age, when more boys than girls cease the practice. Co-sleeping in Sweden is perceived as a normal family activity, which differs from other Western cultures.[91]

Children during an illness, particularly if it is terminal, may seek reassurance from parents at night, particularly when they are fearful. Other approaches should be considered if the child is not receiving end-of-life care and is expected to live more than one month. Having the child continue to sleep in his or her own bedroom with the parent available, although not sleeping in the same bed, is a more sustainable compromise. Parents also demonstrating love, care, and their ability to provide safety and protection to their child will also be important in this context (Fig. 30-6).

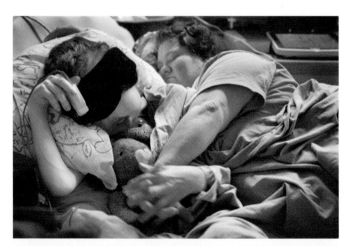

Fig. 30-6 A patient and his mother share their night-time ritual of cuddling in his hospital bed. He holds his stuffed rabbit, Mr. Browney. *(Photography by Monica Lopossay. Courtesy the Baltimore Sun Company, Inc., All rights reserved.)*

Complementary and Alternative Medicine Treatments

Given the preponderance of patients who may be employing complementary and alternative medicine (CAM) treatments and techniques for insomnia, it is important that clinicians be familiar with these approaches.[92] Research into pharmacologic complementary and alternative substances to treat sleep disturbances in patients, both adult and pediatric, is almost nonexistent. There is insufficient evidence to recommend valerian for insomnia.[5] There is also interest in the effectiveness of traditional Chinese medicine, massage, and acupuncture in managing sleeping problems in adults.[93,94] Another study that explored the effectiveness of hypnosis treatment in children experiencing loss, such as the death of a parent or sibling, showed promise by concluding that young children can be taught self-hypnosis to manage their sleeping problems effectively.[95]

Clinical Vignettes

Amy, 8, had a primary diagnosis of relapsed rhabdomyosacroma involving her lungs and sacrum (Fig. 30-7). She developed back and abdominal pain on the fourth day of a bone marrow transplant. Patient-controlled analgesia using fentanyl was commenced to manage her pain. Subsequently to this, she developed bright and vivid dreams, which were distressing. These dreams were characteristic of the dreams associated with opioid analgesia. Her analgesia was changed to hydromorphone and her dreams settled. She also had diazepam to assist with sleep initiation for three nights at this time.

Her sleep continued to be disturbed, with frequent waking related to diarrhea, urination, itch, and pain. Ten days later her dreams recurred. They were less bizarre and vivid. They related to her transplant and included themes of not being able to walk and people wanting to hurt her. At the same time her

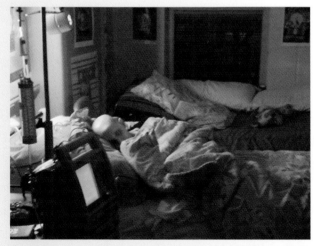

Fig. 30-7 Amy has a respite from her bone marrow transplant while sleeping.

mother noted increased sadness, increased anger, and social withdrawal.

An interdisciplinary team approach to assessment and therapy was undertaken. This included a social worker, play therapist, physiotherapist, psychiatrist, occupational therapist, and teacher. She had lost hearing as a result of chemotherapy and was offered a pocket talker that allowed her to better hear what people were saying and facilitated communication. A play therapist allowed her to engage in craft and artwork during the day and gave her some sense of control. This also allowed the psychiatrist to engage with her and talk about operations and procedures which had caused pain during previous treatments.

Medical management included ongoing analgesia and a 3-day course of promethazine to assist with sleep and itch. A diagnosis of a reactive depression related to prolonged hospitalization and loss of control was made and consideration given to using an antidepressant. Her parents were not keen for this intervention. With supportive counseling her sleep improved. The play therapist helped her create "Tweety Bird" expression cards so that she could show how she was feeling. She also used a worry doll, which she would talk to before going to sleep and then place under her pillow to place her worrying thoughts to rest. Her brother also used this because he was anxious and experiencing difficulty sleeping. The play therapist also helped her make a dream catcher, which helped to catch her bad dreams. In summary, she was given assistance to communicate and a safe space to talk and express her feelings. This improved her sleep.

An 8-month-old boy with Pelizaeus-Merzbacher syndrome had severe cerebral irritability and sleeping difficulties. Other problems included developmental delay, a movement disorder, sensorineural deafness and blindness. He had persistent seizures despite receiving intensive therapy of phenobartitone, clobazam, and vigabatrin. He required frequent doses of buccal midazolam for breakthrough seizures. He would settle somewhat with touch and being cuddled by his mother but she was becoming fatigued nursing him around the clock.

There was no pattern to his sleep disturbance. He had minimal sleep during the day.

An MRI of his brain showed complete loss of myelination and an abnormal pituitary gland. A trial of melatonin was started particularly in relation to his blindness and abnormal MRI findings.

Unfortunately, a dose of 3 mg of melatonin did not make a significant improvement. His irritability was treated with chloral hydrate, which was titrated to a dose 50 mg/kg every 6 hours. This sedative was rotated to diazepam 3 months later when the chloral hydrate became less effective. His parents were able to accommodate his irregular sleeping patterns and irritability at home using nonpharmacologic measures and reserved medications for occasions when his symptomatology was severe. His case was severe and responded poorly even to medications.

Summary

Insomnia is an important symptom to be aware of when caring for children with life-threatening conditions. Poor sleep has an impact on quality of life, including daytime and emotional functioning, for the entire family. The etiology of sleeping problems can be complex and multifaceted and include the child's specific medical condition, other intrinsic factors such as pain and cerebral irritability, environmental and psycho-social factors. Assessment and treatment is best achieved by an interdisciplinary team. Nonpharmacologic approaches to managing sleep problems are critical and include relaxation techniques, cognitive behavioral strategies and establishing a bedtime routine and sleeping environment that is safe and conducive to rest. Medications may be required to treat pain, anxiety, depression, and other symptoms, which affect sleep. Medications may also be required for sleep problems when they are severe or non-responsive to other measures. Educating hospital and hospice staff about how to improve the sleep conduciveness of the hospital or hospice environment is also important to consider.

Acknowledgments

We extend our appreciation to Dr. John Collins for his assistance in conceptualizing this clinical review and to Carmel Mason for assistance in manuscript preparation.

REFERENCES

1. Hippocrates, Aphorism LXXI in Sateia MJ, Nowell PD: Insomnia, *Lancet* 364(9449):1959–1973, 2004.
2. Splaingard M: Sleep medicine, *Pediatr Clin North Am* 51:xiii–xiv, 2004.
3. Blask DE: Melatonin, sleep disturbance and cancer risk, *Sleep Med Rev* 13(4):257–264, 2009.
4. Rosen GM: Sleep in children who have cancer, *Sleep Med Clin* 2: 491–500, 2007.
5. Bartlett DJ, Paisley L, Desai AV: Insomnia diagnosis and management, *Medicine Today* 7(8):14–21, 2006.
6. American Academy of Sleep Medicine: *The International Classification of Sleep Disorders, Revised—Diagnostic and Coding Manual*, American Academy of Sleep Medicine, Westchester, 2001.
7. American Psychiatric Association: *Diagnostic and statistical manual of mental disorders* (Revised ed 4). Washington, DC, 2000, American Psychiatric Association.
8. Rosen G: Evaluation of the patient who has sleep complaints: a case-based method using the sleep matrix process, *Prim Care Clin Office Pract* 32:319–328, 2005.
9. Lee KA: Continuing education program integrating and understanding of sleep knowledge into your practice, *Am Nurse* 26–27, 1995.
10. Iglowstein I, Jenni OG, Molinari L, et al: Sleep duration from infancy to adolescence: Reference values and generational trends, *Pediatrics* 111:302–307, 2003.
11. Yang C, Kim JK, Patel SR, et al: Age-related changes in sleep/wake patterns among Korean teenagers, *Pediatrics* 115:250–256, 2005.
12. Dollman J, Ridley K, Olds T, et al: Trends in the duration of school-day sleep among 10- to 15-year-old South Australians between 1985 and 2004, *Acta Paediatr* 96(7):1011–1014, 2007.
13. Richman N: Sleep problems in young children, *Arch Dis Child* 56(7):491–493, 1981.
14. Klackenberg G: Sleep behaviour studied longitudinally. Data from 4-16 years on duration, night-awakening and bed-sharing, *Acta Paediatr Scand* 71(3):501–506, 1982.
15. Dahl RE, Carskadon MA: Sleep and its disorders in adolescence. In Ferber R, Kryger MH, editors: *Principles and practice of sleep medicine in the child*, Philadelphia, 1995, Saunders, pp 19–27.
16. Smaldone A, Honig JC, Byrne MW: Sleepless in America: inadequate sleep and relationships to health and well-being of our nation's children, *Pediatrics* 119(Suppl 1):S29–S37, 2007.
17. Ferber R: Childhood sleep disorders, *Neurol Clin* 14(3):493–511, 1996.
18. Naqvi SK, Sotelo C, Murry L, et al: Sleep architecture in children and adolescents with cystic fibrosis and the association with severity of lung disease, *Sleep Breath* 12(1):77–83, 2008.
19. Bandla H, Splaingard M: Sleep problems in children with common medical disorders, *Pediatr Clin North Am* 51:203–227, 2004.
20. Stenekes SJ, Hughes A, Grégoire MC, et al: Frequency and self-management of pain, dyspnea and cough in cystic fibrosis, *J Pain Symptom Manage* 38(6):837–848, 2009.
21. Walz NC, Beebe D, Byars K: Sleep in individuals with Angelman syndrome: parent perceptions of patterns and problems, *Am J Ment Retard* 110(4):243–252, 2005.
22. Young D, Nagarajan L, de Klerk N, et al: Sleep problems in Rett syndrome, *Brain Dev* 29(10):609–616, 2007.
23. Fraser J, Gason AA, Wraith JE, et al: Sleep disturbance in Sanfilippo syndrome: a parental questionnaire study, *Arch Dis Child* 90(12): 1239–1242, 2005.
24. Zucconi M, Bruni O: Sleep disorders in children with neurologic diseases, *Semin Pediatr Neurol* 8(4):258–275, 2001.
25. Rosen GM, Bendel AE, Neglia JP, et al: Sleep in children with neoplasms of the central nervous system: case review of 14 children, *Pediatrics* 112(1 Pt 1):e46–e54, 2003.
26. Collins JJ, Byrnes ME, Dunkel IJ, et al: The measurement of symptoms in children with cancer, *J Pain Symptom Manage* 19(5):363–377, 2000.
27. Collins JJ, Devine TD, Dick GS, et al: The measurement of symptoms in young children with cancer: the validation of the Memorial Symptom Assessment Scale in children aged 7-12, *J Pain Symptom Manage* 23(1):10–16, 2002.
28. Hinds PS, Hockenberry M, Rai SN, et al: Clinical field testing of an enhanced-activity intervention in hospitalized children with cancer, *J Pain Symptom Manage* 33(6):686–697, 2007.
29. Miser A, McCalla J, Dothage J: Pain as a presenting symptom in children and young adults with newly diagnosed malignancy, *Pain* 29: 85–90, 1987.
30. Berger AM, Parker KP, Young-McCaughan S, et al: Sleep wake disturbances in people with cancer and their caregivers: state of the science, *Oncol Nurs Forum* 32(6):E98–E126, 2005.
31. Chalkiadis GA: Management of chronic pain in children, *MJA* 175: 476–479, 2001.
32. Herbert A, De Lima J, Seton C, et al: A survey of sleeping patterns in children admitted to hospital, *Sleep and Biological Rhythms* 6(Suppl 1):A49, 2008.
33. Lewin DS, Dahl RE: Importance of sleep in the management of pediatric pain, *J Dev Behav Pediatr* 20(4):244–252, 1999.
34. Gedaly-Duff V, Lee KA, Nail L, et al: Pain, sleep disturbance, and fatigue in children with leukemia and their parents: a pilot study, *Oncol Nurs Forum* 33(3):641–646, 2006.
35. Rose M, Sanford A, Thomas C, et al: Factors altering the sleep of burned children, *Sleep* 24(1):45–51, 2001.
36. Raymond I, Nielsen TA, Lavigne G, et al: Quality of sleep and its daily relationship to pain intensity in hospitalized adult burn patients, *Pain* 92(3):381–388, 2001.
37. Roehrs T, Hyde M, Blaisdell MS, et al: Sleep loss and REM sleep are hyperalgesic, *Sleep* 29(2):145–151, 2006.
38. Theunissen PMH: Symptoms in the palliative phase of children with cancer, *Pediatr Blood Cancer* 49(2):160–165, 2007.
39. Drake R, Frost J, Collins JJ: The symptoms of dying children, *J Pain Symptom Manage* 26(1):594–603, 2003.
40. Wolfe J, Grier HE, Klar N, et al: Symptoms and suffering at the end of life in children with cancer, *N Engl J Med* 342(5):326–333, 2000.
41. Pelayo R, Chen W, Monzon S, et al: Pediatric sleep pharmacology: you want to give my kid sleeping pills? *Pediatr Clin North Am* 51:117–134, 2004.
42. Vella-Brincat J, Macleod AD: Adverse effects of opioids on the central nervous system of palliative care patients, *J Pain Palliat Care Pharmacother* 21(1):15–25, 2007.
43. Hagemann V: Night sleep of children in a hospital. Part I: sleep duration, *Matern Child Nurs J* 10(1):1–13, 1981.
44. Hagemann V: Night sleep of children in a hospital. Part II: sleep disruption, *Matern Child Nurs J* 10(2):127–142, 1981.
45. Corser NC: Sleep of 1- and 2-year-old children in intensive care, *Issues Compr Pediatr Nurs* 19(1):17–31, 1996.
46. Naughton F, Ashworth P, Skevington SM: Does sleep quality predict pain-related disability in chronic pain patients? The mediating roles of depression and pain severity, *Pain* 127(3):243–252, 2007.

47. Widger K, Davies D, Drouin DJ, et al: Pediatric patients receiving palliative care in Canada: results of a multicenter review, *Arch Pediatr Adolesc Med* 161(6):597–602, 2007.

48. Sadeh A, Raviv A, Gruber R: Sleep patterns and sleep disruptions in school-age children, *Dev Psychol* 36(3):291–301, 2000.

49. Dinges DF, Pack F, Williams K, et al: Cumulative sleepiness, mood disturbance and psychomotor vigilance performance decrements during a week of sleep restricted to 4-5 hours per night, *Sleep* 20:267–277, 1997.

50. Alfano CA, Beidel DC, Turner SM, et al: Preliminary evidence for sleep complaints among children referred for anxiety, *Sleep Med* 7: 467–473, 2006.

51. Hudson JL, Gradisar M, Gamble A, et al: The sleep patterns and problems of clinically anxious children, *Behav Res Ther* 47:339–344, 2009.

52. Forbes EE, Bertocci MA, Gregory AM, et al: Objective sleep in pediatric anxiety disorders and major depressive disorder, *J Am Acad Child Psy* 47:148–155, 2008.

53. Forbes EE, Williamson DE, Ryan ND, et al: Peri-sleep-onset cortisol levels in children and adolescents with affective disorders, *Biol Psychiatry* 59(1):24–30, 2006.

54. Hudson JL, Rapee RM: Parental perceptions of overprotection: Specific to anxious children or shared between siblings? *Behav Change* 22(3):185–194, 2005.

55. van der Bruggen CO, Stams GJ, Bögels SM: Research Review: the relation between child and parent anxiety and parental control: a meta-analytic review, *J Child Psychol Psyc* 49(12):1257–1269, 2008.

56. Adair R, Bauchner H, Philipp B, et al: Night waking during infancy: role of parental presence at bedtime, *Pediatrics* 87:500–504, 1991.

57. Meltzer LJ, Mindell JA: Nonparmacologic treatments for pediatric sleeplessness, *Pediatr Clin North Am* 51:135–151, 2004.

58. Benca RM, Obermeyer WH, Thisted RA, et al: Sleep and psychiatric disorders. A meta-analysis, *Arch Gen Psychiatry* 49(8):651–668, 1992.

59. Liu X, Buysse DJ, Gentzler AL, et al: Insomnia and hypersomnia associated with depressive phenomenology and comorbidity in childhood depression, *Sleep* 30(1):83–90, 2007.

60. Ferber R: The Sleepless Child. In Guilleminault C, editor: *Sleep and its disorders in children*, New York, 1987, Raven Press, pp 141–163.

61. Cross SJ: Assessment of sleep in hospital patients: a review of methods, *J Adv Nurs* 13:501–510, 1988.

62. Owens JA, Dalzell V: Use of the "BEARS" sleep screening tool in a pediatric residents' continuity clinic: a pilot study, *Sleep Med* 6(1): 63–69, 2005.

63. Owens JA: Epidemiology of sleep disorders during childhood. In Sheldon SA, editor: *Principles and practice of pediatric sleep medicine*, Philadelphia, 2005, Saunders, pp 27–33.

64. Sadeh A: Evaluating night wakings in sleep-disturbed infants: a methodological study of parental reports and actigraphy, *Sleep* 19(10):757–762, 1996.

65. Waters K: Interventions in the paediatric sleep laboratory: The use and titration of respiratory support therapies, *Paed Resp Rev* 9: 181–192, 2008.

66. Stojanovski SD, Rasu RS, Balkrishnan R, et al: Trends in medication prescribing for pediatric sleep difficulties in US outpatient settings, *Sleep* 30(8):1013–1017, 2007.

67. Mindell JA, Emslie G, Blumer J, et al: Pharmacologic management of insomnia in children and adolescents: consensus statement, *Pediatrics* 117(6):e1223–e1232, 2006.

68. Zinman R, Corey M, Coates AL, et al: Nocturnal home oxygen in the treatment of hypoxemic cystic fibrosis patients, *J Pediatr* 114:368–377, 1989.

69. Collins JJ, Fitzgerald DA: Palliative care and paediatric respiratory medicine, *Paediatr Respir Rev* 7:281–287, 2006.

70. Simonds AK: Nocturnal ventilation in neuromuscular disease: when and how? *Monaldi Arch Chest Dis* 57:373–376, 2002.

71. Meltzer LJ, Mindell JA, Owens JA, et al: Use of sleep medications in hospitalized pediatric patients, *Pediatrics* 119(6):1047–1055, 2007.

72. Merenstein D, Diener-West M, Halbower AC, et al: The trial of infant response to diphenhydramine: the TIRED study: a randomized, controlled, patient-oriented trial, *Arch Pediatr Adolesc Med* 160(7):707–712, 2006.

73. France KG, Blampied NM, Wilkinson P: Treatment of infant sleep disturbance by trimeprazine in combination with extinction, *J Dev Behav Pediatr* 12(5):308–314, 1991.

74. France KG, Blampied NM, Wilkinson P: A multiple-baseline, double-blind evaluation of the effects of trimeprazine tartate on infant sleep disturbance, *Exp Clin Psychopharmacol* 7(4):502–513, 1999.

75. Holbrook AM, Crowther R, Lotter A, et al: Meta-analysis of benzodiazepine use in the treatment of insomnia, *CMAJ* 162:225–233, 2000.

76. Herman JH, Sheldon SH: Pharmacology of sleep disorders in children. In Sheldon SH, Ferber R, Kryger MH editors: *Principles and practice of pediatric sleep medicine*, 2005, Saunders, pp 327–328.

77. Smits MG, van Stel HF, van der Heijden K, et al: Melatonin improves health status and sleep in children with idiopathic chronic sleep-onset insomnia: a randomized placebo-controlled trial, *J Am Acad Child Adolesc Psychiatry* 42(11):1286–1293, 2003.

78. Wasdell MB, Jan JE, Bomben MM, et al: A randomized, placebo-controlled trial of controlled release melatoning of delayed sleep phase syndrome and impaired sleep maintenance in children with neurodevelopmental disabilities, *J Pineal Res* 44:57–64, 2008.

79. Drake R, Longworth J, Collins JJ: Opioid rotation in children with cancer, *J Palliat Med* 7(3):419–422, 2004.

80. Wiggs K, France L: Behavioural treatments for sleep problems in children and adolescents with physical illness, psychological problems or intellectual disabilities, *Sleep Med Rev* 4(3):299–314, 2000.

81. Jan JE, Owens JA, Weiss MD: Sleep hygiene for children with neurodevelopmental disabilities, *Pediatrics* 122(6):1343–1350, 2008.

82. Morin CM, Vallières A, Guay B, et al: Cognitive behavioral therapy, singly and combined with medication, for persistent insomnia: a randomized controlled trial, *JAMA* 301(19):2005–2015, 2009.

83. Espie CA, MacMahon KM, Kelly HL, et al: Randomized clinical effectiveness trial of nurse-administered small-group cognitive behavior therapy for persistent insomnia in general practice, *Sleep* 30(5): 574–584, 2007.

84. Bélanger L, Morina CM, Langloisa F, et al: Insomnia and generalized anxiety disorder: effects of cognitive behavior therapy for GAD on insomnia symptoms, *J Anxiety Disord* 18(4):561–571, 2004.

85. Culbert T, Kajander R: *Be the boss of your sleep*, Minneapolis, 2007, Free Spirit Publishing.

86. Jenni OG, Fuhrer HZ, Iglowstein I, et al: A longitudinal study of bed sharing and sleep problems among Swiss children in the first ten years of life, *Pediatrics* 115(Suppl 1):233–2240, 2005.

87. Li S, Jin X, Yan C, Wu S, Jiang F, Shen X: Factors associated with bed and room sharing in Chinese school-aged children, *Child Care Health Dev* 35(2):171–177, 2009.

88. Chng SY: Sleep disorders in children: the Singapore perspective, *Ann Acad Med Singapore* 37(8):706–709, 2008.

89. Javo C, Rønning JA, Heyerdahl S: Child-rearing in an indigenous Sami population in Norway: a cross-cultural comparison of parental attitudes and expectations, *Scand J Psychol* 45(1):67–78, 2004.

90. Lozoff B, Wolf AW, Davis NS: Co-sleeping in urban families with young children in the United States, *Pediatrics* 74:171–182, 1984.

91. Welles-Nystrom B: Co-sleeping as a window into Swedish culture: considerations of gender and health care, *Scand J Caring Sci* 19(4): 354–360, 2005.

92. Kierlin L: Sleeping without a pill: nonpharmacologic treatments for insomnia, *J Psychiatr Pract* 14(6):403–407, 2008.

93. Zhou Y, Wei Y, Zhang P, et al: The short-term therapeutic effect of the three-part massotherapy for insomnia due to deficiency of both the heart and the spleen: a report of 100 cases, *J Tradit Chin Med* 27(4):261–264, 2007.

94. Zhong ZG, Cai H, Li XL, et al: Effect of acupuncture combined with massage of sole on sleeping quality of the patient with insomnia, *Zhongguo Zhen Jiu* 28(6):411–413, 2008. [Article in Chinese.]

95. Hawkins P, Polemikos N: Hypnosis treatment of sleeping problems in children experiencing loss, *Contemporary Hypnosis* 19(1):18–24, 2002.

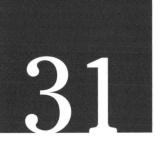

31 Pain Assessment and Management

JOHN J. COLLINS | CHARLES B. BERDE | JUDITH A. FROST

There is no nobler goal than achieving the relief of pain and suffering. —Ronald Melzack[1]

Pain is one of the most common symptoms experienced by children receiving palliative care and one of the most feared by children and their families. The severity of this symptom may increase with time, especially when the terminal phase is reached. Palliative therapeutics should generally be implemented once the underlying causative mechanisms have been established, because therapies directed at the primary cause may ultimately have a more effective outcome for symptom management.

The goals of this chapter are to describe the role of the interdisciplinary team (IDT), the importance of quality improvement, the epidemiology of pain in children with life-limiting illnesses, pain assessment and measurement, the myths surrounding pain management, and pain management guidelines. The reader is referred to other references for more detailed discussion of pediatric analgesic pharmacology.[2,3]

Pain Management, The Interdisciplinary Team, and The Child with a Life-Threatening Illness

In the context of living with a life-threatening illness, the experience of pain is potentially the result of a complex interplay among physical, psychological, social, spiritual, and other factors. The severity of a child's pain, for example, may be exacerbated by anxiety, depression, or suffering, which may be of the spiritual realm. All these factors must be considered, assessed, and treated in order to effectively alleviate suffering related to the experience of pain. Pain assessment and treatment may therefore be complex and access to an IDT may therefore be needed.

The World Health Organization (WHO) mandates that a certain standard of pain management be available to every child receiving palliative care irrespective of location.[4] As an extension of the WHO document, individual countries and groups of countries are declaring standards of pain management related to pediatric palliative care. Quality of life is often related to a child's experience of pain and is therefore vital that the child receive excellent pain assessment and management. Successful pain management often needs the combined efforts of an IDT within the palliative care team of the medical, nursing, social work, play therapy, physiotherapy, occupational therapy disciplines, among others.

The degree to which the child or caretaker believes pain is well managed can influence other outcomes, such as where a family might choose to care for their child for the end-of-life phase. Poorly controlled pain can militate against a family caring for a child at home. Good pain control, on the other hand, can mean the difference between memories of distress and angst or memories that soften the inevitable transition from life to death. Communication and flexibility are foundation stones of good management of pain in children. These two factors provide firm foundations for all other building blocks in the construction of a successful pain management plan.

COMMUNICATION

Whatever the source and intensity of the child's pain, communication is central to successful pain management. Communication among all parties involved in the child's care ensures continuity, concordance, and a feeling of safety for the child and family. A pediatric palliative care service supports families in their choice of location for end-of-life care. These locations can include home, hospital, or a pediatric in-patient hospice unit. Home may provide a sense of familiarity and comfort that may lessen the need for medications to manage physical pain. Conversely, hospital or hospice may provide a sense of security in having access to doctors and nurses and a variety of medications not necessarily available at home.

In the hospital, one role of the palliative care team is to provide pain management for the child in collaboration with the primary care team as well as supportive care to the family. Once the child and family leave the hospital, the palliative care nurse often establishes the link to community services and becomes the link between the family and the primary care team. Communication, consultation, and feedback to the family enhances a feeling of safety and ensures them that they have not been abandoned by health professionals who have been involved in the child's care for months or years. This communication can improve pain control and reduce unnecessary admissions to hospital.

The role of a pediatric palliative care team is often that of a consultant-liaison team who take responsibility for both symptom management and family support. A palliative care service that provides successful pain management can facilitate collaboration and a strengthening of professional relationships among the palliative care and other care teams within a hospital. It also diminishes the notion that palliative care teams are the harbingers of death. Just as important as dialogue between teams and the family is communication with the child. Time should be spent listening to the child, to his or her complaint of pain, in an effort to determine not only pain severity but the meaning of the pain to the child.

FLEXIBILITY

Successful pain management requires flexible care provision from all healthcare providers. Flexibility is needed when pain escalates and is difficult to manage; when parents try unproven therapies; when families suddenly choose to go for a family holiday providing little notice to clinicians; when the location for terminal care is changed at short notice. Flexibility is also needed by clinicians when extraordinary doses or unusual therapies are needed for pediatric symptom management.

The Interdisciplinary Team and the Alleviation of Suffering

Suffering as a contributing factor to pain must also be considered. Suffering is a multifaceted entity. Frequently this component of care may be helped by first trying to gauge an understanding of the meaning of suffering to each child and family. Some children, for example, may be experiencing great sadness at the knowledge of their impending death and the loss of their future. Others may be suffering because the family is silent about the progression of illness, and are unable to share their fears and anxieties with family members. For others it may be long periods of hospitalization and missing familiar environments or friends. Some children suffer from the loss of body image, from their inability to participate in sports or other activities, or the unrelenting nature of their symptoms. This suffering can amplify the experience of pain.

Support for parents includes education about anticipated potential symptoms. Knowledge will increase a sense of control. This in turn lessens anxiety and this may positively affect the child's pain experience. Competent and compassionate care can alleviate a child's pain and suffering. This can be achieved through a trusting, consistent, and honest relationship among all involved in providing care, and the family and the child. Because children are especially vulnerable and depend on adults to act as their advocates we must support the humane and competent treatment of pain and suffering at all times (Table 31-1).

Clinical Vignette

Peta was a 7-year-old girl with disseminated neuroblastoma metastatic to the long bones of her lower limbs and significant left-sided auxiliary lymphadenopathy causing mild lymphedema of the left arm. At the referral to palliative care, four months before her death, she had no pain complaint. Peta was the only child of Mark and Tricia. Her mother was 8 months' pregnant. The interdisciplinary palliative care team met the family and discussed its role in the management of symptoms and support with psychological, social, and spiritual issues, should they arise. While the parents' primary goal was for Peta to die free of pain at home, they expressed an interest in the possibility of Peta dying in an in-patient hospice facility if home care became too difficult. The team contacted the local pediatric in-patient hospice unit and facilitated Peta's admission with her family for respite care. The family were impressed by their visit and made a reservation for Peta to stay

for respite care when the baby was born. During these admissions, professional relationships were developed with the palliative care social worker, nurses, doctors, and play therapist. One outcome was that the pediatric in-patient hospice unit was viewed as a viable alternative to home for terminal care.

Bone, auxiliary and left arm pain became symptom management issues during the last two months of life. Pain management became complex because of presumed infiltration of the left brachial plexus with tumor and significant lymphedema of the entire left arm. The bone pain was initially treated successfully with localized palliative radiation. Long-acting oral morphine and supplementary short-acting morphine for breakthrough pain and gabapentin as an adjuvant analgesic were prescribed for the management of neuropathic pain related to brachial plexus infiltration by tumor.

Helpful nonpharmacological interventions were lymphedema massage of the left arm and play therapy. Of all the clinicians on the interdisciplinary team, the child life therapist was the one with whom Peta most eagerly engaged. Play as part of an overall strategy for pain management was helpful because it permitted Peta to more easily express her feelings. The financial situation was difficult as the father became unemployed and the mother needed to give up her work to devote time to Peta. The family had great anxiety related to finances and the involvement of the palliative care social worker became critical.

Peta's pain severity rapidly increased during her last week of life. As the oral route of administration was becoming more difficult, the morphine dose was converted to the intravenous equivalent dose and administered as a continuous infusion with a bolus option using a patient controlled analgesia (PCA) pump via a central line. The palliative care nurse educated the family in the care and management of the PCA pump. She also educated the local community nurses by providing an in-service program and educational materials on pain management for children.

A brachial plexus block was considered for Peta's neuropathic pain. A consulting anesthetist's review of MRI studies and ultrasound examination indicated that, because of distortion of landmarks and tissue planes by tumor, it would not be technically feasible to position a brachial plexus catheter proximal (medial and rostral) to the site of tumor, as needed to provide analgesia. Unfortunately, Peta developed thrombocytopenia and no form of nerve block was possible. A drug switch to methadone was made, which substantially improved pain control. Peta's condition deteriorated quickly and she died peacefully and free of pain at home in the presence of her family; the family's wishes being fulfilled.

Supporting a Culture of Quality Improvement in Pediatric Pain Management Related to Palliative Care

Internationally, there has been a rapid growth in the number of pediatric palliative care services. Many children's hospitals throughout the world have dedicated pain services, and in tandem with this development is the evolution of dedicated pediatric palliative care services. While the latter may be in a children's hospital or a pediatric department of a larger adult hospital, many pediatric palliative care services have evolved

TABLE 31-1 Clinical Background and Responsibilities in Pediatric Pain Management for Children Receiving Palliative Care

Professional background	Contribution toward pain management
Pediatric palliative care physician	Primarily responsible for the assessment, diagnosis, and management of physical pain, including the prescription of pharmacologic, and non-pharmacologic management. May have a role in the alleviation of the psychological and existential components of pain.
Pediatric palliative care nurse	Primarily responsible for implementing and monitoring pain management through ongoing assessment and measurement. Also has a role in advocating for the child's pain management and a role in the alleviation of the psychological and existential components of pain.
Pediatric palliative care social worker	Primarily responsible for the social domain of care of the child and family, especially when affecting pain management. Has a major role advocating for the child and family, including pain management.
Pediatric palliative care child-life therapist	Primarily responsible for the use of play as a therapeutic means of self-expression. This may include the expression of pain severity and suffering through therapeutic play.
Pediatric palliative care spiritual care provider	Primarily responsible for assessing and managing the spiritual components of patient receiving palliative care and the existential suffering related to dying. Suffering related to the spirit may be related to the experience of physical pain.

for children receiving care at home or in an in-patient hospice unit. The continued advancement of these important areas of pediatric clinical practice can be achieved only through the development of pediatric palliative care quality programs and improved research output in these areas.

Part of quality measurement involves the use of outcome measures. These may be clinical indicators, as in measures of clinical outcomes; process indicators such as measures of clinical processes; and qualitative reflective review. Outcome measures are designed to identify the rate of occurrence or non-occurrence of an event, which in turn reflects the care that was or was not provided. They are aggregated data from all patients receiving the service that can highlight areas that need improving, and can be used to measure the service against particular standards. Indicators can be collected over a number of settings and used as a way of benchmarking or comparing like services.

Clinical indicators concerning pain management at the end of life may include care planning and symptom management, patient and family education, and the provision of holistic care. For example, a high number of patients whose distressing symptoms were addressed may indicate a provision of high-quality education, symptom assessment, care planning and implementation. Conversely, a high number of children being admitted to hospital for symptom management at end of life may reflect a poor quality of symptom management at home.

Epidemiology of Pain in Children with Life-Threatening Illnesses

PAIN AND OTHER SYMPTOMS AT THE END OF A CHILD'S LIFE

Pain and other physical and psychological symptoms are highly prevalent in children at the end of life. The proxy report of nurses documented the symptoms of dying children, using a modified Memorial Symptom Assessment Scale.[5] A mean of 11.1 ± 5.6 symptoms was documented per child. At least half of the children had six symptoms; the most frequent ones being lack of energy, pain, drowsiness, skin changes, irritability, and extremity swelling. Lack of energy was the most distressing symptom for nearly one-third of the children. Nervousness, worry, and dysesthetic extremities were notably distressing, although not frequent. Most children were described in the health professionals' notes as being "always comfortable" to "usually comfortable" in the last week (64%), day (76.6%), and hour (93.4%) of life. A retrospective chart review documented the signs and symptoms occurring at the end of life in 28 children dying from cancer in Japan. All children experienced anorexia, 82.1% had dyspnea, and 75% had pain. Other symptoms included fatigue (71.4%), nausea and/or vomiting (57.1%), constipation (46.4%), and diarrhea (21.4%).[6] This symptom profile parallels that of the North American reviews of the symptoms of dying children.[7-9]

PAIN SYNDROMES RELATED TO TUMORS IN CHILDREN WITH CANCER

Despite the predominance of treatment-related pain, a number of children have pain related to a tumor, despite the initial response of their pain to treatment. One-third of the pain experienced by patients in the hospital setting was tumor-related pain, but less than 20% of the pain experienced by outpatients was caused by tumor.[10] Direct tumor involvement of bone, hollow viscera, or nerves are more common causes of pain in adult patients with cancer than in children. Such tumor involvement commonly results in somatic, visceral, and neuropathic pain, respectively. Somatic pain is typically well-localized and is frequently described as aching or gnawing. Examples of somatic pain include pain associated with primary or metastatic bone disease or postsurgical incision pain. Visceral pain results from the infiltration, compression, distension, or stretching of thoracic and abdominal viscera by primary or metastatic tumor. This pain is poorly localized, often described as deep squeezing and pressure and may be associated with nausea, vomiting, and diaphoresis, particularly when acute. An example of visceral pain includes pain associated with tumor of the liver, either primary such as hepatoblastoma, or metastatic, such as neuroblastoma. Neuropathic pain most commonly results from tumor compression or infiltration of peripheral nerves or the spinal cord. Chemical- or radiation-induced injury also may result in this sort of pain. The clinical features of pain resulting from neural injury include:

- Abnormal or unfamiliar unpleasant sensations, such as dysesthesias frequently having a burning or electrical quality,
- A paroxysmal brief shooting or stabbing component,
- Allodynia, or pain that is induced by stimuli that are not normally painful such as light touch of the skin,
- Or pain that may be felt in the region of a sensory deficit.

The pattern of symptoms, based on the self-reports of children aged 10 to 18 treated for cancer, was studied.[11] Children were surveyed across the spectrum of illness and included newly diagnosed patients, those receiving a bone marrow transplant, and those receiving palliative care. It showed that children with cancer are very symptomatic and are often highly distressed by their symptoms. A prevalence rate greater than

35% was noted for the symptoms of pain, drowsiness, nausea, cough, anorexia, lack of energy, and psychological symptoms. In-patients reported being more symptomatic than their out-patient cohorts. Children with solid tumors were more symptomatic than children with other malignancies. Pain, nausea, and anorexia were clustered as being highly distressing symptoms.[11] Children 7 to 12 years of age, also treated for cancer, similarly self-reported their symptoms. The most prevalent symptoms were pain, difficulty sleeping, itch, nausea, fatigue, and anorexia.[12]

PAIN IN CHILDREN WITH CYSTIC FIBROSIS AT THE END OF LIFE

A retrospective chart review at a tertiary-care hospital summarized the end-of-life care of patients more than 5 years of age and dying from cystic fibrosis in the United States.[13] Increasing pain for this patient population may signal advanced, progressive disease.[14] Twenty-five percent of these patients had been receiving opioids for the treatment of chronic headache and/or chest pain for more than their last 3 months of life. When opioids were used for the treatment of breathlessness and/or chest pain, the proportion increased to 86%. Chest, head, extremity, abdomen, and back pain were the most common pain locations during end-of-life care.[14]

PAIN AND OTHER SYMPTOMS IN CHILDREN WITH NEURODEGENERATIVE ILLNESSES

Pain, breathlessness, and oral symptoms such as secretions were highlighted as the most common symptoms by caregivers proxy reports for children in the last month of life at an in-patient hospice.[15] Half of the children were noncommunicative. Neurodegenerative illness was the major diagnostic category in this in-patient hospice population. Common sources of pain in children with cognitive and physical impairment include muscle spasticity and problems of the musculoskeletal system, such as hip dislocation or kyphoscoliosis.

PAIN AND OTHER SYMPTOMS IN CHILDREN WITH HIV/AIDS

HIV/AIDS is known to cause pain and other symptoms for multiple reasons, including primary treatments, associated infections, and other complications.[16] Possible causes of pain include bowel dysfunction, cachexia, pancreatitis and sequelae of infection. In a U.S.,-based study, 59% of HIV-infected children reported that their pain impacted negatively on their lives.[17]

Pain Mechanisms: Implications for Treatment

Nociception, or the sensation of tissue injury or inflammation, is an important biologic function that alerts an individual to potential or ongoing injury and prompts the avoidance or limitation of further injury. Lack of protective sensation can lead to a variety of medical complications, including compartment syndromes or decubitus ulcers. Conversely, there is often no protective significance to other types of pain, such as that of metastatic cancer or migraine.

Nociceptors in deep and superficial tissues can be activated by chemical, thermal, or mechanical stimuli to send afferent impulses through thinly myelinated A-d fibers or unmyelinated C fibers. Primary afferents synapse in the dorsal horn of the spinal cord. Secondary fibers then convey impulses rostrally through a number of tracts, especially the anterolateral spinothalamic tracts. Descending control systems modulate and inhibit pain perception. Endogenous opioids, serotonin, and norepinephrine all appear to be involved in these descending pain-inhibiting systems. In neonates there is a relative excess of excitatory mechanisms for pain transmission with immature inhibitory mechanisms and large receptive fields. All of these factors contribute to a more generalized response to lower intensity pain stimulation in the neonate.

Nociceptive pain refers to pain associated with intact neurons detecting and transmitting impulses associated with tissue injury or inflammation. *Neuropathic pain* refers to pain associated with abnormal excitability in peripheral or central neurons. Neuropathic pain may persist even after tissue injury or inflammation has subsided. Neuropathic pain often is described as burning, shooting, or stabbing, and it is often associated with paresthesias. *Allodynia* refers to a condition in which pain can be elicited by normally nonpainful stimuli, such as light stroking of the skin. In the absence of acute inflammation of the skin, allodynia generally implies the existence of an underlying neuropathic condition.

Pathophysiology of Tumor-Related Pain in Childhood Cancer

Tumor commonly causes pain from involvement of bone, viscera, and nerves. Visceral stretch, compression, or ischemia activates nociceptive endings that evoke pain. Visceral pain is typically more poorly localized than somatic pain. Animal studies have demonstrated primary visceral afferents that discharge maximally only to apparent noxious stimuli and have small myelinated or unmyelinated axons. Possible mechanisms that may cause pain from bone metastases include stimulation of nerve endings in the endosteum by chemical agents released from the destroyed bone tissue, such as prostaglandins, bradykinin, substance P, or histamine; stretching of the periosteum; fractures; and tumor growth into surrounding nerves and tissues. The periosteum is more sensitive than bone marrow and cortex.

Mechanisms for persistent neuropathic pain after damage to peripheral tissues include:

- Deafferentation-induced hyperactivity of dorsal horn pain transmission cells,
- Loss of central inhibition by loss of myelinated primary afferents,
- Ectopic impulse generation in damaged nociceptive primary afferents,
- Sympathetic efferent activation of damaged or intact primary afferents,
- Changes in autonomic reflexes.

Pain Assessment in Children with Life-Threatening Illnesses

The pain assessment of the child receiving palliative care may be a complex process. Regular pain assessment of the child receiving post-operative pain management is standard practice at most children's healthcare facilities. It is a less-established practice that the child with progressive illness receives a regular pain assessment. Pain may still not be thought of or asked about when the child's condition is rare, poorly understood, and/or impairs cognition; and clinicians may erroneously believe that if patients do not volunteer information about pain, then it is not a relevant clinical issue.[18] In addition, children and their caregivers may not volunteer information about pain due to a fear that it may indicate progressive disease. Continually assessing a child's pain is an essential component of competent pain management in pediatric palliative care.

Assessment necessitates finding out what language is used by the child to describe pain and a pain history including: location, radiation, duration, quality, exacerbating or relieving factors, and impact on the usual activities of play and mobility. A physical examination should also be performed where appropriate. History and physical examination are of critical importance in determining a diagnosis. It is possible that therapies directed at the primary cause of pain, such as antibiotics for infection as a cause of pain, will be ultimately more effective than the administration of analgesics. Assessment is sometimes made indirectly by quantifying the type, frequency, and dosing of medications. The report from someone other than the child is frequently relied upon for a proxy measure of pain in children who are cognitively impaired.

PAIN MEASUREMENT AS PART OF PAIN ASSESSMENT

Measuring pain is one component of the assessment of pain in children. Measurement relies on a metric applied to a specific aspect of the pain experience, usually pain severity.

Unidimensional Self-Report Measures

Self-report measures of pain in children have largely focused on the assessment of acute pain severity. Generally the data support the use of visual analogue scales (VAS) or faces scales for children over the age of 5.[19] VAS have been used in the assessment of pediatric cancer pain; frequently they have anchors of no pain and the worst pain possible. To use such scales, children must understand proportionality, to be able to conceptualize their pain experience along a continuum and be able to translate that understanding to the visual representations on the line and the anchors (Fig. 31-1).

Similar strategies, such as Likert scales with anchor points of 1, no pain, and 5, extreme pain, have been used to assess pain in children with cancer.[20] However, research on the use of verbal rating scales with children 9 years and older has not clearly established the utility of this approach over visual analog scales.[21] Other investigators have used visual cues, such as different pictures of a child's face that are graded from neutral or happy expressions for no pain to sad or distressed expressions for extreme pain.[22,23]

Behavioral Observation Measures

A child in pain may exhibit some of the following behaviors: irritability and uncooperativeness, lethargy, excess activity, being unusually quiet, loss of appetite, disturbed sleep, anger, flat effect, withdrawn, and paucity of movement. Actions, especially in babies and/or toddlers that are less common than those above but nevertheless can demonstrate pain, include: pulling at ears, banging the head, lying with knees flexed, holding themselves rigid, and clenching fists.

The subjective distress of acute pain, particularly after traumatic medical procedures, often manifests itself in certain facial expressions, verbal, and motor responses. Behavioral methods for assessing pain in children require independent raters recording the physical behaviors of children in pain, as well as the frequency of the occurrence.[24] Behavioral measures of pain in children consist of observation checklists in which a trained observer records the occurrence of certain behaviors. The frequency and duration of the behaviors that occur during the medical procedures are scored to produce a numerical value that represents the child's overall distress. This value is an integrated index of a child's anxiety, fear, distress, and pain, but children's behavioral scores have been interpreted as their global pain scores.[25]

The Gauvain-Piquard rating scale[26] is an observation scale designed to assess chronic pain in pediatric oncology patients aged 2 to 6 years. The lack of operational definitions and the low kappa coefficients question the utility of this scale. The scale consists of 17 items:

- 7 are related to pain assessment: antalgic rest position, spontaneous protection of painful areas, somatic complaints, the child points out painful areas, antalgic behavior during movement, control exerted by child when moved, and emotional reactions to medical examination of painful regions.
- 6 are related to depression: child retires into his shell, lack of expressiveness, lack of interest in surroundings, slowness and rarity of movements, signs of regression, social withdrawal.
- 4 assess anxiety: nervousness and/or anxiety, ability to protest, moodiness and/or irritability, tendency to cry.

Pain Measurement in Children with Neurocognitive Impairment

A substantial number of children who die have an illness that results in cognitive impairment. Many neurodegenerative

 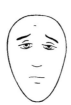 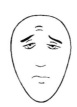 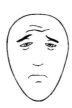 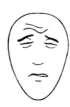 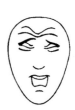

Fig. 31-1 **Visual Scale for Assessment of Pediatric Pain.** (Hicks CL, von Baeyer CL, Spafford P, van Korlaar I, Goodenough B. Faces Pain Scale-Revised: Toward a Common Metric in Pediatric Pain Measurement. Pain 2001; 93:173-183. With the instructions and translations as found on the website: www.painsourcebook.ca. This figure has been reproduced with permission of the International Association for the Study of Pain® [IASP®].)

diseases impact profoundly on the child's ability to verbally communicate. The physical aspects of certain illnesses, such as grimacing or hypertonia, can mimic features or behaviors commonly attributed to pain. In one post-operative pain study, 24 children aged 3 to 19 years with cognitive impairment were rated by their caregivers and researchers as to their perceived intensity of the child's pain pre- and post-surgery.[27] Familiarity with an individual child was not necessary for observers to have congruent pain measurements. Pain cues reported by 29 caregivers of non-communicative children aged 2 to 12 years with life-threatening conditions were compared against a checklist of 203 items. This study yielded a common core set of six pain cues. These are screaming and/or yelling, crying, distressed facial expression, tense body, difficult to comfort, and flinching when touched.[28]

MultiDimensional Symptom Assessment Scales

The Memorial Symptom Assessment Scale 10-18, modified from an adult version, was developed for children aged 10 to 18 years with cancer. In a mean of 11 minutes, the majority of children were able to answer questions about how severe, frequent, and distressing they found their symptoms.[11] For the younger child with cancer, the scale was modified and trialed in 7 to 12 year olds.[12] On this scale, pain is one of many symptoms assessed in 3 dimensions: severity, frequency, and distress.

Adequate Pain Management at the End of Life is Achievable

GOALS FOR PAIN MANAGEMENT

The goals for pain management for the child receiving palliative care are:

- To be pain-free or as near as pain-free as possible,
- To be able to move with minimal discomfort,
- To have minimal or no side effects from medications,
- To maintain the ability to interact with others to the extent, that this is a child and family priority.

Pain relief with what would be considered conventional analgesic doses and routes is achievable to fulfill these goals for the vast majority of children facing pain as a consequence of advanced illness. This was well documented in a 1995 study of a pediatric oncology population, where the records of 199 children and young adults dying of malignancy were reviewed. Only 6% of these patients required what would be considered massive doses of an opioid infusion, defined as 100-fold the usual post-operative opioid requirement.[29] Of that small proportion of patients, there were a few instances where extraordinary doses of analgesia, the use of unusual routes such as opioid infusions given via the subarachnoid route, or the provision of sedation was required to ensure comfort at end of life.[29] Similarly, regional anesthetic techniques are infrequent in treating pain at end of life for children with cancer diagnoses.[30] A review conducted over a 5-year period assessed the opioid doses used in children (n = 42) dying at a pediatric hospice. The parental morphine equivalents ranged from 0.001-73.9 mg/kg/hr, with a median of 0.085 mg/kg/hr.[31]

Since the publication of these reports, practice has become better informed by subsequent research and a greater understanding of the management of the pediatric pain crisis. Practice also now includes the calculation of opioid rescue dosing and dose escalation, opioid switching, greater understanding of the management of opioid side effects to permit greater opioid dose escalation, the NMDA antagonists as new therapeutic options, and a better understanding of invasive approaches to pain management in children. Given the change in therapeutics, it may be that fewer children need to be sedated to reduce conscious awareness of intractable symptoms.

MYTHS AND MISPERCEPTIONS ABOUT PAIN IN CHILDREN

The myth that children either do not experience pain, or do not experience pain as much as adults, has until recently inhibited progress in pain management for children. Since the 1980s there has been a growing movement toward improved pain control for infants, children, and adolescents. This movement was partly a response to the weight of evidence indicating that poor pain control negatively influenced outcome in post-operative neonates.[32] It was also partly due to improved measures of pain severity in infants and children and a critical mass of clinicians with developing expertise in this area. This latter has seen the development of interdisciplinary pain services in many pediatric centers around the world. In most cases centers have a close professional affiliation with pediatric palliative care services.

Although there is an increasing consciousness toward improved pain control for children in general, there are some particular issues pertaining to children receiving palliative care. For example, the meaning of increasing pain severity for some families may be as a marker of disease progression. Some children and families defer opioid dose increases because of the meaning associated with increasing pain. The names of the opioids have certain meanings for some families. Methadone, for example, can sometimes be an appropriate analgesic for children. However, the mention of methadone can cause anxiety for some families and clinicians because of its association with the treatment of opioid drug addiction.

Confusion exists about the term's tolerance, dependence, and drug addiction. Analgesic tolerance refers to the progressive decline in potency of an opioid with chronic use, so that increasingly higher doses are required to achieve the same analgesic effect. Parents are sometimes reluctant to increase opioid doses in their child because of a fear that tolerance will make opioids ineffective later. Reassurance should be given that tolerance, in the majority of cases, can be managed by simple dose escalation, use of adjuvant medications, or perhaps by an opioid switch in the setting of dose-limiting side effects. Physical dependence is a physiologic state characterized by withdrawal, or abstinence syndrome, after dose reduction or discontinuation of the opioid, or administration of an opioid antagonist. Initial manifestations of withdrawal include yawning, diaphoresis, lacrimation, coryza, and tachycardia.

Addiction is a psychological and behavioral syndrome characterized by drug craving and aberrant drug use. Some parents fear that exposure to an opioid will result in their child subsequently becoming a drug addict. The incidence of opioid addiction was examined prospectively in 12,000 hospitalized adult patients who received at least one dose of a strong opioid.[33] There were only four documented cases of subsequent addiction in patients who did not have a history of drug abuse. These data suggest that iatrogenic opioid addiction is an uncommon problem in adults. This observation is also consistent with a large worldwide experience with opioid treatment of cancer pain in childhood.

ANALGESIC STUDIES AT THE END OF A CHILD'S LIFE

The need to improve pain management in dying children is demonstrated by data indicating that pain is often not adequately assessed and treated effectively.[7] Improvement in pain management will be dependent not only on advances in pediatric analgesic therapeutics but also on strategies to correct the barriers to the adequate treatment of pain in these children. Few analgesic studies have been performed in children receiving palliative care. One reason pertains to the heterogeneous nature of pain in this population, and that children with cancer tend to receive therapies directed at control of their tumors until very late in the course of their illnesses. They are frequently very ill and highly symptomatic. These variables make it less likely that a subpopulation of children receiving palliative care exists who have a stable, chronic pattern of pain amenable to evaluation in a trial. The lack of an appropriate analgesic study design to account for small numbers of subjects is a further impediment to progress in pain management for these children.

The standard designs of analgesic clinical trials in adults generally involve randomization between test drug and placebo. This design would generally be regarded as ethically and practically unacceptable for children in palliative care. One variant of this design is to randomize between active drug and placebo with both groups having immediate access to PCA with a standard opioid such as morphine. In this design, morphine-sparing has been used as a surrogate measure of analgesic effect of the test drug. While this method is widely used in pediatric postoperative trials, it still does not solve the problem of small numbers and heterogeneous populations in pediatric palliative care.

The Evidence from Analgesic Studies

Given the difficulties of performing analgesic studies in children receiving palliative care, most pediatric analgesic studies have been performed using other pain models, such as postoperative pain or musculoskeletal pain. Although the pharmacokinetic and the major pharmacodynamic properties, analgesia and sedation, of most opioids have been studied in pediatrics and previously documented, little information is available about oral bioavailability, potency ratios, and other pharmacodynamic properties in children. In addition, there have been no controlled clinical trials of adjuvant analgesic agents in pediatrics.

Of the few analgesic studies performed in the setting of life-threatening illness, most have conformed to one of the following two objectives:

1. The evaluation of a drug proved efficacious in adult pain models but now targeted to the pediatric cancer pain population.

Most of the analgesic studies of opioids performed in children with cancer[34–42] have been previously performed in adults. Most of these studies had small numbers of subjects, few were controlled studies, and did not use validated pain severity assessment scales. Most did not demonstrate differences between pediatric and adult data. Significantly, however, one study[40] demonstrated age differences in morphine pharmacokinetics compared with the adult population and recommended a starting total daily dose of morphine of 1.5 to 2.0 mg/kg/day to provide plasma concentrations >12ng/ml in

children with cancer pain unrelieved by analgesics used for mild to moderate pain.

2. The evaluation of novel approaches to opioid delivery or analgesic study design in this population.

Historically, the status of pediatric analgesic studies has improved, as have psychometric data for measures of pain severity. This has resulted in a greater sophistication of pediatric analgesic studies in this patient population. For example, PCA morphine was compared with continuous infusion morphine for the relief of mucositis pain in patients aged 12 to 18 years. This study used randomized controlled trial methodology.[43] Less morphine intake and fewer opioid side effects were demonstrated in the morphine PCA group.

With small patient numbers, a novel pediatric analgesic study used randomized, double-blind, three period cross-over methodology.[44] The safety and efficacy of a clinical protocol for the administration of opioids by PCA for mucositis pain after bone marrow transplantation was demonstrated. In this small study, hydromorphone was not superior to morphine in terms of analgesia or the side-effect profile. The clearances of hydromorphone and morphine in the children studied were generally greater than those previously recorded, but this finding may be related to disease or treatment variables. Apart from clearance, the morphine pharmacokinetics in the study population were similar to those previously recorded. In addition, hydromorphone may be less potent in this population of children than indicated by adult equipotency tables.[45]

Pain Management Guidelines

Guidelines for the management of pain in children with life-threatening conditions need to be created at a local level. The extent to which clinical guidelines promote improvement is unknown. However, a recent Swedish questionnaire surveyed all the pediatric departments about their pain management practices for cancer.[46] It showed that 63% of physicians follow the analgesic ladder approach recommended in the World Health Organization (WHO) guidelines.[46]

ANALGESICS

Analgesics can be divided into three groups of drugs: nonopioid analgesics, opioid analgesics, and adjuvant analgesics. The prescription of these drugs for children with cancer pain is based on the WHO analgesic ladder, which emphasizes pain intensity as the guide to choice of analgesic, rather than etiologic factors. In other words, the prescription of analgesics should be according to pain severity, ranging from acetaminophen and non-steroidal anti-inflammatory drugs for mild pain to opioids for moderate to severe pain. The choice of analgesics is individualized to achieve an optimum balance between analgesia and side effects (Table 31-2).

Acetaminophen

Acetaminophen is one of the most commonly used nonopioid analgesics in children with cancer. It has a potential for hepatic and renal injury,[47] but this is uncommon in therapeutic doses. Unlike aspirin, acetaminophen does not have an association with Reye Syndrome. The antipyretic action of acetaminophen may be contraindicated in neutropenic patients in whom it is important to monitor fever. Pediatric dosing of acet-

TABLE 31-2 Opioid Analgesic Initial Dosage Guidelines*

Drug	Equilanalgesic doses		Usual starting IV or SC doses and intervals		Parenteral/ oral dose ratio	Usual starting oral doses and intervals	
	parenteral	oral	Child < 50 kg	Child >50 kg		Child < 50 kg	Child >50 kg
Codeine	120 mg	200 mg	N/R	N/R	1:2	0.5-1 mg/kg every 3-4 hrs	30-60 mg every 3-4 hours
Morphine	10 mg	30 mg (chronic dosing)	Bolus: 0.1mg/kg every 2- 4 hrs Infusion: 0.03 mg/ kg/hr	Bolus: 5-8 mg every 2-4 hrs Infusion: 1 mg/hr	1:3 (chronic)	Immediate release: 0.3 mg/kg every 3-4 hrs Sustained release: 20-35 kg: 10-15 mg every 12 hrs 35-50 kg: 15-30 mg every 12 hrs	Immediate release: 15-20 mg every 3-4 hrs Sustained release: 30-45 mg every 12 hrs
Oxycodone	N/A	15-20 mg	N/A	N/A	N/A	0.1-0.2 mg/kg every 3-4 hrs	5-10 mg every 3-4 hrs
Methadone	10 mg	10-20 mg	0.1 mg/kg every 4-8 hrs	5 mg	1:2	0.2 mg/kg every 4-8 hrs	10 mg every 4-8 hrs
	Methadone requires additional vigilance, because it can accumulate and produce delayed sedation. If sedation occurs, doses should be withheld until sedation resolves. Thereafter, doses should be substantially reduced and/or the dosing interval should be extended to 8-12 hrs.						
Fentanyl	100 mcg (0.1 mg)	N/A	Bolus: 0.5-1 mcg/kg every 1-2 hrs Infusion: 0.5-2 mcg/kg/hr	Bolus: 25-50 mcg every 1-2 hrs Infusion: 25-100 mcg/hr	N/A	N/A	N/A
Hydromorphone	1.5-2 mg	6-8 mg	Bolus: 0.02 mg/kg every 2-4 hrs Infusion: 0.006 mg/kg/hr	Bolus: 1 mg Every 2-4 hrs Infusion: 0.3 mg/hr	1:4	0.04-0.08 mg/kg every 3-4 hrs	2-4 mg every 3-4 hrs
Meperidine (pethidine)	75-100mg	300 mg	Bolus: 0.8-1 mg/kg every 2-3 hrs	Bolus: 50-75 mg every 2-3 hrs	1:4	2-3 mg/kg every 3-4 hrs	100-150 mg every 3-4 hrs
	Meperidine should generally be avoided if other opioids are available, especially with chronic use, because its metabolite can cause seizures.						

Data from Cancer Pain Relief and Palliative Care in Children. WHO Press, Geneva, 1998[4].
N/A, Not available; N/R, Not recommended.
*Doses refer to patients older than 6 months. In infants younger than 6 months, initial doses/kg should begin approximately 25% of the doses/kg recommended here. All doses are approximate and should be adjusted according to clinical circumstances.

aminophen has been based on the antipyretic dose-response. Oral dosing of 15 mg/kg every 4 to 6 hours is recommended, with a maximum daily dose of 60 mg/kg/day for patients of normal or average build.

There are no data on the safety of chronic acetaminophen administration in children. In Australia, New South Wales Health Policy mandates that paracetamol, or acetaminophen, should not be administered to children for more than 48 hours without a medical review.[48] Intravenous paracetamol is available as a therapeutic analgesic option in some countries. Its use has been documented in the context of pediatric post-operative pain management[49] and practice guidelines are evolving.[50]

Aspirin and Nonsteroidal Anti-inflammatory Drugs (NSAID)

Aspirin and NSAIDs are frequently contraindicated in pediatric oncology patients who are often at risk of bleeding due to thrombocytopenia. In a comparative study of aspirin and ibuprofen in children with juvenile rheumatoid arthritis, the drugs were equally efficacious, but the drop-out rate caused by side effects was significantly higher in the aspirin group.

Choline magnesium trisalicylate (Trilisate) has been widely recommended because of reports in adults of minimal effects on platelet function in vitro and experimental studies showing minimal gastric irritation in rats, in contrast to aspirin.[51] The studies do not include medically frail patients with thrombocytopenia or other morbidities.

The cyclooxygenase-2 (COX-2) inhibitors target a specific isoenzyme involved in the generation of prostanoids, which contribute to pain and inflammation. Although celecoxib and meloxicam have undergone some limited trials in children with rheumatoid arthritis and post-operative pain,[52,53] their role in pediatric pain management is unclear. Rofecoxib was removed from the international market because of increased risk of cardiovascular events in adults.[54]

Codeine

In pediatrics, codeine is commonly administered via the oral route and in combination with acetaminophen. It is prescribed for mild to moderate pain. Codeine is typically administered in pediatrics in oral doses of 0.5-1 mg/kg every 4 hours for children older than 6 months. Pharmacogenetic studies have demonstrated that 4% to 14% of the population lacks the hepatic enzyme responsible for the conversion of codeine to morphine. A pediatric study has shown that 35% of children showed inadequate conversion of codeine to morphine.[55] The prescription of codeine as an analgesic in pediatrics is declining.

Tramadol

Tramadol may be a useful analgesic for the management of moderate cancer pain and is thought to cause less respiratory depression than morphine. While tramadol has been studied for postoperative pain in children, there are few data on the safety and efficacy of tramadol for children with pain due to cancer or chronic illness.

Oxycodone

Oxycodone is used for moderate to severe pain in children with cancer. Oxycodone may be available only as an oral preparation in combination with acetaminophen in some countries. The total daily acetaminophen dose may be the limiting factor in dose escalation of these products. Oxycodone has a higher clearance value and a shorter elimination half life, $t_{1/2}$, in children aged 2 to 20 years than adults.[56,57] Oxycodone is available as a long-acting preparation in some countries.

Morphine

Morphine is one of the most widely used opioids for moderate to severe cancer pain in children. Evolving data indicate that a variable human analgesic response of morphine may be explained in part by genetic variation and different μ-opioid receptor neurotransmitter responses.[58]

The binding of morphine to plasma protein is age dependent. In premature infants, less than 20% is bound to plasma proteins.[59,60] Within the neonatal period for term infants, the volume of distribution is linearly related to age and body surface area,[59–61] but after the neonatal period the values are approximately the same as adults.[62,63]

Morphine clearance is delayed in the first 1 to 3 months of life. The half-life of morphine, $t_{1/2}$, changes from values of 10 to 20 hours in preterm infants to values of 1 to 2 hours in preschool aged children.[62,63] Therefore starting doses in very young infants should be reduced to approximately 25% to 30% on a per kg basis relative to dosing recommended for older children.

Following oral dosing, morphine has a significant first-pass metabolism in the liver. An oral-to-parenteral potency ratio of approximately 3:1 is commonly encountered during chronic administration.[64] A typical starting dose for immediate release oral morphine in opioid-naive subjects is 0.3 mg/kg every 4 hours. Typical starting intravenous infusion rates are 0.02-0.03mg/kg/hr beyond the first 3 months of life, and 0.015mg/kg/hr in younger infants. Sustained release preparations of morphine are available for children and permit oral dosing either twice or three times daily. Crushing sustained-release tablets produces an immediate release of morphine. This limits its use in children who must chew tablets.

Hydromorphone

Hydromorphone is an alternative opioid when the dose escalation of morphine is limited by side effects or volume restriction is needed for parenteral administration. It is available for oral, intravenous, subcutaneous, epidural, and intrathecal administration. Adult studies indicate that intravenous hydromorphone is 5 to 8 times as potent as morphine. A double-blind, randomized crossover comparison of morphine to hydromorphone using PCA in children and adolescents with mucositis following bone marrow transplantation showed that hydromorphone was well tolerated and had a potency ratio of approximately 6:1 relative to morphine in this setting.[44] Because of its high potency and aqueous solubility, hydromorphone is convenient for subcutaneous infusion. Little is known about the pharmacokinetics of hydromorphone in infants.

Fentanyl

Fentanyl is a synthetic opioid that is approximately 50 to 100 times more potent than morphine during acute intravenous administration. The half-life of this opioid is prolonged in preterm infants undergoing cardiac surgery,[65] but comparable values with those of adults are reached within the first months of life.[66–69] The clearance of fentanyl is higher in toddlers and children than in adults. (For younger infants, including those undergoing abdominal surgery, the clearance is not higher than in adults.[68,69]) Fentanyl may also be used for continuous infusion for selected patients with dose-limiting side effects from morphine. Rapid administration of high doses of IV fentanyl may result in chest wall rigidity and severe ventilatory difficulty.

Oral transmucosal fentanyl produces a rapid onset of effect and escapes first-pass hepatic clearance. Oral transmucosal fentanyl for sedation and/or analgesia during bone marrow biopsy and/or aspiration and lumbar puncture was found safe and effective, although the frequency of vomiting may be a limiting factor in its tolerability.[70] Its use for breakthrough cancer pain in adults has been described.[71]

In a small study using a clinical protocol, the utility, feasibility, and tolerability of transdermal fentanyl was demonstrated in children with cancer pain.[39] The mean clearance and volume of distribution of transdermal fentanyl are the same for both adults and children, but the variability is higher in adults.[39] A subsequent larger study confirmed the effectiveness of this analgesic for children.[72]

Meperidine

Meperidine has been used for procedural and postoperative pain in children. It is a short half-life synthetic opioid. Neonates have a slower elimination of meperidine than children and young infants.[73–77] Normeperidine is the major metabolite of meperidine. This can cause CNS excitatory effects, including tremors and convulsions,[78] particularly in patients with impaired renal clearance. Meperidine is therefore not generally recommended for children with chronic pain but may be an acceptable alternative to fentanyl for short painful procedures.

Methadone

Methadone is a synthetic opioid that has a long and variable half-life. Following single parenteral doses, its potency is similar to that of morphine. In children receiving post-operative analgesia, methadone produced a more prolonged analgesia than morphine.[79,80] Because of its prolonged half-life, methadone has a risk of delayed sedation and overdose occurring several days after initiating treatment.

The oral:parenteral potency ratio of methadone is approximately 1.5 to 2:1. Frequent patient assessment is the key to safe and effective use of methadone. If a patient becomes comfortable after initial doses, the dose should be reduced or the interval extended to reduce the likelihood of subsequent somnolence. If a patient becomes oversedated early in dose escalation, it is recommended to stop dosing, not just reduce the dose, and to observe the patient until there is increased alertness. Although as needed dosing is discouraged for most patients with cancer pain, some clinicians find this approach a useful way to establish a dosing schedule for methadone.[79,80] Methadone remains a long-acting agent when administered either as an elixir or as crushed tablets. Unique issues with conversion between other opioids and methadone are detailed below in the section on "Opioid Switching."

ROUTES AND METHODS OF ANALGESIC ADMINISTRATION

Oral

Oral administration of analgesics is the first choice for the majority of children and young patients. Analgesics should generally be administered to children by the simplest, safest, most effective and least painful route. Oral dosing is generally predictable, inexpensive, and does not require invasive procedures or technologies.

Topical

The eutectic mixture of local anesthetics, EMLA, is a topical preparation that provides local anesthesia to the skin, dermis, and subcutaneous tissues if applied under an occlusive dressing for at least one hour. It has been shown to be useful for procedural pain, including lumbar puncture[81] and central venous port access[82] in children with cancer. Preliminary studies of topical amethocaine for percutaneous analgesia before venous cannulation in children have demonstrated promising safety and efficacy data.[83] The newer generation of topical local anesthetics promise a quicker onset of action and are being reviewed.[84]

Intravenous

Intravenous administration has the advantage of rapid onset of analgesia, easier opioid dose titration, bioavailability, and continuous effect when infusions are used. The intravenous route of administration is often an option in children with cancer because many have indwelling intravenous access.

Subcutaneous

The subcutaneous route is an alternative route of administration for children with either no or poor intravenous access. Solutions are generally concentrated so that infusion rates do not exceed 1-3 ml/hr.[85] An application of a topical local anesthetic agent is recommended prior to the placement of a subcutaneous needle. A small catheter or butterfly needle (27 gauge) may be placed under the skin of the thorax, abdomen, or thigh, with sites changed approximately every 3 days.

Intramuscular

Intramuscular administration is painful and may lead to the under-reporting of pain. This route of administration does not permit easy dose titration or infusion and should be avoided.

Rectal

Rectal administration is discouraged in the pediatric cancer population because of concern regarding infection and because of the great variability of rectal absorption of morphine.[86] It may be useful in the home care of the dying child when no other route is available. Slow-release morphine tablets can be administered via the rectum.

Patient-Controlled Analgesia

Patient-controlled analgesia (PCA) is a method of opioid administration that permits the patient to self-administer small bolus doses of opioid within set time limits. PCA caters to an individual's variation in pharmacokinetics, pharmacodynamics, and pain intensity. It allows appropriate children to have control over their analgesia and allows them to choose a balance between the benefits of analgesia versus the side effects of opioids. In patients with severe mucositis, for example, opioid dosing can be timed with routine mouth care and other causes of incidental mouth pain.

PCA has been used successfully for the management of prolonged oropharyngeal mucositis pain following bone marrow transplantation in children and adolescents.[43,44,87] A controlled comparison of staff-controlled continuous infusion (CI) of morphine and PCA in adolescents with severe oropharyngeal mucositis found that the PCA group had equivalent analgesia but less sedation and less difficulty concentrating.[43]

The Pediatric Pain Crisis

A pain crisis in a child is an emergency and may require treatments beyond conventional means. A specific diagnosis must be made, as therapies directed at the primary cause may be more effective in the long term. Management requires the clinician to be at the patient's bedside to titrate incremental intravenous opioid doses every 10 to 15 minutes until effective analgesia has been attained. The analgesic effect of opioids increase in a log-linear function, with incremental opioid dosing required until either analgesia is achieved or somnolence occurs.[64] A continuous infusion of opioid may need to be commenced to maintain this level of analgesia. The initial infusion rate is often based on the opioid administered as a loading dose rather than the starting doses typically referred to in practical reference manuals.[64] An alternative to a continuous infusion of opioid is intermittent parenteral opioid, especially in the setting of an unpredictable pain syndrome.

BREAKTHROUGH PAIN IN CHILDREN

Breakthrough or rescue doses are additional doses of opioid incorporated into the analgesic regime to allow for additional analgesia if required by the patient. Breakthrough doses of opioid may be calculated as approximately 5% to 10% of the total daily opioid requirement and may be administered orally every hour.[64] Given the frequency with which additional analgesia may be required for severe pain, it may be convenient for some children to self-administer breakthrough opioid doses using a PCA device. Data suggest that 7-year-old children of normal intelligence can use PCA effectively to provide analgesia post-operatively.[88]

A prospective study determined the prevalence, characteristics, and impact of breakthrough pain in children with cancer.[44] Twenty-seven pediatric inpatients with cancer aged 7 to 18 years who had severe pain requiring treatment with opioids participated in this study. The children responded to a structured interview, Breakthrough Pain Questionnaire for Children, designed to characterize breakthrough pain in children. Measures of pain, anxiety, and depressed mood were completed. Fifty-seven percent of the children experienced one or more episodes of breakthrough pain during the preceding 24 hours, each episode lasting seconds to minutes, occurring three of four times a day and most commonly characterized as sharp and shooting by the children. Younger children, those 7 to 12 years, had a significantly higher risk of experiencing breakthrough pain compared to teenagers. No statistical difference could be shown between children with and without breakthrough pain in regard to anxiety and depression. The most effective treatment of an episode of breakthrough pain was a PCA opioid bolus dose. It is clear that further studies of breakthrough pain in children and more effective treatment strategies in this age group are necessary.[89]

OPIOID DOSE ESCALATION

If pain can be controlled by the opioid loading technique described previously, then the subsequent intravenous opioid dose escalation may be calculated as follows:

- If greater than approximately 4 to 6 breakthrough doses of opioid are required in a 24-hour period, then the hourly average of this total daily rescue opioid should be added to the baseline opioid infusion. An alternative would be to increase the baseline infusion by 50%.[64]
- Breakthrough doses are kept as a proportion of the baseline opioid infusion rate and with dose titration, are recalculated as between 50% and 200% of the hourly basal infusion rate.[64]

OPIOID SWITCHING

The usual indication for switching to an alternative is dose-limiting opioid side effects that prevent dose escalation. An observation is that a switch from one opioid to another is often accompanied by change in the balance between analgesia and side effects.[90] A favorable change in opioid analgesia to side-effect profile will be experienced if there is less cross-tolerance at the opioid receptors mediating analgesia than at those mediating adverse effects.[91] An opioid switch may permit better analgesia with less opioid side effects.[92] There are emerging pediatric data on the practice of opioid rotation in children with cancer. Following a review of opioid prescription at a pediatric hospital for the above indications, opioid rotation was employed in 9% of all opioid prescriptions, with a positive impact on side-effect control and without a significant change in pain scores.[93]

Following a prolonged period of regular dosing with one opioid, equivalent analgesia may be attained with a smaller dose of a second opioid than that calculated from an equianalgesic table. An opioid switch is usually accompanied by a reduction in the equianalgesic dose, approximately 50% for short half-life opioids. In contrast to short half-life opioids, the doses of methadone required for equivalent analgesia after switching may be of the order of 10% to 20% of the equianalgesic dose of the previously used short half-life opioid. Protocols for methadone dose conversion and titration have been documented in adults.[94,95] These protocols have been incorporated into a very convenient opioid dose conversion program available on the web at www.globalrph.com/narcoticonv.htm. Methadone is both extremely useful and challenging to titrate, both because of its variable metabolism and because of its combined action as a mu-opioid and as an NMDA receptor antagonist. In our view, if there is a pain emergency and pain remains difficult to manage despite a rapid and aggressive opioid dose escalation, a trial of methadone should be strongly considered in many cases.

SIDE EFFECTS OF OPIOIDS

Children do not necessarily report opioid side effects such as constipation, pruritus, and dreams voluntarily and should be asked specifically about these problems. All opioids can potentially cause the same constellation of side effects. Tolerance to some opioid side effects such as sedation, nausea and vomiting, and pruritus often develops within the first week of starting opioids. Children do not develop tolerance to constipation and concurrent treatment with laxatives should be provided. Myoclonus is a rare complication of opioid therapy and is usually seen with rapidly escalating opioid dosage or with high-dose opioid prescription. Treatment consists of either switching to an alternative opioid or treating with a benzodiazepine such as clonazepam.

If opioid side effects limit dose escalation, then consideration should be given to an alternative opioid. Young children may not understand the rationale that tolerance to opioid side effects may resolve with time. To ensure ongoing trust and the child's overall comfort, any potential side effects must be anticipated and proactively managed.

Many symptoms are commonly assumed to be generated by opioids without adequate consideration of other causes. It is appropriate to consider these other causes as guided by the history and physical examination, and by consideration of the child's overall situation. For example, urinary retention may be caused by opioids, but could also arise from a variety of other causes, such as anticholinergic effects of medications, neurogenic bladder due to epidural spinal cord compression, cauda equina syndrome or involvement of the sacral plexus. Similarly, nausea and vomiting can be caused by opioids but also be a large number of other processes.

Treatment of opioid side effects is commonly based on custom, on extrapolation from adult clinical trials, or on extrapolation from pediatric clinical trials in other settings, such as postoperative care. There is a need for more research on optimal methods to prevent and treatment opioid side effects. Opioid side effects can be a significant barrier to achieving good pain control, and may result in the child or caregivers being reluctant to give adequate dosing of opioids to achieve pain relief.

Children with many life-threatening conditions commonly experience the overlapping symptoms of fatigue, mental clouding, sleep disturbance, depressed mood, and daytime somnolence. Evaluation and treatment of these symptoms should be broad-based and not limited to a narrow medical model. A recent study suggested that as pain in children with advanced illness is more aggressively treated with opioids, the complex of fatigue-associated symptoms becomes more common.[96]

In some cases, fatigue and somnolence may be improved by simplifying regimens to reduce the cumulative burden of sedating medications. Antihistamines have minimal evidence for efficacy for the treatment of opioid-induced pruritus, and they do contribute to sedation. We have been unable to identify controlled studies of the less-sedating antihistamines for pruritus or for many of the common uses of antihistamines, such as for premedication prior to administration of blood products. Data on the effectiveness of stimulants for the treatment of fatigue and somnolence in children with advanced cancer is limited to one case series.[97]

Although constipation is eminently treatable, studies from adult hospices with formal and fairly aggressive bowel regimens still report refractory constipation as a common problem. Oral naloxone has been studied in adults with refractory constipation, with some variability in recommended dose and in response rates. Two novel opioid antagonist drugs have been designed to provide a more mechanism-based approach to treatment of opioid-induced bowel dysfunction.[98] Methylnaltrexone is a quaternized derivative of the opioid antagonist naltrexone that is excluded from the central side of the of blood-brain barrier. It can be given by intravenous or subcutaneous routes. Alvimopan is an orally-administered enterally constrained opioid antagonist. Methylnaltrexone is now available in the United States, albeit at a retail cost of approximately $40 per dose. Pediatric experience to date is limited, though anecdotally the safety and efficacy has appeared quite good. Methylnaltrexone may be especially useful for the child receiving high dose opioids with refractory constipation who cannot tolerate an enteral laxative regimen. Based on favorable anecdotal experience, methylnaltrexone may also be considered for two other situations:

- A child receiving opioids for pain caused by pancreatitis, because it should be expected to block opioid actions on the biliary and pancreatic sphincters,
- A child or adult with cystic fibrosis and meconium ileus equivalent with severe abdominal pain for whom co-administration of methylnaltrexone along with systemic opioids may possibly permit analgesia while reducing the risks of opioid-induced worsening of the bowel dysfunction.

NMDA RECEPTOR ANTAGONISTS

NMDA-receptor antagonists depress central sensitization to painful stimuli in animal experiments and in humans.[99–102] Dextromethorphan, dextrorphan, ketamine, memantine, and amantadine, among others, have been shown to have NMDA-receptor antagonist activities. The clinical usefulness of some of these medications is compromised by a high adverse side effect to analgesic ratio. There are limited data of their utility in pediatrics, other than procedural pain management. Clinical usage is increasing, particularly for severe neuropathic pain and rapid opioid dose escalation and perceived tolerance. A small case series described low-dose ketamine infusions for children with poorly controlled pain due to cancer.[103]

In our experience, ketamine may be worth considering for the small subgroup of patients with pain, often with neuropathic characteristics, that has responded poorly to the usual measures of opioid dose escalation, opioid switching, a trial of methadone, and other adjuvants. We generally recommend starting an infusion at a rate of 0.1 mg/kg/hr and titrating up to approximately 0.2 mg/kg/hr. Although some clinicians recommend initial boluses or loading doses, we have seen some cases of significant dysphoria and hallucinations with bolus doses as small as 10 mg in a 70 kg adolescent, approximately 0.15 mg/kg. Based on this occurrence, our preference is generally to avoid rapid boluses, and to give small loading doses relatively slowly if a patient is having a pain emergency. A general impression is that dysphoria is rare with infusion rates up to 0.2 mg/kg/hr, and occasional patients are quite clear-headed at rates up to 0.3 mg/kg/hr. Dosing recommendations for oral ketamine are more provisional. Most of the available information about oral

and/or parenteral ratios in pediatrics is based on single doses for preoperative or pre-procedural sedation, and these ratios probably do not account adequately for accumulation of the active metabolite norketamine with chronic dosing. Our limited anecdotal impression is that with chronic dosing, some patients report benefit from dosing of oral ketamine in a dose range of around 2 mg/kg approximately 3 times daily.

OTHER APPROACHES TO INTRACTABLE PEDIATRIC CANCER PAIN

The experience of using regional anesthesia for children with intractable pain is limited. A retrospective study of children with terminal cancer[30] showed that regional anesthesia may be appropriate in a highly select subset of children. The indications for regional anesthesia in this group were mostly related to either dose-limiting side effects of opioids or opioid unresponsiveness in patients where pain was confined to one region of the body. Rapid intravenous opioid dose reduction was required in some cases.[30] In the years since publication of that case series, some technical aspects of regional anesthesia in this setting have evolved.[104]

At Children's Hospital Boston, our general preference is to use subarachnoid catheters rather than epidural catheters, even when the desired position of catheter tips is at mid-thoracic levels. In addition, the preference is to place indwelling ports, rather than a tunneled catheter, to improve skin care and reduce the chances for infection or dislodgment. Ports are placed under general anesthesia, in a lateral decubitus position, and using fluoroscopic guidance to ensure proper cephalad advancement of catheter tips to the appropriate dorsal horn levels innervating the predominant sites of the patient's pain. Coagulopathy is managed by infusions of blood components during the procedure, and perioperative antibiotics are maintained for an extended period, particularly in the setting of neutropenia. In adults, there is widespread use of fully implanted magnetically driven pumps, which require refills at intervals ranging from several weeks to several months. The experience in Boston is that for most children and adolescents with cancer, local anesthetics form a crucial component of the mixture, PCA-like boluses are often required, and both of these features favor use of ports with small external infusion pumps rather than fully implanted systems. Conversely, fully implanted pumps have been used in palliative care for administration of the GABA agonist medication baclofen, or baclofen in combination with morphine or other opioids, for children with refractory spasticity and pain associated with neurodegenerative disorders, including metachromatic leukodystrophy, spinocerebellar ataxia, and Friedrich's ataxia.

For an occasional child or adolescent whose pain arises entirely from the territory of a plexus or peripheral nerve, a tunnelled perineural catheter or plexus catheter may be used for prolonged local anesthetic infusion. In considering peripheral perineural infusions, it is important to know that the catheter can be placed proximal to the tumor or previous surgery, so that local anesthetic can gain access to intended sites of action. Ultrasound guidance is rapidly emerging as a preferred approach to placement of plexus and peripheral perineural catheters.

Neurodestructive approaches to pain management are very rarely used for children. In most situations, a large number of peripheral nerves innervate the area where pain originates, and it would be undesirable to produce sensory or motor deficits. One exception is neurolytic blockade of the celiac plexus, which may be useful for a very small number of patients with massive tumor involving upper abdominal viscera, but not extending beyond these organs to the peritoneum or paraspinous areas. When considering this procedure, the preference is to perform it in collaboration with an interventional radiologist using computed tomographic guidance.

With proper consideration of the child's and family's wishes and consideration of the trajectory of illness, in invasive procedures for pain management for a child with a life-threatening illness have the potential for improved pain relief, especially with movement, improved alertness, and improved quality of life. Conversely, specific expertise is required for both the technical and management issues, which differ in several respects from those used in pediatric perioperative regional anesthesia and in adult chronic pain management. Expert consultation and attention to communication among team members can help in the implementation of these approaches, especially in the home setting.

OTHER MODALITIES OF PAIN MANAGEMENT

Although prominent in clinical practice, there is little in the published literature about such modalities as radiotherapy, radiopharmaceuticals, and transcutaneous electrical nerve stimulation (TENS), generally used concurrently with other pain management techniques. A case series reported some benefit for 29 children with symptomatic metastatic neuroblastoma sites treated with palliative radiotherapy.[105] Similarly, the use of strontium-89 was reported for pain relief in children treated for metastatic cancer but the numbers were too small to make suggestions for clinical care.[106]

Adjuvant Analgesics

Adjuvant analgesics are a heterogeneous group of drugs that have a primary indication other than pain but are analgesic in some painful conditions.[107] Adjuvant analgesics are commonly, but not always, prescribed with primary analgesic drugs. Common classes of these agents include antidepressants, anticonvulsants, neuroleptics, psychostimulants, antihistamines, corticosteroids, and centrally acting skeletal muscle relaxants.

Antidepressants Data from adult studies have guided the use of antidepressants as adjuvant analgesics in pediatrics. Tricyclic antidepressants have been used for a variety of pain conditions in adults, including postherpetic neuralgia,[108] diabetic neuropathy,[109] tension headache,[110] migraine headache,[111] rheumatoid arthritis,[112] chronic low back pain,[113] and cancer pain.[114] Antidepressants are potentially effective in relieving neuropathic pain. With very similar results for anticonvulsants, it is still unclear which drug class should be the first choice.[115]

Baseline hematology and biochemistry tests, including liver function tests, and an electrocardiogram (ECG) to exclude Wolff-Parkinson-white syndrome or other cardiac conduction defects have been recommended prior to starting treatment with tricyclic antidepressants.[116] The measurement of antidepressant plasma concentration allows confirmation of compliance and ensures that optimization of dosage has occurred before discontinuing. An ECG is recommended periodically during long-term use or if standard mg/kg dosages are exceeded.[117]

Psychostimulants Dextroamphetamine potentiates opioid analgesia in postoperative adult patients[118] and methylphenidate counteracts opioid-induced sedation[119] and cognitive dysfunction[120] in advanced cancer patients. Psychostimulants may allow dose escalation of opioids in patients who have somnolence as a dose-limiting side effect.[107] The potential side effects of methylphenidate include anorexia, insomnia, and dysphoria. The use of dextroamphetamine and methylphenidate was reported in a retrospective survey of 11 children receiving opioids for a variety of indications, including cancer pain.[97] Somnolence was reduced in these patients without significant adverse side effects.

Corticosteroids Corticosteroids may produce analgesia by a variety of mechanisms, including anti-inflammatory effects and reduction of tumor edema. It may potentially produce analgesia by a reduction of spontaneous discharge in injured nerves.[121] Dexamethasone tends to be used most frequently because of its high potency, longer duration of action, and minimal mineralocorticoid effect. Corticosteroids may have a role in bone pain due to metastatic bone disease,[122] cerebral edema due to either primary or metastatic tumor,[123] or epidural spinal cord compression.[124]

Anticonvulsants The mechanism of action of anticonvulsants in controlling lancinating pain is not known but is probably related to reducing paroxysmal discharges of central and peripheral neurons. Anticonvulsants are effective in relieving neuropathic pain. With very similar results for antidepressants, it is still unclear which drug class should be the first choice.[115] The use of phenytoin, carbamazepine, and valproate may be problematic in the pediatric cancer population due to their potential adverse effects on the hematological profile. Gabapentin and pregabalin have a generally good safety profile, and may benefit some children with neuropathic pain. Some children experience adverse effects on mood with gabapentin, pregabalin, or any other of the anticonvulsants.

Neuroleptics Methotrimeprazine, a phenothiazine, has been reported as being analgesic for adult cancer pain.[126] Methotrimeprazine is not considered to be a substitute for opioid analgesia. The mechanism by which methotrimeprazine produces analgesia, and its role as an adjuvant agent in pediatric cancer pain, is unclear. It may be useful as an adjuvant analgesic in a patient disseminated cancer who also experiences pain associated with anxiety, restlessness, or nausea[107] (Table 31-3).

Sedation in Pediatric Palliative Care

The European Association for Palliative Care (EAPC) has reviewed the use of sedation in palliative care including the indications, risks, benefits and potential for abuse, injudicious use and substandard clinical practice in 2009.[127] (See Chapter 23 for more information.) The guidelines given may inform clinical services in the development of policies and procedures to promote ethical decision making and promote and protect the interests of patients, their families and healthcare providers. Many of the principles in this review may be applicable to pediatric practice (Box 31-1).

The use of sedation for refractory pain generally assumes that therapies beyond the conventional have been used or

TABLE 31-3 Dosage Guidelines for Commonly Used Adjuvant Analgesics

Adjuvant analgesic	Starting dose	Dose guideline
Amitriptyline	5 mg	0.5 - 1.0 mg/kg/day
Nortriptyline	5 mg	0.5 -1.0 mg/kg/day
Gabapentin	10 mg/kg/day	Increasing dose every day until maximum 30 mg/kg/day reached. Then reassess.
Gabapentin	100 mg at night for patients > 50 kg	Increase dose every 2 to 7 days depending on the clinical setting. In 2 days begin twice daily dosing. Escalate to 3 times daily dosing, with half the daily dose at night, as tolerated or until reaching a full TID dose of 600 mg / 600 mg / 1200 mg
Pregabalin	25 mg BID for patients > 50 kg	Increase dose every 2 to 7 days, depending on the clinical setting, as tolerated or until reaching 150 mg BID

BOX 31-1 Framework for the Development of Sedation Guidelines

- Recommend pre-emptive discussion of the potential role of sedation in end-of-life care and contingency planning.
- Describe the indications in which sedation may be considered or should be considered.
- Describe the necessary evaluation and consultation procedures.
- Specify consent requirements.
- Indicate the need to discuss the decision-making process with the family.
- Present direction for selection of the sedation method.
- Present direction for dose titration, patient monitoring and care.
- Guide decisions regarding hydration and nutrition and concomitant medications.
- Support the family and provide information.
- Care for the clinicians involved in delivering care.

Adapted from Ozen, S et al. EULAR/PRINTO/PRES criteria for Henoch-Schönlein purpura, childhood polyarteritis nodosa, childhood Wegener granulomatosis and childhood Takayasu arteritis: Ankara 2008. Part II: Final classification criteria. Ann Rheum Dis. 2010 May; 69(5):798–806.

are impractical and that there is no acceptable means of providing analgesia without compromising consciousness. Given the principles of pain management outlined above, this is an extremely rare practice in pediatrics. Continuous deep sedation should be considered only if the patient is in the very terminal stages, with an expected prognosis of hours or days at most.[127] Transient respite sedation may be considered earlier in the illness trajectory to provide temporary relief while waiting for more effective analgesic therapies to take effect.

The trade-off between sedation and inadequate pain relief requires the consideration of the wishes of the child, as appropriate, and his or her family. The ethical issues surrounding prolonged sedation in pediatrics, including the principle of double effect, have been previously discussed.[128–130] The continuation of high-dose opioid infusions in these circumstances is recommended to avoid situations in which a patient may have unrelieved pain but inadequate clarity to express pain perception. A variety of drugs have been used in this setting, including barbiturates, benzodiazepines, and phenothiazines.[129,131]

Summary

Adequate pain management, even for intractable pain, can be achieved if the principles of pain assessment and management are applied to every child needing palliative care services. The context of pain management for pediatric palliative care practice should impel clinicians toward a standard of excellence. In addition there are increasing international and national political forces supported by quality programs demanding excellence in pain management. As a consequence, the need for sedation to reduce conscious awareness, even in the setting of intractable pain, should be an extremely rare entity in pediatric clinical pain management practice.

REFERENCES

1. Wall PD, Melzack R: *Textbook of pain*, ed 5, London, 2006, Elsevier Churchill Livingstone.
2. Collins JJ, Stevens MM, Berde CB: Pediatric cancer pain. In Sykes N, Bennett MI, Yung KK, editors: *Cancer pain*, ed 2, London, 2008, Hodder and Stroughton, pp 345–358.
3. Greco C, Berde CB: Acute pain management in children. In Ballantyne J, Rathmell J, Fishman S, editors: *Bonica's pain management in children*, ed 4, Philadelphia, 2009, Lippincott Williams and Wilkins.
4. *Cancer pain relief and palliative care in children*, Geneva, 1998, WHO. Ref Type: Pamphlet.
5. Drake R, Frost J, Collins JJ: The symptoms of dying children, *J Pain Symptom Manage* 27(7):6–10, 2003.
6. Hongo T, Watanabe C, Okada S: Analysis of the circumstances at the end of life in children with cancer: symptoms, suffering and acceptance, *Pediatr Int* 45:60–64, 2003.
7. Wolfe J, Grier HE, Klar N, et al: Symptoms and suffering at the end of life in children with cancer, *N Engl J Med* 342(5):326–333, 2000.
8. McCallum DE, Byrne P, Bruera E: How children die in hospital, *J Pain Symptom Manage* 20(6):417–423, 2000.
9. Belasco J, Danz P, Drill A, Schmid W, Burkey E: Supportive care: palliative care in children, adolescents, and young adults, *J Palliat Care* 16:39–46, 2000.
10. Miser AW, Dothage P, Wesley RA, et al: The prevalence of pain in a pediatric and young adult population, *Pain* 29:265–266, 1987.
11. Collins JJ, Byrnes ME, Dunkel I, Foley KM, Lapin J, Rapkin B, et al: The Memorial Symptom Assessment Scale (MSAS): validation study in children aged 10-18, *J Pain Symptom Manage* 19(5):363–367, 2000.
12. Collins JJ, Devine TB, Dick G, Johnson EA, Kilham HK: The measurement of symptoms in young children with cancer: the validation of the Memorial Symptom Assessment Scale in children aged 7-12, *J Pain Symptom Manage* 23(1):10–16, 2002.
13. Robinson WM, Ravilly S, Berde CB, Wohl ME: End-of-life care in cystic fibrosis, *Pediatrics* 100:205–209, 1997.
14. Ravilly S, Robinson W, Suresh S, Wohl ME, Berde CB: Chronic pain in cystic fibrosis, *Pediatrics* 98:741–747, 1996.
15. Hunt AM: A survey of signs, symptoms and symptom control in 30 terminally ill children, *Dev Med Child Neurol* 32:347–355, 1990.
16. Oleske JM, Czarniecki L: Continuum of palliative care: lessons from caring for children infected with HIV-1, *Lancet* 354:1287–1290, 1999.
17. Hirschfeld S, Moss H, Dragisic K, Pizzo PA: Pain in pediatric immunodeficiency virus infection: incidence and characteristics in a single-institution pilot study, *Pediatrics* 98:449–452, 1996.
18. McGrath PJ, Frager G: Psychological barriers to optimal pain management in infants and children, *Clin J Pain* 12:135–141, 1996.
19. Bieri D, Reeve RA, Champion GD, Addicoat L, Ziegler JB: The Faces Pain Scale for the self-assessment of the severity of pain experienced by children: development, initial validation, and preliminary investigation for ratio scale properties, *Pain* 41(2):139–150, 1990.
20. LeBaron S, Zeltzer L: Assessment of acute pain and anxiety in children and adolescents by self-reports, observer reports and a behavior checklist, *J Consult Clin Psychol* 52:729–738, 1984.
21. Savedra M, Gibbons P, Tesler M, et al: How do children describe pain? A tentative assessment, *Pain* 14:95–104, 1982.

22. Kuttner L, Bowman M, Teasdale M: Psychological treatment of distress, pain and anxiety for children with cancer, *Dev Behav Pediatr* 9:374–381, 1988.

23. Manne SL, Bakeman R, Jacobsen P, et al: Adult and child interaction during invasive medical procedures: sequential analysis, *Health Psychol* 11:241–249, 1992.

24. Jay SM, Ozolins M, Elliott C, Caldwell S: Assessment of children's distress during painful medical procedures, *J Health Psych* 2:133–147, 1983.

25. Shacham S, Daut R: Anxiety or pain: what does the scale measure? *J Consult Clin Psychol* 49(468):469, 1981.

26. Gauvain-Piquard A, Rodary C, Rezvani A, Lemerle J: Pain in children aged 2-6 years: a new observational rating scale elaborated in a pediatric oncology unit: a preliminary report, *Pain* 31:177–188, 1987.

27. Breau LM, Finley GA, McGrath PJ, Camfield CS: Validation of the Non-communicating Children's Pain Checklist-Postoperative Version, *Anesthesiology* 96(3):523–526, 2002.

28. Stallard P, Williams A, Velleman R, Lenton S, McGrath PJ: Brief report: behaviors identified by caregivers to detect pain in noncommunicating children, *Pediatr Psychology* 27:209–214, 2002.

29. Collins JJ, Grier HE, Kinney HC, Berde CB: Control of severe pain in terminal pediatric malignancy, *J Pediatr* 126(4):653–657, 1995.

30. Collins JJ, Grier HE, Sethna NF, Berde CB: Regional anesthesia for pain associated with terminal malignancy, *Pain* 65:63–69, 1996.

31. Siden H, Nalewajek P: High dose opioids in pediatric palliative care, *J Pain Symptom Manage* 25(5):397–399, 2003.

32. Anand KJ, Hansen DD, Hickey PR: Hormonal metabolic stress response in neonates undergoing surgery, *Anesthesiology* 73:661–670, 1990.

33. Porter J, Lick J: Addiction is rare in patients treated with narcotics [letter], *N Engl J Med* 302:123, 1980.

34. Miser AW, Moore L, Greene R: Prospective study of continuous intravenous and subcutaneous morphine infusions for therapy-related or cancer-related pain in children and young adults with cancer, *Clin J Pain* 2:101–106, 1986.

35. Miser AW, Dothage JA, Miser JS: Continuous intravenous fentanyl for pain control in children and young adults with cancer, *Clin J Pain* 2:101–106, 1987.

36. Miser AW, Miser JS: The use of oral methadone to control moderate and severe pain in children and young adults with malignancy, *Clin J Pain* 1:243–248, 1985.

37. Miser AW, Miser JS, Clark BS: Continuous intravenous infusion of morphine sulfate for control of severe pain in children with terminal malignancy, *J Pediatr* 96(5):930–933, 1980.

38. Miser AW, Davis DM, Hughes CS, Mulne AF, Miser JS: Continuous subcutaneous infusion of morphine in children with cancer, *Am J Dis Child* 137(4):383–385, 1983.

39. Collins JJ, Dunkel I, Gupta SK, et al: Transdermal fentanyl in children with cancer: feasibility, tolerability, and pharmacokinetic correlates, *J Pediatr* 134:319–323, 1999.

40. Hunt AM, Joel S, Dick G, Goldman A: Population pharmacokinetics of oral morphine and its glucuronides in children receiving morphine as immediate-release liquid or sustained-release tablets, *J Pediar* 135(1):47–55, 1999.

41. Noyes M, Irving H: The use of transdermal fentanyl in pediatric oncology palliative care, *Am J Hosp Palliat Care* 18(6):411–416, 2004.

42. Hunt AM, Goldman A, Devine TB, Phillips M: Transdermal fentanyl for pain relief in a paediatric palliative care population, *Palliat Med* 15(5):405–412, 2001.

43. Mackie AM, Coda BC, Hill HF: Adolescents use patient controlled analgesia effectively for relief from prolonged oropharyngeal mucositis pain, *Pain* 46:265–269, 1991.

44. Collins JJ, Geake J, Grier HE, et al: Patient-controlled analgesia for mucositis pain in children: a three-period crossover study comparing morphine and hydromorphone, *J Pediatr* 129(5):722–728, 1996.

45. Cherny NI, Chang V, Frager G, Ingham JM, Tiseo PJ, Popp B, et al: Opioid pharmacotherapy in the management of cancer pain, *Cancer* 76(7):1283–1292, 1995.

46. Ljungman G, Kreuger A, et al: Treatment of pain in pediatric oncology: a Swedish nationwide survey, *Pain* 68:385–394, 1996.

47. Sandler DP, Smit JC, Weinberg CR, et al: Analgesic use and chronic renal disease, *N Engl J Med* 320:1238–1243, 1989.

48. *Paracetamol use*, 2009, NSW Health. Available from: URL: www.health.nsw.gov.au/policies/pd/2006/PD2006_004.html. Accessed June 25, 2010.

49. Wurthwein G, Koling S, Reich A, et al: Pharmacokinetics of intravenous paracetamol in children and adolescents under major surgery, *Eur J Clin Pharmacol* 60:883–888, 2005.

50. NSW Therapeutic Advisory Group I: *IV paracetamol—where does it sit in hospital practice?* NSW, Australia, 2005 Sep.

51. Stuart JJ, Pisko EJ: Choline magnesium trisalicylate does not impair platelet aggregation, *Pharnatheraoeutica* 2:547, 1981.

52. Foeldvari I, Burgos-Varos R, Thon A, Tuerck D: High response rate in the phase 1/11 study of meloxicam in juvenile rheumatoid arthritis, *J Rheumatol* 29:1079–1083, 2002.

53. Stempak D, Gammon J, Klein J, et al: Single-dose and steady-state pharmacokinetics of celecoxib in children, *Clin Pharmacol Ther* 72:490–497, 2006.

54. Mukherjee D, Nissen SE, Topol EJ: Risk of cardiovascular events associated with selectiev COX -2 inhibitors, *JAMA* 286:954–959, 2001.

55. Williams D, Patel A, Howard RF: Pharmacogenetics of codeine metabolism in an urban population of children and its implication for analgesic reliability, *Br J Anaesth* 89:839–845, 2002.

56. Poyhia R, Seppala T: Lipid solubility and protein binding of oxycodone in vitro, *Pharmacol Toxicol* 74:23–27, 1994.

57. Pelkonen O, Kaltiala EH, Larmi TKL: Comparison of activities of drug metabolizing enzymes in human fetal and adult liver, *Clin Pharmacol Ther* 14:840–846, 1973.

58. Ross J, Riley J, Welsh K: Genetic variation in the catechol-o-methyltransferase gene is associated with response to morphine in cancer patients. In Flor H, Kalso E, Dostrovsky JO, editors: *Proceedings of the 11th World Congress on Pain*, Seattle, 2006, IASP Press, pp 461–467.

59. McRorie TI, Lynn A, Nespeca MK: The maturation of morphine clearance and metabolism, *Am J Dis Child* 146:972–976, 1992.

60. Bhat R, Chari G, Gulati A, et al: Pharmacokinetics of a single dose of morphine in pre-term infants during the first week of life, *J Pediatr* 117:477–481, 1990.

61. Pokela ML, Olkkala KT, Seppala T: Age-related morphine kinetics in infants, *Dev Pharmacol Ther* 20:26–34, 1993.

62. Stanski DR, Greenblatt DJ, Lowenstein E: Kinetics of intravenous and intramuscular morphine, *Clin Pharmacol Ther* 24:52–59, 1978.

63. Olkkola KT, Maunuksela EL, Korpela R, Rosenberg PH: Kinetics and dynamics of postoperative intravenous morphine in children, *Clin Pharmacol Ther* 44(2):128–136, 1988.

64. Cherny NI, Foley KM: Nonopioid and opioid analgesic pharmacotherapy of cancer pain. In Cherny NI, Foley KM, editors: *Hematol Oncol Clin North Am* 1996, pp 79–102.

65. Collins C, Koren G, Crean P, et al: Fentanyl pharmacokinetics and hemodynamic effects in preterm infants during ligation of patent ductus arteriosus, *Anesth Analg* 64:1078–1080, 1985.

66. Koren G, Goresky G, Crean P, et al: Unexpected alterations in fentanyl pharmacokinetics in children undergoing cardiac surgery: age related or disease related? *Dev Pharmacol Ther* 9:183–191, 1986.

67. Koren G, Goresky G, Crean P, et al: Pediatric fentanyl dosing based on pharmacokinetics during cardiac surgery, *Anesth Analg* 63:577–582, 1984.

68. Johnson K, Erickson J, Holley F, Scott J: Fentanyl pharmacokinetics in the pediatric population, *Anesthesiology* 61(3A):A441, 1984.

69. Gauntlett IS, Fisher DM, Hertzka RE, et al: Pharmacokinetics of fentanyl in neonatal humans and lambs: effects of age, *Anesthesiology* 69:683–687, 1988.

70. Schechter NL, Weisman SJ, Rosenblum M, et al: The use of oral transmucosal fentanyl citrate for painful procedures in children, *Pediatrics* 95:335–339, 1995.

71. Payne R, Coluzzi P, Hart L, Simmonds M, Lyss A, Rauck R, et al: Long-term safety of oral transmucosal fentanyl citrate for breakthrough cancer pain, *J Pain Symptom Manage* 22(1):575–583, 2001.

72. Hunt A, Goldman A, Devine T, Phillips M: Transdermal fentanyl for pain relief in a paediatric palliative care population, *Palliat Med* 15(5):405–412, 2001.

73. Tamsen A, Hartvig P, Fagerlund C, et al: Patient-controlled analgesic therapy, part 1: pharmacokinetics of pethidine in the pre- and postoperative periods, *Clin Pharmacokinet* 7:149–163, 1982.

74. Hamunen K, Maunuksela EL, Seppala T, et al: Pharmacokinetics of IV and rectal pethidine in children undergoing ophthalmic surgery, *Br J Anaesth* 71:823–826, 1993.

75. Koska AJ, Kramer WG, Romagnoli A, et al: Pharmacokinetics of high dose meperidine in surgical patients, *Anesth Analg* 60:8–11, 1981.

76. Pokela ML, Olkkala KT, Kovisto M, et al: Pharmacokinetics and pharmacodynamics of intravenous meperidine in neonates and infants, *Clin Pharmacol Ther* 52:342–349, 1992.

77. Mather LE, Tucker GT, Pflug AE, et al: Meperidine kinetics in man: intravenous injection in surgical patients and volunteers, *Clin Pharmacol Ther* 17:21–30, 1975.

78. Kaiko RF, Foley KM, Grabinsky PY, et al: Central nervous system excitatory effects of meperidine in cancer patients, *Ann Neurol* 13:180–185, 1983.

79. Berde CB, Sethna NF, Holzman RS, Reidy P, Gondek EJ: Pharmacokinetics of methadone in children and adolescents in the perioperative period, *Anesthesiology* 67:A519, 1987.
80. Berde CB, Beyer JE, Bournaki MC, Levin CR, Sethna NF: Comparison of morphine and methadone for prevention of postoperative pain in 3- to 7-year-old children, *J Pediatr* 136–141, 1991.
81. Kapelushnik J, Koren G, Solh H, et al: Evaluating the efficacy of EMLA in alleviating pain associated with lumbar puncture: comparison of open and double-blinded protocols in children, *Pain* 42:31–34, 1990.
82. Miser AW, Goh TS, Dose AM, et al: Trial of a topically administered local anesthetic (EMLA cream) for pain relief during central venous port access in children with cancer, *J Pain Symptom Manage* 9(4):259–264, 1994.
83. Van Kan HJM, Egberts ACG, Rijnvos WPM, Ter Pelkwijk NJ, Lenderink AW: Tetracaine versus lidocaine-prilocaine for preventing venipuncture-induced pain in children, *Am J Obstet Gynecol* 54:388–392, 1997.
84. Houck CS, Sethna NF: Transdermal analgesia with local anesthetics in children: review, update and future directions, *Expert Rev Neurother.*
85. Bruera E, Brenneis C, Michaud M, et al: Use of the subcutaneous route for the administration of narcotics in patients with cancer pain, *Cancer* 62:407–411, 1988.
86. Gourlay G: Fatal outcome with use of rectal morphine for postoperative pain control in an infant, *Br Med J* 304:766–767, 1992.
87. Dunbar PJ, Buckley P, Gavrin JR, Sanders JE, Chapman CR: Use of patient-controlled analgesia for pain control for children receiving bone marrow transplants, *J Pain Symptom Manage* 10:604–611, 1995.
88. Berde CB, Lehn BM, Yee JD, et al: Patient controlled analgesia in children and adolescents: a randomized, prospective comparison with intramuscular morphine for postoperative analgesia, *J Pediatr* 118:460–466, 1991.
89. Friedrichsdorf S, Finney D, Bergin M, Stevens M, Collins JJ: Breakthrough pain in children with cancer, *J Pain Symptom Manage* 34(2):209–216, 2007.
90. Galer BS, Coyle N, Pasternak GW, et al: Individual variability in the response to different opioids: report of five cases, *Pain* 49:87–91, 1992.
91. Portenoy RK: Opioid tolerance and responsiveness: research findings and clinical observations. In Gebhart GF, Hammond DI, Jensen TS, editors: *Progress in pain research and management*, Seattle, 1994, IASP Press, pp 615–619.
92. Indelicato RA, Portenoy RK: Opioid rotation in the managment of refractory cancer pain, *J Clin Oncol* 21:87–91, 2003.
93. Drake R, Longworth J, Collins JJ: Opioid rotation in children with cancer, *J Palliat Med* 7(3):419–422, 2004.
94. Inturrisi CE, Portenoy RK, Max M, Colburn WA, Foley KM: Pharmacokinetic-pharmacodynamic relationships of methadone infusions in patients with cancer pain, *Clin Pharmacol Ther* 47:565–577, 1990.
95. Ripamonti C, Groff L, Brunelli C, et al: Switching from morphine to oral metahadone in treating cancer pain: what is the equianalgesic dose ratio? *J Clin Oncol* 16:3216–3221, 1998.
96. Ullrich C, Dusel V, Hilden J, et al: Recognition and treatment of fatigue in children with advanced cancer, *Pediatr Blood Cancer* 52(6):2009.
97. Yee JD, Berde CB: Dextroamphetamine or methylphenidate as adjuvants to opioid analgesia for adolescents with cancer, *J Pain Symptom Manage* 9:122–125, 1994.
98. Berde CB, Nurko S: Opioid side effects: mechanism-based therapy, *N Engl J Med* 358(22):2332–2343, 2008.
99. Eide PK, Jorum E, Stubhaug A, et al: Relief of post-herpetic neuralgia with the N-methyl-D-aspartic acid receptor antagonist ketamine: a double-blind cross-over comparison with morphine and placebo, *Pain* 58:347–354, 1994.
100. Persson J, Axelsson G, Hallin RG, et al: Beneficial effects of ketamine in a chronic pain state with allodynia, *Pain* 60:217–222, 1995.
101. Nelson KA, Park KM, Robinovitz E, et al: High dose dextromethorphan versus placebo in painful diabetic neuropathy and postherpetic neuralgia, *Neurology* 48:1212–1218, 1997.
102. Eisenberg E, Pud D: Can patients with chronic neuropathic pain be cured by acute administration of the NMDA-receptor antagonist amantadine? *Pain* 74:37–39, 1994.
103. Finkel JC, Pestieau SR, Quezado ZM: Ketamine as an adjuvant for treatment of cancer pain in children and adolescents, *J Pain* 8(6):515–521, 2007.
104. Carullo V, Carpino E, Weldon C, Berde CB: *Intraspinal analgesia via implanted ports for refractory pain in paediatric advanced cancer*, 2010, ISPP Publications. In press.
105. Paulino AC: Palliative radiotherapy in children with neuroblastoma, *Pediatr Hematol Oncol* 20(2):111–117, 2003.
106. Charron M, Brown M, Rowland P, Mirro J: Pain palliation with strontium-89 in children with metastatic disease, *Med Pediatr Oncol* 26(6):393–396, 1996.
107. Lussier D, Portenoy RK: Adjuvant analgesics in pain management. In Hanks GWC, Cherny NI, Christiakis NA, Fallon M, Kaasa S, Portenoy RK, editors: *Oxford textbook of palliative medicine*, ed 4, 2009, Oxford University Press, pp 706–733.
108. Watson C, Evans R, Reed K, et al: Amitriptyline versus placebo in postherpetic neuralgia, *Neurology* 32:671–673, 1982.
109. Max MB: Antidepressants as analgesics. In Fields HL, Liebeskind JC, editors: *Progress in pain research and pain management*, Seattle, 1994, IASP Press, pp 229–246.
110. Diamond S, Baltes B: Chronic tension headache treatment with amitriptyline: a double blind study, *Headache* 11:110–116, 1971.
111. Couch J, Ziegler D, Hassanein R: Amitriptyline in the prophylaxis of migraine: effectiveness and relationship of antimigraine and antidepressant effects, *Neurology* 26:121–127, 1976.
112. Frank R, Kashani J, Parker R, et al: Antidepressant analgesia in rheumatoid arthritis, *J Rheumatology* 15:1632–1638, 1988.
113. Ward N: Tricyclic antidepressants for chronic low back pain: mechanisms of action and predictors of response, *Spine* 11:661–665, 1986.
114. Magni G: The use of antidepressants in the treatment of chronic pain, *Drugs* 42(5):730–748, 1991.
115. McQuay HJ, Tramer M, Nye BA, et al: A systematic review of antidepressants in neuropathic pain, *Pain* 68:217–227, 2003.
116. Heiligenstein E, Gerrity S: Psychotropics as adjuvant analgesics. In Schechter NL, Berde CB, Yaster M, editors: *Pain in infants, children, and adolescents*, Baltimore, 1993, Williams and Wilkins, pp 173–177.
117. Biederman J, Baldessarini RJ, Wright V, et al: A double-blind placebo controlled study of desipramine in the treatment of ADD:II. Serum drug levels and cardiovascular findings, *J Am Acad Child Adolesc Psychiatry* 28:903–911, 1989.
118. Forrest WH, Brown BW, Brown CR, et al: Dextroamphetamine with morphine for the treatment of postoperative pain, *N Engl J Med* 296(13):712–715, 1977.
119. Bruera E, Miller MJ, Macmillan K, Kuehn N: Neuropsychological effects of methylphenidate in patients receiving a continuous infusion of narcotics for cancer pain, *Pain* 48:163–166, 1992.
120. Bruera E, Faisinger R, MacEachern T, Hanson J: The use of methylphenidate in patients with incident pain receiving regular opiates: a preliminary report, *Pain* 50:75–77, 1992.
121. Watanabe S, Bruera E: Corticosteroids as adjuvant analgesics, *J Pain Symptom Manage* 9:442–445, 1994.
122. Tannock I, Gospodarowicz M, Meakin W, et al: Treatment of metastatic prostatic cancer with low-dose prednisone: evaluation of pain and quality of life as pragmatic indices of response, *J Clin Oncol* 7(5):590–597, 1989.
123. Weinstein JD, Toy FJ, Jaffe ME, Goldberg HI: The effect of dexamethasone on brain edema in patients with metastatic brain tumors, *Neurology* 23:121–129, 1973.
124. Greenberg HS, Kim J, Posner JB: Epidural spinal cord compression from metastatic tumor: results with a new treatment protocol, *Ann Neurol* 8:361–366, 1980.
125. Khurana DS, Riviello J, Helmers S, et al: Efficacy of gabapentin therapy in children with refractory partial seizures, *J Pediatr* 128:829–833, 1996.
126. Beaver WT, Wallenstein S, Houde RW: A comparison of the analgesic effects of methotrimeprazine and morphine in patients with cancer, *Clin Pharmacol Ther* 7:436–446, 1966.
127. Cherny NI, Radbruch L: European Association for Palliative Care (EAPC) recommended framework for the use of sedation in palliative care, *Palliat Med* 23(7):581–593, 2009.
128. Truog RD, Berde CB, Mitchell C, Grier HE: Barbiturates in the care of the terminally ill, *N Engl J Med* 327:1678–1682, 1992.
129. Kenny NP, Frager G: Refractory symptoms and terminal sedation in children: ethical issues and practical management, *J Palliat Care* 12:40–45, 1996.
130. Truog RD, Burns JP, Shurin SB, Emanuel EJ: Ethical considerations in pediatric oncology. In Pizzo PA, Poplack DG, editors: *Principles and practice of pediatric oncology*, ed 4, Philadelphia, 2002, Lippincott Williams & Wilkins, pp 1411–1430.
131. Siever BA: Pain management and potentially life-shortening analgesia in the terminally ill child: the ethical implications for pediatric nurses, *J Pediatr Nurs* 5:307–312, 1994.

Respiratory Symptoms

DAWN DAVIES

And by and by Christopher Robin came to an end of things, and he was silent, and he sat there, looking out over the world, just wishing it wouldn't stop. —A.A. Milne

Of all symptoms that very ill children experience, perhaps the most dreaded and disturbing to patients, parents, and caregivers are pain and difficulty breathing. With regard to the latter, common respiratory difficulties encountered are related to a wide spectrum of conditions. These include illnesses that cause systemic problems such as weakness, anemia, or cystic fibrosis. Other times, localized problems such as airway abnormalities, swallowing problems, aspiration of secretions, or pneumonia may cause breathing difficulties. Metastases from cancer may cause widespread disease within the entire thorax, including multiple tumors, pleural effusions, pneumothorax, or airway compression. This list is by no means exhaustive, but gives some idea as to the variety of causes that can lead to disturbing respiratory symptoms in children, particularly toward the end of life. However, not all respiratory symptoms are necessarily progressive, and are sometimes transient as children recover from other life-threatening illnesses (Fig. 32-1).

Apart from physical or mechanical derangements that lead to breathing problems, anxiety can also compound feelings of shortness of breath and/or difficulty swallowing. There is clearly a role for many specific skills of different health professionals and caregivers to maximize a patient's comfort. These include numerous psychological strategies,[1] careful positioning of the patient, artificial ventilatory supports, and medications. Additionally, children require clear explanations for these distressing symptoms, and reassurance that we will work together to alleviate them.

Psychosocial disciplines such as child life specialists, social workers, spiritual care, and psychology are key to providing care to all of these children, who often have frequent and prolonged hospitalizations with chronic respiratory symptoms. Very often, children don't want to talk about it, whatever it is. And yet many will have fears, questions or concerns that go unaddressed unless we can find non-threatening ways to engage them in assuring their comprehension and expressing their thoughts and emotions about their health. Child life specialists develop trusting relationships with patients by use of normalizing activities as well as therapeutic interventions. This is extremely important for children who require mechanical support for assisted breathing, and helps combat some of the isolation that can accompany requiring such therapy. The normalizing activities include a variety of interactions, from going on walks to engagement through crafts and hobbies that diminish boredom and promote fun. They also encourage

sustained connection between the patient and friends and family while children are hospitalized. Therapeutic interventions include art therapy, pre-operative teaching, medical play, diversion, and distraction.

This interdisciplinary approach to care becomes even more important over time, because as technology continues to develop more children who would have died because of their underlying illness now survive. In this context, some of the therapies used to assist with respiratory symptoms also extend life, but with residual respiratory symptoms or limitations lingering in the background. Examples of these therapies range from treating pneumonia with new generation antibiotics to receiving a lung transplant for cystic fibrosis. In other situations, children who cannot be cured of their disease might have their lives extended by months or years by noninvasive ventilation, such as facemask or nose cradle, or tracheostomy, with or without chronic mechanical ventilation. The number of children who live in the hospital or at home requiring respiratory support by biphasic positive airway pressure (BiPAP), continuous positive air pressure (CPAP) or continuous mechanical ventilation by way of tracheostomy has grown significantly in the past decade.[2] Despite this, there are some who believe these procedures are underused in pediatric populations.[3] In addition to the array of medical equipment and operative procedures that may alleviate respiratory symptoms, there are also many medical therapies that may be employed, which will be described later in more detail.

Even with the evolution of respiratory aids and treatments for children, there are still many respiratory symptoms that children experience, which adversely affect their quality of life. In the case of high tech treatment such as ventilation, a child's ability to return home is also adversely affected. This chapter will delve into the many respiratory symptoms that children may experience, as well as the interactive treatments that are offered by nurses, respiratory therapists, physicians, and psychosocial professionals to alleviate these symptoms. The ethical implications of some of these therapies will also be discussed.

Dyspnea

Dyspnea is "a distressful subjective sensation of uncomfortable breathing that may be caused by many disorders, including certain heart and respiratory conditions, strenuous exercise, or anxiety."[4] The differential diagnosis is vast, and the causes can perhaps best be organized by anatomic location. Dyspnea can result from:

- Fixed or intermittent airway obstruction such as congenital abnormalities of the airway, asthma, external compression, and/or invasion by tumor,

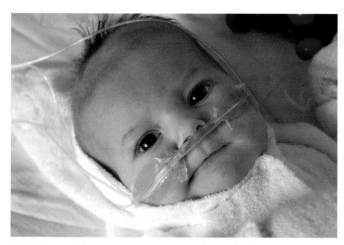

Fig. 32-1 An infant receiving oxygen via nasal cannula. (Provided courtesy of infant's parents.)

- Intrathoracic extra-parenchymal pathologies such as pneumothorax, hemothorax,
- Intrathoracic lung parenchyma abnormalities such as pneumonia, tumor, pulmonary hemorrhage, cystic fibrosis.

This list is by no means all-encompassing, but gives some idea as to the spectrum of conditions that can lead to dyspnea. Focusing on the underlying pathology and directing treatment to reversing the cause of dyspnea is possible in some cases. Modalities that target reversing or ameliorating the underlying pathology may include medications, surgery, and/or radiotherapy.

In terms of assessing dyspnea, two self-report tools could be located.[5,6] One has been tested only in hospitalized patients with asthma, and the other has been limited to small focus groups of children with cystic fibrosis or asthma, compared to normal children. They were found to be reliable in children 6 or 8 years of age, respectively, but not younger. In the absence of any validated tool for dyspnea in other diseases, visual analogue scales (VAS) can also be used for children in these age ranges.

There are many studies evaluating both pharmacologic and non-drug treatment of this distressing problem. Results from meta-analyses in the Cochrane Database of systematic reviews are mixed:[7]

"Studies showed that these interventions can help to relieve shortness of breath: vibration of patient's chest wall, electrical stimulation of leg muscles, walking aids and breathing training. There are mixed results for the use of acupuncture/acupressure. Further interventions identified were counseling and support, either alone or in combination with relaxation-breathing training, music, relaxation, a handheld fan directed at a patient's face, case management, and psychotherapy. There are several non-drug methods available to relieve shortness of breath in incurable stages of cancer and other illnesses. There is currently not enough data to judge the evidence for these interventions. Most studies were conducted in participants with chronic lung disease. Only a few studies included participants with heart failure, cancer, or neurological disease."

Many children anecdotally do respond positively to practicing deep, slow breathing, singing, or blowing bubbles or pinwheels when they are feeling anxious and short of breath. The use of self-hypnosis in children to manage dyspnea has also been found to be beneficial.[8] This may be directed for younger children by a professional skilled in hypnotherapy. Pediatricians and others can learn to help their patients learn self-hypnosis, which gives the child more immediate and constant access to this form of therapy, through the Society for Developmental and Behavioral Pediatrics. Maintaining a calm and quiet environment is also important, and can be accentuated by use of machines that create light patterns on the ceiling, relaxation carts such a Snoezelen, and favorite music being played quietly.

As for drug treatment of dyspnea, the mainstay medications are opioids and benzodiazepines, titrated to minimal effective dose (Table 32-1). There is sometimes an exaggerated concern on the part of health professionals and parents that initiating opioids to treat dyspnea may cause respiratory depression. Very often, the dose of opioid required for the treatment of dyspnea is a quarter to half that required for the treatment of pain. A recent Cochrane review did report benefits of opioid therapy in ameliorating breathlessness in patients due to both malignant and non-malignant disease.[9] Although the number of studies was small, the results were significant when these medications were given via the enteral or parenteral route. Educating families and colleagues that judicious use of opioids have been found to be safe and beneficial often allays these fears. Also, opioids can sometimes be used transiently, while other therapies aimed at ameliorating the cause of the dyspnea can be employed and given time to take effect. In addition to systemic administration of opioids, there have been many studies evaluating the possible role of inhaled opioid agonists, the theory being that this might confer a direct benefit by stimulating mu receptors in the lungs themselves, thereby reducing systemic side effects such as pruritis, somnolence, and constipation. A recent meta-analysis reveals that this mode of therapy is not beneficial, even in dose ranges from 1 to 40 mg morphine equivalent,[10] despite isolated case reports showing positive effects.

There is no meta-analysis that evaluates the use of benzodiazepines for relief of dyspnea, though the Cochrane Database has a published protocol for such a study. Other published clinical trials in adults have demonstrated that use of midazolam, in addition to morphine, can further diminish the sensation of dyspnea.[11] There are no similar trials in children, but the combination of morphine or another opioid in conjunction with benzodiazepines are frequently used to treat this symptom in children despite the paucity of data for both children and adults. Occasionally, suffering from symptoms such as dyspnea becomes intractable, despite multiple combined treatments. In this event, many patients and/or families agree to a course of sedation as a last resort to provide comfort, although conscious awareness may be very diminished as a consequence.[12] This treatment might be continued until death occurs, but certainly not always if other treatments such as radiotherapy alleviate the symptom over time in such a way that sedation can be lessened or discontinued. In one study, such sedation was eventually discontinued in a quarter of adult patients.[13]

Other medications that may provide relief, depending on the underlying disease, are bronchodilators, inhaled steroids, or mucolytics.[14] Many patients suffer from orthopnea, and occupational therapists and physiotherapists can often combine their skills to devise modifications to beds and seating such

TABLE 32-1 Common Pharmacologic Management of Respiratory Symptoms in Children

Symptom	Medication	Dosing	Comment
Dyspnea[*, †]	*Opioids:*		
	Morphine	0.02-0.05 mg/kg/dose IV	¼ to ½ the dose used for analgesia.
		0.06-0.15 mg/kg/dose PO	
	Hydromorphone	0.005-0.01 mg/kg/dose IV	
		0.01-0.02 mg/kg/dose PO	
	Benzodiazepines:		
	Lorazepam	0.02-0.05 mg/kg/dose IV/PO	Start with low dose in combination with opioid.
	Midazolam	0.1-0.2 mg/kg/dose IV/IM	Intermittent dose can be given intranasal, but can cause burning sensation.
		OR	3mg/kg made up to 50 mL with D5W at 1-4 mL per hour to deliver this dose.
		Continuous IV/SC infusion 1-4 microgram/kg/MINUTE	
Bronchospasm	Salbutamol	2.5-5 mg/dose by nebulizer	Can cause jitteriness, increased heart rate.
Secretions	*Anticholinergics*[‡]:		
	Glycopyrrolate	0004-0.01 mg/kg/dose IV	Need ten-fold dose if given enterally; titrate to effect; give BID-QID.
	Atropine 10% eyedrops	0.04-0.1 mg/kg/dose PO	
	Scopolamine patch	1-2 drops SL titrate to effect	
		½-1 patch transdermally to skin behind ear	
Cough	Dextromethorphan[§]	0.2-0.4 mg/kg/dose	Or see dosing on over-the-counter formulations by age.
	Hydrobromide	0.5-1 mg/kg/dose	
	Codeine	0.06-0.15 mg/kg/dose	
	Morphine	PO0.005-0.01 mg/kg/dose IV	
	Hydromorphone	0.01-0.02 mg/kg/dose PO	

[*]Consider treating all identified underlying causes of dyspnea: antibiotics for infection, transfusion for anemia, drainage and/or pleurodesis or tunneled catheter for pneumothorax or pleural effusion, and radiotherapy for metastases.
[†]Any other potent opioid can be used at ¼ to ½ the dose ordinarily used for analgesia.
[‡]Watch for increased anticholinergic effects: urinary retention, constipation.
[§]No longer recommended for simple URI children younger than 6 years old.

that the patient can maintain a comfortable position even during sleep. Other helpful therapies that may assist with dyspnea include use of a fan for increased air movement in the room. Patients experiencing dyspnea also often feel less symptomatic at an incline of 30 degrees to 90 degrees.

The role of oxygen has been controversial in the management of dyspnea. However, in a 2008 study, patients dying of metastatic lung disease and receiving oxygen therapy were no less dyspneic than those receiving only room air.[15] However, oxygen therapy may have a symbolic role for families, particularly if their child has required oxygen frequently throughout his or her life. Therefore, many patients and families do request that oxygen be provided, particularly in home settings. Having oxygen to provide often seems to enhance patient and parental sense of control, and can be important from that point of view.

Cough

A very aggravating symptom is cough. Cough interferes with activities as basic as eating and sleeping, and also as far-reaching as social isolation that prevents one from attending concerts, movies, etc. Moreover, cough leads to fatigue, abdominal or chest pain, and even vomiting and rib fractures. Persistent cough is a serious problem that healthcare professionals sometimes minimize, perhaps because everyone has had a cough at one time or other. Again, medical treatment to this point is somewhat limited, given that mechanical factors such as secretions in the alveoli and bronchi, and irritation of the carina, are potent stimuli of the cough reflex. No meta-analysis looking at treatment of cough in palliative care could be located. Cough may respond to N-methyl-D-aspartate (NMDA) receptor antagonists, such as dextromethorphan. This is often available in low-dose formulations in over-the-counter

cough preparations. There are no controlled trials in children evaluating its role in cough due to progressive respiratory illness. However, one study demonstrated more improvement in parent-report of cough compared with placebo when used for viral upper respiratory infection, though not as effective as ingesting honey.[16] Some patients get a measure of relief from a relatively small dose of opioid.[17] However, for those with a lesion in the bronchi, cough can be fairly intractable without more intense treatments, such as radiotherapy or surgery. With regard to radiotherapy, an area of lung or total lung can be targeted when there is diffuse parenchymal disease, but in the case of bronchial tumors, this can be administered by endobronchial brachytherapy. This is accomplished by delivering a radioactive treatment via an endoscopically placed catheter, which is left in place for a few minutes, then removed.[18,19]

SECRETIONS

Some children develop noisy breathing due to the movement of secretions in an uncontrolled airway as they lose consciousness prior to death. While there is no evidence of distress to the patient, this situation can be intolerable for parents and other caregivers. Alerting families to the possibility of this occurring is very helpful in terms of anticipatory guidance.

For children who have excessive or difficult-to-manage secretions, suction equipment is often the first line treatment for airway maintenance. In the home, portable suction is easily provided by respiratory equipment vendors, at relatively low cost, or through local home care programs.

When loss of airway control is caused by imminent death, and causes caregivers distress, it can be treated by a variety of anticholinergic medications, although the evidence for these strategies is quite weak.[20] One noninvasive strategy is to use 10% atropine eyedrops sublingually, titrated to effect.

Another is to use a scopolamine patch applied transdermally behind the patient's ear. Systemic medications such as glyco-pyrrolate can also be used, either enterally or parenterally, and this particular medication has the added advantage of not crossing the blood-brain barrier. These medications need to be carefully titrated such that secretions do not become too thick or tenacious. If this complication arises, secretions may become much harder to move within the airways, leading to the formations of large, solid mucous plugs, which can then worsen the child's respiratory symptoms. In these situations, families and caregivers also need to be alert to other anti-cholinergic symptoms, such as urinary retention, which some-times requires indwelling urinary catheterization, dry mouth, and worsening constipation.

Pulmonary Hemorrhage

At the mild end of the spectrum, patients may have blood-tinged sputum, progressing to frank hemoptysis. On the other end, one might experience sudden life-threatening pulmonary hemorrhage. Bleeding from the airways is almost always a terrifying event for the patient, family, and healthcare profes-sionals. Causes include a combination of pulmonary disorders exacerbated by bleeding diatheses. In the pediatric popula-tion, significant pulmonary hemorrhage commonly arises from complications of advanced lung disease, sepsis, or end-stage liver disease, but also in critically ill patients of any etiology who are mechanically ventilated. For patients in whom pulmo-nary bleeding might be anticipated, this possibility should be explained to the patient and/or parents and other care providers. In order to diminish the visual impact of bleeding, the patient should as much as possible wear darker clothing and be cared for using darker bed linens, towels, etc. In situations in which the patient is distressed, a dose of subcutaneous, intravenous, or intramuscular, midazolam can be given, titrated to a mini-mal level of sedation that allows comfort and reduces memory of the event. Initially, midazolam can be given as a bolus dose during the acute event, but if bleeding is recalcitrant, the patient may benefit from a continuous midazolam infusion, given the very short duration of effect from intermittent dosing.

Pleural Effusions and Pneumothorax and/or Hemothorax

A pleural effusion, accumulation of fluid between the lung and chest wall, or pneumothorax, collection of air between the lung and the chest wall, may be asymptomatic when it is small. However, as they enlarge, they often cause increasing dyspnea. Depending on the child's overall disease trajectory, more conservative attempts to control symptoms might be lim-ited to medications if the child is believed to be very advanced in the course of the underlying disease. On the other hand, if the child is relatively well overall, it often is reasonable to consider other options, including surgery and/or radiotherapy. For malignant pleural effusion, it is not worthwhile to place a chest tube as a sole therapy only transiently, as the effu-sion will doubtlessly re-accumulate, often within days. Many patients complain of increased pain at the chest tube site for the entire time it is in place, and this discomfort needs to be anticipated and weighed against the benefit that might be con-ferred by its placement. Surgeries undertaken often include the insertion of pigtail catheters or chest tubes for emergency

drainage, and sometimes pleurodesis once the effusion is drained. Pleurodesis is a process by which the pleural surfaces of the chest wall and the lung can be intentionally inflamed by reaction to placement of foreign material in this space, with the goal that the two pleural surfaces permanently adhere to each other, avoiding recurrence of the pneumothorax or pleu-ral effusion. A recent review in adult patients did show that pleurodesis is preferentially done thorascopically rather than by thoracotomy, given the more minimal nature of the former therapy, and that talc is the material of choice to seal the pleu-ral surfaces together.[21]

A more recent innovation is the insertion of a tunneled catheter for control of malignant pleural effusion. These are increasingly being used for ambulatory adult patients, and can often be inserted by a thoracic surgeon as an outpatient pro-cedure.[22] This procedure involves placing a tunneled catheter under the skin and subcutaneous tissue, through the thorax, and into the pleural collection of fluid. The exterior portion of the catheter can then be attached to a sterile collection bottle to perform serial drainages of the effusion as it re-accumulates, to maintain comfort. A 2006 local study[23] of 250 insertions in adults suggested that this approach is superior compared with talc pleurodesis, due primarily to the avoidance of a days-long hospital admission and long duration of result, usually until patients' deaths (Fig. 32-2).

WEAKNESS OF RESPIRATORY MUSCULATURE

Many inherited diseases cause systemic weakness, but it is the extreme weakness of the respiratory musculature that leads to dyspnea and/or respiratory failure in infants and children. Of these, spinal muscular atrophy type 1 (SMA 1), and Duchenne (DMD) and other muscular dystrophies are frequently dis-cussed in the pulmonary literature.

Children with such diseases are highly symptomatic from a respiratory standpoint. The degree and timing of weakness is variable, depending upon the underlying condition. Symptoms caused by these diseases include dyspnea, swallowing difficul-ties, resultant excessive oral secretions, and aspiration of feeds and secretions. Recently, more and more families have been advocating for significant respiratory intervention for these chil-dren, including long-term CPAP, BiPAP, or tracheostomy and ventilation. With the first two forms of noninvasive ventilation support, children with diseases such as SMA 1 might have life expectancy lengthened from a few months to somewhere into

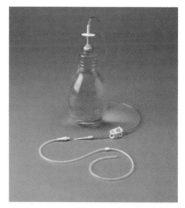

Fig. 32-2 PleurX catheter. (Courtesy Cardinal Health, Inc. All rights reserved.)

the first decade of life. For many parents, these forms of respiratory supports cannot be emphasized enough in terms of their importance in their child's care. To that end, many parents correspond through a variety of websites, including www.curesma. org, and have become strong advocates for parents newly adjusting to this serious diagnosis. This has certainly resulted in globalization of medical advice. It is not uncommon for families from around the world to be corresponding with each other, or even with clinicians. This can sometimes be problematic, as parents seek to be involved in clinical trials for their children in other cities, or even foreign countries, but find that practical limitations of their child's ability to travel, or insurance and other issues, will preclude their participation.[24–26] Parents often feel over time that they would be better off in other treatment centers, and this can lead to feelings of frustration and distrust of local care providers, despite the fact that the day-to-day care will include all proven therapies for these incurable diseases.

Recent consensus suggests that combination therapy of non-invasive ventilation, gastrostomy feeding and fundoplication, and use of a mechanical insufflation/exsufflation machines that mimic cough, extend life.[27] The Cough Assist® machine mimics a cough. When a healthy person coughs, it is preceded by a deep inspiration. With insufflation/exsufflation machines, this is mechanically simulated by applying positive pressure to the airways, followed by rapid switch to a negative pressure through a facemask. This often moves secretions higher into the airway or pharynx to allow for improved suctioning of deeper or inspissated secretions.[28] However, despite the advances demonstrated in this most recent consensus statement, the same publication contends that it remains unclear as to which is ethically the more correct path; extension of life through these technologies, or providing care directed at comfort only, but resulting in much earlier death (Fig. 32-3).

Many parents now opt for the treatment path. This is a complex journey for the child and his or her family, which is hard for them to imagine at diagnosis, especially when the condition is SMA 1. Parents and caregivers alike are profoundly affected by the conundrum of making eye contact with these young infants, noting their initially normal facial expressions and evident alertness and normal neurodevelopment, in the context of the baby's unmoving body. Long hospitalizations in infancy frequently occur, and eventual transfer to home or home community means the highest level of devotion of the family to maintain the lives of these very dependent handicapped children. These children, although cognitively intact, have little means to make their wishes and experiences known. Frequent and sometimes prolonged re-hospitalizations for episodes of deterioration are often the norm when the child is usually cared for at home.

The advent of advanced computerized communication technology has alleviated this isolation, for example, by allowing the child to respond to questions via activation of a thumb switch. However, not every family has access to this expensive technology. In either event, parents are left to guess as to their child's innermost thoughts and emotions. The benefit of the child's extended life and enjoyment of life comes at some real but unarticulated and unknown costs, at least from the patient's perspective. The application of a mask for hours at a time, or even constantly, may be uncomfortable for the child. Even in situations where the child easily accepts the mask or nasal cannula, skin breakdown and pressure points can be an uncomfortable side effect. Also, over the period of months or years, frequent use of a facemask can lead to mid-face deformities, caused by ongoing pressure to the nasal bridge and surrounding tissues. Parents often note a sense of distance created by the mask, which impairs visualization of their child's whole face, and obstructs the child's visual field as well. Often, parents will ask if there is any other way, short of tracheostomy, to provide breathing support without obscuring their child's face, which feels like a barrier to interaction. Furthermore, because of the child's often very precarious respiratory status, children are not held by their parents nearly as often as parents want, or as babies need, because parents often report desaturations and/or bradycardias in the most fragile of these infants. Parents often fear that attempting to hold or cuddle will cause the child to suffer, and this only enhances the sense of isolation for the parent, and likely the child.

With regard to benefit versus burden of these treatments, the proportionality of each is very difficult to ascertain. These children are non-verbal due to their extreme weakness, so one really doesn't have a way to determine the child's symptom experience, nor cognitive, emotional, and spiritual dimensions and development in ways adequate for them to inform their own treatment decisions. Some parents have been able to articulate this very well with statements reflecting ambiguity around decision-making. In the words of one mother: "Would we have chosen all this if we could have seen her lying in this bed years later? We did, and I don't regret it, but I wonder if meeting us would help other families to see what life will be like if they choose this for their babies." Another related issue that is likely embedded in these choices is the hope for eventual cure of spinal muscular atrophy and other neuromuscular diseases. The advent of stem cell research has been very topical and pervasive in the media, and many families will volunteer that part of their decision making to pursue significant respiratory intervention is the hope that their child will be cured, regardless of the obstacles and time that stretches between their child and this potential therapy. Some parents have been quite pragmatic about banking the cord blood of subsequent babies in the faint hope that a cure will be achieved for their child, however unlikely they know this may be.[29,30] Numerous families have requested stem cell transplant in China, and have raised funds in that hope, despite having been counseled that there are no published studies as to outcomes of this therapy, nor any way for their child to be transported that distance. All of these actions suggest their spoken and unspoken desperation in caring for these children.

With regard to resource use, there are also questions of distributive justice in allocation of scarce resources including equipment, prolonged hospitalizations, overnight awake caregivers, and education modifications. While these factors should never influence care or decision making at the bedside, organizations and funders may have to consider parameters by which to guide these decisions systemically. For those of us who

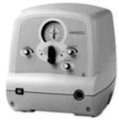

Fig. 32-3   **Cough Assist machine.** (Courtesy Philips Respironics, Cough Assist Manual.)

work in a universally funded healthcare system, cost containment and deficit reduction have become the order of the day. Somehow, governments are seeking the implausible combination of spending reductions in the order of hundreds of millions of dollars, while preserving quality of and access to the highest level of care. The dilemma that does not go publicly discussed is the virtual explosion of diagnostic tests and treatments that drive costs and often extend length of life through prolonged hospital or intensive care unit stays, which previously would have been impossible. Physicians are often left in the uncomfortable position of providing every possible feasible treatment, in the context of trying to be good stewards of limited healthcare resources, without any guidance or mandate from society or government funders as to how this should be done.

Children with diseases such as Duchenne (DMD) and other forms of muscular dystrophy present with similar symptoms in the advanced stages of the disease to children with SMA 1. However, the disease trajectory that leads them to this point is often very different. When a child has DMD, he or she becomes gradually weaker, deteriorates from full ambulation in a seemingly normal early childhood, to using a wheelchair, to the point of extreme respiratory muscle weakness that often requires mechanical ventilation by mid-adolescence.[31] Child life specialists, and other psychosocial disciplines, are essential in the care of these patients in helping them find a voice, share their feelings, and cultivating their ability to learn strategies to cope with their chronic and progressive illness.

In this situation, the disease trajectory is often well known to the parents, and most often also to the adolescent patient. That said, when patients with DMD present with a sudden severe deterioration in their health, perhaps resulting in ICU admission, it sometimes becomes obvious that these patients and their families have either had little conversation about advance care planning, or have heard mixed messages such that decision making has not occurred prior to the crisis.[32] This situation often leads to the sudden addition of BiPAP to the care of these patients. Sometimes, sudden reliance on ventilatory support is the jarring introduction to a more advanced stage of illness as depicted in the drawing by a 9-year-old patient (Fig. 32-4). This can then lead to crisis-oriented decision making, and leave patients and/ or families feeling as if they are contributing to the patient's eventual death if a decision to forgo ventilation is later considered.

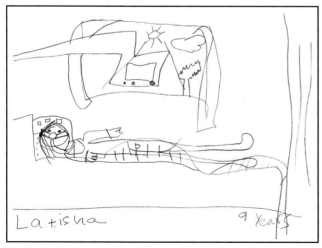

Fig. 32-4 Original art courtesy of patient and guardian.

Consideration of Tracheostomy

All of the situations in which a child becomes chronically or repeatedly critically ill cause significant angst and distress to children, their families and healthcare professionals. These illnesses often have a high rate of mortality, and therefore the implication is that treatments should not be unduly burdensome, and offer some tangible benefit.[33,34] However, because so many of these situations are rare, either the underlying disease itself is rare, or confounding serious complications of a more common primary disease make the constellation of problems rare, there is often virtually no clear evidence on which to base decisions. Many decisions are undertaken with a sense of ambiguity, because of the uncertainty as to whether treatments will lead to a positive outcome. The clinical entities of chronic critical illness and frailty are starting to be explored in the adult intensive care literature, but not yet substantially in the pediatric literature. Therefore, in the case of tracheostomy for the chronically critically ill child, or for those with end-stage neuromuscular disease, it is not always straightforward to ascertain the relative proportionality of burdens and benefits, nor in whose interest decision makers are acting when the child has never been able to speak to his or her own interests. As stated by the Canadian Pediatric Society,[35]

"There is a dearth of information regarding advance care planning in the paediatric population compared with the adult population, in which there is much clinical experience and research. A number of factors contribute to this gap. The emphasis on beneficence rather than patient autonomy in parental substitute decision-making leads to a prima facie bias toward curative rather than palliative options. This bias is consistent with parental obligation to protect children and societal predisposition in favour of life."

Some children have isolated anatomical problems with their airways, or may have diseases that involve airway abnormalities as part of a constellation of symptoms, as in the case of Pierre-Robin or Treacher-Collins syndromes. While these are not always life-threatening conditions, others may be. Whether the tracheostomy is done for airway conditions that do not result in the need for artificial ventilation, or for systemic conditions in which ventilation is required in addition, these patients require a high level of care in order to protect their airways. Although there is no clear consensus as to the standard of care, many children are cared for by an awake caregiver at night. Obviously, this ongoing role is beyond the capability of any family for the long term, and thus caregivers, often a series of strangers, are present in the family home for months and years at a time. Regardless of the plan, there will always be unexpected disruptions to this care, including the illnesses and other absences of paid caregivers, or outright cessation of services when a caregiver quits. In addition to parents' responsibilities to the ill child, there are often other children in the home to consider and employment demands. The other realities of embarking upon this treatment choice is the almost-universal need for one parent to stay at home with the ill child for a prolonged time, and thus cease their employment, very often adversely affecting the family's economic security.

Our duty, then, as physicians, nurses, and respiratory therapists, is to educate ourselves as to what day-to-day life looks like for these families, in order that parents are fully informed as to the ramifications of taking this decision. Unfortunately, this type of disclosure does not always occur in advance, and sometimes families who have been left to decide about a simple trach come to learn that there is really no such thing. One suggestion for healthcare professionals, and for physicians in particular given their strong role in medical decision making, is mandatory exposure to home care and chronic illness during their training.[36] Sometimes, one visit to a family home can suddenly make sense of decisions made by patients or parents that didn't seem to be clear when they were seen only in a clinical setting. Some European countries, and increasingly North American schools, ensure that all medical students have exposure to home settings, and the role of nursing. The schools require students work as a nurse during their junior clinical training,[37] perform interprofessional learning projects,[38] and/or by having medical students and residents spend clinical rotations in home care and community care in other sites such as respite centers or hospices.[39–41] The first of these cited papers has even advocated short-term hospitalizations of medical students to experience the patient role. The reality that families face after hospital discharge is often overwhelming as they seek to return home and build a new normal life, and this remains foreign to healthcare providers unless we make a concerted effort to educate ourselves as a matter of course about community and home care. There are many assumptions made by us as caregivers, which are communicated to families about the amount and cost of support at home. These discussions often overestimate care provision, such as the amount of available respite, homemaking, night time care, and underestimate costs that families will encounter in caring for their ill child at home.[42] Even with the best teaching and preparation that we can offer, families caring for a child with a tracheostomy often leave the hospital after many months, greatly anticipating their return home, only to express despair and fatigue a few months after discharge (personal communication).[57] Realistically, disease and treatment management are often very different between a hospital setting and home setting, particularly if the family lives in a rural area.

Finally, a very significant disclosure that healthcare professionals need to make is that the patient will lose his or her usual speaking voice if the tracheostomy is undertaken. In the case of chronically critically ill patients, use of one's voice and communicating freely gives a sense of control in day-to-day life. Similarly, for patients with progressive neuromuscular disease, it is imperative that the perspective of the child be sought as able. The child should understand what is being proposed and the hoped-for benefits, but also the likely burdens, such as possible limitations in the care setting, voice impairment, probable lengthy hospitalization, and finally, having someone watch every night while the child sleeps upon returning home.

In recent years, more and more adolescent or young adult patients living with DMD have undergone tracheostomy and continuous ventilation, in order to pursue goals when they feel their quality of life is relatively good. However, even with optimal medical therapy, more than 50% of those aged 15 to 19 years are dependent on ventilation, and the long-term survival is still limited to early adulthood.[43] As this decision is often faced by adolescent patients, it is critical that they be active participants in the decision-making process, and be well informed as to what their future care and illness might be like.

Another group of children have systemic weakness caused by chronic critical illness, and this is perhaps a new group in the past decade for whom significant respiratory symptoms are developing.[44] Chronic critical illness can be identified by the patient needing to be managed by way of tracheostomy and ongoing mechanical ventilation, because of myriad underlying conditions, often multiorgan dysfunction, that prevent a patient from being weaned from a ventilator in the short term.[45] These children often have complex chronic illnesses that lead to multifactorial respiratory symptoms. These factors include months of being bedbound, leading to generalized polyneuropathy and myopathy.[46] This weakness is compounded by intrinsic lung and airway disease, caused by factors such as previous pneumonia or adult respiratory distress syndrome (ARDS) and ongoing barotrauma. These children may also be symptomatic from a variety of other organ failures and treatments, as well as from emotional symptoms arising from existential distress, chronic hospitalization, hopelessness, and fear and anxiety.[47] The role of psychosocial care providers is essential in reducing some of these psychological symptoms. Child life specialists devise activities that provide a reprieve from the seriousness of the acute care setting in which patients reside for sometimes many months at a time.

Special Considerations for Patients with Cystic Fibrosis

Cystic fibrosis is a common multisystem disease from which children, adolescents, and adults suffer. Over time, progressive respiratory symptoms such as dyspnea, recurrent pneumonias, chronic cough, and hypercarbic headaches are accompanied by other distressing symptoms, such as weight loss, diabetes mellitus, and limited mobility. Aside from being a life-threatening disease, this is a progressive chronic disease that can physically limit the child due to impaired pulmonary function. School absences for appointments, or hospitalization for pneumonia or a so-called CF tune-up are common. This disease also requires compliance to constant daily respiratory treatment regimens, including ingestion of multiple enzymes and medications, inhalation treatment, and chest physiotherapy/postural drainage, all of which are time-consuming, and may be a challenge to maintain. A wonderful example of creativity on the part of a mother to enhance adherence was to devise a marshmallow blower instead of an incentive spirometer, which the child loved to use. Lastly, these children are often of small stature for their age, and therefore they might stand out as different from their healthy peers if they are fairly symptomatic in childhood or adolescence. This combination of factors sometimes leads to social isolation of the child, and more school absences because of psychosocial issues that compound already compromised attendance and involvement. Coupled with these physical symptoms are often fear and anxiety around the possibility of death and dying, fear of symptom progression, and feelings of loss and separation from daily routines and comforts, family and friends. In some situations, children and their families have to make difficult decisions about whether or not to embark on the path to undergo lung transplant. A decision to proceed with transplant often takes them out of their home community to a transplant center for prolonged periods of time, during which they may also have to undergo fairly strenuous pulmonary and general rehabilitation to optimize the chances of successful transplant. To this point, the decision is not an easy one, given the paucity of pediatric data, and controversies about wait-list mortality, etc.[48-50]

Apnea

In some instances, central nervous system disease can cause apnea, which is often very distressing for parents and caregivers, but is occasionally very distressing for the aware patient, who has a normal sensorium but severe brainstem disease, such as pontine glioma.

Another condition that frequently causes apnea is trisomy 18. Management of these apneas and/or supporting the weak infant with trisomy 18 by modalities such as CPAP or high-flow nasal cannulae are becoming a more common request from parents.[51,52] While many centers offer comfort-directed therapy to these babies, other centers are offering increasing supportive therapies such as CPAP or BiPap, and invasive interventions such as open heart surgery for correction of congenital heart disease.[53,54] It is true that many conditions would be lethal, were all therapies to be withheld. This is the argument raised by some parents advocating treatment for their babies: that trisomy 18, and even trisomy 13, cause death in infancy and early childhood because nothing has been done therapeutically for these children. On the other hand, most parents still consider the ramifications of trisomies 13 and 18 to be inconsistent with what they believe to be a good life for their child, and the majority choose noninvasive intervention for management of the child's airway and breathing.

Abnormal breathing patterns

Patients often have erratic breathing patterns toward the end of their lives, sometimes called Cheyne-Stokes respirations. In this situation, the patient may develop very long pauses between breaths, to the extent that caregivers often believe that the patient has died. After the long pause, the patient then compensates with a series of relatively rapid breaths. This is most often described in adult patients with brainstem injury or tumors, and severe congestive heart failure.[55] However, this exaggeration of periodic breathing is often seen as pediatric patients approach death from many other types of disease, and the mechanism for it is not fully elucidated. It is helpful for families to know that this breathing irregularity may occur, and that it is a very common finding at the end stages of illness. However, it is important not to make absolute predictions about survival based on this alone, as some patients have had very irregular respirations with apneas for days or weeks before death.

ADVANCE CARE PLANNING FOR THE CHILD WITH RESPIRATORY SYMPTOMS

In the larger context of the patient's life, a significant burden of respiratory symptoms often heralds the realization that a child is seriously ill, regardless of the etiology. Perhaps because of the technical and medical supports that can be instituted to ease breathing, parents sometimes seem to be unaware of the gravity of the situation when new options are exhausted. It is not uncommon for parents of chronically ill children to be very focused on how the patient is being ventilated when the child becomes more ill, in their search to make their child more comfortable. Sometimes, the underlying disease and its potential

for worsening seem less obvious to parents than faults of the machines as the child's condition worsens. Often, there is still a huge element of shock when children with profound respiratory compromise and symptoms do succumb to their disease. There are probably many reasons patients and their parents may not choose to embark on conversations about what they want if the situation becomes worse. These likely include deferring the conversation while there are still other things to try, or while a child is seemingly well despite chronic ventilation. Parents may also perceive a lack of consensus among care providers, integrating the most hopeful messages, and not focusing on less optimistic messages they've received.

Most parents want physicians to discuss advance care planning with them and help them make decisions. Effective communication skills are required, including familiarity with developmentally appropriate language if the child is included in the discussions. Rather than asking parents whether they want everything to be provided for their child, it is better to be clear and decide on individual interventions that are feasible within the context of the child's illness. It is important to be sensitive to emotions that may surface including fear, guilt, anger, denial, and surprise. In anticipation of these reactions, it may help to be explicit about the shift in focus from cure and survival to comfort and well being. The benefits for parents include knowing that they have assured the best care for their child, including preserving quality of life and avoiding unnecessary pain or suffering.[35]

Another concern is the frequent absence of the child's wants in these discussions about treatment options and decisions.[56] It is hoped that this situation will become less and less common, as more familiarity with the concept and practice of advance care planning evolves. Certainly, some children and adolescents will decline to hear information about, or participate in, decisions related to their care, but it is likely that these are in the minority.

These sentiments are expressed in another excerpt from the previously cited document from the Canadian Paediatric Society:

"There may be a role for paediatric health care practitioners to lobby for legislative change that is uniform across Canada and other countries so that advance directives expressed by or on behalf of minors become legally valid. In the meantime, capable children and youths can still express their wishes in the hope that adults will take them into account.

"We should encourage them to make their wishes known widely and consider having them put in writing as 'advance directives,' which in practice are being accepted more commonly, despite legislative gaps. We should also advocate for research on advance care planning with paediatric patients with life-threatening conditions, including but not limited to research on decisional capacity, to substantiate our efforts to effect legislative change."

Summary

Although there have been significant advances in the development of medications and technologies to treat respiratory symptoms in children, there is still a relative deficit of high-quality research to evaluate them in pediatric patients. Many treatments are extrapolated from studies of adult patients.

Furthermore, medications used for the treatment of dyspnea are largely systemic medications of only two major categories, opioids and benzodiazepines, that work mainly by affecting central nervous system perception, rather than medications that target the lungs directly, leaving further basic science study of dyspnea as an important issue given the high prevalence of this symptom at the end of life. Importantly, even with limitations in current knowledge, in working collaboratively, the interdisciplinary team can ease dyspnea and other distressing symptoms in children with advanced illness (Fig. 32-5).

Clinical Vignette

A very difficult situation arose when a 14-year-old girl was deemed to have end-stage pulmonary disease related to cystic fibrosis. Her situation was further complicated because she lived three hours from the referral center, and she had been non-adherent to much of her therapy. She also was truant from school, despite a stated wish to attend, and with

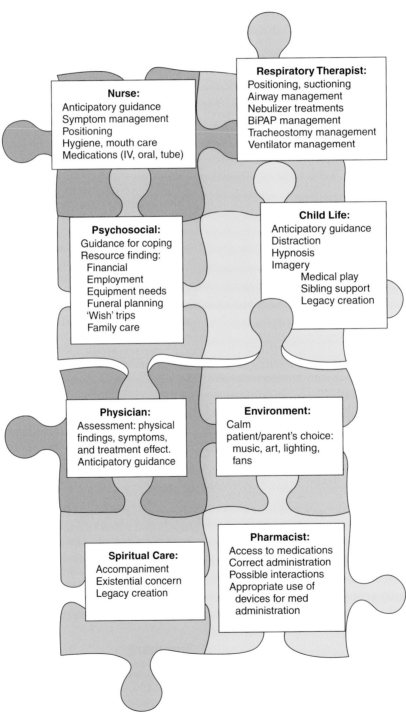

Fig. 32-5 Diagram depicting team contribution to management of respiratory symptoms.

many conveniences put into place to make this easily possible. She suffered from a variety of symptoms, including episodes of moderate dyspnea, anxiety, and occasional hypercarbic headaches. Our team was involved prior to her admission at outpatient meetings with regard to non-adherence to treatment, which had resulted in extreme weight loss and worsened respiratory illness. Ultimately, she shouted at the treating team, "What do you think I am, stupid? I don't want to _____ die." I calmly returned her exact words to her, that we didn't want her to _____ die, either, and that was why so many of us had gathered. That public exchange of profanity seemed to cement the relationships with the larger team, from her perspective. Over what would become a hospitalization of about 6 months, her behavior gradually improved, as did her adherence to treatment, such that she did become a candidate for lung transplant. However, her health condition continued to deteriorate over this time: she lost weight despite many efforts to improve her nutrition with gastrostomy feeds, her cough became quite bothersome to her despite treatment with chest physio, spirometry, salbutamol, tobramycin nebules, and codeine. Eventually, her hypercarbic headaches and her dyspnea were best treated with BiPAP, first at night, and then at all times. During this period, she had moments in which she would discuss her wishes for her funeral, should that occur, and did embark on some legacy projects with the child life specialist's assistance. The call was then received that the lungs were available. This young woman was extremely distraught the morning of her transplant surgery, by then second-guessing whether or not she could or should go through with it. However, with repeated discussion from her attending pulmonologist, child life specialist, palliative care nurse, and physician, and most importantly, her parents, she did consent. Fortunately, the story has a happy ending. We only see her now when she visits the teen room to check on old friends, but mostly she visits the child life team members who were so instrumental to her during her long stay, and longer journey.

Acknowledgments

Many thanks to Terry Fraser, child life specialist, and Tara Wren, palliative care nurse coordinator, for their contributions and review of this manuscript.

REFERENCES

1. Anbar RD, Geisler SC: Identification of children who may benefit from self-hypnosis at a pediatric pulmonary center, *BMC Pediatr* 5(1):6, 2005.
2. Hadfield PJ, Lloyd-Faulconbridge RV, Almeyda J, Albert DM, Bailey CM: The changing indications for paediatric tracheostomy, *Int J Pediatr Otorhinolaryngol* 67(1):7–10, 2003.
3. Principi T, Morrison GC, Matsui DM, Speechley KN, Seabrook JA, Singh RN, et al: Elective tracheostomy in mechanically ventilated children in Canada, *Intensive Care Med* 34(8):1498–1502, 2008.
4. *Mosby's Medical Dictionary*, 2009. http://medical-dictionary.thefreedictionary.com/Dyspnea. Accessed December 11, 2009.
5. Khan FI, Reddy RC, Baptist AP: Pediatric Dyspnea scale for use in hospitalized patients with asthma, *J Allergy Clin Immunol* 123(3):660–664, 2009.
6. McGrath PJ, Pianosi PT, Unruh AM, Buckley CP: Dalhousie dyspnea scales: construct and content validity of pictorial scales for measuring dyspnea, *BMC Pediatr* 5:33, 2005.
7. Bausewein C, Booth S, Gysels M, Higginson I: Non-pharmacological interventions for breathlessness in advanced stages of malignant and non-malignant diseases, *Cochrane Database Syst Rev* (2):005623, 2008.
8. Mize WL: Clinical training in self-regulation and practical pediatric hypnosis: what pediatricians want pediatricians to know, *J Dev Behav Pediatr* 17(5):317–322, 1996.
9. Jennings AL, Davies AN, Higgins JP, Broadley K: Opioids for the palliation of breathlessness in terminal illness, *Cochrane Database Syst Rev* (4):002066, 2001.
10. Polosa R, Simidchiev A, Walters EH: Nebulised morphine for severe interstitial lung disease, *Cochrane Database Syst Rev* 2, 2009.
11. Navigante AH, Cerchietti LC, Castro MA, Lutteral MA, Cabalar ME: Midazolam as adjunct therapy to morphine in the alleviation of severe dyspnea perception in patients with advanced cancer, *J Pain Symptom Manage* 31(1):38–47, 2006.
12. Krakauer EL, Penson RT, Truog RD, King LA, Chabner BA, Lynch TJ Jr: Sedation for intractable distress of a dying patient: acute palliative care and the principle of double effect, *Oncologist* 5(1):53–62, 2000.
13. Elsayem A, Curry I, Boohene J: Use of palliative sedation for intractable symptoms in the palliative care unit of a comprehensive cancer center, *J Pain Symptom Manage* 31(1):38–47, 2006.
14. Twycross R, Wilcock A: *Respiratory Symptoms*, 2009. www.palliative-drugs.com/palliative-care-formulary.html. Accessed December 11, 2009.
15. Cranston JM, Crockett A, Currow D: Oxygen therapy for dyspnoea in adults, *Cochrane Database Syst Rev* (3):004769, 2008.
16. Paul IM, Beiler J, McMonagle A, Shaffer ML, Duda L, Berlin CM Jr: Effect of honey, dextromethorphan, and no treatment on nocturnal cough and sleep quality for coughing children and their parents, *Arch Pediatr Adolesc Med* 161(12):1140–1146, 2007.
17. Morice AH, Menon MS, Mulrennan SA, Everett CF, Wright C, Jackson J, et al: Opiate therapy in chronic cough, *Am J Respir Crit Care Med* 175(4):312–315, 2007.
18. Klopp AH, Eapen GA, Komaki RR: Endobronchial brachytherapy: an effective option for palliation of malignant bronchial obstruction, *Clin Lung Cancer* 8(3):203–207, 2006.
19. *High-dose rate endobronchial brachytherapy*. www.upmccancercenteres.com/radonc/internal/lung_endobronchial.html. Accessed July 11, 2009.
20. Wee B, Hillier R: Interventions for noisy breathing in patients near to death, *Cochrane Database Syst Rev* (1):005177, 2008.
21. Shaw P, Agarwal R: Pleurodesis for malignant pleural effusions. *Cochrane Database Syst Rev* (1):002916, 2004.
22. Efthymiou C, Masoudi T, Thorpe J, Papagiannopoulos K: Malignant pleural effusion in the presence of trapped lung. Five-year experience of pleurX tunnelled catheters, *Interact Cardiovasc Thorac Surg* July 28, 2009 (e-pub).
23. Tremblay A, Michaud G: Single-center experience with 250 tunneled pleural catheter insertions for malignant pleural effusion, *Chest* 129(2):362–368, 2006.
24. Mercuri E, Bertini E, Messina S, Solari A, D'Amico A, Angelozzi C, et al: Randomized, double-blind, placebo-controlled trial of phenylbutyrate in spinal muscular atrophy, *Neurology* 68(1):51–55, 2007.
25. Brahe C, Vitali T, Tiziano FD, Angelozzi C, Pinto AM, Borgo F, et al: Phenylbutyrate increases SMN gene expression in spinal muscular atrophy patients, *Eur J Hum Genet* 13(2):256–259, 2005.
26. Tsai LK, Yang CC, Hwu WL, Li H: Valproic acid treatment in six patients with spinal muscular atrophy, *Eur J Neurol* 14(12):e8–e9, 2007.
27. Wang CH, Finkel RS, Bertini ES, Schroth M, Simonds A, Wong B, et al: Consensus statement for standard of care in spinal muscular atrophy, *J Child Neurol* 22(8):1027–1049, 2007.
28. Fauroux B, Guillemot N, Aubertin G, Nathan N, Labit A, Clement A, et al: Physiologic benefits of mechanical insufflation-exsufflation in children with neuromuscular diseases, *Chest* 133(1):161–168, 2008.
29. Gross L: Stem cell promise, interrupted: how long do US researchers have to wait? *PLoS Biol* 5(1):e32, 2007.
30. Nayak MS, Kim YS, Goldman M, Keirstead HS, Kerr DA: Cellular therapies in motor neuron diseases, *Biochim Biophys Acta* 1762(11–12):1128–1138, 2006.
31. Hyde SA, Steffensen BF, Floytrup I, Glent S, Kroksmark AK, Salling B, et al: Longitudinal data analysis: an application to construction of a natural history profile of Duchenne muscular dystrophy, *Neuromuscul Disord* 11(2):165–170, 2001.
32. Levetown M: American Academy of Pediatrics Committee on, Bioethics, *Pediatrics* 121(5):e1441–e1460, 2008.

33. Devictor D, Latour JM, Tissieres P: Forgoing life-sustaining or death-prolonging therapy in the pediatric ICU, *Pediatr Clin North Am* 55(3):791–804, 2008; xiii.

34. Giannini A, Messeri A, Aprile A, Casalone C, Jankovic M, Scarani R, et al: End-of-life decisions in pediatric intensive care. Recommendations of the Italian Society of Neonatal and Pediatric Anesthesia and Intensive Care (SARNePI), *Paediatr Anaesth* 18(11):1089–1095, 2008.

35. Advance care planning for paediatric patients, *J Paediatr Child Health* 13(9):793–796, 2008.

36. Kleinman A: Medicine and morality: Health care's missing care, *Globe and Mail* A13, 2009.

37. Hylin U, Nyholm H, Mattiasson AC, Ponzer S: Interprofessional training in clinical practice on a training ward for healthcare students: a two-year follow-up, *J Interprof Care* 21(3):277–288, 2007.

38. Sternas KA, O'Hare P, Lehman K, Milligan R: Nursing and medical student teaming for service learning in partnership with the community: an emerging holistic model for interdisciplinary education and practice, *Holist Nurs Pract* 13(2):66–77, 1999.

39. Wilkes M, Milgrom E, Hoffman JR: Towards more empathic medical students: a medical student hospitalization experience, *Med Educ* 36(6):528–533, 2002.

40. Blasco PA, Kohen H, Shapland C: Parents-as-teachers: design and establishment of a training programme for paediatric residents, *Med Educ* 33(9):695–701, 1999.

41. Engelke MK, Britton BP, Burhans L, Hall S: Is there a doctor in the house? Integrating medical education and home health care, *Home Care Provid* 3(5):260–265, 1998; quiz 266-267.

42. Carnevale FA, Alexander E, Davis M, Rennick J, Troini R: Daily living with distress and enrichment: the moral experience of families with ventilator-assisted children at home, *Pediatrics* 117(1):e48–e60, 2006.

43. Jeppesen J, Green A, Steffensen BF, Rahbek J: The Duchenne muscular dystrophy population in Denmark, 1977-2001: prevalence, incidence and survival in relation to the introduction of ventilator use, *Neuromuscul Disord* 13(10):804–812, 2003.

44. Marcin JP, Slonim AD, Pollack MM, Ruttimann UE: Long-stay patients in the pediatric intensive care unit, *Crit Care Med* 29(3):652–657, 2001.

45. Camhi SL, Mercado AF, Morrison RS, Du Q, Platt DM, August GI, et al: Deciding in the dark: advance directives and continuation of treatment in chronic critical illness, *Crit Care Med* 37(3):919–925, 2009.

46. Schweickert WD, Hall J: ICU-acquired weakness, *Chest* 131(5):1541–1549, 2007.

47. Melnyk BM, Alpert-Gillis L, Feinstein NF, Crean HF, Johnson J, Fairbanks E, et al: Creating opportunities for parent empowerment: program effects on the mental health/coping outcomes of critically ill young children and their mothers, *Pediatrics* 113(6):e597–e607, 2004.

48. Huddleston CB, Bloch JB, Sweet SC, de la Morena M, Patterson GA, Mendeloff EN: Lung transplantation in children, *Ann Surg* 236(3):270–276, 2002.

49. Liou TG, Adler FR, Cox DR, Cahill BC: Lung transplantation and survival in children with cystic fibrosis, *N Engl J Med* 357(21):2143–2152, 2007.

50. Liou TG, Adler FR, Cahill BC, Cox DR: Correction: Lung transplantation and survival in children with cystic fibrosis, *N Engl J Med* 359(5):536, 2008.

51. McGraw MP, Perlman JM: Attitudes of neonatologists toward delivery room management of confirmed trisomy 18: potential factors influencing a changing dynamic, *Pediatrics* 121(6):1106–1110, 2008.

52. Goc B, Walencka Z, Wloch A, Wojciechowska E, Wiecek-Wlodarska D, Krzystolik-Ladzinska J, et al: Trisomy 18 in neonates: prenatal diagnosis, clinical features, therapeutic dilemmas and outcome, *J Appl Genet* 47(2):165–170, 2006.

53. Graham EM, Bradley SM, Shirali GS, Hills CB, Atz AM, Pediatric Cardiac Care C: Effectiveness of cardiac surgery in trisomies 13 and 18 (from the Pediatric Cardiac Care Consortium), *Am J Cardiol* 93(6):801–803, 2004.

54. Kaneko Y, Kobayashi J, Yamamoto Y, Yoda H, Kanetaka Y, Nakajima Y, et al: Intensive cardiac management in patients with trisomy 13 or trisomy 18, *Am J Med Genet A* 146A(11):1372–1380, 2008.

55. Cherniack NS, Longobardo G, Evangelista CJ: Causes of Cheyne-Stokes respiration, *Neurocrit Care* 3(3):271–279, 2005.

56. Harrison C, Kenny NP, Sidarous M, Rowell M: Bioethics for clinicians: 9. Involving children in medical decisions, *CMAJ* 156(6):825–828, 1997.

57. DeVlaming D: Personal communication, professional practice lead, children's services homecare, Edmonton, Alberta, Canada.

33 Gastrointestinal Symptoms

STEFAN J. FRIEDRICHSDORF | ROSS DRAKE | M. LOUISE WEBSTER

Digestion, of all the bodily functions, is the one which exercises the greatest influence on the mental state of an individual.

—Jean-Anthelme Brillat-Savarin

Palliative care no longer means helping children die well, it means helping children and their families to live well, and then, when the time is certain, to help them die gently.

—Mattie Stepanek

A 16-year-old girl with cystic fibrosis and advanced but stable lung disease was hospitalized with severe abdominal pain, nausea, and anorexia following viral gastroenteritis. There was an initial belief that she may have a partial bowel obstruction but this was ruled out after multiple investigations failed to show any significant organic factors. She adamantly denied anxiety or depressive symptoms.

The gastrointestinal symptoms did not improve with standard psychological and pharmacologic strategies, and her lung function began to deteriorate further secondary to weight loss and immobility. A family meeting involving the psychosocial team, the teen, and her parents provided a forum for her parents to discuss their spiritual beliefs and the teen's acceptance that she would die from her condition at some stage. This was distressing for the teen to hear and allowed her to talk about her own anxieties about death, her fear that her symptoms represented a terminal illness, and that her death would be sudden and unexpected and that her family could not be present because of that. She had been reluctant to discuss these matters with her parents as she believed they would be disappointed in her.

These revelations opened the way for her primary pediatrician to discuss with her the likely modes of death from cystic fibrosis, and the expectation that her death was not imminent given good nutrition and mobilization. The pediatrician also promised to talk openly and honestly with her when her lung function declined to the point that her death was near. Within several days the young woman was eating well, mobilizing, communicating more openly with her family, and her pain levels were manageable. She lived with a good quality of life for an additional 14 months before dying at home with her family present.

This vignette highlights a number of important concepts of pediatric palliative care and pediatric medicine in general. Arguably, the most important of these is the existence of a strong, inextricable link between the physical and the psychological, or the mind-body link. This link brings into sharp relief the need to work in an interdisciplinary fashion, as no one person and no one discipline has the full skill set to adequately address the needs of a child, and his or her family, with a life-threatening condition.

Adherence to a purely mechanistic and/or biological approach to care provides some degree of success and, in controlling troublesome symptoms, can open the door to address the wider emotional, psychosocial, and spiritual issues that are present. Not addressing these appropriately ultimately means lost opportunities and inferior care. In this example, symptoms were not amenable to a pharmacologic approach and should stand as a warning that properly investigated and treated symptoms that remain uncontrolled indicates the need to deal with an underlying psychological, emotional, and/or spiritual issue.

A well-functioning interdisciplinary team is critical to the management of gastrointestinal symptoms in pediatric palliative care. The nature of the interdisciplinary work in a specific team is often shaped by the members of the team and the range of disciplines included. In addition to the holistic child and family focused skill set expected of all team members, there are some particular skills that are more specific to nurses, medical practitioners, or psychosocial clinicians.

Nurses often provide overall case management that incorporates ongoing symptom assessment, medication management, and psychosocial care, but they also have unique skills in the assessment and provision of physical care and comfort to the dying child. Some of these skills include providing and/or teaching family members developmentally appropriate strategies for feeding, toileting, wound care, line management, medication administration, and positioning and pressure area care.

Physicians have particular skills and training in diagnostic assessment, particularly where there are complex symptoms, in palliative treatment and/or management planning, and in pharmacologic interventions.

Psychosocial or mental health clinicians may come from a variety of disciplines including psychology, psychotherapy, social work, child life, chaplaincy, and psychiatry. Specific skills include the assessment of more complex mental health issues for children and family members and of challenging family interaction or communication difficulties. They can provide psychotherapeutic input such as play therapy, cognitive behavioral therapies for such things as anxiety, depression, pain, nausea, hypnosis training, focused family and couple work, and in some instances, systems interventions where communication difficulties are present among teams involved in the child's care.

Gastrointestinal symptoms and distress are relatively common in children and are not limited to those receiving palliative care. Tummy-aches and vomiting are integral to the childhood portrayed by Shakespeare with his 'mewling and puking' infant, and the nursery rhymes and songs of childhood where 'Miss Polly had a dolly that was sick, sick, sick' and on the good ship Lolly-pop where 'if you eat too much, oh, oh, you'll awake with a tummy-ache.' As many as 30% of otherwise healthy children will experience recurrent abdominal pain during childhood, one in six adolescents report functional gastrointestinal symptoms consistent with irritable bowel syndrome (IBS),[1] and abdominal discomfort maybe the primary presenting symptoms for the child with anxiety and emotional difficulties.

Gastrointestinal symptoms are prominent among children receiving palliative care. Six studies examining the prevalence of distressing symptoms in a total of 592 children with malignant and non-malignant diseases reveal that the majority of dying children experience pain, 53% to 92%, and fatigue, 52% to 97%, during their end-of-life period. In addition, a large percentage suffer from gastrointestinal symptoms such as vomiting and/or nausea, 40% to 63%, constipation, 27% to 59%, and diarrhea, 21% to 40%.[2–7]

Many of these children will have previously experienced abdominal pain, nausea and vomiting, anorexia, and disturbed bowel function in association with their primary disease, or as a consequence of treatment and treatment complications. The result is that they and their parents may be particularly anxious and sensitized to any recurrence of symptoms, as this may be perceived as a heralding event to deterioration and the onset of the final stages of the child's illness. In addition, any alteration or loss of the normal bodily rhythms of eating and toileting is disquieting for families; the inability to feed and nourish their child may symbolize failure of the most fundamental parenting role, and loss of bowel control may be humiliating and seem like the final insult for a young person with a life-threatening illness. For these reasons alone, the evaluation and management of the many potential contributors to gastrointestinal distress is challenging and requires a holistic approach.

This chapter aims to provide treatment algorithms for individual gastrointestinal symptoms as originally proposed in 2000.[8] The evidence for any recommendations made is often poor due to the lack of randomized controlled trials (RCTs) in pediatric palliative care and, unfortunately, pediatrics continues to be hampered by the common, unacceptable problem of many medications not being approved for use in children or for the specified indication resulting in off-label use.

Nausea and Vomiting

Nausea and vomiting is one of the most distressing symptoms for ill children and their caregivers. Gastrointestinal, central nervous system (CNS), metabolic, pharmacologic, and psychological factors may all contribute, and prolonged episodes of nausea and vomiting may themselves contribute to the development of anticipatory nausea and conditioned vomiting. Treatment approaches are best based on the presumed, following careful assessment, underlying pathophysiology and management should include integrative therapies, such as cognitive behavioral therapies, aromatherapy, and acupressure, where appropriate.

PATHOPHYSIOLOGY

Vomiting is controlled by two distinct brain centers, the vomiting center and the chemoreceptor trigger zone (CTZ). Both are located in the medulla oblongata with the CTZ lying outside the blood-brain barrier in the area postrema at the floor of the fourth ventricle, while the vomiting center is located inside the blood-brain barrier.

Excitation of the vomiting center results in nausea and vomiting and the reflex may result from the following input:

- Direct activation of the CTZ. Responds to metabolic products or medications in the blood or cerebrospinal fluid.
  - Dopamine type 2 (D_2)-receptors in the area postrema are stimulated by emetogenic substances such as calcium, uremia products, opioids, and digoxin.[9]
  - 5-Hydroxytryptamine ($5HT_3$)-receptors, also located at the area postrema, respond to many cancer-directed chemotherapy drugs and uremia.
- Stimulation via the vestibular apparatus.
  - Muscarinic acetylcholine (ACh_m).
  - Histamine (H_1) excitatory receptors.
- Gut wall and vagal and/or splanchnic afferents. Both carry $5HT_3$-receptors, the former also has $5HT_4$ and D_2-receptors.
  - All play an important emetic role and are activated by distention in the gut lumen, abdominal radiotherapy, and chemotherapy when serotonin (5HT) is produced by the enterochromaffin cells lining the lumen epithelium.
  - Peripheral or central afferents. Emetogenic stimuli reaches the central nervous system via afferent pathways with the nucleus tractus solitarii probably playing a coordinating role.
  - Sensory stimuli such as smells that have previously been associated with episodes of vomiting can become triggers for anticipatory nausea and so-called conditioned vomiting.

Toxins commonly associated with nausea and vomiting during the pediatric end-of-life period include medications such as chemotherapeutic agents, antibiotics, and opioids, and metabolic byproducts of uremia or hepatic failure.[10]

The majority of receptors in the vomiting center and CTZ are excitatory, that is, they induce nausea and vomiting with stimulation. An important exception is the presence of the μ-opioid receptor in the vomiting center. Opioids seem to have a dose-dependent interaction on emesis. At standard doses, opioids may cause nausea by stimulating D_2-receptors in the area postrema but at high doses opioids are often not emetic. This is postulated to be due to an antiemetic or inhibitory effect at the μ-opioid receptor in the vomiting center.[9,11]

Opioid-Induced Nausea

Although individual patients may tolerate one opioid better than another, data suggest that prevalence of these side effects differ greatly among the commonly used opioids. Children usually develop tolerance to nausea, however this may take days to occur. From experience the single most helpful approach to opioid-induced nausea in the Minneapolis pediatric pain and palliative care patients represents a rotation or a switch to another opioid at an equianalgesic dose.[12]

Alternatively, low-dose naloxone infusions, at 0.25–1 mcg/kg/h, can reduce the frequency and severity of nausea without antagonizing analgesia in children who receive opioids.[13] Infusion rates used are several-fold lower than infusion rates typically used to produce measurable reversal of analgesia or respiratory depression.

If neither an opioid rotation nor low-dose naloxone infusion are effective or feasible in the disease trajectory, then the addition of a dopamine (D_2)-receptor antagonists such as metoclopramide and antiemetics of other classes should be considered, see later in this chapter.

TREATMENT ALGORITHM

Step 1: Evaluation and Assessment

Every child suffering from nausea and/or vomiting in palliative care needs to be thoroughly evaluated by taking a careful history and performing a focused clinical examination. Questions of clinical importance include possible correlation with eating, medication administration, and association with other symptoms such as pain or sensory stimuli. Undertreated pain can cause nausea and vomiting. Other considerations are the presence or absence of raised intracranial pressure, sub-ileus, constipation, or seizures.

Step 2: Treatment of Underlying Causes

Any consideration to treat an underlying cause needs to take into account each child's situation with a key element of these deliberations being the maintenance or improvement of the child's quality of life. Common pathophysiologies are constipation, reflux, sub-ileus, infections such as gastroenteritis, metabolic disorders including hypercalcemia and renal failure, seizure, and anxiety. Drug adverse effects are common and include side effects to antibiotics, anticholinergics, corticosteroids, non-steroidal anti-inflammatory drugs, opioids, palliative chemotherapy, and tricyclic antidepressants.

Step 3: Implement Integrative and Supportive Therapies

The combination of supportive and integrative modalities with pharmacologic management should be seen as a gold standard to any pain and symptom management approach in the twenty-first century.[14] Integrative and supportive approaches include the provision of small meals chosen by the child, frequently offering favorite drinks, good oral care, and the avoidance of discomforting smells.

Management of anxiety for the child and his or her family is paramount and should start with careful explanation of the likely factors contributing to the symptoms. A number of therapeutic techniques can be used to help the child to relax, feel calmer, and have a greater sense of control. These include cognitive behavioral strategies such as simple relaxation exercises, controlled breathing, and focusing on positive self messages and imagery. Younger children may need a parent to cue them and help them with guided imagery and stories, while older children can be taught self-hypnosis to manage symptoms. Pleasant masking aromas of the child's choosing can also be used if there are particular odors that trigger nausea. Scheduling enjoyable distracting activities including music, or acupressure or acupuncture may also be useful for some children.[9,15–20]

An 11-year-old boy with a previous history of severe chemotherapy-associated nausea and vomiting was troubled by persistent nausea during the palliative phase of management for relapsed osteosarcoma. Although no longer receiving chemotherapy, the smell of the hospital antiseptic and the smell of his overnight enteral feed triggered bouts of intense nausea. Working with the team psychologist, he was able to use a combination of muscle relaxation, calm breathing and thinking about his favorite television program hero to reduce his nausea and associated anxiety. He also found that the smell of citrus and eucalyptus oils helped mask the hospital smell during clinic visits, and at his nighttime feed at home.

Step 4: Pharmacology

The selection of an antiemetic for treatment of nausea and/or vomiting requires a rational approach based on the assessed pathophysiology (see previous text) and, because both nausea and vomiting can have multiple etiologies in any individual, initially directed at the major cause. In the event of a single agent being ineffective, then a combination of antiemetics, where each targets different receptors, should be considered. Several randomized controlled trials (RCTs) exist only in children with cancer and postoperative nausea, and may not be applicable for children with non-malignant conditions in palliative care. However, the rational approach of first targeting the assessed major etiology followed by the introduction of an agent with a different receptor action profile, if needed, should be seen as good practice.

5-HT₃-Receptor Antagonists Several RCTs showed that the serotonin (5-hydroxytryptamine-3) antagonist ondansetron (Zofran) provides a good antiemetic effect in children with cancer after chemotherapy administration or bone marrow transplant,[21–24] compared with placebo and other antiemetics such as metoclopramide plus dexamethasone[25] or metoclopramide plus diphenhydramine.[26] Other 5-HT₃ antagonists, such as tropisetron (Navoban)[27,28] and granisetron (Kyrtec)[29] show a similar effect.

A common adverse effect of this class is constipation. They may also cause headaches, and nausea at higher doses, especially when administered above the recommended doses. Anecdotal experience also suggests 5-HT₃-receptor antagonists are effective for nausea and vomiting in children with non-malignant palliative conditions.

D₂-Receptor Antagonists Dopamine₂-receptor antagonists such as metoclopramide (Reglan) and haloperidol (Haldol) are prokinetic and have been clinically effective in treating nausea and vomiting in pediatric palliative and hospice care. Stress, anxiety, and nausea via peripheral dopaminergic receptors at the plexus myentericus may cause a slowing of gastrointestinal passage, the so-called dopamine break. This effect is antagonized by metoclopramide (Reglan) and domperidone (Motilium).[30] Other D₂-receptor antagonists may have a similar effect.

They may, however, be underused due to an overemphasis on possible extrapyramidal reactions. Metoclopramide has been associated with a dyskinetic syndrome and reported to occur with an incidence of 1:5000 in teenagers.[31] Any such reaction can be treated with either a centrally acting antihistamine, such as diphenhydramine (Benadryl), or central anticholinergic, such as benztropine. This concern extends to a lesser extent to phenothiazine derivates (psychotropics) such as haloperidol (Haldol), prochlorperazine (Compazine), and chlorpromazine (Thorazine). Chlorpromazine and prochlorperazine are also H_1- and ACh_m- receptor antagonists.

Domperidone does not cross the blood-brain barrier and therefore does not cause extrapyramidal side effects. The intravenous form of domperidone was discontinued following reports of cardiovascular adverse effects.

Prokinetics should not be administered concurrently with antimuscarinic agents, such as diphenhydramine or scopolamine, as these block the final common pathway for prokinetic agents. The concurrent administration of diphenhydramine and metoclopramide to prevent a dyskinetic syndrome, as practiced in some centers, will therefore result in the loss of metoclopramide's prokinetic effect, however not of its antiemetic effect. The concurrent intravenous administration with 5-HT$_3$-receptor antagonists increases the risk of cardiac arrhythmia. Droperidol (Inapsine), a butyrophenone neuroleptic similar to haloperidol, can no longer be recommended because of the risk of QT prolongation.

H_1- and ACh_m- Receptor Antagonists

Histamine-1 and muscarinic acetylcholin receptor antagonists are effective antiemetics in daily clinical practice though there are no pediatric RCTs. These medications have an astounding regional preference without any head-to-head comparison. The first-generation antihistamine diphenhydramine (Benadryl) has a significant anticholinergic, especially sedating, side effect and is hardly used as a first-line medication outside North America. Promethazine (Phenergan), commonly used in Australia, is similarly sedating. In central Europe the preferred pediatric antiemetic is dimenhydrinate (Dramamine), which in clinical practice rarely causes over-sedation. The most commonly used antinausea drug in the UK on the other hand is cyclizine.

Scopolamine, an ACh_m but not H_1, receptor antagonist with stronger anticholinergic side effects than dimenhydrinate or cyclizine, can also be administered as a transdermal patch.

Medications that also have D_2-receptor antagonistic properties include chlorpromazine, prochlorperazine, and levomepromazine. The latter, in our experience, is particularly helpful in refractorary nausea in pediatric palliative care and is not available in the United States.

NK$_1$-Receptor Antagonists

Aprepitant (Emend), a neurokinin-1 receptor antagonist, possesses antidepressant, anxiolytic, and antiemetic properties. NK$_1$ receptors can be found in the central and peripheral nervous system, as well as the gastrointestinal tract. RCTs indicated it to be superior to ondansetron 24 to 48 hours post-surgery when given as a single pre-operative dose[32,33] but, in general, pediatric data is scarce.[34] One RCT ($n = 46$) in adolescents with chemotherapy-induced nausea and vomiting showed the combination of aprepitant (125 mg IV TID), dexamethasone, and ondansetron to be superior to dexamethasone and ondansetron alone.[35]

Cannabinoids

The activation of the endocannabinoid system suppresses behavioral responses to acute and persistant noxious stimulation, and D-9-tetrahydrocannabinol (THC) has been shown to have an antiemetic effect.[36] THC can also stimulate appetite in addition to minimizing nausea.

Two types of cannabinoid receptors have been identified, CB$_1$ and CB$_2$. CB$_1$ receptors are found in the central nervous system, including periaqueductal gray, rostral ventro-medial medulla and in peripheral neurons, where activation produces a suppression in intestinal neurotransmitter release.[37] Dronabinol and nabilone do not fully replicate the effect of total cannabis preparations[38] but a meta-analysis of 30 RCTs ($n = 1366$ patients)[39] showed cannabinoids to be effective for controlling chemotherapy-related sickness in adults. Adverse effects included dizziness, dysphoria, depression, hallucinations, paranoia, and arterial hypotension.

Corticosteroids

Nausea caused by raised intracranial pressure secondary to a brain tumor may show dramatic short- to medium-term improvement with corticosteroid administration. Agents such as dexamethasone are thought to act by reducing the peritumor edema. In addition, corticosteroids inhibit prostaglandin synthesis, which may also play an antiemetic role. Because of the significant side effect profile, including mood swings and excessive weight gain, associated with this class of drugs use in palliative care is controversial.[40]

Benzodiazepines

Low-dose benzodiazepines, such as midazolam, lorazepam, or diazepam, can be a part of an effective antiemetic drug treatment in pediatric palliative care. However, there is only limited pediatric data with RCTs showing effectiveness for postoperative nausea[41,42] and chemotherapy-induced nausea.[43,44]

Propofol

Propofol possesses antiemetic properties at subhypnotic doses.[45,46] The mechanism of action of this short-acting hypnotic and general anesthetic is not well defined and possibly includes potentiation of GABA-A receptor activity,[47] sodium channel blocking activity,[48] and activation of the endocannabinoid system.[49] One adult case study reports successful nausea management in palliative cancer care at 0.6–1 mg/kg/h intravenously.[50] Little pediatric data is published[51] but the experience of the program in Minnesota with low-dose propofol in 12 children and teenagers[52] points to it having an important role in managing refractory pain and nausea at the end-of-life when other agents fail (Table 33–1).

Summary

A multimodal approach to controlling nausea and/or vomiting should be directed toward the most likely assessed pathophysiology. Uni-modal approaches including pharmacology alone have a high risk of treatment failure in pediatric palliative care. The evidence does not allow for a step-by-step approach when the underlying mechanism remains unclear but clinical experience would suggest the following pharmacologic approach can work well. The palliative care teams in Minneapolis as well as in Auckland usually schedule a single medication and add another scheduled agent acting on a different receptor group if ineffective, not infrequently requiring two, three, or even four scheduled around-the-clock antiemetics.

First Line

1. 5-HT$_3$-receptor antagonist, such as ondansetron; and/or
2. D$_2$-receptor antagonist, such as metoclopramide; and/or
3. H$_1$ & ACh$_m$-receptor antagonist, such as dimenhydrate

Second Line

1. Consider adding corticosteroid, such as dexamethasone as a short-term pulse.
2. Add a low-dose benzodiazepine such as midazolam.

TABLE 33-1 Medications in the Treatment of Nausea and Vomiting

Receptor activity	Medication	Dose	Route of administration	Comments and side effects
5-HT₃-receptor antagonists	Ondansetron (Zofran)	0.1-0.2 mg/kg Q6-8h; max. 4-8 mg/dose	IV, PO, SL	Induces nausea and constipation at higher doses
	Granisetron (Kyrtec)	0.01-0.05 mg/kg Q8h; max.3 mg/dose	IV, PO, transdermal patch	Induces nausea and constipation at higher doses
Dopamine(D₂)-receptor antagonists	Metoclopramide (Reglan)	0.15-0.3 mg/kg (max. 10-15 mg) Q6h	IV, PO, PR	Extrapyramidal side effect. Prokinetics not to be given concurrently with antimuscarinics
	Haloperidol (Haldol)	0.01-0.1 mg/kg Q12h (slowly titrated to max. of 1-2 mg/kg, max. 100 mg/dose)	IV, PO	Class: Butyrophenone; extrapyramidal side effect
	Domperidone	0.2-0.4 mg/kg Q4-8h; max. 10 mg	PO, PR	Does not cross blood-brain barrier, and no extrapyramidal side effects
Histamine (H₁)/ muscarinic acetylcholine (AChm) receptor antagonists	Dimenhydrinate (Dramamine)	1-2 mg/kg Q8h IV; 2-5 mg/kg Q6-12h	IV, PO, PR	Anticholinergic side effects including constipation, sedation
	Cyclizine	1 mg mg/kg Q8h	PO, IV	Anticholinergic side effects
	Diphenhydramine (Benadryl)	0.5-1 mg/kg Q6h (max. 50mg)	PO, IV	Anticholinergic side effects, including significant sedation
	Promethazine (Phenergen)	0.2-0.5 mg/kg Q6h	IV, PO	Anticholinergic side effects, including significant sedation
	Scopolamine (Transderm Scop)	0.01 mg mg/kg Q6h IV; Patch: 0.33 mg/24h or 0.5 mg/24h: > 10 years Q72h	IV, transdermal	Antimuscarinic, not an antihistamine. Anticholinergic side effects
Dopamine(D₂)- and histamine (H₁)/ muscarinic acetylcholine (AChm) receptor antagonists	Chlorpromazine (Thorazine)	PO, PR: 0.5-2 mg/kg; IV: 0.25-1 mg/kg slow infusion	PO, PR, IV	Phenothiazine: psychotropic effect. Extrapyramidal and anticholinergic side effects, agranulocytosis
	Prochlorperazine (Compazine)	0.1-0.2 mg/kg Q8h	PO	Phenothiazine: psychotropic effect. Extrapyramidal and anticholinergic side effects, agranulocytosis
Neurokinin-1 receptor antagonists	Aprepitant (Emend)	> 12 years preoperative dose 40 mg (not per kg) once 125 mg (not per kg once, then 80 mg once per day during chemotherapy)	PO	Chemotherapy-associated nausea. Side effects: Constipation, headaches, fatigue, sinus tachycardia
Cannabinoid (CB₁) receptor agonist	Nabilone (Cesamet)	Adult dose: 1-2 mg BID	PO	May stimulate appetite Side effects: dizziness, dysphoria, hallucinations, arterial hypotension
	Dronabinol (Marinol)	5 mg/m² Q2-4h, max. 4-6 doses/day	PO	Dizziness, dysphoria, hallucinations, arterial hypotension

3. Substitute first-line drugs of same class, such as rotation to granisetron, haloperidol, diphenhydramine.
4. Consider substituting phenothiazine, such as chlorpromazine, for both antihistamine and dopamine receptor antagonist.

Third Line

1. Consider aprepitant.
2. Add cannabis, such as dronabinol.
3. Consider low-dose propofol.

Considerations in the setting of bowel obstruction include octreotrid (see following text).

Constipation

Hardly any other topic in palliative care provokes more discussion than the treatment of constipation. This could be in part due to it being such a common symptom, at 27% to 59%

in children at the end of life, that healthcare workers feel sufficiently knowledgeable about its treatment to have an opinion. Yet, constipation can be quite difficult to manage, resulting in a significant impact on the child and their family. This makes prevention of constipation of utmost importance in pediatric palliative care.

Normal stool frequency varies in children from three times per day to once every 3 days, and in the case of a breast-fed infant, up to once every 2 weeks. Common reasons for constipation in pediatric palliative care include dietary changes, a decrease in fluid and/or food intake, and a decrease in mobility and activity as colon peristalsis is, in part, stimulated by activity.

Chronic constipation is common in children with underlying neurologic impairments related to longstanding poor tone and immobility, while in children with cancer intra-abdominal tumors can cause direct compression of the gut or spinal cord compression.[10]

TREATMENT ALGORITHM

Step 1: Evaluation and assessment

Constipation commonly results in abdominal pain, bloating, flatulence, nausea and vomiting. The presence of sloppy, foul-smelling feces and soiling should be an alert to the presence of constipation with overflow incontinence.

As with the evaluation of any symptom, a thorough history is required and focused examination must be completed. Adolescents in particular may not volunteer important information about changes in bowel habit because of embarrassment, so it is important to tactfully check for specific changes.

Examination includes a rectal examination, using the small finger for small children, to evaluate whether the rectum contains stool and what consistency it is. There are a number of circumstances where this part of the examination may not be advisable, particularly when the child is neutropenic or thrombocytopenic. The exam can be helpful in ruling out local pain from anal fissures or hemorrhoids as a cause for constipation.

Attention needs to be paid to warning signs indicating neurologic compromise, such as: lower extremity motor weakness, paresthesisias, urinary retention, and fecal incontinence.

If the diagnosis is in question, then an abdominal radiograph or an ultrasound may be helpful in the assessment of stool content and to rule out an obstruction.

Step 2: Treatment of Underlying Causes

Underlying causes of constipation should be treated, if possible. In addition to the previously mentioned common reasons for constipation, consideration should be given to management of anorexia (see following text), weakness, decreased abdominal muscle tone, inconvenient toilet access, poor posture, and psychological factors such as depression. More specific pathologies to consider are hypothyroidism, hypokalemia, hypercalcemia, bowel obstruction (see later text), and adverse effects of medication.[53]

Step 3: Implement Integrative and Supportive Therapies

Whenever possible, integrative and supportive approaches need to be implemented to manage a child's constipation, and include:

- The establishment of a regular bowel routine should be supported: The strongest propulsive contractions occur postprandial, especially after breakfast. Access to a toilet or potty, with privacy for older children, daily at this time may be beneficial.
- Encourage the increase of activity, which may include the help of physical therapy or child life specialist, outside of a bed if possible.
- Increase fluid intake of the child's favorite drinks.
- Increase dietary fiber. Prune juice is often well liked.
- Consider abdominal massage in clockwise fashion.
- Carefully review medications and their constipating side effects, including opioids (see following text), tricyclic antidepressants, phenothiazines, diuretics, antihistamines and/or anticholinergics, and iron supplements. Self-hypnosis, biofeedback and cognitive-behavioral therapy may be effective in children with neurogenic bowel.

Step 4: Pharmacologic Management

A stool softener without a stimulant is mush without push.

A rational approach usually seems to include the scheduled administration of a stool softener and, if ineffective, the addition of a stimulant. However, with distressing constipation, especially when the rectal exam reveals hard stool in the ampulla in conjunction with abdominal pain, children may have to be unplugged first with the use of a rectal suppository or an enema. A manual evacuation would be usually reserved for adult-sized teenagers, if the former approaches fail.

Stool Softener

Stool softeners include liquid osmotic laxatives, such as lactulose, sorbitol, and polyethylene glycol, which draw water into the bowel by osmotic effect and surfactant laxatives including docusate sodium, which increase water penetration.

Outside the United States, the most commonly used stool softener in pediatrics appears to be the sugar lactulose, a combination of galactose and fructose (Enulose).[54,55] Lactulose does not affect the management of diabetes mellitus. In North America, polyethylene glycol (Miralax) is frequently used instead, and has also shown to be effective and safe.[54,56–58] Lactulose's advantage over polyethylene glycol is the much smaller volume, which is beneficial in the pediatric palliative care setting, where children often have trouble taking medication orally. All laxatives, including stool softeners, may cause abdominal pain and meteorism.

Stimulant laxatives

Children with a full rectum containing soft feces, or those for whom stool softeners were ineffective as a single approach, may be treated with a stimulant laxative such as senna[59] or bisacodyl, to stimulate bowel motility. These medications act by stimulation of the myenteric plexus. However, stimulants alone can be dangerous when there is obstruction or impaction.[53]

Contrary to conventional wisdom, that stool softeners should be administered with stimulants, one recent RCT ($n = 60$ adults) treating opioid-induced constipation, showed that sennosides alone were superior than sennosides plus docusate.[60]

Of note, the brand name Dulcolax in the United States refers to three medications: the stimulant bisacodyl and the stool softeners docusate sodium or polyethylene glycol, supporting the notion of avoiding brand names in medication.

Prokinetics

If gastrointestinal hypoactivity is a presumed pathophysiology, then prokinetics such as low-dose metoclopramide or low-dose erythromycin,[61] 5 mg/kg QID, may be considered.

Suppositories and Enemas

As mentioned previously, in cases of severe impaction a child may need to receive a rectal suppository or enema for relief. Some young people are acutely embarrassed and resistant to even the thought of using a suppository or enema. This may be a particular issue in early adolescence when bodily concerns, increased self-consciousness, and concerns about privacy are prominent. Careful explanation of the choices and reasons for use of enemas or suppositories is needed, along with negotiation about who the young person would feel most comfortable with to assist them. In cancer patients with neutropenia and/or thrombocytopenia, the rectal administration needs to be weighed against the risk of infection and/or bleeding. Glycerine suppositories promote defecation by softening and lubricating the mass as well as stimulating defecation. The Pain & Palliative Care team in Minneapolis has gathered good experience with the polyphenolic bisacodyl suppositories, which act principally by promoting colonic peristalsis.

Enemas may be required if the constipation is unresponsive to combined scheduled stool softeners and stimulant laxatives. Adult data shows that sodium phosphate/sodium biphosphate enemas, or saline rectal laxatives, and docusate sodium/glycerin mini-enemas, or surfactant rectal laxatives, are equal in efficacy.[62] However, the latter is usually preferred in pediatrics because of its much smaller enema volume of 2.5–5 mL compared with 130 mL.

If a manual evacuation is considered, adequate analgesia and sedation would be the expected standard of care.

Opioid-Induced Constipation The mantra in adult medicine "the hand who writes the opioids without writing for laxatives is the hand who disimpacts the patient's bowel" should serve at least as a warning in pediatrics. Unless diarrhea or other specific contraindication is present, laxatives should be prescribed routinely whenever more than one opioid dose per day is administered. The previous principles of a stool softener, possibly complemented with a stimulant and/or suppository, holds true as well.

Opioid-Antagonists The administration of opioid-antagonists has shown to be rather effective in the management of opioid-induced constipation in adults. Pediatric studies have not yet been published.

Naloxone The oral administration of naloxone anecdotally seems to have good effect in adult palliative care. Dose suggestions include 20% of oral morphine equivalent divided into one or several doses.[63] There is no published data about the intravenous administration of ultra-low-dose naloxone for constipation management, however the Minneapolis team has had several pediatric cases with very good results in their pediatric palliative care population with a dose of 0.25–1 mcg/kg/hr.

Alvimopan Alvimopan (Entereg) is a peripherally acting μ-opioid antagonist, with limited ability to cross the blood-brain barrier. One adult RCT showed good effect without evidence of opioid analgesia antagonism, with an adult dose of 0.5 mg BID PO.[64]

Methylnaltrexone Methylnaltrexone (Relistor) is a quaternary amine μ-opioid-receptor antagonist, and has restricted ability to cross the blood-brain barrier. An adult RCT showed good effect and treatment did not affect central analgesia or precipitate opioid withdrawal with an adult dose of 0.15 mg/kg every other day subcutaneously.[65] It is unclear, whether or not this medication may be administered intravenously. Pediatric trials, although undertaken, have not yet been published (Table 33-2).

Diarrhea

A significant number of children (21% to 40%) experience diarrhea during their end-of-life period. Fecal incontinence is often particularly humiliating for older children and adolescents who have been previously independent in their personal cares.

TREATMENT ALGORITHM

Step 1: Evaluation and Assessment

A child suffering from diarrhea in palliative care needs to be evaluated, which includes taking a careful history and performing

TABLE 33-2 Medications in the Treatment of Constipation

Class	Medication	Dose	Route of administration	Comments and side effects
Stool softener				
Liquid osmotic laxatives	Lactulose (Enulose) 15g/10 mL	Infants: 0.8-3.5 mL (not per kg) TID Children: 10-30 mL (not per kg) TID	PO	Dose titration to effect beyond these doses possible. Side effects: Bloating, diarrhea, nausea, abdominal pain
	Polyethylene glycol 3350 (Miralax)	8.5-17 g dissolved in 120-240 mL fluid (water, soda, juice) once per day	PO	Side effects: Diarrhea, nausea, abdominal pain
Surfactant laxatives	Docusate sodium (Colace)	>3 yrs: 10-40 mg/day divided in 1-4 doses 3-6 yrs: 20-60 mg/day divided in 1-4 doses 6-12 yrs: 40-120 mg/day divided in 1-4 doses >12 yrs: 50-200 mg/day divided in 1-4 doses	PO	Side effects: Diarrhea, nausea, abdominal pain
Stimulants				
	Senna	Standardized Senna Concentrate 1-5 yrs: 109-218 mg (not per kg) QHS 5-15 yrs: 218-436 mg (not per kg) QHS Sennoside 6 mo-2 yrs: 3.75 mg (not per kg) QHS 3-10 yrs: 7.5-15 mg (not per kg) QHS >10 yrs: 15-30 mg (not per kg) QHS	PO (also as tea), PR	Side effects: Nausea, abdominal pain, cramping
	Bisacodyl	6-11 yrs: 5 mg (not per kg) once daily >12 yrs: 5-15 mg (not per kg) once daily	PO, PR	Side effects: Nausea, abdominal pain, cramping

a clinical exam. Common causes of diarrhea include gastroenteritis, malabsorption, laxative overuse, overflow constipation, fecal impaction, adverse effects to medication such as antibiotics or chemotherapy, radiation therapy, or concurrent illness, such as colitis. Anal leakage may occur following surgical or pathological injury to the anal sphincter.[66]

Step 2: Treatment of Underlying Causes

Severe diarrhea resulting in dehydration may require oral rehydration with electrolyte/glucose solution. If possible and feasible in the individual child, underlying causes of diarrhea should be treated. Frequent treatable causes include:[67,68]

- Overflow incontinence caused by constipation or fecal impaction.
- Anxiety.
- Enteral feeding and/or feeding intolerance.
- Laxative overuse.
- Radiation-induced gastrointestinal damage.
- Irritable bowel syndrome.
- Inflammatory bowel disease, such as ulcerative colitis or Crohn's disease.
- Malabsorption and steatorrhea from decreased pancreatic function Bacterial infections: Antibiotic therapy, usual after stool sensitivity testing, is rarely indicated. Exceptions include presence of *Shigella*, *Salmonella typhi/paratyphi,* or *Clostridium difficile toxine*, the latter usually preceded be antibiotic administration. In severe clinical causes antibiotic treatment would be indicated with infections by *camphylobacter*, enteropathogen *E. coli* or *Yersinia*. In patients with AIDS, *Mycobacterium avium-intracellulare* may be causative in diarrhea.
- Viral infections: Pathogens include adenovirus, cytomegalovirus (CMV), ECHO-Virus, human immunodeficiency virus (HIV), Norwalk virus, and rotavirus. A specific therapy is available only for CMV, and rotavirus vaccination is effective.[69]
- Enteric protozoal infections, prevalent in immunocompromised patients, such as those with AIDS: Possible pathogens include *Cryptosporidium*, *Giardia lamblia*, and *Microsporidium.*
- Carcinoid syndrome.
- Vasoactive intestinal peptide tumor (VIPoma).
- Rule out celiac disease, cystic fibrosis, and lactate intolerance.

Step 3: Implement Integrative and Supportive Therapies

Integrative and supportive therapies in the management of diarrhea in pediatric palliative care may include:[67]

- Encourage oral rehydration with glucose/electrolyte solution, if possible.
- Consider decrease of milk intake: Bacterial gastroenteritis may result in transient lactase deficiency.
- Consider decrease of enteral intake, either solid dietary intake including bran and fruit or reduction of rate and/or osmolarity of nutrition formula.
- Prevention of skin breakdown with frequent skin care of perianal area, including application of barrier creams or zinc oxide paste.
- Assistance with toileting and washing and the use of continence aids, which need to be sensitively handled. Young people may worry especially about the possibility of

incontinence while in the presence of friends and peers, and this may lead to them avoiding contact. Adopting an active problem solving approach may help to examine all possible ways of handling potentially embarrassing situations, including use of disposable pads and/or continence pants, timing of visits, and enlisting a close friend or family member as support.

Step 4: Pharmacologic Management

RCT in the management of diarrhea in pediatric palliative care do not exist, however some studies include children with life-limiting conditions.

Loperamide Loperamide is a potent μ-receptor opioid agonist and, although well absorbed from the gastrointestinal tract, it is almost completely metabolized by the liver and excreted via the bile. Loperamide does not cross the blood-brain barrier. As a result this agent acts via a local effect in the GI tract. However, it may take 16 to 24 hours for loperamide to show maximum effect in diarrhea treatment.[70] As with morphine and other opioids, loperamide decreases propulsive activity, but unlike other opioids also has an antisecretory effect.[71] If toxic substances are the pathophysiologic basis of diarrhea and need to be excreted, then the use of loperamide is not recommended.

Although three pediatric trials ($n = 95$) did not show a significant lorapamide effect,[72–74] four other trials were able to demonstrate a decrease in stool frequency and duration of diarrhea.[75–78] A case series of 15 children with chronic diarrhea following resection of advanced abdominal neuroblastoma, possibly resulting from disruption of the autonomic nerve supply to the gut during clearance of tumor from the major vessels of the retroperitoneum, demonstrated that loperamide reduces but did not abolish symptoms.[79]

Adverse effects, such as constipation or bloating, were uncommon in these trials and case reports. However children, especially infants, occasionally demonstrated central nervous side effects such as opioid over-sedation. Of note, inhibitors of P-glycoprotein such as ketoconazole, omeprazole, quinidine, and verapamil allow loperamide to cross the blood-brain barrier and as a result manifest central opioid effects.[80] An overdose of loperamide in 216 cases has not resulted in life-threatening adverse effects or deaths with doses up to 0.94mg/kg.[81]

Bismuth subsalicylate The mechanism of bismuth subsalicylate (Pepto-Bismol) is not well understood. A decrease in length of acute diarrhea symptoms could be shown in children with acute[82,83] and chronic[70,84] diarrhea. To prevent Reye's syndrome, this medication and other salicylates should not be administered in children with viral infections.[85] The administration of bismuth subsalicylate may result in black stools.

Colestyramine Colestyramine (Questran) is a bile acid sequestrant, which binds bile in the gastrointestinal tract to prevent its reabsorption. Cholestyramine is primarily administered in the management of hypercholesterolemia, but also in the treatment of pruritus induced by liver failure and chronic diarrhea. Three pediatric trials[74,86,87] ($n = 78$) resulted in a reduction in the duration of diarrhea. Case reports in the successful management of chronic pediatric diarrhea have been published.[88–91] One study (n = 39 infants and children) showed treatments with cholestyramine and bismuth sub-salicylate were equally effective in decreasing stool frequency in patients with green diarrhea, such as following partial illeocolectomy or *Candida albicans* overgrowth, however children with brown stools had an insignificant response to therapy.[70] Because cholestyramine is not absorbed systemically, there are no severe systemic side effects. Possible adverse effects, such as abdominal pain, flatulence, and constipation, were not reported in the pediatric literature.

Octreotride In the management of secretory diarrhea, including carcinoid-associated, vasoactive intestinal peptide (VIP) tumors, or AIDS, the administration of the somatostatin analogue octreotride may represent a successful approach. The secretory effect of several gastrointestinal active hormones. such as gastrin, colecystokinine, secretine, VIP, and motiline/ may be inhibited. Four case reports (*n* = 6 children) showed a successful approach in the treatment of chronic diarrhea caused by intestinal graft vs. host disease, cryptosporidium enteritis, and status post ileum resection.[92–95] See Bowel Obstruction later in this chapter (Table 33-3).

Anorexia and Cachexia

At its simplest, anorexia is a loss of appetite, while the definition of cachexia has been disputed until recently. In 2008 a consensus definition for cachexia emerged as "a complex metabolic syndrome associated with underlying illness and characterized by loss of muscle with or without loss of fat mass."[96] Anorexia and cachexia are two interrelated symptoms that are often acknowledged together as the anorexia-cachexia syndrome.

The symptoms of anorexia and cachexia, assuming weight loss is a marker of cachexia, appear to be highly prevalent in children with life-limiting conditions of both malignant[3,6,97] and non-malignant origin.[3] In a study[97] of 164 children and young people who died of progressive malignant disease, 48% had anorexia and 41% had weight loss on entering the study and these symptoms increased to just more than 67% in the last month of life, indicating anorexia and weight loss were not responsive to any treatments used. They were significantly more evident in children with CNS tumors when compared with leukemia and/or lymphoma or solid tumors. Similarly, a study[6] reported a high prevalence of anorexia in

children dying from cancer. However, this did not seem to result in a high level of suffering, but neither was it successfully treated.

A lower prevalence in the last week and day of life for anorexia, 33% and 24%, respectively, and weight loss, 20% and 21%, respectively, was found in 30 children dying in the hospital environment; 12 children had non-malignant conditions.[6] They were not believed to cause undue distress to the child, but in more than half the children with the symptom were of moderate to severe intensity.

Anorexia-cachexia syndrome characterized by anorexia, involuntary weight loss, tissue wasting, weakness and poor physical function is a condition of advanced protein calorie malnutrition that inevitably leads to death[98] if the underlying condition cannot be treated. In contrast to adults, children may manifest this problem as growth failure rather than weight loss.

For many parents the sight of their child visibly losing weight may intensify feelings of impotence and failure as parents, and lead to misunderstanding and blame within the extended family.

> *The mother of a teenage girl who had severe lung and liver disease as a result of cystic fibrosis became tearful and distressed by the sight of her daughter's "stick-like legs." After years of intense focus on weight gain and enhanced calorie intake in the management of the cystic fibrosis, the mother believed that she was failing as a mother and allowing her daughter to "starve to death."*

PATHOGENESIS

The process of anorexia-cachexia syndrome is complex, but what is clear is anorexia, alone, is inadequate for the syndrome to develop. In normal circumstances the reduced caloric intake from anorexia results in a loss of fat stores, which stimulates an adaptive response to maintain the fat stores. This response is driven by declining levels of leptin, a hormone secreted by adipose tissue. The consequence of low levels of leptin in the brain is for the hypothalamus to increase orexigenic signals such as neuropeptide-Y (NPY) to stimulate appetite and repress energy expenditure and decrease anorexigenic signals, corticotrophin-releasing factor and melanocortin, to achieve the same effect.[98]

TABLE 33-3 Medications for the Treatment of Diarrhea

Medication	Dose	Route of administration	Comments and side effects
Loperamid (Imodium)	0.03-0.27 mg/kg TID	PO	Bloating, constipation; occasionally, central nervous side effects (especially in infants); inhibitors of P-glycoprotein (such as ketoconazole, omeprazole, quinidine, verapamil) allow loperamide to cross the blood-brain barrier and as a result manifest central opioid effects
Bismut subsalicylate (Pepto-Bismol)	15-25 mg/kg 5-6 times/day	PO	Limited pediatric data, caution: Reye's syndrome; stool colored black
Colestyramine (Questran)	0-6 years: 1-2 g BID (-QID) >6 years: 2-4 g BID (-QID)	PO	Few documented adverse effects; dose NOT per kg
Octreotid (Sandostatin)	Starting dose: 1-2 mg/kg BID-TID, titration to effect to >10 mg/kg/dose	IV, SC	Limited pediatric evidence; side effects: nausea, worsening of pre-existing arterial hypertonus; cholelithiasis, gallbladder hypercontractility

There is increasing evidence that the cachectic process is established by an acute phase response mediated by several cytokines of which tumor necrosis factor-α, interleukin-1, interleukin-6 and interferon-γ have been implicated. The evidence to date would suggest these cytokines stimulate the expression and release of leptin and/or mimic the hypothalamic negative feedback signaling from leptin and, in so doing, prevent the normal compensatory mechanisms in the face of reduced food intake and decreasing weight.

This abnormal response has been suggested in a study[99] that reported on the possible role of leptin and NPY levels as prognostic indicators in children with cancer. The study revealed a mean NPY level of 82.32 pmol/L and mean leptin level of 6.60 ng/mL at diagnosis in children who achieved complete remission, vs. a mean NPY and leptin level of 430.16 pmol/L and 0.192 ng/mL, respectively in those children who died with disease during the follow-up period. Furthermore, the mean NPY level declined and mean leptin level increased during the course of chemotherapy in the 23 children studied.

Other factors indicated in this syndrome include hypermetabolism or an elevation in resting energy expenditure and changes in carbohydrate, protein, and fat metabolism.

EVALUATION AND ASSESSMENT

There are no specific diagnostic criteria for this syndrome, but this is not required as knowledge of the disease process, clinical history and focused physical examination makes for an uncomplicated clinical diagnosis. This basic evaluation can be augmented with measures such as body weight, skin fold thickness, and body composition. These are often not necessary in the clinical setting, especially when one keeps in mind the lack of tolerance sick, debilitated children have to even the simplest procedure and that they are likely to receive the majority of their care at home.

Body weight can be useful in establishing a broad measure of the rate of deterioration either by detecting a frank weight loss or failure to grow over time. If, for example, there was a rapid decline in weight, then changes in fluid balance are much more likely to be the cause and it may be reasonable, depending on the overall situation, to intervene and correct the problem.

Laboratory tests evaluating nutritional depletion are of limited value[100] and because they often cause a great deal of apprehension in children and young people cannot be recommended as routine. Albumin is the most common to measure because of its low cost and accuracy when liver and renal disease is absent.[101] However, judicious testing for potentially reversible causes such as hypercalcemia are warranted.

TREATABLE CAUSES

The presence of anorexia-cachexia syndrome in the palliative setting would suggest an unavoidable deterioration to death. However, the presence of anorexia and cachexia together or alone can represent a number of readily correctable causes that should be kept in mind during assessment. Consideration needs to be given to:
- Adverse effects of medication including cancer-related therapies,
- Dehydration,
- Mouth problems, such as oral thrush, xerostomia,
- Gastrointestinal dysfunction, such as dysphagia, gastroesophageal reflux (GER), constipation, intestinal obstruction,
- Infection, either local or systemic,
- Nausea and vomiting,
- Pain,
- Psychological factors, such as anxiety, fear, depression.

INTEGRATIVE AND SUPPORTIVE THERAPIES

Management of anorexia-cachexia syndrome includes, preferably pre-emptive, acknowledgment that this is not unexpected. The provision of information and education to the child and his or her family is extremely important and should not be underestimated. Allowing for anticipatory exploration of emotional and spiritual subjects offers a forum to air out and deal with the commonly held beliefs that may be destructive to the therapeutic relationship if left unaddressed.

Beliefs include feeling it is necessary to feed the child in the face of reduced food intake. These feelings are very powerful and innate while others, such as their child receiving inadequate care when the wasting process relentlessly progresses, can be borne of feelings of frustration and helplessness.

The profit from such deliberations may be the ability to arrange, in advance, strategies to help empower the child and family and by this means improve appetite and food intake. This will not necessarily improve survival, but has the opportunity to enhance the quality of life and feelings of comfort for the child and their family. Strategies that may increase food intake are:

- Offering the child favorite foods and nutritional supplements he or she enjoys,
- Eliminating dietary restrictions,
- Reducing portion sizes and increasing the number of meals,
- Making food look more enticing,
- Avoiding disliked food odors.

This approach can be supported by sufficient evidence[102] that hypercaloric feeding does not increase lean tissue mass and there is no significant improvement in survival. Hypercaloric feeding particularly does not increase skeletal muscle mass, the loss of which is a defining[96] event in cachexia.

There has been significant interest in the influence that more specific nutritional factors can have on cachexia with much of the focus on omega-3 fatty acids such as eicosapentaenoic acid (EPA). There has been a general trend in favor of EPA use from studies with a 2009 prospective, randomized; open-label study[103] finding a decrease of cancer-induced weight loss in 33 children with cancer. The patients were fed a protein- and energy-dense nutrition supplement containing EPA when compared with 19 children who did not receive the supplements. However, a 2007 Cochrane review[104] had concluded there was insufficient data to establish whether EPA was better than placebo in adults. This finding has been further supported by the publication of preliminary results of a randomized phase III clinical trial[105] of 475 adult patients with cancer-related anorexia-cachexia syndrome who received one of five treatment arms (95 patients per arm) including pharmaco-nutritional support containing EPA. This arm of the study was withdrawn after analysis of 125 patients (25 each arm) indicated a worsening of lean body mass, resting energy expenditure, and fatigue compared with the other groups.

Psychological approaches should be seen as an extension of the exploration of emotional and spiritual issues and could include:[100]

- Encouraging child and family interaction to reduce psychological distress,
- Supporting the family to distinguish between things they can and cannot control, such as normal disease progression vs. helping their child find comfort,
- Exploring the emotional components and the meaning of their child not eating and losing weight,
- Assessing the impact of symptoms on the child and his or her family,
- Assessing the quality of life of the child and his or her family.

PHARMACOLOGY

Pharmacologic management of anorexia-cachexia syndrome is adjunctive to the integrative and supportive measures highlighted previously. This statement is supported by the finding that both anorexia and weight loss occur in high frequency and respond poorly to treatment in children and/or young people with progressive malignant disease.[97] This suggests that available pharmacologic agents are not successful in alleviating these symptoms and this is further reflected in the large number of existing and experimental agents reported to be helpful (Tables 33-3 and 33-4). The data supporting the majority of medications are limited in adults and nonexistent in children. Arguably, the most studied medications are those of the progestational group of which Megestrol acetate has received the most scrutiny. This has culminated in a Cochrane review in 2005[106] and an update in 2007. Megestrol acetate was demonstrated to improve appetite and weight gain in adult patients with cancer although this is largely due to fat rather than muscle mass, the tissue lost in cachexia. No overall conclusion could be drawn on quality of

life because of statistical and clinical heterogeneity. Similarly, patient numbers and methodological shortcomings allowed no recommendations to be made about megestrol acetate use in patients with AIDS or other underlying pathologies.

Megestrol acetate has been trialed in a small number of children with cachexia, not necessarily at a time of palliation, due to cancer,[107–109] cystic fibrosis,[110,111] and HIV disease[112] and reported to improve nutritional status by increasing appetite and weight. Adverse effects were significant, with most children studied reported to have adrenal suppression, with one child manifesting clinical hypoadrenalism with hemodynamic collapse requiring ionotropic support.[108] This effect was shown to be transient[109] as a normal adrenocorticotropic hormone (ACTH) stimulation test was returned once megestrol acetate was discontinued. However, replacement glucocorticoid therapy was advised during times of severe stress.

Cyproheptadine hydrochloride has been used in children with cancer and/or cancer treatment-related cachexia and shown[113] to improve average weight gain by 2.6 kg and significantly enhance mean weight-for-age z-scores in 50 of 66 children. The main side effect was drowsiness. Seven of the nonresponding children then received megestrol acetate with five demonstrating an average weight gain of 2.5 kg with one child developing low cortisol levels and hyperlipidemia.

A preliminary report[114] on the use of recombinant human growth hormone in four HIV infected children with failure to thrive suggested mean fat-free mass and weight gain were increased with no deleterious effect on disease control.

SUMMARY

Anorexia and cachexia are common symptoms that increase near the end of life. Both symptoms and the anorexia-cachexia syndrome respond poorly to treatment, although there is some evidence for improved appetite and weight with the progestational agent, megestrol acetate. However, this comes at the expense of potentially significant adrenal suppression and no data to support improvement in quality of life.

In view of this, management should embrace an integration of information, education and psychological support to the child and his or her family with medication being considered but not being unduly favored.

Distressing Symptoms of Mouth and Throat

MOUTH CARE

The care of a child's mouth during palliative care is an essential element of his or her overall care and one in which an informed child and family can take a lead role. This can be associated with an improved quality of life, create a sense of control and prevents mouth care from being overlooked. This aspect of palliative care for children has been well documented[115] with respect to children with cancer, with many of the recommendations applicable to children with life-limiting illnesses of non-malignant origin.

Evaluation and Assessment

The majority of problems will be readily diagnosed with nothing more than a good history and a look inside the mouth. A number of oral assessment tools have been reviewed[115] with

TABLE 33-4 Existing and Experimental Pharmacologic Agents for Anorexia and Cachexia

Pharmacologic agents		Pharmacologic agents	
Anabolic agents	Testosterone and analogues Growth hormone	Cytokines	IL-10 IL-12
Anti-cytokine agents	Antibodies Antisense therapy Pentoxifylline Thalidomide	Hormones	Insulin Melatonin Erythropoetin
Anti-depressants	Mirtazepine	Metabolic inhibitor	Hydrazine
Anti-inflammatory agents	Ibuprofen Indomethacin	Porcine extract	
Anti-psychotic agents	Olanzepine	Prokinetic agents	Metoclopramide Cisapride
Appetite stimulants	Progestational agents Corticosteroids Cannabinoids	Serotonin antagonists	Cyproheptadine Ondansetron
Beta-adrenergic agonists	Clenbuterol	Suramin	

only one tool, Eiler's Oral Assessment Guide,[116] being identified as user-friendly and appropriate for everyday clinical use in children and adults. This guide covers the assessment of voice, ability to swallow, lips, tongue, saliva, mucous membrane, gingival, and teeth and/or dentures.

Treatable Conditions

There are a number of potential conditions and/or symptoms that may require management, including:

- Poor oral hygiene, including halitosis
- Oral candidiasis, or thrush
- Mouth ulceration, including mucositis
- Xerostomia, or dry mouth
  - Mouth breathing
  - Air and/or oxygen with and without humidification
  - Drugs
  - Dehydration
  - Local infection
  - Disease-related, such as graft vs. host disease
  - Treatment-related, such as from surgery or radiotherapy
- Bleeding gums
  - Hematological cancers
  - Liver disease or dysfunction
  - Clotting disorders

Integrative and Supportive Therapies

The mainstay of preventing the development of mouth problems is maintaining the twice-daily routine of careful and gentle cleaning of the teeth and gums with a fluoride toothpaste.[115] This should also apply to cooperative severely disabled children. Mouth-care sponges dipped in mouthwash can be applied to the gums and teeth in the unconscious or less-cooperative child. This has the added advantage of keeping the mouth moist. Cream or soft white paraffin can be applied to the lips to prevent dryness and cracking.

Where children have much longer palliative needs, regular dental review and oral assessment by a dentist or dental unit with specific training should be a standard part of their pediatric care. There are no recommended preventative therapies in the palliative care setting for the highlighted conditions.

Pharmacology

Pharmacological management is detailed in Table 33-5. Management of xerostomia is dealt with in Table 33-6.

TABLE 33-5 Pharmacologic Measures for Common Mouth Problems

Condition	Pharmacologic management
Candidiasis	Use absorbed or partially absorbed anti-fungal agent such as fluconazole for visible thrush[117,118]
Ulceration	For aphthous ulcers, use local orobase agents For traumatic ulcers, consider dental review if recurrent If severe mucositis, use appropriate pain control There is only weak, unreliable evidence for specific therapies to improve or eradicate cancer-related mucositis[119]
Bleeding gums[120]	Use tranexamic acid mouthwashes Use hemostatic agents, including Gelfoam and Gelfilm Platelet transfusions may be required, depending on stage of palliation

TABLE 33-6 Management of Non-Specific Xerostomia

Supportive measures	Pharmacologic measures
Regular oral hygiene	KY Jelly can be very effective and well tolerated[120]
Avoid oral drying agents	Artificial saliva
Food and fluids with high sugar content	*Pilocarpine[121]
Rinses with an alcohol content	
Offer crushed ice, unsweetened pineapple chunks/juice, and sugarless chewing gum	
Use a moisturizing lip balm regularly	

*Pilocarpine use in children is limited to a case study of one child receiving this drug to prevent xerostomia.

XEROSTOMIA

Xerostomia, or dry mouth, has a reported prevalence[3] of about 40% during the last week of life and causes quite a bit to very much distress at a similar level as pain. It results from a reduction in saliva secretion, particularly the serous component. This can lead to difficulties with eating and speaking and contribute to anorexia, changes in taste, and increase the risk of oral infections.

Evaluation requires a thorough review of the possible causes (see previous) with a review of medication essential. The list of medications implicated with xerostomia is large, but anticholinergics, tricyclic antidepressants, antipsychotics, anticonvulsants, antihistamines, and diuretics are more commonly involved. Alternative therapies should be asked about.

Identified specific causes should be managed as is appropriate for the stage of the child's palliation. For instance, depending on the level of distress caused, connected medications may be reduced in dose or changed. In the case of dehydration, the underlying reason could be corrected and the oral fluid intake of the child increased, if appropriate. Equally, the use of subcutaneous and intravenous fluid administration could be considered a legitimate intervention.

THROAT PROBLEMS

Dysfunction of the throat, esophagus, and upper stomach in the form of dysphagia and gastroesophageal disease (GERD) are not uncommon in the palliative care of children, with the most affected group being those with neurological impairment. This group has been reported[122] to have an aspiration prevalence of 68% to 70% and a silent aspiration rate of 94%.[123] They generally enter services with these conditions identified and managed but these symptoms can develop or, in the case of GERD, be unrecognized.[120]

Troublesome hiccups are a less common problem but can be a source of considerable challenge.

Dysphagia

Swallowing is a complex process in which a bolus of food or fluid is prepared in the mouth and propelled to the stomach without entering the trachea, which would cause aspiration. This requires the coordination of oral musculature for the preparatory and transport phase, pharyngeal musculature, and esophageal musculature. Swallowing difficulties or dysphagia results when there is interference to the nerves involved in the process or there is damage along the pathway.

The prevalence of dysphagia has been reported[3,97] to be a significant problem in 23% to 30% of dying children during the last month of life, and in the palliative cancer population the prevalence increases with time.[97]

Dysphagia can be the result of disease process, previous treatment, or symptoms associated with progressive disease. Treatment-related swallowing difficulties can result from surgery, radiotherapy, chemotherapy, and other drugs. Diseases progression results in dysphagia through:

- Damage to brain and/or nervous system from cerebral palsy, neurodegenerative disorders, metabolic disorders, brain tumors or congenital and genetic disorders,
- Structural problems of the swallowing pathway that are secondary to obstruction, infiltration or compression from solid tumors of the head and neck,
- Muscular damage such as that from muscular dystrophy.

Evaluation and Assessment Evaluation of dysphagia and other throat symptoms to be discussed requires a holistic approach that goes beyond observation of feeding[123] and, in children at the end of life, may not require action once the wishes of the child and/or his or her family are considered.

The diagnosis can be made clinically and improves with experience.[122] However, comparison of a therapist's judgment to a videofluoroscopic swallowing study (VFSS) only indicated a sensitivity of 80%, specificity of 42% and positive and negative predictive values of 65% and 60%, respectively, for clinical evaluation to detect penetration of liquids. Disturbingly, the sensitivity, 70%, specificity, 55%, and positive, 41%, and negative, 80%, predictive values were inferior when detection of penetration of solids by clinical evaluation were analyzed.

Suggestive Symptoms

Symptoms associated with eating and/or drinking that may herald the presence of dysphagia include:

- Infants with poor coordination of their suck and swallow
- Back arching
- Children taking a long time to eat
- Difficulty in chewing food
- Trying to swallow a single mouthful of food several times
- Gagging
- Food or liquids coming out of the nose during or after feeding
- The presence of drooling, vomiting, and/or coughing
- Frequent sneezing after feeding
- Inability to coordinate breathing
- A feeling that food or liquids are sticking in the throat or esophagus, or that there is a lump in these areas
- Discomfort in the throat or chest
- Chest congestion
- Wet or raspy sounding voice during or after feeding
- Tiredness or shortness of breath during feeding
- Color change during feeding, such as becoming blue or pale
- Change in voice before or after eating
- Recurrent pneumonia
- Weight loss

A retrospective analysis[124] of various signs and symptoms of aspiration and dysphagia revealed wet voice, OR 8.9, wet breathing, OR 3.35, and cough, OR 3.3, to be good clinical markers for children aspirating on thin fluid, but not on purée. Age and neurological status influenced the significance of these clinical markers. The significant predictive qualities of cough for fluid aspiration and penetration had previously been determined.[122] This same study also indicated the aspiration risk factor increased when other features such as voice changes, color changes, and/or delayed swallow were also present.

Further evaluation should be considered necessary only if the investigation is likely to change the diagnosis or management for the child. Investigations to be considered are:

- Videofluoroscopic swallowing studies
- Barium swallow/upper GI series
- Endoscopy
- Esophageal manometry
- Laryngoscopy

The appropriateness of these assessments depends on what course of action is being contemplated and must be individualized to the child and his or her situation. Debatably, if a single study were used to determine the presence of dysphagia and aspiration, then VFSS, where the child's swallow is examined by a series of x-rays after they take a small amount of liquid and/or solid containing barium, would be that study.

Treatable Conditions

Dysphagia in children under palliative care, by definition, suggests a disease process that is not curative and unlikely to be treatable. The exception would be where a palliative procedure was able to reverse a process to improve quality of life, such as radiotherapy to a tumor mass or widening a stricture under anesthetic. Likewise, treatment-related dysphagia is liable to be irreversible unless the cause was an adverse drug effect that could be resolved by discontinuing the medication.

More potential exists for dysphagia caused by symptoms associated with disease progression, such as:

- Xerostomia
- Infection of the mouth, throat, or esophagus
- GERD
- Pain
- Psychological factors including anxiety, fear, and depression

Integrative and Supportive Therapies The extent to which dysphagia is managed is dependent on the stage of the child's palliation and the goals of the child and/or the family. A speech therapist's involvement is advisable from the time of evaluation through to the child's management. They are able to provide specific exercises to improve coordination and muscle strength or suggest individualized strategies to compensate for impaired swallowing function and enhance the ease and safety of oral intake[125] (Table 33-7).

However, there will be situations where it will be appropriate for children to have nutrition administered through an enteral feeding device such as a nasogastric (NG) tube or gastrostomy (GT).

Feeding Devices

A 2006 clinical report[126] on the nutrition support for neurologically impaired children recommended, among other things, that enteral tube feedings be initiated early in children who are unable to feed orally or who cannot achieve sufficient oral

TABLE 33-7 Strategies for Impaired Swallowing

General strategies	During feeding
Postural changes	Taking smaller mouthfuls
Changes in rate of food presentation	Chewing on the stronger side
Use of modified feeding tools	Double-swallowing
Modifications to amount and texture of food-softer consistencies, thickened fluids	Suctioning, when necessary

intake to maintain adequate nutritional or hydration status. It also recognized that parental concerns and family issues have a role in the decision to provide aggressive nutritional support. The latter reflection, questionably, becomes even more valid when considering an interventional approach in the palliative care setting.

Both NG and GT are common pieces of equipment used to feed and/or administer medication in medically fragile children when there are undue risks with oral intake. However, NG or nasojejunal (NJ) tube feedings should be reserved for short-term nutritional intervention and GT or gastrojejunostomy (GJ) tube feedings may be used when long-term nutritional rehabilitation is required.[126]

NG requires the placement of, usually, a silicone-based tube, down the nasopharyngeal airway into the stomach and in the case of NJ tubes into the jejunum. Success of placement can be measured by the drawing back of acidic stomach contents in the case of NG insertion or, as with NJ tubes, radiological visualization. Removal is a reversal of the process.

GT requires a surgical procedure where an opening through the abdomen into the stomach is made through which a feeding device is inserted. This bypasses the mouth and throat of the child and allows for feeds directly into the stomach. There are a variety of devices on the market, with three main types: percutaneous endoscopic gastrostomy (PEG), Malecot tube, and a tube or button balloon device.

The pros and cons for each device are relative to the situation and include the child's medical condition, age, previous and future operations, and preference of the surgeon. The Malecot device is typically considered temporary, being replaced by a balloon device after 1 to 2 months, and removal does not require surgery. Removal of a balloon device requires only deflation of the balloon, but a PEG removal requires endoscopic extraction. Care of all feeding devices is important and has been well detailed in a 2003 best practice guideline from Scotland.[127]

In a study[128] on the effects of tube feeding on 26 children, with 13 NG, 10 NG changing to GT, and 3 GT, for a mean of 23 months indicated a significant improvement from 73% to 94% in mean percent ideal body weight for height-age for the whole group. Seventeen parents perceived an enhanced mood in their child and they spent less time in caring for their child after NG or GT feedings began. No hospitalizations due to tube-feeding complications were reported.

A 2004 Cochrane review[129] that highlighted the considerable uncertainty about the effects of gastrostomy for children with cerebral palsy remains because of the lack of well designed and conducted randomized controlled trials. Despite the lack of these trials an improvement in body weight was confirmed in a review[130] of the benefits and risks for GT or GJ feeding in comparison to oral feeding for children with cerebral palsy. On the downside, there was an approximately fourfold increase in risk of death reported in one cohort of GT-fed children and many complications were reported, including potential for increased gastroesophageal reflux and fluid aspiration into the lungs. In 2006,[131] published evidence refuted an increased respiratory risk to children with cerebral palsy following GT insertion.

Similarly, a prospective cohort study[132] of 57 caregivers of Caucasian children with cerebral palsy detailed a significant, measurable (short-form 36 version II) quality of life at 6 months and 12 months after GT insertion. Improvements were noted in social functioning, mental health, energy and/or vitality, and general health perception. When compared to baseline data and values at 12 months, results were not significantly different from the normal reference data. The value of gastrostomy placement has conceivably been enhanced further by a prospective controlled study of children[133] that found significant clinical benefit at no significant extra cost. The cost of food did increase post surgery from $65 to $78 per week with the mean net cost difference being $41 per week per child inclusive of food and surgery. Community service costs were significantly lower post surgery and few parents reported personal costs at either time point, although many had reduced or stopped paid work to care for the child.

Unfortunately, enhancements in the quality of life of neurological impaired children through use of feeding devices have not been so evident. A recent prospective report[134] of 50 neurologically impaired children receiving either GT or GJ feeding noted the mean weight-for-age z-score and ease of medication administration increased significantly over time but there was no improvement in either their quality of life or health related quality of life over a 12-month period. Also, the eight children with a progressive neurological disorder had a significantly lower quality of life over time. Nonetheless, caregivers were of the opinion that GT and GJ tube feeding had a positive impact on their child's health at 6 months (86%), and 12 months (84%).

Gastroesophageal Reflux Disease (GERD)

In GERD, food or liquid travels backward from the stomach to the esophagus, resulting in symptoms from irritation of the esophagus. It is a common diagnosis in neurologically impaired children and infants, ranging from 15% to 75% of children,[120] and children with cystic fibrosis and children nearing the end of life, especially when cachexia, general debility and restriction to the supine position are evident.

Suggestive Symptoms[120] The clinician should have a high index of suspicion for the possibility of GERD, particularly in the previously mentioned group of children. A thoughtful history and focused examination can go a long way toward determining the diagnosis with suggestive symptoms being:

- Gastrointestinal
  - Food refusal vomiting, especially during or after feedings or when supine
  - Dysphagia
  - Weight loss or failure to thrive
  - Hematemesis or melena secondary to esophagitis
- Respiratory
  - Excessive secretions
  - Aspiration pneumonia

- Recurrent respiratory tract infections
- Bronchitis
- Cough
- Wheeze
- Choking and/or gagging
- Other symptoms, often having a temporal relationship to feeding
  - Irritability, more so when supine
  - Pain
  - Hyperextended posturing
  - Sandifer's syndrome: neck extension and head rotation during or after meals in infant or young child often associated with iron deficiency anemia and severe esophagitis

As with other issues in pediatric palliative care, further investigation warrants careful consideration of the risks and benefits of the procedure on the child's management, and these deliberations will have a different outcome depending on where the child is in their palliative journey. It would not be too controversial to suggest that investigations for GERD could be relegated to a time when a trial of therapy had failed or when symptoms were out of keeping with the expected progression of the child's condition. The common investigations to be considered are:

- 24-hour esophageal pH study

  This study measures the pH in the esophagus over a 24-hour period thereby providing a direct measurement of how much acid from the stomach reaches the esophagus while symptoms are recorded on a time chart. The data can then be analyzed to determine reflux frequency and any relationship with symptoms over time. However, the study can fail to diagnose GERD or associated problems.

- Barium swallow

  This study overlaps with the analysis of dysphagia and gives a more direct assessment of the anatomy and, to a degree, the function of the upper GI tract. Reflux can be visualized but this, while suggestive, is not sufficient to provide a diagnosis of GERD as there is no information about frequency and relationship to symptoms.

- Upper GI endoscopy

  Direct visualization of the upper GI tract allows for the visualization of the upper GI tract and the diagnosis of inflammation, bleeding and altered anatomy. A study can be conducted in situations where there is concern about the presence of esophagitis and/or gastritis, other symptoms such as pain, dysphagia and/or persistent vomiting, or an unexpected development in the case of a child with cancer.

Integrative and Supportive Therapies The presence of GERD in children and infants regularly leads to a number of lifestyle and nutritional change recommendations (Table 33-8). These have, most commonly, been considered in the context of relatively healthy children or infants with mild symptoms. They are unlikely to be successful as the sole modality of management for children with life-threatening conditions and/or moderate to severe symptoms.

There have been a limited number of studies even in the healthy pediatric population and two Cochrane reviews[135,136] could find no evidence to support or refute the efficacy of

TABLE 33-8 Common Recommendations to Reduce GERD

Recommended lifestyle and nutritional changes	
Adjust posture • Elevate the head of the bed/cot by using blocks of wood under the legs of the bed or a foam wedge under the mattress • Avoid lying down after eating or lie left side down	Uses gravity to prevent reflux by having the head and shoulders higher than the stomach Extra pillows are not helpful, can worsen reflux • Children/infants can slip off • Can cause a bend in the body increasing pressure on the stomach
Minimize exposure to tobacco smoke • Including second hand smoke	Smoke promotes GERD by: • Reducing saliva (acid neutralizing qualities) in the mouth and throat • Lowering the pressure in the lower esophageal sphincter • Provoking cough
Avoid reflux inducing foods • Caffeine, chocolate, alcohol, peppermint and acidic beverages including cola and orange juice	These foods can cause relaxation of the lower esophageal sphincter
Alter feeds and feeding regimen • Thicken feeds • Check for overfeeding • Decrease feed/meal frequency and volume of feed/meal • Allow for longer time before going to bed	In NG/GT feeding • Consider overnight/continuous feeds • Give more slowly, even to point of allowing gravity feed

feed thickeners in newborn infants with GERD. However, between the ages of 1 month and 2 years this strategy was deemed helpful in reducing GERD symptoms,[135] but elevation of the head of the cot was not supported as a helpful strategy.

The adult literature has been reviewed in 2006[137] with the evidence for the effect lifestyle measures had on GERD in adults pointed toward an improvement in the overall time esophageal pH was less than 4.0 through bed head elevation and left lateral decubitus position, while weight loss improved pH profiles and symptoms. Furthermore, there was physiologic evidence that exposure to tobacco smoke, alcohol, chocolate, and high-fat meals decreased lower esophageal sphincter pressure but cessation of tobacco smoking and alcohol, and other dietary measures did not directly support betterment in GERD.

Surgical management of GERD may be a consideration for a child with a life-limiting illnesses and troublesome GERD that has not responded to medical management, although there is no evidence to support this claim.[138] The most frequent surgery performed is the Nissen fundoplication, either as an open (ONF) or laparoscopic (LNF) procedure. It involves wrapping the upper part of the stomach around the lower end of the esophagus, allowing the lower esophageal sphincter to close more completely, reducing reflux.

This can be seen as a safe procedure with a median duration of 70 minutes and in a retrospective study[139] comparing Nissen, Thal, and Toupet fundoplications for 238 children without neurological impairment, all three procedures were found to be equally effective with an overall 5% intra-operative and 5.4% post-operative complication rate. Only 2.5% of children required second operations, and all but 9 children were free of symptoms 5 years out from their operation.

Earlier, retrospective analysis[140] of fundoplication for GERD in 52 neurologically impaired and 25 unimpaired children indicated that impaired children had significantly fewer hospital admissions and total days of hospitalization during the first 6-month post-operative period and a short-term weight gain improvement in those with failure to thrive (FTT). However, longer term (1 and 2 years post-operation) weight gain and weight gain in unimpaired children with FTT was not improved.

The advent of the laparoscopic approach made for a faster, safer procedure with a smooth postoperative recovery and similar failure rates.[141] A retrospective review[142] of 456 children with GERD who underwent ONF ($n = 150$) or LNF ($n = 306$) concluded that the majority of re-operations occurred in the first year after operation with LNF having a significantly higher rate than ONF; 10.5% vs. 4%. The probability for a further operation increased with co-morbidities, particularly prematurity and chronic respiratory conditions.

How this and other data translates to the pediatric palliative care population is not certain, although the study populations have included children with severe neurological problems. This must be tempered with a lack of good, prospective information on the long-term efficacy, risks, and benefits of this surgery. Advice for caregivers and healthcare providers to carefully weigh the potential risks and benefits for the child remains very relevant.

Pharmacology

Drug management of moderate to severe GERD should be seen as standard care, and there are three approaches:

- Altering the viscosity of the feeds with alginates,
- Altering the gastric pH with antacids, histamine H_2 receptor antagonists (H_2RA), proton pump inhibitors (PPIs),
- Altering the motility of the gut with prokinetic agents.

Antacids +/− Alginate Antacids provide only short-term stomach acid neutralization with each dose taken making them less effective, other than for short-term relief of symptoms. They contain aluminum, calcium, or magnesium or a combination of these chemicals, and as such long-term use cannot be recommended because it introduces the risk of toxicity. Toxicity examples include diarrhea with magnesium containing antacids, or the reported case[143] of phosphate depletion-induced osteopenia in an infant on prolonged aluminum and magnesium hydroxide gel therapy for colic.

Aluminum/magnesium trisilicate (Gaviscon) has the added effect of serving as a protective barrier for the esophagus. It produces a viscous, demulcent antacid foam that floats on the stomach contents and in addition to reducing the frequency of reflux episodes, the alkaline foam aids the neutralization of refluxed gastric acids. Aluminum/magnesium trisilicate infant sachets were recently reported[144] to be safe and able to improve symptoms of reflux.

Histamine H_2 Receptor Antagonists (H_2RA) This group of agents reduces acid production in the stomach by antagonism of the H_2 histamine receptor. A comprehensive evidence-based review[145] stated ranitidine to be safe and effective in infant GERD and the early use of H_2RA's was supported

in older children. These medications are usually taken by mouth once or twice a day with intravenous, oral syrup and effervescent tablet forms available. The effervescent ranitidine tablets may be dissolved in water, fruit juice, and carbonated drinks and one tablet dissolved in 100 mL of water is stable for 24 hrs and a tablet is soluble in water volumes down to 15 mL.

Oral dosing for ranitidine:

- Neonates: 2 mg/kg/DOSE every 12 hours
- Infants and children: 2-4 mg/kg/DOSE every 8-12 hours (max 150 mg/DOSE)

Oral dosing for famotidine:
- Infants and children: 0.5 mg/kg/DOSE every 12 hours (max 20 mg/DOSE)

Proton Pump Inhibitors (PPIs) PPIs are highly selective and effective in their action of blocking the production of acid in the stomach at the final common metabolic pathway of gastric parietal cells. In a Cochrane review[145] of adults with GERD symptoms, PPIs were found to be more effective than H_2RAs (RR 0.66, 95%; CI 0.60 to 0.73) and prokinetics (RR 0.53, 95%; CI 0.32 to 0.87). In children they were found to be highly effective, have a very good tolerability profile and have few short- and long-term adverse effects.[146] The safety and efficacy of omeprazole and lansoprazole were confirmed in a 2009 evidence-based systematic review.[144] Both also promoted symptomatic relief and endoscopic and histological healing of esophagitis in infants with GERD. The evidence also supported the early use of proton pump inhibitors in older children.

The oral dosages recommended for infants and children are:

- Omeprazole
  - Under 10 kg: 5 mg once daily
  - 10-20 kg: 10 mg once daily (max 20 mg/DAY)
  - Over 20 kg: 20 mg once daily (max 40 mg/DAY), or 0.7-1.4 mg/kg/DAY (max 60 mg/DAY)
- Lansoprazole
  - 0.73-1.66 mg/kg/DAY (maximum 30 mg/DAY)

When children cannot swallow tablets or capsules, then omeprazole capsules can be opened and the granules mixed with an acidic drink and swallowed without chewing. In the case of PEG and NG tubes, the granules can be mixed with 10 mL of 8.4% sodium bicarbonate and left to stand for 10 minutes until a turbid suspension is formed. The suspension is then given immediately and flushed with water. Lansoprazole fastabs dissolve very well in water and are less likely to block tubes.[120]

Prokinetic Agents Prokinetic agents such as metoclopramide and domperidone have been used in GERD and their action discussed in the section on nausea and vomiting. Unfortunately, two reviews[135,147] could suggest only some benefit for infants under the age of 2 years with GERD from metoclopramide in comparison with placebo, but pointed out there was insufficient evidence to support or oppose use.

Hiccups

Hiccups are a physiological process involving a reflex[148] consisting of the following:

- Afferent limb, the phrenic and vagus nerves and sympathetic chain arising from T6-12
- Hiccup center, a nonspecific location between C3 and C5
- Connections to the respiratory center, phrenic nerve nuclei, medullary reticular formation, and hypothalamus
- Efferents
  - Phrenic nerve (C3-5)
  - Anterior scalene muscles (C5-7)
  - External intercostals (T1-11)
  - Glottis, the recurrent laryngeal component of vagus
  - Inhibitory autonomic processes
  - Decreasing esophageal contraction tone
  - Lower esophageal sphincter tone

The purpose of hiccups remains a mystery and the reflex results in irregular, involuntary contractions of the diaphragm and accessory respiratory muscles, with an associated noise from sudden closure of the glottis.

Treatable Conditions The history, examination, and any investigation are directed to elucidating the cause of the hiccup as the diagnosis of the symptom is readily apparent. Gastrointestinal mechanisms are common with gastric distention and GERD often implicated. There are many other potential considerations:

- Metabolic disorders, including hypocapnia, uremia, hypocalcaemia
- Local nerve damage and central nervous system disorders
- Anxiety
- Surgical complications
- Drugs including digoxin, corticosteroids, anti-depressants

The cause in children and infants is rarely found.[148]

Integrative and Supportive Therapies Nonpharmacologic therapies including well-known traditional remedies, medical interventions and complementary therapies all work on sound physiological principles and can succeed by effecting components of the hiccup reflex. These have been well detailed:[148]
- Traditional remedies
  - Stimulation of nasopharynx by forcible traction on the tongue, swallowing granulated sugar, gargling with water, sipping ice water, drinking from the far side of a glass, biting on a lemon, inhaling noxious agents such as ammonia
  - C3-5 dermatome stimulation, including tapping or rubbing back of the neck, coolant sprays, acupuncture
  - Direct pharyngeal stimulation with a nasal or oral catheter, which is 90% effective
  - Direct uvular stimulation with a spoon or cotton-tip applicator
  - Removal of gastric contents by emetics, NG tube
- Vagal stimulation (only one technique at a time is recommended)
  - Iced gastric lavage
  - Valsalva maneuver
  - Carotid sinus massage, but only by experienced personnel after exclusion of contraindications
  - Digital ocular globe pressure, but only by experienced personnel after exclusion of contraindications
  - Digital rectal massage
- Interference with normal respiratory function
  - Breath holding

- Hyperventilation
- Gasping, such as by fright
- Breathing into a paper bag, which increases partial pressure of carbon dioxide
- Pulling knees up to chest and leaning forward
- Continuous positive airway pressure
- Rebreathing 5% carbon dioxide
- Mental distraction
- Other
  - Behavioral conditioning
  - Hypnosis
  - Acupuncture
  - Phrenic nerve or diaphragmatic pacing
  - Phrenic nerve block surgery
  - Microvascular decompression of the vagus nerve
  - Prayer

Pharmacology

A large array of pharmacologic agents can potentially be used to treat hiccups[149] promoting the adage that the larger the variety of agents available to treat a symptom, the less likely they are to be helpful. The most positive evidence has arisen for the muscle relaxant, baclofen[149,150] and, more recently, the anticonvulsant, gabapentin[151–153] has been receiving favorable attention.

Summary

Mouth and throat symptoms are often interrelated and a measured evaluation is required, which should include a critical review of the child's current drug therapies. In the case of a symptom such as GERD, a high index of suspicion should be held for its presence, particularly in certain populations of children with life-limiting illness.

Assessment will often provide a rational management approach but for dysphagia, xerostomia, and intractable hiccups, resolution may not be possible. This should encourage the practitioner to use an encompassing approach of integrative, supportive, and pharmacologic techniques and, where appropriate, seek a considered surgical opinion for a more interventional approach.

Bowel Obstruction

The frequency, incidence or prevalence of bowel obstruction among children with life-limiting conditions has yet to be detailed. Clinical experience would indicate this to be an infrequent event that is most likely to be seen in children with incurable cancers of the abdomen or pelvis such as lymphoma, rhabdomyosarcoma, or Ewing's sarcoma.

PATHOGENESIS

Obstruction in this setting occurs when the lumen of the bowel is sufficiently occluded to prevent the movement of intestinal contents along the gastrointestinal tract. In a report by the Working Group of the European Association of Palliative Care,[154] several pathological mechanisms were detailed for adults with end-stage cancer and are likely to be the process for children. These are:
- Mechanical obstruction
- Extrinsic occlusion of the lumen

- Intraluminal occlusion of the lumen
- Intramural occlusion of the lumen
- Adynamic ileus or functional obstruction
- Intestinal motility disorders from tumor infiltration of the mesentery or bowel muscle and nerves or malignant involvement of the celiac plexus
- Intestinal motility disorders from paraneoplastic neuropathy

It is important to note that even in the adult patient with end-stage cancer, benign causes such as adhesions, post-irradiation bowel damage, inflammatory bowel disease, and hernia can be the cause of the obstruction in around half of the cases.[155]

EVALUATION AND ASSESSMENT

The presentation of bowel obstruction is site-dependent, with symptoms determined by the sequence of distention-secretion-motor activity of the obstructed bowel.[154] The symptoms most likely to occur involve a combination of pain, both continuous and/or colicky; nausea and/or vomiting; and constipation with or without overflow diarrhea. Vomiting is more likely to be a feature of, and develop earlier in, small bowel obstruction particularly that of the stomach and duodenum. Large bowel involvement tends to involve deeper pain of less severity, occurring at longer intervals.[156]

Good clinical acumen including a careful examination along with knowledge of the natural history of the disease can often be sufficient to make an accurate diagnosis of bowel obstruction. Examination findings that add credibility to the diagnosis include the presence of a distended bowel, palpable mass, tympanic percussion and abnormal bowel sounds such as high pitched, tinkling sounds. These do not have to be present for a diagnosis to be made.

The symptoms of obstruction can be mimicked by the absence or impairment of gastrointestinal motility, a pseudo-obstruction. Indicators for this include absent or reduced bowel sounds and other signs of constipation, peritonitis, septicemia, or spinal cord compression. These require specific treatment and management.

Investigations are not a prerequisite to confirm a diagnosis and would seem to be an unnecessary burden to the child and his or her family particularly, when the patient is very ill, desires a conservative approach to care, and there is no doubt as to the presence of a bowel obstruction.

If further investigation is warranted, then a plain abdominal x-ray could show the presence of bowel distension and more than six gas-fluid levels on supine and erect films. In suspected small bowel obstruction, plain supine and standing films are required and have been reported[157] to be as sensitive as computed tomography (CT) in adults. However, plain films are less sensitive for detection of low grade or partial obstruction. CT scan adds a more global assessment of disease and can assist in the choice of intervention: surgical, endoscopic, or pharmacologic palliation.[154]

Contrast studies provide information on the site and extent of obstruction, particularly partial obstructions, and can evaluate problems with motility. Barium, while it gives good definition, can cause problems with impaction because it is often not absorbed. Hyperosmolar water-soluble contrast mediums, such as Gastrografin, are safe and have a therapeutic role in that they are a predictive test for non-operative resolution of adhesive small-bowel obstruction with a pooled sensitivity of 97% and specificity of 96%.[158] This review also indicated contrast did not reduce the need for surgical intervention but it did reduce hospital stay compared with placebo.

INTEGRATIVE AND SUPPORTIVE THERAPIES

Management of bowel obstruction is primarily aimed toward the relief of symptoms and this does vary according to the presence of a partial or complete obstruction.[159]

Feeding and Hydration

In the majority of situations, good pharmacologic management precludes the need for intravenous hydration and total parenteral nutrition as the child can satisfy their appetite and thirst with sensible oral intake.

Oral feeding can continue in cases of partial and intermittent obstruction by using small, frequent meals of a low-residue, low-fiber diet. Complete and continuous obstructions do not exclude oral intake with a trial of occasional, small snacks and sips allowable.

Xerostomia may be especially troublesome as the medications used to manage pain, nausea and vomiting can be associated with this symptom.

Nausea and Vomiting

Nausea and vomiting usually requires very active management with medication directed toward a goal of no to minimal nausea and two or fewer vomits in a 24-hour period. The main agents to be considered are anti-secretory and anti-emetic agents.

If a partial obstruction without colic is present, then a prokinetic agent such as domperidone or metoclopramide can be initiated and titrated to effect. Any worsening of symptoms necessitates this approach be discontinued and an anti-secretory agent commenced. The mainstay of treatment is hyoscine butylbromide (Buscopan), with or without an anti-emetic agent that acts to slow intestinal transit such as cyclizine or methotrimeprazine. The somatostatin analogue octreotide can then be introduced if required.[154] Hyoscine butylbromide is not available in the United States, the alternative is hyoscyamine (Levsin).

Corticosteroids have been used to provide temporary symptom relief and resolution of the obstruction through their edema-reducing and anti-secretory effects. However, two systematic reviews[160,161] were unable to show statistical significance because of methodological weakness in existing studies but another study[160] commented on a trend toward resolution of bowel obstruction with corticosteroid use.

Nasogastric Suction

The use of intravenous hydration and nasogastric suction fail to control the symptoms of inoperable bowel obstruction in around 90% of adults.[162,163] It should be considered only a short term measure to deal with excessive secretions while pharmacologic treatment is established.

Long-term use may be necessary when pharmacologic management fails, surgical interventions are not appropriate and gastrostomy cannot be performed.

Gastrostomy

A venting gastrostomy can be considered when pharmacologic management has not been able to manage vomiting. This is more likely to occur in small-bowel obstruction. The intermittent venting of the gastrostomy provides the child with the chance to maintain an oral intake and more active lifestyle.

Gastrostomy placement can be operative or by percutaneous endoscopy. PEG placement can be done under CT guidance when there are concerning complicating factors, such as carcinomatosis, portal hypertension, or ascites. PEG is a superior technique to both NG and operative gastrostomy for palliation of small bowel obstruction,[164] and overall this approach can control nausea and vomiting in more than 90% of cases of bowel obstruction.

Constipation

All laxatives should be stopped in complete bowel obstruction. However, the presence of a partial and intermittent block does allow for a trial of a softening agent such as docusate and the dose titrated to produce a comfortable stool without colic.[159]

Pain

Pain associated with bowel obstruction can be continuous, colicky and, in higher abdominal masses, involve the celiac plexus. Continuous pain frequently requires the use of a strong opioid, which may also alleviate colic. However, if colic is not satisfactorily managed by a strong opioid, then the addition of an anti-secretory drug is warranted.[154]

Surgery

The role of surgery in malignant bowel obstruction in adults with advanced gynecological or gastrointestinal cancer remains controversial with no firm conclusions by a systematic review.[165] The literature lacked appropriate and validated outcome criteria, but prognostic criteria[154] are available to select patients who are more likely to benefit from surgical intervention.

Unfortunately, there are no such guidelines for children, but a compassionate and considered surgical opinion that takes into account all the individual factors should be seen as part of the decision-making process.

PHARMACOLOGY

Hyoscine butylbromide (Buscopan) and octreotide are the mainstays of pharmacologic management. In the United States, it is hyoscyamine (Levsin) and octreotide. In a qualitative systematic review of the limited data available[161] octreotide was evidenced to be superior to hyoscine butylbromide in relieving gastrointestinal symptoms from inoperable malignant bowel obstruction in a total of 103 adult patients.

Hyoscine Butylbromide

This anti-secretory agent acts by blocking muscarinic cholinergic receptors at the parasympathetic ganglia in the walls of the viscera, relaxing the bowel and reducing gastric and intestinal secretions. It has a low-lipid solubility so it does not readily cross the blood-brain barrier resulting in the absence of central adverse effects such as somnolence and hallucinations.

In children the anti-spasmodic dose is 0.5mg/kg/DOSE with a maximum dose of 20 mg every 6 hours to 8 hours[179] or a continuous infusion dose of 0.6–1.2mg/kg/24hr.[40] The maximum continuous infusion dose has not been determined in children.

Hyoscine butylbromide (Buscopan) is not available in the United States. Possible alternatives include hyoscyamine (Levsin).

Octreotide

Octreotide is a long-acting synthetic analogue of endogenous somatostatin and a potent inhibitor of growth hormone, glucagon, and insulin. It also modulates gastrointestinal function by slowing intestinal motility, reducing gastric acid secretion, decreasing bile flow, increasing mucous production, and reducing splanchnic blood flow.[166,167]

In adults, octreotide reaches peak serum concentrations within 30 minutes of either an intravenous or subcutaneous injection, has a half-life of around 90 minutes and duration of action of approximately 12 hours, allowing for twice daily-administration. Elimination is prolonged in renal failure; it is metabolized and excreted unchanged. It can interact with cyclosporine to reduce serum concentrations and prolong the corrected QT interval at therapeutic doses.[167]

In children it has been reported to assist in the management of a range of gastrointestinal conditions,[94,168–170] including chronic gastrointestinal bleeding[171,172] and non-gastrointestinal disorders such as chylothorax[167] and reversing hypoglycemia.[173] Octreotide has also been described[174] to improve the quality of life of a 12-year-old boy with malignant bowel obstruction by abating symptoms and improving appetite.

Dosing recommendations depend on the condition being treated, but usually range from 1-10 mcg/kg/dose every 8 hours with a maximum dose of 500 mcg. Octreotide has been given as a continuous infusion of 1-5 mcg/kg/hour[175] for acute variceal bleeding and in children being treated for chylothorax infusions have been titrated up to 10 mcg/kg/hr with the duration of treatment ranging from 3 to 29 days.[167]

SUMMARY

Bowel obstruction in children under palliative care is a relatively unusual clinical event and this is reflected in the paucity of evidence-based recommendations for managing this condition. Borrowing from the adult literature on bowel obstruction and the pediatric literature describing the medications used in bowel obstruction to treat other conditions suggests octreotide to be the first line agent although, if resourcing demands, hyoscine butylbromide can be an able substitute. The addition of corticosteroids probably, at best, aids by providing temporary relief.

Feeding Intolerance

A large number of children with non-malignant life-limiting diseases receive part or all their feeding by tube, often by gastric and/or jejunal tube (PEG-tube). Data shows that a subgroup of those children develop a progressive intolerance to their feeds, clinically manifesting as worsening reflux, vomiting, abdominal bloating, ileus, irritability, and pain (in non-verbal children often described as "episodes of inconsolability" or "screaming of unknown origin"). This intolerance persists despite modifications to the artificial feeding rate or route, modifications to formula composition, and the addition of medications.[176] These children have repeated episodes of intolerance to feeds before the end-of-life phase of their illness.

If a thorough workup does not reveal a pathophysiology, visceral hyperalgesia should be considered. The enteric nervous system contains more than 100 million neurons, both myenteric and submucosal ganglionated plexi, transmitting nociception via dorsal horn neurons, vagal afferents at the medulla, and thalamus to the sensory cortex. Viceral hyperalgesia may be based on alterations in response to bowel sensory input, which result in recruitment of previously silent nociceptors, resulting in sensitization of visceral afferent pathways. There is very limited pediatric data in the management of feeding intolerance and/or retching.[177] Successful treatment strategies in our pediatric palliative care patients seem to include the administration of analgesics following the WHO ladder from non-opioids such as acetaminophen and/or ibuprofen, to weak opioid such as tramadol or strong opioid such as morphine, oxycodone, hydromorphone. The addition of tricyclic antidepressants such as amitriptyline, calcium-channel ligands such as gabapentin, and/or less frequently 5-HT3 receptor antagonists such as ondansetron seems effective in our experience. Integrative, nonpharmacologic therapies include cognitive behavioral therapy for parents and affected child, aromatherapy, massage, and/or music therapy.

Before making the diagnosis, a trial of changing the formula type or route of administration should be considered. The decrease of feeding volume may be particularly helpful; however it may cause parental resistance with parental fears of starving the child. A careful discussion about the treatment goal of improving distressing symptoms by decreasing feeding volume may be helpful. It may also be helpful to propose a short-term trial, such as decreasing daily feeding volume by 25% to 50% for 3 days to establish treatment effectiveness and parental rapport.

FORGOING NUTRITION AND HYDRATION

Discussions about the possibility of forgoing medical nutrition and hydration in a child continues to be one of the most challenging conversations that pediatric palliative care professionals may have with parents and medical colleagues. Providing nutrition and hydration is appropriate in most cases, but it is recognized that circumstances exist in which the goals of care change and that providing nutrition and/or hydration may not be appropriate. The following considerations are relevant to patients such as those with neurologic devastation, total irreversible intestinal failure, also known as "terminal feeding intolerance," and those for whom death from any cause is expected soon. These discussions are difficult to parents and health staff because offering of nutrition and hydration is a basic component of human interaction that in most instances provides sustenance and comfort.

In Minneapolis a pediatric statement on forgoing medically provided nutrition and hydration by the ethics committee[178] is used, which discusses the following issues:

Oral Nutrition and Hydration

If oral nutrition and hydration would provide more harm than benefit to a patient, it can be permissible to discontinue offering them. The harms and benefits of oral nutrition and hydration should be specifically discussed in the context of decisions about and goals of medical treatments. Decisions regarding medically provided nutrition and hydration should be placed in the context of all other treatment and life values decision of the patient, and should be consistent with decisions about levels of other medical support, provision of comfort cares, and other experiences, including social, educational, and family needs. Open communication of all involved in treatment planning about the issues of medical provision nutrition and hydration is strongly endorsed. The patient, family, and caregivers are encouraged to share any concerns or information regarding medically provided nutrition and hydration with the others most closely involved in the patient's care. Decisions about providing nutrition and hydration should be made on the best available information. There are cases in which decisions must be delayed because of inadequate information; it is also permissible in some cases to forgo medically provided nutrition and hydration even if there is some degree of uncertainty regarding prognosis or benefit.

For most children, the parents or other legal guardians are the primary decision makers, but the decision to forgo medically provided nutrition and hydration requires the concurrence of the healthcare team most closely involved in the patient's care.

Children have the same rights as adults to have treatment provided or not provided based on how the treatment affects their interests. It is an emotionally difficult situation to make a decision about medically provided nutrition and hydration for another person, especially when that person is a child. It is ethically permissible for the person deciding for the child to choose among the full range of treatment decisions.

Feeding Through a Medical Device

The provision of nutrition and hydration through any medical device is considered a medical treatment and is in a different category than oral nutrition and hydration. These medical treatments include NG feedings and fluid, GT feedings and fluid, and IV fluid, including total parenteral nutrition (TPN).

The medical provision of nutrition and hydration may or may not be a comfort measure, and in some situations may increase or prolong suffering. Like all treatments, the use of medically provided nutrition and hydration is governed not by the nature of the treatment, but whether the treatment advances the patient's interests and whether the benefits of providing the treatment outweigh the burdens of the treatment.

It can be ethically permissible to forgo medically provided nutrition and hydration when hope for recovery is low or non-existent if the parents, with the concurrence of the healthcare team, believe that forgoing treatment is in the child's best interest.

There is no ethical obligation to continue a treatment that is no longer advancing the interests of the patient. It is therefore permissible in some cases to stop medically providing nutrition and hydration after it has been started.

The use of an ethics and/or palliative care consultation for further discussion and clarification of these issues if uncertainty or disagreement exists for the family or healthcare providers is recommended.

Loving families who have decided to forgo medically provided nutrition and hydration need to be reminded that they are not starving their child. Overwhelming experience shows that children very rarely need comfort medications, such as sublingual morphine or benzodiazepines in non-sedating doses, and usually do not show distress during their last days or weeks of life. Excellent mouth care, with the goal to keep the mouth moist, is paramount.

REFERENCES

1. Hyams JS, Burke G, Davis PM, Rzepski B, Andrulonis PA: Abdominal pain and irritable bowel syndrome in adolescents: a community-based study, *J Pediatr* 129(2):220–226, 1996.
2. Friedrichsdorf SJ, Brun S, Zernikow B, Dangel T: Palliative Care in Poland: The Warsaw Hospice for Children, *Europ J Pall Care* 13(1):35–38, 2006.
3. Drake R, Frost J, Collins JJ: The symptoms of dying children, *J Pain Symptom Manage* 26(1):594–603, 2003.
4. Goldman A: Symptoms and suffering at the end of life in children with cancer, *N Engl J Med* 342(26):1998, 2000.
5. Hongo T, Watanabe C, Okada S, Inoue N, Yajima S, Fujii Y, et al: Analysis of the circumstances at the end of life in children with cancer: symptoms, suffering and acceptance, *Pediatr Int* 45(1):60–64, 2003.
6. Wolfe J, Grier HE, Klar N, Levin SB, Ellenbogen JM, Salem-Schatz S, et al: Symptoms and suffering at the end of life in children with cancer, *N Engl J Med* 342(5):326–333, 2000.
7. Wolfe J, Hammel JF, Edwards KE, Duncan J, Comeau M, Breyer J, et al: Easing of suffering in children with cancer at the end of life: is care changing? *J Clin Oncol* 26(10):1717–1723, 2008.
8. Lipmann A, Jackson II K, Tylor L: *Evidence based symptom control in palliative care*, New York, 2000, Pharmaceutical Products Press.
9. Twycross R, Back I: Nausea and vomiting in advanced cancer, *Europ J Pall Care* 5(2):39–44, 1998.
10. Santucci G, Mack JW: Common gastrointestinal symptoms in pediatric palliative care: nausea, vomiting, constipation, anorexia, cachexia, *Pediatr Clin North Am* 54(5):673–689, 2007.
11. Ventaffrida V, Oliveri E, Caraceni A, Spoldi E, De Conno F, Saita L, et al: A retrospective study on the use of oral morphine in cancer pain, *J Pain Symptom Manage* 2(2):77–81, 1987.
12. Drake R, Longworth J, Collins JJ: Opioid rotation in children with cancer, *J Palliat Med* 7(3):419–422, 2004.
13. Maxwell LG, Kaufmann SC, Bitzer S, Jackson EV Jr, McGready J, Kost-Byerly S, et al: The effects of a small-dose naloxone infusion on opioid-induced side effects and analgesia in children and adolescents treated with intravenous patient-controlled analgesia: a double-blind, prospective, randomized, controlled study, *Anesth Analg* 100(4):953–958, 2005.
14. Friedrichsdorf SJ, Kuttner L, Westendorp K, McCarty R: *Integrative pediatric palliative care*. In Culbert T, Olness K, editors: Integrative Pediatrics. 2010, Oxford University Press.
15. Lebaron S, Zeltzer L: Behavioral intervention for reducing chemotherapy-related nausea and vomiting in adolescents with cancer, *J Adolesc Health Care* 5(3):178–182, 1984.
16. Cotanch P, Hockenberry M, Herman: Self-hypnosis as antiemetic therapy in children receiving chemotherapy, *Oncol Nurs Forum* 12(4):41–46, 1985.
17. Hockenberry MJ, Cotanch PH: Hypnosis as adjuvant antiemetic therapy in childhood cancer, *Nurs Clin North Am* 20(1):105–107, 1985.
18. Jacknow DS, Tschann JM, Link MP, Boyce WT: Hypnosis in the prevention of chemotherapy-related nausea and vomiting in children: a prospective study, *J Dev Behav Pediatr* 15(4):258–264, 1994.
19. Zeltzer L, LeBaron S, Zeltzer PM: The effectiveness of behavioral intervention for reduction of nausea and vomiting in children and adolescents receiving chemotherapy, *J Clin Oncol* 2(6):683–690, 1984.
20. Vickers AJ: Can acupuncture have specific effects on health? A systematic review of acupuncture antiemesis trials, *J R Soc Med* 89(6):303–311, 1996.
21. Brock P, Brichard B, Rechnitzer C, Langeveld NE, Lanning M, Soderhall S, et al: An increased loading dose of ondansetron: a North European, double-blind randomised study in children, comparing 5 mg/m2 with 10 mg/m2, *Eur J Cancer* 32A(10):1744–1748, 1996.
22. Stiakaki E, Savvas S, Lydaki E, Bolonaki I, Kouvidi E, Dimitriou H, et al: Ondansetron and tropisetron in the control of nausea and vomiting in children receiving combined cancer chemotherapy, *Pediatr Hematol Oncol* 16(2):101–108, 1999.
23. Parker RI, Prakash D, Mahan RA, Giugliano DM, Atlas MP: Randomized, double-blind, crossover, placebo-controlled trial of intravenous ondansetron for the prevention of intrathecal chemotherapy-induced vomiting in children, *J Pediatr Hematol Oncol* 23(9):578–581, 2001.
24. Orchard PJ, Rogosheske J, Burns L, Rydholm N, Larson H, DeFor TE, et al: A prospective randomized trial of the anti-emetic efficacy of ondansetron and granisetron during bone marrow transplantation, *Biol Blood Marrow Transplant* 5(6):386–393, 1999.
25. Dick GS, Meller ST, Pinkerton CR: Randomised comparison of ondansetron and metoclopramide plus dexamethasone for chemotherapy induced emesis, *Arch Dis Child* 73(3):243–245, 1995.
26. Koseoglu V, Kurekci AE, Sarici U, Atay AA, Ozcan O: Comparison of the efficacy and side-effects of ondansetron and metoclopramide-diphenhydramine administered to control nausea and vomiting in children treated with antineoplastic chemotherapy: a prospective randomized study, *Eur J Pediatr* 157(10):806–810, 1998.
27. Uysal KM, Olgun N, Sarialioglu F: Tropisetron in the prevention of chemotherapy-induced acute emesis in pediatric patients, *Turk J Pediatr* 41(2):207–218, 1999.
28. Ozkan A, Yildiz I, Yuksel L, Apak H, Celkan T: Tropisetron (Navoban) in the control of nausea and vomiting induced by combined cancer chemotherapy in children, *Jpn J Clin Oncol* 29(2):92–95, 1999.
29. Aksoylar S, Akman SA, Ozgenc F, Kansoy S: Comparison of tropisetron and granisetron in the control of nausea and vomiting in children receiving combined cancer chemotherapy, *Pediatr Hematol Oncol* 18(6):397–406, 2001.
30. Klaschik E: In Husebø S, Klaschik E, editors: *Schmerztherapie und Symptomkontrolle in der Palliativmedizin*, ed 3, Berlin, Heidelberg, New York, 2003, Springer.
31. Bateman DN, Rawlins MD, Simpson JM: Extrapyramidal reactions with metoclopramide, *Br Med J (Clin Res Ed)* 291(6500):930–932, 1985.
32. Diemunsch P, Apfel C, Gan TJ, Candiotti K, Philip BK, Chelly J, et al: Preventing postoperative nausea and vomiting: post hoc analysis of pooled data from two randomized active-controlled trials of aprepitant, *Curr Med Res Opin* 23(10):2559–2565, 2007.
33. Diemunsch P, Gan TJ, Philip BK, Girao MJ, Eberhart L, Irwin MG, et al: Single-dose aprepitant vs ondansetron for the prevention of postoperative nausea and vomiting: a randomized, double-blind phase III trial in patients undergoing open abdominal surgery, *Br J Anaesth* 99(2):202–211, 2007.
34. Smith AR, Repka TL, Weigel BJ: Aprepitant for the control of chemotherapy induced nausea and vomiting in adolescents, *Pediatr Blood Cancer* 45(6):857–860, 2005.
35. Gore L, Chawla S, Petrilli A, Hemenway M, Schissel D, Chua V, et al: Aprepitant in adolescent patients for prevention of chemotherapy-induced nausea and vomiting: a randomized, double-blind, placebo-controlled study of efficacy and tolerability, *Pediatr Blood Cancer* 52(2):242–247, 2009.
36. Hall W, Degenhardt L: Medical marijuana initiatives: are they justified? How successful are they likely to be? *CNS Drugs* 17(10):689–697, 2003.
37. Nocerino E, Amato M, Izzo AA: Cannabis and cannabinoid receptors, *Fitoterapia* 71(Suppl 1):S6–S12, 2000.
38. Williamson EM, Evans FJ: Cannabinoids in clinical practice, *Drugs* 60(6):1303–1314, 2000.
39. Tramer MR, Carroll D, Campbell FA, Reynolds DJ, Moore RA, McQuay HJ: Cannabinoids for control of chemotherapy induced nausea and vomiting: quantitative systematic review, *BMJ* 323(7303):16–21, 2001.
40. Goldman A, Burne R: *Symptom management*. In Goldman A, editor: Care of the dying child. Oxford, New York, 1999, Oxford University Press.
41. Riad W, Altaf R, Abdulla A, Oudan H: Effect of midazolam, dexamethasone and their combination on the prevention of nausea and vomiting following strabismus repair in children, *Eur J Anaesthesiol* 24(8):697–701, 2007.
42. Ozcan AA, Gunes Y, Haciyakupoglu G: Using diazepam and atropine before strabismus surgery to prevent postoperative nausea and vomiting: a randomized, controlled study, *J AAPOS* 7(3):210–212, 2003.
43. Kearsley JH, Williams AM, Fiumara AM: Antiemetic superiority of lorazepam over oxazepam and methylprednisolone as premedicants for patients receiving cisplatin-containing chemotherapy, *Cancer* 64(8):1595–1599, 1989.
44. Bishop JF, Olver IN, Wolf MM, Matthews JP, Long M, Bingham J, et al: Lorazepam: a randomized, double-blind, crossover study of a new antiemetic in patients receiving cytotoxic chemotherapy and prochlorperazine, *J Clin Oncol* 2(6):691–695, 1984.
45. Gan TJ, Ginsberg B, Grant AP, Glass PS: Double-blind, randomized comparison of ondansetron and intraoperative propofol to prevent postoperative nausea and vomiting, *Anesthesiology* 85(5):1036–1042, 1996.

46. Borgeat A, Wilder-Smith OH, Saiah M, Rifat K: Subhypnotic doses of propofol possess direct antiemetic properties, *Anesth Analg* 74(4):539–541, 1992.

47. Krasowski MD, Hong X, Hopfinger AJ, Harrison NL: 4D-QSAR analysis of a set of propofol analogues: mapping binding sites for an anesthetic phenol on the GABA(A) receptor, *J Med Chem* 45(15):3210–3221, 2002.

48. Haeseler G, Karst M, Foadi N, Gudehus S, Roeder A, Hecker H, et al: High-affinity blockade of voltage-operated skeletal muscle and neuronal sodium channels by halogenated propofol analogues, *Br J Pharmacol* 155(2):265–275, 2008.

49. Fowler CJ: Possible involvement of the endocannabinoid system in the actions of three clinically used drugs, *Trends Pharmacol Sci* 25(2):59–61, 2004.

50. Lundstrom S, Zachrisson U, Furst CJ: When nothing helps: propofol as sedative and antiemetic in palliative cancer care, *J Pain Symptom Manage* 30(6):570–577, 2005.

51. Glover ML, Kodish E, Reed MD: Continuous propofol infusion for the relief of treatment-resistant discomfort in a terminally ill pediatric patient with cancer, *J Pediatr Hematol Oncol* 18(4):377–380, 1996.

52. Hooke MC, Grund E, Quammen H, Miller B, McCormick P, Bostrom B: Propofol use in pediatric patients with severe cancer pain at the end of life, *J Pediatr Oncol Nurs* 24(1):29–34, 2007.

53. Beckwith C: Constipation in Palliative Care Patients. In Lipmann A, Jackson IIK, Tylor L, editors: *Evidence based symptom control in palliative care*, New York, 2000, Pharmaceutical Products Press, pp 47–57.

54. Gremse DA, Hixon J, Crutchfield A: Comparison of polyethylene glycol 3350 and lactulose for treatment of chronic constipation in children, *Clin Pediatr (Phila)* 41(4):225–229, 2002.

55. Pitzalis G, Deganello F, Mariani P, Chiarini-Testa MB, Virgilii F, Gasparri R, et al: [Lactitol in chronic idiopathic constipation in children], *Pediatr Med Chir* 17(3):223–226, 1995.

56. Pashankar DS, Bishop WP, Loening-Baucke V: Long-term efficacy of polyethylene glycol 3350 for the treatment of chronic constipation in children with and without encopresis, *Clin Pediatr (Phila)* 42(9):815–819, 2003.

57. Pashankar DS, Loening-Baucke V, Bishop WP: Safety of polyethylene glycol 3350 for the treatment of chronic constipation in children, *Arch Pediatr Adolesc Med* 157(7):661–664, 2003.

58. Tolia V, Lin CH, Elitsur Y: A prospective randomized study with mineral oil and oral lavage solution for treatment of fecal impaction in children, *Aliment Pharmacol Ther* 7(5):523–529, 1993.

59. Sondheimer JM, Gervaise EP: Lubricant versus laxative in the treatment of chronic functional constipation of children: a comparative study, *J Pediatr Gastroenterol Nutr* 1(2):223–226, 1982.

60. Hawley PH, Byeon JJ: A comparison of sennosides-based bowel protocols with and without docusate in hospitalized patients with cancer, *J Palliat Med* 11(4):575–581, 2008.

61. Bellomo-Brandao MA, Collares EF, da-Costa-Pinto EA: Use of erythromycin for the treatment of severe chronic constipation in children, *Braz J Med Biol Res* 36(10):1391–1396, 2003.

62. Sykes N: Constipation. In Doyle D, Hanks G, Cherny N, Calman K, editors: *Oxford textbook of palliative medicine*, ed 3, Oxford, 2004, Oxford University Press, pp 483–490.

63. Sykes NP: An investigation of the ability of oral naloxone to correct opioid-related constipation in patients with advanced cancer, *Palliat Med* 10(2):135–144, 1996.

64. Webster L, Jansen JP, Peppin J, Lasko B, Irving G, Morlion B, et al: Alvimopan, a peripherally acting mu-opioid receptor (PAM-OR) antagonist for the treatment of opioid-induced bowel dysfunction: results from a randomized, double-blind, placebo-controlled, dose-finding study in subjects taking opioids for chronic non-cancer pain, *Pain* 137(2):428–440, 2008.

65. Thomas J, Karver S, Cooney GA, Chamberlain BH, Watt CK, Slatkin NE, et al: Methylnaltrexone for opioid-induced constipation in advanced illness, *N Engl J Med* 358(22):2332–2343, 2008.

66. Driscoll CE: Symptom control in terminal illness, *Prim Care* 14(2):353–363, 1987.

67. Beckwith C: Diarrhea in Palliative Care Patients. In Lipmann A, Jackson IIK, Tylor L, editors: *Evidence based symptom control in palliative care*, New York, 2000, Pharmaceutical Products Press, pp 91–108.

68. Friedrichsdorf S, Wamsler C, Zernikow B: Diarrhö. In Zernikow B, editor: *Palliativversongung von Kindern, Jugendlichen und jungen Erwachsenen*, Heidelberg, 2008, Springer, pp 169–180.

69. Soares-Weiser K, Goldberg E, Tamimi G, Pitan OC, Leibovici L: Rotavirus vaccine for preventing diarrhea, *Cochrane Database Syst Rev* (1): CD002848, 2004.

70. Gryboski JD, Kocoshis S: Effect of bismuth subsalicylate on chronic diarrhea in childhood: a preliminary report, *Rev Infect Dis* 12(Suppl 1):S36–S40, 1990.

71. Twycross R, Wilcock A: *Hospice and Palliative Care Formulary USA*, ed 2, Nottingham, 2008, Palliativedrugs.com Ltd.

72. Ghisolfi J, Baudoin C, Charlet JP, Olives JP, Ghisolfi A, Thouvenot JP: [Effects of loperamide on fecal electrolyte excretion in acute diarrhea in infants], *Arch Fr Pediatr* 44(7):483–487, 1987.

73. Owens JR, Broadhead R, Hendrickse RG, Jaswal OP, Gangal RN: Loperamide in the treatment of acute gastroenteritis in early childhood. Report of a two centre, double-blind, controlled clinical trial, *Ann Trop Paediatr* 1(3):135–141, 1981.

74. Vesikari T, Isolauri E: A comparative trial of cholestyramine and loperamide for acute diarrhea in infants treated as outpatients, *Acta Paediatr Scand* 74(5):650–654, 1985.

75. Kaplan MA, Prior MJ, McKonly KI, DuPont HL, Temple AR, Nelson EB: A multicenter randomized controlled trial of a liquid loperamide product versus placebo in the treatment of acute diarrhea in children, *Clin Pediatr (Phila)* 38(10):579–591, 1999.

76. Turck D, Berard H, Fretault N, Lecomte JM: Comparison of racecadotril and loperamide in children with acute diarrhea, *Aliment Pharmacol Ther* (Suppl 6):27–32, 1999.

77. Karrar ZA, Abdulla MA, Moody JB, Macfarlane SB, Al Bwardy M, Hendrickse RG: Loperamide in acute diarrhea in childhood: results of a double blind, placebo controlled clinical trial, *Ann Trop Paediatr* 7(2):122–127, 1987.

78. Diarrhoeal Diseases Study Group (UK): Loperamide in acute diarrhea in childhood: results of a double blind, placebo controlled multicentre clinical trial, *Br Med J (Clin Res Ed)* 289(6454):1263–1267, 1984.

79. Rees H, Markley MA, Kiely EM, Pierro A, Pritchard J: Diarrhea after resection of advanced abdominal neuroblastoma: a common management problem, *Surgery* 123(5):568–572, 1998.

80. Heykants J, Michiels M, Knaeps A, Brugmans J: Loperamide (R 18 553), a novel type of antidiarrheal agent, *Arzneim-Forsch/Drug Res* 24:1649–1653, 1974.

81. Litovitz T, Clancy C, Korberly B, Temple AR, Mann KV: Surveillance of loperamide ingestions: an analysis of 216 poison center reports, *J Toxicol Clin Toxicol* 35(1):11–19, 1997.

82. Figueroa-Quintanilla D, Salazar-Lindo E, Sack RB, Leon-Barua R, Sarabia-Arce S, Campos-Sanchez M, et al: A controlled trial of bismuth subsalicylate in infants with acute watery diarrheal disease, *N Engl J Med* 328(23):1653–1658, 1993.

83. Soriano-Brucher H, Avendano P, O'Ryan M, Braun SD, Manhart MD, Balm TK, et al: Bismuth subsalicylate in the treatment of acute diarrhea in children: a clinical study, *Pediatrics* 87(1):18–27, 1991.

84. Gryboski JD, Hillemeier AC, Grill B, Kocoshis S: Bismuth subsalicylate in the treatment of chronic diarrhea of childhood, *Am J Gastroenterol* 80(11):871–876, 1985.

85. Hurwitz ES, Barrett MJ, Bregman D, Gunn WJ, Pinsky P, Schonberger LB, et al: Public Health Service study of Reye's syndrome and medications. Report of the main study, *JAMA*. 257(14):1905–1911, 1987.

86. Isolauri E, Vahasarja V, Vesikari T: Effect of cholestyramine on acute diarrhea in children receiving rapid oral rehydration and full feedings, *Ann Clin Res* 18(2):99–102, 1986.

87. Isolauri E, Vesikari T: Oral rehydration, rapid feeding, and cholestyramine for treatment of acute diarrhea, *J Pediatr Gastroenterol Nutr* 4(3):366–374, 1985.

88. Bujanover Y, Sullivan P, Liebman WM, Goodman J, Thaler MM: Cholestyramine treatment of chronic diarrhea associated with immune deficiency syndrome, *Clin Pediatr (Phila)* 18(10):630–633, 1979.

89. Coello-Ramirez P: [Cholestyramine in a case of a prolonged diarrhea after a partial ileocolectomy], *Bol Med Hosp Infant Mex* 34(2):325–328, 1977.

90. Kreutzer EW, Milligan FD: Treatment of antibiotic-associated pseudomembranous colitis with cholestyramine resin, *Johns Hopkins Med J* 143(3):67–72, 1978.

91. Liacouras CA, Piccoli DA: Whole-bowel irrigation as an adjunct to the treatment of chronic, relapsing *Clostridium difficile* colitis, *J Clin Gastroenterol* 22(3):186–189, 1996.

92. Beckman RA, Siden R, Yanik GA, Levine JE: Continuous octreotide infusion for the treatment of secretory diarrhea caused by acute

intestinal graft-versus-host disease in a child, *J Pediatr Hematol Oncol* 22(4):344–350, 2000.

93. Guarino A, Berni Canani R, Spagnuolo MI, Bisceglia M, Boccia MC, Rubino A: In vivo and in vitro efficacy of octreotide for treatment of enteric cryptosporidiosis, *Dig Dis Sci* 43(2):436–441, 1998.

94. Lamireau T, Galperine RI, Ohlbaum P, Demarquez JL, Vergnes P, Kurzenne Y, et al: Use of a long acting somatostatin analogue in controlling ileostomy diarrhea in infants, *Acta Paediatr Scand* 79 (8–9):871–872, 1990.

95. Smith SS, Shulman DI, O'Dorisio TM, McClenathan DT, Borger JA, Bercu BB, et al: Watery diarrhea, hypokalemia, achlorhydria syndrome in an infant: effect of the long-acting somatostatin analogue SMS 201–995 on the disease and linear growth, *J Pediatr Gastroenterol Nutr* 6(5): 710–716, 1987.

96. Evans WJ, Morley JE, Argiles J, Bales C, Baracos V, Guttridge D, et al: Cachexia: a new definition, *Clin Nutr* 27(6):793–799, 2008.

97. Goldman A, Hewitt M, Collins GS, Childs M, Hain R: Symptoms in children/young people with progressive malignant disease: United Kingdom Children's Cancer Study Group/Paediatric Oncology Nurses Forum survey, *Pediatrics* 117(6):e1179–e1186, 2006.

98. Inui A: Cancer anorexia-cachexia syndrome: current issues in research and management, *CA Cancer J Clin* 52(2):72–91, 2002.

99. Caglar K, Kutluk T, Varan A, Koray Z, Akyuz C, Yalcin B, et al: Leptin and neuropeptide Y plasma levels in children with cancer, *J Pediatr Endocrinol Metab* 18(5):485–489, 2005.

100. Mason P: Anorexia-cachexia: the condition and its causes, *Hospital Pharmacist* 14:249–253, 2007.

101. Inui A: [Feeding-related disorders in medicine, with special reference to cancer anorexia-cachexia syndrome], *Rinsho Byori* 54(10): 1044–1051, 2006.

102. Kotler DP: Cachexia, *Ann Intern Med* 133(8):622–634, 2000.

103. Bayram I, Erbey F, Celik N, Nelson JL, Tanyeli A: The use of a protein and energy dense eicosapentaenoic acid containing supplement for malignancy-related weight loss in children, *Pediatr Blood Cancer* 52(5):571–574, 2009.

104. Dewey A, Baughan C, Dean T, Higgins B, Johnson I: Eicosapentaenoic acid (EPA, an omega-3 fatty acid from fish oils) for the treatment of cancer cachexia, *Cochrane Database Syst Rev* (1): CD004597, 2007.

105. Tanca F, Madeddu C, Macciò A: New perspective on the nutritional approach to cancer-related anorexia/cachexia: preliminary results of a randomised phase III clinical trial with five different arms of treatment, *Mediterr J Nutr Metab* 2:29–36, 2009.

106. Berenstein EG, Ortiz Z: Megestrol acetate for the treatment of anorexia-cachexia syndrome, *Cochrane Database Syst Rev* (2): CD004310, 2005.

107. Azcona C, Castro L, Crespo E, Jimenez M, Sierrasesumaga L: Megestrol acetate therapy for anorexia and weight loss in children with malignant solid tumours, *Aliment Pharmacol Ther* 10(4):577–586, 1996.

108. Orme LM, Bond JD, Humphrey MS, Zacharin MR, Downie PA, Jamsen KM, et al: Megestrol acetate in pediatric oncology patients may lead to severe, symptomatic adrenal suppression, *Cancer* 98(2):397–405, 2003.

109. Meacham LR, Mazewski C, Krawiecki N: Mechanism of transient adrenal insufficiency with megestrol acetate treatment of cachexia in children with cancer, *J Pediatr Hematol Oncol* 25(5):414–417, 2003.

110. Marchand V, Baker SS, Stark TJ, Baker RD: Randomized, double-blind, placebo-controlled pilot trial of megestrol acetate in malnourished children with cystic fibrosis, *J Pediatr Gastroenterol Nutr* 31(3):264–269, 2000.

111. Eubanks V, Koppersmith N, Wooldridge N, Clancy JP, Lyrene R, Arani RB, et al: Effects of megestrol acetate on weight gain, body composition, and pulmonary function in patients with cystic fibrosis, *J Pediatr* 140(4):439–444, 2002.

112. Stockheim JA, Daaboul JJ, Yogev R, Scully SP, Binns HJ, Chadwick EG: Adrenal suppression in children with the human immunodeficiency virus treated with megestrol acetate, *J Pediatr* 134(3):368–370, 1999.

113. Couluris M, Mayer JL, Freyer DR, Sandler E, Xu P, Krischer JP: The effect of cyproheptadine hydrochloride (periactin) and megestrol acetate (megace) on weight in children with cancer/treatment-related cachexia, *J Pediatr Hematol Oncol* 30(11):791–797, 2008.

114. Pinto G, Brauner R, Goulet O, Clapin A, Blanche S: *Recombinant human growth hormone therapy for cachexia in HIV infected children*, Program Abstr 4th Conf Retrovir Oppor Infect Conf 1997. p. (abstract 690).

115. UKCCSG-PONF. *Mouth care for children and young people with cancer: Evidence-based guidelines*, Guideline report version 1.0 February 2006. 2006; Available from: http://www.cclg.org.uk/treatment and research/content.php?3id=28&2id=19 Last accessed June 15, 2010.

116. Eilers J, Berger AM, Petersen MC: Development, testing, and application of the oral assessment guide, *Oncol Nurs Forum* 15(3):325–330, 1988.

117. Worthington HV, Clarkson JE, Eden OB: Interventions for treating oral candidiasis for patients with cancer receiving treatment, *Cochrane Database Syst Rev* (2): CD001972, 2007.

118. Pienaar ED, Young T, Holmes H: Interventions for the prevention and management of oropharyngeal candidiasis associated with HIV infection in adults and children, *Cochrane Database Syst Rev* 3: CD003940, 2006.

119. Clarkson JE, Worthington HV, Eden OB: Interventions for treating oral mucositis for patients with cancer receiving treatment, *Cochrane Database Syst Rev* (2): CD001973, 2007.

120. Jassal S, editor: *Basic symptom control in paediatric palliative care—The Rainbows Children's Hospice Guidelines*, ed 7, 2008.

121. Deutsch M: The use of pilocarpine hydrochloride to prevent xerostomia in a child treated with high dose radiotherapy for nasopharynx carcinoma, *Oral Oncol* 34(5):381–382, 1998.

122. DeMatteo C, Matovich D, Hjartarson A: Comparison of clinical and videofluoroscopic evaluation of children with feeding and swallowing difficulties, *Dev Med Child Neurol* 47(3):149–157, 2005.

123. Arvedson JC: Assessment of pediatric dysphagia and feeding disorders: clinical and instrumental approaches, *Dev Disabil Res Rev* 14(2):118–127, 2008.

124. Weir K, McMahon S, Barry L, Masters IB, Chang AB: Clinical signs and symptoms of oropharyngeal aspiration and dysphagia in children, *Eur Respir J* 33(3):604–611, 2009.

125. *Care and communication: The role of the speech pathologist in palliative care—Infants and Children: Dysphagia.* Available from: www.latrobe.edu.au/careandcommunication/children.htm Last accessed June 15, 2010.

126. Marchand V, Motil KJ: Nutrition support for neurologically impaired children: a clinical report of the North American Society for Pediatric Gastroenterology, Hepatology, and Nutrition, *J Pediatr Gastroenterol Nutr* 43(1):123–135, 2006.

127. Scotland NQI: *Nasogastric and gastrostomy tube feeding for children being cared for in the community: best practice statement*, Edinburgh, 2003. Available from: www.nhshealthquality.org/nhsqis/394.html Last accessed June 15, 2010.

128. Naureckas SM, Christoffel KK: Nasogastric or gastrostomy feedings in children with neurologic disabilities, *Clin Pediatr (Phila)* 33(6):353–359, 1994.

129. Sleigh G, Sullivan PB, Thomas AG: Gastrostomy feeding versus oral feeding alone for children with cerebral palsy, *Cochrane Database Syst Rev* (2): CD003943, 2004.

130. Sleigh G, Brocklehurst P: Gastrostomy feeding in cerebral palsy: a systematic review, *Arch Dis Child* 89(6):534–539, 2004.

131. Sullivan PB, Morrice JS, Vernon-Roberts A, Grant H, Eltumi M, Thomas AG: Does gastrostomy tube feeding in children with cerebral palsy increase the risk of respiratory morbidity? *Arch Dis Child* 91(6):478–482, 2006.

132. Sullivan PB, Juszczak E, Bachlet AM, Thomas AG, Lambert B, Vernon-Roberts A, et al: Impact of gastrostomy tube feeding on the quality of life of carers of children with cerebral palsy, *Dev Med Child Neurol* 46(12):796–800, 2004.

133. Townsend JL, Craig G, Lawson M, Reilly S, Spitz L: Cost-effectiveness of gastrostomy placement for children with neurodevelopmental disability, *Arch Dis Child* 93(10):873–877, 2008.

134. Mahant S, Friedman JN, Connolly B, Goia C, Macarthur C: Tube feeding and quality of life in children with severe neurological impairment, *Arch Dis Child* 94(9):668–673, 2009.

135. Craig WR, Hanlon-Dearman A, Sinclair C, Taback S, Moffatt M: Metoclopramide, thickened feedings, and positioning for gastro-oesophageal reflux in children under two years, *Cochrane Database Syst Rev* (4): CD003502, 2004.

136. Huang RC, Forbes DA, Davies MW: Feed thickener for newborn infants with gastro-oesophageal reflux, *Cochrane Database Syst Rev* (3): CD003211, 2002.

137. Kaltenbach T, Crockett S, Gerson LB: Are lifestyle measures effective in patients with gastroesophageal reflux disease? An evidence-based approach, *Arch Intern Med* 166(9):965–971, 2006.

138. Vernon-Roberts A, Sullivan PB: Fundoplication versus post-operative medication for gastro-oesophageal reflux in children with neurological impairment undergoing gastrostomy, *Cochrane Database Syst Rev* (1): CD006151, 2007.

139. Esposito C, Montupet P, van Der Zee D, Settimi A, Paye-Jaouen A, Centonze A, et al: Long-term outcome of laparoscopic Nissen, Toupet, and Thal antireflux procedures for neurologically normal children with gastroesophageal reflux disease, *Surg Endosc* 20(6):855–858, 2006.

140. Rice H, Seashore JH, Touloukian RJ: Evaluation of Nissen fundoplication in neurologically impaired children, *J Pediatr Surg* 26(6):697–701, 1991.

141. Rothenberg SS: Experience with 220 consecutive laparoscopic Nissen fundoplications in infants and children, *J Pediatr Surg* 33(2):274–278, 1998.

142. Diaz DM, Gibbons TE, Heiss K, Wulkan ML, Ricketts RR, Gold BD: Antireflux surgery outcomes in pediatric gastroesophageal reflux disease, *Am J Gastroenterol* 100(8):1844–1852, 2005.

143. Chesney RW: A new form of Rickets during infancy: phosphate depletion-induced osteopenia due to antacid ingestion, *Arch Pediatr Adolesc Med* 152(12):1168–1169, 1998.

144. Tighe MP, Afzal NA, Bevan A, Beattie RM: Current pharmacological management of gastro-esophageal reflux in children: an evidence-based systematic review, *Paediatr Drugs* 11(3):185–202, 2009.

145. van Pinxteren B, Numans ME, Bonis PA, Lau J: Short-term treatment with proton pump inhibitors, H2-receptor antagonists and prokinetics for gastro-oesophageal reflux disease-like symptoms and endoscopy negative reflux disease, *Cochrane Database Syst Rev* 3: CD002095, 2006.

146. Gibbons TE, Gold BD: The use of proton pump inhibitors in children: a comprehensive review, *Paediatr Drugs* 5(1):25–40, 2003.

147. Hibbs AM, Lorch SA: Metoclopramide for the treatment of gastroesophageal reflux disease in infants: a systematic review, *Pediatrics* 118(2):746–752, 2006.

148. Wilkes G: *Hiccups*, 2009. Available from: http://emedicine.medscape.com/article/775746-overview. Last accessed June 15, 2010.

149. Karwacki MW: Gastrointestinal symptoms—Hiccup. In Goldman A, Hain R, Liben S, editors: *Oxford textbook of palliative care for children*, Oxford, 2003, Oxford University Press, p 361.

150. Walker P, Watanabe S, Bruera E: Baclofen, a treatment for chronic hiccup, *J Pain Symptom Manage* 16(2):125–132, 1998.

151. Smith HS, Busracamwongs A: Management of hiccups in the palliative care population, *Am J Hosp Palliat Care* 20(2):149–154, 2003.

152. Porzio G, Aielli F, Narducci F, Varrassi G, Ricevuto E, Ficorella C, et al: Hiccup in patients with advanced cancer successfully treated with gabapentin: report of three cases, *N Z Med J* 116(1182):U605, 2003.

153. Tegeler ML, Baumrucker SJ: Gabapentin for intractable hiccups in palliative care, *Am J Hosp Palliat Care* 25(1):52–54, 2008.

154. Ripamonti C, Twycross R, Baines M, Bozzetti F, Capri S, De Conno F, et al: Clinical-practice recommendations for the management of bowel obstruction in patients with end-stage cancer, *Support Care Cancer* 9(4):223–233, 2001.

155. Spears H, Petrelli NJ, Herrera L, Mittelman A: Treatment of bowel obstruction after operation for colorectal carcinoma, *Am J Surg* 155(3):383–386, 1988.

156. Mercadante S: Bowel obstruction in home-care cancer patients: 4 years experience, *Support Care Cancer* 3(3):190–193, 1995.

157. Maglinte DD, Reyes BL, Harmon BH, Kelvin FM, Turner WW Jr, Hage JE, et al: Reliability and role of plain film radiography and CT in the diagnosis of small-bowel obstruction, *AJR Am J Roentgenol* 167(6):1451–1455, 1996.

158. Abbas S, Bissett IP, Parry BR: Oral water soluble contrast for the management of adhesive small bowel obstruction, *Cochrane Database Syst Rev* (3): CD004651, 2007.

159. Regnard C, Hockley J: Other Symptoms—Bowel obstruction. In Regnard C, Hockley J, editors: *A guide to symptom relief in palliative care*, ed 5, Oxford, 2003, Radcliffe Medical Press, pp 71–74.

160. Feuer DJ, Broadley KE: Systematic review and meta-analysis of corticosteroids for the resolution of malignant bowel obstruction in advanced gynaecological and gastrointestinal cancers. Systematic Review Steering Committee, *Ann Oncol* 10(9):1035–1041, 1999.

161. Mercadante S, Casuccio A, Mangione S: Medical treatment for inoperable malignant bowel obstruction: a qualitative systematic review, *J Pain Symptom Manage* 33(2):217–223, 2007.

162. Glass RL, LeDuc RJ: Small intestinal obstruction from peritoneal carcinomatosis, *Am J Surg* 125(3):316–317, 1973.

163. Bizer LS, Liebling RW, Delany HM, Gliedman ML: Small bowel obstruction: the role of nonoperative treatment in simple intestinal obstruction and predictive criteria for strangulation obstruction, *Surgery* 89(4):407–413, 1981.

164. Malone JM Jr, Koonce T, Larson DM, Freedman RS, Carrasco CH, Saul PB: Palliation of small bowel obstruction by percutaneous gastrostomy in patients with progressive ovarian carcinoma, *Obstet Gynecol* 68(3):431–433, 1986.

165. Feuer DJ, Broadley KE, Shepherd JH, Barton DP: Surgery for the resolution of symptoms in malignant bowel obstruction in advanced gynaecological and gastrointestinal cancer, *Cochrane Database Syst Rev* (4): CD002764, 2000.

166. Mercadante S: The role of octreotide in palliative care, *J Pain Symptom Manage* 9(6):406–411, 1994.

167. Buck ML: *Octreotide for the management of chylothorax in infants and children*, Pediatr Pharm 2004; 10(10) Available from: http://www.healthsystem.virginia.edu/internet/pediatrics/education/pharm-news.cfm Last accessed June 15, 2010.

168. Ohlbaum P, Galperine RI, Demarquez JL, Vergnes P, Martin C: Use of a long-acting somatostatin analogue (SMS 201–995) in controlling a significant ileal output in a 5-year-old child, *J Pediatr Gastroenterol Nutr* 6(3):466–470, 1987.

169. Couper RT, Berzen A, Berall G, Sherman PM: Clinical response to the long acting somatostatin analogue SMS 201–995 in a child with congenital microvillus atrophy, *Gut* 30(7):1020–1024, 1989.

170. Wallace AM, Newman K: Successful closure of intestinal fistulae in an infant using the somatostatin analogue SMS 201–995, *J Pediatr Surg* 26(9):1097–1100, 1991.

171. Totapally BR, Copaescu GM, Glover ML: Use of octreotide in children with bleeding from esophageal varices, *J Pediatr Gastroenterol Nutr* 26(5):585, 1998.

172. Zellos A, Schwarz KB: Efficacy of octreotide in children with chronic gastrointestinal bleeding, *J Pediatr Gastroenterol Nutr* 30(4):442–446, 2000.

173. Rath S, Bar-Zeev N, Anderson K, Fahy R, Roseby R: Octreotide in children with hypoglycaemia due to sulfonylurea ingestion, *J Paediatr Child Health* 44(6):383–384, 2008.

174. Watanabe H, Inoue Y, Uchida K, Okugawa Y, Hiro J, Ojima E, et al: Octreotide improved the quality of life in a child with malignant bowel obstruction caused by peritoneal dissemination of colon cancer, *J Pediatr Surg* 42(1):259–260, 2007.

175. Schell D, Chin C, Chin R, editors: *Drug doses for children*, ed 2, Sydney, 2005, The Children's Hospital at Westmead, p 34.

176. Siden H, Tucker T, Derman S, Cox K, Soon GS, Hartnett C, et al: Pediatric enteral feeding intolerance: a new prognosticator for children with life-limiting illness? *J Palliat Care* Autumn 25(3):213–217, 2009.

177. Zangen T, Ciarla C, Zangen S, Di Lorenzo C, Flores AF, Cocjin J, et al: Gastrointestinal motility and sensory abnormalities may contribute to food refusal in medically fragile toddlers, *J Pediatr Gastroenterol Nutr* 37(3):287–293, 2003.

178. *Children's Hospitals and Clinics of Minnesota Health Care Ethics Committee: Statement on Forgoing Medically Provided Nutrition and Hydration*, 1998.

179. Schell D, Chin C, Chin R, editors: *Drug doses for children*, ed 2, Sydney, 2005, The Children's Hospital at Westmead, p 26.

34 Hematologic Symptoms

MARY ELIZABETH ROSS | PEDRO A. DE ALARCÓN

Request

You, in white

who maintains the healthy attitude,

Respond to my mood.

Persevere the facts,

Chart efficiently,

But don't discard feeling from a patient's history.

A sentimental phrase

or a known truth

solemnly spoken

is not required or desired.

Just feel

outwardly.

You see,

symptoms and contraindications

make dreadful memories

relieved when recalled.

A slow, soft eye-blink,

thoughtful, unhurried pauses—

lips pursed in silence—

Evoked responses, unsuppressed,

become meanings most cherished,

for they are evidence

of empathy—

(and) human understanding. —Karen Godecke

Many patients develop hematologic symptoms requiring medical intervention. As suggested in the poem, the manner in which we go about attending to these symptoms can be as important as relief of the symptoms. From a pathophysiology standpoint, patients fall into two general categories: those who are symptomatic as a result of a primary hematologic disorder, and those with hematologic symptoms secondary to an underlying disease or treatment for the disease, such as cancer. Broad categories of hematologic symptoms include anemia, thrombocytopenia, neutropenia, bleeding disorders, and thrombosis. In this chapter, we address anemia, thrombocytopenia, and bleeding disorders.

Anemia

PRIMARY ANEMIA

Primary anemias result from production of red blood cells that have a structural defect, leading to increased red cell destruction such as in sickle cell anemia, beta-thalassemia, and others (Box 34-1). Primary anemias are no longer strictly childhood illnesses. The ability to replace defective red blood cells with transfusion or partial exchange transfusion has revolutionized the care of these children, extending life expectancy well into the sixth decade or beyond. As these diseases have been converted into chronic illnesses, patients suffering from these diseases are rarely included in the dialogue of palliative care.

Frequent transfusions have brought new challenges to the care of children and young adults affected by primary anemias. During the 1980s and 1990s, blood-borne infection with Hepatitis B and C, and HIV infected many people who received transfusions due to primary anemia. Although the risk of transfusion-associated infection is now decreased to approximately 1 in 2 million transfusions,[1,2] relieving symptoms of primary anemia continues to carry a significant cost in the form of iron overload. The deposits of iron in tissues, especially the liver and heart, ultimately compromises end-organ function leading to heart failure and death. Development and clinical use of first intravenous and more recently oral iron chelators are once again revolutionizing delivery of care to patients with primary anemia. Nonetheless, significant challenges and opportunities for improving palliative care to this often overlooked population remain. David Nathan has written a poignant description of one patient's journey navigating the waves of innovation in care for patients with thalassemia. He discusses the burdens of subcutaneous desferoxamine infusion and how much his patient hated it, to the extent of refusing to take the desferoxamine. That decision resulted in repeated episodes of heart failure. Dr. Nathan talks about the development of the oral chelator, desferisirox and the positive impact on quality of life for his patient to be free of the iron-chelator infusion pump.[3]

SECONDARY ANEMIA

The most common cause of secondary anemia is exposure to marrow-suppressive chemotherapy and radiation therapy in the course of treatment for childhood cancer. Overall survival for childhood cancer has improved significantly during the past 30 years and is 80%.[4] Cure rates of some childhood cancers, such as low-risk acute lymphoblastic leukemia (ALL), Hodgkin Lymphoma, and low stage Wilms tumor are 95 percent or better.[4] However, many chemotherapeutic agents used in the treatment of childhood cancers have bone marrow suppression or transient bone marrow aplasia as a side effect. Children receiving intensive chemotherapy are frequently at risk for development of anemia, bleeding, and infection. For many modern chemotherapy regimens, transfusions of packed red blood cells (pRBC) and apheresed platelets are an integral and anticipated component of supportive care.

BOX 34-1 Common Causes of Anemia

Primary

- Sickle cell disease, Hemoglobin SS, SC, S thalassemia
- Thalassemia
- Pyruvate kinase deficiency
- Hereditary spherocytosis
- Hereditary elliptocytosis
- Diamond-Blackfan anemia
- Glucose-6-dehydrogenase deficiency

Secondary

Lack of production

- Bone marrow failure syndromes, Fanconi anemia, aplastic anemia
- Bone marrow failure due to previous and/or concurrent cytotoxic drugs and/or radiation therapy
- Encroachment of marrow space with tumor
- Bone overgrowth, osteopetrosis
- Lack of marrow due to immobility, nonweight bearing
- Nutritional deficiencies including iron, folic acid, vitamin B_{12}, protein
- Anemia of chronic disease, including suppressive cytokines
- Infectious myelosuppression, most characteristically parvovirus
- Erythropoietin deficiency, such as renal failure

Increased loss and/or destruction:

- Acute and/or chronic hemorrhage due to primary disease
- Hemolysis
- Acquired antibodies from transfused products
- Autoimmune antibodies
- Hepatorenal failure
- Hemophagocytosis
- Drug induced

BOX 34-2 Symptoms of Anemia

- Pallor
- Difficulty feeding
- Decreased appetite
- Fussiness in infants and toddlers
- Irritability
- Increased number of hours spent sleeping
- Fatigue
- Tachycardia
- Headache
- Increased awareness of heartbeat
- Lightheadedness on sitting or standing quickly
- Orthostatic hypotension
- Hypotension
- Poor tissue oxygenation
- Cardiomegaly
- Decreased urine output
- Muscle weakness

Progressive or recurrent malignancy may be accompanied by even greater bone marrow insufficiency as a result of cumulative toxicity to the bone marrow. Extreme cases may result in therapy-associated bone marrow aplasia. Cancer progression may result in marrow space infiltration by tumor. Both bone marrow aplasia and marrow infiltration can result in increased transfusion frequency.

In contrast, children receiving palliative care for medical conditions other than cancer may have a completely different etiology for anemia. An immobile child with neurologic deficits may also be anemic. Absence of weight-bearing activity weakens bones and leads to fatty replacement of bone marrow. These children may have deficiencies of iron, folic acid, or biotin, which can lead to anemia. In this situation, transfusion is rarely required. Appropriate steps should be taken to detect and to the extent possible, correct the underlying cause of anemia.

SYMPTOMS ASSOCIATED WITH ANEMIA

Fatigue during treatment for malignancy, in part related to anemia, is the most frequently reported symptom for adults with cancer. A survey of major pediatric hematology-oncology centers in Europe documented more than 80 percent of children with cancer as being anemic.[5] For children, symptoms related to anemia can extend far beyond a complaint of fatigue (Box 34-2). Children manifest different symptoms of anemia in different age groups. Many young school-age and toddler-age children appear very active and apparently feel well with moderate anemia where hemoglobin is in the 8 g/dL range. For infants and toddlers, symptomatic anemia may be expressed by a decreased ability to nurse, take a bottle, or eat. Many a mother has made the simple statement that their infant or toddler "probably needs to be transfused" because the child

just isn't eating as well as usual. Administration of a transfusion can be the difference between a child who is able to eat consistently with his or her personal baseline and one who is not eating well. For other children, anemia may be recognized by longer nap times, change in temperament or limitations in ability to engage in activities or play. All of these are important issues of quality of life for families of children with life-threatening illness, whether they are pursuing curative therapy or during terminal care.

Teenagers are more likely to present with classic symptoms associated with anemia. While fatigue, or need for increased hours of sleep may be a part of their symptoms, they may also experience headaches, fast heart rate, feeling like their heart is pounding, or lightheadedness when rising to sit or stand. For teens, symptoms related to anemia can be apparent when the hemoglobin drops below 9 gm/dL, a level where younger children are often apparently asymptomatic. Other parameters that affect symptoms from anemia include:

- How quickly the anemia has developed,
- Whether a person is beginning therapy or has experienced multiple cycles of chemotherapy,
- Anticipated time to recovery of adequate marrow function to resolve the anemia,
- Which chemotherapeutic agents have been administered,
- Psychosocial context such as whether the child is well enough to attend school or participate in social functions important to them.

As with secondary anemias, symptoms of primary anemia are varied. Fatigue, tiredness, increased requirements for sleep, and decreased tolerance for activity are common. However, children who are chronically anemic have a lower threshold hemoglobin for symptoms. Sequelae of uncorrected severe chronic anemia include cardiomegaly, progressive decrease in exercise endurance, congestive heart failure, growth abnormalities, and pulmonary hypertension. Patients with uncorrected β-thalassemia major suffer bone deformities and massive hepatosplenomegaly from ineffective hematopoiesis. Those with sickle cell disease suffer avascular osteonecrosis, and can suffer debilitating central nervous system ischemia or acute chest syndrome as consequence of vasocclusion from deformed red blood cells.

DIAGNOSTIC EVALUATION

Hemoglobinopathies are frequently identified because of presence of family history or newborn screening. However, some defects of red cell structure, such as hereditary spherocytosis, may cause sufficiently mild anemia to go undetected into adulthood in otherwise healthy parents. Diagnostic evaluation includes a thorough patient and family history, physical exam, examination of the blood smear, hemoglobin electrophoresis, evaluation of nutritional status, and osmotic fragility studies to name the most frequently used tests. A detailed diagnostic algorithm is beyond the scope of this text. Readers are referred to other resources such as *Practical Algorithms in Pediatric Hematology and Oncology* for more information.[6]

For patients experiencing secondary anemia, the depth to which a diagnostic evaluation is pursued is dependent upon where the child is in their illness trajectory. A child who develops anemia from a chemotherapy regimen that is known to be myelosuppressive may not need any further evaluation. However, it is appropriate to pursue more aggressive diagnostic evaluation of a child with anemia greater than anticipated for the chemotherapeutic regimen used. Conversely, the cause of worsening anemia for a child receiving terminal care may be of minimal relevance. Foregoing further evaluation may be appropriate when the focus of care is on provision of relief from symptoms no matter the cause.

Guidelines for Transfusion

PRIMARY ANEMIA

The most recent recommendations for medical management of sickle cell disease are available from the National Heart, Lung, and Blood Institute of the National Institutes of Health (NIH).[7] General indications for transfusion of children with sickle cell anemia include hemoglobin less than 5 to 6 g/dL, development of acute chest syndrome, aplastic crisis, preoperative prophylaxis, or to resolve protracted pain crises. Similarly, transfusion goals for patients with β-thalassemia major is to maintain a hemoglobin in the range of 9 to 9.5 g/dL.[8,9]

SECONDARY ANEMIA

Several transfusion guidelines exist.[8,9] While many centers use a guideline of hemoglobin less than 7 to 8 g/dL as a parameter for transfusion, the ultimate indication for transfusion is a symptomatic patient who is unlikely to correct the anemia in a timely manner without medical intervention. Symptoms of anemia include: tachycardia, tiredness, orthostatic hypotension, increased fatigue, and sleeping more hours per day (see Box 34-2).

Specifications of the Product

Leukoreduced ABO and D blood group appropriate and cross-matched pRBC are used in primary as well as secondary anemia to decrease alloimmunization and febrile transfusion reactions. Contaminating white blood cells, especially lymphocytes, are responsible for the majority of allergic transfusion reactions. Leukocyte reduction can be achieved either during processing soon after collection of the product or before administration to a patient. The American Association of Blood Bank Standards requires leukoreduced units to have less than 5 million leukocytes per unit.[10] Packed RBC for immunocompromised individuals should be leukoreduced. In some geographic regions, blood banks provide exclusively leukoreduced red cells or platelets.

PRIMARY ANEMIA

Extensive transfusion exposure in this largely immunocompetent population leads to alloimmunization and development of antibodies to minor blood group antigens. The blood bank should be made aware of the primary anemia history, blood transfusion history, and the need for more extensive blood antigen typing, such as E, C, Kell, and Duffy. As children with primary anemias receive increased numbers of transfusions, finding an appropriate donor unit becomes more challenging. Alloimmunization and iron overload are two of the reasons efforts are made to minimize transfusions in children with sickle cell disease. Children and teens with sickle cell disease should receive sickle negative blood so that determinations of hemoglobin S are solely reflective of the patient and can be used to reliably guide management of exchange transfusion. Because patients with primary anemias are in large part immunologically intact, there is less concern about transfusion associated graft-versus-host disease GVHD. Therefore, irradiation of pRBC is not routinely used. However, irradiation of blood products should be considered for primary anemia patients who are candidates for stem cell transplantation in the near future.

SECONDARY ANEMIA

Neonates and CMV negative immunocompromised recipients are at risk for blood-borne transmission of cytomegalovirus (CMV). While leukoreduction decreases the risk of transmission of CMV, pRBC from CMV-negative donors are recommended for these most vulnerable patients.

Even with leukoreduction, small T lymphocytes, which have a diameter similar to erythrocytes, can pass through the filter and ultimately into the recipient. These lymphocytes have the potential in immunocompromised individuals to cause GVHD.[11] To prevent transfusion-associated GVHD, pRBC are irradiated at 25 to 50 Gy.[10] In large urban areas, hospital blood banks have their own blood product irradiators. Smaller urban areas may rely on a single unit centrally located at the local Red Cross Center. More rural areas may have to special order irradiated units from distant Red Cross Centers, creating a delay in availability of the product of hours to days.

To raise the hemoglobin 1 gm/dL requires 3 to 5 mL/kg pRBC. For a child with hemoglobin in the range of 7 to 9 g/dL, a reasonable transfusion is 10 to 15 mL/kg. This volume of pRBC should be administered over 2 to 4 hours. Repeat transfusions may be required to adequately improve hemoglobin levels for children with poor red cell production or ongoing red cell destruction. For more profound anemia, or for a patient with chronic anemia, transfusion of smaller aliquots of 5 mL/kg pRBC each transfused over 4 hours may help prevent development of congestive heart failure.

Transfusion Side Effects

ACUTE

The most common complications of transfusions include fluid overload, allergic reaction including hives and bronchospasm, febrile reactions, and hemolysis. Patients who are particularly sensitive to fluid loading may require diuresis during or after transfusion to maintain a good fluid homeostasis. Administration of furosemide 0.5 to 1.0 mg/kg immediately following a transfusion is frequently effective.

Minor allergic reactions vary from appearance of few to abundant hives. Minor allergic reactions usually respond quickly to 0.5 to 1 mg/kg diphenhydramine administered intravenously or orally. Alternatively, hydroxyzine 0.5 to 1 mg/kg intravenously or 2 mg/kg orally can be used. Allergic reactions leading to shortness of breath and bronchospasm are more common with transfusion of platelet products, due to the greater volume of donor plasma, which contains antibodies. Anaphylaxis may require administration of hydrocortisone 1 to 5 mg/kg/day intravenously or, in severe cases, epinephrine according to resuscitation protocols. Patients with a history of allergic reaction may do better with prophylactic diphenhydramine or hydroxyzine before transfusion.[7] Washing pRBC may lessen the amount of plasma in the product, decreasing allergic and hemolytic reactions, at the cost of also decreasing the number of RBC in the unit. The most severe form of allergic reaction is transfusion-related acute lung injury (TRALI), which occurs during or immediately after transfusion and is characterized by difficulty breathing and pulmonary infiltrates on chest x-ray. Patients experiencing TRALI may require intubation and ventilator support.

Profoundly neutropenic patients who develop febrile reactions during a transfusion are generally committed to a minimum of 24 to 48 hours of intravenous antibiotic therapy, until it is clear the fever is not due to bacterial contamination of the product or other bacterial infection in the patient. Culturing the transfusion product bag is ideal. In practice though, febrile reactions often occur after completion of the transfusion, at which point the product bag has been discarded. Many clinicians have reasoned that administration of prophylactic acetaminophen should decrease the febrile inflammatory response to the blood product. If we could decrease the incidence of febrile transfusion reaction, we may be able to spare immunocompromised patients from hospital admission and empiric antibiotics. However, several studies have failed to demonstrate benefit.[12,13] Therefore, routinely administering acetaminophen before transfusion is not recommended unless the child has a personal history of transfusion reaction.

Hemolytic transfusion reactions can also start with fever accompanied by abdominal or flank pain. Patients may experience a general sense of feeling unwell or agitation. Tea-colored or cola-colored urine is a supportive finding of intravascular hemolysis. The product infusion should be stopped and returned to the blood bank with new patient samples so evaluation for a hemolytic reaction can be pursued. Routine blood counts demonstrate a decreased hemoglobin. Other supporting laboratory studies include increased haptoglobin levels. Urinalysis may demonstrate urine hemoglobin in the absence of red blood cells. When these symptoms occur in a patient with sickle cell disease, it can be challenging to sort out the presence of a hemolytic transfusion reaction from underlying pathophysiology of hemolysis due to vaso-occlusive crisis. The hallmark of a transfusion reaction is that the patient becomes Coombs positive. Additionally, patients with sickle cell disease can experience delayed transfusion reactions with a fall in hemoglobin below their personal baseline days to weeks after a transfusion. Adding to the challenge of managing these patients is that both acute and chronic transfusion reactions can precipitate an acute vaso-occlusive pain crisis or acute chest syndrome.[7]

Because of the potential for a variety of transfusion-associated reactions, patients receiving supportive care for primary anemia or those with secondary anemia who are still pursing curative therapy should receive transfusions in a setting that can provide infusion services and respond in a timely manner to any transfusion reactions. This generally means an inpatient setting or outpatient infusion clinic.

CHRONIC

Other adverse events associated with transfusions include transmission of infectious agents, particularly viruses. Risks of known viral infectious agents such as hepatitis B, hepatitis C, and HIV are approximately 1 in 2 million units.[1,2]

Those who are regularly transfused, especially for primary anemia, battle with chronic complications of transfusion. For adults transfused pre-1990, transfusion-acquired viral infection may add additional complexity to their healthcare. Teenagers and young adults with extensive transfusion histories may develop extensive alloimmunization that makes finding an appropriately matched unit challenging. The incidence of alloimmunization in patients with sickle cell disease is 25%, higher than the general population.[7] The higher incidence of alloimmunization is due in part to the difference in surface expression of red cell antigens between sickle cell patients who are predominantly African American and blood donors, who are predominantly Caucasian.[14] Additionally, alloimmunization makes allergic, acute, and chronic hemolytic transfusion reactions much more frequent in this population than in children receiving transfusions for chemotherapy-induced anemia.

For children and young adults with any primary anemia who receive frequent pRBC transfusions, the major complication is from iron overload. Iron deposition leads to end organ dysfunction, particularly in the heart and liver. Patients receiving regular transfusions should be monitored closely for elevated ferritin levels, our closest noninvasive surrogate measure for assessing iron deposition in tissue. Other noninvasive measures, such as cardiac and liver MRI to measure organ iron loads, are under investigation. Introduction of desferoxamine, an iron chelator, revolutionized care of patients with thalassemia and sickle cell anemia.[15] However, desferoxamine must be administered intravenously or through subcutaneous injections or subcutaneous continuous infusion. These methods are cumbersome and problematic for many patients. Administration of desferoxamine was identified as a source of discomfort and decreased quality of life in several studies.[16–18] Nearly 50% of patients identified iron chelator injections as the most disliked component of therapy. More than 40% identified missed work or school as a quality of life issue whether receiving transfusions or not.[16] In one study, quality of life measures were higher for Malaysian patients with β-thalassemia who were receiving optimal desferoxamine regimens compared with patients receiving suboptimal desferoxamine.[18] Healthcare providers would identify frequent transfusions with a greater medical burden as compared with transfusion independence. One study used the Dartmouth primary care cooperative information chart system (COOP) questionnaire found reported complaints of moderate pain in both transfused and nontransfused patients. Interestingly, 27% of transfused patients reported moderately impaired overall health versus 42% of transfusion independent patients.[17] Additionally, physical fitness and better performance of daily activities were reported by patients receiving regular transfusions. Despite the complication of iron overload, regular transfusions appear to improve the quality of life in at least some populations of patients with primary anemia.

INTERDISCIPLINARY TEAM CONSIDERATIONS

Each institution has its own policy regarding infusion of blood components, though there are common themes. Some issues relate to safety of administration, including confirmation of appropriate blood type of unit to be transfused, confirmation of identity of recipient, appropriateness of intravenous access and frequent monitoring for signs of transfusion reaction. For details on infusion protocols, the reader is referred to their institutional transfusion policy and *Essentials of Pediatric Oncology Nursing*.[19] Nurses contribute to team assessment of the patient's and family's religious or cultural beliefs, which may affect transfusion administration. Nurses also have an important ongoing role in educating patients and families with regard to symptoms of anemia, what to expect from a transfusion, and signs of transfusion reactions. Some individuals have very strong visceral reactions to the sight of blood, whether their own or someone else's. In the context of blood transfusion, both nursing and child life specialists have helped address these concerns by finding creative ways to disguise transfusions, such as decorating a pillowcase to cover the pRBC bag.

Alternatives to Transfusion

Erythropoietin is produced by the kidney in response to anemia. Hematopoietic stem cells differentiate along the erythroid lineage in response to erythropoietin. Erythropoietin was first licensed in 1989 for treatment of anemia associated with chronic renal failure. There are two erythropoietin formulations, epoetin alpha is marketed by Amgen as Epogen and by Ortho Biotech as Procrit. Epoetin alpha is administered 2 to 3 times a week. The second formulation, Darbepoetin, is longer acting and is marketed by Amgen as Aranesp. These agents are frequently used in adults receiving chemotherapy. In fact they have become the first and second ranked expenditures for individual drugs by Medicare Part B. However, recent studies have led to FDA warnings about increased thromboembolic events and increased risk for cardiovascular events.[20] Poorer survival in some studies where epoetin was used has again raised questions about whether epoetin may be a growth factor for some types of cancer. The American Society of Hematology/American Society of Clinical Oncology clinical practice update cautions against the use of epoetins in patients with malignancy who are not receiving either chemotherapy or radiation therapy.[21]

There are fewer randomized studies using erythropoietin in pediatric cancer patients. Epoetin alpha has been shown to be well tolerated by pediatric oncology patients and results in increased hemoglobin levels.[22,23] However, results differed with respect to affecting the number of transfusions administered or quality of life parameters. In one study of patients with solid tumors receiving platinum-based chemotherapy regimens, epoetin alpha decreased transfusion requirements.[22] Another study reported 224 patients receiving chemotherapy for nonmyeloid malignancy who were randomized to receive either epoetin alpha or placebo. The group receiving epoetin alpha had greater improvement in hemoglobin and a higher percentage of the patients were independent of transfusions at 4 weeks. Pediatric Quality of Life Inventory Generic Core Scales (PedsQL-GCS) did not differ between treatment groups.[23] However, further analysis demonstrated correlation between PedsQL-GCS and improved hemoglobin.[24] Use of epoetin alpha in combination with granulocyte colony stimulating factor (G-CSF) for children with high-risk neuroblastoma resulted in an increased number of transfusions compared with patients in the control group receiving G-CSF without epoetin alpha.[25] After reviewing these studies and others, the French National Cancer Institute's evidenced-based practice guideline does not recommend systematic administration of erythropoietin for prevention of chemotherapy associated anemia in children with cancer.[26]

Although FDA warnings and mixed results in pediatric oncology studies raise concerns, erythropoietin may be useful for patients who object to blood transfusions on ethical or religious grounds, as do many of the Jehovah's Witness faith.[5] Indeed, patients of the Jehovah's Witness faith have taught us that much more severe anemia can be tolerated than was initially supposed.[27–31] Additionally, they have helped drive the interest in development of blood conservation programs and blood alternatives. Blood alternatives such as human and bovine hemoglobin based oxygen carriers (HBOC), which are acellular cross-linked hemoglobin molecules, have been described as bridging the gap between life-threatening anemia and recovery of normal red cell mass after trauma.[32] These products are in clinical trials in Africa and other countries. As yet, none are available for clinical use in the United States, but may have a future role in palliation of anemia.

Caring for patients of the Jehovah's Witness faith who refuse transfusion may cause ethical conflicts for medical personnel who feel strongly that transfusion is medically indicated.[33] The moral distress caused by discordance between the values and goals of the medical staff and the values and goals of the patient can be destructive to delivery of patient-centered care as well as to the medical team striving to provide care. It can take considerable emotional and ethical work for the team to honor a patient's autonomy and freedom to refuse specific treatments without destroying staff-patient or staff-staff relationships. At times it may be necessary to use the experience and expertise of resources such as patient advocates, the hospital ethics committee, and human resources for the staff.

In sickle cell anemia, administration of hydroxyurea switches on production of fetal hemoglobin, decreasing percentage of hemoglobin S. Some patients experience a significant decrease in acute vaso-occlusive and acute chest syndrome episodes, therefore decreasing the need for transfusion.[7]

BLOOD CONSERVATION STRATEGIES

While not strictly an alternative to transfusion, attention paid to limiting iatrogenic blood loss can decrease the frequency of transfusion. Whenever blood is drawn from a heparin-locked venous access device, be it Broviac, Hickman, Mediport, or another, that is heparin locked, 3 to 10 mL of blood and heparin mixture are drawn out and discarded to prevent dilution of the blood sample, leading to erroneous laboratory results. Relatively simple maneuvers, such as making sure to draw all desired blood tests at one time rather than at different times throughout the day, may minimize that discard volume. Frequent blood tests such as CBC and chemistries can become more a matter of routine than medical management. Careful consideration of the frequency of laboratory studies needed to manage a patient may also result in significant decreases in blood loss. Obtaining finger-stick or venopuncture blood samples, when the central line is not going to be accessed that day for any other reason decreases blood loss by eliminating the need for a waste volume. Use of smaller-volume microtainer tubes can similarly result in a savings of 2 to 9 mL of blood per blood test. These measures can result in decreased transfusion needs in small children. Indeed, many NICUs have implemented blood-conservation strategies. These measures are less routine for chemotherapy infusion, but are worth consideration when limiting the number of transfusions is an important goal for the individual patient.

DONOR DIRECTED TRANSFUSIONS

Faced with their child's need for transfusions, many families inquire about having blood provided by family donors or friends of the family. It is often useful to check the motivation behind the request. For some it is a fear of unknown donors and potential transmission of infection. For others it is a way for extended family to do something useful during a crisis. It is often sufficient to educate them with regard to general issues such as the need for blood types to match, the safety of the blood supply, and the need for complete testing even when the blood donation is directed. Additionally, there are many situations where family members are not the ideal donors or may even increase the chance for complications for the child.

The ideal donation scenario for family members to fully meet the transfusion needs of the child would be where infrequent transfusions were required, and the transfusions can be anticipated days if not weeks ahead. When donated blood is directed to a specific recipient, the blood bank has an increased administrative burden tracking and storing the blood. The Red Cross does have procedures in place to meet this need. A direct donation unit is still required to undergo thorough testing and processing, which takes days. Direct donation for urgent and emergent transfusion is often technically challenging due to the time required for processing.

For patients with primary anemia, family members are often not suitable donors. For example, in sickle cell anemia each parent has at least sickle trait, if not sickle cell disease themselves. This makes the parents and most siblings an inappropriate candidate for directed donation. Similarly, the frequency of transfusions for children with primary anemias can be more often than an individual is allowed to make blood donations. Additionally, the physical demands of frequent blood donation may put additional burden on a family already under stress simply from caring for an ill child.

Families of children diagnosed with cancer also often inquire about direct donation. Here, too, the frequency of required transfusions is generally too often for any one parent

or family member to safely donate. For patients with either malignant disorders or with primary hematologic failure disorders who are candidates for hematopoietic stem cell transplantation (HCST), transfusions from family members are strongly discouraged. Siblings and, in some cases, parents are potential HSCT donors. Family-member blood transfusions before HSCT sensitize the patient to minor histocompatibility antigens, which increases the risk of graft failure. Similarly, because of shared histocompatibility antigen, related donor transfusions carry a risk of inducing transfusion associated graft versus host disease even in immunocompetent individuals. Therefore, all transfusions from a donor related to the recipient must be irradiated, adding cost to the transfusion. Finally, due to the emotional incentives for family and friends to donate for a specific patient, there may be a higher risk of transfusion-related infections than from a blood bank unit. A safer product is likely to come from a donor who has donated multiple times and therefore been frequently screened.[34]

Many friends and family do want to donate blood in an effort to help. Once the reasons why those donations should not be designated for a specific patient, it is prudent to encourage friends and family to donate blood without specifying a recipient. In this way the precious resources can be built up and donors receive a sense of having helped someone in need. In fact, having a blood drive is an often-employed way for a community group to show support for a community member fighting illness.

Palliative Care Considerations in Secondary Anemia

I'm not afraid of dying, I'm afraid of not living.
—KERRI COSTELLO

Despite the incredible improvement in disease-free survival achieved with modern chemotherapy and multimodality treatment, nearly 20% of all children diagnosed with childhood cancer will die of their malignancy. In fact, among all children with life-limiting illness, cancer remains the leading cause of disease-related death.[35,36] Early in the trajectory of treatment of malignancy, transfusion may be largely a matter of supportive care, allowing administration of more myelosuppressive or more frequent chemotherapy. When cure is not possible, transfusion may be used to maintain the quality of life rather than prolong life. During the days, weeks, or months after the realization that cure can no longer be the endpoint, many short- and long-term goals are reassessed. Transfusion frequency varies considerably during this phase of illness. Transfusions may not be required or may be infrequent for a patient with a solid tumor that is not invading the bone marrow space. Conversely, for a child with a bone marrow failure syndrome or malignancy that involves the marrow space, transfusions may become increasingly frequent. Reassessing the goals with regard to transfusion is an important discussion to have with the patient and family.

In this part of the illness trajectory as in others, we need to tailor the approach to the needs and priorities of the patient and his or her family. A child who is no longer pursuing curative therapy may have days, weeks, or months of feeling relatively well. They may be able to engage in legacy making, in accomplishing short-term goals that are important to themselves and their families. For example, it may be important to a teenage patient to walk across the stage at high school graduation. If there are symptoms from anemia, continuing regular transfusions may help them achieve short-term goals and decrease symptoms from anemia, allowing them to enjoy these important activities. Supporting children who are symptomatic from anemia with transfusions supports their own definitions of quality of life.

Open and frank discussion about goals should include discussion of what changes should be expected in even such basic components of care as frequency of laboratory studies. Frequent monitoring of laboratory studies may be a recognizable portion of the routine of care that is comfortable and expected by families. Even when decreased laboratory monitoring is meant to limit results that wouldn't be acted on or to conserve blood, a sudden decrease in laboratory frequency without open dialog is easily misinterpreted by patients and families as abandonment of the child by the medical system. For other patients, particularly ones without central access devices, a decrease in laboratory frequency may be a very welcome change in management. Both venipuncture and finger sticks can be distressing events for children, even if measures such as topical anesthetic cream or freezing solution are used.

Some healthcare providers may believe that transfusions should end when curative therapy ends. By this point in therapy, transfusions can be a familiar and accepted part of medical care. Both patients and families quickly become adept at recognizing signs and symptoms of anemia. They will likely have well-developed expectations about what level of hemoglobin requires transfusion. Transfusion may be as basic a component of therapy for them as acetaminophen is for an otherwise healthy child who has fever. To be told to stop transfusions would be undesirable. It may even be perceived as abandonment by the healthcare team. These decisions, like so many others during illness, need to be arrived at together, with the family perceiving and receiving support for their decisions from the healthcare team.

Continuing transfusion support may complicate other decisions as a family prepares for end-of-life care such as enrollment in hospice care. Although attitudes and practices are changing, some hospice programs still do not support such services as transfusion, parenteral nutrition, or continuing chemotherapy.[37] In recent years, the attitude toward providing transfusions for patients enrolled in hospice has begun to shift. In some hospice organizations, transfusion is now allowable if the motivation for administration of the transfusion is solely for relief of symptoms.

Clinical Vignette

Jay was an 11-year-old boy, the only child of a single mother. He developed secondary acute myeloid leukemia while receiving therapy for T cell acute lymphoblastic leukemia. He and his mother had been intensely private throughout their battle against cancer. Although there were some extended family members, mother and son were the main social support for each other. In fact, during uncomplicated admissions for scheduled chemotherapy of uncomplicated fever and neutropenia, she continued to work. He spent the day in the hospital alone, without complaint. When it became clear that the

leukemia was not responding adequately to chemotherapy, they chose to enroll in hospice and forgo further chemotherapy. He had a number of weeks where his main complaint was limited to low back pain. While at home he was able to pursue activities that he enjoyed. Intermittently, he was seen in the clinic. Jay and his mother both believed that his quality of life was reasonable and decided to pursue transfusions because he would get tired and cranky when his hemoglobin dropped below 7 or 8. Initially, we transfused him in the pediatric hematology-oncology clinic. After a few additional clinic visits, his mother requested a decrease in the time spent in the clinic. Couldn't home health draw labs? Was there any way to have transfusions done at home? In the area where he lived, we were able to accomplish transfusion at home through home health and hospice. In a later clinic visit, she indicated that eliminating the hours in clinic for labs to be drawn, waiting for results, and infusing blood was very important to them. They wanted to be at home. Being in their own surroundings for those additional hours was very important to both of them.

Several programs have demonstrated successful administration of transfusions at home.[38,39] However, in many areas, providing transfusion with blood or platelets at home remains technically challenging, if not impossible. In some regions, even if a child is enrolled in hospice with Do Not Resuscitate (DNR) or Allow Natural Death (AND) directives in place, there are no agencies willing to provide transfusions in the patient's home. This means families must go to an outpatient infusion center or be admitted to the hospital for transfusion. When admission is required to provide a transfusion, some third-party payers require discharge from hospice during the time the child is admitted to the hospital. Upon discharge from the hospital, nursing resources are then questionably used to repeat paperwork for readmission to hospice. For families in more rural areas, many hours may be spent traveling to and from the site for transfusion, receiving a transfusion, and repeating paperwork to resume hospice care. Further efforts are needed for development and dissemination of procedures and protocols for delivery of transfusions at home. Administrative support will be necessary for a personnel intensive investment for home transfusion programs. Payer mechanisms will also have to see the benefit and provide reimbursement commensurate with skill level.

On the other side of the equation are families for whom a transfusion is a physical, emotional, or social burden. For such families, decreasing or even ending transfusion therapy may be very desirable. It may also be reasonable to consider erythropoietin use in the clinical scenario of a child or young adult who is no longer pursuing a curative goal, but continues to have a relatively high level of function for what is anticipated to be a limited time. Goals such as decreased transfusion frequency, decreased travel time to obtain transfusions, and decreased time in the hospital to receive transfusions may be of considerable importance to the patient and family. Clearly, in light of recent FDA warnings, the decision to use an erythropoietin must include disclosure of the concerns for potentiating tumor growth. Given concerns for thromboembolic events and potential tumor growth, erythropoietin should be discontinued once a beneficial effect on hemoglobin levels can no longer be demonstrated.

Palliative Care Considerations for Primary Anemia

Children with primary anemias are not typically included in the discussion of palliative care. Now that children with hemoglobinopathies can expect to reach adulthood and have the potential to live into their fifth decade and beyond, we are met with new challenges for providing high-quality palliative care for this population. The principles of palliative care offer new opportunities to address the evolving needs of these patients.[40,41]

The hemoglobinopathies are characterized by largely unpredictable episodic acute pain from vaso-occlusion. Adequately addressing these painful episodes remains a challenge to the medical system. Many physicians are uncomfortable managing both acute and chronic episodes of pain.[41] The problem is compounded by an often adversarial patient-physician relationship.[41] Parents of children with sickle cell disease are more frequently dissatisfied with their child's care in the hospital.[42] The care of this population is complicated by decreased access to care, resulting in increased emergency room use, and therefore inconsistent care.[41,43] New models of care such as the "Day Hospital" design used by the Bronx Sickle Cell Center are needed to provide rapid and consistent access to pain medications.[41] Additionally, when children with sickle cell disease are not followed by a hematologist, they miss out on the benefit of preventative care.[44]

Children with cancer often carry physical reminders of their disease on their bodies, including hair loss, pallor, anorexia, limb deformities, surgical scars, and deformities from tumors or the therapy to rid them of the tumor. Children with primary anemias, especially sickle cell disease, often suffer without outwardly obvious reminders. Pain, the major debilitating symptom for children with sickle cell disease, cannot be seen at all. It is an internal experience. Even a major symptom of anemia, pallor, can be difficult or impossible for classmates, teacher, nurses, and doctors with lighter skin pigmentation to appreciate.

Contrast as well the social experience of the child with cancer who is in school. Often the school and even the broader community rallies around this child, celebrating each day he or she is in school, working hard to arrange alternate education plans for the days, weeks, or months when therapy or illness prevents school attendance. The child with sickle cell disease doesn't receive that community and school support. Missed school days are difficult to make up. Where patients with cancer may miss school in large blocks of time, patients with primary hematologic disease miss smaller blocks of time but multiple times throughout the year and throughout their school career. There are relatively few studies examining the impact of sequelae of sickle cell disease on school and school performance. Several small studies suggest that adolescents with sickle cell disease miss an average of 12% to 21% of school days.[45,46] In a recent study, 35% of the children followed missed a month of school from one school year.[46] Children with sickle cell disease miss more days of school than their siblings.[47] Falling behind in schoolwork missed because of pain, hospitalization, and clinic follow-up may develop into a pattern of school avoidance for some. Many missed days can leave the child who has primary anemias socially alienated and educationally delayed. There are only limited studies evaluating healthcare quality of life in children with sickle cell disease.

However, in two studies using the health related quality of life questionnaire (HRQOL) parent report form, parents identified their children as being more limited in physical, psychological, and social well-being and having more limitations on schoolwork and interaction with peers than healthy children.[48,49]

There are simple practical challenges for children with sickle cell anemia in school. Maintaining adequate hydration is a very basic component of self care. Water fountains, if they exist, are located in hallways, but children spend most of their time in classrooms. They are not allowed free access to the water fountains except at appointed times of the day. It often takes a letter from the physician for a child to be allowed to carry a water bottle to class. Even with the letter, the effort is not always successful. Access to water is only half of the equation. If a child is drinking more water than the average classmate, he or she will need to use bathroom facilities more often as well. For a busy teacher with a classroom full of children to teach and discipline, structured bathroom times are a necessity. Increased water consumption will lead to the need for bathroom facilities outside the normally structured time. It only takes a few conflicts or embarrassing interactions for the child to learn to avoid drinking the extra water to avoid the need to use the bathroom. Ultimately these experiences thwart basic lessons in self care and are counterproductive to the child learning that they can have some control and ownership over this disease. Lessons learned in childhood, including not drinking sufficient water, are difficult to undo in adulthood.

Truly challenging are the issues of ready access to pain medications, at times including opioids, while children are at school. Schools have legitimate concerns about children having and controlling their own medications. In our society, it is not a stretch to understand that a child with opioids in his or her own possession may be in physical danger. Similarly, where medications are kept and who at school has access to them are very real and often challenging issues. Yet, prompt access to oral pain medications and simple interventions such as rest and oral hydration are key components of care to prevent mild pain from progressing to more extensive vaso-occlusive crises or acute chest syndrome.

We need more school programs to educate the educators and classmates about why children with sickle cell disease miss school. We need to develop innovative and novel ways to keep children engaged in education and to help them keep up with studies despite hospitalizations. One such program might be a mentoring program pairing young teens struggling with the challenges of a chronic disease and its unwanted and uninvited effects on their lives with an adopted medical role model, a medical version of Big Brothers Big Sisters or a medical grandparent. The role model could be someone who also struggles with chronic disease of any sort but continues to be productive in the community and job force despite the medical challenges. There are scholarship programs for survivors of childhood cancer and young adults with hemophilia. More scholarship programs designated for children with primary anemias could help them access and complete higher levels of education and thereby obtain jobs with healthcare benefits.

Cancer affects 14 to 16 in 100,000 children. Sickle cell disease affects 500 in 100,000 African American children, and African American children are 18% of the population. Hemophilia affects 1 child in every 5000 male births, which translates to 10 in 100,000 children. There are 141 federally funded hemophilia treatment centers for children and adults;

the listing is available at www.cdc.gov/ncbddd/hbd/htc_list. htm. Funding for these centers is specifically focused on provision of medical care. Comprehensive hemophilia treatment centers were first established in 1973. There were 10 funded Comprehensive Sickle Cell Centers for treatment of children and adults with sickle cell disease. Only a portion of affected children received care in centers specialized in providing treatment for those affected by sickle cell anemia. Recently, these programs have been eliminated and are now converted to funded Basic Translation Research Programs for sickle cell centers primarily engaged in clinical research. After reorganization, funding for provision of care to patients with sickle cell disease is through HRSA and the CDC on a limited and competitive basis. Children not treated by specialists are often missing the opportunity for the preventive care so essential for preventing life-altering complications from end organ damage, such as stroke.[44] The most effective management occurs in the context of a consistent albeit unique interdisciplinary approach. Within the medical field we need to continue to build and strengthen medical homes for not only children but also adults with chronic anemias.

What accounts for the difference between the approach to treatment for hemophilia and treatment for sickle cell disease? In part, the existence of the National Hemophilia Foundation (NHF) established 1948. NHF is a very strong advocate for patients with hemophilia, and lobbies for healthcare legislation that improves care for those who suffer from hemophilia. Goals of NHF are: to increase lifetime insurance caps, increase funding for hemophilia treatment centers, and eliminate any travel ban for people with HIV (www.hemophilia.org/nhfweb). NHF is an organization of consumers, that is people with hemophilia, with an advisory board of providers. There are numerous sickle cell foundations that are more recently formed, smaller, and generally local or regional organizations. These foundations primarily focus on community education and testing for sickle cell trait and disease. As yet, they do not have as extensive private-sector funding or federal lobbying influence. Such efforts on behalf of patients with sickle cell disease would result in more resources focused on addressing the palliative care needs of these patients.

Public education, treatment and palliative efforts in sickle cell disease could benefit from a well-known celebrity or sports figure that championed the cause of children and adults affected with sickle cell disease. Recently, Michael J. Fox has raised public awareness, participated in raising money for research and lobbying the federal government to increase the investment in Parkinson disease research. Similarly, Lance Armstrong's "LiveStrong" foundation and the Susan G. Komen Foundation raise public awareness and billions of dollars in cancer research support. Examples of more long-term celebrity champions include Jerry Lewis, whose 2009 telethon raised $60.5 million dollars for the Muscular Dystrophy Association, which supports research, provision of care and services, and education (www.mda.org).

Thrombocytopenia and Functional Platelet Disorders

Platelet failure may be due to abnormal numbers or abnormal function (Box 34-3). Both of these may be primary, due to an intrinsic platelet disorder or secondary to underlying disease, such as malignancy. As with secondary anemia, poor bone

---

BOX 34-3 Causes of Thrombocytopenia

Primary

- Amegakaryocytic thrombocytopenia
- Thrombocytopenia and absent radii syndrome
- Platelet dysfunction
- Glanzmann thrombasthenia
- Bernard-Soulier syndrome
- Exposure to aspirin
- Renal failure

Secondary

- Aplastic anemia
- Autoimmune destruction
- Bone marrow failure due to previous and/or concurrent cytotoxic drugs and or radiation therapy
- Encroachment of marrow space with tumor
- Bone overgrowth, osteopetrosis
- Lack of marrow due to immobility and/or nonweight bearing
- Infectious myelosuppression
- Increased destruction associated with infection and fever

---

marrow reserve and hematopoietic toxicities from chemotherapeutic agents can lead to thrombocytopenia. Frequent platelet transfusion can lead to development of alloimmunization against platelet antigens, which in turn can worsen thrombocytopenia due to increased platelet destruction.

PRIMARY THROMBOCYTOPENIA

Severe primary thrombocytopenia occurs principally in four disorders. Three are primary failures of platelet production while the fourth is primarily an increased destruction process. Aplastic anemia is an autoimmune disorder leading to failure of production of all three hematopoietic cell lines. Infection and hemorrhage are the leading causes of death for patients with aplastic anemia. Platelet transfusions are essential for survival and to provide a reasonable quality of life in patients who await definitive therapy with HSCT or immunosuppressive therapy. Equally important is the transfusion support of patients for whom disease-directed therapy does not succeed. In the initial phase awaiting therapy, maintaining a platelet count greater than 20,000/uL can improve quality of life. However, a major risk is platelet sensitization, and transfusions must be used with care. In fact, graft rejection is seen more frequently in patients who have received many blood products prior to HSCT. In patients for whom primary therapy was not successful, platelet transfusions for symptomatic hemorrhage is better than the prophylactic use because it decreases the use and cost and is just as effective. It is prudent to have a specific plan in place for accessing transfusions when needed, because prolonged bleeding such as nose or gum bleeding can be very disturbing to patients even when it is not life-threatening.

Amegakaryocytic thrombocytopenia is a rare inherited failure of platelet production due to mutations in c-mpl, the thrombopoietin receptor, in about 50% of cases.[50] The disorder has a tendency for malignant transformation. Platelet transfusions are essential in the support of these patients as they await definitive therapy with HSCT.

Thrombocytopenia and absent radii (TAR) syndrome is an inherited autosomal recessive disorder with characteristic radial abnormalities not involving the thumbs and thrombocytopenia. The disorder presents at birth and, in most cases, the platelet count improves so that most patients achieve a platelet count sufficient to suppress hemorrhage by 1 year of age. Therefore platelet transfusion support to maintain platelet count greater than 20,000/uL is both life saving and greatly improves quality of life of these children. The requirement for transfusion usually decreases during the first year of life.

Primary Platelet Dysfunction

Primary platelet dysfunction in general causes mild bleeding problems. Only two disorders, Glanzmann thrombasthenia and Bernard-Soulier Syndrome, could be classified as life threatening.[51] Both are genetic defects affecting the critical platelet receptors for fibrin and von Willebrand factor, respectively. Infants with severe Glanzmann thrombasthenia present early in life including the neonatal period. Severe hemorrhages are responsive to platelet transfusion, but sensitization to platelet antigens makes the long term use of platelet transfusion therapy difficult. Judicious use of platelet transfusion allows these children to have a reasonably normal life. Because of the risk of platelet sensitization, definitive therapy with hematopoietic stem cell transplantation is indicated for children with the severe form of Glanzmann thrombasthenia. Bernard-Soulier syndrome is less severe and patients have a reasonable quality of life when supported with the judicious use of platelet support.[52]

Hemorrhage secondary to platelet dysfunction is best exemplified by renal disease. As renal function decreases and blood urea nitrogen levels increases to above 50 mg/dL, platelet dysfunction becomes clinically significant.[53] Menorrhagia and nosebleeds are the most common clinical manifestation and the most disturbing to the quality of day to day living. Several strategies can improve these patients' quality of life. The hematocrit has an inverse relation to the bleeding time in renal disease. Thus, improving hemoglobin levels with erythropoietin not only improves quality of life from disease fatigue but also decreases the risk of hemorrhage. Clinical hemorrhage can also be treated by increasing the levels of von Willebrand factor with desmopressin acetate (DDAVP) therapy or by transfusions of cryoprecipitate. Finally, anti-fibrinolytic therapy with ε-amino caproic acid or tranexemic acid can decrease both nasal hemorrhage as well as menorrhagia.

SYMPTOMS OF THROMBOCYTOPENIA

Thrombocytopenia first manifests with skin and mucosal membrane petechiae, which can coalesce into purpuric lesions. Gum and nosebleeds can result from thrombocytopenia. Other bleeding manifestations can include hematuria, menorrhagia, scleral hemorrhage, and retinal hemorrhage. Intracranial hemorrhage is the most significant and life-threatening bleeding (Box 34-4).

DIAGNOSTIC EVALUATION

Diagnostic evaluation for primary thrombocytopenia includes past medical history, family history, physical exam, complete blood counts, evaluation of the blood smear, and may include a bone marrow aspirate as well as genetic testing. Specifics of the differential diagnostic evaluation of primary thrombocytopenia is beyond the scope of this chapter, and for further diagnostic algorithms the reader is referred to other sources.[6]

In secondary thrombocytopenias, patients experiencing disproportionate thrombocytopenia while receiving chemo-

---

BOX 34-4 Symptoms of Thrombocytopenia

- Petechiae
- Easy bruisibility
- Purpura
- Nosebleeds
- Gums bleeding
- Menorrhagia
- Hematuria
- Sclera hemorrhage
- Retinal hemorrhage
- Intracranial hemorrhage

---

therapy in a curative pursuit should certainly be evaluated for other causes of thrombocytopenia. It may be informative to review a blood smear from before the administration of any blood products and chemotherapy to evaluate platelet morphology.

GUIDELINES FOR TRANSFUSION

A general transfusion guideline has been to transfuse for platelets less than 20,000/uL. This guideline was initially derived from a study correlating the frequency of spontaneous bleeding and platelet count. It was done in the era of administration of aspirin for fever. Because aspirin interferes with platelet function, some institutions have dropped transfusion guidelines to less than 10,000/uL.

Active bleeding, especially intracranial hemorrhage, should be considered an indication for transfusion in any patient with thrombocytopenia regardless of the platelet count. Patients who are expected to receive a HSCT for aplastic anemia or Glanzmann thrombasthenia may benefit from a conservative transfusion approach, limiting transfusions to symptomatic bleeding rather than prophylaxis based on any platelet count.

Specification of the Product

Apheresed platelet units provide a greater number of platelets than the platelet fraction separated from a single unit of whole blood. Apheresed platelets are obtained using a continuous circuit that allows repetitively removing a volume of blood, separating out the platelets, and returning the red cells and plasma to the donor. An apheresis unit contains approximately 10^{10} platelets. Transfuse 10 mL/kg of body weight. Platelets can be transfused over 30 to 60 minutes or at a rate of 10 mL/kg/hr.

When administering platelets to immunocompromised patients, platelets should be leukoreduced and irradiated to minimize risks of transfusion reactions and transfusion-related GVHD, respectively. CMV naive or severely immunocompromised patients can be transfused with platelets from CMV-negative donors to limit transmission risks. If alloimmunization develops, platelets from ABO, Rh, and HLA-matched donors can be used to improve platelet response by decreasing immune-mediated destruction.

Transfusion Side Effects

Platelet transfusions are associated with a higher incidence of allergic transfusion reactions because there is a greater amount of donor plasma and donor immunoglobulin in a platelet product than with packed red blood cells. For treatment of allergic reactions, see Transfusion Side Effects in the Anemia section.

With the development of skin cleansing protocols and closed circuit systems for processing of donated products, bacterial contamination is low. Platelet apheresis units are stored at room temperature, which makes growth of any contaminating bacterial agent more likely than in a pRBC unit. As with pRBC, profoundly neutropenic patients who develop fever during or soon after platelet transfusions should be hospitalized and treated with intravenous antibiotics until it can be proved that no bacteremia exists.

Interdisciplinary Considerations

As with pRBC, every medical facility has its own policy regarding infusion of blood components. The reader is referred to their institutional transfusion policy and *Essentials of Pediatric Oncology Nursing*.[19] Nurses educate patients with severe thrombocytopenia to consider not flossing teeth and using soft toothbrushes to minimize gum bleeding. When a nosebleed happens, the patient is advised to sit up and lean forward so blood loss can be more accurately monitored. Also, this decreases the amount of swallowed blood. Rectal bleeding can occur with the passage of hard stool, so stool softeners are encouraged to decrease bleeding with constipation. Encourage patients to avoid use of rectal thermometers in thrombocytopenic and neutropenic infants. Counsel teens to avoid high-impact sports, and activities associated with high G-forces or high impact such as rollercoasters, mountain biking, and paintball.

ALTERNATIVES TO TRANSFUSION

DDAVP

An alternative to platelet transfusions in mild platelet disorders is the use of desmopressin acetate (DDAVP). DDAVP can be dosed intravenously or subcutaneously at a dose of 0.03 mg/kg. DDAVP can also be administered intranasally, one puff for children and two puffs for adults. It is important that the correct nasal preparation, Stimate, be used for bleeding because it has a much higher concentration than the preparation available for the treatment of diabetes insipidus or enuresis. DDAVP should not be used for children younger than 1 year of age. It can cause severe hyponatremia and seizures because infants cannot easily control their liquid intake. Older children should be instructed to limit their liquid intake and drink only if very thirsty after being treated with DDAVP.

Antifibrinolytics

Antifibinolytics can also be a useful product to stop mild bleeding or to prevent bleeding in patients with hemorrhagic disorders resulting from platelet failure or plasma coagulation failure. Tranexemic acid is no longer available in the United States. Epsilon amino caproic acid comes in tablets, liquid, and intravenous preparations. A loading dose of 200 mg/kg of body weight followed by 100 mg/kg every 4 to 6 hours is the recommendation commonly found in text. However, experience suggests that a loading dose is not necessary and a dose of 25 to 50 mg/kg every 6 hours is effective with less gastrointestinal adverse effects such as nausea, vomiting and abdominal pain, and headaches and dizziness that are frequently seen with higher doses, especially in older children and teenagers.

BLEEDING IN TERMINAL CARE

Bleeding, particularly visible bleeding, is a very distressing event for families particularly for those involved in terminal care. A United Kingdom Hospice delivered platelet transfusions at home for children with cancer in terminal care, who had known thrombocytopenia and bleeding lasting more than 1 hour.[39] There is greater potential for transfusion-related reactions with platelets than with pRBC because of the greater plasma volume associated with a unit of apheresed platelets. However, the authors were encouraged by a low frequency of transfusion reactions, most of which were mild hives or mild lip swelling. Of all their pediatric oncology patients that died at home, less than 20% received platelet transfusions. The transfusion was effective in stopping the bleeding most times.

Where home transfusion of platelets is not available or not desired by the family, a few simple maneuvers can help minimize the distress of terminal bleeding should it occur. First and most importantly, the caregivers should be warned of the possibility of terminal bleeding and plans discussed. They should be encouraged to remain calm and remain with the child rather than leave to seek help or supplies. Minor gum bleeding may be lessened by application of a dampened tea bag to the child's gums. Dark colored towels and linens may make the amount of blood lost less distressing for anyone present.

Bleeding Disorder

PRIMARY

Primary plasma coagulation disorders are best represented by hemophilia. A discussion of the care of patients with hemophilia and of subjects suffering from rare factor deficiencies is beyond the scope of this chapter and readers are referred to other sources.[54–56] However, the principles of therapy of hemophilia as life-saving and improving quality of life are worth discussing.

In the past 70 years, we have moved from a potentially lethal disorder to a chronic illness, with a marked improvement of quality of life and almost achieving life span comparable to the general population. Until 1950, the average life expectancy of patients with hemophilia was about 11 years of age. With the advent of transfusion therapy of plasma in 1950s, cryoprecipitate in 1964 and factor concentrate use in the early 1970s, the expected average life span increased to 68 years. The introduction of effective therapy for hemophilia lead to the understanding that care not only relates to correction of the deficiency of a clotting factor, but also to the attempt of normalization of life. Home care programs as understood by hemophilia providers began in the 1970s. Although more expensive, having factor replacement products at home vastly improved the quality of life of the patients as well as provided prompt care. Still a pediatric disease, hemophilia care became an interdisciplinary collaborative effort. Comprehensive hemophilia treatment centers now bring together social workers, educators, nurses, dentists, physical therapists, orthopedic specialists, and hematologists. In 1989, with the first reported cases of HIV infection in hemophilia, a new challenge for the care team made those providing care for patients with hemophilia concentrate on the quality of life of our patients.

The advent of recombinant factors and viral inactivation strategies for clotting factor concentrates has improved safety during the past 20 years. Once again, prophylaxis with factor replacement became possible and has improved the quality of life of people with hemophilia. This generation of children with hemophilia can expect freedom from infusion-acquired viral infection and good joint health, in addition to a life expectancy nearly equivalent to the general population.[57] Arthropathy, pain, arthritis, school performance, employment, and psychological adjustment to a chronic illness are cultural aspects of hemophilia care that are becoming the focus of hemophilia centers. The hemophilia growth and development study outlined the school problems of children with hemophilia.[58] Early intervention and educational consultations are critical in the well being of children with hemophilia. Dutch children with hemophilia are more likely to participate in sports than their peers.[59] How do we prepare these children and families to cope with sports and the tendency for risk-taking behavior in children with hemophilia? Arthropathy is still a problem with pain. Hemophilia programs have developed techniques to improve pain, and use arthroscopy to improve pain and function and cryo-cuffs to provide pain relief, decrease swelling, and inflammation.

With improved life, people with hemophilia are becoming adults and need to cope with social pressures: employment, social adjustment, sexual function, and problems that come with aging, such as coronary artery disease, diabetes, and Alzheimer's. These are a few of the challenges that face hemophilia treatment centers, their new focus is the quality of life of the patient they can now cure of what was a lethal disorder 80 years ago.

SECONDARY

Secondary failure of the plasma coagulation system, manifested by multiple factor deficiencies, is seen in severe liver disease. Initially it may be due to vitamin K deficiency with low levels of factors II, VII, IX, and X, but may progress to include all coagulation factors produced in the liver including I, V, and XI. The hemorrhage due to liver disease may respond to vitamin K early in the course of liver failure. Severe liver failure requires infusion of plasma. The use of activated factor VII is not approved by FDA but can be effective in controlling hemorrhage. Because it is degraded in the liver, the dose may last longer in patients with liver disease. The manufacturer's recommendation for factor VIIa is a dose of 90 mcg/kg of body weight repeated every 2 hours. However, a single dose may be all that is required in liver failure.

Secondary failure of the plasma coagulation system may also be seen in acute promyelocytic leukemia or acute myelomonocytic leukemia, where the leukemia cells release enzymes leading to consumption of coagulation factors. Infusion of both fresh frozen plasma and cryoprecipitate are often required.

Guidelines for Transfusion

PRIMARY

Primary plasma coagulation disorders are now treated by transfusion of specific factors to replace the deficient factor. A discussion of the particular products and dosing of these factors is beyond the scope of this chapter and the interested reader is referred to several excellent recent reviews.[54,55,60] However, there are two principles of the use of these factors that are important when we discuss palliative care in the broader sense. The contamination of these factors with HIV created not only a devastating medical crisis but also left the families of patients with primary plasma coagulation disorders with fear and often distrustful of their care providers. For these patients it is important that their providers are familiar with the products and transparent regarding side effects, particularly transfusion-transmitted infections. The safety of the product becomes very important. The second concept is the purity of the factor. Although often both go together, they are not necessarily the same.

SECONDARY

Secondary plasma coagulation disorders are often treated with transfusions of fresh frozen plasma because they involve many coagulation factors. Fresh frozen plasma (FFP), 20 mL/kg body weight infused over 2 hours, is frequently enough to provide hemostasis. Alternatively, it can be used as a continuous infusion. Monitor PT, PTT, and fibrinogen. Goals to minimize clinical bleeding, normalize prothrombin time (PT) and activated partial thromboplastin time (PTT), and maintain fibrinogen greater than 50 ng/mL. In clinical scenarios, where there is not only poor synthetic function of clotting factors but also consumption of fibrinogen and clotting factors, cryoprecipitate may be infused. Relative to FFP, cryoprecipitate has a greater content of fibrinogen. A unit of cryoprecipitate per 5 kg of body weight is sufficient to raise the fibrinogen level.

Mentoring

Palliative care has not traditionally been taught in medical school or residency programs. These programs are only now being developed. An important role of physicians caring for patients in palliative care is to mentor young physicians. When considering a patient who is symptomatic from anemia, we teach about transfusion guidelines. We must encourage young physicians to grow a step further, to consider the guidelines as just a guideline. It takes an active dialog with the trainee to encourage him or her to think critically about each individual patient and the patient's unique circumstances. Is he or she symptomatic despite having a hemoglobin higher than the guideline, and therefore a good candidate for transfusion anyway? Is this patient expected to recover bone marrow function eminently and therefore does not need, or does not want, a transfusion despite meeting guideline criteria for transfusion? The medical art of implementing practice guidelines while tailoring therapy for an individual takes time to teach. With increasing demands on physicians and nurses' time, it is an easy component to overlook. Both our profession as a whole and our patients as individuals stand to gain from this priceless investment of our time.

Clinical Vignette

A 4-year-old girl who had recently been internationally adopted was brought to the clinic. Limited translations of available records indicated she had received blood transfusions approximately monthly. The average hemoglobin pretransfusion was 3 to 5 gm/dL. On initial presentation, she was pale and jaundiced with frontal bossing and midface bony overgrowth characteristic of thalassemia major.

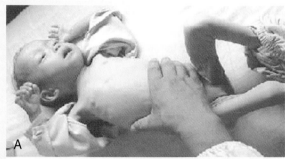

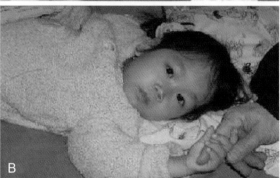

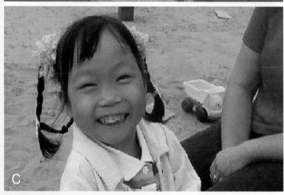

Fig. 34-1 The same child suffering with β-thalessemia at different timepoints. **A,** In the orphanage at 16 months of age. Note the contrast in color between the same ethnicity adult's well perfused and pink hand versus the child's pallor. **B,** Age 4 years, just as she is arriving in the United States. Her hemoglobin is 4 g/dL. She is somewhat jaundiced. She appears tired. Contrast her pallor especially in fingernail beds and jaundice with the pink caucasian adult's hand. **C,** Age 4 years, approximately 2 months after photograph in B. Hemoglobin is 10 g/dL. She is an energetic, smiling child now tan, consistent with her ethnic background, rather than jaundiced. Note less contrast between child's color and adult's arm despite different ethnic backgrounds.

She was tachycardic with a palpable thrill and heart rate of 110 and greater with 6-cm hepatomegaly and 8-cm splenomegaly (Fig. 34-1). She was a quiet, polite little girl. Although she cried with IV starts, everyone was impressed with the fact that she was so well behaved and really didn't offer much resistance. She sat in clinic for hours entertaining herself with coloring and puzzles. She showed little interest in television. She did not walk about to explore the clinic. We assumed that was due to recent changes of environment, unfamiliar people, and even recently new caretakers, her newly adoptive parents. In her new home, she also preferred to sit and play with crayons and small toys.

Sometimes she fell asleep on the floor while playing. She refused to walk more than 10 feet before she would sit down and cry. She went to the second floor of the house only when carried. She did not participate in running or playing games with the other children. In fact, there wasn't much interaction with the other six children in the household. When they were out of the house, she rode in a stroller. Mom had been told prior to the adoption that the girl's activity level was low. Because she had an international change of surroundings and caretakers, the parents assumed the quiet behavior was due partly to the adjustment to new surroundings and partly to her unique personality. They had a picture of her in the orphanage at age 16 months.

Over the ensuing weeks, she came to the clinic at least weekly. She remained polite, quiet and easy to interact with. Her English vocabulary increased. She continued to cry with starting IVs though she fought relatively little and was easily calmed afterward. Despite receiving 20 to 25 mL/kg transfusions, her hemoglobin remained in the 3 to 4 range in 2 weeks. She also had initial worsening of splenomegaly, which extended to 12 cm below the left costal margin and was very firm. Evaluation by cardiology demonstrated cardiomegaly but otherwise adequate function. During this period of time, she continued to walk very little. She arrived at clinic in a stroller because the distance from parking garage to clinic is approximately a quarter mile. When she did walk, she walked with a slow, wide-based gait. Her protuberant abdomen gave her the appearance of a pregnant 4 year old. Mom indicated that she walked inside the house but sometimes stumbled while walking. She did not go up stairs. She did not seem interested in joining the other children with outdoor play.

After several weeks, her hemoglobin before transfusion was 8. Her heart rate was under 100 for the first time since we had begun her care. Her spleen had returned to 8 cm. Her murmur was less prominent and she no longer had a palpable thrill. We proceeded with the transfusion as scheduled. At the end of the transfusion, her heart rate had finally improved to an age-appropriate rate in the 80s. A follow up hemoglobin a few days later was 10 (Fig. 34-1). On the next clinic visit, her mother excitedly described how she was a "totally different" little girl. She had walked much more that week. In fact, she had run for the first time since arriving in the United States. She had engaged in pillow fights with the siblings. She had engaged in a game of her own making called "monster" with the other children. For the next visit to the clinic, she walked through the door. The nurses were struck with how much more physical resistance she put up when they started her IV. Over the next several clinic visits her parents continued to comment on being aware of how much more active she was now that her hemoglobin was higher. They also repeatedly commented on how she now appeared tan consistent with her ethnic heritage rather than pale and yellow. The child also no longer complained of being cold.

This little girl's experience powerfully illustrates the impact anemia can have on a child's activity level. Until her chronic anemia was resolved to a level of moderate rather than severe anemia, she did not have the energy to engage in physically active play. Because of her otherwise quiet manner and recent entry into this family unit, even the medical team underestimated how much the anemia contributed to her restricted activity until after she became more active. We attributed some of her tendency to pursue quiet activities to personality and adjustment to a new environment. Indeed, she remains a child who is quiet mannered. She also continues to prefer crayons and small toys to television. Once the anemia was improved from severe anemia to mild anemia, she clearly began to feel better. The jaundice resolved and was replaced by pink lips and ethnically appropriate tan coloration. She became more interactive, of course she is also learning more English words by now, too. She walks around the clinic and explores as would be expected of a 4 year old. Truly the quality of her life and ability to participate in play has drastically improved with correction of the chronic anemia.

Summary

For children experiencing secondary anemia, thrombocytopenia, and bleeding disorders due to malignancy and chemotherapy, guidelines have been developed to help address these symptoms. Our patients changing needs throughout the disease trajectory challenges us to continually reassess and tailor how we address the hematologic symptoms of individual patients. The transition of primary anemia, primary thrombocytopenia, and primary bleeding disorders to chronic illnesses where children survive and can lead productive lives well into adulthood presents both new problems and ever broadening opportunities for palliative care.

Acknowledgments

We thank the many patients who have entrusted their care to us. We consider it a great privilege. Thank you to Susan Gaitros and Jane Hankins for critical reading of the manuscript and constructive suggestions.

REFERENCES

1. Kleinman S, Chan P, Robillard P: Risks associated with transfusion of cellular blood components in Canada, *Transfus Med Rev* 17:120–162, 2003.
2. Busch MP, Glynn SA, Stramer SL, et al: A new strategy for estimating risks of transfusion-transmitted viral infections based on rates of detection of recently infected donors, *Transfusion* 45:254–264, 2005.
3. Nathan DG: Lessons from an unexpected life: a doctor, a patient, and a formerly fatal disease, *Harvard Magazine* 36–41, 2009.
4. Horner MJRL, Krapcho M, Neyman N, Aminou R, Howlader N, Altekruse SF, Feuer EJ, Huang L, Mariotto A, Miller BA, Lewis DR, Eisner MP, Stinchcomb DG, Edwards BK, editors: *SEER Cancer Statistics Review, 1975–2006*, Bethesda, Md, 2009, National Cancer, Institute.
5. Michon J: Incidence of anemia in pediatric cancer patients in Europe: results of a large, international survey, *Med Pediatr Oncol* 39:448–450, 2002.
6. Sills RH, editor: *Practical algorithms in pediatric hematology and oncology*, New York, 2003, Karger.
7. *The Management of Sickle Cell Disease*, 4th edition, June 2002, National Institutes of Health: National Heart, Lung, and Blood Institute.
8. Miller Y, Bachowski G, Benjamin R, et al: *Practice guidelines for blood transfusion: a compilation from recent peer-reviewed literature*, 2007, American National Red Cross.
9. Liumbruno G, Bennardello F, Lattanzio A, Piccoli P, Rossetti G: Recommendations for the transfusion of red blood cells, *Blood Transfus* 7:49–64, 2009.
10. Roseff S: *Pediatric transfusion, a physicians handbook*. In Triulzi D, editor: Bethesda, 2003, American Association of Blood Banks.
11. Ruhl H, Bein G, Sachs UJ: Transfusion-associated graft-versus-host disease, *Transfus Med Rev* 23:62–71, 2009.
12. Sanders RP, Maddirala SD, Geiger TL, et al: Premedication with acetaminophen or diphenhydramine for transfusion with leucoreduced blood products in children, *Br J Haematol* 130:781–787, 2005.
13. Geiger TL, Howard SC: Acetaminophen and diphenhydramine premedication for allergic and febrile nonhemolytic transfusion reactions: good prophylaxis or bad practice? *Transfus Med Rev* 21:1–12, 2007.
14. Vichinsky EP, Haberkern CM, Neumayr L, et al: A comparison of conservative and aggressive transfusion regimens in the perioperative management of sickle cell disease. The Preoperative Transfusion in Sickle Cell Disease Study Group, *N Engl J Med* 333:206–213, 1995.
15. Brittenham GM, Griffith PM, Nienhuis AW, et al: Efficacy of deferoxamine in preventing complications of iron overload in patients with thalassemia major, *N Engl J Med* 331:567–573, 1994.
16. Telfer P, Constantinidou G, Andreou P, Christou S, Modell B, Angastiniotis M: Quality of life in thalassemia, *Ann N Y Acad Sci* 1054:273–282, 2005.
17. Pakbaz Z, Treadwell M, Yamashita R, et al: Quality of life in patients with thalassemia intermedia compared to thalassemia major, *Ann N Y Acad Sci* 1054:457–461, 2005.
18. Dahlui M, Hishamshah MI, Rahman AJ, Aljunid SM: Quality of life in transfusion-dependent thalassaemia patients on desferrioxamine treatment, *Singapore Med J* 50:794–799, 2009.
19. Kline NE, O'Neill JEB, Hooke MC, Norville R, Wilson K, editors: *Essentials of Pediatric Oncology Nursing*, ed 2, Glenview, Ill, 2004, Association of Pediatric Oncology Nurses.
20. Steinbrook R: Erythropoietin, the FDA, and oncology, *N Engl J Med* 356:2448–2451, 2007.
21. Rizzo JD, Somerfield MR, Hagerty KL, et al: Use of epoetin and darbepoetin in patients with cancer: 2007 American Society of Hematology/American Society of Clinical Oncology clinical practice guideline update, *Blood* 111:25–41, 2008.
22. Buyukpamukcu M, Varan A, Kutluk T, Akyuz C: Is epoetin alfa a treatment option for chemotherapy-related anemia in children? *Med Pediatr Oncol* 39:455–458, 2002.
23. Razzouk BI, Hord JD, Hockenberry M, et al: Double-blind, placebo-controlled study of quality of life, hematologic end points, and safety of weekly epoetin alfa in children with cancer receiving myelosuppressive chemotherapy, *J Clin Oncol* 24:3583–3589, 2006.
24. Hinds PS, Hockenberry M, Feusner J, Hord JD, Rackoff W, Rozzouk BI: Hemoglobin response and improvements in quality of life in anemic children with cancer receiving myelosuppressive chemotherapy, *J Support Oncol* 3:10–11, 2005.
25. Wagner LM, Billups CA, Furman WL, Rao BN, Santana VM: Combined use of erythropoietin and granulocyte colony-stimulating factor does not decrease blood transfusion requirements during induction therapy for high-risk neuroblastoma: a randomized controlled trial, *J Clin Oncol* 22:1886–1893, 2004.
26. Marec-Berard P, Chastagner P, Kassab-Chahmi D, et al: Standards, options, and recommendations: use of erythropoiesis-stimulating agents (ESA: epoetin alfa, epoetin beta, and darbepoetin) for the management of anemia in children with cancer, *Pediatr Blood Cancer*, 2009. 53:7–12, 2007.
27. Howell PJ, Bamber PA: Severe acute anaemia in a Jehovah's Witness. Survival without blood transfusion, *Anaesthesia* 42:44–48, 1987.
28. Penson RT, Amrein PC: Faith and freedom: leukemia in Jehovah Witness minors, *Onkologie* 27:126–128, 2004.
29. Knuti KA, Amrein PC, Chabner BA, Lynch TJ Jr, Penson RT: Faith, identity, and leukemia: when blood products are not an option, *Oncologist* 7:371–380, 2002.
30. Varela JE, Gomez-Marin O, Fleming LE, Cohn SM: The risk of death for Jehovah's Witnesses after major trauma, *J Trauma* 54:967–972, 2003.
31. Collins SL, Timberlake GA: Severe anemia in the Jehovah's Witness: case report and discussion, *Am J Crit Care* 2:256–259, 1993.
32. Gannon CJ, Napolitano LM: Severe anemia after gastrointestinal hemorrhage in a Jehovah's Witness: new treatment strategies, *Crit Care Med* 30:1893–1895, 2002.
33. Bodnaruk ZM, Wong CJ, Thomas MJ: Meeting the clinical challenge of care for Jehovah's Witnesses, *Transfus Med Rev* 18:105–116, 2004.
34. Wong EC, Baxter CA, Frey C, Criss VR, Luban NL: Transfusion transmitted viral disease and deferral rates in parental, directed and community donors for pediatric patients, *Transfusion* 41:114S, 2001.
35. Friebert S: *NHPCO Facts and Figures: Pediatric Palliative and Hospice Care in America*, Alexandria, Va, 2009, National Hospice and Palliative Care Organization.
36. Field MJ, Behrman REE: *When children die: improving palliative and end-of-life care for children and their families*. Washington, D.C., 2003,

Institute of Medicine of the National Academies; National Academies Press.

37. Fowler K, Poehling K, Billheimer D, et al: Hospice referral practices for children with cancer: a survey of pediatric oncologists, *J Clin Oncol* 24:1099–1104, 2006.

38. Benson K: Home is where the heart is: do blood transfusions belong there too? *Transfus Med Rev* 20:218–229, 2006.

39. Brook L, Vickers J, Pizer B: Home platelet transfusion in pediatric oncology terminal care, *Med Pediatr Oncol* 40:249–251, 2003.

40. McClain BC, Kain ZN: Pediatric palliative care: a novel approach to children with sickle cell disease, *Pediatrics* 119:612–614, 2007.

41. Benjamin L: Pain management in sickle cell disease: palliative care begins at birth? *Hematology Am Soc Hematol Educ Program* 466–474, 2008.

42. Brousseau DC, Mukonje T, Brandow AM, Nimmer M, Panepinto JA: Dissatisfaction with hospital care for children with sickle cell disease not due only to race and chronic disease, *Pediatr Blood Cancer* 53:174–178, 2009.

43. Raphael JL, Dietrich CL, Whitmire D, Mahoney DH, Mueller BU, Giardino AP: Healthcare utilization and expenditures for low income children with sickle cell disease, *Pediatr Blood Cancer* 52:263–267, 2009.

44. Hankins J, Wang W: The painful face of poverty, *Pediatr Blood Cancer* 52:157–158, 2009.

45. Shapiro BS, Dinges DF, Orne EC, et al: Home management of sickle cell-related pain in children and adolescents: natural history and impact on school attendance, *Pain* 61:139–144, 1995.

46. Schwartz LA, Radcliffe J, Barakat LP: Associates of school absenteeism in adolescents with sickle cell disease, *Pediatr Blood Cancer* 52:92–96, 2009.

47. Ogunfowora OB, Olanrewaju DM, Akenzua GI: A comparative study of academic achievement of children with sickle cell anemia and their healthy siblings, *J Natl Med Assoc* 97:405–408, 2005.

48. Palermo TM, Schwartz L, Drotar D, McGowan K: Parental report of health-related quality of life in children with sickle cell disease, *J Behav Med* 25:269–283, 2002.

49. Panepinto JA, O'Mahar KM, DeBaun MR, Rennie KM, Scott JP: Validity of the child health questionnaire for use In children with sickle cell disease, *J Pediatr Hematol Oncol* 26:574–578, 2004.

50. Geddis AE: Congenital amegakaryocytic thrombocytopenia and thrombocytopenia with absent radii, *Hematol Oncol Clin North Am* 23:321–331, 2009.

51. Nurden AT: Glanzmann thrombasthenia, *Orphanet J Rare Dis* 1:10, 2006.

52. Simon D, Kunicki T, Nugent D: Platelet function defects, *Haemophilia* 14:1240–1249, 2008.

53. Borawski J, Rydzewski A, Mazerska M, Kalinowski M, Pawlak K, Mysliwiec M: Inverse relationships between haemoglobin and ristocetin-induced platelet aggregation in haemodialysis patients under erythropoietin therapy, *Nephrol Dial Transplant* 11:2444–2448, 1996.

54. Tarantino MD, Aledort LM: Advances in clotting factor treatment for congenital hemorrhagic disorders, *Clin Adv Hematol Oncol* 2:363–368, 2004.

55. Srivastava A: *Guideline for the Management of Hemophilia: World Federation of Hemophilia*, Montréal, Québec, 2005, World Federation of Hemophilia.

56. Acharya SS, Coughlin A, Dimichele DM: Rare bleeding disorder registry: deficiencies of factors II, V, VII, X, XIII, fibrinogen and dysfibrinogenemias, *J Thromb Haemost* 2:248–256, 2004.

57. Tarantino M, Ma A, Aledort L: Safety of human plasma-derived clotting factor products and their role in haemostasis in patients with haemophilia: meeting report, *Haemophilia* 13:663–669, 2007.

58. Su Y, Wong WY, Lail A, Donfield SM, Konzal S, Gomperts E: Long-term major joint outcomes in young adults with haemophilia: interim data from the HGDS, *Haemophilia* 13:387–390, 2007.

59. Heijnen L, Mauser-Bunschoten EP, Roosendaal G: Participation in sports by Dutch persons with haemophilia, *Haemophilia* 6:537–546, 2000.

60. Manco-Johnson M: Hemophilia management: optimizing treatment based on patient needs, *Curr Opin Pediatr* 17:3–6, 2005.

35 Dermatologic Conditions and Symptom Control

KIMBERLY A. BOWER | GERIT D. MULDER |
ANKE REINEKE | SHIREEN V. GUIDE

Beauty is not in the face; beauty is light in the heart.
—Kahlil Gibran

Skin disorders are often encountered in pediatric palliative care patients and can have both significant physical and emotional impact on a child's well being. The skin is the largest organ in the body and accounts for 15% of a person's body weight. Its major function is to provide protection from the external environment. This protection allows intimacy through the ability to touch and be touched. The skin is visible to the external world and its appearance can strongly affect a child's self-image and a parent's perception of the child. It is critical to identify dermatologic disorders and use an interdisciplinary team to take a whole-person approach to the treatment (Table 35-1).

Psychosocial Impact of Dermatologic Conditions

Dermatologic disorders in pediatric palliative care patients have traditionally been viewed from the perspective of their medical management, rather than their psychosocial impact. Because children with palliative care needs face so many other distressing problems, it is perhaps not surprising that so little research exists concerning the psychosocial impact of skin disorders.

In order to understand the psychosocial impact of skin disorders on pediatric palliative care patients, it is important to understand how skin disorders affect body image. Body image is a central part of self-concept and self-esteem, which is broadly defined as "the composite of thoughts, values, and feelings that one has for one's physical and personal self at any given time."[1] Reactions to physical changes in the body often depend on whether the change involves an emotionally loaded body part or function or whether it results in a visible disfigurement. Physical appearance and attractiveness are major issues confronting adolescents, and their body image becomes a central aspect of their identity development.[2] As a result of physical changes in appearance, others may stare or avoid looking at a child. Thereafter, the affected child may suffer emotionally and may withdraw socially. Although psychosocial research has been limited, studies have suggested that altered body image can interfere with daily functioning and has been associated with grief, anxiety, depression, social introversion, social avoidance behaviors, negative self-esteem, and avoidance of intimate relationships.[3,4]

A common diagnosis causing dermatologic symptoms in pediatric palliative care patients is cancer. The diagnosis of cancer is frequently associated with psychosocial and emotional issues. Studies indicate that children of all ages experience distress due to the effects of cancer treatment.[5] A diagnosis of cancer often leads to multiple changes in physical appearance. These changes frequently include hair loss, presence of a central venous catheter, weight changes, and scars from surgery. The body-altering side effects of cancer have been reported by adolescents as the worst aspect of their disease.[6] The adolescents' sense of self-worth can be affected to such a degree that they withdraw socially from their friends and family. Physical changes due to cancer or its treatment can be devastating to a child's self-image and can place the child at an increased risk for psychological and adjustment issues.[7-9]

Regardless of the underlying medical diagnosis, intact skin allows for intimacy and the ability to touch and be touched. Many teams that provide palliative care include massage or healing touch treatments to provide moments in which the child feels relaxed. Furthermore, touch is an important means for a child's family to express their emotions and care. Any change in a child's body image is likely to change closeness and intimacy through touch. Loss of intimacy may elicit psychological responses that become enduring and pathological, such as depressive symptoms and social anxiety. It should, however, be kept in mind that psychological responses subsequent to the development of dermatological conditions may not be simply the result of the skin condition, but be part of the child dealing with a life-threatening illness.[10]

Another important consideration is the psychological impact of pain that can be caused by the treatment of skin conditions. Painful treatments may include such things as changing wound dressings and physical therapy. The wound is a constant reminder that one's body has been changed and nurses need to be attentive and sensitive to patient responses during wound care.[11] Moreover, patients with wounds often report symptoms of depression and anxiety due to the pain.[12] Another important factor to consider is that effects of dermatologic conditions such as pain, skin breakdown, and scarring may lead to limitation of motion and activity. These limitations may become a major cause of distress for the child.[13] Young children particularly cope with distressing situations by engaging in play therapy. If the child's play routine is limited due to a skin symptom, coping may be limited, too.

A skin disorder may also affect a child's sense of self-competence as well as relationships with parents, siblings, or friends. Children and adolescents rely on different sources of social support. Children rely more on their parents and siblings, whereas adolescents obtain much of their support from peers. Peers are influential in the adolescents' self-definition and self-evaluation. If adolescents become isolated from their

TABLE 35-1 The Roles of Team Members in the Treatment of Wounds

Discipline	Role
Psychosocial clinician	Identify that there is a wound or that there is emotional distress related to a wound
Psychologist	Provide presence and support to the patient and family
Social worker	Assess the emotional impact of the wound on the child
	Assess the emotional impact of the wound on the child's family members
	Provide therapy and counseling to the patient
	Provide therapy and counseling to the family
	Provide education and support in the patient's school for the child's classmates
	Provide activity therapies to the patient and family, such as art, music, and play
Child life specialist	Identify that there is a wound or that there is emotional distress related to a wound
	Provide presence and support to the patient and family
	Provide activity therapies to the patient and family, such as art, music, and play
	Prepare the patient for what to expect during a dressing change
	Provide distraction during a dressing change
Spiritual counselor	Identify that there is a wound or that there is emotional distress related to a wound
	Provide presence and support to the patient and family
	Assess whether the wound is causing spiritual distress to the patient
	Address the spiritual distress that may be caused by the wound
	Identify and address the spiritual needs of the patient's family
	Perform spiritual rituals that may support the patient and family
Nurse	Identify that there is a wound or that there is emotional distress related to a wound
	Provide presence and support to the patient and family
	Assess the physical signs and symptoms associated with the wound
	Provide hand on medical care including dressing changes, medication administration, and repositioning
	Educate the family about wound care and wound prevention
	Educate the school nurse about the patient's medical and emotional needs
Certified nurses assistant	Identify that there is a wound or that there is emotional distress related to a wound
	Provide presence and support to the patient and family
	Provide repositioning and skin care
Physician	Identify that there is a wound or that there is emotional distress related to a wound
	Provide presence and support to the patient and family
	Assess the physical signs and symptoms associated with the wound
	Provide medical care including dressing changes, medication administration, and repositioning
	Prescribe a treatment plan
Psychiatrist	Identify that there is a wound or that there is emotional distress related to a wound
	Provide presence and support to the patient and family
	Assess the emotional impact of the wound on the child
	Assess the emotional impact of the wound on the child's family members
	Make a psychiatric diagnosis such as anxiety disorder or depression
	Prescribe a treatment plan including medications
Wound care specialist	Identify that there is a wound or that there is emotional distress related to a wound
	Provide presence and support to the patient and family
	Make recommendations to the team about the best management plan to treat the wound

peers, this may contribute to a sense of social deprivation and can put the adolescent at increased risk for depressive symptoms. Also, older adolescents facing changes in body image may be less likely to establish intimate relationships.[14] If children or adolescents have less social contact, this may have significant implications on their ability to cope with the skin disease and their overall quality of life. It is important to facilitate and encourage connections between family members and peers. This can be done by open communication and by encouraging interactions with friends. These interactions may be face to face, through e-mails or social networking websites, or by phone calls between the child and his or her friends.

Adjustment to dermatologic symptoms is influenced by individual needs and coping behaviors, family support, palliative medicine treatment team, sex, age, and location of the injury.[15] A powerful mediator of psychological problems is good communication among the care team, family, and child.[16] Many of the problems experienced by the child require a combination of psychosocial and integrative medicine interventions. Possible psychological interventions are assisting the child to explore activities in which he or she is able to expose thoughts and feelings without feeling vulnerable. This includes validating their feelings, rationalizing, and developing a sense of acceptance. The treatment could be a combination of counseling and art therapy. Further, it may be helpful to allow the family to incorporate integrative modalities, such as guided imagery, healing touch, hypnosis, acupuncture, aromatherapy, or other mind-body skills. However, keep in mind that caring for children with skin conditions should not be separated from educating and helping families cope with the impact of the conditions.

There is a large range of psychosocial impacts of dermatologic symptoms in pediatric palliative care patients, and this makes generalizations difficult. Unfortunately, only a limited empirical database exists and little is known regarding the experiences that children encounter with dermatological symptoms. Possible psychosocial problems include coping with grief, change in body image, functional losses, depressive symptoms, and social anxiety. Despite the limited research, the palliative care team can guide children in adjusting to the changes in their physical appearance by providing verbal and nonverbal messages that validate the experience and help them to develop a sense of acceptance. Further, the palliative care team can offer integrative treatments, as well as educating the family on how to support their child. Greater attention to understanding the impact and effective interventions for children with skin disease in palliative care are needed to ease the suffering and increase the child's' overall well-being.

Generalized Pruritus

Pruritus is an unpleasant cutaneous sensation that provokes the desire to scratch. It can be distressing and sometimes difficult to treat. It may lead to sleep disturbance, difficulty concentrating, anxiety, depression, and agitation. Left inadequately managed, it can have a significantly negative impact on a child's quality of life.[1]

A recent position paper by the International Forum for the Study of Itch identifies six categories for the classification of pruritus based on its etiology: dermatologic disease, systemic disease, neurologic, psychiatric, and/or psychosomatic, mixed, and others.[2] The causes of pruritus are numerous, and an extensive list is included in the paper published by the International Forum. Identifying the etiology of pruritus can be helpful when formulating a therapeutic approach. This chapter will address only the most common causes of pruritus in the palliative care setting.

PATHOPHYSIOLOGY OF PRURITUS

The neuronal pathways for the transmission of pruritus are thought to be closely related to, but distinct from, pain pathways. The skin is densely innervated by afferent C-fibers. These C-fibers transmit signals that lead to both the perception of pain and pruritus. About 80% of the C-fibers are activated by mechanical stimuli, being mechano-sensitive, while the remaining 20% are activated by chemical stimuli, including histamine, called mechano-insensitive. It is likely that some combinations of mechano-insensitive and mechano-sensitive C-fibers are responsible for the transmission of the itch signal to the dorsal root ganglia.[3] Dorsal horn neurons then carry the itch signal up the spinal cord to the thalamus. Functional MRI imaging of the brain has shown activity in multiple areas of the brain, which encode sensory, emotional, attention-dependent, cognitive, and motivational aspects of itch.[4] The perception of itch causes the response of scratching. Scratching creates a mild pain stimulus, which activates fast-conducting low-threshold nerve fibers that inhibit itch. It is believed that itch is under tonic inhibitory control of pain-related signals. It has also been demonstrated that μ-opioid receptor antagonists can have antipruritic effects but may intensify pain (Fig. 35-1).[5-8]

When pruritus is caused by dermatologic disease, peripheral C-fibers must be activated to transmit an itch signal. Histamine is the itch-stimulating substance, pruritogen, that is most typically targeted when treating itch, but there are other substances that stimulate itch including acetylcholine, bradykinin, endothelins, interleukins, leukotrienes, neurotrophins, prostaglandins, proteases, and kallikreins. These pruritogens can be released from various intracutaneous cell types. When these substances stimulate C-fibers, neuropeptides, such as substance P, are released. The neuropeptides then act on a variety of non-neuronal cell types, such as mast cells, which release further pruritogens thus creating a positive feedback loop and increases itch. Itch leads to scratching, which causes

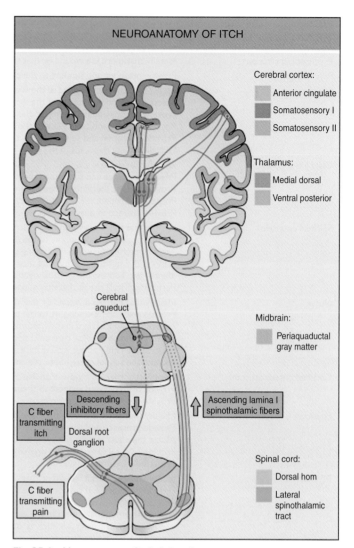

Fig. 35-1 Neuroanatomy of itch. Itch and pain transmission occurs via unmyelinated C nerve fibers that excite the lamina I subset of neurons in the dorsal horn of the spinal cord. Studies have demonstrated specific C fibers that convey itch. Information on both itch and pain is conducted through the lateral spinothalamic tract, with projections to the thalamus and subsequently the cerebral cortex. Processing of itch activates several regions of the brain that are similar to those involved in pain, such as the primary somatosensory cortex, the anterior cingulate cortex, and the premotor cortex. The latter validates the clinical observation that itch is inherently linked to a desire to scratch. Of note, some studies on the central processing of itch have failed to demonstrate stimulation of somatosensory areas. Unlike itch, pathways of pain perception activate the secondary as well as primary somatosensory cortex. Concomitant painful stimuli can reduce the sensation of itch, possibly by a descending inhibitory mechanism resulting from activation of the periaqueductal gray matter. (Adapted from Yosipovitch G. Pruritis: an update. Curr Probl Dermatol. 2003;15:137-64. In Bolognia, Jorizzo, editors: *Dermatology*, ed 2, Saunders: an Imprint of Elsevier Science, 2008, Fig 6-1.)

inflammation and the release of more pruritogens. Breaking this itch-scratch cycle can be particularly challenging. Recently investigators have identified ion channels, called transient receptor potential channels, that when stimulated, desensitize sensory afferents by depleting neuropeptides such as substance P. This interrupts the interplay between sensory neurons and mast cells and is a promising focus for the development of future therapies for pruritus.[3] Capsaicin, which is being used in adults to treat pruritus, is an example of a medication that works through this mechanism.

The pathophysiology of pruritus caused by systemic disease is not fully understood, but it is often caused by increased levels of pruritogens, including endogenous and exogenous opioids. Itch of the neurological classification arises secondary to damage of nerves anywhere along the afferent pathway. Nerve damage can be seen in peripheral neuropathies, nerve compression or cerebral processes such as tumors, abscess, or thrombosis. Itch caused by psychiatric and/or psychosomatic disease can occur in disorders such as obsessive-compulsive disorder and parasitophobia. It is believed that both acute and chronic stress can trigger or enhance pruritus.[9]

ASSESSMENT

In the palliative care setting the most likely etiologies of a pruritus include underlying medical disorders, drug therapy, and dry skin. The etiology of pruritus can frequently be determined by history and physical exam. History should include localized versus generalized location, description, temporal profile, provoking factors, effect of medications, current medication list, atopic history, and travel history. Physical exam should include evaluation for dry skin, scabies, icteric conjunctivae, weight loss, and mental status changes. Radiologic and laboratory workup can be considered based on clinical presentation and goals or care.

There are few assessment tools to evaluate the severity of pruritus in children. The tools that do exist are designed to be used in specific conditions, such as atopic dermatitis.[10] In older children visual analog scales can be used to evaluate itch intensity. In the research setting a quantitative measure of pruritus can be obtained by a device that is able to measure the vibrations of the fingernails in the act of scratching.[11]

Management of Specific Conditions

The most effective treatment for pruritus is treating the underlying cause of the itch. This is not always possible, and even when it is possible the itch often does not resolve immediately. For this reason it is important to identify treatments specifically aimed at quickly and effectively relieving itch regardless of the state of patient's underlying condition. In this section we will review the management of pruritus that is caused by conditions frequently seen in pediatric palliative care.

Some simple practical steps can be taken in the treatment of pruritus regardless of the etiology. Simple interventions such as restricting time in the bath or shower, bathing in cool or lukewarm water instead of hot water, and applying emollients to the skin after bathing and on a regular basis can be helpful. Some children may find oatmeal baths to be soothing to itchy skin. High skin surface pH has been noted in several skin disorders, including atopic dermatitis and uremia. Using low pH cleanser and moisturizers can address this issue. Baths can also be prepared with sodium bicarbonate added to the bath water. Using a humidifier, maintaining a cool ambient temperature and avoiding rapid changes in environmental temperature and humidity can all be helpful general measures.

It can be quite difficult to keep children from scratching areas that itch. Children often scratch irritated areas in their sleep or without thinking about it. It is crucial to keep a child's fingernails cut short to prevent significant damage to the skin from scratching. Gloves or mittens can be place on children's hands but they are often difficult to keep in place and can limit the child's function. Case reports have suggested that hypnosis can be effective in reducing pruritus. This therapy may be a helpful adjuvant therapy for itch that is difficult to treat.[12–14]

XEROSIS

Children with serious medical conditions can be predisposed to the development of dry skin related to dehydration. Dry skin can be the primary cause of pruritus or can exacerbate pruritus of a different etiology. In any patient with pruritus, it is important to keep the skin moist by applying emollients on a regular basis. Common over-the-counter emollients may contain water and alcohol; for serious xerosis, products that are predominately oil applied immediately after bathing when skin is moist will be most effective.

OPIOID-INDUCED PRURITUS

Generalized pruritus that may localize to the face and trunk is a common complication of parenteral or neuraxial opioid administration. Pruritus can also be seen with the administration of oral opioids. It is difficult to estimate the incidence of opioids-induced pruritus in children for several reasons including limited data, variation between opioids and routes of administration, and lack of uniformity in methods of evaluation of pruritus. The incidence has been reported to be as high as 77% with parenteral administration of opioids in the postoperative setting.[15] Among children with cancer-related pain, the incidence has been reported to be 28% with administration of oral or parenteral opioids.[16] It is generally accepted that the incidence of pruritus is higher in neuroaxial administration of opioids than in parenteral administration. One 2006 study shows an incidence of 18% with parenteal opioids and 30% with epidural opioids.[8]

The mechanism of opioid-induced pruritus is not fully understood. It is known that orally and parenterally administered morphine can cause the release of histamine from mast cells, but fentanyl does not.[17–19] Because both morphine and fentanyl are known to cause pruritus, this argues against histamine playing a significant role in opioid-induced pruritus. Furthermore, in studies done in primates, the administration of a histamine antagonist did not attenuate scratch induced by morphine.[20] Any reported benefit of the use of H1-antihistamines in the treatment of opioid-induced pruritus is most likely related to the sedative properties of the medication. It is likely that opioid-induced pruritus is mediated centrally through μ-opioid receptors.[20]

In the initial management of pruritus caused by morphine, it may be helpful to change from morphine to an alternative opioid such as hydromorphone or fentanyl. If this is not effective, an opioid receptor antagonist can be administered in conjunction with the patient's opioid. It is important, however, that the opioid antagonist be used in a low enough dose that it does not reverse the analgesia achieved by the opioid. Both naloxone and naltrexone have been studied. Naloxone can be administered at a starting dose of 0.25 mcg/kg/hr to 1 mcg/kg/hr. It is believed that doses of more than 2 mcg/kg/hr are likely to cause an unacceptable degree of reversal of the analgesic effect of the opioid. A pilot study done in children in sickle cell crisis found that patients tolerated co-administration of naloxone and morphine.[5] A second study of 46 pediatric postoperative patients found that concomitant administration of low-dose naloxone and morphine PCA significantly reduced opioid-associated pruritus.[15]

Opioid agonist-antagonists, including nalbuphine and butorphanol, have also been studied as agents to reduce pruritus. Results of these studies have been mixed and studies are limited in the pediatric population. One study of 184 pediatric patients found that nalbuphine 50 mcg/kg IV given as a one-time dose was not effective in the treatment of postoperative opioid-induced pruritus.[8] Nonetheless, additional studies are warranted. While these drugs have conceptual advantages over pure opioid antagonists in that they do not reverse the analgesic effect to the opioid, in combination with pure agonist opioids, they risk the precipitation of an opioid withdrawal syndrome and worsened pain. These medications act as antagonists at the μ-receptor and as agonists at the kappa-receptor. It appears that activation of kappa receptors attenuates morphine-induced itch without interfering with analgesia.[21]

Opioid-induced pruritus remains difficult to treat, and new approaches are being evaluated. Along with opioid receptors, serotonin receptors, dopamine D_2 receptors, and prostaglandins have been implicated in the mechanism of opioids-induced pruritus. For this reason serotonin 5-HT$_3$ receptor antagonists, such as ondansetron and mirtazapine, are being studied. D_2 receptor antagonists, such as droperidol and prostaglandin-blocking non-steroidal anti-inflammatory agents, are also being studied as possible treatments for opioid-induced pruritus. Studies of these agents in adults have not shown dramatically positive results. Few studies have been done in children and many trials have included only subjects receiving intrathecal or epidural opioids. These two factors make it difficult to predict the effect that these medications may have in the treatment of opioid-induced pruritus in children in the palliative care setting.

CANCER-SPECIFIC

Many children with cancer experience pruritus. In order to be able to choose the most appropriate treatment, it is important to carefully consider the cause of the symptom. The pruritus may be a direct result of the cancer or may be a side effect of the child's treatment. Children with cancer may experience xerosis, radiation desquamation, drug reactions, side effects from chemotherapy and biologic agents, or graft versus host reactions, all of which can cause pruritus.

The most common types of cancers that cause pruritus in the pediatric population are leukemias and lymphomas. Hodgkin lymphoma often causes burning and itching in localized areas, while other leukemias and lymphomas cause more generalized pruritus. Adenocarcinoma and squamous cell carcinoma of various organs, as well as carcinoid tumors, are less common in children, but may also cause pruritus. The exact mechanism by which cancer causes pruritus is unknown, but it is likely that it is mediated through the release of pruritogenic substances, including histamine, leukopeptidase, kininogen, bradykinin, and serotonin.

The most effective treatment for cancer-related pruritus is anticancer therapy. In palliative care, however, many patients are responding poorly to or are no longer receiving disease-modifying therapies. In these patients, other approaches to the treatment of the pruritus must be identified. There is very limited data on the treatment of pruritus associated with cancer. In Hodgkin lymphoma there are case reports suggesting that the H$_2$-receptor antagonist, cimetidine, is effective in treating pruritus.[22] Corticosteroids typically given in conjunction with palliative chemotherapy can also relieve itch in late-stage Hodgkin

lymphoma. Case series that have included pediatric patients suggested that pruritus caused by solid tumors may respond to the serotonin selective reuptake inhibitor paroxetine.[23] While paroxetine's antidepressant effects can take weeks to see, its antipruritic effects may be seen in as little as 24 hours after administration. In carcinoid tumors, blocking serotonin with a 5-HT$_3$ receptor antagonist, such as odansetron, may be helpful.

CHOLESTASTIS

Cholestasis occurs in children of all ages, but it is particularly common in the neonatal period. The incidence of neonatal cholestasis is estimated to be approximately 1 in 2500 live births.[24] The mechanism by which cholestasis causes pruritus is unclear, but elevated levels of circulating bile acids and endogenous opioids are both believed to play a role. It is also probable that the serotonin neurotransmitter system is involved. Recently the role that the serotonin neurotransmitter system plays in pruritus caused by cholestasis has been explored. There are studies in adults suggesting that the the 5-HT$_3$ receptor antagonist ondansetron, the selective serotonin reuptake inhibitors paroxetine and sertraline, and the noradrenalin and specific serotonin antagonist mirtazapine can be effective therapies.[25–29] The pruritus of cholestasis is not thought to be mediated by histamine. Any relief that patients perceive with the administration of antihistamines is likely related to the sedating effects of the medication. It is of interest to note that if a patient progresses to liver failure, then pruritus often resolves.

First line therapy for pruritus caused by cholestasis is typically a medication directed at decreasing the level of circulating bile acids. Medications that can be used to achieve this result include nonabsorbable anion exchange resins such as cholestyramine, the hydrophilic bile acid ursodeoxycholic acid, and the hepatic enzyme inducers rifampin and phenobarbital.[26,30–33] Nonabsorbable anion exchange resins are not effective in the case of complete biliary obstruction because the bile acids must reach the intestine for the medication to be effective. They are usually avoided in infants with portoenterostomy for biliary atresia because of concern about accumulation of the drug at the anastomosis causing obstruction.

If decreasing the level of circulating bile acids is ineffective or only partially effective, an opioid antagonist can be administered. The opioid antagonists naloxone, nalmefene, and naltrexone have all been shown to be helpful.[34–37] Tolerance to these medications may develop over time, requiring dose escalation. Patients may experience symptoms of opioid withdrawal if they are treated with opioids; this can limit the medications' usefulness.

Surgical interventions may also be helpful if medical management has not been successful and surgery makes sense within the goals of care. Procedures including partial external biliary diversion and terminal ileal exclusion have been shown to decrease pruritus in some children with intrahepatic cholestasis.[38,39] In pruritus caused by extrahepatic disease, stenting the bile duct is often the best treatment for pruritus. In extreme cases of pruritus that is refractory to treatment and that is causing significant negative effects on a patient's quality of life, liver transplant can be considered.

UREMIA

Pruritus from uremia is seen in patients with chronic renal failure, but rarely in those with acute renal failure. The rate of pruritus is higher in patients receiving dialysis than in those not receiving dialysis. In adults, the presence of severe uremic pruritus is a predictive factor for death.[40] The mechanism by which uremia causes pruritus is not fully understood, but as in other systemic illnesses it is likely caused by the accumulation of pruritrogens in the blood.

There is very little research that has been done in the pediatric population on pruritus secondary to uremia, so the treatment options are based on the adult literature. Initial management in patients on dialysis includes enhancing the dialysis regimen and correcting the patient's calcium, phosphorus, and magnesium. Xerosis, which is very common in uremic patients, should be aggressively treated.[41] If a patient is found to have hyperparathyroidism secondary to renal failure, pruritus can sometimes completely resolve after parathyroidectomy.[42] Beyond these steps, UV-B therapy has been shown to be effective, but it has potential carcinogenic side effects.[43] In recent studies, gabapentin has been shown to be a helpful treatment.[44] Kappa-opioid receptor agonists have shown promise, but they have not been studied in children.[45] As in pruritus caused by most other systemic diseases, the only role that antihistamines play in treatment are as sedatives.

Pruritus caused by renal failure can frequently be localized. This fact may allow for the use of topical agents. There has been recent interest in the use of capsaicin cream because it has been shown to deplete substance P from C-fibers when repeatedly applied.[46] Its use may be limited in young children because it causes a burning sensation for the first few days it is applied. To make capsaicin more tolerable the skin can be anesthetized with a topical anesthetic, such as eutectic mixture of local anesthetics (EMLA), before the capsaicin is applied. Other topical agents, as well as systemic medications, are being studied for the treatment of pruritus caused by uremia, but the lack of clarity about the pathogenesis of the condition makes identifying new treatments difficult.

HIV/AIDS

Pruritus is very common in patients with HIV infection. It can be secondary to multiple etiologies, including infection, infestation, peripheral neuropathy, xerosis, a primary skin condition, systemic disease, drug reaction, or elevated levels of cytokines. A thorough evaluation for the most likely causes of the pruritus should be done and should direct treatment. Idiopathic HIV pruritus is uncommon and is diagnosed by the exclusion of other causes. Phototherapy can be an effective treatment, and one study in adults suggests that indomethacin may also be helpful[47] (Table 35-2).

MUCOSITIS

Oral and gastrointestinal mucositis, referred to collectively as alimentary tract mucositis, is very common in children receiving chemotherapy and/or radiation to areas encompassing the gastrointestinal tract including the head and neck. Younger patients develop both oral mucositis more frequently and heal more quickly than older patients receiving similar treatments. This is thought to be secondary to an increased rate of basal cell turnover in children as compared to adults. Mucositis of the alimentary tract increases morbidity and mortality by predisposing the affected child to bleeding, local infections, and sepsis. It is often the dose-limiting factor in the administration of chemotherapy.

TABLE 35-2 Treatment of Pruritus by Cause

Cause	Treatment
Xerosis	Oil-based emollients
Opioid induced	Opioid rotation
	Opioid receptor antagonist
	Opioid receptor agonist-antagonists
	5-HT$_3$ receptor antagonists
	D$_2$ receptor antagonists
	Non-steroidal anti-inflammatory agents
Cancer-specific	Anticancer therapy
Hodgkin lymphoma	H$_2$ receptor antagonists
Solid tumors	Corticosteroids
Carcinoid tumors	Serotonin selective reuptake inhibitors
	5HT$_3$ receptor antagonists
Cholestastis	
Extrahepatic cholestasis	Stenting of the bile duct
Intrahepatic cholestasis	Surgical intervention
Partial biliary obstruction	Nonabsorbable anion exchange resins
Any cause	Hydrophilic bile acid ursodeoxycholic acid
	Hepatic enzyme inducers
	Opioid antagonists
	5HT$_3$ receptor antagonists
	Selective serotonin reuptake inhibitors
	Noradrenalin and specific serotonin antagonist mirtazapine
Uremia	Enhance dialysis regimen
	Correct calcium, phosphorus, and magnesium
	Treat hyperparathyroidism
	UV-B therapy
	Gabapentin
	Kappa-opioid receptor agonists
	Capsaicin cream
HIV/AIDS	Phototherapy
	Indomethacin

Mucositis of the oral cavity and esophagus can lead to considerable oral pain, while mucositis of the gastrointestinal tract can lead to abdominal pain, diarrhea, and bloating. These symptoms can compromise both a patient's nutritional status and quality of life. Because mucositis causes serious complications, limits treatment, and leads to significant symptom burden, increasing attention has been paid to how best to prevent and manage it. Most studies have focused on how to prevent the development of or minimize the severity of mucositis in chemotherapy and radiation. Few studies have focused on how to treat the symptoms associated with mucositis.

In 2004 the Multinational Association of Supportive Care in Cancer and the International Society for Oral Oncology published evidence-based guidelines on the treatment of cancer therapy-induced oral and gastrointestinal mucositis. These guidelines were then revised in 2006.[48,49] Recommendation for the prevention of mucositis in patients receiving 5-fluorouracil, bolus doses of edatrexate, and high-dose melphalan included the use of oral cryotherapy. Unfortunately, very few recommendations about symptomatic treatment of oral mucositis could be made because of the limited evidence base. The group was able to recommend the use of patient-controlled analgesia with morphine for oral mucositis pain in those undergoing high-dose chemotherapy with hematopoietic stem cell transplantation. Because of the paucity of evidence, clinical experience is the primary basis for treatment of mucositis.

Gastrointestinal mucositis primarily causes diarrhea, and it is important to ensure that adequate hydration is maintained. Diarrhea can be treated with standard anti-diarrheal medications including loperamide. If loperamide is not effective, then octreotide can be used.

Particular attention has been paid to the prevention and treatment of oral mucositis. In patients receiving chemotherapy that is likely to lead to mucositis, cryotherapy can be used to minimize mucositis. This involves having the child suck on ice for 20 to 45 minutes while receiving chemotherapy. The ice cools the mucosal tissue and leads to vasoconstriction, decreasing the exposure of the tissue to the chemotherapeutic agent. The approach has been found to be modestly effective.

The mainstay of treatment of oral mucositis, regardless of the cause, is the use of systemic opioids. Opioids can be very helpful, but they frequently do not completely control the pain and their use may be limited by side effects. For this reason many oral rinses have been used as adjuvant therapy. Topical agents are often mixed in different combinations and referred to by various colloquial names such as magic mouthwash. Topical agents that have been tried include anesthetics such as viscous lidocaine, and benzocaine. Anesthetics are frequently combined with other analgesic drugs such as morphine, diphenhydramine, and anti-inflammatory agents such as topical benzydamine hydrochloride, which is not FDA approved in the United States, or dexamethasone. Coating agents such as aluminum hydroxide and magnesium hydroxide containing liquid antacids are also frequently included in oral rinses. Some combination of these agents are often combined and ordered for topical use by swishing the solution around the oral cavity and then spitting it out. Caution needs to be taken when considering the use of topical anesthetics due to the theoretical concern over an increased risk of aspiration secondary to the numbing effects of the drugs and concern over systemic absorption through damaged mucosal surfaces. Topical ketamine has shown promise as an effective treatment for oral pain. In one study, topical ketamine and morphine were shown to be safe, easy to use, and effective treatments for post-tonsillectomy pain in children 3 to 12 years of age.[50]

The most promising therapy being investigated for the prevention and treatment of oral mucositis is low-level laser therapy. Laser therapy has trophic, anti-inflammatory, and analgesic effects. One pilot study showed that laser therapy in children with chemotherapy-induced oral mucositis resulted in decreased severity of the mucositis and marked pain relief.[51] Another study showed a significant decrease in the duration of chemotherapy-induced oral mucositis in children.[52]

One of the major complications of mucositis is secondary infection, which often causes increased oral pain. Oral cultures from one study of children with lymphoblastic leukemia and oral mucositis showed that fungal organisms were isolated in 39% of episodes and bacterial organisms were isolated 28% of the episodes. Herpes serology from the same patients was positive in 16% of the episodes as compared with 2% of controls. In patients with mucositis, evaluation should be done for any signs of infection. Identified infections should be treated appropriately. Frequently an antifungal, such as nystatin or fluconazole, and/or an antibiotic, such as tetracycline, is added to the oral rinse. It is unclear if this is effective. In immunosuppressed patients, including patients on systemic steroids, topical treatment of oral infections is typically not sufficient and systemic treatment should be considered.

Finally, there is consensus among experts that oral care is critical in the management of oral mucositis. Its goal is to reduce the impact of oral microbial flora, prevent infection of the oral soft tissues and help alleviate bleeding and pain. Basic oral care includes brushing teeth with a soft toothbrush, flossing, using mouth moisturizers, and rinsing with bland agents such as sterile water, normal saline and sodium bicarbonate. It is helpful to follow an oral care protocol and to provide education about appropriate oral care to patients and their families.

DIAPER DERMATOSIS

Children with chronic and life-threatening diseases are often especially prone to diaper dermatosis due to long-term bed rest, illness-related incontinence, and/or immunosupression. Irritant contact dermatitis is probably one of the most commonly seen dermatoses in this group and presents with erythematous papules and plaques, characteristically sparing the folds. If skin breakdown occurs, then this area is at risk for development of secondary infection. Both fungal and bacterial infections are common and early recognition and treatment can prevent complications and serious life-threatening sequelae. Candidiasis commonly presents as erythematous papules or plaques with satellite pustules. Microscopic slide examination (KOH) or fungal smear and culture can aid with diagnosis. Usually if the patient is afebrile without systemic symptoms, cutaneous infectious can be easily treated with topical nystatin cream. Combination barrier creams, such as zinc oxide with antifungal creams, can also be helpful for prophylaxis in predisposed individuals. Bacterial infections in the diaper area can also present with vesiculopustular lesions often mistaken for fungal infection. For instance, bullous impetigo most commonly caused by *Staphylococcus aureus* often presents as large bullae that break down, leaving collarettes of scale behind. Newborns are especially prone to development of bullous impetigo, and this can be treated with appropriate antibiotic therapy tailored to bacterial culture results and organism susceptibility profiles. Allergic contact dermatitis (ACD) may also occur due to sensitivity to topical creams or their components. ACD may occur to topical medications including neomycin, antifungals, and steroids. Components of creams such as the lanolin in aquaphor or the formaldehyde releasers in moisturizers can also cause ACD. Even preservatives such as benzalkonium chloride used in baby wipes can cause an allergic or irritant contact dermatitis.

For erosions and/or ulcerations of perineal area, the mainstay of treatment is barrier creams, such as zinc oxide. That can be combined with creams, such as silver sulfadiazine, to help encourage re-epitheliazation and prevent secondary infection. Combination products such as Vusion, or topical miconazole, zinc oxide, and petrolatum, as well as creams, such as Biafine, containing growth factors may also be good treatment choices.

Immunocompromised states may predispose children to perianal abscesses. Palpation may be necessary to detect the abscess. In some cases these lesions drain on their own and in other cases incision and drainage is required.

For persistent dermatoses that present in the diaper area, and are unresponsive to conventional treatment, dermatologic consultation along with skin biopsy might be indicated. Skin diseases such as inverse psoriasis or inverse pityriasis rosea as well as viral exanthems may present with prominent groin involvement. It is also important to exclude eruptions such as Langerhan cell histiocytosis (LCH), which generally presents as scaly papules or plaques with a predilection for intertriginous and scalp areas (Fig. 35-2).

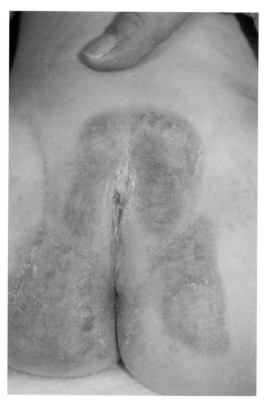

Fig. 35-2 Diaper dermatitis.

Wounds

There are several causes for wounds that occur in children receiving palliative care. Pressure ulcers, malignant wounds, and wounds caused by blistering skin conditions are the most common. Only minimal literature is available regarding treatment of pediatric versus adult wounds, because the majority of data has focused on the compromised and elderly patient. Lack of scientific data has contributed to ongoing use of modalities that are not optimal in managing wounds in the pediatric population, including saline gauze and leaving wounds open to air so that they can breathe.[8]

Unlike wound management in the general population, the first determination that should be made when managing a wound in a child receiving palliative care is the goal of the treatment. Frequently the goal is to heal the wound, but in some cases, particularly when the child is near the end of life, there may not be time to heal the wound. The goal then becomes to stabilize the wound and control the symptoms associated with the wound including pain, odor, bleeding, and excessive exudate.

TYPES OF WOUNDS

Pressure Ulcers

Pressure ulcers in the pediatric population, while not as prevalent as in adults, are still a significant dermatologic occurrence that must be appropriately addressed. The incidence of pressure ulcers in the pediatric population ranges from 20% to 43% in outpatients with spina bifida to 23% in children in neonatal intensive care.[1–4] Minimal data is available on the overall incidence of pediatric pressure ulcers. The exception is a national survey of healthcare institutions[5] that suggests

a pressure ulcer incidence of 0.29% and a prevalence rate of 0.47%, while Dixon and Ratcliff list incidence and prevalence of pressure ulcers in pediatric patients as between 7% to 27% and 0.47% to 6.5%, respectively.[6] Data on the incidence and point prevalence of pediatric pressure ulcers in different care settings, such as the home setting versus the hospital, are not available.

Children who are bed or chair bound or who have limited ability to reposition themselves are at particularly high risk for developing pressure ulcers. Poor nutritional status and conditions leading to moist skin, such as incontinence, are also compounding risk factors. It is very important to identify patients who are at high risk and take steps to prevent ulcer formation. If a child is identified as being high risk for ulcer formation his or her skin should be inspected daily so that issues can be identified before they become problematic. A bed-bound patient should be repositioned every two hours and a chair-bound patient every hour. Pressure-reducing mattresses and chair cushions should also be used. Donut-type cushions should be avoided because they reduce blood flow to the tissue within the donut. Children should be lifted with the help of a draw sheet or trapeze when repositioned to prevent shearing forces. Pillows or foam wedges should be used to prevent boney prominences such as the heels and ankles from coming into contact with each other. A pressure-reducing device such as a gel pad should be placed below the child's heels, or a pillow should be placed under the calf to raise the heels off of the bed. When patients are in a side-lying position, pressure directly on the trochanter should be avoided. When a child is incontinent, an absorbent diaper or brief should be used and it should be changed as soon as the child becomes wet or soiled. In addition, a barrier cream should be used to protect the skin from moisture. Prevent excessively dry skin by using emollients and humidifying air. When a child is being cared for at home it is important that the parents and other caregivers are educated on how to prevent pressure ulcers and how to identify ulcers at their earliest stage.

Pressure ulcers occur in similar locations in both adults and children. The most common locations are the heels, neck, sacrum, and scalp. Spina bifida and other diseases requiring immobilization may result in wounds over bony protrusions and popliteal areas.[7]

The primary concern, regardless of location of the ulcer, is addressing and eliminating the source of the pressure. Pressure-relieving mattresses and other devices are designed to assist with reducing pressure but may not always be effective. Examination of pressure sources includes evaluation of support surfaces, splints, braces, clothing, and any other material or device that come in contact with the skin. Failure to address the source of pressure will result in the failure of adjunctive treatments and may lead to continued tissue damage. Whenever using any product on a child, whether a pressure reducing surface, device, or other product, it is important to review the information related to age-specific use.

When a child complains of pain from a cast, splint, or other supportive device, the complaint should always be taken seriously pending complete review of the source of the pain. If in doubt, the supportive device should always be removed to allow for a full assessment. Sources of pressure that may require removal include but are not limited to casts, other immobilization devices and boards, masks, pressure cuffs and tubing.

Identification of the ulcer etiology is critical to optimal outcomes. When treating pressure ulcers it is important to rule out other potential etiologies. These etiologies include fluid extravasation; surgery-related wounds; electrical, thermal, and chemical burns, incontinence-related lesions; congenital abnormalities; trauma from dressings, adhesives, and clothing; and systemic diseases. Abuse should also be included in the differential diagnosis based on the presentation and history. Failure to treat underlying pathophysiology will delay or prevent closure of the wound.

Malignant wounds

Malignant wounds can be caused by a primary skin cancer, invasion of a primary or metastatic tumor through the skin, or the cutaneous infiltration of a tumor via the bloodstream or lymphatics. Many of the cancers in adults that most commonly cause these types of wounds include skin, breast, lung, head and neck, melanoma, colorectal, cervical and ovarian. Sarcomas can also cause fungating malignant wounds and are more common in children than the other cancers typically associated with malignant wounds.

Malignant wounds alter the perfusion of the involved tissue. There is often significant tumor necrosis. Necrotic tissue can become infected with anaerobic bacteria leading to pain and odor. The challenges in the management of a malignant wound are controlling the infection, exudate, odor and bleeding, and addressing the psychological impact of the wound on the child. Malignant wounds may affect the child's body image and the associated odor may be embarrassing and lead to isolation because family and friends are repulsed.

Generally, the principles of management of malignant wounds are the same as those for advanced pressure ulcers. In malignant wounds there may be a role for antineoplastic treatments in reducing tumor size and managing symptoms. Radiation may be used to reduce bleeding, pain, and exudate. These wounds are not expected to heal and the focus of treatment should be on controlling the symptoms associated with the wound.

Blistering Dermatoses

Genetic inherited blistering disorders, such as epidermolysis bullosa (EB), present a spectrum of disease severity and prognosis depending on type and defect in cell adhesion molecules. EB simplex is due to defects in keratin 5 and 14 represents a mild phenotype, which does not usually affect patients' lifespan, whereas patients with junctional or dystrophic EB have significant morbidity and mortality associated with their diseases. The emphasis in these patients is adequate nutrition and wound care along with infection prophylaxis when necessary.

An attempt to minimize the formation of wounds is important in this group of patients. Minor trauma and shearing forces can cause blistering. Using gentle handling techniques is critical. The seams of clothing and elastic on disposable diapers can cause trauma. Loose clothing should be chosen and should be turned inside out when worn. Cloth diapers can be used or the elastic can be cut out of disposable diapers. Fusion of the digits can be a problem in children with EB and children's figures and toes can be individually wrapped in an attempt to prevent this from occurring. It is important to avoid adhesives that are frequently used to attach medical devices, such as cardiac monitors and pulse oximeters,

to the skin. When necessary, children should be bathed in a tub and gently patted dry or allowed to air dry. Breast feeding and bottle feeding can cause trauma to the lips. Petroleum should be used to lubricate lips prior to feeding, or syringe or dropper feeds should be considered. Trauma to the anal area caused during bowel movements can be minimized by keeping the child's stools soft. Controlling the child's environment by avoiding heat and high humidity can also be helpful in preventing blister formation.

When large blisters do form they may need to be aspirated without removal of the roof of the blister, which provides a natural dressing. When there are open wounds the general principles of wound care discussed in this chapter can be applied. Open wounds are often treated with an antibiotic cream and covered with a non-adherent dressing. Dressings can be held in place with stretchy tubular gauze netting (Figs. 35-3 and 35-4).

DOCUMENTATION AND EDUCATION

An important component of the treatment of problematic pediatric wounds is the documentation of the findings, the treatment applied, and the family education provided. Documentation in conjunction with family and patient education is an intrinsic component of the care process, and may be more difficult and time consuming than care of the wound itself. Initial documentation requires measurements, a description including unusual characteristics, photos, staging, past treatments, and response to treatments. A thorough history including a review of systems, past medical history, and history of past therapies is a requirement for the development of an appropriate treatment plan. Subsequent documentation should reflect a complete evaluation done at each examination. Risk assessment is also part of documentation.

Family education may be difficult as the expectations for rapid recovery and optimal outcomes may be unreasonable. Underestimation of time to closure, lack of clarity about expected outcomes and non-disclosure of treatment complications and their advantages and disadvantages may lead to frustration on the part of the patient and family. A clear, concise, compassionate explanation of the treatment and the expected outcome establishes credibility and collaboration.

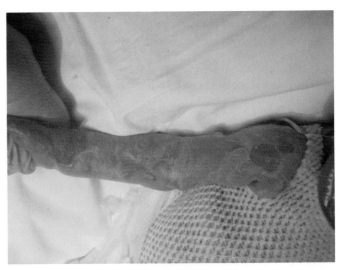

Fig. 35-3 Epidermolysis bullosa of the arm.

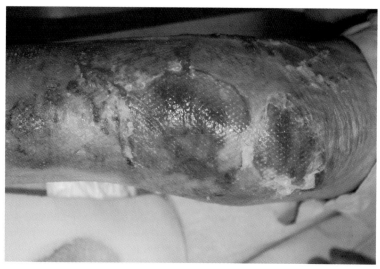

Fig. 35-4 Epidermolysis bullosa of the leg.

Risk assessment and prevention practices are outlined by various associations, organizations, and publications.[9-11]

Staging of pressure ulcers is the same in adult and pediatric populations. The accepted stages presented by the National Pressure Ulcer Advisory Panel (NPUAP) are listed in Box 35-1. The description and identification listed for each stage has not been modified for the pediatric population.

Treatment

Six primary general principles of wound care can be applied when initiating the treatment of any wound.

- Identify and treat underlying pathophysiology if possible
- Debride non-viable tissue if healing is expected
- Provide nutritional support if healing is expected
- Identify and treat infection
- Use appropriate topical therapy
- Consider advanced modalities

Along with managing the wound it is also crucial to manage the symptoms that are often associated with wounds including pain, odor, bleeding, and exudate. When these symptoms are left untreated they have the potential to affect a child's quality of life by leading to anxiety, embarrassment, and social isolation.

When formulating a treatment plan there must be a clear definition about whether the goal is to heal the wound or control the symptoms associated with the wound. For example,

---

BOX 35-1 Pressure Ulcer Staging System from the National Pressure Ulcer Advisory Panel (NPUAP)

Stage I: Intact skin with non-blanchable redness of a localized area, usually over a bony prominence. Darkly pigmented skin may not have visible blanching; its color may differ from surround area.

The area may be painful, firm, soft, warmer or cooler as compared with adjacent tissue. Stage I may be difficult to detect in individuals with dark skin tones. May indicate at risk persons.

Stage II: Partial-thickness loss of epidermis or dermis presenting as a shallow open ulcer without slough. May present as an intact or open and/or ruptured serum-filled blister.

Presents as a shiny or dry shallow ulcer without slough or bruising, which would indicate a suspected deep-tissue injury. This stage should not be used to describe skin tears, tape burns, perineal dermatitis, maceration, or excoriation.

Stage III: Full-thickness tissue loss. Subcutaneous fat may be visible but bone, tendon, or muscle are not exposed. Slough may be present, but does not obscure the depth of tissue loss. May include undermining and tunneling.

The depth of a stage III pressure ulcer varies by anatomic location. The bridge of the nose, ear, occiput, and malleolus do not have subcutaneous tissue and stage III ulcers can be shallow. In contrast, areas of significant adiposity can develop extremely deep stage III pressure ulcers. Bone and/or tendon is not visible or directly palpable.

Stage IV: Full-thickness tissue loss with exposed bone, tendon, or muscle. Slough or eschar may be present on some parts of the wound bed. Other characteristics often include undermining and tunneling.

The depth of a stage IV pressure ulcer varies by anatomic location. The bridge of the nose, ear, occiput and malleolus do not have subcutaneous tissue and these ulcers can be shallow. Stage IV ulcers can extend into muscle and/or supporting structures such as the fascia, tendon or joint capsule, making osteomyelitis possible. Exposed bone and/or tendon is visible or directly palpable.

DTI (Suspected Deep Tissue Damage): Purple or maroon localized area of discolored intact skin or blood-filled blister due to damage of underlying soft tissue form pressure and/or shear. The area may be preceded by tissue that is painful, firm, mushy, boggy, warmer, or cooler compared with adjacent tissue.

Deep-tissue injury may be difficult to detect in individuals with dark skin tones. Evolution may include a thin blister over a dark wound bed. The wound may further evolve and become covered by thin eschar. Evolution may be rapid exposing additional layers of tissue even with optimal treatment.

Unstageable: Full-thickness loss in which the base of the ulcer is covered by yellow, tan, gray, green, or brown slough and/or tan, brown, or black eschar in the wound bed.

Until enough slough and/or eschar is removed to expose the base of the wound, the true depth, and therefore stage, cannot be determined. Stable, that is dry, adherent, and intact without erythema or fluctuance, eschar on the heels serves as the body's natural cover and should not be removed.

From National Pressure Ulcer Advisory Panel. Updated Staging System 2007. Accessed June 28, 2010. www.npuap.org/pr2.htm.

when the goal is to heal a wound, debridement is critical to allow wound healing. When the goal is to control symptoms associated with a wound, debridement is only important to the extent that it is required to control odor. Nutritional support is also critical to wound healing, but when a wound won't heal, the child is near the end of life, and the goal is to control the symptoms associated with the wound, then nutrition is not important. Children who are close to the end of life may have poor appetites. In these cases there is no need to encourage any more nutritional intake than the child can comfortably tolerate.

DEBRIDEMENT

Extensive literature discusses the importance of removing non-viable or infected tissue from a wound bed because it may delay wound closure and contribute to infection.[18–20] The data is largely derived from adult literature, but the principles can be applied to the pediatric population. Unless surgical debridement is necessary due to extensive damage that is not easily addressed by conservative approaches, topical wound debridement outside the operating room may be successfully performed by application of a topical anesthetic such as EMLA followed by gentle curettage or cautious debridement with a sharp instrument. Enzymes have also been used successfully in cases where sharp or more aggressive debridement may not be possible or indicated. As with many products related to wound care, minimal data is available establishing safety and efficacy of enzymes in the pediatric population. Establishing the risk-benefit ratio and reviewing the patient medical history is imperative prior to prescription of any enzyme. No documentation is available regarding use of this drug category in neonates, therefore, application in this population cannot be recommended.

The primary enzyme available on the U.S. market is collagenase, because papain-urea products are not available. Use of medicinal honey as an antimicrobial and debridement-promoting agent has been documented for pediatric use, although not in well-designed randomized controlled and adequately powered trials. It appears to have been well tolerated and effective in the limited data presented.[21]

Autolytic debridement, the use of occlusion and a moist environment to promote debridement through the body's own macrophages, presents an alternative approach to topical drug or medication therapy. In the presence of normal cell and immune response activity, preventing desiccation of the wound bed allows for a natural debridement accomplished by macrophage activity, wound bed enzymes and subsequent autolytic activity. Thin films, hydrocolloids, hydrogels, and other dressings that maintain a moist environment may benefit the autolytic process.

NUTRITION

The adverse effects of poor nutritional status on tissue repair, infection rates, morbidity and mortality are well documented in the literature.[25–27] Understanding the overall nutritional status of the pediatric patient by reviewing markers, including but not limited to albumin and pre-albumin levels, is a key component of wound healing. Despite relieving pressure, addressing the underlying wound etiology and choosing an adequate dressing, tissue repair may not occur in the absence of adequate nutrition. Including a nutritionist in the interdisciplinary team caring for the patient may be useful.

TOPICAL THERAPY

Myriad topical dressings, ointments, and treatment modalities are available. The variety of products and manufacturers' claims creates confusion rather than clarity as to which treatment is most appropriate and effective. It is important to explore in greater depth the information provided with each product, particularly indications and contra-indications, before product selection. This overview is intended to categorize each of the primary dressing types. Table 35-3 provides a concise list of advantages and disadvantages of each product in a category. The data listed are meant as a guideline since individual medical status needs and considerations will vary among patients. Similar products within each category have never been compared with each other in any published Level I or credible trial. Based on the lack of research, it may be justly assumed that the major differences between products within a dressing category are based on cost considerations, qualitative features, patient tolerance, availability, and educational support provided by the industry. Each patient's wound requirements, medical status, tolerance to product components, reaction to adhesives, and other features should be considered before choosing a product in any category.

Thin Film

Thin film dressings are primarily polyurethane-based and are designed to permit vapor transmission. Their primary purpose is to seal and protect superficial wounds, reducing the risk of external contamination or abrasion. This particular category of products are adhesive in nature and if removed prematurely, or less than 48 hours after application, may damage newly formed and periwound tissue. Even when left intact for up to one week, they should be removed with caution. Thin film dressings are not designed for use with heavily exudating or full thickness wounds.

Hydrocolloid

Hydrocolloid dressings usually contain guar gum and carboxymethylcellulose in varying degrees and are designed for use on partial- and full-thickness wounds that are low to moderately exudating. They may be left intact on clean, non-infected low-exudate wounds for up to a week. Caution must be exerted when removing adhesive dressings from the skin because continued adhesion may damage surrounding tissue. Thin hydrocolloid dressings may allow limited routine bathing and hygiene because they are water impermeable. This category of products is of particular benefit to the pediatric patient because they conform well to irregular surface areas and are generally well-tolerated. Dressing residue may be present on removal, so this type of dressing should be avoided in very deep wounds with tunneling or sinus tracts where the residue cannot be removed. They should also be avoided when high levels of exudate are present or when friable and fragile tissue is present.

Foam Dressings

Foam dressings are minimally traumatic to tissue while being one of the most versatile categories of products on the market. Especially versatile are the configurations without adhesive backings or borders. Other than sensitivity to adhesives or

TABLE 35-3 Wound Dressings

Classification or description	Indications	Contraindications	Advantages and disadvantages	Helpful hints
Transparent Films Transparent Polyurethane film Gas permeable Moisture vapor permeable Impermeable to bacteria and liquids Adhesive	Dry to minimally exudating wounds Partial thickness Granular or necrotic, ideal for softening eschar Skin tears May use over absorptive wound fillers or hydrogels on full-thickness wounds	Infected wounds Wounds with heavy exudate Fragile surrounding skin	Advantages: Protection Autolysis, especially eschar Allows visual assessment Waterproof Flexible Pain reducing Moist environment Up to 7-day wear time Disadvantages: Not absorptive Excess drainage may cause maceration of surrounding skin May strip fragile skin upon removal May be difficult to apply	Use a large enough dressing to cover at least 1 inch of surrounding skin. Application of skin sealant to surrounding skin improves seal Change dressing when exudate leaks onto intact skin around the wound to avoid maceration
Hydrocolloids Wafer dressing that interacts with wound exudate to form a moist gel on wound bed Impermeable to oxygen (occlusive) Impermeable to bacteria Adhesive	Wounds with low to moderate exudate Partial or full thickness Granular or necrotic Pressure ulcers Venous ulcers May be used over absorptive wound fillers, alginates, or hydrogels depending on amount of drainage	Infected wounds Third-degree burns Diabetic ulcers Arterial ulcers Wounds with heavy exudate Fragile surrounding skin	Advantages: Protection Autolysis Waterproof Flexible Pain reduction Moist environment 3- to 7-day wear time Insulates wound Disadvantages: Odor May strip fragile skin upon removal Excess drainage can cause maceration of surrounding skin Potential for sensitivity to adhesive	Consider patch test to check for allergy to adhesive when using over venous ulcers Cover at least 1 inch of surrounding skin for improved adhesion Change the dressing before it leaks Educate families in advance of the odor and drainage associated with this product
Foams Polyurethane foam Varying degrees of thickness and gas permeability Adhesive and nonadhesive forms	Wounds with moderate to high exudate Partial or full thickness Granular or necrotic Pressure ulcers Venous ulcers Diabetic ulcers Arterial ulcers Infected wounds if changed daily Can be used over hydrogels, absorptive wound fillers, or alginates	Stage I wounds Dry wounds Fragile surrounding skin	Advantages: Protection Autolysis Conforms to shape Moist environment Insulates wound May decrease excess granulation tissue 4- to 7-day wear time Disadvantages: Some require tape or other securing method Adhesive foams may strip skin upon removal Cavity foams may harm tissue if over-packed	Tape nonadhesive foams across dressing rather than picture-framing with tape; this keeps the foam in contact with the wound Cover at least 1 inch of surrounding skin Most foams should be changed when strike-through of drainage is within 1 inch of the edge. Read package instructions
Absorptive Wound Fillers Sheets, ropes, pastes, granules, or powders that absorb exudate Two main types: *Starch Copolymers Alginates:* Naturally occurring polymer of seaweed; gel is formed when fibers interact with wound fluid Some products are fillers, but do not absorb much exudate. Read product insert	Moderate to high exudate Partial or full thickness Granular or necrotic Pressure ulcers Venous ulcers Diabetic ulcers Arterial ulcers Used as a filler with other dressings Infected wounds if changed daily	Dry or low exudating wounds Deep tunneling wounds or deep undermining Alginates not recommended for third-degree burns	Advantages: Autolysis Conforms to shape Moist environment Absorbs exudate Nonadherent Pain reducing No reinjury at removal Up to 7-day wear time Alginates are mildly hemostatic Disadvantages: Requires secondary dressing Alginates may dry out and adhere to wound, requiring saline soak to remove	For very high-draining wounds, cover with gauze or abdominal (ABD) pad and change when drainage strikes through to outside May cover with foam, hydrocolloid, or film, depending on amount of exudate Some starch copolymers should be packed to fill the wound only ⅓ to ½ full. Read product insert. Absorption capacity varies among fillers.

Continued

TABLE 35-3　Wound Dressings—cont'd

Classification or description	Indications	Contraindications	Advantages and disadvantages	Helpful hints
Hydrogels Sheets or amorphous gels that have 20%-90% water Some have starch copolymers that absorb small amounts of exudate Some products are dehydrated gels that offer more absorption Nonadhesive Gas permeable	Dry to minimally exudating wounds Partial thickness, use sheet gel Full thickness, use amorphous gel Granular or necrotic Pressure ulcers Diabetic ulcers Arterial ulcers, leave dry if there is no healing potential. Amorphous gels may be used on infected wound if changed daily	Wounds with heavy exudate Stage 1 wounds Sheet hydrogels are not recommended on infected wounds	Advantages: Autolysis Conforms to wound bed Moist environment Nonadhesive Pain reduction No trauma upon removal Disadvantages: Potential to macerate surrounding skin May require secondary dressing Some products may dehydrate in wound	Saturate gauze pad with amorphous gel to pack into wounds with depth Change dressing based on amount of drainage. If wound is drying out after one day, change daily; if wound is staying moist longer, change less often if wound not infected Sheet hydrogels work well on skin tears—change only 1 to 2 times a week
Contact Layers Exudate-permeable sheets that are applied directly over wound to prevent dressing adherence to wound Used commonly under gauze	Wounds in which dressings are adhering Petrolatum-impregnated contact layers may help keep dry wounds moist Used over skin substitutes and extracellular matrices	No major contraindications	Advantages: Provides for atraumatic removal of dressings Disadvantages: Some contact layers may still adhere to wound bed Petrolatum-based contact layers may contribute to peri-wound maceration in higher draining wounds	Overlap onto surrounding skin by 1-2 cm to protect fragile wound edges
Antimicrobial Dressings Sheets, pastes, foams, films, or gauze dressings with nontoxic antimicrobials that maintain a moist environment, although gauze product may dry out	Indicated to decrease colonization of microbes and reduce the risk of infection in partial- and full-thickness wounds Absorptive capacity varies among products	Sensitivity to ingredients	Advantages: Provides nontoxic alternative to antiseptics in patients at risk for infection Broad-spectrum coverage Reduces wound odor Film dressings provide bacterial barrier Disadvantages: Expensive Some products require secondary dressing	Match dressing to exudate level
Gauze Linen fiber dressing Some are woven, some are nonwoven	Wounds with minimal to heavy exudate Partial or full thickness Granular or necrotic Pressure ulcers Venous ulcers Diabetic ulcers Arterial ulcers May be used on infected wounds Use over topical antibiotics, growth factors, or enzymes	None	Advantages: Universally available Easy to use Ribbon gauze packs deep tunnels Facilitates mechanical debridement Disadvantages: Nonselective debridement, will harm healthy tissue Readily dries out wound Must be kept continually moist with saline to provide moist wound healing Usually requires multiple dressing changes per day Cotton fibers left in wound may cause prolonged inflammation and may interfere with wound healing	Avoid use of wet-to-dry dressings if possible because of pain and tissue damage upon removal For continuously moist dressing, remove secondary dressing and reapply saline to packing every 4-6 hrs Use ribbon gauze for packing deep sinus tracts Pack wounds lightly to prevent pressure on tissue

This list is not all-inclusive of every dressing on the market. No inferences should be made regarding the inclusion or exclusion of products on this list.

©2009 Susie Seaman

products, there are no major contraindications. Depending on the level of exudate and bacterial burden, the dressing may be left in place for up to one week. Absorption of fluid on low to moderately exudating wounds is good, allowing for the wicking of excess fluid. Foam products tend to be easy to apply, well tolerated by the patient, and painless when removed. Abdominal, back and scalp wounds as well as those on relatively flat surfaces are easily covered with smaller or larger size dressings. When adhesive is not desired, they may be held in place with a burn net or gauze wraps. Modified foams are available for irregularly shaped surfaces, including the buttocks, elbows, and heels. Foams, although giving the impression of reducing pressure, do not provide any significant pressure reduction or relief. Foams are also available with a silver antimicrobial component.

Alginate, Collagen-Alginate, and Composite Dressings

Products combining varying levels of collagen, alginate and/ or seaweed, or oxidized reduced collagen are optimal in moderate to heavily draining wounds and deeper undermined tissue. As with all products, caution is needed in deep tracts and cavities to avoid allowing product or residue remaining in areas that cannot be cleaned well between dressing changes. This category of product usually requires change once a day. Fortunately, the products dissolve and can be removed with gentle rinsing or cleansing as part of normal bathing; they don't need to be rubbed or peeled off. Products left on low-exudate wounds for extended periods of time may desiccate and be difficult or painful to remove.

Hydrogel Dressings

These are available in amorphous or sheet configurations. They consist of varying degrees of water, polymers, humectants, and preservatives. Their primary use is in maintaining moisture in low-exudate wounds while assisting with debridement through autolysis. Hydrogel dressings and topical hydrogels require a minimum of daily applications. Application of hydrogels to moderate- or heavily exudating wounds may contribute to maceration of the wound edges. Maceration decreases tissue tensile strength and, in the presence of shear, friction or ongoing pressure, may contribute to further tissue breakdown.

Silver and Antimicrobial Dressings

Silver and antimicrobial dressings are available in versions of almost all of the above products. They are also readily available topically, as in silver sulfadiazine cream. There is no Level I study or other significant data related to antimicrobial dressing use and improved outcomes in pediatric pressure ulcers. Patients with heavy colonization of a wound, high risk of wound infection, or an immunosuppressive disorder are at risk of developing a clinical infection requiring oral or systemic antibiotic therapy. Reducing or controlling the level of pathogens in a chronic wound to below a critical level in high-risk scenarios may ultimately benefit the patient. However, antimicrobial products, while not contraindicated in the presence of infection, are not meant to be used as the primary treatment for a true clinical infection. Except for in an immunocompromised individual, the host immune system may be expected to be successful at eradicating bacteria at a local level. Products with high silver content, above 2 parts per million have not been well studied in the pediatric patient and should be used with caution, particularly in the neonatal population. High concentrations of silver in clean wounds may impede new cell formation.[12]

Zinc is another heavy metal with antimicrobial properties. While some benefit has been suggested when applied topically,[13] pediatric data is not available. There is no reason to suspect that limited use of a product with topical zinc on a superficial lesion poses any risk, yet caution is still warranted. Topical antimicrobials, including Neosporin, are commonly prescribed and are also available over the counter. Neosporin and similar agents are known to cause sensitizing reactions.[14] Available data suggests they may be of benefit in reducing surface colonization, however simple daily cleansing with a liquid antimicrobial cleanser and water, followed by occlusion with gauze, is inexpensive and effective.[15] A comparative study on incision and drainage of simple lesions in adults randomized to either an oral antibiotic or placebo showed no difference in outcomes, thereby suggesting that good wound cleaning is effective in preventing infection in the non-compromised patient.[16]

Topical gels with metronidazole offer the benefits of a hydrogel as listed above, while assisting with odor control caused by anaerobes. Other antimicrobial ointments, including mupirocin ointment, address gram-positive organisms in the wound environment. A review of the literature[17] reviews differences in effectiveness and cytotoxicity levels of different topical antimicrobial agents. The data presented are from studies in the adult population and should be interpreted with caution when applied to the pediatric wound patient.

INFECTION CONTROL

All wounds are colonized by bacteria, fungi, and other infectious agents. It is not until the infectious agent is present in sufficient quantities that the wound is considered infected. *Staphylococcus epidermis* and *Corynebacterium* are the most common wound colonizers while *Proteus, Klebsiella, Pseudomonas,* and *Candida* are the most common infectious agents. The presence of pathogens at critically colonized levels are known to delay the tissue repair process.[22,23] They can also lead to purulent exudate, pain, and odor. Clinical and systemic signs of infection must be carefully reviewed to ensure the wound and peri-wound skin condition is consistent with infection. Swabs and wound cultures are most accurate when taken post debridement or following gentle cleansing with a non-antimicrobial agent. Use of antimicrobial agents may result in no growth from the culture. Unless superficial debris and contaminants have been removed, the swab culture may not be indicative of deep-tissue pathogens.[24] Simple contamination may be addressed through superficial debridement and wound cleansing and may not require the use of antibiotic therapy. Antimicrobial dressings may be used with caution as previously mentioned. The larger the wound surface area, the greater the need becomes to determine risk of systemic absorption of any agent that may be incorporated into a dressing, including silver, polyhexamethybutylene, iodine, or other antimicrobial. Antibiotic selection will be based on numerous factors, including identification of pathogens, spectrum of coverage of the antibiotic, and patient tolerance.

Ancillary, Advanced, and New Technologies

Modalities that have been developed in the last decade include the use of growth factors, acellular matrices, cell-based products, topical drugs and mechanical devices, such as electrical stimulation, moisture vapor therapy and ultrasound, all designed to assist with wound closure in the lesion that is more difficult to heal. Studies related to these products have all been conducted on the adult population. Product application, indications, and contraindications must be carefully reviewed to determine if the benefit justifies their risks. There is an abundance of literature on all of these product categories for treatment of problematic wounds in the adult population although, except for biological materials, most of the evidence is Level II or usually Level III. Virtually no literature may be found that discusses the same application of any of these materials in the pediatric population.

Of the ancillary treatment modalities, Negative Pressure Wound Therapy (NPWT) has become one of the most commonly used. NPWT is indicated for full-thickness wounds of most etiologies, including pressure ulcers. Reading the manufacture's recommendations for pediatric use and any available literature is a requirement before use of any of the devices. A review of the literature finds no data showing any advantage of using one manufacturer's NPWT product over another's. NPWT is of greatest benefit in larger defects to assist with granulation. The few studies that have been done looking at the use of NPWT in the pediatric population suggest that NPWT is safe and may assist in rapid granulation and successful wound closure.[28,29] Limited availability of data does not mean that the products may not be used; rather it strongly suggests that the treating clinician review the evidence for use and contact the manufacturer for any additional information concerning safety and outcomes in the pediatric population (Table 35-4; see also Table 35-3).

Symptom Control

Whether or not the goal is to heal a wound, it is critical to assess for and treat the symptoms associated with the wound. Poor control of symptoms may have both adverse physical and psychological impacts on children.

PAIN

There is frequently significant pain associated with wounds. The pain may be constant or it may be associated only with dressing changes. When the pain is constant, an evaluation should be done for treatable factors that may be causing or contributing to the pain, such as wound infection, tissue reaction, or increased pressure, particularly that over a bony prominence. Pain associated with wounds can be either nociceptive or neuropathic. For constant pain, the principles of pain management discussed in previous chapters can be applied. This might include treatment with systemic medications including opioids and pain adjuvants. Non-steroidal anti-inflammatory drugs (NSAIDs) can be particularly helpful in managing wound pain, but if the goal of care is to heal the wound then it should be noted that NSAIDs may interfere with angiogenesis and delay wound healing.[53]

Topical treatments can also be effective in controlling wound pain. It is known that opioid receptors are not only present in the central nervous system but also in the periphery.[54] Topical opioids can be placed directly on wounds to block these receptors. In case studies the use of morphine-infused IntraSite gel has been shown to be effective in controlling wound pain.[55]

If the patient has pain only with dressing changes, then an evaluation should be made to ensure that the dressing has been carefully selected to minimize tissue adherence. If there is pain with removal of the dressing, then a 2% to 4% solution of lidocaine can be used to moisten the dressing and the wound as the dressing is being removed. It is important to allow enough time for the lidocaine to take effect as the dressing is being removed.

Finally, debridement causes acute pain that will be present only as long as the procedure lasts. If there is eschar that requires debridement, the eschar can be scored and EMLA cream can be applied in a thick layer, then covered with an occlusive dressing and allowed to sit for 30 to 60 minutes before the procedure. It there is slough and debris to be removed, then a 2% to 4% lidocaine solution can be applied to the wound. If there is likely to be pain in the tissue surrounding the wound it can be injected with lidocaine before the procedure. If local anesthesia is insufficient for pain associated with debridement or dressing changes, a short-acting systemically administered opioid can be used. The patient might also need light sedation with nitrous oxide, ketamine, or a short-acting benzodiazepine.

ODOR

Odor associated with wounds is caused by putrefying tissue and infection. *Pseudomonas* or anaerobic bacteria are the most frequent causes. To minimize odor, the wound should first be gently debrided to remove putrefying tissue. If there is a superficial anaerobic infection, then treatment with topical metronidazole or silver sulfadiazine may be sufficient to neutralize the odor. For deeper infections, systemic metronidazole may be required. If the goal is simply to control symptoms and not to heal the wound, then cytotoxic cleansers such as iodine can be used. For *Pseudomonas*, 0.0025% acetic acid may be helpful. Dressings can be placed over the wound to contain the odor. An odor-absorbing dressing, such as charcoal dressings, can be helpful.

There are also several adjustments that can be made to the child's environment to minimize odor. First the child's room should have adequate ventilation. Cat litter or activated charcoal can be placed in a flat container, such as a cookie tray, with large surface area and placed under the child's bed or close to the child to absorb odor. Introducing an alternate odor such as coffee, vanilla, vinegar or using aromatherapy may be helpful. If this approach is used, then it is important to make sure that the aroma is acceptable to the child and does not cause an adverse reaction, such as nausea.

BLEEDING

Bleeding is more common in malignant tumors than in pressure ulcers. The surface of malignant tumors is often very friable. Dressings should be removed carefully. If the dressing adheres to the wound surface, then it should be wet with normal saline before the removal to minimize bleeding. If the wound is particularly friable it may be necessary to apply an inert, nonstick, nonabsorbent synthetic polymer mesh as the first dressing. This type of dressing does not need to be removed and can be covered with other dressings that can be changed regularly. Alternately alginate dressings are hemostatic and can be left in place for several days. They turn to jelly when exposed to liquid

TABLE 35-4 Choosing the Appropriate Dressing

Wound characteristic	Goal of therapy	Dressing examples
High exudate	Exudate absorption	Absorptive wound fillers Foams (high MVTR) Gauze
Low to moderate exudate	Maintain moisture Provide some absorption as needed	Hydrocolloids Thin foams or foams with lower MVTR Island dressings (dressings with absorptive island, covered with and surrounded by a transparent film) Gels, creams, ointments, contact layers
Minimal to no exudate	Add moisture	Hydrogels Amorphous for wounds with depth Sheet for superficial wounds Transparent films—add small amount of amorphous hydrogel under film for rapid hydration Hydrocolloids—slower than hydrogels and/or films at hydration
Clinically infected	Systemic treatment of infection Wick away exudate Wound cleansing	Use dressing appropriate for amount of exudate, but change dressing daily Avoid occlusive dressings Antimicrobial dressings may be used Saline irrigation (35-cc syringe/19-g needle)

High infection
    risk—immunosuppression
Ischemic ulcer
Diabetic foot ulcer
	Prevent infection	Use dressing appropriate for amount of exudate, but change dressing every
		    1-3 days
		Antimicrobial dressings may be used
		Utilize occlusive dressings with caution

Wound location	Prevent wound contamination
	Prevent maceration on plantar foot
		Use adhesive dressings, such as films over filler, hydrocolloids, foams, in the
		    sacral area to protect from incontinence
		Avoid dressings that will compress with ambulation and ooze onto surrounding
		    skin, such as hydrocolloids and paste wound fillers

Skin quality	Fragile skin Risk of contact sensitivity Peri-wound maceration	Avoid adhesive dressings; use a sheet hydrogel on skin tears secured with gauze wrap or netting Avoid adhesive dressings or products with sensitizing preservatives Use skin sealants on surrounding skin for protection

and can be easily washed off with normal saline with minimal trauma. If there is significant oozing from the wound, then low-dose topical thromboplastin can be sprayed onto the wound. A 0.5% to 1% silver nitrate solution may also be effective. For frank bleeding, silver nitrate sticks, electrocautery, or gentle pressure may be effective. A single fraction of radiation directed to the skin will sclerose most vessels and stop bleeding within just a few days. Interventional radiology may also be able to stop bleeding from a large vessel by sclerosing it.

EXUDATE

Exudate can be significant, especially in malignant wounds and Stage IV pressure ulcers. When the amount of exudate is substantial, consideration should be given as to whether edema or infection may be contributing. Both foam and alginate dressings are highly absorptive and can be very useful in keeping clothes, intravascular lines, and the surrounding healthy skin dry. The goal is to control the exudate without desiccating the wound bed.

Clinical Vignette

Matt is a 13-year-old boy with hereditary sensory autonomic neuropathy type II. He presents as significantly younger than his stated age and academically is at a first grade level. His ability to sense pain is very limited, and for this reason he has developed multiple wounds throughout his life. He has also been treated several

times for osteomyelitis and has had his left leg amputated below the knee. He was recently admitted to the PICU for sepsis. He is wheelchair bound and incontinent of urine and stool. His appetite is poor and his albumin is 2.5. He has three large Stage III wounds on his coccyx. There is an unpleasant odor coming from the wounds. Matt is very self conscious and is reluctant to have anyone other than his mother look at his wounds.

Matt lives with his mother, 11-year-old brother and 9-year-old sister. The family is Catholic and has limited resources. Matt has not attended school for the last year because his mother believes that his wounds get worse when he is at school. He does not leave the house very frequently because he is self conscious.

An interdisciplinary palliative care team consisting of a nurse, social worker, spiritual counselor, bereavement counselor, physician, psychiatrist, wound care nurse, and dietitian started working with Matt and his family. A treatment plan for the wounds was devised. The odor from the wounds resolved, and the wounds slowly began to decrease in size. The wound care nurse ensured that Matt had a pressure-relieving mattress on his bed and a pressure-relieving cushion for his wheelchair. The palliative care nurse did regular dressing changes while the social worker provided Matt with distraction and emotional support during the procedure. The nurse also educated his mother on wound care and prevention. The dietitian worked with the patient to identify ways to improve his nutritional status. The psychiatrist diagnosed Matt with depression and started him on an antidepressant medication. The social worker helped to identify resources for the family and provided emotional support to the patient and his siblings. The patient's mother worked with a bereavement counselor to address her fear around the possibility of Matt dying prematurely and the spiritual counselor provided prayer and addressed Matt's mother's questions about why God had made her son sick.

With support from the team Matt's mood improved and he started to leave the house and go on outings more frequently. In fact, he became restless and started to look for any excuse to leave the house. The team started to work with Matt's school on a plan to allow Matt to return to school.

Given Matt's underlying medical condition, he will always have wounds and a risk of osteomyolitis, sepsis, and death. Matt's medical condition will continue to affect him physically and emotionally. Exacerbation of his physical symptoms will likely cause new emotional and spiritual distress. Matt's siblings will be significantly affected by Matt's illness and Matt's mother will continue to benefit from help locating resources and from counseling and spiritual support. Matt's story highlights the need for a family-centered interdisciplinary approach to the care of children with chronic medical conditions and wounds.

Acknowledgments

Portions of the wound section of the text under the symptom management heading were modified from Ferris FD: Management of pressure ulcers and fungating wounds. In Berger AM, Shuster JL, Von Roenn JH, editors: *Principles and practice of palliative care and supportive oncology*, ed 3. Philadelphia: Lippincott Williams & Wilkins, 239–252, 2007.

REFERENCES

1. Weisshaar E, et al: Itch intensity evaluated in the German Atopic Dermatitis Intervention Study (GADIS): correlations with quality of life, coping behaviour and SCORAD severity in 823 children, *Acta Derm Venereol* 88(3):234–239, 2008.
2. Stander S, et al: Clinical classification of itch: a position paper of the International Forum for the Study of Itch, *Acta Derm Venereol* 87(4):291–294, 2007.
3. Biro T, et al: TRP channels as novel players in the pathogenesis and therapy of itch, *Biochim Biophys Acta* 1772(8):1004–1021, 2007.
4. Valet M, et al: Cerebral processing of histamine-induced itch using short-term alternating temperature modulation: an FMRI study, *J Invest Dermatol* 128(2):426–433, 2008.
5. Koch J, et al: Pilot study of continuous co-infusion of morphine and naloxone in children with sickle cell pain crisis, *Am J Hematol* 83(9):728–731, 2008.
6. Metze D, et al: Efficacy and safety of naltrexone, an oral opiate receptor antagonist, in the treatment of pruritus in internal and dermatological diseases, *J Am Acad Dermatol* 41(4):533–539, 1999.
7. Wolfhagen FH, et al: Oral naltrexone treatment for cholestatic pruritus: a double-blind, placebo-controlled study, *Gastroenterology* 113(4):1264–1269, 1997.
8. Nakatsuka N, et al: Intravenous nalbuphine 50 microg x kg(-1) is ineffective for opioid-induced pruritus in pediatrics, *Can J Anaesth* 53(11):1103–1110, 2006.
9. Arck PC, et al: Neuroimmunology of stress: skin takes center stage, *J Invest Dermatol* 126(8):1697–1704, 2006.
10. Carel K, et al: The Atopic Dermatitis Quickscore (ADQ): validation of a new parent-administered atopic dermatitis scoring tool, *Ann Allergy Asthma Immunol* 101(5):500–507, 2008.
11. Molenaar HA, Oosting J, Jones EA: Improved device for measuring scratching activity in patients with pruritus, *Med Biol Eng Comput* 36(2):220–224, 1998.
12. Ruckridge JJ, Saunders D: The efficacy of hypnosis in the treatment of pruritus in people with HIV/AIDS: a time-series analysis, *Int J Clin Exp Hypn* 50(2):149–169, 2002.
13. Ruckridge JJ, Saunders D: Hypnosis in a case of long-standing idiopathic itch, *Psychosom Med* 61(3):355–358, 1999.
14. Sampson RN: Hypnotherapy in a case of pruritus and Guillain-Barre syndrome, *Am J Clin Hypn* 32(3):168–173, 1990.
15. Maxwell LG, et al: The effects of a small-dose naloxone infusion on opioid-induced side effects and analgesia in children and adolescents treated with intravenous patient-controlled analgesia: a double-blind, prospective, randomized, controlled study, *Anesth Analg* 100(4): 953–958, 2005.
16. Mashayekhi SO, et al: Pharmacokinetic and pharmacodynamic study of morphine and morphine 6-glucuronide after oral and intravenous administration of morphine in children with cancer, *Biopharm Drug Dispos* 30(3):99–106, 2009.
17. Flacke JW, et al: Histamine release by four narcotics: a double-blind study in humans, *Anesth Analg* 66(8):723–730, 1987.
18. Hermens JM, et al: Comparison of histamine release in human skin mast cells induced by morphine, fentanyl, and oxymorphone, *Anesthesiology* 62(2):124–129, 1985.
19. Rosow CE, et al: Histamine release during morphine and fentanyl anesthesia, *Anesthesiology* 56(2):93–96, 1982.
20. Ko MC, et al: The role of central mu opioid receptors in opioid-induced itch in primates, *J Pharmacol Exp Ther* 310(1):169–176, 2004.
21. Ko MC, et al: Activation of kappa-opioid receptors inhibits pruritus evoked by subcutaneous or intrathecal administration of morphine in monkeys, *J Pharmacol Exp Ther* 305(1):173–179, 2003.
22. Aymard JP, et al: Cimetidine for pruritus in Hodgkin's disease, *Br Med J* 280(6208):151–152, 1980.
23. Zylicz Z, Smits C, Krajnik M: Paroxetine for pruritus in advanced cancer, *J Pain Symptom Manage* 16(2):121–124, 1998.
24. Venigalla S, Gourley GR: Neonatal cholestasis, *Semin Perinatol* 28(5):348–355, 2004.
25. Muller C, et al: Treatment of pruritus in chronic liver disease with the 5-hydroxytryptamine receptor type 3 antagonist ondansetron: a randomized, placebo-controlled, double-blind cross-over trial, *Eur J Gastroenterol Hepatol* 10(10):865–870, 1998.
26. O'Donohue JW, et al: A controlled trial of ondansetron in the pruritus of cholestasis, *Aliment Pharmacol Ther* 21(8):1041–1045, 2005.
27. Zylicz Z, et al: Paroxetine in the treatment of severe non-dermatological pruritus: a randomized, controlled trial, *J Pain Symptom Manage* 26(6):1105–1112, 2003.
28. Browning J, Combes B, Mayo MJ: Long-term efficacy of sertraline as a treatment for cholestatic pruritus in patients with primary biliary cirrhosis, *Am J Gastroenterol* 98(12):2736–2741, 2003.
29. Davis MP, et al: Mirtazapine for pruritus, *J Pain Symptom Manage* 25(3):288–291, 2003.
30. Bachs L, et al: Comparison of rifampicin with phenobarbitone for treatment of pruritus in biliary cirrhosis, *Lancet* 1(8638):574–576, 1989.
31. Cynamon HA, Andres JM, Iafrate RP: Rifampin relieves pruritus in children with cholestatic liver disease, *Gastroenterology* 98(4): 1013–1016, 1990.
32. El-Karaksy H, et al: Safety and efficacy of rifampicin in children with cholestatic pruritus, *Indian J Pediatr* 74(3):279–281, 2007.
33. Ghent CN, Bloomer JR, Hsia YE: Efficacy and safety of long-term phenobarbital therapy of familial cholestasis, *J Pediatr* 93(1):127–132, 1978.
34. Bergasa NV, et al: Effects of naloxone infusions in patients with the pruritus of cholestasis: a double-blind, randomized, controlled trial, *Ann Intern Med* 123(3):161–167, 1995.
35. Bergasa NV, et al: Open-label trial of oral nalmefene therapy for the pruritus of cholestasis, *Hepatology* 27(3):679–684, 1998.
36. Mansour-Ghanaei F, et al: Effect of oral naltrexone on pruritus in cholestatic patients, *World J Gastroenterol* 12(7):1125–1128, 2006.
37. Chang Y, Golkar L: The use of naltrexone in the management of severe generalized pruritus in biliary atresia: report of a case, *Pediatr Dermatol* 25(3):403–404, 2008.
38. Ekinci S, et al: Partial external biliary diversion for the treatment of intractable pruritus in children with progressive familial intrahepatic cholestasis: report of two cases, *Surg Today* 38(8):726–730, 2008.

39. Hollands CM, et al: Ileal exclusion for Byler's disease: an alternative surgical approach with promising early results for pruritus, *J Pediatr Surg* 33(2):220–224, 1998.

40. Narita I, et al: Etiology and prognostic significance of severe uremic pruritus in chronic hemodialysis patients, *Kidney Int* 69(9):1626–1632, 2006.

41. Morton CA, et al: Pruritus and skin hydration during dialysis, *Nephrol Dial Transplant* 11(10):2031–2036, 1996.

42. Hampers CL, et al: Disappearance of "uremic" itching after subtotal parathyroidectomy, *N Engl J Med* 279(13):695–697, 1968.

43. Gilchrest BA, et al: Ultraviolet phototherapy of uremic pruritus. Long-term results and possible mechanism of action, *Ann Intern Med* 91(1):17–21, 1979.

44. Razeghi E, et al: Gabapentin and uremic pruritus in hemodialysis patients, *Ren Fail* 31(2):85–90, 2009.

45. Wikstrom B, et al: Kappa-opioid system in uremic pruritus: multicenter, randomized, double-blind, placebo-controlled clinical studies, *J Am Soc Nephrol* 16(12):3742–3747, 2005.

46. Cho YL, et al: Uremic pruritus: roles of parathyroid hormone and substance P, *J Am Acad Dermatol* 36(4):538–543, 1997.

47. Smith KJ, et al: Pruritus in HIV-1 disease: therapy with drugs which may modulate the pattern of immune dysregulation, *Dermatology* 195(4):353–358, 1997.

48. Rubenstein EB, et al: Clinical practice guidelines for the prevention and treatment of cancer therapy-induced oral and gastrointestinal mucositis, *Cancer* 100(Suppl 9):2026–2046, 2004.

49. Barasch A, et al: Antimicrobials, mucosal coating agents, anesthetics, analgesics, and nutritional supplements for alimentary tract mucositis, *Support Care Cancer* 14(6):528–532, 2006.

50. Canbay O, et al: Topical ketamine and morphine for post-tonsillectomy pain, *Eur J Anaesthesiol* 25(4):287–292, 2008.

51. Abramoff MM, et al: Low-level laser therapy in the prevention and treatment of chemotherapy-induced oral mucositis in young patients, *Photomed Laser Surg* 26(4):393–400, 2008.

52. Kuhn A, et al: Low-level infrared laser therapy in chemotherapy-induced oral mucositis: a randomized placebo-controlled trial in children, *J Pediatr Hematol Oncol* 31(1):33–37, 2009.

53. Jones MK, et al: Inhibition of angiogenesis by nonsteroidal anti-inflammatory drugs: insight into mechanisms and implications for cancer growth and ulcer healing, *Nat Med* 5(12):1418–1423, 1999.

54. Stein C: The control of pain in peripheral tissue by opioids, *N Engl J Med* 332(25):1685–1690, 1995.

55. Twillman RK, et al: Treatment of painful skin ulcers with topical opioids, *J Pain Symptom Manage* 17(4):288–292, 1999.

36 Easing Distress When Death is Near

JOANNE WOLFE

Music, when soft voices die,
Vibrates in the memory,
Odours, when sweet violets sicken,
Live within the sense they quicken.
Rose leaves, when the rose is dead,
Are heaped for the beloved's bed;
And so thy thoughts, when thou art gone,
Love itself shall slumber on.—Percy Bysshe Shelley

What is a good death? When asked, many adults facing the end of life hope to control pain and other distressing symptoms, have a sense of preparation for death, and achieve a sense of completion; however, other factors important to quality at the end of life differ by the individual.[1] For some, a child's death can never be good. Nevertheless, as palliative care clinicians, we can aspire to enable a better death experience for the child and family when we are faced with the inevitability of a child dying. This chapter will review strategies aimed at trying to achieve this outcome.

Importantly, when a child is dying, all care goals may not be uniformly focused on easing suffering. Recent studies affirm the common clinical experience that even when a child's illness is said to be incurable, parents will hope to extend life concurrent with ensuring comfort.[2,3] Family values will differ: While some aspire for a peaceful end of life experience for their child, others value another approach, as stated by one father:

"The battle with the dragon, or the intent and the need, or the struggle to come to grips with him, or just coexist with him even, threatened to consume our lives. In the sense that the battle against the illness and all the circumstances—logistical and practical, and medical, and financial, and interpersonal…that became all consuming, just like the dragon's fiery breath…just like his fiery breath is understood to be all consuming, literally obliterating either an individual, or a number of individuals, or a whole village."[4]

In other words, it is a fight to the bitter end. As clinicians, however, it is critical to remember that whatever the primary goal of care and setting, care should never be at the exclusion of ensuring comfort.

Of note, studies that assess quality of life at the very end of life in children are limited. Thus clinical experience based upon consensus and the existing literature guide the content of this chapter.

Interdisciplinary Caring

During this most intimate of clinician-family experiences, the care of a dying child, exquisite collaboration among all involved is required to meet the needs of the child and family. Table 36-1 highlights key roles and activities of the interdisciplinary team. No matter where the child is being cared for, short huddles or meetings among team members may be helpful to maintain open lines of communication.

Recognizing When Death Is Imminent

Dying is a dynamic process. Though the process is influenced by many factors, it is remarkable how similar it can be despite very different underlying illnesses. Clinical experience suggests that when approaching death, a child typically experiences the following constellations of findings. The child is often bedridden, semiconscious, with little or no oral intake, and changes in pulse, respiration and peripheral circulation may also be apparent (Box 36-1).[5]

LETTING THE FAMILY KNOW WHEN DEATH IS IMMINENT

Parents and other family members are often fearful that if they step away from the bedside, they will not be present at the time of the child's death. As such, it is often helpful to let family and loved ones know about the signs of impending death both to achieve a sense of preparedness about what to expect and to try to judge when presence at the bedside is helpful. To introduce this topic, simply ask whether it would be helpful to know more about what to expect as the child is dying. If a parent agrees to be informed, it is important to be clear and to provide short pieces of information, and then subsequently check if it is all right to continue.

It is also critical to warn parents that it may not be possible to know the exact moment of when the death will occur. Some families find comfort in knowing that children sometimes choose to die when their parent is not present as a last effort to protect the parent from further suffering, if such a choice is indeed possible.

BRAIN DEATH

Typical signs of dying may not be present when a child is brain dead and is still receiving cardiorespiratory support. In children, brain death most commonly arises from traumatic brain injury due to child abuse, motor vehicle accidents, or asphyxia.[6] Though there is general acceptance of the definition of brain

TABLE 36-1 Interdisciplinary Roles in the Care of the Imminently Dying Child

Clinician	Discipline specific roles	Interdisciplinary roles
Primary physician/ Nurse practitioner	• Leads discussions related to establishing and re-evaluating goals of care and care plans • Therapeutic recommendations to relieve distress • Request for organ donation and autopsy	• Presence • Anticipatory guidance • Assessment and relief of child and family distress • Respond to questions and/or concerns • Perform little acts of kindness
Nurse	• Administration of distress relieving interventions • Ensure the setting is equipped to meet child's and family's needs with regard to staff, medications and equipment • Gatekeeper when requested by family • Communicator with larger team regarding bedside experiences of child and family	
Psychosocial clinician	• Provide individual or family psychotherapy as a continuation of an ongoing process, or as needed on a crisis basis • Facilitate legacy-building opportunities • Assist with advanced care planning regarding after-death steps such as wake and/or funeral arrangements • Consider larger family and community needs such as siblings and school	
Child life specialist	• Play activities to allow legacy-building opportunities • Play activities for child if able, siblings and other children to promote expression of feelings regarding child's death • Play activities for siblings and other children to create opportunities to escape from the intensity of being with a dying child	
Chaplain	• Assess and respond to spiritual needs of child and family • Ensure that clinicians are familiar with and respectful of family rituals related to death and dying • Meet with community spiritual leader as indicated	
Pharmacist	• Advise about distress-relieving medications • Ensure adequate supply of distress-relieving medications	

death, it may still be difficult for parents and other loved ones to grasp this reality because the child may not appear dead. The clinical neurological examination remains the standard for the determination of brain death and has been adopted by most countries. The declaration of brain death requires not only a series of careful neurologic tests but also the establishment of the cause of coma, the ascertainment of irreversibility, the resolution of any misleading clinical neurologic signs, the interpretation of the findings on neuroimaging, and the performance of any confirmatory laboratory tests that are deemed necessary (Box 36-2).[6] Despite medical consensus of the definition of brain death, not all religions officially accept this definition of death.[7] Depending on the family's beliefs and those of spiritual or religious advisers, families rarely disagree with this death pronouncement but conflict resolution may require ethics consultation and/or judicial involvement. Nonetheless, a thorough understanding of brain death can aid

in conversations with families. Once cardiorespiratory support is discontinued, the typical signs of dying ensue.

KEY COMMUNICATION TOPICS

Several communication topics are discussed in detail in Section 2, and will therefore not be covered in this chapter. Notably, however, anticipatory guidance can help prepare families for the child's end-of-life course and ease the child's and family's

---

BOX 36-1 Signs of Impending Death

- Profound progressive weakness
- Sleeping much of the time
- Little interest in food and drink
- Difficulty swallowing
- Disorientation to time, with increasingly short attention span
- Urinary incontinence or retention
- Oliguria or anuria
- Dropping blood pressure not related to hypovolemia, with rising, weak pulse
- Changes in respiratory rate and pattern, which may include a Cheyne-Stokes pattern characterized by oscillation of ventilation between apnea and tachypnea with a crescendo-decrescendo pattern in the depth of respirations
- Noisy breathing, airway secretions
- Mottling and cooling of skin
- Mental status changes, such as delirium, restlessness, agitation, and coma

Adapted from Bicanovsky L. Comfort Care: Symptom Control in the Dying. In Walsh, D et al Palliative Medicine 1st Edition, Saunders, An imprint of Elsevier Science, 2009.

BOX 36-2 Clinical Criteria for Brain Death in Adults and Children

Coma
Absence of motor responses
Absence of pupillary responses to light and pupils at midposition with respect to dilatation (4-6 mm)
Absence of corneal reflexes
Absence of caloric responses
Absence of gag reflex
Absence of coughing in response to tracheal suctioning
Absence of sucking and rooting reflexes
Absence of respiratory drive at a $PaCO_2$ that is 60 mm Hg or 20 mm Hg above normal base-line values*
Interval between two evaluations, according to patient's age
Term to 2 months old, 48 hours
>2 months to 1 year old, 24 hours
>1 year to <18 year old, 12 hours
>18 year old, interval optional
Confirmatory tests[†]
Term to 2 months old, 2 confirmatory tests
>2 month to 1 year old, 1 confirmatory test
>1 year to <18 year old, optional
>18 year old, optional

*$PaCO_2$ denotes the partial pressure of arterial carbon dioxide
[†]Confirmatory tests include cerebral angiography, electroencephalography, transcranial Doppler ultrasonography and cerebral scintigraphy
Adapted from Wijdicks E. The Diagnosis of Brain Death. *N Engl J Med* 2001;344:1215–1221.

distress. Proposed timing for key communication topics in children with advanced life-threatening illness is as follows:

- In advance of clear decline:
  - Considerations about resuscitation status (Chapter 22)
  - Discussions related to preferred location of care (Chapters 7 and 21)
- During clear decline:
  - Discussion related to preferred location of child's death and who will pronounce the child's death (Chapters 7 and 21)
- When death appears to be within days:
  - Discussion related to organ and tissue donation and autopsy (Chapters 24 and 25)
  - Funeral and commemoration planning
- Following death:
  - Bereavement guidance. (Chapter 5) Parents have reported finding face-to-face visits following the child's death to be very helpful in their bereavement.[8,9]

There are several key principles in managing the child's final days. An analytical approach to symptom control continues, but usually relies on clinical findings rather than investigation. Drugs should be reviewed with regard to need and route of administration. Some patients manage to take oral drugs until near their death, but many require an alternative route. Finally, it is essential that the care team maintains effective communication and ensures that support is in place for the family. A daily visit for inpatients or a daily phone call at a planned time can be very reassuring for families. Experience suggests that clinician home visits from the hospital-based team are greatly appreciated throughout the entire palliative care course, and data suggest that this is especially valued at the end of a patient's life.[10]

Importantly, even when the child may be comfortable and symptoms are well controlled, a caregiver's mere presence during the final period can be very comforting to family members. Such a presence reinforces that the dying patient's welfare remains important, and it provides support and guidance to the family at a time of extreme stress. It is critical to inform the family that although death may be imminent, the time frame may be hours to days. It is essential to ensure that someone will be available to pronounce the child's death, especially when the child is not in the hospital.

Easing Child Distress

When a child is actively dying, and there is consensus that the primary focus of care should be on comfort, there is much that the interdisciplinary team can do to permit a more natural death experience. Continued medical interventions, including vital sign assessments, pulse oximetry, nonessential medications and blood work, may be disruptive and no longer beneficial to the child's care. However, discussion of discontinuing these procedures is delicate and can be perceived as no longer caring for the child. This is especially true among families who are used to vigilantly monitoring their child. Parents should be made aware that discontinuing these procedures allows them time to be with the child without interference from intermittent procedures, wires and tape, and/or sounds from alarms. Gentle suggestions can be made that discontinuing monitors would enable the family to focus entirely on the child, rather than the surrounding medical equipment. As always, flexibility is essential. Some families may simply not want to forgo what they are used to and will often state that the vital sign assessment and/or the monitor will help them know when the child's time has come.

SYMPTOMS THAT NEED NOT BE TREATED

Importantly, when a child is actively dying, comfort can be achieved without a focus on reversing the underlying causes of symptoms. For example, it may no longer be indicated to directly treat severe constipation if the child is not expected to live more than a few days. Rather, abdominal discomfort from constipation could be treated symptomatically with opioids, even though opioids may exacerbate constipation. Similarly, continued dressing changes for bedsores may be more painful and disruptive than opting for a more general approach of titrating symptom-relieving medications. Most importantly, when a symptom is not a priority for the child and the parent, this should guide treatment decisions. Again, these decisions should be individualized and discussed with parents so that they understand that it represents a change in care strategy rather than a decrease in care provided.

DRAWING INWARD

The endpoint of the terminal phase is often marked by a turning inward, away from the external world, by the child. Cognitive and emotional horizons narrow, as all energy is needed simply for physical survival. A generalized irritability is not uncommon. The child may talk very little, and may even retreat from physical contact. Although such withdrawal is not universal, a certain degree of quietness is almost always evident. The child is pulling into himself or herself, not away from others. It is critical to explain this behavior as a normal and expectable precursor to death to the parents so that they do not interpret it as rejection.[11,12]

DROWSINESS AND ALTERED CONSCIOUSNESS

Diminished wakefulness is also very common during the last days of life[13] and is often desirable for the child and family. However, it is also not uncommon for parents and loved ones to want to hold onto every wakeful moment possible. At times this desire can hinder titration of pain-relieving medications because of the worry of further limiting wakefulness. The team should continue efforts to try for a careful balance of comfort and an ability to interact, while at the same time encourage the family to continue their own interactions, such as gentle hugging or touching, talking or singing, with the hope that the child perceives such gestures. One family reread aloud the first book of the Harry Potter series to their dying child, hoping that the story would bring as much joy to him as it had previously.

ESCALATING PAIN, DYSPNEA, AND AGITATION

Three highly common symptoms that may require intensive treatment efforts are escalating pain, dyspnea, and agitation during the final days of life. Full details for management of these distressing symptoms can be found in Chapters 28, 31, and 32. One challenge to successful management is variability among providers in the approach to medication titration. Children's Hospital Boston examined adequate symptom management in children with cancer at the end of life and found the following barriers to care:[14]

- Availability of nurses and physicians
- Identification of the team responsible for the patient
- Physician relying on the nurse at the bedside to recommend adequate pain medication to relieve symptoms of distress

- Delay in turn-around time from pharmacy in providing opioids to caretakers upon short notice
- Lack of knowledge and fear of opioid use in rapid escalation of doses
- Lack of understanding of the principle of double effect
- Fear on the part of the physicians and nurses of respiratory depression, addiction, hastening the death, and so-called euthanasia
- Variability in attitudes, practices, and experience of physicians and other members of the care team

In response to these findings, an interdisciplinary taskforce developed guidelines and a standardized order set to achieve greater consistency in medication titration and symptom management outcomes (Box 36-3). When a patient experiences a refractory symptom that cannot be captured through appropriate titration of symptom-relieving medications as described, then sedation to unconsciousness, or palliative sedation, may be indicated. Full details related to consideration, discussion and administration of palliative sedation can be found in Chapter 23.

BOX 36-3 Guidelines for Management of Escalating Pain, Dyspnea, or Agitation at the End of Life

These guidelines are intended for a patient at the end of life with a "Do Not Resuscitate" order in place, and with escalating pain, dyspnea, or agitation. Palliative sedation may be considered, with experienced guidance.

With escalating pain, dyspnea, agitation:

Identify the doctor or nurse responsible for prescribing for patient.

Care nurse to remain at bedside, and prescriber to remain on unit until symptoms controlled.

Charge nurse or designee will be available to assist as needed until symptoms controlled.

Nurse will notify pharmacy of expected need for increased opioid use. A back-up continuous infusion supply will be maintained. Nurse will call for new infusion each time back-up solution is started.

No ceiling dose exists for symptom management at the end of life. The correct dose is the one that relieves the symptoms.

Loading Dose:

For patient already on opioids: administer loading dose of same opioid equal to 10% of total opioid dose from preceding 24 hours.

For patients not already receiving opioids: administer loading dose IV x1 as follows:

Morphine 0.1 mg/kg IV x 1 dose

Hydromorphone 0.015 mg/kg IV x 1 dose

Fentanyl 1 mcg/kg IV x 1 dose

Subsequent Dosing:

Doses may be given Q10 minutes prn end of life symptoms.

Begin intermittent dosing, increasing every third dose, as indicated below:

If pain/dyspnea not relieved: Doses given Q 10 min. prn	Example:
Dose #1 is starting/loading dose	10 mg
1 x previous dose	10 mg
Increase to 1.5 x previous dose	15 mg
1 x previous dose	15 mg
Increase to 1.5 x previous dose	22.5 mg

If inadequate relief from first dose, give second dose.

If inadequate relief from second dose, notify prescriber of need for additional orders.

If good relief from either dose after 30 minutes, obtain order to begin and/or adjust continuous infusion.

If inadequate relief, continue the same sequence prn: 1x, 1.5x, 1x, 1.5x, 1x, 1.5x previous dose.

Pain Assessment may be by pain scale or be descriptive, such as crying, grimacing, moaning when moved.

Continuous Infusion Instructions:

Recommended Hourly Rate = total opioid dose administered during rapid titration phase ÷ 6 (which is 2x half-life in hours).

Adjustments for Moderate Increase in Symptoms:

If at any time symptoms recur, resume intermittent dosing as recommended above, and then increase hourly continuous infusion dose accordingly.

For a patient who has been stabilized on Patient Controlled Analgesia and then experiences a mild to moderate increase in symptoms, increase continuous infusion and intermittent dose by 1.3-1.5 x current dose.

Always consider use of adjunctive therapy (see guidelines). If morphine equivalent > 5 mg/kg/hour, or hydromorphone > 0.8 mg/kg/hour, adjunctive therapy is strongly recommended.

Adjunctive Therapy:

For Anxiety/Agitation: (Recommended Starting Dose)

Intermittent Lorazepam: 0.05 mg/kg IV Q4h prn anxiety/agitation

Intermittent Haloperidol: 0.01-0.03 mg/kg/day, IV divided Q8h or Q12h prn hallucinations/agitation (adult dosing: 0.5-5 mg/dose)

For excess respiratory secretions:

Glycopyrrolate: 4-10 mcg/kg/dose IV every 3 hours prn secretions

Hyocyamine:

Children 2-12 years: 0.0625-0.125 mg PO/SL every 4 hours as needed; maximum daily dosage 0.75 mg

Children >12 years to Adults: 0.125-0.25 mg PO/SL every 4 hours as needed; maximum daily dosage 1.5 mg

Scopalomine:

Children >12 years and Adults: Apply 1 disc behind the ear every 3 days as needed

---

Adapted from Children's Hospital Boston Guidelines for Management of Escalating Pain/Dyspnea/Agitation at the End of Life. Boston, Mass. Revised 9/2000. All rights reserved.

NOISY BREATHING

Breathing can become particularly noisy when death is imminent and is often described as the death rattle. This is more common in patients with primary lung disease or brain tumors.[15] It is critically important to prepare family members for this possibility. Because this symptom is often present when the child is already unconscious, the child may not experience this as uncomfortable. However, transdermal scopolamine, L-hyoscyamine drops for smaller patients and glycopyrrolate can be helpful in drying secretions and diminishing this symptom.[16-18] Treatment of what the family perceives as suffering should be a priority, even if there are differences of opinion within the care team.

TERMINAL EMERGENCIES

Rare circumstances can result in the child experiencing sudden high distress and some are best treated using more invasive strategies. Patients should be assessed for their risk of experiencing these complications so that effective interventions can be readily available. Such emergencies include:

Tension Pneumothorax

Sudden gasping can develop in a child who experiences a tension pneumothorax, which can occur in pulmonary metastases, for example. It results from a progressive deterioration and worsening of a simple pneumothorax associated with the formation of a one-way valve at the point of a rupture in the lung. Air becomes trapped in the pleural cavity between the chest wall and the lung and builds up, putting pressure on the lung and keeping it from fully inflating. Rapid titration of opioids alone is often insufficient to relieve suffering. Thus management should involve needle thoracostomy, the insertion of a large-bore needle into the second intercostal space on the midclavicular line, thereby releasing the pressure in the pleural cavity and converting the tension pneumothorax to a simple pneumothorax. Hemothorax can result in the same symptoms and can be treated similarly.

Upper Airway Obstruction

Acute stridor resulting from sudden upper airway obstruction is one of the most feared end-of-life symptoms. Death is near when this occurs, and emergency tracheotomy is not indicated. Instead, rapid initiation of opioids and benzodiazepines or initiation of palliative sedation are, at times, indicated.

Urinary Retention

Urinary retention is a known side effect of opioids, and if time permits, then opioid rotation should be considered. Crede's maneuver, the application of manual pressure over the lower abdomen, can also promote emptying of the bladder. However, depending on how imminent death is, or if retention is due to an irreversible cause, such as neurologic compromise or obstruction, then bladder decompression via catheterization can provide tremendous symptomatic relief. In such instances, decisions should be made regarding whether to continue with intermittent straight catheterization or Foley catheter placement depending on child and family preference.

Bowel Obstruction

Similarly there are effective strategies for the medical management of bowel obstruction, as delineated in Chapter 33; however, placement of nasogastric suctioning can provide the most immediate and sustained relief.

Hemorrhage

Massive hemorrhage is a catastrophic event. Dark towels should be made available if the event is anticipated. The only effective medical intervention is rapid initiation of sedation.

Myoclonus and Seizure

Myoclonus is often experienced in association with the use of high-dose opioids and can evolve into overt seizure. Early recognition and treatment with benzodiazepines can effectively treat this symptom. If seizure occurs either as a result of high-dose opioids or other underlying etiologies, it is critical to have anti-seizure medications available that can be administered intravenously, such as lorazepam, or rectally, such as diazepam.

Delirium and/or Hallucinations

It is common for the child to become less coherent toward the end of life, however, overt hallucinations and agitation can be extremely distressing for both the child and family. Chapter 28 provides an extensive review of assessment and management of delirium. In truly end-of-life instances, the child may respond well to intermittent doses of haloperdol, which can be administered intravenously.

ENSURING COMFORT DURING SPECIAL CIRCUMSTANCES

There are times at the end of a child's life when the process of either discontinuing certain medical interventions, such as fluids and nutrition, or beginning acts such as initiation of cardiopulmonary resuscitation, affect the experience of the child and family. When these special circumstances arise it is again helpful to prepare the family and child, if he or she is conscious.

When Fluids and Nutrition are Discontinued

Typically, as a child approaches end of life, there is little drive for drinking and eating, and older patients have indicated that this is not experienced as hunger or thirst.[19] It is not uncommon, however, for children to be receiving medically administered fluid and/or nutrition near the end of life, and this may prolong dying without providing benefit in terms of comfort. Continued fluids and nutrition may even contribute to discomfort. For example, in a child dying from an advanced brain tumor, continued fluids can increase cerebral edema and headache. In a child with end-stage lung disease, continued fluid can increase secretions, and at times pulmonary edema, both of which can exacerbate dyspnea. In such circumstances, clinicians and parents may opt to discontinue medically administered fluid and nutrition. However, once discontinued and depending on how long a child is likely to survive, the child's appearance may change over time. Anticipatory guidance is critical to helping the family through this end-of-life period. The following key considerations should be discussed:

Duration Before embarking on this conversation, the clinician should assess how long the child is likely to survive without hydration and nutrition. Estimates should be given in terms of hours, days, or weeks, rather than an exact amount of time. The duration that a child may survive depends on multiple factors. One consideration is the condition of internal organs, especially the heart and kidneys. For example, if fluids and nutrition are discontinued in a child in a persistent vegetative state, but without other end-organ damage, the child may live for days to weeks. However, in a child with multisystem organ involvement, the duration is likely to be considerably shorter. One sign that can indicate that death is near is when the child becomes aneuric. It is uncommon for a child to live more than a few days once the kidneys have stopped functioning. Importantly, though a decision may have been made to discontinue supplemental fluid and nutrition if the child is receiving intravenous medications, especially as continuous infusions, these include some fluid and can greatly impact the duration of the child's life. Estimates in these cases are much more difficult to make.

Change in Appearance With discontinuing fluids and nutrition, the child will appear increasingly dehydrated and this can be difficult to bear. In infants, the fontanel will become sunken. Eye sockets will become sunken in all children. Depending on how malnourished the child was to start, the abdomen may become concave. Mucous membranes become increasingly dry and secretions very thick. The skin will become looser. Though changes are likely, this does not mean the child is feeling uncomfortable. Nonetheless, the physical appearance of the child may invoke images of malnourished children, and although parents may understand that the child is not suffering, emotionally the changes may be unacceptable to them. As such, it is important to offer parents the opportunity to express their worries, and it may be even helpful to reinstitute some hydration at times.

What Can and Should Be Done As noted, most children do not express discomfort when not receiving medically administered fluid and nutrition, especially as consciousness lessens. Nonetheless, simple measures can be helpful to both the child and family. Sips of desired liquid and small bites of any food requested can provide a great deal of comfort. Administration of artificial tears can prevent painful cornea abrasions as the eyes become dryer. Gentle moistening of the mouth with water-soaked toothettes or ice chips can also be extremely comforting, as is moistening of the lips with a damp cloth or petroleum hydrolatum. Gentle repositioning to prevent bedsores is also helpful. Finally, as described in Chapter 31, opioids should be titrated appropriately in response to any expression of distress.

When the Ventilator Is Discontinued One of the most common ways a child typically dies in the intensive care unit (ICU) is through the discontinuation of ventilator support.[20–22] Though difficult to know with certainty, this decision is typically made when there is consensus that the underlying cause of ventilator dependence is irreversible, and continued ventilatory support will not result in a meaningful quality of life. The following considerations are important when the patient, when involved, the family, and the healthcare team reach consensus that ventilator support will be discontinued.

The counseling of families[23] is a critical aspect of care for the patient who is to be removed from a ventilator. Before withdrawal, the following issues should be discussed:

- **Potential outcome of ventilator withdrawal:** Clinical experience suggests that even when there is clear consensus that the child will not survive for long following discontinuation of ventilator support, at times a child will unexpectedly breathe on his or her own. This is especially possible in the newborn who was initially intubated for apnea. Thus preparing the family for the possibility that the child may survive is essential. In most situations, however, when all other life-sustaining treatments have been stopped, including artificial hydration and nutrition, outcomes include rapid death within minutes, that is when patients are on maximal respiratory support, or death in hours to days. More specific prognostication is often not possible.
- **Assurances about comfort:** It is important to prepare the family for the possibility that breathlessness may occur, but that it can be managed. Confirm that medication will be available to manage any discomfort and that the patient will likely need to be kept asleep to control symptoms. It is helpful to further explain that involuntary moving or gasping does not reflect suffering if the patient is properly sedated or in a coma. Explain that the family can be at the bedside throughout withdrawal of the ventilator.
- **Reinforce the decision:** Even though a family is able to make a definite decision for ventilator withdrawal, such a decision is always emotionally difficult. It is helpful to provide reassurance they have made the best decision possible for their child.

Options for Ventilator Withdrawal Two methods have been described for ventilator withdrawal:[24] immediate extubation and terminal weaning. The clinician's and patient's comfort, and the family's perceptions, should influence the choice. In immediate extubation, the endotracheal tube is removed after appropriate suctioning. Humidified air or oxygen is given to prevent the airway from drying. This is the preferred approach to relieve discomfort if the patient is conscious, the volume of secretions is low, and the airway is unlikely to be compromised after extubation. A patient likely to experience significant hemoptysis, for example, may benefit from a terminal wean with the gradual reduction in oxygen and/or ventilator rate at a pace not faster than pharmacologic sedation is administered to treat objective signs of distress from the effects of hypoventilation and hypoxia. In terminal weaning, the ventilator rate, positive end-expiratory pressure (PEEP), and oxygen levels are decreased while the endotracheal tube is left in place. Terminal weaning may be carried out over a period of as little as 30 minutes, or it can be longer. If the patient survives and it is decided to leave the endotracheal tube in place, a Briggs T-piece can be placed.

The following are suggested steps to ensure smooth withdrawal of ventilator support:

- Encourage family members to make arrangements for clergy, special music or rituals that may be important to them.
- Document clinical findings, discussion with family and plan of care.
- Turn off all monitors and alarms, when agreed upon by family.
- Remove any unnecessary medical paraphernalia, such as the nasogastric tube.
- Maintain intravenous access for administration of palliative medications.

- Suction patient and set the oxygen to 0.21; observe for signs of respiratory distress.
- Adjust medications as needed to relieve distress before proceeding further.

Neuromuscular Blockade (NMBA)

Neuromuscular blocking drugs have no sedative or analgesic properties and may mask symptoms of suffering at the end of life. As a general rule, therefore, pharmacologic paralysis should be avoided at the end of life. In most cases, the effect of these agents can be reversed or allowed to wear off within a short period of time, allowing for the withdrawal of mechanical ventilation in the absence of the confounding effects of paralysis. Patients who have been receiving NMBAs chronically for management of their ventilatory failure occasionally can present a more difficult ethical dilemma. In some situations, restoration of neuromuscular function may not be possible for several days or even weeks. When faced with this problem, the clinician must choose between withdrawing the ventilator while the patient is paralyzed versus continuation of life support well beyond the point at which the patient and family have determined that the burdens of such treatments outweigh the probable benefits. In this circumstance, it may be preferable to proceed with withdrawal of life support despite the continued presence of neuromuscular blockade.

Symptom Control

The most common symptoms related to ventilator withdrawal are breathlessness and anxiety. Opioids and benzodiazepines are the primary medications used to provide comfort, typically requiring doses that cause sedation to achieve good symptom control. The dose needed to control symptoms will depend on the neurological status of the patient and the amount of similar medication used up to the time of extubation. In unconscious patients, it should not be assumed that they will not experience distress, and symptom-relieving medications should be administered in advance of planned extubation. Patients who are awake at the time extubation or in whom significant amounts of opioids and benzodiazepines have been used previously will require greater dosages or a change to a barbiturate to achieve symptom control.[25] Medication titration should proceed according to guidelines discussed in Chapter 23.

Clinical Vignette

Jamal was a 3-year-old boy with a history of hypoxic ischemic encephalopathy who was admitted to the intensive care unit with aspiration pneumonia requiring intubation. This was the fourth intensive care unit admission in 6 months. After 3 weeks of care in the ICU, and several unsuccessful attempts at extubation, the family was approached about tracheostomy placement and chronic ventilation. After extensive consultation with the pediatric palliative care team, his parents came to the decision that Jamal had been through enough, that despite the doctors' best efforts his condition continued to deteriorate. They expressed the desire that he be allowed to die. They also expressed the hope that he die at home, despite the fact that they lived 3 hours away in a rural area.

Extensive discussions were held with the ICU staff about the following concerns:

- *How could the ICU team be sure that he would be comfortable if extubation were to take place at the home?*

- *What if the family changed their minds and asked for him to be reintubated?*
- *Is it fair to use hospital resources, such as the transport team, to transfer the child home if these same resources might be needed to save a child's life?*

Many interdisciplinary conversations were held to ease the worries of the ICU team. Arrangements for support at home were made in advance of the transport. Ultimately, Jamal was taken home by the transport team and the palliative care physician. He was stable during the journey. His extended family was at his home when he arrived. They said their farewells, and Jamal received the sacrament of the sick from his local priest. Also present were his pediatrician and two nurses from a local hospice. Jamal received 2 mg morphine and 1 mg midazolam, and was then removed from the ventilator. He was given four morphine rescue doses and two midazolam rescue doses through his pump for respiratory rate of greater than 50 breaths per minutes and increased work of breathing as assessed by clinicians or his parents. He died peacefully in his mother's arms 75 minutes after extubation. The family was extremely grateful that he was home to die.

Easing Family Distress

DURING A RESUSCITATIVE EFFORT

Approximately 75% of children who experience pulseless cardiac arrest in the hospital, and 90% of those who experience an out-of-hospital arrest will die.[26,27] Most hospitals are instituting efforts to pre-empt unexpected cardiorespiratory arrest by instituting protocols to promote early transfer to the ICU.[28] Despite these efforts, codes continue to occur and efforts should be made to attend to the family's distress. Such efforts include identifying a point person for the family, who can serve as a constant presence during the resuscitative effort, provide regular updates, answer questions and make every effort to meet the family's needs. Families are now regularly invited to be present during resuscitative efforts. The data suggest that when they are present, there is less anxiety, litigation, and second-guessing regarding the efforts and competence of the staff providing that care.[29]

THE LINGERING CHILD

Clinical experience suggests that it is not uncommon for families to express distress regarding the length of time it is taking for the child to die when active dying lasts for hours or days. It is impossible to imagine the enormity of the distress associated with this period of time, the ambivalence of feelings related to wanting to hold on to every moment versus not being able to bear a moment longer at the child's bedside. Anticipatory guidance aimed at preparing families for this period can be helpful. Further, suggesting ways to be with the child can also ease family distress. Communication strategies include:

- Touch, such as lying beside the child, gentle massage, and hugging,
- Sound, family's spoken words, including reading favorite books, reflecting on memories, music, and prayer, much of which depends on family background and communication style,

- Sight, such as looking at photos and other memorabilia, and adjusting the lighting to family preference,
- Smell, depending on family culture incense and other familiar smells may be calming,
- Doing, continuing with caring through application of damp cloths to forehead, moistening lips, or gentle suction when helpful is also part of the process.

Management of visitors is a key role of the healthcare team. For some families, being surrounded by extended family and friends is critical, for others it is unbearable. Inquiring about what is most comforting is essential.

Throughout this period, attention to the child's comfort remains the top priority and if suffering is perceived by loved ones and clinicians, medications should be further titrated.

HASTENING DEATH

Rarely, a parent will overtly request that the child's death be intentionally hastened,[30] and this is most commonly associated with parental fears about child suffering. Euthanasia is legal only in the Netherlands[22,31,32] and is for children either younger than 1 year old or older than 12 and who are considered able to provide assent. Euthanasia for minors is also under consideration in Belgium.[33] There are no legal hastening options for minors in North America. Yet, if the parent requests hastening, it is important to respond with more than just a statement that hastening is not legally permissible. Just as other requests should be explored to identify underlying meaning and fears, so should this type of request. Explanation of legal and effective alternatives, such as further titration of symptom-relieving medications and palliative sedation, is helpful.

Clinical Vignette

Eddie was 6-year-old boy with advanced metastatic alveolar rhabdomyosarcoma. The primary lesion involved his face and neck, and he also had pulmonary and bone marrow metastases. His parents wanted to be prepared for what to expect for his end-of-life course and the palliative care team offered the following information. One significant concern was that Eddie's tumor would progress locally faster than in his lungs and bone marrow and, as a result, he was at high risk for upper airway obstruction and suffocation at the end of life. The family was also told about progressive dyspnea and fatigue, should other sites of disease progress faster. Upon hearing these possibilities his father, Charlie, asked whether Eddie's life could be intentionally ended when he reached a stage when his life was no longer worth living. Rather than focusing on the illegal nature of such an action, Charlie was asked more about his worries and he described immense concerns about Charlie's experience of suffering. In response, the physician gently informed him that we may not be able to tell when life was not worth living from Eddie's perspective, but that every effort would be made to try to ensure his comfort. Eddie's father was told about strategies for intensive symptom management and palliative sedation, if necessary.

Eddie did not suffer from dyspnea or upper airway obstruction. He simply became less and less responsive, and required minimal pain-relieving medications. He died peacefully surrounded by family, friends, and clinical caregivers. Several weeks following his death, Charlie reflected that had Eddie's life been intentionally ended, it would have been treating his own suffering, and not Eddie's.

PARTICIPATING IN PRAYER WITH FAMILIES

Clinicians are, at times, asked to pray for a child or to lead a family in prayer. This may be an indication of unmet spiritual needs and further exploration of whether it would be helpful to involve the chaplain, if he or she is not already involved, may be warranted. Regardless, the clinician may feel conflicted about whether to participate in or lead a prayer on behalf of the patient because of considerations of professional-personal boundaries and his or her own religious beliefs or spirituality. Consideration of the following options, which attempt to respect the integrity of the clinician's beliefs and to be supportive of the family's needs, may be helpful.[34,35]

1. Praying for the patient: It may be suitable for clinicians to pray if they feel comfortable doing so and such prayer is consistent with their own beliefs.
2. Sit with patient and family while the family prays: A clinician who is uncomfortable praying with the family may choose instead to sit quietly in supportive company while they pray. In this way, clinicians lend support to the patient and family without explicitly endorsing a particular belief system.
3. Respectfully decline: Clinicians may also respectfully decline to pray with the family. To avoid the patient feeling rejected, the clinician may want to say, "Because of my own values, I am unable to participate; however, please know that you will be in my thoughts."

MEMORY MAKING

There are numerous activities that families can take part in during the final periods of the child's life that contribute to the legacy and family memories. The following activities are commonly gently offered to families:

- Prints of the hands and feet, or making molds
- Obtaining a lock of hair
- Making of a memory box or book
- Photographing and videotaping
- Journaling

It is important to offer a variety of possibilities, because activities will appeal to different family members. At the same time, respecting the family's decision to decline is also critically important.

At the Time of Death

There is no true standard for declaring that a patient has died. When a clinician enters the room and is not known to the family, an introduction and explanation of his or her purpose is warranted. Empathetic statements, such as "I am sorry for your loss," can ease the distress, as can telling the family that they are welcome to stay while their loved one is examined.

THE PRONOUNCEMENT[36]

Consider the following steps to pronounce the death:

1. Identify the patient by the hospital ID tag.
2. Note the general appearance of the body; ensure that the patient is not overtly hypothermic at the time of this assessment.
3. Ascertain that the patient does not rouse to verbal or tactile stimuli. Avoid overtly painful stimuli such as deep sternal pressure.
4. Listen for the absence of heart sounds; feel for the absence of carotid pulse.
5. Look and listen for the absence of spontaneous respirations.

   There is no standard amount of time for steps 4 and 5; at Children's Hospital Boston it is recommended to observe for 60 seconds.

6. Record the position of the pupils and the absence of pupillary light reflex.
7. Record the time at which assessment is completed.
8. Once completed, it is considerate to again make an empathetic statement acknowledging the family's loss.

DOCUMENTATION IN THE MEDICAL RECORD

A simple statement in the medical record is all that is required, "Called to pronounce (name); chart the findings of physical examination and note the date and time of death." The following additional items should also be noted:

- If attending physician and family, if not present, were notified
- If the organ bank was notified, which is required in the United States
- If the coroner or medical examiner was notified, which is required in some states for a child death regardless of cause

DEATH CERTIFICATE COMPLETION

There is tremendous variability in diagnoses used for completion of the death certificate; however, experience suggests that what is written can hold great importance for family members. Guidelines are readily available. In the United States, the National Association of Medical Examiners provides the following guidelines:[37]

1. Make every effort to report an etiologically specific underlying cause of death.
2. Try to use a Sequential Part I Format, if possible.
3. Err on the side of reporting too much rather than too little.
4. Do not report mechanistic terminal events such as:
   - Cardiac arrest
   - Asystole
   - Cardiopulmonary arrest
   - Respiratory arrest
   - Electromechanical dissociation
   - Ventricular fibrillation
5. Do not report symptoms or signs.
6. Do not report a condition if its existence in the patient is obvious based on another reported condition.
7. Do not oversimplify.
8. Do not use abbreviations.

After Death Care

The most important message to relay to parents is that nothing needs to be done in a hurry when their child dies. This is very much a private time for family to say their individual goodbyes. Saying goodbyes and performing rituals are important because they enable parents, siblings, and other family members to express their love, sorrow, relief, regrets, and share precious memories. Many will be guided by religious practices, which can vary considerably (Table 36-2). Washing the child for the last time, dressing the child in special clothes, taking photos, playing favorite music, praying together, touching and cuddling the child, talking to the child, taking foot and handprints, cutting a lock of hair and writing a message or poem for the child are all examples of rituals that families have found helpful and necessary.

Clinical Vignette

Laila was a 2-month-old girl with junctional epidermolysis bullosa, an often fatal disorder involving fragility of the skin and mucous membranes. Laila was being cared for in the neonatal intensive care unit, and with time, the primary hopes of her parents became focused on ensuring her comfort. Laila's parents were newly arrived immigrants from China and they were living with paternal grandparents, also first generation immigrants. All family members were often present at the bedside. Laila's mother, Hua, sought support from the pediatric palliative care team social worker to help reconcile two concerns. The first was that related to the families' cultural background, photographs were not permitted. Hua felt caught between respecting tradition and her elders and wanting to have an image of her daughter. Through strategizing with the care team, she decided to seek permission from the family to obtain a passport for Laila. The family agreed, hoping that should Laila's condition improve she could be brought to China for herbal remedies. The social worker arranged for representatives from the passport agency to come to the hospital to complete the application, which included taking a photograph. The passport was expedited and arrived just prior to Laila's death.

Hua also said her in-laws had told her that she would need to leave Laila at the hospital following her death and they would not permit burial. They believed that if Laila were to be buried, her spirit would interfere with Hua being able to attach to future children. Despite this advice, Hua was desperate to know the place where Laila would be buried. Arrangements were made to bury her in the hospital's burial grounds, where Hua could visit without the knowledge of her family.

When the family is ready, they need to phone the funeral home. If preparation for death has been encouraged, then most families will have already chosen the funeral director they wish to use. Parents need to inform the funeral director of the time they wish for the child's body to be collected. It is very important that parents remain in control of the timing and they are not hurried. Funeral directors are on call 24 hours a day and parents can phone at any time. There may be an extra cost if the child needs to be taken after normal working hours.

TABLE 36-2 Examples of Religion and Care at the Time of Death

This information is an introduction to specific religious traditions, and is meant to help clinicians understand variations in religious practice. Providers are cautioned not to over-generalize or characterize all members of a religious group as being alike. A person's spiritual and religious profile is unique and can only be determined when trust has been established, and open-ended assessment questions are asked.

Religion	Concepts about death	Rituals near and at time of death	Routine postmortem care	Body disposal	Mourning rituals
Buddhism	Death is seen as a process in the cyclical continuum, which includes birth, sickness, old age, death, rebirth, sickness, old age, death, and so on.	Because death is associated with rebirth, great importance is attributed to the state of mind, which should be calm and clear. This means that serene surroundings are important at the time of death. No formal rituals are customary at the time of death. The family may wish to contact a monk who will pray for the deceased. Prayers do not need to be performed in the presence of the body.	In general, Buddhism does not oppose autopsies. Many Tibetan Buddhists believe that the dead body should not be cut or embalmed until 3 days have passed. Routine postmortem care is generally acceptable.	Cremation is typical.	The first 7 days after death are the most important for final and funereal prayer. Prayers are then said weekly, during a 49-day funeral period. It is during this period that the prayers of the mourners are believed to help the deceased during the post-death transformation and awaken their spirit to the true nature of death.
Greek and Eastern Orthodox	Orthodox Christians believe death is a necessary consequence of human life due to original sin. Death is necessary to achieve everlasting life.	When a person nears death, it is customary for the priest of the church to be called. The priest in the family's parish is preferred. If the family does not have its own clergy locally, the chaplain may assist in contacting an Orthodox priest through the local Greek Orthodox Diocese. If the patient is awake, Holy Communion can and should be offered to the dying person. The Orthodox priest may also anoint the ill person on the forehead, cheeks, chest, and hands with holy oil in a ritual of spiritual and bodily healing known as the Sacrament of Holy Unction. There are no Last Rites in the Orthodox Church. When the patient has died, the priest will read special prayers for the dead, as well as provide emotional and spiritual support to the bereaved.	Orthodox persons usually decline autopsies, although they are permitted if there are compelling medical reasons to do so, if the body is treated with dignity and if all the tissues and organs are returned to the body for burial. When a child dies, it is customary to dress him or her in white as a groom or bride of Christ, and great care is taken in the selection of burial clothing.	Burial is preferred but the Orthodox Church allows cremation if the law of the country requires it.	The Eastern Orthodox hold a special vigil over the dead called the parastasis or panikhida, as a time of contemplation on death. The funeral service includes hymns, chants, and Bible readings.

Continued

TABLE 36-2 Examples of Religion and Care at the Time of Death—cont'd

This information is an introduction to specific religious traditions, and is meant to help clinicians understand variations in religious practice. Providers are cautioned not to over-generalize or characterize all members of a religious group as being alike. A person's spiritual and religious profile is unique and can only be determined when trust has been established, and open-ended assessment questions are asked.

Religion	Concepts about death	Rituals near and at time of death	Routine postmortem care	Body disposal	Mourning rituals
Hinduism	Hindus believe that although the physical body dies, the soul of a person has no beginning or end (*Samsara*). Death marks a passage rather than the end of life. At death, the soul may be reborn into another living being. The nature of subsequent rebirth is a consequence of actions taken in this life.	The family may wish to keep vigil at the bedside, and play recordings of sacred Indian music to help the patient detach from pain or other worldly things. While the burning of incense is not permitted in the hospital, special arrangements may be made for the use of incense in the hospital chapel or prayer room. The ashes from the incense are often placed on the forehead of the patient, as a blessing. Hindu clergy is not usually requested; although when present, may tie sacred threads around the wrists or neck of the body. Clinical staff should not remove these threads.	Autopsy is permissible. After death, the family may wish to place drops of holy water and basil leaves in the mouth of the deceased, as well as wash or dress the body. The clinician should wear disposable gloves to show respect in closing the eyes and wrapping the body. The deceased's arms should be straightened.	Cremation is preferred, usually within 24 hrs of death. In preparation for cremation, the body is bathed, laid in a coffin, adorned with sandalwood paste and garlands, and wrapped in white cloth. Embalming is not customary.	Survivors may choose to fast until the cremation takes place. If so, families may appreciate advocacy to ensure prompt cremation. Family members sometimes choose to delay the cremation until the arrival of extended family. The remains are usually scattered in the Ganges River in India or another body of water. In the cremation ceremony, the body is carried three times counterclockwise around the pyre, then placed upon it. The chief mourner hits the cremation switch. The days of mourning are considered a time of ritual impurity. Mourners cover all religious pictures in the house and do not attend festivals or visit swamis or take part in marriage ceremonies. Mourning period length varies, though Hindu scriptures caution against excessive mourning. A bereavement ceremony to assist the well being of the soul takes place in the home between 10 and 30 days after death, often on the 13th day. The first year anniversary and subsequent anniversaries of death are very important to surviving family members and involves sacred religious rites.
Islam	Muslims believe that there is another world after death for which believers should prepare during their lives on earth.	The family of a dying Muslim may ask that the patient face the east, with his or her head elevated. At the time of death, the Muslim call to prayer is recited by friends, and a chapter of the Koran is read aloud. An imam is not customarily present at the time of death, but will come if asked.	The body is considered sacred, thus autopsies are forbidden except in cases of compelling legal or medical reasons. If an autopsy must be done, it should be as non-invasive and minimally disfiguring as possible, such as tissue biopsy, and all body parts and fluids returned to the body for burial. Healthcare providers should speak with the family or the Muslim chaplain before giving postmortem care. Many may prefer that another Muslim of the same sex prepare the body. If no Muslim is present, a non-Muslim should use gloves so as to not touch the body. The body should be draped to ensure privacy at all times. Washing will be done in a ritual way at the funeral home. When doing the postmortem care, the head should be turned to the right, and the arms are laid by the patient's side. No locks of hair should be cut.	Burial is performed as soon as possible because embalming is not customary. Cremation is forbidden. The corpse is bathed and wrapped in a plain cloth called a kafan. The deceased is buried in the ground after the funeral service. Only burial in the ground is allowed according to Shari'ah, Islamic law.	Mourners gather and offer Janazah, prayers for the forgiveness of the deceased. Once the body is buried, Muslim mourners offer one final Janazah prayer.

| Judaism | Judaism defines death as occurring when respiration and circulation are irreversibly stopped. Brain death is not generally acknowledged among the most Orthodox, and is a source of debate among Conservatives. Euthanasia and withdrawal of care that hastens death are strictly forbidden. In some cases, extraordinary care may be withheld. There are precise rabbinical guidelines called *Responsa* for such situations, and consultation with the Rabbi around such matters is often sought by the family. Jews believe death in this life will eventually lead to resurrection in a world to come. | At the time of death, the family may wish to gather at the bedside, read psalms and recite the *vidui*, the last prayer of confession. It is not customary for a rabbi to be present at the time of death, although one may be requested. | Some Orthodox and Conservative Jews do not approve of autopsy, unless required by law or the life of a specific person, such as other family members in the case of a hereditary illness, can be saved by information from the autopsy.

If an autopsy is done, the more limited the disfigurement, the better. Needle biopsy, limited autopsy, or in situ examination are preferred. All body parts and fluids need to be returned for burial. Some Orthodox families may request their rabbi to be present to observe the autopsy.

Postmortem care is very important to observant Jews. Medical personnel should consult the family before washing the body. The nurse should provide routine care of the body wearing gloves. The arms are not crossed in postmortem care. Any clothing, dressings, or medical equipment with the patient's blood must be buried with the patient.

The Jewish community may use designated individuals to wash the body at a later time, and prefer funeral homes who are familiar with Jewish faith and ritual.

In the Jewish traditions, the body may not be left alone until the burial. Family may wish to station someone outside the morgue to sit with the body until it is removed from the hospital. | Cremation is forbidden. Burial is required to be done as soon as possible; embalming is not permitted unless legally required. The dead are buried as soon as possible. The body is washed to purify it, dressed in a plain linen shroud. The casket, a plain wooden coffin, remains closed after the body is dressed. The body is watched over from time of death till burial, as a sign of respect. The kaddish, a prayer in honor of the dead, is said. | Jews do not make funeral arrangements on the Sabbath or major holidays. A mourning period follows the funeral for the immediate family (*shiva*). Friends and hospital staff who have come to know the family well are welcome to visit the home in the mourning period. It is customary to make charitable contributions rather than send flowers. There is an intense 7-day mourning period, called *shiva*, following the burial. Mourners traditionally rent their garments as a symbol of grief. Today, people often wear a black ribbon instead of tearing their clothes. Mourners also cover mirrors, sit on low stools, and avoid wearing leather. The full mourning period lasts a year, after which mourners observe the dead's yahrzeit, or yearly anniversary, of the death. |

Continued

TABLE 36-2 Examples of Religion and Care at the Time of Death—cont'd

This information is an introduction to specific religious traditions, and is meant to help clinicians understand variations in religious practice. Providers are cautioned not to over-generalize or characterize all members of a religious group as being alike. A person's spiritual and religious profile is unique and can only be determined when trust has been established, and open-ended assessment questions are asked.

Religion	Concepts about death	Rituals near and at time of death	Routine postmortem care	Body disposal	Mourning rituals
Protestantism	Conservative Protestants believe that everyone has the gift of eternal life. The body dies, but the soul lives forever. The larger question is where each person will spend eternity. Heaven is a glorious location where there is an absence of pain, disease, sex, depression, etc. and where people exist in the presence of Jesus Christ. Hell is a location where its inmates will be punished without any hope of relief, for eternity. The level of punishment will be the same for everyone. A second major belief is that most humans will be sent to hell after they die. Only those few who have been saved will go to heaven. Salvation requires repentance of sins and trusting Jesus as one's Lord and Savior. Believers who have done many good deeds will be rewarded more in heaven; believers who have led an evil life will be rewarded less.	If a child is critically ill, the nurse may want to ask the family about baptism. If the family wishes to baptize their child in the hospital, the Protestant chaplain can be paged or the church pastor called. The family usually prefers to be present, and often finds the pastor to be a reassuring companion at such a time. Providers should inquire if families would like their pastor or chaplain called. There are no essential end-of-life sacraments, although some Episcopalian, Lutheran, and Pentecostal persons may request anointing. Reading of scripture, bedside prayers that are personalized to the particular situation, and singing are common.	There are no special concerns for postmortem care. Organ donation and autopsy are a matter of personal preference.	No restrictions or special concerns.	Funerals, memorial services and burials are scheduled at the family's convenience because embalming and/or cremation are common.
Roman Catholicism	The Catholic church has a high regard for the preservation and dignity of life, including the sick, disabled, and unborn. The church does not obligate persons to pursue gravely burdensome or ineffective life-sustaining interventions. Analgesics may be used in sufficient amounts to relieve pain even if life is thereby shortened, so long as death is not the intended effect. Catholics see death as a passage from this life to the new, everlasting life promised by Christ. The soul of the deceased goes on to the afterlife, which includes purgatory as well as heaven and hell. According to Catholic belief, the bodies of the dead will be resurrected at the end of time.	Because the priest is viewed as an intermediary between the believer and God, and one whose prayers have special merit, the priest is often requested at the time of death. Even when all sacramental care has been provided earlier, families may request that the priest be present. Families may request an emergency baptism, or sacrament of the sick before death.	There are no special concerns for postmortem care. Organ donation and autopsy are a matter of personal preference.	No restrictions or special concerns. The Church encourages Catholics to be buried in Catholic cemeteries. In 1963, the Vatican lifted the ban on cremation for Catholics. However, the cremains must be interred, not scattered or kept at home.	The Catholic funeral service is called the Mass of the Resurrection. During it, Jesus Christ's life is remembered and related to that of the deceased. Eulogies are not generally allowed during the funeral mass, but may be delivered at a wake or other non-religious ceremony. There is also a final graveside farewell, and additional traditions depending on the region.

Adapted from Children's Hospital Boston practitioner information pages:
Religious Traditions - Buddhism Copyright (c) 1997 Children's Hospital, Boston, Mass. Revised 9/2000 All rights reserved.
Greek (and Eastern) Orthodox Copyright (c) 1999 Children's Hospital, Boston, Mass. All rights reserved.
Religious Traditions - Hinduism Copyright (c) 1998 Children's Hospital, Boston, Mass. All rights reserved.
Religious Traditions - Islam (the faith of Muslims) Copyright (c) 1997 Children's Hospital. Boston, Mass. Revised 10/2002. All rights reserved.
Religious Traditions - Judaism Copyright (c) 1998 Children's Hospital. Boston, Mass. All rights reserved.
Religious Traditions - Protestantism (Christian) Copyright (c) 1997 Children's Hospital. Boston, Mass. All rights reserved.
Religious Traditions - Roman Catholicism Copyright (c) 1998 Children's Hospital. Boston, Mass. All rights reserved.

If the family plans to be with the child's body for a prolonged duration, then it may be helpful to gently prepare them for how the body will change over time.

LIVOR MORTIS

One of the early changes that can be observed is livor mortis, also referred to as *lividity, postmortem hypostasis, vibices, and suggilations.*[38] This is a physical process. While the individual is alive, the heart circulates the blood. When death occurs, circulation stops and the blood begins to settle, by gravity, to the lowest portions of the body. This results in a discoloration of those lower, dependent parts of the body. Although beginning immediately, the first signs of livor mortis are typically seen about 1 hour following death, with full development being observed 2 to 4 hours following death.[38]

RIGOR MORTIS

Rigor mortis is a chemical change resulting in a stiffening of the body's muscles following death, resulting from changes in the myofribrils of the muscle tissues. Immediately following death, the body becomes limp and is easily flexed.[38] As ATP is converted to ADP and lactic acid is produced lowering the cellular pH, locking chemical bridges are formed between actin and myosin resulting in formation of rigor. Typically, the onset of rigor is first observed 2 to 6 hours following death and develops over the first 12 hours. The onset begins with the muscles of the face and then spreads to all of the muscles during the next 4 to 6 hours. Rigor typically lasts from 24 to 84 hours, after which the muscles begin once again to relax.

DEATH IN THE HOSPITAL

Once the family has left the hospital, nurses typically prepare to do postmortem care by two staff members who can support one another. Preparation of the body will vary depending on hospital policy, religious and cultural preference, and whether or not the body will be examined by the medical examiner and/or an autopsy will be performed (see Table 36-2). When the body is formally examined, all indwelling lines and tubes must remain intact. Appropriate pads should be placed over puncture or wound sites and under the perineum to contain body fluids if necessary. The body should be dressed in a hospital gown or clothing designated by family.

Non-Medical Examiner Cases

If permission for autopsy is anticipated, all indwelling lines and tubes must remain intact, depending upon type of autopsy. This enables the pathologist to perform a more accurate examination. Parents who object to this practice may communicate their wishes for modifying the autopsy consent form. After consulting with the family as to specific religious or cultural practices:

- Consider warming lights to assist in maintaining some of the body's warmth.
- Bathe the body and attempt to restore as normal an appearance as possible. Some parents may wish to participate in bathing and dressing their child. This should be offered.

- Families may request special handling or positioning.
- Contact the appropriate chaplain for assistance, if indicated.

In most hospitals, the body is transported to the morgue in anticipation of being picked up by the funeral home. Body bags and special stretchers are used so that others will not recognize that a body is being transported. At times families object to the child's body being transported to the morgue and every effort should be made to accommodate such requests. In addition, certain religious observances require different handling of the body (see Table 36-2).

DEBRIEFING STAFF

No matter how common or rare it is for staff to care for a child through death, it is always helpful to create a safe and nonjudgmental forum for staff to reflect on the experience. As a example, in one setting staff bereavement rounds take place biweekly and each child who died during the period is discussed. The goals of such discussions are fourfold:

1. To reflect on the care delivered to the child and family regarding what went well and what could be improved upon,
2. To report on the bereavement experience of the family to ensure that their support needs are being met,
3. To celebrate the life of the child,
4. To support one another.

Because of role modeling by senior staff, these rounds are generally well attended.

STAFF COMMEMORATION

With the death of a child, whether that child has been cared for by staff for a short or long time, there are various ways in which to commemorate the child. At the same time, these actions often provide opportunities for self-care. In a study of more than 200 pediatric critical care specialists, 79% contacted families following the death at least sometimes, 72% attended funerals, and only 2.5% thought that it was inappropriate for clinicians to attend funerals. A total of 76% agreed that follow-up contact helps the family, whereas 47% agreed that follow-up contact helps the physicians.[39] For a more detailed description of staff commemorative activities see Chapter 18.

The condolence letter or card is one of the simplest gestures that can be made by a clinician and is typically highly valued by family members. Personal experience suggests that these notes are kept indefinitely and become a part of the child's legacy. A good condolence letter has two goals: to offer tribute to the deceased and to be a source of comfort to the survivors. One of the greatest hurdles to writing these letters is simply finding the right words. Bedell and colleagues offer some concrete suggestions:[40] One can begin the letter with a direct expression of sorrow about the death, such as "I am writing to send you my condolences on the death of your son." Typical themes to include in the letter are:

- A personal memory of the patient and family,
- Specific references to qualities of the child, such as courage, humor, and kindness, can bring life to the letter,
- An acknowledgment of all the family did for the child,

- A statement that it was a privilege to have participated in the child's care,
- Let the family know that it is fine to contact caregivers with questions or concerns,
- Conclude with a statement that the child will be remembered, which can also be very comforting.

Clinician acts of kindness and commemoration following a child's death should not be taken lightly. In a qualitative study[41] of bereaved parents whose child was in the care of the ICU three critical themes were identified:[41]

1. Parents place great importance on the hospital's memorial service, and on staff presence at such a service.
2. Parents often find it difficult to return to the hospital after the child's death, but attending the memorial service is common and helps with their bereavement.
3. Parents greatly appreciate receiving cards and clinician efforts to telephone, visit and attend the funeral and these little acts of kindness are recalled months, even years, later. Conversely, parents express disappointment when clinicians did not engage in these activities.

It is increasingly common for palliative care programs to offer longer-term bereavement support to families and these efforts are described in detail in Chapter 5.

Summary

Caring for a dying child is a truly intimate experience and a privilege that brings with it great sadness, but also enormous gifts, especially when clinicians are prepared to participate in this process and are given the opportunity to provide unhurried, compassionate care. The following case exemplifies such an experience.

Clinical Vignette

Mary was a 16-year-old girl with an advanced brain tumor and spinal metastases. Together with her family, her goals were to continue to strive for cancer control, but at the same time enjoy as much time at home in her community, which was several hours away from the hospital. She was passionate about attending school, being with family and friends, and painting (Fig. 36-1). Comprehensive support was put into place at home and Mary's many symptoms were managed proactively. Her medication regimen was extensive including the following:

Oral Medication	Indication
Dexamethasone 2 mg qid	*Cerebral edema*
Omeprazole 20 mg bid	*Gastric prophylaxis*
Bisacodyl 2 tabs bid	*Constipation*
Ondansetron 8 mg tid	*Nausea*
Metoclopramide 10 mg tid	*Nausea*
Methadone 15 mg tid	*Pain*
Methylphenidate 15 mg qam, 15 mg qnoon	*Daytime drowiness*
Celecoxib 100 mg bid	*Antiangiogenic agent*
Nortryptiline 20 mg qhs	*Neuropathic pain*
Gabapentin 300 mg tid	*Neuropathic pain*
Baclofen 15 mg tid	*Muscle spasm*
Sertraline 100 mg qhs	*Depression, anxiety*
Trazadone 25 mg qhs	*Depression, insomnia*

Fig. 36-1 Painting by Mary in the last year of her life.

Unfortunately, 1 month before death, Mary was admitted to the hospital in pain crisis and it took 3 days before her distress could be eased. The team was concerned that the only way to achieve comfort would be through palliative sedation, and Mary's family was prepared for this possibility. But in true Mary fashion, despite substantial escalation of symptom-relieving medications, she woke up and was comfortable. The next phase of conversation related to whether it would be possible to transition Mary back home. Unfortunately, her home hospice team believed that they could not manage her complex regimen. Instead, she resided in the hospital's homelike suite, "The Comfort Care Room," for the final weeks of life. Fortunately, her community came to her. Mary continued to be involved in decision making. One such decision was related to her continuing to take food by mouth. Despite many hours of being asleep a day, Mary would regularly wake up in the morning and asked to be wheeled down to the cafeteria for a breakfast of bacon, eggs, and potatoes. However, her ability to swallow effectively was diminishing and she was at high risk for aspiration. Nonetheless, she chose to continue her passion of eating breakfast. Comfort was achieved through a modified medication regimen.

Intravenous Medication	Indication
Dexamethasone 4 mg qid	*Cerebral edema*
Ondansetron 8 mg tid	*Nausea*
Methadone 10 mg qid	*Pain*
Fentanyl 225 mcg/h PCA with 180 mcg bolus q6min	*Pain*
Ativan 1.75 mg IV q4h, 1 mg IV q1h prn	*Anxiety*

| Haldol 1 mg IV q6h | Anxiety, agitation, hallucinations |
| Scopolamine patch | Excess secretions |

Three days before death, Mary experienced an aspiration event and progressive respiratory distress. Opioids were further titrated to comfort. She died surrounded by family, friends, and the care team. As stated by Mary's mother, "To me, the comfort corner room was beyond words in our last days with Mary. To have the safety of the hospital (doctors, nurses, all caregivers, Father Nee) and for all of us to be with her until the end was the ultimate blessing."

Consistent with her passion for education and generous spirit, Mary's family agreed to an autopsy. In her usual manner, the neuropathologist, Dr. Hannah Kinney, extensively reviewed Mary's record and spoke with many clinicians in advance of performing the autopsy. Her discoveries inspired the following poem.

In Honor of Mary
By Hannah Kinney

What does courage look like
Under the microscope?
I want to know,
Me, the disease detective
Who entrusts in the power
Of the microscope
To reveal the truth.

Here is tumor
Deep in the eye's pathways
That transmit the faces we love;
Here is tumor
Deep in the hypothalamus
That generates the daily rhythms
Of vitality;
And here is tumor
Destroying the spinal cord
Beyond recognition,
No chance ever to stand again.

But looking down the microscope
I see the young woman
Who refused to sit in a wheelchair
At the special class picture
As she was losing strength in both legs
Forever.
I see the young woman
Who painted pink-tipped flowers
On brilliant blue water
With a background
Of life's greenery
Just before dying.

The pathologist's job
Is to integrate

Microscopic findings
With clinical history:
Looking down the microscope,
I correlate the devastation
Of the spinal cord
With the joyful spirit
Of the doomed woman
To stand anyway,
And I see courage.

May 1, 2003

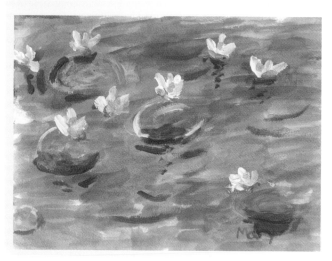

Fig. 36-2 Painting by Mary in the last weeks of her life.

REFERENCES

1. Steinhauser KE, Christakis NA, Clipp EC, McNeilly M, McIntyre L, Tulsky JA: Factors considered important at the end of life by patients, family, physicians, and other care providers, *JAMA* 284(19):2476–2482, 2000.
2. Bluebond-Langner M, Belasco JB, Goldman A, Belasco C: Understanding parents' approaches to care and treatment of children with cancer when standard therapy has failed, *J Clin Oncol* 25(17):2414–2419, 2007.
3. Wolfe J, Klar N, Grier HE, et al: Understanding of prognosis among parents of children who died of cancer: impact on treatment goals and integration of palliative care, *JAMA* 284(19):2469–2475, 2000.
4. Davies B, Gudmundsdottir M, Worden B, Orloff S, Sumner L, Brenner P: "Living in the dragon's shadow": fathers' experiences of a child's life-limiting illness, *Death Stud* 28(2):111–135, 2004.
5. Bicanovsky L: Comfort Care: Symptom control in the dying. In Walsh D, Caraceni AT, Fainsinger R, et al: *Palliative medicine*, Philadelphia, 2009, Saunders.
6. Wijdicks EF: The diagnosis of brain death, *N Engl J Med* 344(16):1215–1221,2001.
7. Bulow HH, Sprung CL, Reinhart K, et al: The world's major religions' points of view on end-of-life decisions in the intensive care unit, *Intensive Care Med* 34(3):423–430, 2008.
8. Kreicbergs UC, Lannen P, Onelov E, Wolfe J: Parental grief after losing a child to cancer: impact of professional and social support on long-term outcomes, *J Clin Oncol* 25(22):3307–3312, 2007.
9. Meert KL, Eggly S, Pollack M, et al: Parents' perspectives regarding a physician-parent conference after their child's death in the pediatric intensive care unit, *J Pediatr* 151(1):50–55, 55 e51–55 e52, 2007.
10. Cherin DA, Enguidanos SM, Jamison P: Physicians as medical center "extenders" in end-of-life care: physician home visits as the lynch pin in creating an end-of-life care system, *Home Health Care Serv Q* 23(2):41–53, 2004.
11. Sourkes BM: *The deepening shade: psychological aspects of life-threatening illness*, Pittsburgh, 1982, University of Pittsburgh Press.
12. Sourkes BM: *Armfuls of time : the psychological experience of the child with a life-threatening illness*, Pittsburgh, 1995, University of Pittsburgh Press.

13. Drake R, Frost J, Collins JJ: The symptoms of dying children, *J Pain Symptom Manage* 26(1):594–603, 2003.

14. Houlahan KE, Branowicki PA, Mack JW, Dinning C, McCabe M: Can end of life care for the pediatric patient suffering with escalating and intractable symptoms be improved? *J Pediatr Oncol Nurs* 23:45–51, 2006.

15. Morita T, Tsunoda J, Inoue S, Chihara S: Risk factors for death rattle in terminally ill cancer patients: a prospective exploratory study, *Palliat Med* 14(1):19–23, 2000.

16. Wildiers H, Menten J: Death rattle: prevalence, prevention and treatment, *J Pain Symptom Manage* 23(4):310–317, 2002.

17. Bennett M, Lucas V, Brennan M, Hughes A, O'Donnell V, Wee B: Using anti-muscarinic drugs in the management of death rattle: evidence-based guidelines for palliative care, *Palliat Med* 16(5):369–374, 2002.

18. Back IN, Jenkins K, Blower A, Beckhelling J: A study comparing hyoscine hydrobromide and glycopyrrolate in the treatment of death rattle, *Palliat Med* 15(4):329–336, 2001.

19. Dalal S, Del Fabbro E, Bruera E: Is there a role for hydration at the end of life? *Curr Opin Support Palliat Care* 3(1):72–78, 2009.

20. Finan E, Bolger T, Gormally SM: Modes of death in neonatal intensive care units, *Ir Med J* 99(4):106–108, 2006.

21. Sands R, Manning JC, Vyas H, Rashid A: Characteristics of deaths in paediatric intensive care: a 10-year study, *Nurs Crit Care* 14(5):235–240, 2009.

22. Verhagen AA, Dorscheidt JH, Engels B, Hubben JH, Sauer PJ: End-of-life decisions in Dutch neonatal intensive care units, *Arch Pediatr Adolesc Med* 163(10):895–901, 2009.

23. von Gunten C, Weissman DE: *Fast Fact and Concept #033: Ventilator Withdrawal Protocol (Part I).* www.aahpm.org/cgi-bin/wkcgi/view?status=A%20&search=182&id=174&offset=0&limit=25. Accessed March 20, 2010.

24. Campbell ML: How to withdraw mechanical ventilation: a systematic review of the literature, *AACN Adv Crit Care* 18(4):397–403, 2007; quiz 344–395.

25. Truog RD, Berde CB, Mitchell C, Grier HE: Barbiturates in the care of the terminally ill, *N Engl J Med* 327(23):1678–1682, 1992.

26. Nadkarni VM, Larkin GL, Peberdy MA, et al: First documented rhythm and clinical outcome from in-hospital cardiac arrest among children and adults, *JAMA* 295(1):50–57, 2006.

27. Topjian AA, Nadkarni VM, Berg RA: Cardiopulmonary resuscitation in children, *Curr Opin Crit Care* 15(3):203–208, 2009.

28. Parshuram CS, Hutchison J, Middaugh K: Development and initial validation of the Bedside Paediatric Early Warning System score, *Crit Care* 13(4):R135, 2009.

29. Nibert L, Ondrejka D: Family presence during pediatric resuscitation: an integrative review for evidence-based practice, *J Pediatr Nurs* 20(2):145–147, 2005.

30. Dussel V, Joffe S, Hilden JM, Watterson-Schaeffer J, Weeks JC, Wolfe J: Considerations about hastening death among parents of children who die of cancer, *Arch Pediatr Adolesc Med* 164(3):231–237, 2010.

31. Verhagen AA, Sauer PJ: End-of-life decisions in newborns: an approach from the Netherlands, *Pediatrics* 116(3):736–739, 2005.

32. Vrakking AM, van der Heide A, Arts WF, et al: Medical end-of-life decisions for children in the Netherlands, *Arch Pediatr Adolesc Med* 159(9):802–809, 2005.

33. Pousset G, Bilsen J, De Wilde J, et al: Attitudes of adolescent cancer survivors toward end-of-life decisions for minors, *Pediatrics* 124(6):e1142–e1148, 2009.

34. Cadge W, Ecklund EH: Prayers in the clinic: how pediatric physicians respond, *South Med J* 102(12):1218–1221, 2009.

35. *Fast Fact and Concept #120: Physicians and prayer requests* www.aahpm.org/cgi-bin/wkcgi/view?status=A%20&search=151&id=554&offset=0&limit=25. Accessed March 22, 2010.

36. *Fast Fact and Concept #004; Death Pronouncement in the Hospital.* www.aahpm.org/cgi-bin/wkcgi/view?status=A%20&search=126&id=95&offset=0&limit=25. Accessed March 22, 2010.

37. National Association of Medical Examiners: http://thename.org/index.php?option=com_content&task=view&id=113&Itemid=58. Accessed March 17, 2010.

38. Lee Goff M: Early post-mortem changes and stages of decomposition in exposed cadavers, *Exp Appl Acarol* 49(1–2):21–36, 2009.

39. Borasino S, Morrison W, Silberman J, Nelson RM, Feudtner C: Physicians' contact with families after the death of pediatric patients: a survey of pediatric critical care practitioners' beliefs and self-reported practices, *Pediatrics* 122(6):e1174–e1178, 2008.

40. Bedell SE, Cadenhead K, Graboys TB: The doctor's letter of condolence, *N Engl J Med* 344(15):1162–1164, 2001.

41. Macdonald ME, Liben S, Carnevale FA, et al: Parental perspectives on hospital staff members' acts of kindness and commemoration after a child's death, *Pediatrics* 116(4):884–890, 2005.

SECTION 4 | Illness and Treatment Experience

Enough
When they came to take you
in that dark night, their hands
gathering up what was left of you
as you lay in your mother's arms,
the blood going to your brain
without sufficient oxygen to keep you,
we said: If she can live….

A mother whose 11-month-old child had lived with dilated cardiomyopathy and then underwent heart transplant wrote these lines. As her poem continues, it articulates the experience of so many parents of children with life-threatening illness: times of hope intermixed with times of despair, and a course all too unpredictable.

The first chapter in this book, on the language of interdisciplinary pediatric palliative care, distinguished between the illness experience and the underlying disease or condition. The aim of this section is to describe selected life-threatening *diseases and conditions*, how the child's experience transforms them into *illnesses*, and how pediatric palliative care emerges as the overarching framework for clinical intervention. The very nature of the interdisciplinary team is ideally suited to address these complex disorders as they are *lived* by a broad diversity of children and their families.

The chapters in this section introduce the reader to life-threatening illnesses in childhood, from their epidemiology and disease-specific characteristics and treatments to illness-specific guidance and communication. The knowledge of – and appreciation for – the unique qualities of each clinical entity (or grouping) are an essential foundation for the pediatric palliative care team, as they contribute their language and skills to the optimal care of the child and family.

And when they carried you
to the airplane and lifted
their tiny cargo up
into the sky, we said: If they
can carry her safely.

And when they opened
your delicate rib cage to reveal
the overgrown bird struggling
inside to be free of you, we said:
If she can lose her worn heart.

And when the child, your secret brother,
gave up his heart, when it entered the cave
of your body, we pledged: We will always
remember your secret brother.

But the new heart rested
like a hibernating creature, barely
fluttering within you, and you grew
cold, first your feet and then
your legs. We promised:
Whatever it takes.

And when the heart began
to awaken, to send the blood strongly
along all its channels like a great engine
dreaming of air, we said:
She must live.

When that heart
pumped oxygen hungrily
through the great vessels
of your body, when you saw us with
your eyes and your hands,
when you asked your father
if it was night and he carried you
to the window, we said: Now there are
mornings and evenings.

And when the world began
to breathe again, we said all
those things you might say
when a child is born
and you are planning
the long life ahead of her.

It is never enough. —MYRA SKLAREW[1]

REFERENCE

1. Poem reprinted from Cross SN, Berlin R, Jo Blank D, et al. Illness: A Collection of Poems. *J Med Humanit.* (2010) 31:176–178. With kind permission of Springer Science and Business Media.

37 Prenatal and Neonatal Palliative Care

RENEE BOSS | KAREN KAVANAUGH | KATHIE KOBLER

Having the baby was a surreal experience; it was entering a world of unknowns and uncertainties. Would he be born alive? Would he live for minutes, hours, days, or months? —a mother

For most, pregnancy is a time filled with joyful anticipation of welcoming a new life into the family. Technological advances provide early confirmation of pregnancy, thus allowing parents to share their news with others, often just weeks after conception. Technology also permits clinicians to detect life-threatening fetal complications. Each year in the United States, more than one million pregnancies will end in fetal death, many due to genetic abnormalities. More than 26,000 babies between 20 and 40 weeks' gestation will be stillborn, and nearly 18,000 neonates will die within the first 28 days of life, with nearly half of these deaths due to congenital diseases and/or prematurity.[1] Gestational risk factors such as a family history of genetic diseases or maternal chronic illness can result in repeated losses.

Families may learn that their baby has a life-threatening fetal diagnosis early in pregnancy, in the prenatal period just prior to delivery, or in the neonatal period after birth. As parents learn of a life-threatening fetal condition, they bear the difficult task of shifting from joyful welcoming of new life to comprehending the ramifications of their baby's diagnosis. Palliative care in each scenario is targeted to families' unique needs after diagnosis, when families begin to grieve the loss of a "normal" pregnancy or infant.[2] Fetal-neonatal conditions that would benefit from the interventions and support of palliative care can include rare syndromes such as anencephaly and Potter's syndrome, all extremely premature infants, and infants with severe birth injuries. We will describe how interdisciplinary clinicians can deliver integrated, compassionate, and evidence-based services for these infants and families.

In this chapter, we discuss prenatal-neonatal palliative and end-of-life care. Often the term *perinatal* is used to describe care around the time of birth; we will use prenatal and neonatal to be more precise. We will highlight the unique contributions of interdisciplinary team (IDT) clinicians, as related to four distinct periods (Fig. 37-1):

- Early prenatal period: the life-threatening fetal diagnosis is made weeks to months before birth
- Late prenatal period: the life-threatening fetal diagnosis is made hours to days before birth
- Early neonatal period: the neonatal death occurs in the first hours to days of life
- Late neonatal period: the neonate's or infant's death occurs in the first weeks to months of life

A general overview of concepts and issues common to all periods will be presented first, followed by more specific information pertinent to each of the four periods. In this chapter, we conclude with information specific to end-of-life care and bereavement. Whenever available, data from relevant clinical research across disciplines are referenced. Because of the ethical and logistical limitations to research with pregnant women, women in labor, and parents of critically ill newborns, data are sometimes limited or absent. Where data are lacking, our recommendations are drawn from historical and current texts, and from the clinical experience of interdisciplinary experts.

IDT Clinicians and Roles

The diagnosis and management of a life-threatening condition for an infant can span the prenatal and neonatal periods, and may require the involvement of unique interdisciplinary team clinicians not found in other areas of pediatric palliative care (Fig. 37-2). Not uncommonly, IDT clinicians work in different clinics, hospitals, or even cities due to the nature of regionalized neonatal care. For example, a life-threatening fetal diagnosis may be made by a community obstetrician, with subsequent management of both mother and baby by multiple subspecialists at a large referral center. Particular effort must be made to communicate well and to provide seamless care to families throughout this trajectory of care.

SUPPORTING FAMILIES' PRACTICAL NEEDS

Mothers with a high-risk pregnancy are often hospitalized for a prolonged period before birth. The mother's hospitalization can profoundly disrupt the life of the family, and mothers often worry about this burden on their loved ones.[3] Distance from home to the regional hospital may be significant, with the associated costs of travelling and parking. Families with a limited income may be forced to visit during late hours when parking is free, which can affect communication with daytime care providers.

Environments that are conducive to and promote family presence are essential. Privacy and lenient visitation hours are important to women hospitalized prenatally.[3] When private rooms are not available, strategies are needed to maintain confidentiality during parent-provider discussions. Parents are very cognizant of and appreciative for those clinicians who go out of their way to enable family members to be present with them at their time of distress.[4]

Fathers, in particular, may need to balance multiple demands to be physically present at the hospital, care for other children, and work to provide for the family. Grandparents

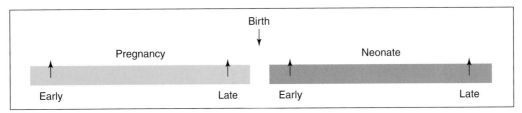

Fig. 37-1   Periods of prenatal and neonatal palliative care.

may not know how to support their children through something that they themselves have never experienced. Staff can help families with simple tasks such as obtaining a food tray for the visiting father or informing the family about parking discounts, to ensure that families' most basic needs are being addressed.

Siblings may be aware of a baby's expected arrival before the life-threatening fetal diagnosis is made. Siblings have their own feelings of anticipation, excitement, sadness, or ambivalence. IDT clinicians may need to provide families with strategies to allow siblings to maintain closeness with their mother during her hospitalization while maintaining as normal of a home routine as possible. Parents may need suggestions about how to include their children in the events surrounding the baby's birth and death.[5] Child life specialists can offer creative avenues of art, play, and interactive therapies to assist these children as they meet and say good-bye to their baby brother or sister.

COMMUNICATION

When families learn of a life-threatening fetal or neonatal condition, providers may feel an urgency to communicate essential information quickly, without careful attention to the way it is presented. Whenever possible, providers should anticipate the impact of the information on a family already under significant stress. Priority should be placed on asking parents who else should be present for discussions regarding treatment decisions. Meeting times should not be restricted to routine morning or evening rounds, and should allow for extended family presence. Family members often assist the parent to recall information given during these meetings. If a discussion must occur with the mother or father alone, a nurse or other clinician should be assigned to help the parent interpret the information.

Sequential discussions are often needed. Parents should be encouraged to write down information and questions, and should be provided with a means to do so.

The importance of clear, honest, and compassionate communication is central to prenatal and neonatal palliative care.[6-9] Clinicians can convey empathy through careful listening and anticipation of the family's needs. Respect is apparent when clinicians refer to the baby by his or her given name. Respect extends to colleagues when conflicting opinions, which often arise in prenatal and neonatal decision-making, are approached in a professional manner. A family's confidence and trust in the healthcare team are eroded if they witness disrespectful behavior among members of the team. An example of disrespectful behavior is when clinicians are openly critical of the competency of their colleagues because of a disagreement with a medical diagnosis and/or a management decision. These conversations should never occur in the family's presence or where the conversations could be overheard. A family needs to know that clinicians work collaboratively as a team and with the family to identify a plan of care.

DECISION-MAKING

Families who receive a diagnosis of a potentially lethal fetal or neonatal condition face decisions that are unparalleled in other areas of pediatrics, and range from pregnancy termination to experimental fetal surgery. The level of uncertainty is also unparalleled, as decisions are often necessary before birth when diagnosis and prognosis are rarely definite. This can create moral dilemmas for providers and parents as they consider options.

Internationally, there is significant variation in the process of decision-making for these infants. In countries with paternalistic models of medical care, physicians decide which

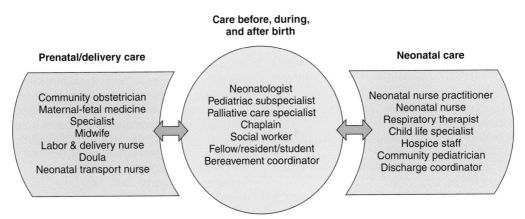

Fig. 37-2   Potential interdisciplinary team members.

infants will receive life-sustaining therapies, without family input.[10] In the United States, parent-provider collaboration in shared decision-making has become increasingly important. Neonatologists acknowledge that, at times, family autonomy in decision-making may even surpass the authority of the medical team.[11-13] For instance, a neonatologist may not feel comfortable limiting delivery room resuscitation for an infant born at 22 5/7 weeks' gestation if the family requests that "everything be done," even when the likelihood of survival is extremely low.

Best practices for engaging in shared decision-making before, during, and after birth are not clear. Ideally, multiple interdisciplinary discussions would occur with families over time while minimizing the stressors of maternal illness, pain, and disruption of the family's home life. But this rarely occurs. While data about these interactions are limited, retrospective data suggest that parent-provider collaboration in these scenarios is incomplete. A study interviewing the parents and neonatologists within 24 hours of counseling showed there was only 59% agreement that a management plan had been formulated.[14]

Parents and providers may come to these conversations with very different priorities. Neonatologists often emphasize predictions of morbidities and mortality,[15-17] yet families often focus on emotions, hope, and religious and spiritual beliefs.[18,19] Those who became pregnant through assisted reproduction or who have suffered repeated losses may be particularly committed to continuing a pregnancy, regardless of predictions of illness or death.[20] Families may possess unrealistic expectations for their infant based on media portrayal of "miracle babies."

As with older children, parents have the right to act as surrogate decision makers for their infants. But surrogate decision-making for infants is unique in several ways. The concept of prior preferences does not apply to newborns. Parents and providers may differ significantly in their perceptions of a "good" quality of life for infants; in one study, parents were more likely than providers to believe that attempts should be made to save all infants, regardless of projected outcomes.[21] New parents already expecting to bring home a totally dependent infant may underestimate the consequences of decisions that may extend this dependence indefinitely.

Shared decision-making requires IDT clinicians to assist families in expressing their values and goals while focusing on the infant's best interests. Families should be asked about what the pregnancy or the infant means to them, and what they believe is a good quality of life. They should be encouraged to talk with important extended family members and religious leaders. They should be asked about their preferred decision-making role, and reminded that the IDT is there to support them regardless of the decision.

Families must be cautioned that, once a decision is made, diagnostic and prognostic uncertainty may translate into unexpected outcomes. The family who makes a carefully detailed birth plan involving out-of-state family members and religious rituals may suffer a fetal death before birth. Families who opt for non-resuscitation of an extremely premature infant to prevent infant suffering may deliver a vigorous baby weighing 200 g more than predicted. Providers and families alike should prepare for the possibility that management decisions may need to be altered quickly based on new information.[22-24]

Finally, it should be noted that not all management options are equally available to families. Hospital and state policies can impact provider willingness to offer the options of pregnancy termination, non-initiation of resuscitation, and withdrawal of therapy.[25,26]

HOPE

Redefining hope is critical during prenatal and neonatal palliative care. Families are often unprepared for the diagnosis of a potentially lethal fetal or neonatal condition. Physicians may worry that talking about hope will create unrealistic expectations, yet parents who have gone through this have emphasized that, regardless of the infant's prognosis, parents need providers to give them hope for something.[18,19,27] One study found that physicians who provided more hope to families were not necessarily more likely to predict survival, but they did express emotion and showed parents that they were touched by the tragedy of the situation.[18] Adult patients with a terminal diagnosis said providers can provide hope by shifting the focus to what can be realistically achieved versus what can only be wished for.[28] For the IDT that is counseling a family, this might mean openly acknowledging the grief and pain of the situation, reassuring the family that the team will join in their hope that the infant's outcome will be a good one, and helping them to imagine how they might want events to proceed if the outcome is death or severe disability.

It is helpful to talk with families about what is meaningful to them, such as the possibility of holding a baby who is alive, or making sure that the infant does not experience pain. Hope for a good outcome may need to be redefined repeatedly over time in a way that helps families to cherish what is possible with their infant. For parents expecting multiple babies, parental hope for each of the developing fetuses in utero may hang in a delicate balance, especially if one is diagnosed with a life-threatening condition. When the death of a multiple occurs, parents must simultaneous maintain hope for the surviving babies while experiencing grief for their loss.[29]

CULTURAL, RELIGIOUS, AND SPIRITUAL ISSUES

Families often struggle to make meaning of a child's death in the context of their cultural, religious, spiritual, or existential beliefs. This struggle may inform the decisions families make regarding their infant. A 2010 text[30] provides an excellent reference for neonatal end-of-life care issues as related to a number of religious traditions. Several aspects of religion and prenatal and/or neonatal end-of-life care should be noted. In some traditions, a fetus is not recognized as a person until it is born alive. Parents from these traditions who experience a miscarriage or stillbirth may feel abandoned by their communities, and may need additional resources from the IDT. In other traditions, families may struggle to reconcile pregnancy termination or withdrawal of neonatal care with religious doctrine. Talking with their own religious leader and/or a hospital chaplain can be invaluable, both by alleviating family guilt and by helping the medical team to better understand the parents' values. Obstetric and neonatal wards often limit visitors; accommodations need to be made for families' cultural or religious end-of-life rituals. One advantage of home hospice for infants is the opportunity for families to more freely participate in religious and cultural rituals.

Studies of adults who face end-of-life decisions for themselves or their family members suggest that race and ethnicity impact choices about life-sustaining therapies. While this issue has not yet been evaluated for prenatal and neonatal end-of-life care, IDT clinicians should be prepared to assess the role that race or ethnicity may play in parents' decisions.

Professional Caregiver Suffering and Moral Distress

As in other areas of pediatric palliative care, being with families throughout their baby's dying can be deeply rewarding but can also lead to suffering by the professional caregiver. Suffering is intensified in situations involving moral distress, which often characterizes the uncertainty of prenatal and neonatal prognosis.[31] Tragic infant deaths and cumulative losses can make it difficult for a clinician to create meaning in his or her profession. clinicians who themselves are childbearing or childrearing may closely identify with families, particularly when clinicians have a long-term relationship with the family. Though such sensitivity can promote empathy in the clinician, it can also cause death anxiety and grief. A dual-process model of clinician's grief has been described: clinicians will simultaneously experience grief reactions by focusing on the loss and avoiding grief reactions by focusing on other aspects of a patient's care.[32,33]

Infant deaths often occur in environments that do not support clinicians' needs. Prenatal deaths may occur in birth centers, where care is focused on healthy births, often evidenced by names such as the New Life Center. Clinicians in birth centers may struggle to care for bereaved families while simultaneously caring for parents who are birthing healthy infants.[34] Neonatal deaths often occur in intensive care units, which rarely emphasize the sacredness of the end-of-life experience. Though clinicians may join in annual rituals to honor deceased patients and their own grief, support during acute losses may not be available.

IDT clinicians from varying disciplines have unique experiences with families at the end of life. For example, while neonatal nurses rarely feel involved in decision-making, neonatal physicians feel very responsible for end-of-life decision-making.[35] These differences may make it difficult for providers to fully support each other. IDT clinicians, such as chaplains, with expertise in addressing suffering could facilitate self-care for others.

Strategies for minimizing professional caregiver suffering must also take place at the organizational level. An educational intervention in end-of-life care, which included content on prevention of compassion fatigue, has been shown to increase the comfort of neonatal nurses who care for a dying infant.[36] Other strategies might include a core group of clinicians to serve as a resource on all shifts, case reviews of each death for all disciplines, engaging mental health liaisons for debriefing, and providing meaningful gestures to clinicians, such as massages. Co-creation of ritual may provide clinicians with opportunities to both support bereaved families and facilitate their own grief work[30] (Fig. 37-3).

The Four Periods of Prenatal and Neonatal Palliative Care

In this section, we discuss considerations for patients and families in each of four periods: early prenatal period, late prenatal period, early neonatal period, and late neonatal period. Case studies are followed by recommendations for specific interventions for each patient population.

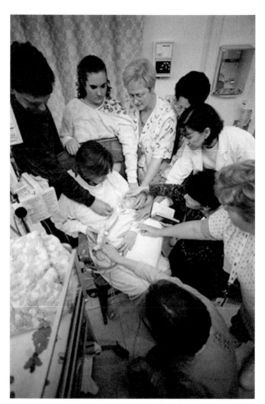

Fig. 37-3 IDT clinicians join parents in a ritual of thanksgiving and blessing for baby Logan before his death. (Photograph provided courtesy of Todd Hochberg.)

EARLY PRENATAL PALLIATIVE CARE

Mr. and Mrs. Chang are expecting their fourth baby, with prenatal care provided by a community obstetrician who speaks the family's primary language, Korean. A routine ultrasound at 18 weeks' gestation reveals the baby has probable cardiac, renal, and neural tube defects. The obstetrician recommends further testing at an urban medical center 60 miles away.

Hesitantly, the Changs travel to the medical center, where further testing reveals a diagnosis of trisomy 18 and multiple anomalies. Without an interpreter, the medical center team shares the diagnosis, offering Mrs. Chang the option to terminate her pregnancy. Upon hearing this news, Mr. and Mrs. Chang decline to discuss other options for their baby's care, and return home. No further communication occurs among the medical center staff, the community obstetrician, or the family.

At 37 weeks' gestation, Mrs. Chang presents at the community hospital in active labor. As she is admitted to the labor and delivery ward, her 12-year-old daughter translates, telling the nurse, "My mother is very scared because my father is at work right now and they think the baby may be sick."

Before a thorough history can be obtained, the baby is born. He requires immediate intubation, chest compressions, umbilical line placement, and medications. Within 30 minutes of birth, the baby is stabilized, and transport is arranged for the baby to a Level 3 NICU at a regional medical center.

Mrs. Chang briefly views her son before signing consents for the transfer of his care. Mr. Chang arrives at the community hospital just minutes after the ambulance's departure with his son.

Upon arrival at the NICU, the neonatologist suspects a chromosomal disorder, and orders genetic testing. Aggressive intervention is provided to sustain the baby until a diagnosis can be confirmed. With aid of an interpreter, the baby's current condition and suspected diagnosis is shared with Mr. and Mrs. Chang over the phone. Mr. Chang tells the staff to "do everything" for their baby.

Twelve hours later, Baby Chang's condition deteriorates. He does not respond to resuscitation, and dies. His parents receive a phone call in Mrs. Chang's postpartum room, notifying them of their son's death.

The delivery of palliative care in the early prenatal period (EPP) presents a unique challenge in planning for a patient who is not yet born. As a life-threatening condition is identified in utero, both parents and providers must transition care goals in preparation for a baby who may die shortly after birth. The provision of palliative care subsequently unfolds during three distinct phases: in the prenatal period, during labor and delivery, and eventually throughout the baby's living and dying.

Setting

As illustrated in the case study, EPP palliative care may begin in the obstetrician's office. Further evaluation may involve specialist consultations at a regional hospital far from the family's home. In some instances, diagnosis of a specific prenatal condition, such as twin-to-twin transfusion or monoamniotic twins, may require the parents to travel out of state for specialized prenatal care. The emergence of hospital-based fetal care programs affords each IDT clinician the opportunity to initiate palliative care throughout the trajectory of care.[37] If the baby survives past delivery and beyond the time of the mother's discharge from the hospital, palliative and hospice care may be provided in the family's home. Some families may opt for home birth, with care provided by a hospice and midwife team.

Interdisciplinary Team Clinicians

Parents who receive a life-threatening fetal diagnosis may interact with numerous IDT clinicians at multiple sites of care. In fact, each discipline represented in Fig. 37–2 could interact with the family throughout pregnancy, delivery, and the baby's birth and death. Therefore, it is of utmost importance that a key point person be identified who can facilitate continuity throughout the trajectory of care. As one mother reported to the advanced practice nurse who filled such a role on the palliative care team: "You were our safe, familiar center in the middle of this frightening storm."

Communication

In addition to the principles of communication discussed in this chapter's introduction, there are particular considerations during the EPP.

IDT clinicians should establish and maintain a relationship with the family as the pregnancy continues, supporting the family and facilitating attachment to the baby. Clinicians can help parents anticipate questions from bystanders about the pregnancy. It may be helpful to schedule prenatal visits before or after regular office hours. Some sites may offer separate childbirth education sessions separate from classes for families expecting healthy babies.[38]

Throughout the EPP, clinicians may find themselves reviewing test results and other prognostic information with parents on multiple occasions. Patience and compassionate listening skills are important. Clinicians should explore with parents how best to provide updates on the baby's status before, during, and after birth. Parents may worry about how their baby will tolerate labor. Clear expectations should be established about the management plan should fetal distress occur during labor. When the plan is for non-initiation of delivery room resuscitation, good communication among the obstetric, neonatal, and pediatric teams can help make this experience the least obtrusive as possible for families, so that they can cherish the time that they have with their infant. A palliative care order set or protocol can be a helpful communication tool, and should specify orders for vital signs, medications, fluids and/or nutrition, and who should be called to declare death and complete post-mortem documentation (Box 37-1). Staff training and preparation is important, as obstetric and newborn nursery staff who typically care for healthy infants may be unfamiliar with and uncomfortable with neonatal end-of-life care.

Creation of a Birth Plan and Advance Directive

The use of a written birth plan and advance directive can facilitate communication during the EPP.[38–40] The co-creation of a birth plan between parents and clinicians provides an opportunity for parents to be actively involved in their baby's care. As one mother eloquently stated, "this is a special kind of nesting I can do to prepare for my son."

A well-crafted planning tool should effectively communicate the parents' wishes for care of the mother during labor and delivery, and should be partnered with advance directives outlining appropriate medical and palliative interventions for the baby. Box 37-2 highlights possible components of a palliative care birth plan and advance directives. It is important to note that this tool is effective only if it is shared, discussed, and readily accessible to all IDT clinicians before the baby's birth.

BOX 37-1 Sample Palliative Care Order Set for Neonate Following Delivery

1. Admission Diagnosis: _____
2. Birth Weight _____ kg
3. Do Not Resuscitate (Refer to DNR order form)
4. Admit to ___ NICU ___ Newborn Nursery for comfort care
5. Infant to stay in mother's postpartum room at all times. If respite care needed, may transfer to NICU per parents' request
6. No cardiorespiratory monitoring. Assess for breathing/heart beat prn, per patient status changes.
7. Nutrition/Hydration: Per family's request (e.g., breastfeeding prn as tolerated. No formula supplementation).
8. Provide non-pharmacologic measures prn for irritability or mild pain:
   ☐ Swaddle in warm blankets
   ☐ Holding
   ☐ Pacifier
   ☐ Sucrose
9. For moderate pain and/or dyspnea control:_____ (e.g., morphine)
10. With cessation of breathing/heart rate, page _____ for death pronouncement.
11. Expiration paperwork to be initiated by _____.

BOX 37-2 Components of a Prenatal Palliative Birth Plan and Neonatal Advance Directive

Opening Statement
Summarizes parents' overall goal for their baby
Example: *We would like to honor our son's living, minimize his suffering, and share as many meaningful moments with him as possible.*

Care of Mother and Baby During Labor and Delivery
- Timing, route and location of the baby's delivery
- Management of mother's pain during labor
- Extent of monitoring baby's heart beat during labor
- If parents have strong desire to meet the baby alive, possible interventions for fetal distress
- Presence of family members or friends
- Faith traditions, prayers or rituals to be initiated soon after baby's birth

Initial Care Management of the Baby
- Extent of desired resuscitation measures, or clear DNR/Limitation of emergency treatment orders
- Drying baby thoroughly after birth and placing on warm, clean blankets
- Use of warmth to maximize comfort and minimize unwanted symptoms
- Use of suctioning and free flow oxygen
- Management of pain, dyspnea, seizures or other symptoms

Care for the Family Following Delivery
- Opportunities to maximize family's time together, including sibling presence, memory making and keepsake activities, ritual, and photographs
- Plan for communicating baby's status to family and friends not at the hospital

Ongoing Care Management for the Baby
- Comfort measures, including warmth, mouth and lip care, kangaroo care, skin care
- Potential initiation of nutrition: breast and/or bottle feeding, formula via dropper, gavage feedings
- Use of suctioning and free flow oxygen
- Management of pain, dyspnea, seizures or other symptoms
- Plan for extent of diagnostic testing, such as no x-rays, ultrasounds, or blood draws
- Plan for if baby will stay in mother's postpartum room, newborn nursery, or NICU

Discharge Plan for Infants Who Survive the Postpartum Period
- Anticipatory plan for baby's care when mother ready to be discharged from the hospital
- Care of the baby in the NICU, home palliative and/or hospice care, community hospice

End-of-Life Care Needs
Some families may not want to address these issues prior to baby's death.
- Location of death
- Family's preferred funeral director
- Autopsy, Post mortem biopsy, and/or special genetic testing
- Organ or tissue donation plans if appropriate

Contact Information
For the following as needed: Palliative care coordinator or primary IDT contact, consulting physicians, family's clergy or pastor, photographer, local prenatal, pediatric palliative care, or hospice program.

Decision Making

The process of decision making in the EPP begins at diagnosis. As reflected in the case study, parents may be offered the option to terminate the pregnancy. Clinicians presenting such options should be clear about any institutional policies related to terminations, such as family counseling, ethical review, or committee approval. Decisions about termination often reflect parents' moral, ethical and religious views. Data are limited regarding pregnancy outcome following a lethal fetal diagnosis, with two programs reporting 60 percent of parents opting to terminate the pregnancy.[37,41] Termination decisions may be further complicated if the family has experienced infertility, or

with the diagnosis of a life-threatening condition with one fetus of a multiple pregnancy.

For those parents who choose to continue the pregnancy, subsequent decision making is guided by the certainty of diagnosis, the certainty of prognosis, and the meaning of that prognosis to the parents.[39] Together, IDT clinicians and parents work to determine those interventions that are of best interest for the baby, weighing treatment benefits and burdens. There are several congenital conditions for which neonatal resuscitation at birth is not recommended, including anencephaly and trisomy 13. In addition, the American Academy of Pediatrics (AAP)[23] and the Neonatal Resuscitation Program[42] confirm that resuscitation may be forgone in any scenario if infant survival is unlikely. It is important to note that the number of conditions for which there are clear recommendations for non-resuscitation has decreased steadily over time, as medicine and technology diminish the chance that a disease will be lethal.[43]

Providers should be aware that death at very early gestational age may present unique issues regarding hospital practices and disposition options. In most states, pregnancies ending before 20 weeks' completed gestation do not require reporting or the generation of a fetal death certificate. Therefore, parents experiencing an early pregnancy loss are not legally bound to make any disposition choice, and most states do not require clinicians to notify parents that they have a choice in the disposition of their tiny baby's body. If and when a fetal death occurs, IDT clinicians should be mindful of hospital, local and state ordinances and practices regarding options for disposition, and communicate these to parents in an appropriate, considerate and consistent manner.

For infants who survive birth, decision-making is an ongoing process guided by the infant's status during critical transition points, including the immediate postpartum period and the maternal hospital discharge. Together, IDT clinicians work to promote maximum comfort for the family and infant while accommodating evolving needs and preferences. If a mother requests hospital discharge soon after birth and before the baby's death, staff may have little time to adequately provide information and address all of the parents' needs. Routine follow-up after hospital discharge is essential as decision making unfolds.

Redefining Hope

Families in the EPP face the daunting task of understanding their unborn child's poor prognosis while simultaneously waiting to meet their baby face-to-face. IDT clinicians must always be mindful that some parents may maintain seemingly unrealistic hope that the diagnosis will be proved false upon the baby's birth. Facilitating choices in care for both mother and child can nurture a sense of control, provide meaning, and foster hope for the family in the midst of chaos and heartbreak.[44] Parental hopes may shift throughout the EPP care trajectory, and IDT clinicians should be prepared to address these preferences accordingly.

Management of Infant Suffering

IDT clinicians should anticipate and prepare for potential symptoms of infant suffering after birth. Table 37-1 presents pharmacological and non-pharmacological options for pain and symptom management. Table 37-2 presents medication dosing appropriate for term newborns and infants.

TABLE 37-1   Strategies to Minimize Infant Suffering

Site of Care	Pharmacologic	Nonpharmacologic
In the delivery room	**Oral or rectal:** Acetaminophen chloral hydrate, also intranasal Midazolam Morphine sucrose	Warmth Minimal stimulation Swaddling Kangaroo care Non-nutritive sucking
NICU care	**IV bolus or IM:** Midazolam Lorazepam (no IM dosing) Morphine Fentanyl **IV continuous infusion:** Midazolam Morphine Fentanyl **Oral or rectal:** Acetaminophen Sucrose Chloral hydrate, also intranasal Midazolam Morphine Furosemide Midazolam Glycopyrrolate **Topical:** Fentanyl patch EMLA	Warmth Minimal stimulation Minimal painful procedures Swaddling Non-nutritive sucking Noise reduction Light reduction Nesting Kangaroo care Massage Music
Home care	**Oral or rectal:** Acetaminophen Sucrose Chloral hydrate, also intranasal Midazolam Morphine Furosemide Midazolam Glycopyrrolate **Topical:** Fentanyl patch EMLA	Warmth Swaddling Nutritive or Non- nutritive sucking Kangaroo care Massage Music

Case Study Revisited

Care for the Chang family could have been improved by the following palliative care measures:

* Establish what is most important to this family, their understanding of the diagnosis and what it means

to them. Also identify the family's wishes and preferences for the baby's care, and work to honor those wishes.
* Identify cultural needs that may affect the Changs' understanding of their baby's condition.
* Learn how the Changs prefer to receive information and prepare the family for a life-threatening diagnosis.
* Use a professional medical translator throughout the trajectory of care.
* Establish clear lines of communication between the community hospital and regional medical center.
* Creat a birth plan.
* Provide opportunities for the parents and siblings to connect with the baby and make memories, including honoring cultural and religious traditions and/or rituals.

LATE PRENATAL PALLIATIVE CARE

Mrs. Reynolds is admitted at 23½ weeks' gestation with bulging membranes and preterm labor. She had been monitored closely during prenatal care because of bleeding in the first trimester. A cerclage was placed early on in her pregnancy because of a history of preterm labor 3 years because prior. For that pregnancy, she selected a rescue cerclage at 20 weeks' gestation over termination, and gave birth to a premature infant at 36 weeks' gestation who suffered no major complications.

For the current pregnancy, Mrs. Reynolds' membranes ruptured shortly after admission. It seemed as if many different doctors gave her information, but none asked her to make any decisions. Mr. Reynolds was not able to be present for any of these discussions. Within 2 days of hospital admission, she delivered a stillborn infant girl who weighed 525 g.

Mrs. Reynolds had not expected her infant to be born so soon, and thought she would be able to "hold on to this baby like her first one." She and her husband selected hospital

TABLE 37-2   Dosing for Term Neonates and Infants

	Route					
	PO	**PR**	**Intranasal**	**IV bolus**	**IM**	**IV gtt**
Medication						
Acetaminophen	12-15 mg/kg q6hr	12-18 mg/kg q6hr	X	X	X	X
Chloral hydrate	25-75 mg/kg/dose	25-75 mg/kg/dose	X	X	X	X
Fentanyl	X	X	X	0.5-4 mcg/kg q2-4hr	X	1-5 mcg/kg/hr
Furosemide	1-6 mg/kg q12hr	X	X	1-2 mg/kg q12hr	1 mg/kg q12hr	X

Glycopyrrolate	0.04-0.1 mg/kg q4-8hr			0.004-0.01 mg/kg
				  q4-8hr
					0.004-0.01 mg/kg
					  q4-8hr	

Lorazepam	X	X	X	0.05-0.1 mg/kg/dose	X	X

Midazolam	0.25 mg/kg q2-4hr	X	0.2-0.3 mg/kg
			  q2-4hr
				0.05-0.15 mg/kg
				  q2-4hr
					X	0.01-0.06 mg/kg/hr

Morphine	3-5x the IV dose	X	X	0.05-0.2 mg/kg q4hr	0.05-0.2 mg/kg q4hr	10-20 mcg/kg/hr
Sucrose 24%	Max 2mL/dose via pacifier	X	X	X	X	X

X, does not apply.
Adapted from Neofax, 2009, 22nd ed. Montvale: Thomson Reuters, 2009. Please refer to most recent edition for dosing in premature infants.

burial because of financial reasons, and were given pictures of their baby. At her request, Mrs. Reynolds was discharged the same day as the birth, before their families could come to the hospital to see her and the infant. Mrs. Reynolds was instructed to call and schedule a postpartum visit for 6 weeks post discharge.

Palliative care in the late prenatal period (LPP) is focused on those families who face an acute delivery of an infant with a life-threatening condition. Examples include mothers with a previously uncomplicated pregnancy who suddenly develop extremely premature labor, or mothers who develop their own life-threatening condition, such as pre-eclampsia, so that delivery of the infant must occur emergently. Other families who may benefit from palliative care in the LPP are those who have known about a potential fetal complication for weeks but who have not developed close relationships with providers and have not made any decisions for their infant's care.

Setting

A pregnant woman's medical complications may be diagnosed during a routine prenatal visit, or she may present to a local hospital. Mothers are not always aware of the signs of preterm labor and premature rupture of membranes,[4] and may delay seeking care. Mothers who present with urgent medical conditions to local hospitals that lack expertise in high-risk pregnancies may receive inaccurate prognostic information or outdated medical management. If the mother can be stabilized, she may be quickly transferred to a regional medical center far from home. If she cannot be transferred, she may deliver at the local hospital.

Typically, the antepartum unit or the labor and delivery unit do not practice palliative care, as the focus of care on these units is the birth of a healthy infant. Families who deliver a critically ill infant may have a heightened sensitivity to the sights and sounds of the unit, such as cries of other healthy babies or jingles that play over the hospital intercom each time a baby is born. Clinicians need to modify environments to promote privacy and family togetherness and to support grief. One such strategy is to use door markers that signify the special care that the mother and her family need.

Interdisciplinary Team Clinicians

The IDT varies depending on the presence of a palliative care team and the institutional practice of including neonatal clinicians in prenatal decision-making. Figure 37-2 highlights typical IDT clinicians in the LPP, which can include obstetricians, nurse midwives, labor room and/or triage nurses, antepartum nurses, neonatal physicians, nurse practitioners, social workers, and chaplains. If the mother was transported, a transport nurse may be the person to spend the most amount of time with the mother and may best get to know her and her family. IDTs that do not include neonatal clinicians in the LPP can lead to distress and frustration among obstetric and neonatal nurses.

Communication

Communication during the LPP is often rushed and easily fragmented. Multiple providers speak with the family about the mother's and infant's conditions. A maternal-fetal medicine specialist may be the first to meet a woman after she has been transferred to a regional medical center with imminent delivery. If involved, neonatologists or neonatal nurse practitioners typically provide prognostic information to the parents regarding infant survival and morbidity. Regardless of the discipline involved, the clinicians must be knowledgeable about local and national data for infant outcome. This is especially critical because treatment decisions made by physicians have been shown to be influenced by their knowledge of outcome and the type of information that is available.[45]

Data suggest that women may experience a profound sense of responsibility for preventing preterm birth.[46] Providers should choose their words carefully to avoid enhancing mothers' guilt. For example, phrases such as "hold on for two more weeks" should be avoided. Mothers may also fault themselves for somehow causing premature birth. Providing accurate information is critical to reassure mothers who did nothing to cause the events.

The benefits of a prenatal tour to the NICU during a high-risk pregnancy have been documented.[47] However, the practice of giving a prenatal tour is not consistent and may be dependent on the institution's philosophy of care regarding involvement of neonatal clinicians. For mothers restricted to bed rest, information about the NICU can be presented in a variety of innovative ways, including photo albums and/or digital recordings.

Parents who rely on other sources, such as the internet, to supplement healthcare information may feel hampered by limited availability or access to these external resources in the hospital setting. Families who do access the internet may develop unrealistic expectations for their infant's outcome. Parents who access chat rooms with other parents can become frustrated with limited options offered at their site of care if they hear of other possible care practices. Providers must listen carefully to the families to understand their ongoing need for information and care options.

Decision Making

For diagnoses made in the LPP, termination is generally not an option. Instead, decisions include:

- Tocolysis vs. induction of labor,
- Whether to monitor for fetal well-being,
- The use of antenatal steroids,
- Whether to perform a cesarean section for fetal distress,
- Whether to initiate resuscitation in the delivery room,
- How many neonatal interventions and treatments should be at birth and in the first days of life,
- Withdrawal of neonatal therapies.

In reality, decisions for life-threatening fetal conditions diagnosed in the LPP are often rushed and chaotic, with inadequate time to explore parents' authentic values and goals. This may partially explain why only 36% of neonatologists say that they would defer to parent wishes for infants born in the grey zone of 23 to 24 weeks' gestation, where prognostic uncertainty is high.[48]

Despite an attempt to account for prognostic indicators beyond gestational age,[49] the ability to give an accurate prognosis in the LPP is limited.[22] Therefore, the AAP recommends that providers guide families through a process of deciding whether to initiate life-sustaining therapies in the delivery room.[23,24] A clinician skilled in newborn care should be present at delivery to evaluate the infant. Ideally, this clinician will have been a part of the management plan. The World Health Organization's definition of "live born" should be used to document infant condition at birth.[50] Parents will notice any signs of life in the infant at birth, and may need help to understand that a weak cry or reflexive movement do not change the infant's prognosis. If the infant's condition is the same as what was anticipated, then the plan of care can be followed. If the infant's condition is different than anticipated or the parent requests, then treatment decisions may change from the earlier plan.

Because decision making in the LPP is often rushed and many families are unprepared for the possibility that their infant could die, recent recommendations have called for the introduction of "antenatal advanced directives."[51,52] With these recommendations, all expectant parents would receive information about extreme prematurity and be advised to consider the management options. While such directives might assist parents to be informed, it is unknown how the directives would impact the actual decisions at the time of birth.

Redefining Hope

There may not be an opportunity for hope to be redefined by parents in the LPP because of the short time between diagnosis and birth. Clinicians may feel reluctant to even begin a preliminary discussion about hope with parents because of the high probability of infant death.[27,53] Clinicians can mistakenly equate hope with intact survival of an infant. In an attempt to avoid giving false hope, clinicians overemphasize poor prognostic data to try to convince parents of the gravity of the condition. Discussions about hope are most easily started by asking families what they value, and reframing hope within those parameters, such as hoping that the baby can live until a grandmother arrives.

Management of Infant Suffering

In the delivery room, drying and warming the infant are key methods for minimizing infant suffering. Additional measures to reduce infant suffering are in Tables 37-1 and 37-2.

Case Study Revisited

Several interventions might have improved care for the Reynolds family:
- Learning about the parents' past experiences, hopes, and preferred role in decision making
- Making sure the father was involved in communication with the physicians
- Creating a birth plan
- Suggesting ways for the Reynolds to create meaningful memories in the short time they have with their infant
- Providing comprehensive information about burial options
- Providing follow-up after the death, including a phone call within 2 weeks and a chance for the Reynolds to meet with providers to review the death

EARLY NEONATAL PALLIATIVE CARE

Ms. Jones is 20 years old and pregnant for the first time. She is no longer involved with the baby's father, and plans to raise the infant alone. She has an uneventful pregnancy, and goes into labor on her due date. During labor at a local hospital, fetal bradycardia occurs. A stat cesarean section reveals total

placental abruption. The infant is pale, limp, and apneic at birth. A neonatal nurse practitioner begins resuscitation, and first detects the infant's heart rate at 12 minutes of life. He is brought to the special care nursery and placed on a ventilator. He is profoundly acidotic, and within 1 hour he has a seizure. He is transferred by helicopter at 3 hours of life to a regional NICU 100 miles away.

The infant is encephalopathic and hypotensive. An EEG is consistent with hypoxic ischemic encephalopathy and seizures. Ms. Jones is recovering from her surgery at the community hospital, and the NICU team speaks with her by telephone. They tell her the infant's condition is very serious.

When Ms Jones arrives at the NICU on hospital day 2, the on-call resident reports that her son is "doing OK." She tells Ms. Jones that the day team will meet with her in the morning. Ms. Jones asks the nurse for information, and the nurse states this is the first time she has cared for her son. She tells Ms. Jones that the baby has "had a good evening."

The attending physician meets alone with Ms. Jones the next day. He discusses the infant's diagnosis and his current treatments. Ms. Jones is told that should the infant survive, he is very likely to have profound disability. She is also told that, in scenarios like this, some parents do not want their baby to be supported by machines, and they decide to take the baby off the ventilator. "Ms. Jones, do you want us to take your son off the machines?"

Palliative care in the early neonatal period (ENP) targets those families who experience a normal pregnancy, but whose neonate develops a life-threatening condition during birth or in the first few hours of life. Common neonatal diagnoses in this period include birth traumas, overwhelming infections, and previously undiagnosed congenital conditions. These families are generally stunned by the abrupt onset of their infant's condition. The primary surrogate decision maker, the mother, has just given birth. Palliative care is appropriate for all of these families from birth, even as acute care and diagnostic evaluation proceeds.

Setting

Care for critically ill infants in the ENP nearly always occurs in the NICU. Intensive care for newborns was regionalized in the 1970s in an attempt to maximize neonatal outcomes by designating hospitals with special technologies and expertise. Critically ill newborns born at community hospitals are often transferred to regional NICUs. When a neonatal life-threatening diagnosis is certain at birth, and the infant is likely to die during transport or soon after, providers should consider whether palliative care should be given by the local providers, in lieu of neonatal transport.

Providing palliative care in the NICU can be challenging. NICUs are fast-paced and loud, with many staff members. There is often little privacy for families, and restrictions on visits by siblings and extended family members. Successful models for NICU palliative care rooms have included drapes, a bed and a refrigerator for the family, music, disposable cameras, and video cameras for parent use.

For some newborns with life-threatening conditions in the ENP, hospital discharge may be possible. Inpatient hospice is rarely available for newborns, particularly in rural areas. Home hospice is available to some, though not all, families. In one study of 62 infants who died at home, only 20 received home hospice.[54] Although little research has examined parent preferences for place of death for newborns, clinical experience suggests that important family-infant bonding can occur when newborns are allowed to go home. Families often treasure the memories of a newborn sleeping in her own crib, wearing her own clothes, and being held by family members. Bonding between extended family members and the newborn has been found to improve the support of parents by the extended family during the bereavement period.[55]

Interdisciplinary Team Clinicians

IDT clinicians in the ENP include many prenatal and neonatal providers involved in the LPP, as well as pediatric subspecialists, child life providers, and community neonatal providers including pediatricians and the home-hospice team. Fig. 37-2 highlights some of the common roles for these providers. As with other intensive care environments, many NICUs do not integrate palliative care early in medical management. In one study, the median time between NICU palliative care consult and infant death was 2.5 days.[56] A palliative care IDT member who is fully integrated into the NICU team can increase opportunities for initiating palliative care earlier into neonatal care.

Communication

When diagnosis of a life-threatening neonatal condition is made in the ENP, provider coordination and communication must be established quickly. For infants who must be transferred, arrangements should be made for the mother to be transferred as well so that the family can be closer to the infant and communication can improve.

In the ENP, the first hours to days after birth are often filled with tests and subspecialist evaluations. Clear and timely communication among IDT clinicians and the family can be challenging. A central IDT member should be designated as the primary person to deliver information and recommendations to the family. The goal is to integrate information into a big picture and to form goals of care. Providers should avoid the temptation to tell families that their infant is "doing OK" or "having a good day" when the overall status is moribund. This provides families with false hope, and does not allow them time to prepare for the grave reality of their infant's condition.

For infants who are discharged to home, communication between hospital and community providers can be facilitated by the involvement of home hospice. Where home hospice is not available, hospital providers must confirm that the community pediatrician is comfortable with caring for the dying infant, including managing seizures and pain, and can access resources for the family. When appropriate, documentation of resuscitation status should be completed as required by the state and provided to the family before discharge from the hospital.

Decision Making

There are several decisions particular to the ENP, which should be noted.

Because the neonatal diagnosis was not made prenatally, aggressive delivery room resuscitation is typical in these scenarios. In the first hours and days of life, as the prognosis becomes grim, decisions arise regarding whether additional therapies such as extracorporeal membranous oxygenation, should be withheld, or if current life-sustaining therapies, such as mechanical ventilation, should be withdrawn. The withholding of fluid and nutrition is particularly controversial in neonates. Some providers have concerns about withholding nutrition in light of the Baby Doe regulations.[57] The 2009 report of the American Academy of Pediatrics Committee on Bioethics reaffirms that nutrition may be withheld from newborns and infants when their benefit to the infant is outweighed by the burden.[58]

These discussions must center on the parents' values and goals and on the infant's best interest. Although parents should be encouraged to share in decision-making, providers can ease guilt and regret by framing these discussions not in terms of "do you want us to stop the ventilator," but instead focusing on what might be of greatest benefit to the infant in the short- and long-term.

When withdrawal of life-sustaining therapies occurs, providers should prepare families for what they will see, hear, and feel as their infant dies. Sensitive introduction of the concept of autopsy may be necessary before removing central lines or thoracostomy tubes in some hospitals; hospital regulations may require that medical devices remain in place. In the case of a suspected congenital syndrome, which could affect future pregnancies, genetic specialists should advise about neonatal testing needed before death. Many genetic tests can be performed on a post-mortem skin biopsy.

Families should be prepared that, while neonatal death typically occurs within hours of extubation, some infants survive for days. Gasping respirations often occur. The neonatal heart rate may persist for hours after breathing stops. Dying may be prolonged if the infant is not bundled closely and kept warm. IDT clinicians may hear parents questioning their decisions and the plan of care for the baby when the dying process seems to be prolonged, and they should be prepared to answer questions and provide support accordingly.

Redefining Hope

Families in the ENP are understandably overwhelmed by the need to assimilate complicated medical information, understand the prognosis, articulate goals of care, and focus on maximizing the time they have with their infant. Providers can help families focus on what can be realistically achieved in hours or days, and making meaning from those goals. For instance, limiting painful procedures, kangaroo (skin to skin) care, or seeing their baby open her eyes have been important to some families.

Management of Infant Suffering

Nearly all sick newborns in the ENP are exposed to painful intravenous access, phlebotomy, intubation and ventilation. Newborns are often agitated by concomitant exposure to cold, noise, and light. Assessing and managing neonatal pain is a skill that differs from pain assessment of older children.[59] While the motor response to pain evolves and becomes more pronounced near term, perception of pain is present as early as 16 to 18 weeks' gestation. Several scales have been developed to assess pain in infants.[60–64] Only a subset of these scales are appropriate for use with premature infants.[60–62] Facial grimacing is central to most of these scales; brow furrowing, nasolabial bulge, and squeezing the eyes shut also indicate pain. When facial movements are decreased by sedation, then heart rate variability can be a reliable indicator of pain.

There may be reluctance to treat sick newborns with medications that depress the central nervous system, because the neurologic exam is often a critical component of accurate diagnosis and prognosis. There may also be concern that the infant's tenuous cardiorespiratory status will be irrevocably depressed before a clear diagnosis is made. Nevertheless, providers should strive to minimize pain and discomfort with pharmacologic and non-pharmacologic therapies as appropriate. Refer to Tables 37-1 and 37-2.

Case Study Revisited

Several interventions might have improved care for Ms. Jones and her son.

- Concurrent with the infant's transfer, the NICU providers could have facilitated transfer of Ms. Jones' obstetric care to the regional hospital
- A single IDT member could have been designated to speak with Ms. Jones
- Ms. Jones could have been encouraged to have a support person present for discussions regarding withdrawing life-sustaining therapies
- Providers could have avoided using euphemisms to describe her son's status to Ms. Jones
- Providers could have initiated a discussion about Ms. Jones' values and the infant's best interest, and avoided asking her if she wanted the staff to discontinue the ventilator

LATE NEONATAL PALLIATIVE CARE

Anna is born at 24 weeks' gestation. She is very sick from birth with severe lung disease. On day 3, she is diagnosed with large, bilateral intraventricular hemorrhages. The family is told that Anna could die, and that if she survives she may have mental retardation or cerebral palsy. The family is religious, and asks the neonatologist to do everything possible for Anna. They pray for a miracle.

Over the coming weeks, Anna remains critically ill and mechanically ventilated. She has one surgery for a persistent ductus arteriosus, and another surgery to place a ventricular shunt. She develops repeated infections related to her immature immune system. She does not tolerate enteral feeding. The family visits infrequently; they live 90 miles away and have had to return to work. With each crisis, they are told that Anna may die. The parents remain hopeful. Privately, Anna's father is becoming more anxious about his daughter's condition and wonders what they should do.

At 10 weeks of age, Anna remains partially dependent on parenteral feeding, and multiple attempts at extubation have been unsuccessful. She develops seizures, which are poorly controlled; twice she has needed CPR during a seizure. She has bradycardia in response to routine care or being held by her parents.

Because it is an academic hospital, the clinical staff rotates frequently, and no one develops a rapport with the parents. The team worries that Anna is suffering, and several clinicians wonder about the option of withdrawing life-sustaining

therapies. A consulting physician, who has not previously been involved in her care, tells the parents it would be wrong to stop treating Anna. The father has a hard time trusting the medical team, and argues with the mother about what should be done.

One night Anna has a prolonged seizure and goes into cardiac arrest; she dies before her parents arrive at the hospital.

Palliative care in the late neonatal period (LNP) targets families whose infant develops a life-threatening condition in the first weeks to months of life. Common neonatal diagnoses in this period are surgical complications, such as diaphragmatic hernia repair, profound neurologic diseases, and severe sequelae of prematurity, including cor pulmonale. These diseases often manifest as a roller coaster of improvements and decompensations; families endure multiple crises over time. Palliative care is appropriate throughout the disease trajectory.

Setting

Care for critically ill infants in the LNP nearly always occurs in the hospital. In periods of relative stability, the infant may be transferred to a non-acute hospital ward, facility or home. The infant is then often transferred back to a neonatal or pediatric acute-care setting for worsening disease.

As noted previously, providing palliative care in the neonatal or pediatric ICU can be challenging. Both inpatient and home-based hospice is more available for older infants than for newborns, but remains a scarce resource in the LNP.

Interdisciplinary Team Clinicians

Many of the IDT clinicians in the ENP maintain important roles in the LNP. Figure 37-2 highlights some of these roles.

Communication

Continuity of communication with families easily breaks down when infants are hospitalized for weeks to months. Families who live far away may only be able to visit infrequently. Parents may be forced to return to work soon after birth, so that maternity and paternity leave can be saved until the infant is discharged. Parent-infant bonding can be disrupted because of the infant's prolonged illness, and parents may feel a loss of their role as parent. For mothers, postpartum depression can increase feelings of sadness and detachment. Regular meetings with the family throughout the hospitalization can assess their evolving needs.

Poor communication among IDT clinicians, resulting in a loss of focus on the goals of care, can occur. Multiple strategies are needed to improve communication. Regular IDT meetings, with minutes distributed to missing clinicians, are helpful. This is particularly true when multiple subspecialists have recommendations that must be placed in the context of the infant's overall condition. Family satisfaction is improved when IDT clinicians deliver consistent information.[19] In settings with regularly rotating clinicians, a non-rotating IDT member, such as a social worker, may best serve as the primary contact person for the family.

As noted earlier, hospital providers must ensure clear communication with community providers for infants who are discharged to home with or without home hospice. Explicit discussions about pain and symptom control, resuscitation status, and family resources are needed.

Decision Making

There are several decisions particular to the LNP that should be noted.

When infants have been critically ill for weeks to months, families have often been asked to make repeated decisions about life-sustaining therapies. Some families become immune to the gravity of these discussions. They find it difficult to trust providers' judgment of a new crisis as life-threatening when the infant has already survived similar crises in the past. Families may develop conflicting goals at different points during the hospitalization. One parent may wish to pursue all therapies regardless of the outcome, while the other wishes to focus on comfort care. Providers encourage families to talk about their disagreements. Providers should anticipate that parents' goals often evolve over time, and decisions to not withdraw therapies early in the infant's hospitalization may change as parents develop a greater understanding of the prognosis. It is particularly important to elicit the parents' values regarding quality of life, as these may differ from providers'.[21]

Redefining Hope

Parents and providers who have resisted not giving up during earlier medical crisis may have difficulty recognizing that an infant's death is near. It can be helpful to reframe the choice of limiting or withdrawing therapies as not giving up, but as an active choice to limit suffering. Working toward discharge with home hospice, organizing a religious ritual with extended family members, or spending some time in a private room with the infant before extubation may all be goals for which parents can hope.

Management of Infant Suffering

Infants who have had repeated painful experiences may manifest hyperalgesia in response to minor procedures such as heel sticks or immunizations.[65] These older infants may tolerate a wider variety of pharmacologic formulations of analgesia and anxiolytics than newborns, such as patches, sublingual and rectal applications. Older infants may also benefit from help with secretions, gastroesophageal reflux, and anemia. Pharmacologic and non-pharmacologic strategies that reduce infant suffering are in Tables 37-1 and 37-2.

Case Study Revisited

A number of strategies could have improved care for Anna and her family.

- Regularly scheduled family meetings from early in the Anna's hospitalization
- Regular IDT meetings to review the goals of care
- Early discussions with Anna's family to help them anticipate a prolonged hospitalization
- Creative methods for enhancing the parents' bonds with their infant, such as encouraging them to leave a camera for staff to take pictures of Anna when the parents cannot visit
- Inform the family that the social worker should be their primary contact person throughout the hospitalization, as he can always identify the clinicians responsible for their infant's care
- Inquire about disagreement between Anna's parents regarding the goals of care
- Ask the family about their religious beliefs, and involve chaplain support

---

End of Life and Bereavement Care

Though caring for families during their child's dying and throughout bereavement have been described by several other authors in this book, several issues unique to prenatal and neonatal loss should be recognized.

MEMORY MAKING

For families whose infant dies around the time of birth, an entire lifetime of meeting, treasuring, and loving their babies may be wrapped up in mere minutes, hours, or days. Parents value the choice to interact and make memories with their baby during this brief time.[6,8,66] Ritual to acknowledge the baby's living and dying can provide meaning and nurture relationships among the parents, siblings and the baby.[67,68] All IDT clinicians can play an integral role in facilitating such moments between parent and child.

Some families willingly accept opportunities to interact with their baby and make memories. Others may hesitate initially, but may appreciate time to consider the options. Opportunities for memory making and ritual are highlighted in Table 37-3. Families should be encouraged to interact with their baby at a pace and in ways that are most meaningful to them, even if their choices differ from how clinicians believe memories should be made (Fig. 37-4).[69,70]

CARE OF THE FAMILY DURING THE DYING PROCESS

IDT clinicians should ascertain how much information parents wish to know about what death may be like, including anticipated changes in the baby's breathing, level of consciousness, color, and heart rate. Parents should be encouraged to be with their baby during death in ways that are meaningful and comfortable to them. Child life specialists and nurses may help prepare siblings for what they will see and experience before meeting their dying baby, keeping in mind that this is their first time actually seeing and interacting with their baby brother or sister.

Special cultural or religious actions, including proper care of the body, should be determined before the baby's death, and implemented accordingly. A safe, private location should be established, providing families the opportunity to be with their baby's body after death if desired. A time limit should not be imposed, as parental contact with their deceased baby's body poses little risk for infection and also does not impact potential postmortem testing.[71,72] In addition, IDT clinicians should ensure processes are in place should a mother hospitalized on a postpartum unit wish to be with her baby's body again before discharge.[73]

Recognizing that many young parents have never before made arrangements for the care of a loved one's body after death, IDT clinicians should be prepared to provide both verbal and written information on choosing a funeral director. An appropriate IDT member should be knowledgeable on the hospital's process for release of remains, as well as local choices for burial or cremation. In addition, the options for autopsy and organ or tissue donation should be discussed with the parents as appropriate. IDT clinicians may choose to develop a process to notify staff members of a baby's death, thus allowing staff who were not working at the time of the baby's death the opportunity to say goodbye to their tiny patient.

TABLE 37-3 Creating Meaningful Memories

Photographs and Video

Both serve as touchstones to the family's moments of interacting with their baby.

Photography Considerations
- Prenatal photography with pregnancy or family portraits
- Photographs of multiples together, including, if needed, photographing baby who has died with surviving multiples[29]
- Parents encouraged to bring their own cameras to the hospital
- Digital or disposable cameras available on the units for both staff and family use
- Method of providing digital images to family including CD ROM or SD card
- Method of storing digital images should parents decide not to receive the photographs at discharge

Photography Resources

- Now I Lay Me Down to Sleep: A national organization that links volunteer photographers to families experiencing the death of a baby. www.nilmdts.org
- Todd Hochberg Bereavement Photography: Todd Hochberg is a pioneer in the field of photojournalistic style of bereavement photography. His website is a resource for clinicians in utilizing this style of photgraphy. www.toddhochberg.com
- RTS Bereavement Services Guidelines for photographing babies at end of life[69]

Plaster Molds

Molds can be created of a baby's hands and feet using a variety of products
- 3-D mold kits such as Precious Hands or Wedding Hands
- Modeling compound used to make an impression such as Crayola's Model Magic or dental resins

Ink Prints and Other Memories

Prints can be created of baby's hands and feet on the following:
- Complimentary hospital birth certificate, card stock, or in a baby book
- Hats, t-shirts, or other items of clothing for the parents or siblings

Locks of Hair

- Can be carefully collected and placed in a small sealable plastic bag for safe-keeping

Scrapbooking

- Can be done during the prenatal period or after the baby's birth. Some antenatal and neonatal units provide scrapbooking opportunities for parents as a way to connect for support while creating memory pages.[70]

Personal Items

- Can be brought by the family or offered by IDT clinicians. Hospital auxiliary members, church or community service groups may provide donations. Patterns for very small size gowns and blankets can be found online. Examples of personal items include:
  Baptismal gowns and baby clothing in a variety of sizes
  Hand-knit caps and blanket
  Small toys
  Tape recorders of parents' voices talking, reading, or singing
  Baby rings (Fig. 37-4) available from www.bereavementservices.org

Memory Boxes

- Plain boxes can be purchased online or inexpensively at local craft stores and then decorated by siblings

Opportunities to Interact with the Baby

Touching and holding the baby, including kangaroo care
Rituals of blessing, naming, dedication, recognition of life, or baptism
Bathing and caring for the baby's body both while living and after death
Rocking, cuddling or laying down with the baby in a bed
Reading special books or singing to the baby
Taking the baby outdoors, or allowing the baby to experience sunshine

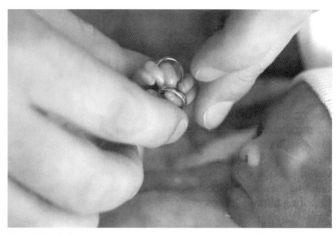

Fig. 37-4 A father gently places baby rings on the hands of his twin babies. (Photograph provided courtesy of Todd Hochberg.)

BEREAVEMENT SUPPORT

Grief support begins with the diagnosis of the life-limiting condition, and continues months after the baby's death.[2] Follow up with these families is essential. Parents' recollections of events surrounding birth and death differ from reality, specifically concerning the infant's condition at birth and the type of treatment that was given. The IDT can review the information with the family, even when there are no autopsy findings to review. The meeting should include IDT clinicians who can review the events around the death, provide recommendations for a subsequent pregnancy, and assess how the parents are working through their grief.

Parents face ongoing challenges when they are back in their community, where the infant's death may not be known or the details misunderstood. When others do not know about the birth and death of the infant, they may approach the mother as if she is still pregnant, thereby creating an uncomfortable situation. Also, it is not uncommon for this type of a loss to be perceived as and called a miscarriage by the lay public. IDT clinicians can help families anticipate the heartbreaking task of returning home to a waiting nursery without their baby. Parents may appreciate the opportunity to consider how they will share the news of the baby's death with their children, other family members, friends, colleagues, and strangers. A packet of supportive literature written specifically for parents experiencing the death of a baby should be provided before discharge from the hospital.

IDT clinicians should create avenues for bereavement follow up tailored to their particular population. Such follow up may occur through phone calls, bereavement mailings, hospital memorial services, or anniversary acknowledgments. Some parents may find comfort from a bereavement support group, or may access similar programs for their surviving children. A full discussion of prenatal and neonatal grief is outside the scope of this chapter. Readers are encouraged to access the following resources for further information:

- Resolve Through Sharing (RTS), www.bereavementservices.org
- National Pregnancy Loss and Infant Death Alliance, www.plida.org
- SHARE Pregnancy and Infant Loss Support, www.nationalshare.org
- MISS Foundation, www.missfoundation.org
- Centering Corporation, www.centering.org
- A Place to Remember, www.aplacetoremember.com

- www.perinatalhospice.org
- www.climb-support.org
- www.compassionatefriends.org
- www.trisomy.org

Conclusion

The needs of families anticipating the birth of a baby with a life-threatening condition offers unique opportunities to implement palliative care measures throughout the prenatal and neonatal periods. IDT clinicians who participate in the provision of such care have the privilege of welcoming new life, creating meaningful moments, and facilitating goodbyes while honoring family's hopes, beliefs, and preferences.

REFERENCES

1. MacDorman MF, Kimeyer S: In *Fetal and perinatal mortality, United States, 2005: National Vital Statistics Reports* (vol 57), Hyattsville, Md, 2009, National Center for Health Statistics.
2. Milstein J: A paradigm of integrative care: healing with curing throughout life, "being with" and "doing to," *J Perinatol* 25:563–568, 2005.
3. Richter MS, Parkes C, Chaw-Kant J: Listening to the voices of hospitalized high-risk antepartum patients, *JOGN Nurs* 36:313–318, 2007.
4. Kavanaugh K: Parents' experience surrounding the death of a newborn whose birth is at the margin of viability, *JOGN Nurs* 26:43–51, 1997.
5. Limbo R, Kobler K: Will our baby be alive again? Supporting parents of young children when a baby dies, *Nurs Women's Health* 13:302–311, 2009.
6. Widger K, Picot C: Parents' perceptions of the quality of pediatric and perinatal end-of-life care, *Pediatr Nurs* 34:53–58, 2008.
7. Williams C, Munson D, Zupancic J, et al: Supporting bereaved parents: Practical steps in providing compassionate perinatal and neonatal end-of-life care. A North American perspective, *Semin Fetal Neonatal Med* 13:335–340, 2008.
8. Gold KJ: Navigating care after a baby dies: A systematic review of parent experiences with health providers, *J Perinatol* 27:230–237, 2007.
9. Moro T, Kavanaugh K, Okuno-Jones S, et al: Neonatal end-of-life care: a review of the research literature, *J Perinat Neonatal Nurs* 20:262–273, 2006.
10. Carnevale FA, Canoui P, Cremer R, et al: Parental involvement in treatment decisions regarding their critically ill child: a comparative study of France and Quebec, *Pediatr Crit Care Med* 8:337–342, 2007.
11. Doron MW, Veness-Meehan KA, Margolis LH, et al: Delivery room resuscitation decisions for extremely premature infants, *Pediatrics* 102:574–582, 1998.
12. Peerzada JM, Richardson DK, Burns JP: Delivery room decision-making at the threshold of viability, *J Pediatr* 145:492–498, 2004.
13. van der Heide A, van der Maas PJ, van der Wal G, et al: The role of parents in end-of-life decisions in neonatology: physicians' views and practices, *Pediatrics* 101:413–418, 1998.
14. Zupancic JA, Kirpalani H, Barrett J, et al: Characterising doctor-parent communication in counseling for impending preterm delivery, *Arch Dis Child Fetal Neonatal Ed* 87:F113–F117, 2002.
15. Bastek TK, Richardson DK, Zupancic JA, et al: Prenatal consultation practices at the border of viability: a regional survey, *Pediatrics* 116:407–413, 2005.
16. Martinez AM, Partridge JC, Yu V, et al: Physician counseling practices and decision-making for extremely preterm infants in the Pacific Rim, *J Paediatr Child Health* 41:209–214, 2005.
17. Partridge JC, Martinez AM, Nishida H, et al: International comparison of care for very low birth weight infants: parents' perceptions of counseling and decision-making, *Pediatrics* 116:e263–e271, 2005.
18. Boss RD, Hutton N, Sulpar LJ, et al: Values parents apply to decision-making regarding delivery room resuscitation for high-risk newborns, *Pediatrics* 122:583–589, 2008.
19. Miquel-Verges F, Woods L, Aucott SA, Boss RD, Donohue PK: Prenatal consultation with a neonatologist for congenital anomalies: parental perceptions, *Pediatrics* 124: 573–576, 2009.
20. Freda MC, Devine KS, Semelsberger C: The lived experience of miscarriage after infertility, *MCN Am J Matern Child Nurs* 28:16–23, 2003.
21. Streiner DL, Saigal S, Burrows E, et al: Attitudes of parents and health care professionals toward active treatment of extremely premature infants, *Pediatrics* 108:152–157, 2001.
22. Chiswick M: Infants of borderline viability: ethical and clinical considerations, *Semin Fetal Neonatal Med* 13:8–15, 2008.
23. American Academy of Pediatrics Committee on Fetus and Newborn, Bell EF: Noninitiation or withdrawal of intensive care for high-risk newborns, *Pediatrics* 119:401–403, 2007.
24. Batton DG, Committee on Fetus and Newborn: Clinical report: antenatal counseling regarding resuscitation at an extremely low gestational age, *Pediatrics* 124:422–427, 2009.
25. Hurst I: The legal landscape at the threshold of viability for extremely premature infants: a nursing perspective, part II, *J Perinat Neonatal Nurs* 19:253–262, 2005; quiz 263–264.
26. Hurst I: The legal landscape at the threshold of viability for extremely premature infants: A nursing perspective, part I, *J Perinat Neonatal Nurs* 19:155–166, 2005; quiz 167–168.
27. Kavanaugh K, Savage T, Kilpatrick S, et al: Life support decisions for extremely premature infants: Report of a pilot study, *J Pediatr Nurs* 20:347–359, 2005.
28. Evans WG, Tulsky JA, Back AL, et al: Communication at times of transitions: how to help patients cope with loss and redefine hope, *Cancer J* 12:417–424, 2006.
29. Pector EA: Views of bereaved multiple-birth parents on life support decisions, the dying process, and discussions surrounding death, *J Perinatol* 24:4–10, 2004.
30. Kenner C, Boykova M: Palliative care in the neonatal intensive care unit. In Ferrell B, Coyle N, editors: *Textbook of palliative nursing*, ed 3, New York, 2010, Oxford University Press, pp 1065–1080.
31. Kain VJ: Moral distress and providing care to dying babies in neonatal nursing, *Int J Palliat Nurs* 13:243–248, 2007.
32. Papadatou D: *In the face of death: professionals who care for the dying and the bereaved*, New York, 2009, Springer.
33. Papadatou D: A proposed model of health professionals' grieving process, *Omega* 41:59–77, 2000.
34. Roehrs C, Masterson A, Alles R, et al: Caring for families coping with perinatal loss, *JOGN Nurs* 37:631–639, 2008.
35. Epstein EG: End-of-life experiences of nurses and physicians in the newborn intensive care unit, *J Perinatol* 28:771–778, 2008.
36. Rogers S, Babgi A, Gomez C: Educational interventions in end-of-life care: Part I: An educational intervention responding to the moral distress of NICU nurses provided by an ethics consultation team, *Adv Neonatal Care* 8:56–65, 2008.
37. Leuthner S, Jones EL: Fetal Concerns Program: A model for perinatal palliative care, *MCN Am J Matern Child Nurs* 32:272–278, 2007.
38. Sumner LH, Kavanaugh K, Moro T: Extending palliative care into pregnancy and the immediate newborn period: state of the practice of perinatal palliative care, *J Perinat Neonatal Nurs* 20:113–116, 2006.
39. Leuthner SR: Palliative care of the infant with lethal anomalies, *Pediatr Clin North Am* 51:747–759, xi, 2004.
40. Munson D, Leuthner SR: Palliative care for the family carrying a fetus with a life-limiting diagnosis, *Pediatr Clin North Am* 54:787–798, xii, 2007.
41. Breeze AC, Lees CC, Kumar A, et al: Palliative care for prenatally diagnosed lethal fetal abnormality, *Arch Dis Child Fetal Neonatal Ed* 92:F56–F58, 2007.
42. Kattwinkel J, editor: *The textbook of neonatal resuscitation*, Elk Grove Village, Ill, 2006, Academy of Pediatrics and the American Heart Association.
43. Koogler TK, Wilfond BS, Ross LF: Lethal language, lethal decisions, *Hastings Cent Rep* 33:37–41, 2003.
44. Milstein JM: Introducing spirituality in medical care: transition from hopelessness to wholeness, *JAMA* 299:2440–2441, 2008.
45. Janvier A, Lantos J, Deschênes M, et al: Caregivers attitudes for very premature infants: What if they knew? *Acta Paediatr* 97:276–279, 2008.
46. MacKinnon K: Living with the threat of preterm labor: women's work of keeping the baby in, *JOGN Nurs* 35:700–708, 2006.
47. Griffin T, Kavanaugh K, Soto CF, et al: Parental evaluation of a tour of the neonatal intensive care unit during a high-risk pregnancy, *JOGN Nurs* 26:59–65, 1997.
48. Singh J, Fanaroff J, Andrews B, et al: Resuscitation in the "gray zone" of viability: Determining physician preferences and predicting infant outcomes, *Pediatrics* 120:519–526, 2007.
49. Tyson JE, Parikh NA, Langer J, et al: Intensive care for extreme prematurity: moving beyond gestational age, *N Engl J Med* 358:1672–1681, 2008.

50. World Health Organization: In *International statistical classification of diseases and related health problems*, vol 2, Geneva, Switzerland, 1993, p 129.
51. Harrison H: The offer they can't refuse: parents and perinatal treatment decisions, *Semin Fetal Neonatal Med* 13:329–334, 2008.
52. Catlin A: Thinking outside the box: Prenatal care and the call for a prenatal advance directive, *J Perinat Neonatal Nurs* 19:169–176, 2005.
53. Reder EA, Serwint JR: Until the last breath: exploring the concept of hope for parents and health care professionals during a child's serious illness, *Arch Pediatr Adolesc Med* 163:653–657, 2009.
54. Leuthner SR, Boldt AM, Kirby RS: Where infants die: examination of place of death and hospice/home health care options in the state of Wisconsin, *J Palliat Med* 7:269–277, 2004.
55. Lauer ME, Mulhern RK, Schell MJ, et al: Long-term follow-up of parental adjustment following a child's death at home or hospital, *Cancer* 63:988–994, 1989.
56. Pierucci RL, kirby RS, Leuthner SR: End-of-life care for neonates and infants: the experience and effects of a palliative care consultation service, *Pediatrics* 108:653–660, 2001.
57. Child Abuse and Prevention Act, 42 U.S.C. § 5101 (1994).
58. Diekema DS, Botkin JR, Committee on Bioethics American Academy of Pediatrics: Clinical report: forgoing medically provided nutrition and hydration in children, *Pediatrics* 124:813–822, 2009.
59. Batton DG, Barrington KJ, Wallman C: Prevention and management of pain in the neonate: an update, *Pediatrics* 118:2231–2241, 2006.
60. Stevens B, Johnston C, Petryshen P, et al: Premature Infant Pain Profile: development and initial validation, *Clin J Pain* 12:13–22, 1996.
61. Grunau RV, Johnston CC, Craig KD: Neonatal facial and cry responses to invasive and non-invasive procedures, *Pain* 42:295–305, 1990.
62. Krechel SW, Bildner J: CRIES: A new neonatal postoperative pain measurement score: initial testing of validity and reliability, *Paediatr Anaesth* 5:53–61, 1995.
63. van Dijk M, de Boer JB, Koot HM, et al: The reliability and validity of the COMFORT scale as a postoperative pain instrument in 0 to 3-year-old infants, *Pain* 84:367–377, 2000.
64. Lawrence J, Alcock D, McGrath P, et al: The development of a tool to assess neonatal pain, *Neonatal Netw* 12:59–66, 1993.
65. Taddio A, Shah V, Gilbert-MacLeod C, et al: Conditioning and hyperalgesia in newborns exposed to repeated heel lances, *JAMA* 288:857–861, 2002.
66. Meert KL, Thurston CS, Briller SH: The spiritual needs of parents at the time of their child's death in the pediatric intensive care unit and during bereavement: a qualitative study, *Pediatr Crit Care Med* 6:420–427, 2005.
67. Kobler K, Limbo R, Kavanaugh K: Meaningful moments: The use of ritual in perinatal and pediatric death, *MCN Am J Matern Child Nurs* 32: 288–295, 2007; quiz 296–297.
68. Fanos JH, Little GA, Edwards WH: Candles in the snow: ritual and memory for siblings of infants who died in the intensive care nursery, *J Pediatr* 154:849–853, 2009.
69. Daley M, Limbo R, editors: *Creating memories. RTS bereavement training in early pregnancy loss, stillbirth, and newborn death*, La Crosse, Wis, 2008, Gundersen Lutheran Medical Foundation.
70. Schwarz B, Fatzinger C, Meier PP: Rush SpecialKare Keepsakes, *MCN Am J Matern Child Nurs* 29:354–361, 2004; quiz 362–363.
71. Pregnancy Loss and Infant Death Alliance: *PLIDA position statement: Infection risks are insignificant*, www.plida.org/pdf/infectionRisks.pdf. Accessed July 26, 2009.
72. Pregnancy Loss and Infant Death Alliance: *PLIDA position statement: Delaying postmortem pathology studies*. www.plida.org/pdf/PostmemPath.pdf. Accessed July 26, 2009.
73. Pregnancy Loss and Infant Death Alliance: *PLIDA position statement: Bereaved parents holding their baby*, www.plida.org/pdf/PLIDA_Statement_Holding_Baby_FINAL.pdf Accessed July 26, 2009.

38 Inherited Life-Threatening Illnesses

SARAH DUGAN | RENEE TEMME

Facing the Future
Every journey begins
With but a small step.
And every day is a chance
For a new, small step
In the right direction.
Just follow your Heartsong. — Mattie Stepanek

Many genetic conditions are inherited, while others are the result of a genetic change in the affected individual. Even in these cases, the condition can be considered inherited in the sense that it is usually caused by a genetic defect in a gamete passed from parent to child.

Inherited medical conditions are often amenable to medical management and frequently do not significantly affect life expectancy. However, such conditions can also be life-threatening and lead to early death. Inherited conditions and their associated cultural constructs often impact patients, families, and medical providers in ways that should be considered part of palliative care. Caring for a child with a life-threatening illness secondary to an inherited condition poses a unique set of challenges best addressed by an interdisciplinary approach. Though a complete review of all inherited life-threatening conditions is beyond the scope of this chapter, the table lists some common examples (Table 38-1).

Specific Care Challenges

The stigma, recurrence risk, and isolation that inherited life-threatening illnesses impart all affect attitudes and goals about the treatment plan.[1] Understanding the specific challenges faced by families and children affected by inherited life-threatening illnesses allows providers to respond to an individual family's needs when broaching the subject of palliative care.

STIGMA, GUILT, AND SHAME

The stigma associated with inherited disease stems from multiple sources. The effect of stigma is heavily influenced by personal, social, and cultural forces and therefore varies significantly from case to case. Understanding the impact of this stigma on individual patients and families is essential for introduction and maintenance of a palliative care plan.

The very concept of having passed on a life-threatening condition is a staggering source of guilt for many parents and grandparents. In conditions inherited through a single parent, this guilt can be unevenly distributed.[2] Feelings of guilt in a parent may influence decisions regarding both care meant to prolong life and care meant to improve quality of life. An overwhelming sense of responsibility may prevent some parents from asking for assistance. Although parental guilt is a normal response to having a child with an inherited illness, medical providers should be alert for signs of caregiver fatigue or family stress related to these feelings. Genetic counselors are specially trained to work with families around the time of initial diagnosis. The responses of family members often stem from a desire to find underlying meaning for the birth of a child with a genetic condition. Some parents may believe that a past action or inaction caused their child to have a birth defect or an inherited condition.[3] Some parents are ashamed for having a child who does not fit the ideals they had prior to, or during, pregnancy.[4] Some children or families who have particular difficulty adjusting to a genetic diagnosis may benefit from psychiatry or psychology consultations to discuss these feelings in greater detail.

Even aside from the issue of parental responsibility, genetic conditions are further stigmatizing society's tendency to view a genetic difference as an inherent personal flaw. Medical staff should do all possible not to propagate this viewpoint. In fact, assessing the families' experiences and listening to responses during initial consultations may give clues regarding feelings of guilt or shame. Patients or families experiencing shame will, at times, withdraw from the situation. Those experiencing an internal sense of responsibility or guilt may blame themselves, rationalize, or intellectualize the situation. Lack of control can be particularly painful for parents experiencing this unrealistic sense of responsibility.[4] Actively engaging in medical decision making may allow families to feel that they have regained some control.

LANGUAGE CHOICE

In this increasingly protocol-driven medical environment, providers are often tempted to rely on shorthand terms such as Downs baby to refer to an infant with Down syndrome or CF-er to refer to a child with cystic fibrosis. By doing so, however, they unintentionally marginalize the affected child and suggest that he or she is defined entirely by the disease. Providers should be sensitive to the use of person-first language and current terminology. Providers may invite the family to provide their preferred terminology. For example, a family may express concern regarding the use of mental retardation and prefer cognitive impairment or static encephalopathy. Use of potentially offensive terminology may impede the relationship with the family and prevent open discussion of sensitive issues such as prognosis and

TABLE 38-1 Life-Threatening Inherited Conditions

Examples, inheritance patterns, and clinical descriptions of several types of life-threatening inherited conditions. The listed categories overlap considerably but are a useful framework for thinking about inherited conditions.

Condition type and examples	Inheritance	Description and clinical course
Metabolic Disease		
MELAS	Mitochondrial	Characterized by mitochondrial encephalomyopathy, lactic acidosis, and strokelike episodes that typically present in mid- to late childhood. Early development is often normal. Seizures and hearing loss are common.
Maple syrup urine disease (MSUD)	Autosomal recessive	Caused by branched-chain alpha-ketoacid dehydrogenase complex deficiency that, without treatment, results in poor feeding, irritability, coma, and central respiratory failure. Manifestations vary with level of enzyme activity.
Multiple Malformations		
Smith-Lemli-Opitz syndrome	Autosomal recessive	Individuals may have multiple anomalies of cleft palate, heart defect, hypospadias, abnormal genitalia, growth retardation. The condition results from mutations in the gene encoding 7-dehydrocholesterol reductase, an enzyme involved in cholesterol metabolism.
Noonan syndrome	Autosomal dominant	Individuals may have congenital heart disease, coagulation abnormalities, cryptorchidism, chest deformities, and developmental delay. There are several genes known to cause the condition; however, a genetic change is not detected in all individuals with a clinical diagnosis.
Chromosomal		
Trisomy 13	Chromosomal	Often presents prenatally or at birth with multiple anomalies, including congenital heart disease and craniofacial malformations. Infants usually die in the first year of life from central apnea, but the clinical course is variable.
Williams syndrome	Chromosomal	Individuals often have cardiovascular disease, endocrine abnormalities, connective tissue differences, and mild mental retardation. A contiguous chromosomal deletion involving 7q11.2 is present in 99% of cases.
Neuromuscular Disease		
Duchenne muscular dystrophy (DMD)	X-linked	Affected males often present with delayed milestones, and progressive muscle weakness and atrophy cause wheelchair dependency by age 13 with early death from respiratory and cardiac failure. DMD represents the severe end of the spectrum of dystrophinopathies.
Neurodegenerative Disease		
Adrenoleukodystrophy	X-linked	The childhood cerebral form typically first presents with attention deficit disorder and progresses to cognitive, motor, vision, and hearing impairment, to complete disability within a few years. Widely variable expression even among individuals in the same family.
Storage Disease		
Hunter syndrome	X-linked	A lysosomal storage disease that results in progressive excess storage of glycosaminoglycans. Symptoms include hepatosplenomegaly, CNS involvement, coarse facial features, and joint contractures. Respiratory and/or cardiac diseases are the major causes of morbidity and mortality. Onset and symptoms vary widely.
Pompe disease	Autosomal recessive	A glycogen storage disease that often presents with feeding difficulty, muscle weakness, hypotonia, and cardiomyopathy in the severe infantile-onset form. Without enzyme replacement therapy (ERT), infants often die in the first year of life.
Skeletal Dysplasia		
Campomelic dysplasia	Autosomal dominant	Most individuals die during the neonatal period from respiratory insufficiency. Symptoms include severe laryngotracheomalacia, Pierre Robin sequence, ambiguous genitalia, club feet, bowed limbs, dislocated hips, and short stature. Cervical spine abnormalities, scoliosis, and kyphosis are common. Many females are found to be 46, XY.

end-of-life care. Conversely, choosing language that personalizes the child can set the tone for a holistic approach to medical care giving. Language implying that the medical team sees the child as a whole person allows patients and families to share their goals with the care team.[5]

RECURRENCE

Families affected by life-threatening inherited illnesses often have the unfortunate distinction of going through the process with multiple family members. Experience with the previously diagnosed individual will likely impact care for the next affected individual, but the specific result is not always predictable. Some families who selected a life-prolonging treatment course for their first affected child may provide only comfort measures for their next affected child. The inverse is also

true, and still other families may follow the same course with subsequent affected siblings. These care decisions are highly personal and depend on far more than critique of the care supplied to the previous child. In instances where they can be assessed, the affected child's treatment goals often influence these decisions.

A mother of two boys who had died of muscular dystrophy at ages 17 and 5 shared that her first affected son wanted his life prolonged as much as possible; he achieved this goal with maximum support and intervention. Her second stated at age 3 that he wanted "no tubes." He also expressed his desire to learn to walk and was able to meet both of these goals, with his parents and treatment team acting as advocates.

While primary care providers generally consider parents to have an expert understanding of their children, this attitude is especially appropriate when conditions recur in the same family. Affected children and their parents may possess expert understanding of the condition at many levels. In very rare conditions, their scientific knowledge of the condition may exceed that of the care team. More importantly, however, their intimate experience with the condition in a previously affected family member gives them an additional kind of expertise. Medical care providers should explore these experiences with families in order to grasp their understanding of the illness and facilitate discussion of a treatment plan. In many cases, providers will be able to adjust or enhance the family's perspective, as when the family of the second affected child is unaware of the condition's variability.

A couple whose first child was diagnosed with maple syrup urine disease (MSUD), a life-threatening inborn error of metabolism, responded to the diagnosis with a seemingly disproportionate degree of despair. Additional conversation revealed that an affected maternal cousin had severe intellectual impairment. The conversation allowed an opportunity to educate the family about the importance of early intervention in this condition.

ISOLATION

Most inherited illnesses are relatively rare and can have an isolating effect on families. The interdisciplinary approach is particularly important in such circumstances because subspecialists, in addition to providing medical expertise, can provide informational and social resource contacts for families of children with rare, life-threatening inherited illnesses. Genetic counselors and other specialists can provide families with contact information for state, national, or international support organizations and can directly connect families of children with the same or similar conditions. They can also often connect families with the center of excellence where a provider or providers may have expertise in caring for patients with the condition. This connection can ameliorate the sense of isolation and also be a source of valuable information about care, resources, and natural history of the condition.

A family whose infant had been diagnosed with Cornelia DeLange syndrome, a rare inherited multiple malformation syndrome, was put in contact with a syndrome-specific support group at the time of diagnosis. By their daughter's one-year follow up visit, the family had more than 40 parent contacts throughout the country. This family shared they had learned a great deal about what to expect from other families.

As always, providers should carefully assess each family's goals and psychosocial milieu before they suggest resources. For some families, the thought of talking to another family with a child with the same condition is overwhelming and frightening at the time of initial diagnosis.

After hearing confirmation that his toddler son had achondroplasia, a father recoiled when we offered resources from Little People of America. He later explained that he could not accept that his son would develop the medical problems and extreme short stature described in the pamphlets we had given him.

Although families should be encouraged to use resources, aggressive promotion of resources can alienate a family still adjusting to a particular diagnosis and prevent future access to care. Some families, though initially reluctant, need time to adjust and accept the diagnosis.

A family whose toddler had been newly diagnosed with Williams syndrome declined an offer to meet a family whose child had the same chromosomal change. As their child prepared to enter school, they began to ask more questions about what to expect in the future. We re-extended the offer and found that they were very interested.

Other families prefer to be prepared for the natural progression of an inherited illness well in advance. One woman whose baby was severely affected by a progressive neuromuscular disorder said she was glad to have met another severely affected child who was later in the course of illness. Although she realized the other child's extreme weakness and ventilator dependence were likely to occur in her child as well, she felt more prepared after meeting that child and his family. Primary care providers, social workers, subspecialists, palliative care specialists, and genetic counselors can all be called upon to evaluate a family's need for resources and education throughout the course of an inherited life-threatening condition.

Still another challenge comes with providing support resources for families and children with inherited conditions predisposing them to infection, such as cystic fibrosis (CF). For infection control reasons, individuals with CF often cannot easily connect face to face; however, there are a growing number of online resources for support.

As isolating as a confirmed diagnosis of an inherited life-threatening illness may be, an unknown diagnosis may be even more isolating. Affected children and their families, in addition to being faced with the life-changing effects of a chronic illness and the stigma associated with inherited disease, also must live with a greater degree of uncertainty than those with a known diagnosis. There may be few support resources available to families beyond family members, friends, providers, and community when a diagnosis is unknown. While subspecialists and support staff can still assist these families, prognosis is often less sure when the underlying diagnosis is unknown, and addressing patient and family goals, as well as recurrence risk, may be more difficult for providers.

Role of Diagnostic Workup

Diagnostic workup is indicated to direct treatment in life-threatening illnesses of all etiologies. In life-threatening illnesses suspected to be inherited, diagnostic workup can be particularly prolonged and expensive. Furthermore, diagnosing an inherited condition often has implications for other family members. The medical care team must anticipate these complications and address them with the family throughout the diagnostic and treatment process. Genetic counseling is essential during this process to help with addressing psychosocial issues, obtaining informed consent, interpreting results, and providing resource and recurrence risk information.

Although some genetic conditions are easily diagnosed based on clinical features, others may be more difficult to classify. Often, a life-threatening condition is suspected to be genetic in origin, but the underlying cause is not obvious. In such cases, medical caregivers must communicate these suspicions openly to help the family come to an informed decision about how exhaustive the workup should be. Communication must occur in the context of a holistic, interdisciplinary approach to a treatment plan that encompasses disease-directed and palliative measures. Care providers are responsible for conveying to the family that a diagnostic workup, which can tax both the child and family, is carried out to guide their child's treatment and to provide answers for the family. Even when parents and children would rather not undergo additional procedures for their own purposes, they may agree to them if they believe it will benefit the larger medical establishment. Medical providers may be unaware of this attitude, blithely performing tests they imagine are desired by the family. The medical risks and benefits, as well as the potential monetary cost to the family, of each diagnostic step should be discussed with the family and, when appropriate, with the child.

When a thorough diagnostic evaluation fails to provide an answer, DNA banking, in which a blood or tissue sample is stored for future studies, is also an option. Banking tissue can provide some comfort for families who fear that their child's death will forever be unexplained. The necessary tissue can be obtained before or after death. Banked DNA can then be sent for studies as advancements in medical science allow.

As diagnostic technology improves, input from geneticists and genetic counselors becomes increasingly important. Genetic testing results are easily misinterpreted. For example, comparative genomic hybridization, a relatively new diagnostic technique that scans the genome for very small losses or gains of DNA, has a high diagnostic yield in children with multiple life-threatening congenital anomalies. However, a genetic specialist's input is essential for interpretation of results to this study. A given result may have few or no reported previous occurrences, and thus its implications for disease-directed and palliative care may be difficult to discern without specific training and a review of the medical literature and genome browsers. A geneticist or genetic counselor is best equipped to discuss such results with families and may be able to provide social and educational resources as well.

Such a specialist is also best able to address the implications of a genetic diagnosis for other family members. Although taking the focus from a patient with a life-threatening illness may seem distasteful, it is essential to family-centered care to consider other family members in the workup and treatment for inherited life-threatening conditions.[6] For some children and families, finding a diagnosis that will facilitate treatment and family planning for relatives is seen as a legacy left by the patient.

A family whose daughter died of a progressive cardiomyopathy, allowing her affected sister to be diagnosed and treated early, found solace in the fact that their child's short life had made a real difference in the life of her sister.

The needs of other family members, including current and future siblings, should be included in discussion of the family's and child's goals for diagnosis and treatment.

At times, the diagnostic workup can include postmortem investigations. If postmortem investigations might be diagnostically useful, the matter should be discussed before death whenever possible. The provider might want to discuss the possibility that postmortem studies may represent the last or only chance to obtain diagnosis in a child who has died of an inherited illness. Diagnosis can answer questions for the family and may also provide information about risk for future siblings. Furthermore, performing a postmortem biopsy can spare a procedure in a dying child who is suspected to have an inherited illness. In certain conditions, such as some metabolic diseases, postmortem investigation can be useful, but specimens should be obtained as soon after death as possible, and the necessary materials and procedures should be set up in advance.

UNCERTAINTY, PROGNOSIS, AND TREATMENT

Although some inherited illnesses have no specific therapy, treatment options are expanding. Children and parents are presented with the difficult task of sorting through these options at the turbulent time of diagnosis. Confirming a genetic change underlying a child's life-threatening illness is usually not sufficient to give a certain prognosis; therefore, an array of treatment options is usually available. An interdisciplinary approach is essential at this point. Treatment and life goals of the child and family should be assessed continually and communicated clearly to the medical team.

Conferring a clear diagnosis of an inherited life-threatening condition would seem to also confer a clear prognosis. However, the phenotypic variability in inherited conditions can be great enough that the affected child's eventual clinical and developmental outcome may not be predictable. The concept of genotype-phenotype correlation must be explored on a case-by-case basis. Genotype-phenotype correlation is highlighted by the example of autosomal aneuploidies such as trisomy 18 and trisomy 21. Specialists will counsel families that infants with trisomy 18 have significant risk for early mortality despite reasonable intervention, whereas infants with trisomy 21 will generally do well. However, counseling always includes the caveat that children affected by either condition may have better or poorer health and development than expected. This uncertainty affects treatment decisions in diverse ways. At times, families may want to proceed with intensive interventions when prognosis seems bleak; in other cases, a family may desire to withdraw life-sustaining interventions despite a seemingly good prognosis. These decisions are highly personal and can confound well-meaning medical providers. Social work, genetic counseling, and interdisciplinary care conferences are helpful in such cases to educate the child and family regarding complex medical issues and to alleviate any fundamental misunderstanding on the part of the family or care team. If cultural differences have contributed to a misunderstanding, a cultural liaison may also be helpful. Ethics consultation and spiritual staff can also be useful in helping guide the family and medical team through this difficult process.

As happens in treating life-threatening illness of any etiology, the line between comfort care and life-prolonging measures is not always clear. Children and families who elect not to pursue curative medical therapies for an inherited illness might still benefit from certain treatments that will probably increase both life span and quality of life.

> *A family with a symptomatic child newly diagnosed with Hunter syndrome chose not to pursue intravenous replacement of the genetically missing enzyme, as replacement does not improve neurological outcome. However, progressing joint stiffness and other medical problems associated with the condition led the family to pursue the treatment one year later.*

Delineation of the molecular basis of inherited disease has ushered in novel therapies, some available only on a research basis. Consulted specialists may know of specific trials for which an affected patient would be eligible. Clinical trials can also be sought through the government-sanctioned website www.clinicaltrials.gov. There may already be some evidence of medical benefit, or lack thereof, of the experimental treatment in question. In other trials, the benefit is less clear. Most families are interested in learning of open trials; some are interested in enrolling and may actually raise the subject. The care team should recognize that participation in these trials may be of greater significance to a patient or family than as last-ditch attempt at treatment; engaging in research-based activities may fulfill the deeper obligation of doing everything to fight an illness. Furthermore, families may be interested in involvement of clinical research studies solely to benefit other families in the future and have comfort in knowing they may be contributing to advancing knowledge about the condition.

Commercially available but non–FDA-approved treatments such as stem cell therapy may also be sought by families. Oftentimes, these treatments are available only outside of the United States, and the medical team may not be able to obtain records or speak with the professionals providing the therapies. Such situations can espouse the worry that these procedures may somehow harm the child. Ethics consultation is indicated where there is reasonable concern for harm or fraud. However, when conventional medicine offers no curative measure for a life-threatening condition, casting aspersions at what a family might consider the only curative treatment can be alienating and ultimately sabotage the family's relationship with the medical team.

Interventions such as stem cell therapy, an offshoot of Western medical practice, are distinct from complementary and alternative medicine forms, which are also important resources for many families. Clinicians should keep track of complementary and alternative treatments and medications as they would any treatment or medication. This step is especially important in treatment of inborn errors of metabolism; certain ingredients in supplements or alternative medications might be contraindicated in children with specific enzyme deficiencies.

Inherited life-threatening illnesses are often associated with medical, developmental, and anatomic differences that are not in and of themselves life-threatening. To medical providers, these differences may seem of relatively low priority. To patients and families, however, these external stigmata of disease may be close to the top of the list of concerns. Facial and hand anomalies, even those that are of primarily cosmetic importance, are particularly upsetting for many families. However, this reaction is not consistent from family to family.

> *A Hmong family referred to hand surgery for their child's postaxial polydactyly was shocked to hear that the surgeon actually wanted to remove what to them was a sign of good fortune. Had they known the purpose of this appointment, they would have declined consultation.*
>
> *The Somali parents of a neonate with Prader Willi syndrome expressed greater anguish over their child's transient inability to eat by mouth than over the high likelihood that she would have cognitive impairment throughout life. This family appreciated a visit from endocrinology ahead of schedule to discuss hormonal treatment for hypotonia.*

Promptly addressing specific parental and patient concerns expresses a commitment to personalize care and fosters trust and respect between the family and the care team.

Introducing the Topic of Palliative Care

The concept of palliative care should be introduced at the outset of treatment for any life-threatening condition. Incorporating this topic into the treatment plan routinely will over time dispel the stereotypical thinking that palliative care is intended for only those children for whom all other treatment options have been exhausted or dismissed. An investigation of a series of complaints[7] from young adults and family members affected by CF revealed they had been taken aback by a palliative care survey. Most of the complaints centered on the idea that any discussion of palliative care was not appropriate given the perceived good health of the affected individual. These reactions, which were not necessarily inappropriate, indicate that the topic was a relatively unfamiliar one to the complainants.

Introduction of palliative care can occur especially early in inherited conditions, as they may be diagnosed prenatally. Discovering prenatal anomalies often prompts consultation with perinatologists and surgical specialists. Prenatal genetic counseling is almost always employed, and a clinical geneticist may also meet with the expecting couple. This is an ideal time to introduce the concept of palliative care as one element of the interdisciplinary approach. Consultation with the palliative care team may be indicated if the expecting parents are interested in formulating a specific palliative care plan prenatally.

Diagnosis may also be made before the onset of illness if a known familial condition is diagnosed in an asymptomatic child. In these cases, the idea of palliative care should be introduced early, couched in the initial discussion of life and treatment goals for the child, and reintroduced each time these goals are reviewed or modified. If the inherited condition does become life-threatening, bringing up the subject of palliative care should be perceived as routine rather than as a declaration of treatment failure.

> *The asymptomatic younger brother of a boy with adrenoleukodystrophy was found to have the same deleterious change in the causative gene. The family was devastated to learn that their younger son might, like his brother, develop*

paralysis and encephalopathy. However, they also told us that this knowledge had led them to prioritize differently. For example, they elected to take their child out of school for an extended family vacation that they would not otherwise have taken.

Summary

Providing holistic care to a child with a life-threatening inherited illness requires discussion of palliative care. The topic should be introduced as early as possible in discussion of the diagnosis or suspected diagnosis. Most children with inherited life-threatening illnesses will require the care of multiple specialists, who should stay in communication with each other regarding the overall plan of care. Periodic interdisciplinary care conferences designed to unify the team and family in working toward common treatment goals are essential. A primary care provider or pediatric practice that provides a medical home is also an important part of care coordination, especially in caring for children on an outpatient or in-home basis.

Genetic counseling and genetics consultation are necessary from both a family-centered and a child-centered perspective. These services facilitate access to resources, interpretation of results, family planning, and specialized diagnosis and treatment.

The psychosocial stress generated for children and families faced with an inherited life-threatening illness can be overwhelming and may hamper communication between the care team and the family. Social work, spiritual care, and psychological or psychiatric consultations should be offered to help families and children cope during the more difficult times. If miscommunication is suspected, ethics consultation or cultural liaison may be helpful.

REFERENCES

1. Knebel A, Hudgings C: End-of-life issues in genetic disorders: summary of workshop held at the National Institutes of Health on September 26, 2001, *Genet Med* 4:373–378, 2002.
2. James C, Hadley D, Holtzman N, et al: How does the mode of inheritance of a genetic condition influence families? A study of guilt, blame, stigma, and understanding of inheritance and reproductive risks in families with X-linked and autosomal recessive diseases, *Genet Med* 8:234–242, 2006.
3. Murray RR Jr: Psychosocial aspects of genetic counseling, *Soc Work Health Care* 2:13–23, 1976.
4. Kessler S, Kessler H, Ward P: Psychological aspects of genetic counseling. III. Management of guilt and shame, *Am J Med Genet* 17:673–697, 1984.
5. Hodgson J, Hughs E, Lambert C: "SLANG"—Sensitive Language and the New Genetics: an exploratory study, *J Genet Couns* 14:415–421, 2005.
6. Quillinn J, Bodurtha J, Smith T: Genetics assessment at the end of life: suggestions for implementation in clinic and future research, *J Palliat Med* 11:451–458, 2008.
7. Braithwait M, Philip J, Finlayson F, et al: Adverse events arising from a palliative care survey, *Palliat Med* 23:665–669, 2009.

39 Neurologic Diseases

JULIE HAUER | HELEN WELLS O'BRIEN

None of us is as smart as all of us. —Japanese proverb

It truly takes a village to meet the complex needs faced by children with neurologic conditions and their families. Front and center to this village are the parents and day-to-day care providers of such children, the ones who see the nuances of how a specific disease or condition manifests in an individual child. Medical teams bring expertise in the spectrum of problems seen in many children with similar conditions; parents often bring expertise in how these problems look in their child. Along with the medical needs of such children, families face myriad challenges that exist in the context of their hopes, fears, beliefs, values, the uncertainty of a their child's condition, and the community where they live. Table 39-1 is an introduction to the expertise available from palliative care and hospice teams to assist with the needs of such children and their families.

Pediatric Palliative Care and Neurologic Conditions

Pediatric palliative care teams are commonly consulted to see children who have diseases and impairments of the nervous system. Of children enrolled in a pediatric palliative care project, 44% were categorized with a primary neurologic condition (24% of those were deemed progressive neurologic, 20% were CNS damage) and 15% frequently have associated neurologic impairment (10% with congenital anomalies and 5% with metabolic).[1] Recent data for the Pediatric Advanced Care Team (PACT) at Children's Hospital Boston and Dana Farber Cancer Institute categorized 37% neurologic and 10% genetic or metabolic.[2] Unfortunately, little has been written about palliative care as it pertains to children with neurologic impairment (NI) and their families.

Families of such children face many challenges, including: lifelong conditions, living with hope and uncertainty, experiencing the sorrow of what is not possible along with the joy of small victories, difficulty in assessing and managing symptoms, and navigating through the care of many specialists. Palliative care teams are well suited to address the myriad psychosocial, spiritual, and physical needs experienced by these children and their families.

The personal challenges experienced by children and their families exist within the larger context of societal debates regarding medical decision making for such children. These discussions are guided and influenced by ethics, morality, religion, personal values, justice, resource usage, and quality of life. Case reports in the literature highlight the variability of this debate with examples of doing everything, possibly so as to not create the impression of discrimination based on disability[3] and not offering treatment out of an assumption of poor quality of life.[4] As society wrestles with these challenges, we must avoid bringing this debate to the bedside and instead be guided by legal and ethical knowledge while providing compassion and support.

Patient Population

There are a broad range of conditions with NI that benefit from pediatric palliative care.[5] The conditions may be:

- Static, such as hypoxic injury or structural malformations of the central nervous system,
- Progressive, including metabolic diseases and muscular dystrophies,
- Primary impairment of the nervous system, such as spinal muscular atrophy and in utero infections,
- Associated impairment, such as genetic and congenital syndromes,
- Involving the central nervous system, including metabolic diseases,
- Involving the lower motor neuron, such as muscular dystrophies, spinal muscular atrophy, and congenital myopathies.

Conditions and suggested timing of palliative care consultation are summarized in Table 39-2; assistance with symptom management can occur at any point in time.

UNIQUE EXPERIENCES AND CHALLENGES

There are a number of unique themes experienced by children with NI and their families, including the lifelong nature of such conditions, limitations in acquiring independence, bereavement that includes loss of the intensive care provider role, lack of evidence for medical decision making, and challenges with symptom management. Support from interdisciplinary teams includes anticipating and exploring how each area affects an individual child and family. This section focuses on the themes that cross psychosocial and spiritual areas of need.

Loss is a recurrent theme, starting from the time of diagnosis. This theme is often repeated when what the child cannot do and the ongoing problems that cannot be fixed are reviewed at medical appointments. This journey often includes chronic sorrow, a phrase used to describe sorrow over time in response to ongoing loss.[6] Examples may include loss of functional ability, loss of ability to meet nutritional and fluid needs through eating, and loss of health. Families are also simultaneously exploring meaning and hope in the context of their values, beliefs, relationships, and supportive networks. They may find

TABLE 39-1 Team Member Expertise

These individual areas of expertise are critical to managing the multidimensional needs encountered. Though an individual of an interdisciplinary team will bring in expertise in one of these areas of need, each member will bring skills in assisting with all areas.

Social workers

Provide emotional support to family, psychosocial assessment and supportive counseling in collaboration with other providers for families adjusting to palliative care issues, link to psychosocial and mental health resources in the local community, anticipate legal and financial needs including guardianship, government programs that cover some medical expenses, and special needs trust, and direct to appropriate resources

Child life specialists

Assist siblings with the fears of having a sister or brother with complex healthcare needs, assist families with memory making and legacy of the child, provide bereavement support, provide education around appropriate grief responses of children

Chaplains

Support faith traditions and spiritual values that promote healing and hope, support families as they face loss and grief, identify religious and cultural factors that can shape how a family faces illness and suffering, provide a supportive presence for sick children and their families, provide support and advice in learning how to respond to the suffering witnessed by medical care teams

Nurses

Assist with bedside assessment of pain and other distressing symptoms, work with families and other care providers to determine what specific features in a nonverbal child with NI indicate specific distressing symptoms such as pain and dyspnea, translate this information into a care plan that is translatable to other care providers, listen in real time during times of emotional and spiritual distress for families

Physicians and advance practice nurses

Expertise in symptom management, serve as mediators between the medical teams and families, assist with advanced directives by working with medical teams and families, assist with translating goals of care to how medical interventions can or cannot meet those goals, review autopsy, tissue and organ donation, and Brain and Tissue Bank with families

---

joy in little victories, outcomes that were not expected, as they navigate hope, meaning, loss, and uncertainty.

Loss of function often includes lifelong dependence on others for physical care and may include the same for decision making. Parents may have unspoken worries, such as what will happen if the child outlives his or her parents, and wonder how to factor this future worry into current decisions. As a child ages, questions of who will provide care, the location of this care, and who will make decisions for the child become relevant. Parents may worry about this child being a burden to another sibling while worrying about the quality of care at other facilities. For children living in facilities, such as medical foster homes, group homes, and long-term medical care facilities, another challenge is created when the legal decision maker is removed from the range of daily experiences, including suffering of the child. This can create conflicts when the child's care provider, with a set of values, beliefs, and direct experience with the child, may judge a decision differently than the recognized decision maker. Other conflicting interests that often go unrecognized include financial interests of care facilities and personal interests of care providers, even when the best care for the child is the goal.

The care needs of children with NI often dominates a parents' day, which may lead to limited emotional, spiritual, and physical reserves. This often leaves little energy to reflect and may result in decisions that are made during a time of crisis. The intensity of the care provider's role can naturally result in this role becoming a prominent part of a parents' identity. This may later impact bereavement when a parent experiences the loss of this role and loss of membership in parent support groups. In addition, being a long-term care provider can create a heightened sense of responsibility over outcome and loss of perspective over the intensive efforts being used to maintain the child's level of health.

In the context of these challenges are the themes of hope and joy. It is not uncommon to identify a family saying, "I wouldn't choose this, but I wouldn't have it any other way"

TABLE 39-2 Neurologic Conditions and Timing of Palliative Care Consults

Category	Conditions	Timing of consultation

Severe disability causing vulnerability to health complications and/or palliative after diagnosis	Indicated by developmental label
	  Cerebral palsy
	A result of an insult to the CNS
	  Hypoxic ischemic encephalopathy
	  In-utero infection with cytomegalovirus (CMV)
	  Anoxic encephalopathy
	Associated with a specific diagnosis
	  Genetic disorder
	  Congenital anomaly
	  Structural brain malformation,
	  Mitochondrial diseases
	  Metabolic disorders, inborn errors of metabolism
		Prenatal consultation for conditions identified during pregnancy
		Recurrent illness, hospitalizations, symptoms, or decline in health and function, such as respiratory exacerbations, feeding intolerance, recurrent or chronic irritability and/or pain
		Consideration of the following interventions: CPAP/BiPAP, tracheotomy, tracheal diversion, anti-reflux surgery for prevention of aspiration pneumonia, esophagogastric disconnection

Intensive long-term treatment aimed at maintaining the child's quality of life	Progressive respiratory failure Muscular dystrophy Spinal muscular atrophy (SMA)	At diagnosis (for conditions that progress early in life such as SMA type I) Consideration of gastrostomy feeding tube placement. This is an opportunity to identify goals of care that will then be relevant to future decision making such as use of mechanical ventilation Introduction of CPAP/BiPAP
Curative treatment intended but may fail	Metabolic diseases Leukodystrophies Mucopolysaccharidoses Other lysosomal storage disorders	Consideration of stem cell transplant Patients enrolling in clinical trials for new therapies such as enzyme replacement

as they share the lessons learned through their child and the important role of this child in their family. Such families often experience simultaneous joy and sorrow that allows us to worry and celebrate with them as we join them and assist them on their journey.

Pediatric palliative care teams provide expertise through knowledge of themes that are universal to all children with life-threatening conditions, along with experience of themes that are unique to certain populations. This expertise allows teams to explore supportive approaches to healing and hope, meaning and values, relationships and connections, and grief and loss. Resiliency is an essential component of this process when a child and family live with a condition that is both lifelong, often experienced over years, and will result in an early death.

> *Leo is a 6-year-old boy with cerebral palsy and intellectual impairment as a result of hypoxic-ischemic encephalopathy. He is nonverbal and nonambulatory, and receives fluid and nutrition by a gastrostomy feeding tube. Associated problems include neuromuscular scoliosis and recurrent pulmonary illnesses. He has experienced an increased frequency of respiratory exacerbations during the past 6 months with two recent hospitalizations. His daily chronic treatment includes: nebulizer treatments with a daily inhaled steroid, and albuterol and atrovent as needed; chest physiotherapy and vest for bronchial drainage; and supplemental home oxygen as needed. He is cared for lovingly by his adoptive parents and his devoted home care nurses. They have always anticipated that Leo would not live into adulthood. They celebrate their time together and describe Leo as a boy who enjoys cuddling, music, being around his siblings and being part of family activities.*

What to Expect: Life Expectancy Literature

Life expectancy data for children with NI, whether that data is related to the disability label, such as cerebral palsy, or related to a specific diagnosis that explains the disability, such as a genetic disorder, congenital syndrome, or metabolic disorder, provides a context but is of limited use for individual prognosis. Health problems that are life threatening can be divided into those related to the severity of the motor disability regardless of the cause, such as oral motor dysfunction and recurrent pulmonary aspiration, or related to the specific diagnosis that explains the disability, such as a genetic disorder with an associated cardiac defect or central apnea.

Information about life expectancy demonstrates a wide variation. The more severe the motor disability, such as the inability to lift the head up when prone, the more likely the child will not survive to adulthood.[7-12] Survival for individuals with CP that includes severe impairment in cognitive function, motor ability, vision and hearing was 50% at 13 years and 25% at 30 years.[9] It is beneficial to understand that CP is not a diagnosis but a developmental label indicating impairment of motor control as a result of non-progressive impairment of the central nervous system acquired at an early age. Information and experience from CP is relevant to any disease that results in severe motor impairment.

Even progressive diseases where decline occurs early in life, such as Tay-Sachs disease, often have a range of survival that may vary by several years. Prognostic information for specific diagnoses often lags the expanded survival from routine pulmonary management that assists with mobilization of secretions and treatment of acute respiratory illnesses. Worry over prognosis is further heightened when there is identification of neurologic impairment with no diagnosis. As palliative care clinicians we can assist through knowledge of the limitations of information that may be provided to families, use our knowledge and experience from all disorders with NI, and help anticipate and prepare for future events.

Framework for Approaching Prognosis, Uncertainty, and Decision Making

Literature and experience demonstrates a wide range in life expectancy, yet has provided limited information on how families approach this uncertainty. Studies[13,14] of the experience of families with children dying from neurodegenerative conditions identify how they navigate uncharted territory and use strategies such as seeking and sharing information, focusing on the child, reframing the experience, and promoting the child's health. Factors influencing parental decisions to limit or discontinue medical interventions include perception of their child's suffering, likelihood of improvement, perception of their child's will to survive, quality of life, previous experience with end-of-life decision making for others, and financial resources.[15,16]

ILLNESS TRAJECTORY AS A GUIDE TO DECISION MAKING

Adult literature describes illness trajectories for cancer, organ failure, and frailty.[17,18] Using the latter two trajectories and experience, Fig. 39-1 provides a hypothetical framework for reflecting on and anticipating the trajectory of a child with NI. The figure is intended to guide families through decision making by using a reflection on the past benefit of interventions to anticipating the probable and possible future benefit by hoping for the best, preparing for the worst.[19]

The hypothetical disease trajectory highlights that many health issues in children with NI progress gradually with initial benefit and return to health and functional baseline with treatment available. Over time, less return to baseline will occur from the interventions available, reflecting the inability to fix the problems that are secondary to the permanent NI. Predicting outcome at the beginning of the trajectory before any decline in health status is seen can result in pressure of past success[20] when the outcome is better than predicted. Asking a parent of a child with NI to make a decision to limit interventions before the child has had any significant decline in health may feel as if the emphasis is on limiting interventions because of the disability. By identifying associated health problems, monitoring for changes in health status, and noting any decreased benefit from treatments, we can identify individuals with NI who are at risk for life-threatening events.

Anticipating benefit also requires knowledge of how offered interventions will alter the clinical course. Some of the more common interventions for children with severe NI include anti-reflux surgery, tracheotomy, and spinal surgery. Most of the information in the literature is case reports or small series

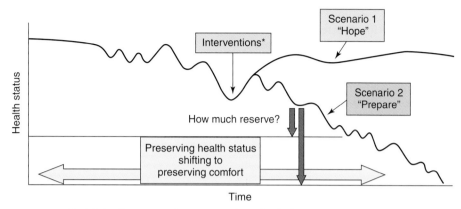

Fig. 39-1   Prognosis and uncertainty—hope for the best, prepare for the rest.

without rigorous evidence to indicate which patient is likely to experience benefit, morbidity greater than the intended benefit, or no alteration in the clinical course. In addition, these interventions are often approached as needed and required for the problems identified, rather than interventions to offer and consider. Fortunately, relevant information can be gained from the literature; a summary of information for these interventions is provided later in this chapter.

Support for the process of decision making is best done through a reflection of the child's history in the context of emotional and spiritual needs that impact this process. Outlined are questions to consider and review with parents and care providers. It is helpful to acknowledge that some may be difficult to answer but help frame what parents are often already worrying about and considering. Such discussions should include opportunities to reflect on the successes and experiences that are enjoyed by the child. In addition, a comprehensive review of emotional coping, sources of stress, spiritual beliefs, and support networks, as examples, should be sought.

Starting the conversation:

- Please share with us what the past few months or years have been like and what you understand about your child's health status.
- What are you worrying about?
- What are you anticipating?
- What are your hopes for your child?
- What do you consider most important for your child as your consider decisions?

Reflective questions with parents and care providers:

- How does a typical day for your child look now compared to the start of these problems and/or symptoms?
- When did you first start worrying about these problems and/or symptoms?
- How does your child's health compare this month to the start of these problems?
- Where would you estimate your child's health baseline to be now compared with 2 years ago?
- Is your child's health baseline 75%, 50%, or less than 50% of where it was? Has your child's health declined by 25%, 50%, or more than 50%?
- How often in a month is your child sick now compared to 12 months ago? Has illness been increasing in frequency?

- What percentage of time in a typical week would you estimate that your child enjoys now compared to 12 months ago? Has this declined over time?
- Are you seeing less benefit from chronic and acute treatments over time with less return to prior baseline, longer duration with each illness, or a shorter time between each illness?
- How much reserve do you estimate for your child?
- Do you worry that your child is suffering?
- What percentage of each day or week is there suffering?

Here are some further questions for families and medical teams after goals have been identified and the child's health trajectory has been reviewed:

- What is the likelihood of the identified interventions bringing an improvement or recovery of the current health and functional baseline? To meeting the goals identified such as improving comfort and quality of life? To prolonging the suffering identified?
- How will the course look with or without the treatment available?
- Are there treatment strategies for the symptoms that are causing distress?

ADVANCE CARE PLANNING: HOW TO HOPE AND PREPARE

Areas of need as a result of slow decline include planning for future problems, avoiding interventions of limited benefit, and assistance for long-term caregivers.[21] A goal is to facilitate planning by giving physicians permission to discuss what-if scenarios while giving parents permission to maintain hope. Palliative care can assist with this process by exploring psychosocial, spiritual, and physical needs that impact on decisions, such as the worry of giving up, a sense of needing to do something, and the fear that treating physical suffering will result in an early death. Given the inherent challenge of determining when goals shift from preserving health status to preserving comfort, medical, and palliative care are ideally integrated together for children with NI.[22,23] Through this process of exploration with families and by integrating symptom-directed treatment into medical care plans, we can minimize the impression of choosing treatment that preserves life vs. comfort care that means giving up.

As palliative care teams attend to spiritual and emotional needs of patients and families, this ideally creates a healthy space for this reflective and anticipatory work. As parents encounter decisions for interventions in children with NI, it is helpful to acknowledge the range of decisions made by families. This naturally creates distress for both parents and medical teams; why is this decision, whether to do or not to do, acceptable when other families would choose differently? Palliative care teams can assist through identification of the details relevant to each family and communication of information to medical teams. Suggestions for follow-up include:

- Define with the family the goals that will guide decisions: A decrease in distressing symptoms? A health improvement? Maintenance of health to a specific event?
- Assess the likelihood of an intervention meeting these goals.
- Know the evidence for the possible benefit and harm for the interventions available.
- Define a time period in which the intervention would be expected to meet a goal.
- Anticipate and discuss if the hoped-for benefit does not occur in this time period, if the benefit is later lost, or if increased suffering occurs. This allows end points to be anticipated before a crisis.

Resuscitation is another important part of advance care planning. Discussing resuscitation requires an honest assessment of the likelihood of benefit and possible burden. It is important that we assume responsibility for this assessment and provide directive guidance so as to not imply parental responsibility for such decisions. Many hospital-based resuscitation order forms now include advance care planning for other medical interventions. This can serve as a prompt to review interventions beyond intubation and cardiac resuscitation. Ideally, these discussions take place grounded by extensive knowledge of the child and family that then allows a comprehensive integration of spiritual, psychosocial, and medical details into care plans.

Several details about resuscitation are important for children with NI:

- Children who are nonambulatory throughout life have a high incidence of osteoporosis, resulting in a high risk that chest compressions could cause fractures.
- Many children with NI, excluding such conditions as Duchenne muscular dystrophy (DMD) with associated cardiomyopathy and congenital syndromes with associated cardiac defects, experience cardiac failure as a result of respiratory failure; focusing decisions on the primary life-threatening event will guide subsequent decisions about cardiac interventions. That includes informing families that there would be no benefit to cardiac interventions when a patient is not intubated, thus eliminating the need for parents to make unnecessary decisions.
- Bagging can become a chronic intervention by default; if it is being considered when intubation will not be used it can be useful to review its historic use as a bridge to intubation.
- Some hospital forms include interventions beyond intubation, such as suctioning, nasal or oral airway, oxygen, and continuous positive end expiratory pressure (CPAP) and/or biphasic positive airway pressure (BiPAP). It is helpful to guide parents to care plans that fit with the child's current use of oxygen and suctioning; and it can

be helpful to discuss the benefit and burden of CPAP and/or BiPAP in a similar manner to intubation, that is, the difference between acute and chronic use.

This is also a time to review that a decline in health is not a result of the care provided at home or a result of decisions made. Rather, it reflects the health problems that cannot be cured or fixed, while providing reassurance that interventions will be used for as long as the parents identify them as meeting goals. Several articles provide further beneficial communication strategies.[24,25]

Leo was admitted to the hospital with another respiratory exacerbation. Soon after admission, he was intubated and identified to have respiratory syncytial virus (RSV). A palliative care consultation was obtained 1 week later. Information identified included an overall decline in health, along with diminishing benefit from chronic treatments and use of antibiotics and steroids during acute exacerbations. Prior evaluation included sleep study negative for obstructive apnea but persistent oxygen desaturation to the mid 80s, a normal upper gastrostomy series (UGI), normal inflammatory markers, and decreased lung volumes noted on chest x-ray. A team meeting was arranged to include Leo's primary physician, pulmonologist, the intensive care physician, as well as the chaplain, social worker, child life specialist, and physician of the pediatric palliative care team. Leo's primary physician wants to give hope to the family by identifying the problem as RSV. Questions identified to facilitate discussion include: Is the prolonged course of ventilation more a result of RSV or chronic changes to the lungs? Would a tracheotomy help? What timeline would be expected to allow recovery to extubation, if this is possible? How much enjoyment or suffering is Leo experiencing between illnesses? Discussion identified that a child of this age would not be expected to require mechanical ventilation from RSV. The RSV was a trigger but the decline to respiratory failure indicates significant lung damage that is likely not reversible. A tracheotomy would not help but would be used if chronic ventilation was used. A timeline of 1 to 1½ weeks was identified as sufficient for recovery.

During this meeting, family and care providers identified goals of comfort, quality of life, and the opportunity to remain home where he is most comfortable. Family and home care nurses continue to hope for recovery and as much time as possible with Leo. They do not anticipate using surgical interventions but need time to consider the options available. A follow-up team meeting is arranged for 1 week later, recognizing that the decisions will depend on whether recovery to extubation occurs.

Documenting, Communicating, and Coordinating Plans of Care

Great care is possible only when information is identified, documented, and communicated to those involved in the child's care. This can ensure that previously defined care plans are carried out, which protects the child from interventions that are anticipated to cause potential harm without long-term benefit. It can be beneficial to others to summarize why certain interventions have been limited. This can lessen a sense of giving up and help direct those involved with the child to what we can do; that there is always care to provide.

Information to consider documenting includes: goals of care and how these goals guide decisions, heathcare and symptom management plans that meet these goals, naming the legal decision maker, the location for acute illness, resuscitation status, care plans for home and school in the event of a life-threatening event, and contact information for individuals with expertise and availability to assist at times of acute events. Those who should receive this information include the family, healthcare proxy or legal decision maker, home care nurses, providers of care in foster care or group homes, school nurses and teachers, respite care providers, bus drivers, healthcare team members, and palliative care and/or hospice teams.

CARE IN THE SCHOOL

Children with NI routinely attend school as assured by the Individuals with Disabilities Education Act (IDEA). Along with educational and socialization opportunities, this has meant that school systems may have children with chronic healthcare needs. For children with a significant compromise to baseline health, this creates the challenge of determining what interventions and monitoring is possible in the school. For children in the community with Do Not Attempt Resuscitation (DNAR) or Allow Natural Death orders, it is necessary to determine state requirements and school policy. This includes meeting with school nurses, teachers, and administrators to develop a plan of care in the event of a life-threatening event. Members of the palliative care team, such as social workers and child life specialists, can work with school systems to assist with the needs of the other children in the classroom. This may involve preparing students prior to a child's return to school if changes have occurred, or assisting following the death of a child.

PRACTICAL CONSIDERATIONS: GUARDIANSHIP AND LONG-TERM FINANCIAL PLANS

Financial issues are a practical concern for families of children with NI. This may be a result of reduced work hours or discontinuing work to stay home and provide care for their child. In addition, overall expenses are often greater for families of children with chronic health care needs. Many families will benefit from assistance with the legal and financial areas of special-needs trusts and guardianship. Government programs can cover some basic medical needs, but for families creating a fund in their child's name for long-term needs, the child will lose eligibility if there is more than $2000 in assets. A special-needs trust is the process that provides financial protection of assets for lifetime care needs and preserves eligibility for Medicaid, Social Security income, and other need-based benefit programs for those with disabilities. For any individual older than 18 years of age unable to participate in decision-making, legal guardianship is the court process of documenting the legal decision maker.

Symptom Management

Children with NI experience pain more frequently than the general pediatric population.[26–29] Caregivers of children with severe cognitive impairment reported 44% experiencing pain

each week over a 4-week interval. Pain frequency was higher in the most impaired group of children.[27] In a study of nonverbal cognitively impaired children, caregivers reported that 62% experienced five or more separate days of pain and 24% experienced pain almost daily.[29] In addition, children with severe-to-profound cognitive impairment were found to have elevated pain scores at baseline on two pain assessment scales.[30]

Other distressing symptoms commonly encountered in children with NI include:[31–33]

* Neurologic, such as spasticity, seizures, and autonomic dysfunction,
* Gastrointestinal, such as vomiting, retching, constipation, and feeding intolerance,
* Respiratory, such as secretions and dyspnea.

In addition, depression and anxiety may be experienced at an increased rate by children with a muscular dystrophy (MD) such as Duchenne MD.[34] Unfortunately, few studies have explored symptom management in children with NI both during life and at the end of life.

GENERAL APPROACH

This section will outline management of distressing symptoms for children with NI (Fig. 39-2). This allows the healthcare provider to consider interventions that may benefit several problems. This can be helpful because it is not always possible to determine which symptoms or problems are the primary source of distress and which ones are the secondary manifestations in these children. Is the nonverbal neurologically impaired child irritable and in distress because of spasticity or is the spasticity secondary to underlying pain? Are the signs and symptoms of dysautonomia caused by pain, mimic the appearance of pain, or do the associated problems of dysautonomia contribute to pain? Given these challenges, it is helpful to focus on all potential sources of distressing symptoms, including neuropathy. The focus of this section will be on nonverbal children with NI given the inherent challenge with this group.

There is regional and international variation in medication selection for the variety of problems and distressing symptoms encountered. Medications provided in the tables indicate mechanisms of action so that medications with similar properties available in different countries can be identified.

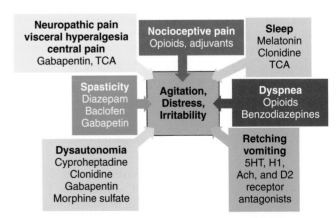

Fig. 39-2 Multidimensional symptom assessment and management. (These symptoms are sources of agitation, distress, and irritability in neurologically impaired children.)

ASSESSMENT

The options for assessing presence and severity of pain include self-report, observational assessment of behaviors in nonverbal children, and assessment of physiological markers. Knowledge of the child's cognitive level allows selection of a validated pain rating tool appropriate for the level of intellectual function such as The Poker Chip tool, the Oucher,[35] and the Wong-Baker FACES pain rating scale[36] for children at a cognitive level of 5 to 6 years.

Observational tools are available for individuals unable to report pain. Specific distress behaviors have been associated with pain and are very helpful in quantifying and monitoring pain in children unable to provide self-report. The reliability and validity of behavioral observations are highest when the pain is acute in nature, such as that associated with medical procedures. Behavioral measurement must be assessed in the context of sources of distress because it may be difficult to distinguish between pain behaviors and those resulting from other types of distress, such as hunger. Observational tools rely on assessing the following items:

- Vocalizations, such as crying and moaning
- Facial expression, including grimacing
- Consolability
- Interactivity, such as being withdrawn
- Mood
- Eating and sleeping
- Protective actions, such as guarding part of the body
- Movement
- Tone and posture, such as arching and stiffening
- Physiological measures

Studies of physiologic measures including vital signs, diaphoresis, and hormone levels such as cortisol have predominantly focused on the pain associated with invasive and surgical procedures. None has proved to be reliable, sensitive, and specific for chronic pain. In addition, such measures may be altered by autonomic dysfunction in children with NI. Physiologic measures may have a role in monitoring pain when used to supplement more reliable information.

Assessment Tools Observational pain assessment tools assist with identifying the presence of pain and monitoring improvement in pain when an intervention is introduced. (Box 39-1).[37-49] In a comparison of the revised-Face, Legs, Activity, Cry, Consolability (r-FLACC) tool, the Non-Communicating Children's Pain Checklist-Postoperative Version (NCCPC-PV), and the Nursing Assessment of Pain Intensity (NAPI), the r-FLACC and NAPI were identified as having a higher overall clinical utility based on complexity, compatibility, and relative advantage.[37] The r-FLACC was the tool most preferred by clinicians in terms of pragmatic qualities.

EVALUATION

This section discusses the sources of pain in neurologically impaired children.

Nocioceptive: Tissue Injury and Inflammation Commonly recognized pain sources in children with NI include acute sources, such as fracture, urinary tract infection, or pancreatitis;[51] and chronic sources, such as gastroesophageal reflex (GER), constipation, feeding difficulties from delayed gut motility, positioning, spasticity, hip pain, or dental pain. (Box 39-2).

BOX 39-1 Pain Assessment Tools for Non-Verbal Neurologically Impaired Children

Face, Legs, Activity, Cry, Consolability (FLACC)[39]
The FLACC tool was revised (r-FLACC) to include behaviors specific to children with cognitive impairment

The Non-Communicating Children's Pain Checklist-Revised (NCCPC-R)[40,41]
30-item standardized pain assessment tool for children with severe cognitive impairment.
Validated to be related to pain intensity ratings provided by caregivers, consistent over time, sensitive and specific to pain, and effective for different levels of cognitive impairment.
Score of 7/90 or above provided 0.84 sensitivity and 0.77 specificity for classifying moderate-severe pain

Paediatric Pain Profile (PPP)[42,43]
20-item behavior-rating scale designed to assess pain in children with severe to profound cognitive impairment
Sensitivity (1.0) and specificity (0.91) optimized at a cut-off of 14/60
Available to download from the web following registration at www.pppprofile.org.uk.

The Individualized Numeric Rating Scale (INRS)[44]
Incorporates parents' knowledge of their cognitively impaired child's pain expression. Parents score severity of pain behaviors using the categories of the FLACC tool based on previous painful experiences

Doloplus-2[49]
An observational pain assessment tool for chronic pain in adults with cognitive impairment

---

Neuropathic: Peripheral Neuropathy and Central Pain
Neuropathic pain conditions are those associated with injury, dysfunction, or altered excitability of portions of the peripheral, central, or autonomic nervous system. It can be caused by compression, transection, infiltration, ischemia, or metabolic injury. Common features of neuropathic pain conditions include: descriptors such as burning, shooting, electric, or tingling; motor findings of spasms, dystonia, and tremor; and autonomic disturbances of erythema, mottling, and increased sweating.[50]

BOX 39-2 Etiology of Pain/Irritability in Nonverbal Neurologically Impaired Children

Head, Eyes, Ears, Nose, Throat (HEENT)
Acute otitis media, pharyngitis, sinusitis, dental abscess and/or gingival inflammation, corneal abrasion, glaucoma, ventriculoperitoneal shunt malfunction
Chest
Pulmonary aspiration and/or pneumonia, esophagitis
Abdomen
Gastrointestinal: gastroesophageal reflux disease, gastritis and/or gastric ulcer, peptic ulcer disease, food allergy, appendicitis, intussusception, constipation, delayed and/or impaired motility, rectal fissure, visceral hyperalgesia
Liver and/or gallbladder: hepatitis, cholecystitis
Pancreas: Pancreatitis
Renal: urinary tract infection, nephrolithiasis, neuropathic bladder, obstructive uropathy
Genitourinary: inguinal hernia, testicular torsion, ovarian torsion and/or cyst, menstrual cramps
Skin
Pressure sore and/or decubitus ulcer
Extremities
Fracture, hip subluxation, osteomyelitis, hair tourniquet
Psychosocial
Loss of caregiver, change in home environment, non-accidental trauma
General
Medication toxicity, sleep disturbance

There are many reasons to consider neuropathic pain in children with NI. Experience shows that a nocioceptive pain source may not be identified or pain may continue despite treatment of an identified source. "Screaming of unknown origin" was used to describe children with neurologic disorders, severe developmental delay, neurodegeneration, or severe motor impairments with persistent agitation, distress, or screaming, acknowledging that evaluation often does not identify a specific nociceptive cause.[52] Pain in children with NI is typically thought to be nociceptive in origin; however, after repeated injury or surgery, neuropathic pain may also occur.[53] In one case series, 6 children with cerebral palsy developed neuropathic pain following multilevel orthopedic surgery.[54] Onset of symptoms ranged from 5 to 9 days. Interventions included gabapentin in 4 children, amitriptyline in 2, and transcutaneous electrical nerve stimulation for 5, with improvement in symptoms over variable periods of time. Although not reported, experience in nonverbal children with NI identifies development of crying spells increasing in intensity weeks to months following major surgery, such as for neuromuscular scoliosis. Medications used for neuropathic pain include opioids, tricyclic antidepressants such as nortriptyline and amitriptyline, and anticonvulsants such as gabapentin, pregabalin, carbamazepine, phenytoin, valproic acid, and lamotrigine.[50]

Visceral Hyperalgesia The gastrointestinal tract is commonly identified by parents as a source of pain in neurologically impaired children. It has been identified as the most frequent source of all episodes of pain in children with severe cognitive impairment.[27,55] Pain of unknown cause was the most intense, followed by pain attributed to the bowels, gastrointestinal tract, and digestive pain. In children with NI, significantly higher rates of pain were reported in those with a gastrostomy tube and those taking medications for feeding, gastroesophageal reflux, or gastrointestinal motility.[28] This association between pain and gastrointestinal symptoms led to the hypothesis that some children with NI experience visceral hyperalgesia that benefits from gabapentin.[56] This potential source of pain is reviewed in more detail in the section on retching and vomiting.

Central Pain Central pain, also referred to as *thalamic pain syndrome*, is a recognized source of pain in adults with insults to the central nervous system such as from multiple sclerosis or following a cerebral vascular accident. Adults describe pain symptoms as burning, aching, throbbing, and the sensation of pins and needles. Associated symptoms include visceral pain, such as an exaggerated sensation of painful fullness from bladder and visceral distention. Symptoms are often poorly localized and constant as well as mixed with brief bursts of intense pain. The mechanisms that result in central pain appear similar but are not identical to peripheral neuropathic pain. Interventions with reported benefit include nortriptyline, gabapentin, lamotrigine, with lack of benefit from carbamazepine.[57,58] Central pain as a source of pain has not been described in children, though is likely a source for consideration in children with NI.

Given the inability to separate these pain syndromes in nonverbal children with NI, the term neuropathy will be used at times to indicate pain as a result of an impaired nervous system. Fortunately, our knowledge of treatment options is similar for each category.

MANAGEMENT

This section outlines management strategies for pain and other common symptoms encountered in neurologically impaired children. Some symptoms are a result of the underlying impairment of the nervous system, may indicate a medical problem to treat, often benefit from interventions that target symptoms, and may be exacerbated by pain. Finally, symptoms such as vomiting and feeding intolerance that persist despite comprehensive evaluation, management of contributing problems, and use of symptom management strategies, may be informing us of an irreversible decline in the child's overall neurological function and health status.

General Approach to Management of Distressing Symptoms in Nonverbal Children with NI

- Center decision making around goals of care
- Assess for the symptom causing distress
- Assess for severity using parental input and assessment tools, if available for the symptom, that are appropriate for the child's age and intellectual level
- Evaluate for potential causes of each symptom
- Treat identified causes when possible and if consistent with goals of care
- Use available symptom management interventions
- Review any prior experience with sedating medications to guide initial dosage selection
- Assess for improvement using appropriate pain assessment tools and parental reporting. Quantitative data is beneficial but assessment tools are not available for all symptoms. It is helpful to not become overly dependent on numbers; practical approaches are outlined.
  - Have the features, such as crying, facial grimacing, spasms, arching, and stiffening, changed to indicate the symptom improved? Has the severity of the symptom improved?
  - Has the frequency and duration of the symptom decreased?
  - How much improvement in the severity or decrease in the frequency and duration would you estimate: is your child 25% improved, 50% improved, greater than 50% improved?
- Follow-up process: Identify the timeline in which an intervention is expected to provided improvement
- Depends on when peak effect is expected and need to titrate medication:
  hours-days: opioid, sucralfate
  1-2 weeks: Proton pump inhibitor (PPI), cyproheptadine
  2-4 weeks: gabapentin, TCA
- Depends on frequency of symptom
  - Shorter trial if symptom occurs daily
  - Longer trial if symptom occurs in a cycle such as several days every other week
- If there is limited to no benefit in that time, then determine if the intervention will be continued or discontinued before initiating other interventions
- If an intervention is discontinued, determine if it requires a titration phase before stopping

Good pain management starts with an assessment for treatable sources of pain, such as urinary tract infection, gastroesophageal reflux, and pancreatitis. For chronic sources of nociceptive pain, such as hip subluxation, pain management is guided by the principles of the World Health Organization (WHO) analgesic ladder.[52,59–61]

In addition to assessment for nociceptive sources of pain, neuropathy should be considered for the reasons previously discussed. For persistent distress that suggests pain, nonverbal children with NI often benefit from a medication trial that targets pain syndromes such as neuropathic pain, visceral hyperalgesia, or central pain. Medications best studied for these sources of nerve pain include gabapentin and tricyclic antidepressants (TCAs) (Table 39-3). There are reasons to start with gabapentin, including a good safety profile and no interactions with other drugs. Gabapentin has been found to be safe in children at doses up to 78 mg/kg/day.[62] Pharmacokinetics indicate that children under 5 years of age require the highest doses.[63] Gabapentin is readily available in an oral solution. Pregabalin is an alternative option known to have higher oral bioavailability compared to gabapentin (90% vs. 33% to 66 %) with a linear increase in plasma concentration with increasing doses compared with gabapentin's decreasing bioavailability at higher doses. At this time there is no data to indicate that this results in a greater clinical benefit for children.

NONPHARMACOLOGIC MANAGEMENT

A critical part of symptom management in children with NI is nonpharmacologic pain management. Parents often become very adept at identifying and sharing tricks through parental support groups. One key area is assistance with identifying supportive equipment that minimizes positional pain. This can include seating systems and supportive pillows. Use of a pool is often found to be very relaxing for such children. Cuddling and physical therapy are commonly used. Although massage

has not been studied in this population, many families report significant benefit for their child. Other modalities for consideration include aromatherapy and acupuncture.

Spasticity

Spasticity is an involuntary, velocity-dependent, increase to muscle tone that results in resistance to movement. Spinal and cortical injury can alter inhibitory and excitatory messages to the motor neuron, resulting in spasticity. Spasticity may be mistaken for seizure activity but is typically not as rhythmic or symmetrical. Factors that can exacerbate spasticity include acute illness, discomfort such as from constipation, and pain. For this reason, neuropathy may be a poorly recognized contributing factor to spasticity in children with NI.

Treatment is intended to reduce the excessive muscle tone, with the goal of improving a patient's functional capacity and comfort. Various therapeutic interventions are available, including physical therapy, medications, and surgery. There are few randomized controlled trials of oral drugs, especially in children. There is weak evidence demonstrating the efficacy of medications such as benzodiazepines, baclofen, dantrolene, and α_2-adrenergic agonists of clonidine and tizanidine.[64,65] There have been only two trials comparing drugs, tizanidine vs. diazepam and tizanidine vs. baclofen, with no significant differences noted between medications in either trial.[66,67] Adverse drug reactions are common, and highest with dantrolene (64% to 91%).[64] Side effects commonly seen with all medications include sedation, drowsiness, and muscle weakness. Side effects tend to be dose related and disappear when doses are reduced. In patients with multiple sclerosis, evidence identifies benefits of treating spasticity with gabapentin without experiencing sedation.[68] This may indicate benefit to children with demyelinating or other neurodegenerative conditions but warrants further study.

Typically, children with NI referred to palliative care are commonly on one of these medications or have an intrathecal baclofen pump. The role of palliative care clinicians can be to search for factors that can exacerbate spasticity, such as pain, and offer therapeutic symptom management trials, rather than increasing or adding other interventions for spasticity.

Autonomic Dysfunction

Autonomic dysfunction, also called *dysautonomia*, is common in children with NI. Other terms used include autonomic storm, sympathetic storm, paroxysmal sympathetic hyperactivity, and paroxysmal autonomic instability with dystonia. In children with NI, dysautonomia typically reflects hypothalamic impairment. Autonomic dysreflexia is used most commonly to describe autonomic dysfunction seen in patients with spinal cord injury above the splanchnic sympathetic outflow, which is at or above T6, though T6-T10 may be susceptible.

The autonomic nervous system regulates body temperature, respiratory rate, heart rate, blood pressure, intestinal motility, urination, salivation, perspiration, and pupillary size. Symptoms that are more commonly seen in children with NI and associated dysautonomia include: tachycardia or bradycardia; hypertension; hyperthermia, or hypothermia; skin changes including pallor, flushing and redness of the face, and/or body; vomiting, retching, bowel dysmotility, and constipation; urinary retention; abnormal sweating; increased salivation; posturing; and agitation.

TABLE 39-3   Medications for Neuropathy and Central Pain

Gabapentin	Day 1-3: 5 mg/kg/dose PO qhs (maximum 250 mg)
	Day 4-6: 2.5 mg/kg/dose am and midday and 5 mg/kg qhs
	Day 7-9: 2.5 mg/kg/dose am and midday and 10 mg/kg qhs
	Day 10-12: 5 mg/kg/dose am and midday and 10 mg/kg qhs
	Increase every fourth day by 5 mg/kg/day until:
	1) effective analgesia occurs titrating to minimum total dose of 30-40 mg/kg/day for children >5 years of age and 40-60 mg/kg/day for children <5 years
	2) side effects experienced
	3) total dose of 75 mg/kg/day is reached (maximum of 3600 mg/day)
	4) give half of the total daily dose as the evening dose
	5) titrate more rapidly for severe pain
Nortriptyline	Day 1-4: 0.2 mg/kg PO qhs
	Day 5-8: 0.4 mg/kg PO qhs
	Increase every fifth day by 0.2 mg/kg/day until
	1) effective analgesia occurs
	2) dosing reaches 1 mg/kg/day (maximum of 50 mg/day)
	3) consider measuring plasma concentration and ECG before further dose escalation beyond 1 mg/kg/day
	4) consider twice daily dosing with 25% in the am and 75% in the pm

Adapted from Hauer JM. Respiratory symptom management in a child with severe neurologic impairment. J Palliat Med. 2007; 10 (5): 1201-1207.

As with other symptoms, evaluation should include a search for factors that may exacerbate the features of dysautonomia, including a review of potential sources of pain. Treatment for dysautonomia in neurologically impaired children has been poorly studied. Treatment options include benzodiazepines, bromocriptine, clonidine, oral and intrathecal baclofen, beta agonists such as metoprolol, and morphine sulfate. Literature is limited to case reports, predominantly in patients with traumatic brain injury. In a review of case reports of hypothalamic dysfunction, cyproheptadine was identified to benefit 4 individuals, including minimizing or eliminating symptoms of temperature instability, diaphoresis, vomiting, and abdominal pain.[69] Other interventions used in patients in this review without benefit included antiepileptics, haloperidol, diazepam, and clonidine. A recent case series of 6 patients following traumatic brain injury identified improvement with gabapentin when symptoms of agitation, dysautonomia, and spasticity persisted despite treatment with bromocriptine, clonidine, ITB pump, metoprolol, morphine, and benzodiazepine.[70] Finally, 13 out of 15 individuals with familial dysautonomia experienced a decrease in symptoms of nausea, retching, tachycardia, and flushing on pregabalin.[71] Most patients were already using clonidine and a benzodiazepine. In children with NI, a therapeutic trial for pain should be considered because it is difficult to determine when features of dysautonomia are indicating underlying pain. In addition to scheduled medications, children with intermittent autonomic storms, often manifested by an acute onset of facial flushing, sweating, tachycardia, retching, agitation, and stiffening, may benefit from use of clonidine, diazepam, and morphine sulfate as needed during these episodes.

Medication Toxicities

Although uncommon, the features of serotonin syndrome and neuroleptic malignant syndrome include autonomic dysfunction and can be a result of medications used in this population. Awareness and monitoring for changes from a child's baseline can alert us to these possible drug effects. Features of serotonin syndrome include tachycardia, hypertension, hyperthermia, diaphoresis, mydriasis, increased bowel sounds, hyperreflexia, clonus, agitation, and rigidity.[72] Drugs commonly implicated include selective serotonin reuptake inhibitors (SSRIs). Other drugs reported, often when used in combination, include: trazadone, fentanyl, tramadol, risperidone, ondansetron, metoclopramide, and valproate. Management includes removal of causative medications, use of cyproheptadine as a 5HT2 antagonist, and supportive care for other associated problems. Features of neuroleptic malignant syndrome are similar and include muscle rigidity, autonomic dysfunction, and altered mental status, most commonly caused by dopamine antagonists such as haloperidol. It has also been associated with tricyclic antidepressants and some anticonvulsants.[73]

Agitation and Delirium

Agitation is considered an unpleasant state of arousal. It may present as loud speech, crying, increased motor activity, increased autonomic arousal of diaphoresis or increased heart rate, inability to relax, or disturbed sleep-rest pattern. Symptoms in agitation overlap with anxiety though are noted to have more motor rather than psychological manifestations.

In contrast, delirium is a disturbance of consciousness with an acute onset over hours to days. Associated features include fluctuating course, disordered thinking, a change in cognition, inattention, altered sleep-wake cycle, perceptual disturbances, and psychomotor disturbances.[74,75] Causes include opioid or anticholinergic medications; metabolic disturbances of infection, dehydration, renal, liver, or electrolyte; pain; and impairment of vision or hearing.

Management of agitation and delirium involves evaluating for treatable medical causes, including medications, metabolic disturbances, and sources of discomfort such as pain, dyspnea, muscle spasms, position, and constipation. It is also helpful to consider conditions that mimic the appearance of agitation, such as akathisia from antidopaminergic medications, myoclonus, withdrawal from opioids, and paradoxical reactions. Medications that can help manage the symptoms include benzodiazepines and neuroleptics.

Seizures

Seizures are frequently identified in children with NI. Such children are typically followed by a pediatric neurologist. Palliative care physicians can assist them through knowledge of side effects with medications and the ketogenic diet such as risk of renal stones. Other events may masquerade as a seizure such as myoclonus, which is a brief, involuntary twitching of a muscle or a group of muscles, and episodes of arching or posturing. We can also assist by working with the child's neurologist to determine a plan for breakthrough seizures using rescue medications. This may include diazepam rectal gel, Diastat, or midazolam, which can be given sublingual and intranasal. There is increasing evidence that midazolam may be more effective than diazepam.[76–78] Finally, we can assist parents if they are experiencing changes in their child's health status occurring in conjunction with refractory epilepsy.

Abnormal Movements: Dystonia and Posturing

Dystonia is a movement disorder that causes the muscles to contract and spasm involuntarily resulting in twisting, repetitive movements and abnormal postures. Dystonia may be a primary disorder of movement, it may be secondary to diseases and insults that injure the central nervous system, or it may be a result of medications such as neuroleptics. Interventions include physical therapy, medications, and botulinum toxin for focal muscle groups. There have been few studies evaluating the effectiveness of medications for secondary dystonia. Those considered include benzodiazepines, baclofen, dopaminergic agents such as bromocriptine and levodopa (Sinemet), and anticholinergics such as trihexyphenidyl (Artane). Palliative care physicians can assist by assessing for distressing symptoms such as pain that can worsen the movement disorder.

Posturing is a term used to describe both findings of abnormal position, such as arching of the back, and clinical exam findings, such as decorticate, decerebrate, and opisthotonos. Lack of nomenclature, assessment tools, and the variability of neurologic impairment results in a variation of assessment, should the movement be labeled dystonia, posturing, or autonomic storm, and approaches to management, as evident by the large number of medications for consideration. Again, palliative care teams can assist by bringing a comprehensive approach to assessment including a thorough consideration of neuropathy as a source of symptoms.

In addition, clinical findings of posturing can be informative as pre-terminal signs of progressive injury to the central nervous system in children with neurodegenerative conditions, indicating loss of inhibitory control. These findings can include: decorticate posturing as indicated by rigid extension of the arms and legs, downward pointing of the toes, and backward arching of the head; decerebrate posturing with rigidity, flexion of the arms, clenched fists, and extended legs; and opisthotonos with rigidity and severe arching of the back, with the head thrown backward. These can also be intermittent findings in children with severe injury of the CNS.

Sleep Disturbance

Treating sources of distress will often improve sleep in children with NI. Pharmacologic treatments to consider include melatonin,[79,80] antidepressants such as tricyclic antidepressants and trazodone,[81–83] clonidine,[84] and antipsychotics, especially for patients with delirium.[85] When using melatonin for children with NI, some advocate that as the severity of disability increases, higher doses, occasionally even up to 15 mg, may be beneficial.[80] Benzodiazepines tend to be overused, leading to dependency and tolerance, and should only be used in a time-limited manner and discontinued or weaned following short-term use.[86] Nonpharmacologic interventions include a consistent bedtime and routine, quiet, a dark environment, and stimulus control.[85] When sleep problems are linked to symptoms such as pain or dyspnea, or correlated with an underlying problem such as obstructive apnea, treatment of the underlying condition may improve sleep.

Benzodiazpines

Common considerations in benzodiazepine use include spasticity, dystonia, dysautonomia, seizures, agitation, irritability, sleep, and dyspnea. They are generally safe and effective in the short term, although cognitive impairments and paradoxical effects such as behavioral disinhibition occasionally occur. Limitations of chronic use are a result of tolerance with a decrease of benzodiazepine-binding sites. This can be prevented by keeping dosages minimal, courses ideally less than four weeks, or intermittent use. Sudden cessation with long-term use can result in a withdrawal syndrome. Ideally, benzodiazepines are used intermittently, such as for a prolonged seizure or autonomic crisis, or as a bridge when other interventions are initiated, such as treating increasing spasticity that is potentially secondary to pain while waiting for titration up to a final dose of gabapentin or nortriptyline. Finally, a few case reports identify clonazepam as a useful adjuvant for neuropathic pain, though these reports are of short duration.

Methadone

Methadone is the only opioid with a prolonged effect that is available as a liquid, a beneficial option for children with NI. The main disadvantages are its biphasic elimination and effect of other medications on metabolism. The initial rapid distribution phase, with a half-life of 2 to 3 hours, followed by a slow elimination phase with a half-life of 4.2 to 130 hours, can result in drug accumulation and toxicity 2 to 5 days after starting or increasing methadone. For this reason, dose adjustments should not occur more often than every 72 hours. Potential drug interactions that may be relevant to children with NI include:

- Medications that decrease the effect of methadone, such as phenobarbital,
- Medications that increase effect of methadone, such as ciprofloxacin, diazepam, metronidazole, TCA, and erythromycin.

Methadone is a beneficial option for symptom management in children with NI. Given some of the complexity, there may be benefit in initiating other medication trials first, such as gabapentin, given its safety and no interactions with other drugs, if suboptimal benefit initiate nortriptyline next, with methadone used as a third-line symptom management intervention. Another reason for this order is the greater benefit with the combination of gabapentin and nortriptyline for neuropathic pain over either one given solely.[87]

Respiratory Health in Children with NI

Children with severe neurologic impairment have a high incidence of respiratory problems.[88] Recurrent respiratory illness leading to respiratory failure is the most common cause of mortality in children with severe cerebral palsy.[10,11] Aspiration is a frequent factor, identified in 31% to 68% of children with cerebral palsy.[89–91] Aspiration pneumonia in neurologically impaired children is best understood as an acute exacerbation resulting from chronic contributing factors. Those factors include:

- Diminished effectiveness of cough,
- Shallow breathing from inactivity and motor impairment,
- Impaired ability to manage routine oral secretions,
- Chronic aspiration of oral secretions resulting in a high enough inoculum of bacteria over time to overcome host defenses,
- Development of inflammation from aspiration of oral secretions,
- Development of mucous plugs with ventilation/perfusion ($\dot{V}/\dot{Q}$) mismatch.

In children with severe NI and recurrent respiratory illnesses, it is misleading to parents to label respiratory exacerbations as pneumonia or aspiration pneumonia because this can give the impression of a reversible problem. Instead, it can be helpful to acknowledge that the goal of chronic and acute treatment is to minimize the effect of these factors and maximize recovery and maintenance of health while we prepare for diminishing benefit.

Other factors that are considered to contribute to a decline in respiratory function include gastroesophageal reflux disease (GERD) and neuromuscular (NM) scoliosis. Evidence for the benefit of interventions is unfortunately limited, but includes:

- Although the improvement in life expectancy for the most medically fragile children with cerebral palsy is believed to be a result of gastrostomy feeding tubes,[92] there are no studies to guide which children benefit.[93] Gastrostomy feeding tubes have not been demonstrated to prevent aspiration pneumonia in adults with advanced dementia.[94]

- Anti-reflux surgery does not routinely alter respiratory symptoms or the frequency of pneumonia, though it is often offered for this purpose.[95–99] As outlined previously, other factors not altered by anti-reflux surgery contribute to respiratory problems. In addition, it can result in or worsen pre-existing retching, a distressing symptom seen in children with NI.[100]
- A review of the indications for tracheotomy identified a mortality of 27% in neurologically impaired patients compared with an 11% or less mortality for conditions of airway obstruction. The review found mortality from upper airway obstruction to be 11%, vocal fold paralysis 8%, and no deaths from craniofacial abnormality.[101] This likely reflects greater benefit for airway obstruction vs. less benefit for children with NI and respiratory compromise from multiple factors, an observation further supported by a recent retrospective review of outcomes following tracheotomy.[102]
- Salivary duct ligation decreases drooling but did not alter the frequency of pneumonia or respiratory symptoms in 62 children with chronic pulmonary aspiration.[103] A more recent study stated benefit but included only 12 children and had a shorter duration of follow-up.[104]
- The outcome following spinal surgery for neuromuscular scoliosis in 288 children with cerebral palsy was reviewed.[105] The average age at time of surgery was 13 years 11 months, with a standard deviation of 3 years 4 months. Mortality included three perioperative deaths, a mean survival of 4.3 years for the 33 other deaths, and a mean estimated survival of 11.2 years for all patients. Missing from this analysis was a stratification of patients based on pulmonary status before surgery and a review of anticipated survival without surgery so as to account for differences in children with multiple factors impacting respiratory health vs. children with restrictive lung disease with no other risk.

Dyspnea

Dyspnea is the experience of shortness of breath, difficulty breathing, or uncomfortable breathing. It is a common symptom of numerous medical disorders. Included are diseases of the lung parenchyma and obstruction of the airway, which can occur from repeated micro-aspiration with resulting infection, inflammation, bronchiectasis, and lung scarring over time.

Measures of respiratory rate, oxygen saturation, blood gas levels, and family perception do not necessarily correlate with the patient's perception of breathlessness. Instruments such as the Respiratory Distress Observational Scale (RDOS) are being evaluated for use in adults unable to report about dyspnea.[106] When assisting parents in assessing for dyspnea in a nonverbal child, strategies are similar to those used in pain assessment of such children. Assessment can include asking a parent if he or she has observed the child to be in distress or appear anxious during a respiratory exacerbation. Behaviors indicating distress may include facial expression, appearing restlessness, or becoming withdrawn. It can also be helpful to instruct parents and care providers to breathe along with the child for 1 minute as an indirect indicator of the child's effort of breathing.

Treating dyspnea is typically focused on identifying and aggressively treating the underlying cause. Evidence is established in adults for using interventions to alleviate dyspnea that persists despite maximum medical management of identified causes. These interventions include an oxygen trial, cool air from a fan or open window, repositioning, lorezepam for associated anxiety, and morphine sulfate. A recent review from the American College of Physicians identified strong evidence for treating adults with dyspnea from chronic lung disease with short-term opioids.[107,108] Evidence includes demonstration of significant improvement in refractory dyspnea in participants completing a randomized, double blind, placebo-controlled crossover study with no significant episodes of sedation.[109] Several studies have demonstrated the safety of using morphine sulfate for management of dyspnea that occurs despite maximum treatment of the underlying cause without development of respiratory depression.[110–112] A suggested starting dose for an opioid naive patient is 25% to 30% of the dose used for pain with a maximum starting dose of 5 mg orally. If the patient is already on an opioid, increase the dose by 30%.

As a decline in respiratory status occurs despite management of these contributing factors, respiratory distress during exacerbations is likely an under-recognized symptom in children with NI. Using evidence for managing dyspnea in adults, children deserve symptom management of respiratory distress incorporated into medical care plans (Table 39-4).[113] For example, the table identifies antibiotics that provide coverage of anaerobic bacteria along with other oral bacteria when treating children who chronically aspirate oral secretions.[114–118] Morphine sulfate is included in Table 39-4 to remind us to ask if there is distress during respiratory exacerbations and to include that information in care plans when distress is identified. This allows integration of symptom management into acute medical care plans in advance of seeing limited benefit from chronic and acute medical interventions. Overall, this will assist with future decisions by assuring that comfort is part of the care plan and avoid decisions to use interventions offered being made solely out of fear of suffering.

Leo was extubated 1 week later, before the next team meeting. The family had discussed what they would want for Leo when the next respiratory illness occurred. They believed they understood what medical interventions in the hospital could and could not do for Leo. A home care plan was outlined and hospice introduced to help assist with the family's goals of maintaining Leo's comfort and care at home. The home care plan included medical interventions to initiate during acute respiratory exacerbations, including several rotating antibiotics and a short course of prednisone. The goal was to use such acute interventions as long as they met the goal of improving Leo's respiratory health status during times of decline without resulting in complications. There was understanding that the benefit of these interventions would lessen over time as they do not eliminate the factors contributing to respiratory decline. The care plan also incorporated symptom management with morphine sulfate. A detailed review identified specific symptoms that indicate when Leo is in distress.

TABLE 39-4   Respiratory Home Management: Medical and Symptom Treatment Strategies

Chronic interventions	
Suctioning	As needed for comfort
Oxygen	Assessed by appearance of patient or by oximeter
Albuterol nebulizer	Every 3-4 hrs for coughing, wheezing, congestion
Ipratropium (Atrovent) nebulizer	Every 3-4 hrs for coughing, wheezing, congestion
Saline or Mucomyst nebulizer	As needed for thick secretions
Chest physiotherapy or vest	2 times/day, increase to 4 times/day with increased symptoms*
Nebulized budesonide (Pulmicort)	2 times/day, increase to 4 times/day with increased symptoms*
Salmeterol (Serevent)	Family history of allergies or benefit from daily albuterol
Acute interventions	
For respiratory exacerbations from chronic aspiration	
Clindamycin, Augmentin or Levofloxacin/Moxifloxacin†	10-14 days
Systemic steroids (prednisone)‡	5 days
Additional interventions	
For symptom management and end-of-life care	
Fan on face	Relieves sensation of breathlessness
Morphine sulfate	Use for respiratory distress§ Starting dose 0.1 mg/kg/dose PO/SL/Gtube (max 5 mg) May increase by 30% until comfortable
Glycopyrrolate (Robinul), scopalamine, hyoscyamine	May contribute to mucous plugging; Decreases oral and respiratory secretions in end-of-life care

Adapted from Hauer JM. Respiratory symptom management in a child with severe neurologic impairment. J Palliat Med 2007; 10(5):1201-1207. Table 39-1. Reprinted with permission from Journal of Palliative Medicine.
*Symptoms include increased coughing, secretions, congestion, respiratory rate and breathing effort.
†Use when respiratory symptoms persist or worsen despite an increase in chronic interventions.
‡Include with third or fourth exacerbation, sooner if symptoms return within two months of antibiotic course.
§Features suggesting respiratory distress include facial expression such as grimacing, appearing restlessness, having an anxious look, stiffening, tears, or becoming withdrawn.

During the next respiratory exacerbation, morphine sulfate was used along with the home treatment plan of an antibiotic and prednisone. Leo's care providers were pleased with how much more comfortable Leo appeared during this illness. They were relieved that they did not need to choose between treatment for medical benefit and treatment for comfort. They are more certain with their goals for Leo and feel prepared for the time when the home treatment plan may no longer benefit him, but are certain they can maintain his comfort throughout life with guidance in dose adjustment as needed.

For such reasons, we likely underuse morphine sulfate when managing respiratory distress, instead reserving its use

for comfort at the end of life. Integrating symptom management earlier can minimize interventions being pursued out of fear of the patient suffering without the intervention. There is a need to study the integration of morphine sulfate into the care plans of neurologically impaired children with recurrent respiratory exacerbations. Waiting until the goal is comfort care rather than treatment focused delays initiation of comfort strategies.

Secretions

Secretions occur for various reasons in children with NI. It is helpful to consider sialorrhea separately from thicker respiratory secretions. Sialorrhea involves thin, watery secretions that can pool out of the mouth as a result of diminished oral sensation of saliva. There is ample evidence of the benefit of medications such as glycopyrrolate and botox or surgical ligation of the salivary ducts in diminishing sialorrhea. In contrast, an increase in respiratory secretions in such children is likely due to multiple factors, including an increase in pulmonary secretions as a result of inflammation from aspiration of oral secretions and mucous that is difficult to mobilize. Management is directed at minimizing the development of such secretions through use of inhaled steroids and assistance with clearance through bronchial drainage techniques and devices such as the pulmonary vest and cough assist. Medications are available to decrease secretions but should be used with caution in this population because they can result in thicker secretions that are more difficult to mobilize. They may have a more beneficial role when comfort is the primary goal of care. Medications with anticholinergic properties that have been used for management of secretions at the end-of-life include scopolamine, hyoscyamine, and atropine, tertiary amines that may cause sedation and delirium as they cross the blood brain barrier. Glycopyrrolate is another option, which may be less sedating. No evidence exists indicating that one is more beneficial than another. Decreasing total fluid intake by 25% or more is another simple intervention to consider for management of excessive respiratory secretions.

Nausea, Retching, Vomiting, and Feeding Intolerance

Gastrointestinal symptoms are common in children with severe NI.[27–29] This includes pain localized to the gut as noted in the pain section. Vomiting in these children is commonly attributed to GERD.[119] Alternatively, stimulation of the emetic reflex is likely an under-reported source of symptoms in these patients.[100,120] Experience and limited evidence suggests the benefit of considering sources beyond GERD. Considerations include visceral hyperalgesia, activation of the emetic reflex, and dysautonomia (Table 39-5).

Tammy is a 9-year-old girl with cerebral palsy and cognitive impairment from an in-utero cerebral vascular accident. She presents with more than 1 year of feeding intolerance, manifested by vomiting and retching. She is receiving 70% of defined nutritional needs and 100% of fluid needs. Any increase in volume causes an increase in the amount of vomiting and retching. Evaluation has

TABLE 39-5 Medications for Retching, Vomiting, Feeding Intolerance in Children with NI

Activation of the emetic reflex		
Medication	**Receptor antagonist**	**Dose**
Ondansetron (Zofran)	5HT3	0.15 mg/kg PO/IV q 8 hr prn (maximum 8 mg)
Metoclopramide (Reglan)	D2—GI tract	0.1-0.2 mg/kg PO/IV q 6 hr (maximum 10 mg)
Haloperidol (Haldol)	D2—CTZ, H1 & Ach	0.01-0.02 mg/kg PO q 8 hr prn (maximum 1 mg)
Promethazine (Phenergan)	H1 & Ach (weak D2)	0.25-0.5 mg/kg PO/IV q 4 hr prn (maximum 25 mg)
Diphenhydramine (Benedryl)	H1	0.5-1 mg/kg PO/IV q 6 hr prn (maximum 50 mg)
Cyproheptadine (Periactin)	5HT2, H1 & Ach	0.08 mg/kg PO q 8 hr (maximum 4 mg) If no improvement within 3-5 days, increase each dose by 0.04-0.08 mg/kg
Scopolamine Hyoscyamine (Levsin)	Ach	Adolescents: 1.5 mg by transdermal patch q 72 hr <u>0.125 mg/ml solution</u> 3-4 kg 4 drops PO q 4 hr prn 10 kg 8 drops PO q 4 hr prn 50 kg 1 ml (0.125 mg) PO q 4 hr prn <u>0.125 mg/5 ml elixir</u> 10 kg 1.25 ml PO q 4 hr prn 20 kg 2.5 ml PO q 4 hr prn 40 kg 3.75 ml PO q 4 hr prn 50 kg 5 ml (0.125 mg) PO q 4 hr prn
Visceral hyeralgesia		
Medication	**Mechanism of action**	**Dose**
Gabapentin	Thought to inhibit excitation by binding to the alpha-2-delta subunit of voltage dependent Ca ion channels in the central nervous system	See Table 39-3
Nortriptyline	Presynaptic reuptake inhibition in the CNS of norepinephrine and serotonin, both inhibitors of pain transmission	See Table 39-3
Dysautonomia		
Medication	**Mechanism of action**	**Dose**
Clonidine	Centrally acting α_2-adrenergic receptor agonist, reducing sympathetic outflow	Day 1-3: 0.002 mg/kg PO qhs (maximum 0.1 mg) Day 4-6: 0.002 mg/kg q 12 hours Day 7-9: 0.002 mg/kg q 8 hours in addition 1) 0.002 mg/kg q 4 hour prn "autonomic storm" 2) doses may be increased to 0.004 mg/kg 3) titrate more rapidly if tolerated
Cyproheptadine	See above	See above
Gabapentin	See above	See above
Morphine sulfate	Binds CNS opioid receptors	0.3 mg/kg PO/SL q 3-4 hr prn "autonomic storm"

been unremarkable and intervention trials have had no benefit including: multiple abdominal x-rays; upper gastrointestinal (UGI) series; upper endoscopy; gastric emptying; multiple blood tests; treatment for GERD, constipation, and delayed motility; formula changes; jejunostomy feedings; and ondansetron and prochlorperazine (Compazine). There have been no other health issues including no significant respiratory illnesses.

PATHWAYS THAT RESULT IN NAUSEA AND VOMITING

An understanding of the pathways, receptors, and neurotransmitters involved in generating nausea, vomiting, and retching is critical to identifying treatment that can alleviate these symptoms.[121–123] The final common pathway resulting in nausea and vomiting is the vomiting center (VC) located in the medulla. The VC is triggered by numerous inputs, including the chemoreceptor trigger zone, cortical inputs, meningeal and ventricular mechanoreceptors, vestibular input, and vagal and glossopharyngeal input.

Visceral Hyperalgesia as a Source of Vomiting, Retching, and Feeding Intolerance

Visceral hyperalgesia is an altered response to visceral stimulation, resulting in a decreased activation threshold for pain in response to a stimulus, such as intraluminal pressure.[124] In a case series of 14 medically fragile children with continued retching and vomiting despite maximal medical treatment and Nissen fundoplication, visceral hyperalgesia was identified in 12 children as a source of symptoms.[125] Tricyclic antidepressants, gabapentin, cyproheptadine, and dicyclomine were used in various combinations depending on evaluation results, with 11 children reported as "better" or "much better" and a decrease in the mean number of retching episodes per day from 14 to 1.5. A case series of nine neurologically impaired children with symptoms indicating pain, feeding intolerance, and disrupted sleep, identified significant improvement following use of gabapentin titrated to standard doses.[56] This suggests that gastrointestinal and pain symptoms may improve with medical management directed toward visceral hyperalgesia when symptoms persist despite management of the more commonly recognized gastrointestinal problems. One report speculates that repeated painful gastrointestinal experiences during infancy contributes to sensitization of visceral afferent pathways.[125] It is interesting to note the higher incidence of pain in children with a gastrostomy feeding tube and taking medications for GERD.[28] Children with NI have an increased frequency of such sensitizing experiences, including GERD, constipation, gastrostomy tube placement, and fundoplication.[119,126]

Information that suggests visceral hyperalgesia in nonverbal children with NI includes:

* Retching indicating a decreased gastric volume threshold with symptom generation from normal distention,
* Pain and feeding intolerance associated with feedings by gastrostomy tube, suggesting decreased gastric volume threshold,
* Pain associated with intestinal gas and feedings by jejunostomy tube, suggesting pain at times of normal intestinal distention,
* Excessive response to a noxious stimulus such as prolonged crying spells associated with GERD,
* Pain associated with flatus and bowel movements, suggesting pain associated with colonic distention.

Retching was identified to benefit from alimemazine, a phenothiazine derivative structurally related to such medication as chlorpromazine.[127] As with other phenothiazine derivatives, various properties may account for this noted benefit with retching, including antihistamine, anticholinergic, antidopinergic, and antiserotonergic. Though alimemazine is not available in the United States, cyproheptadine and other medications that block the receptors that trigger nausea and vomiting may benefit children with NI and retching.

As identified earlier, children with vomiting and symptoms of retching, tachycardia, sweating, or flushing indicating dysautonomia, retching, forceful vomiting, pallor, or sweating indicating activation of the emetic reflex, or pain indicating visceral hyperalgesia likely do not benefit from anti-reflux surgery.[100,120] Esophagogastric disconnection is another surgical intervention that has been proposed for persistent GERD. In two case series reviewing the use of esophagogastric disconnection, morbidity (30% to 43% early complications, 41% to 43% late complications) and mortality (22% to 29%) were high.[128,129] Though used for GERD, patients were also noted to have symptoms of retching, likely indicating a process distinct from GERD. It is essential that medical and symptom management be maximized before considering this surgical intervention and that any surgical intervention for GERD be considered cautiously in neurologically impaired children with retching (see Table 39-5).

INTESTINAL PSEUDO-OBSTRUCTION

Intestinal pseudo-obstruction, also referred to as Ogilvie syndrome, is a clinical picture that suggests mechanical obstruction, but in the absence of any evidence of any obstruction in the intestine. Patients at risk include children with mitochondrial disorders and conditions with significant autonomic

dysfunction, such as autonomic dyreflexia following spinal cord injury. Children with severe NI may be at risk for this clinical picture in the post-operative period with a clinical picture of prolonged ileus.[130] Neostigmine has been reported to benefit some patients with acute intestinal pseudo-obstruction, when it fails to resolve with supportive therapy and management of contributing factors.[131] It must be used with caution, given the potential side effects, including bradycardia, hypotension, increased pain, increased airway secretions and bronchial reactivity. A test dose of 0.01–0.02 mg/kg/dose intravenously can be given in the hospital to allow monitoring, titrated up to 0.08 mg/kg/dose if needed. The oral equivalent is approximately 15 mg oral to 0.5 mg intravenous. Glycopyrrolate has been suggested in conjunction with neostigmine to minimize effects of bradycardia. Children with significant recurrent episodes, as seen with mitochondrial myopathies, may benefit from as needed neostigmine once a dose has been established, though this warrants further study. Other medications that have been considered include 5-HT$_4$ receptor agonists such as tegaserod and somatostatin analogues such as octreotide.

On further review, Tammy was experiencing daily vomiting and retching for 6 months and weekly crying for 2 months. Crying spells range from 2 hours to most of the day with crying averaging 60% of each day. Other symptoms noted at times of distress include sweating, arching, stiffening, and facial flushing. Reflective questions identified that "she has been suffering for over 6 months and is currently suffering every day." Tammy is described as "very social but now unable to enjoy the activities she did before." Visceral hyperalgesia and the role of the nervous system in regulating function of the intestines were discussed in detail. A symptom management plan was outlined: increase gabapentin that was being used for seizure management, initiate cyproheptadine, use morphine sulfate 0.3 mg/kg/dose by G-tube or sublingual as often as every 1 hour, and decrease formula feedings by 25%.

The primary focus of the discussion was Tammy's comfort and the hope for improvement with these interventions. The concept of the G-tube as a life-sustaining technology was introduced with acknowledgment that it is permissible to discontinue any technology that is prolonging suffering. This was approached as an opportunity to inform without any need for a decision. There was "significant improvement" noted within 5 days, described as "the best she has looked in the past year." This included a significant reduction in crying spells, vomiting, retching, and an increase in energy and interaction with her family. Parents were delighted; they hope for continued benefit, but are also prepared for a return of symptoms.

Persistent Feeding Intolerance

Feeding intolerance can be a source of distress for children with severe NI who are receiving fluid and nutrition through a feeding tube. As with recurrent respiratory exacerbations as a result of chronic pulmonary aspiration, the initial benefit from treatment interventions may lessen over time. At such times it can be beneficial to integrate symptom management strategies into medical care plans.

Management includes treating contributing problems such as constipation. As reviewed previously, some children benefit from an empiric trial of gabapentin or nortriptyline for visceral hyperalgesia, cyproheptadine for retching, and ondansetron, or hyoscyamine for vomiting, being mindful of which medication targets which receptor so as to avoid duplication. Because there is limited evidence to guide in such patients, one must be careful from introducing too many trial options. Other intervention strategies include an empiric trial of an elemental formula, an empiric trial of metronidazole or rifaximine for small bowel bacterial overgrowth in children with persistent diarrhea, and a trial of J-tube feedings. Experience shows that J-tube feedings often do not improve pain associated with vomiting. This may reflect irreversible changes in the nervous system with resulting autonomic dysfunction and visceral hyperalgesia.

Some of these children will have persistent problems despite using these options. At such times, some children will benefit from a decrease by 25% or more in the total amount of nutrition and fluids provided by feeding tube. Families benefit at such times from a reflection on primary goals and determining approaches that meet these goals such as feeding to comfort rather than feeding to a required amount, and withholding feedings that are resulting in pain and discomfort.

Medical Nutrition and Hydration

Forgoing medical nutrition and hydration remains one of the more difficult areas given the symbolic significance of nutrition, the myths about dehydration and starvation, and under-recognition of the complications of artificial hydration and nutrition.[132] The American Academy of Pediatrics policy statement recognizes that "Life-sustaining medical treatment encompasses all interventions that may prolong the life of patients. ...includes less technically demanding measures such as antibiotics, insulin, chemotherapy, and nutrition and hydration provided intravenously or by tube."[133] It is permissible to discontinue medical nutrition and hydration when it is prolonging or contributing to suffering.[134–137]

Children with NI receiving medical nutrition and fluids through a feeding tube are vulnerable to complications as health continues to decline. This can include progressive feeding intolerance, development of edema, and increasing oral secretions. It is important to combine knowledge of reversible sources of these problems with an understanding of features that are part of progressive, irreversible decline. This can be challenging in children with NI who live chronically with impairment that is considered static and who often experience decline over a long period, increasing the likelihood of aggressive evaluation and treatment at the end of life. It is helpful to recognize that even children with static conditions experience irreversible decline in organ function, likely a result of ongoing apoptosis in the setting of baseline impairment of the nervous system. This may account for why some children with NI develop feeding intolerance later in life that is not amenable to medical interventions.

It can be helpful to recognize with parents the years of benefit provided by a feeding tube as we consider development of

harm from this intervention. This is a time to inform without expecting a decision; educating on the role of feeding tubes as life-sustaining technology in the same sense as a ventilator and the benefit of considering when technology is becoming more burdensome, even when that technology has been routine and is easy to use. The previous sections are a critical part of this process, by creating a context for understanding the goals of the child and family and through knowledge of the child's health trajectory. It is helpful to estimate for families the length of time that may pass following discontinuation of medical nutrition and hydration until death occurs, often 10 to 14 days, but can be much longer by several weeks when small amounts of fluid are used to flush a feeding tube after medications have been given.

Tammy unfortunately experienced a return of vomiting, retching, and pain 2 months later. Her parents could not imagine allowing suffering to continue but were also distressed over consideration of discontinuing tube feedings. Follow up with the palliative care team included a child life specialist developing a supportive plan for Tammy's younger brother. Decisions were reviewed in the context of the family's faith community and support network. Further adjustments in medications were made and ongoing follow up was arranged including arrangements for home hospice. This provided parents with the time and support they needed as they explored various options. As suffering continued despite adjustments to the care plan, a decision was made to discontinue medical nutrition and hydration. Tammy died 8 days later with ongoing attention to symptom management and family support.

Care Teams to Meet the Complexity of Needs

The goal of palliative care and hospice teams is to meet the needs in the location of care, whether in the hospital, clinic, school, or home. Given the multiple challenges that families of children with NI experience, they benefit from as much anticipation of needs as possible: care in the school setting, symptom management at home, financial planning, and preparing for end-of-life care. One challenge is how to incorporate home-based palliative and/or hospice care into home care plans while preserving established blocks of home care nursing. Some states are eliminating this challenge through waivers that allow both resources to be used, allowing established home nurses to continue. This is of critical importance given the practical day-to-day care needs of such children along with the benefit of early integration of palliative care for such children and their families.

End-of-Life Care

WHAT IS LIFE LIMITING IN SEVERE DISABILITY?

Several categories can be identified that account for shortened life spans in children with NI.

- Impairment of motor control and tone resulting in compromise of pulmonary function,
- Function of the gastrointestinal tract,

- Associated organ impairment such as central apnea or congenital heart disease,
- Sudden death associated with epilepsy.

WHEN DOES CARE BECOME END-OF-LIFE CARE IN CHILDREN WITH NI?

This question is important given the range of interventions available and the variability of choices made by parents. Parents often find themselves struggling with "when will I know when I am doing *to* my child versus *for* my child?" The end of life period for children with NI is most commonly a result of determining when not to use interventions. This can include intubation at times of acute decline; tracheotomy, CPAP or BiPAP, and parenteral nutrition for chronic benefit; and surgery for neuromuscular scoliosis intended to address future problems. In addition to not introducing an intervention, parents may encounter decisions to discontinue chronic interventions if the child is experiencing persistent suffering.

PREPARING AND SUPPORTING FAMILIES THROUGH CARE AT END OF LIFE

Preparing families can be difficult yet tremendously beneficial. Preparation includes: anticipating symptom management needs, reviewing how the child might die, discussing preferred location of death, reviewing physical changes in the child at the end of life, determining who to contact to assist throughout this process, and discussing autopsy or organ and tissue donation.

Hospice and palliative care teams are well suited to support children, parents, and siblings throughout this process. The interdisciplinary team can address the multitude of needs, such as child life specialists providing support for siblings, chaplains exploring spiritual needs in the context of a family's faith community, and social workers addressing emotional and home care support needs. Clinicians can attend to symptoms by creating tailored care plans that use parental input, such as this example for a child with CP and progressive respiratory failure:

1. The following symptoms indicate distress: increased heart rate, working harder to breath, distressed look on face often noted with facial grimacing, increased secretions.
2. When noted give 0.2 mL (4 mg) of morphine sulfate by syringe into the mouth.
3. Vent G-tube if abdomen is distended.
4. If no improvement within 30 minutes, repeat same dose.
5. If no improvement in 15 minutes, give midazolam, 2 mL oral or by G-tube, and call hospice.
6. For increasing secretions give 8 drops hyoscyamine, as often as every 4 hours.
7. Hold feedings until distress remains resolved for 4 hours (as a suggested timeline).

Autopsy, Brain and Tissue Bank, and Organ Donation

The option of autopsy or tissue donation to the Brain and Tissue Bank is ideally discussed with the family by a trusted physician before death. Some families may feel that the child has been through enough while others may feel that this is a way to advance science and help other children who may suffer from the same condition.

The goal of the Brain and Tissue Bank is to advance research on developmental disorders. It serves the critical purpose of collecting, preserving, and distributing human tissues to scientific investigators who are dedicated to the improved understanding, care and treatment of developmental disorders, offering hope to others. The procedure to recover tissue at time of death will not interfere with open casket viewing. The Brain and Tissue Bank covers all expenses related to the recovery of tissue. All donor information remains anonymous and anyone who registers holds the right to withdraw at any time. Further information for families can be found at www.btbankfamily.org.

Increasingly, pediatric hospitals are developing policies that support donation after cardiac death programs. There is increasing awareness of this approach as noted by the number of cases that were initiated by the family.[138,139] Organ donor programs that include donation after cardiac death may have benefit by providing an opportunity for legacy building. Further review is needed on how this impacts end-of-life care and bereavement.

Bereavement

Bereavement often starts before the child's death. Support from palliative care teams can link families to assistance from extended family, friends, or community providers, including faith communities and grief counselors, as families prepare to transition from the specialized healthcare system. Bereavement care also guides the family through the legal requirements and decisions for the care and relinquishment of the body.

Unique areas of bereavement are seen in parents of children with NI. The limited research has not found differences on measures of grief between parents of children with developmental impairment and other parents.[140] Themes identified that are unique to parents of children with NI include: working through two difficult transitions, first when the child was diagnosed with NI and second when the child died; a need to justify their love of their child to others; parents' lack of opportunity to share their grief, resulting in a socially imposed silent grief; loss of an intensive caregiver role and support group membership; conflicting feelings of sadness; and relief over prior fears about the child's future. Bereavement is an essential part of supportive care with importance in attending to the experiences unique to families of children with NI.

Future Directions and Ongoing Challenges

There are many opportunities to better understand how palliative care, as an interdisciplinary team, and palliative medicine, as a medical specialty, can best assist this population. Areas of need include symptom assessment and management and improved understanding of how interventions alter outcomes for these children. There is benefit in exploring how parents approach decision making that is both similar and unique to other groups of children with life-threatening conditions.

Acknowledgments

With gratitude to Melissa Connelly, Elayne Sommers, and Jean Stansbury, members of the palliative care team at Gillette Children's Specialty Healthcare. Through their work they have benefitted countless families and are a source of inspiration to others.

REFERENCES

1. Hays RM, Valentine J, Geyer JR: The Seattle Palliative Care Project: Effects on family satisfaction and health-related quality of life, *J Palliat Med* 9(3):716–728, 2006.
2. Duncan J, Spengler E, Wolfe J: Providing pediatric palliative care: PACT in action, *MCN Am J Matern Child Nurs* 32(5):279–287, 2007.
3. Lohiya GS, Tan-Figueroa L, Crinella FM: End-of-life care for a man with developmental disabilities, *J Am Board Fam Pract* 16(1):58–62, 2003.
4. Tuffrey-Wijne I: The palliative care needs of people with intellectual disabilities: a literature review, *Palliat Med* 17(1):55–62, 2003.
5. Himelstein BP, Hilden JM, Boldt AM, Weissman D: Pediatric palliative care, *N Engl J Med* 350(17):1752–1762, 2004.
6. Scornaienchi JM: Chronic sorrow: one mother's experience with two children with lissencephaly, *J Pediatr Health Care* 17(6):290–294, 2003.
7. Patja K, Iivanainen M, Vesala H, et al: Life expectancy of people with intellectual disability: a 35-year follow-up study, *J Intellect Disabil Res* 44(Pt 5):591–599, 2000.
8. Patja K, Mölsä P, Iivanainen M: Cause-specific mortality of people with intellectual disability in a population-based, 35-year follow-up study, *J Intellect Disabil Res* 45(Pt 1):30–40, 2001.
9. Hutton JL, Pharoah PO: Life expectancy in severe cerebral palsy, *Arch Dis Child* 91(3):254–258, 2006.
10. Hemming K, Hutton JL, Pharoah PO: Long-term survival for a cohort of adults with cerebral palsy, *Dev Med Child Neurol* 48(2):90–95, 2006.
11. Strauss D, Cable W, Shavelle R: Causes of excess mortality in cerebral palsy, *Dev Med Child Neurol* 41(9):580–585, 1999.
12. Katz RT: Life expectancy for children with cerebral palsy and mental retardation: implications for life care planning, *Neuro Rehabil* 18(3):261–270, 2003.
13. Steele R: Navigating uncharted territory: experiences of families when a child is dying, *J Palliat Care* 21(1):35–43, 2005.
14. Steele R: Strategies used by families to navigate uncharted territory when a child is dying, *J Palliat Care* 21(2):103–110, 2005.
15. Meyer EC, Burns JP, Griffith JL, et al: Parental perspectives on end-of-life care in the pediatric intensive care unit, *Crit Care Med* 30(1):226–231, 2002.
16. Sharman M, Meert KL, Sarnaik AP: What influences parents' decisions to limit or withdraw life support? *Pediatr Crit Care Med* 6(5):513–518, 2005.
17. Murray SA, Kendall M, Boyd K, et al: Illness trajectories and palliative care, *BMJ* 330(7498):1007–1011, 2005.
18. Lunney JR, Lynn J, Foley DJ, et al: Patterns of functional decline at the end of life, *JAMA* 289(18):2387–2392, 2003.
19. Back AL, Arnold RM, Quill TE: Hope for the best, and prepare for the worst, *Ann Intern Med* 138(5):439–443, 2003.
20. Graham RJ, Robinson WM: Integrating palliative care into chronic care for children with severe neurodevelopmental disabilities, *J Dev Behav Pediatr* 26(5):361–365, 2005.
21. Dy S, Lynn J: Getting services right for those sick enough to die, *BMJ* 334(7592):511–513, 2007.
22. American Academy of Pediatrics. Committee on Bioethics and Committee on Hospital Care: Palliative care for children, *Pediatrics* 106(2 Pt 1):351–357, 2000.
23. Klick JC, Ballantine A: Providing care in chronic disease: the ever-changing balance of integrating palliative and restorative medicine, *Pediatr Clin North Am* 54(5):799–812, 2007.
24. Levetown M, American Academy of Pediatrics Committee on Bioethics: Communicating with children and families: from everyday interactions to skill in conveying distressing information, *Pediatrics* 121(5):e1441–e1460, 2008.
25. Mack JW, Wolfe J: Early integration of pediatric palliative care: for some children, palliative care starts at diagnosis, *Curr Opin Pediatr* 18(1):10–14, 2006.
26. Perquin CW, Hazebroek-Kampschreur AA, Hunfeld JA, et al: Pain in children and adolescents: a common experience, *Pain* 87(1):51–58, 2000.
27. Breau LM, Camfield CS, McGrath PJ, et al: The incidence of pain in children with severe cognitive impairments, *Arch Pediatr Adolesc Med* 157(12):1219–1226, 2003.
28. Houlihan CM, O'Donnell M, Conaway M, et al: Bodily pain and health-related quality of life in children with cerebral palsy, *Dev Med Child Neurol* 46:305–310, 2004.
29. Stallard P, Williams L, Lenton S, et al: Pain in cognitively impaired, non-communicating children, *Arch Dis Child* 85(6):460–462, 2001.
30. Defrin R, Lotan M, Pick CG: The evaluation of acute pain in individuals with cognitive impairment: a differential effect of the level of impairment, *Pain* 124(3):312–320, 2006 Epub 2006 Jun 14.
31. Drake R, Frost J, Collins JJ: The symptoms of dying children, *J Pain Symptom Manage* 26(1):594–603, 2003.
32. Hunt AM: A survey of signs, symptoms and symptom control in 30 terminally ill children, *Dev Med Child Neurol* 32(4):341–346, 1990.
33. Hunt A, Burne R: Medical and nursing problems of children with neurodegenerative disease, *Palliat Med* 9(1):19–26, 1995.
34. Roccella M, Pace R, De Gregorio MT: Psychopathological assessment in children affected by Duchenne de Boulogne muscular dystrophy, *Minerva Pediatr* 55(3):267–276, 2003.
35. Beyer JE, Aradine CR: Content validity of an instrument to measure young children's perceptions of the intensity of their pain, *J Pediatr Nurs* 1(6):386–395, 1986.
36. Wong DL, Hockenberry-Eaton M, Wilson D, Winkelstein ML, Schwartz P, editors: *Wong's essentials of pediatric nursing*, ed 6, St Louis, 2001, Mosby.
37. Voepel-Lewis T, Malviya S, Tait AR, et al: A comparison of the clinical utility of pain assessment tools for children with cognitive impairment, *Anesth Analg* 106(1):72–78, 2008.
38. Voepel-Lewis T, Merkel S, Tait AR, et al: The reliability and validity of the Face, Legs, Activity, Cry, Consolability observational tool as a measure of pain in children with cognitive impairment, *Anesth Analg* 95(5):1224–1229, 2002.
39. Malviya S, Voepel-Lewis T, Burke C, et al: The revised FLACC observational pain tool: improved reliability and validity for pain assessment in children with cognitive impairment, *Paediatr Anaesth* 16(3):258–265, 2006.
40. Breau LM, Camfield C, McGrath PJ, et al: Measuring pain accurately in children with cognitive impairments: refinement of a caregiver scale, *J Pediatr* 138(5):721–727, 2001.
41. Breau LM, McGrath PJ, Camfield CS, et al: Psychometric properties of the non-communicating children's pain checklist-revised, *Pain* 99(1–2):349–357, 2002.
42. Hunt A, Wisbeach A, Seers K, et al: Development of the paediatric pain profile: role of video analysis and saliva cortisol in validating a tool to assess pain in children with severe neurological disability, *J Pain Symptom Manage* 33(3):276–289, 2007.
43. Hunt A, Goldman A, Seers K, et al: Clinical validation of the paediatric pain profile, *Dev Med Child Neurol* 46(1):9–18, 2004.
44. Solodiuk J, Curley MA: Pain assessment in nonverbal children with severe cognitive impairments: the Individualized Numeric Rating Scale (INRS), *J Pediatr Nurs* 18(4):295–299, 2003.
45. Closs SJ, Barr B, Briggs M, et al: A comparison of five pain assessment scales for nursing home residents with varying degrees of cognitive impairment, *J Pain and Symptom Manage* 27(3):196–205, 2004.
46. Chibnall JT, Tait RC: Pain assessment in cognitively impaired and unimpaired older adults: a comparison of four scales, *Pain* 92(1–2):173–186, 2001.
47. Feldt KS: The checklist of nonverbal pain indicators (CNPI), *Pain Manag Nurs* 1(1):13–21, 2000.
48. Regnard C, Reynolds J, Watson B, et al: Understanding distress in people with severe communication difficulties: developing and assessing the Disability Distress Assessment Tool (DisDAT), *J Intellect Disabil Res* 51(Pt 4):277–292, 2007.
49. Hølen JC, Saltvedt I, Fayers PM: The Norwegian Doloplus-2, a tool for behavioural pain assessment: translation and pilot-validation in nursing home patients with cognitive impairment, *Palliat Med* 19(5):411–417, 2005.
50. Berde CB, Lebel AA, Olsson G: Neuropathic pain in children. In Schechter NL, Berde CB, Yaster M, editors: *Pain in infants, children, and adolescents*, ed 2, Philadelphia, 2003, Lippincott Williams and Wilkins, pp 620–641.
51. Hauer JM: Central hypothermia as a cause of acute pancreatitis in children with neurodevelopmental impairment, *Dev Med Child Neurol* 50(1):68–70, 2008.
52. Greco C, Berde CB: Pain management for the hospitalized pediatric patient, *Pediatr Clin N Am* 52:995–1027, 2005.

53. Oberlander TR, Craig KD: Pain and children with developmental disabilities. In Schechter NL, Berde CB, Yaster M, editors: *Pain in infants, children, and adolescents*, ed 2, Philadelphia, 2003, Lippincott Williams and Wilkins, pp 599–619.

54. Lauder GR, White MC: Neuropathic pain following multilevel surgery in children with cerebral palsy: a case series and review, *Paediatr Anaesth* 15(5):412–420, 2005.

55. Breau LM, Camfield CS, McGrath PJ, et al: Risk factors for pain in children with severe cognitive impairments, *Dev Med Child Neurol* 46(6):364–371, 2004.

56. Hauer J, Wical B, Charnas L: Gabapentin successfully manages chronic unexplained irritability in children with severe neurologic impairment, *Pediatrics* 119(2):e519–e522, 2007.

57. Nicholson BD: Evaluation and treatment of central pain syndromes, *Neurology* 62(5 Suppl 2):S30–S36, 2004.

58. Frese A, Husstedt IW, Ringelstein EB, et al: Pharmacologic treatment of central post-stroke pain, *Clin J Pain* 22(3):252–260, 2006.

59. Berde CB, Sethna NF: Analgesics for the treatment of pain in children, *N Engl J Med* 347(14):1094–1103, 2002.

60. Friedrichsdorf SJ, Kang TI: The management of pain in children with life-limiting illnesses, *Pediatr Clin North Am* 54(5):645–672, 2007.

61. Goldman A, Hain R, Liben S, editors: *Oxford textbook of palliative care for children*, Oxford, 2006, Oxford University Press.

62. Korn-Merker E, Borusiak P, Boenigk HE: Gabapentin in childhood epilepsy: a prospective evaluation of efficacy and safety, *Epilepsy Res* 38(1):27–32, 2000.

63. Haig GM, Bockbrader HN, Wesche DL, et al: Single-dose gabapentin pharmacokinetics and safety in healthy infants and children, *J Clin Pharmacol* 41(5):507–514, 2001.

64. Krach LE: Pharmacotherapy of spasticity: oral medications and intrathecal baclofen, *J Child Neurol* 16(1):31–36, 2001.

65. Montané E, Vallano A, Laporte JR: Oral antispastic drugs in non-progressive neurologic diseases: a systematic review, *Neurology* 63(8):1357–1363, 2004.

66. Bes A, Eyssette M, Pierrot-Deseilligny E, et al: A multi-centre, double-blind trial of tizanidine, a new antispastic agent, in spasticity associated with hemiplegia, *Curr Med Res Opin* 10:709–718, 1988.

67. Medici M, Pebet M, Ciblis D: A double-blind, long-term study of tizanidine ("Sirdalud") in spasticity due to cerebrovascular lesions, *Curr Med Res Opin* 11:398–407, 1989.

68. Cutter N, Scott DD, Johnson JC, et al: Gabapentin effect on spasticity in multiple sclerosis: a placebo-controlled, randomized trial, *Arch Phys Med Rehabil* 81(2):164–169, 2000.

69. Baguley IJ, Heriseanu RE, Gurka JA, et al: Gabapentin in the management of dysautonomia following severe traumatic brain injury: a case series, *J Neurol Neurosurg Psychiatry* 78(5):539–541, 2007.

70. Kloos RT: Spontaneous periodic hypothermia, *Medicine (Baltimore)* 74(5):268–280, 1995.

71. Axelrod FB, Berlin D: Pregabalin: A new approach to treatment of the dysautonomic crisis, *Pediatrics* 2009. Jul 20. [Epub ahead of print].

72. Boyer EW, Shannon M: The serotonin syndrome, *N Engl J Med* 352(11):1112–1120, 2005.

73. Halloran LL, Bernard DW: Management of drug-induced hyperthermia, *Curr Opin Pediatr* 16(2):211–215, 2004.

74. Del Fabbro E, Dalal S, Bruera E: Symptom control in palliative care—Part III: dyspnea and delirium, *J Palliat Med* 9(2):422–436, 2006.

75. Wusthoff CJ, Shellhaas RA, Licht DJ: Management of common neurologic symptoms in pediatric palliative care: seizures, agitation, and spasticity, *Pediatr Clin North Am* 54(5):709–733, xi, 2007.

76. McIntyre J, Robertson S, Norris E, et al: Safety and efficacy of buccal midazolam versus rectal diazepam for emergency treatment of seizures in children: a randomised controlled trial, *Lancet* 366(9481):205–210, 2005.

77. Appleton R, Macleod S, Martland T: Drug management for acute tonic-clonic convulsions including convulsive status epilepticus in children, *Cochrane Database Syst Rev* (3):CD001905, 2008.

78. Mpimbaza A, Ndeezi G, Staedke S, et al: Comparison of buccal midazolam with rectal diazepam in the treatment of prolonged seizures in Ugandan children: a randomized clinical trial, *Pediatrics* 121(1):e58–e64, 2008.

79. Dodge NN, Wilson GA: Melatonin for treatment of sleep disorders in children with developmental disabilities, *J Child Neurol* 16(8):581–584, 2001.

80. Jan JE, Freeman RD: Melatonin therapy for circadian rhythm sleep disorders in children with multiple disabilities: what have we learned in the last decade? *Dev Med Child Neurol* 46(11):776–782, 2004.

81. Collins JJ, Kerner J, Sentivany S, Berde CB: Intravenous amitriptyline in pediatrics, *J Pain Symptom Manage* 10(6):471–475, 1995.

82. Davis MP: Does trazodone have a role in palliating symptoms? *Support Care Cancer* 15(2):221–224, 2007.

83. Pranzatelli MR, Tate ED, Dukart WS, et al: Sleep disturbance and rage attacks in opsoclonus-myoclonus syndrome: response to trazodone, *J Pediatr* 147(3):372–378, 2005.

84. Schnoes CJ, Kuhn BR, Workman EF, et al: Pediatric prescribing practices for clonidine and other pharmacologic agents for children with sleep disturbance, *Clin Pediatr (Phila)* 45(3):229–238, 2006.

85. Sela RA, Watanabe S, Nekolaichuk CL: Sleep disturbances in palliative cancer patients attending a pain and symptom control clinic, *Palliat Support Care* 3(1):23–31, 2005.

86. Rosenberg RP: Sleep maintenance insomnia: strengths and weaknesses of current pharmacologic therapies, *Ann Clin Psychiatry* 18(1):49–56, 2006.

87. Gilron I, Bailey JM, Tu D, Holden RR, Jackson AC, Houlden RL: Nortriptyline and gabapentin, alone and in combination for neuropathic pain: a double-blind, randomised controlled crossover trial, *Lancet* 374(9697):1252–1261, 2009. Epub 2009 Sep 30.

88. Seddon PC, Khan Y: Respiratory problems in children with neurological impairment, *Arch Dis Child* 88:75–78, 2003.

89. Wright RE, Wright FR, Carson CA: Videofluoroscopic assessment in children with severe cerebral palsy presenting with dysphagia, *Pediatr Radiol* 26:720–722, 1996.

90. Mirrett PL, Riski JE, Glascott J, et al: Videofluoroscopic assessment of dysphagia in children with severe cerebral palsy, *Dysphagia* 9:174–179, 1994.

91. Taniguchi MH, Moyer RS: Assessment of risk factors for pneumonia in dysphagic children: significance of videofluoroscopic swallowing evaluation, *Dev Med Child Neurol* 36:495–502, 1994.

92. Strauss D, Shavelle R, Reynolds R, et al: Survival in cerebral palsy in the last 20 years: signs of improvement? *Dev Med Child Neurol* 49(2):86–92, 2007.

93. Sleigh G, Brocklehurst P: Gastrostomy feeding in cerebral palsy: a systematic review, *Arch Dis Child* 89(6):534–539, 2004.

94. Finucane TE, Christmas C, Travis K: Tube feeding in patients with advanced dementia: a review of the evidence, *JAMA* 282(14):1365–1370, 1999.

95. Morton RE, Wheatley R, Minford J: Respiratory tract infections due to direct and reflux aspiration in children with severe neurodisability, *Dev Med Child Neurol* 41(5):329–334, 1999.

96. Jolley SG, Herbst JJ, Johnson DG, et al: Surgery in children with gastroesophageal reflux and respiratory symptoms, *J Pediatr* 96(2):194–198, 1980.

97. Kawahara H, Okuyama H, Kubota A, et al: Can laparoscopic antireflux surgery improve the quality of life in children with neurologic and neuromuscular handicaps? *J Pediatr Surg* 39(12):1761–1764, 2004.

98. Cheung KM, Tse HW, Tse PW, et al: Nissen fundoplication and gastrostomy in severely neurologically impaired children with gastroesophageal reflux, *Hong Kong Med J* 12(4):282–288, 2006.

99. Bui HD, Dang CV, Chaney RH, et al: Does gastrostomy and fundoplication prevent aspiration pneumonia in mentally retarded persons? *Am J Ment Retard* 94(1):16–19, 1989.

100. Richards CA, Milla PJ, Andrews PL, et al: Retching and vomiting in neurologically impaired children after fundoplication: predictive preoperative factors, *J Pediatr Surg* 36(9):1401–1404, 2001.

101. Carron JD, Derkay CS, Strope GL, et al: Pediatric tracheotomies: changing indications and outcomes, *Laryngoscope* 110(7):1099–1104, 2000.

102. Berry JG, Graham DA, Graham RJ, et al: Predictors of clinical outcomes and hospital resource use of children after tracheotomy, *Pediatrics* 124(2):563–572, 2009.

103. Vijayasekaran S, Unal R, Schraff SA, et al: Salivary gland surgery for chronic pulmonary aspiration in children, *Int J Pediatr Otorhinolaryngol* 71(1):119–123, 2007.

104. Raval TH, Elliott CA: Botulinum toxin injection to the salivary glands for the treatment of sialorrhea with chronic aspiration, *Ann Otol Rhinol Laryngol* 117(2):118–122, 2008.

105. Tsirikos AI, Chang WN, Dabney KW, et al: Life expectancy in pediatric patients with cerebral palsy and neuromuscular scoliosis who underwent spinal fusion, *Dev Med Child Neurol* 45(10):677–682, 2003.

106. Campbell ML: Psychometric testing of a respiratory distress observation scale, *J Palliat Med* 11(1):44–50, 2008.

107. Lorenz KA, Lynn J, Dy SM, et al: Evidence for improving palliative care at the end of life: a systematic review, *Ann Intern Med* 148(2): 147–159, 2008.

108. Qaseem A, Snow V, Shekelle P, et al: Evidence-based interventions to improve the palliative care of pain, dyspnea, and depression at the end of life: a clinical practice guideline from the American College of Physicians, *Ann Intern Med* 148(2):141–146, 2008.

109. Abernethy AP, Currow DC, Frith P, et al: Randomised, double blind, placebo controlled crossover trial of sustained release morphine for the management of refractory dyspnoea, *BMJ* 327(7414):523–528, 2003.

110. Clemens KE, Klaschik E: Symptomatic therapy of dyspnea with strong opioids and its effect on ventilation in palliative care patients, *J Pain Symptom Manage* 33(4):473–481, 2007.

111. Allen S, Raut S, Woollard J, et al: Low dose diamorphine reduces breathlessness without causing a fall in oxygen saturation in elderly patients with end-stage idiopathic pulmonary fibrosis, *Palliat Med* 19(2):128–130, 2005.

112. Mazzocato C, Buclin T, Rapin CH: The effects of morphine on dyspnea and ventilatory function in elderly patients with advanced cancer: a randomized double-blind controlled trial, *Ann Oncol* 10(12):1511–1514, 1999.

113. Hauer JM: Respiratory symptom management in a child with severe neurologic impairment, *J Palliat Med* 10(5):1201–1207, 2007.

114. Brook I, Finegold SM: Bacteriology of aspiration pneumonia in children, *Pediatrics* 65(6):1115–1120, 1980.

115. Dreyfuss D: Aspiration pneumonia, *N Engl J Med* 344(24):1868, 2001 (letter).

116. Brook I: Treatment of aspiration or tracheostomy-associated pneumonia in neurologically impaired children: effect of antimicrobials effective against anaerobic bacteria, *Int J Pediatr Otorhinolaryngol* 35(2):171–177, 1996.

117. Allewelt M, Schuler P, Bolcskei PL, et al: Ampicillin + sulbactam vs clindamycin +/- cephalosporin for the treatment of aspiration pneumonia and primary lung abscess, *Clin Microbiol Infect* 10(2):163–170, 2004.

118. Kadowaki M, Demura Y, Mizuno S, et al: Reappraisal of clindamycin IV monotherapy for treatment of mild-to-moderate aspiration pneumonia in elderly patients, *Chest* 127(4):1276–1282, 2005.

119. Del Giudice E, Staiano A, Capano G, et al: Gastrointestinal manifestations in children with cerebral palsy, *Brain Dev* 21(5):307–311, 1999.

120. Richards CA, Andrews PL, Spitz L, et al: Nissen fundoplication may induce gastric myoelectrical disturbance in children, *J Pediatr Surg* 33(12):1801–1805, 1998.

121. Santucci G, Mack JW: Common gastrointestinal symptoms in pediatric palliative care: nausea, vomiting, constipation, anorexia, cachexia, *Pediatr Clin North Am* 54(5):673–689, 2007.

122. Baines MJ: ABC of palliative care. Nausea, vomiting, and intestinal obstruction, *BMJ* 315(7116):1148–1150, 1997.

123. Wood GJ, Shega JW, Lynch B, et al: Management of intractable nausea and vomiting in patients at the end of life: "I was feeling nauseous all of the time ... nothing was working," *JAMA* 298(10):1196–1207, 2007.

124. Delgado-Aros S, Camilleri M: Visceral hypersensitivity, *J Clin Gastroenterol* 39(Suppl 3):S194–S203, 2005.

125. Zangen T, Ciarla C, Zangen S, et al: Gastrointestinal motility and sensory abnormalities may contribute to food refusal in medically fragile toddlers, *J Pediatr Gastroenterol Nutr* 37(3):287–293, 2003.

126. Schwarz SM, Corredor J, Fisher-Medina J, et al: Diagnosis and treatment of feeding disorders in children with developmental disabilities, *Pediatrics* 108(3):671–676, 2001.

127. Antao B, Ooi K, Ade-Ajayi N, et al: Effectiveness of alimemazine in controlling retching after Nissen fundoplication, *J Pediatr Surg* 40(11):1737–1740, 2005.

128. Burrati S, Kamenwa R, Dohil R, et al: Esophagogastric disconnection following failed fundoplication for the treatment of gastroesophageal reflux disease (GERD) in children with severe neurological impairment, *Pediatr Surg Int* 20:786–790, 2004.

129. Danielson PD, Emmens RW: Esophagogastric disconnection for gastroesophageal reflux in children with severe neurological impairment, *J Pediatr Surg* 34(1):84–87, 1999.

130. Gmora S, Poenaru D, Tsai E: Neostigmine for the treatment of pediatric acute colonic pseudo-obstruction, *J Pediatr Surg* 37(10):E28, 2002.

131. Ponec RJ, Saunders MD, Kimmey MB: Neostigmine for the treatment of acute colonic pseudo-obstruction, *N Engl J Med* 341(3):137–141, 1999.

132. Casarett D, Kapo J, Caplan A: Appropriate use of artificial nutrition and hydration: fundamental principles and recommendations, *N Engl J Med* 353(24):2607–2612, 2005.

133. American Academy of Pediatrics Committee on Bioethics: Guidelines on foregoing life-sustaining medical treatment, *Pediatrics* 93(3):532–536, 1994.

134. American Academy of Hospice and Palliative Medicine: *Statement on artificial nutrition and hydration.* www.aahpm.org/positions/nutrition.html. Accessed April 2, 2009.

135. Nelson LJ, Rushton CH, Cranford RE, et al: Forgoing medically provided nutrition and hydration in pediatric patients, *J Law Med Ethics* 23(1):33–46, 1995.

136. Stanley AL: Withholding artificially provided nutrition and hydration from disabled children: assessing their quality of life, *Clin Pediatr (Phila)* 39(10):575–579, 2000.

137. Royal College of Paediatrics and Child Health: *Withholding or withdrawing life sustaining treatment for children: a framework for practice.* www.rcpch.ac.uk/Publications/Publications-list-by-title#W. Accessed December 4, 2008.

138. Pleacher KM, Roach ES, Van der Werf W, et al: Impact of a pediatric donation after cardiac death program. *Pediatr Crit Care Med* 10(2):166–170, 2009.

139. Naim MY, Hoehn KS, Hasz RD, et al: The Children's Hospital of Philadelphia's experience with donation after cardiac death, *Crit Care Med* 36(6):1729–1733, 2008.

140. Reilly DE, Hastings RP, Vaughan FL, et al: Parental bereavement and the loss of a child with intellectual disabilities: a review of the literature, *Intellect Dev Disabil* 46(1):27–43, 2008.

40

Advanced Heart Disease

ELIZABETH D. BLUME | ANGELA GREEN

My daughter has had heart surgery five times. Now the only option is a transplant. She was at home for a while, but now she is in the hospital with a ventricular assist device. She feels better, but being in the hospital is hard. She misses her friends. For us, it is really scary waiting and hoping for a transplant to give her a chance to live. Knowing that even with the transplant, she may not live.

In contrast to adults, severe advanced heart disease is a rare condition in children.[1,2] There are two primary etiologies of pediatric heart failure: cardiomyopathy and congenital heart disease (CHD). The overall incidence of CHD is approximately 8 per 1000 live births,[1] and the incidence of cardiomyopathy is estimated at 0.58 per 100,000 children.[3,4] Yet only a fraction of children diagnosed with either form of pediatric heart disease eventually progresses to advanced heart disease[5] necessitating long-term intensive medical management and/or recurrent hospitalization. Those that do are at high risk for developing end-stage heart disease,[5,6] a clinical syndrome characterized by marked reduction in quality of life, functional status, nutritional deficiency, and respiratory distress. Similar to adults, however, the high mortality associated with pediatric advanced heart disease stems from its sequelae, including low cardiac output, respiratory failure, malignant arrhythmias, stroke, thromboembolism, multi-organ dysfunction, and infection.[5] As such, children with advanced heart disease represent a diverse group ranging from those cared for at home by their parents and still participating in childhood activities to those in hospice care at the end of life. Regardless of the scenario, there is increasing evidence that advanced heart disease impacts not only the physical health of affected children, but also the psychosocial health and quality of life of the child and his or her family across the illness trajectory. Palliative care provides an opportunity to proactively address physical, psychosocial, and spiritual issues in order to maximize the quality of life children with advanced heart disease and their families, as well as prepare families for the complex end-of-life decision making.

Incidence and Epidemiology of Congenital Heart Disease and Pediatric Advanced Heart Disease

The reported prevalence of CHD varies widely, depending on the method of diagnosis and whether the data reflect prenatally detected CHD or live births of children with CHD. In general, the prevalence of CHD is approximately 3 per 1000 for clinically severe defects, 6 per 1000 when including the more moderate defects, and 9 to 20 per 1000 when including smaller septal defects and mild valve stenosis.[1,2] CHD is the leading cause of infant deaths owing to congenital anomalies worldwide.[1,2] Between 1940 and 2002, approximately 2 million infants were born with CHD in the United States.[1] In those same six decades, enormous achievements in medical and surgical care of these infants and children have resulted in improved long-term survival. Despite dramatically improved short- and long-term outcomes, palliated advanced heart disease remains one of the leading causes of non-accidental death in childhood in the United States. During the past 60 years, surgical procedures have been developed to treat most congenital heart defects, including those that were historically uniformly fatal, such as hypoplastic left heart syndrome.[7] During the same time period, major advances have been achieved in intensive care management, ventilatory support, mechanical support, intra-operative management, long-term medical management, and diagnostic imaging.[7,8] These improvements are forcing reassessment of the outcomes and impact of CHD. For example, prenatal diagnosis has led to earlier detection, more controlled perinatal transition, and earlier surgical repair as well as more educated and prepared parents. The traditional statistics of prevalence and outcomes are, therefore of historic value, but may be less helpful in determining the longer term needs of children with advanced heart disease.

Improved survival rates of children with CHD is reported over the past two decades. A review[9] of the multiple-cause mortality files compiled by the National Center for Health Statistics of the Centers for Disease Control and Prevention from all death certificates filed in the United States found that from 1979 through 1997, mortality from heart defects for all ages declined 39 percent, from 2.5 to 1.5 per 100,000. In the last two years of the study, heart defects contributed to 5822 deaths per year. Of these deaths, 51% were infants and 7% were children 1 to 4 years old. In this series, age at death increased over the decade for every heart defect, as more palliated infants are surviving into adolescence and adulthood.[9] Only a small number of children born with CHD will progress to advanced heart disease (Box 40-1). There are no published data on the numbers of children with CHD who meet criteria for advanced heart disease and prognostic indicators to assist with predicting which patients are likely to progress are limited.

BOX 40-1 Pediatric Heart Diseases That May Progress to Advanced Heart Disease

- Single ventricle palliation, such as hypoplastic left heart syndrome
- Pulmonary vein stenosis
- Systemic RV lesions, such as L-TGA
- Post-transplant coronary artery disease
- Cardiomyopathy
- Protein losing enteropathy and/or plastic bronchitis
- Pulmonary hypertension/Eisenmenger's

Evolution of Palliative Care in Advanced Heart Disease in Children

Because of the previously described advances and improved longevity, pediatric cardiac teams now provide long-term care for children for whom previously the only treatment decision was the location of their death. Early efforts necessarily focused on survival. Over time, the focus expanded to include managing medical morbidity and maximizing the quality of life of children with CHD, including those with advanced heart disease. The evolution of palliative care in children with advanced heart disease has occurred slowly in part due to the perception of heart disease as treatable with the focus on surgical cures. This is similar to the evolution of care in adult advanced heart disease as well.[10,11] It is important to recognize that many interactions between families and the healthcare team revolve around the surgical or interventional procedure to fix the child's heart. Even in complex situations where palliative surgery is planned, death is rarely an immediate outcome. Aggressive, highly technological options and treatments are available and offered even in the final stages of advanced disease. Ongoing successes encourage caretakers and families to pursue continued therapies. Also, the progression of heart failure in children is largely variable, and the point at which there is no possibility for long-term survival is often unclear.

Advanced heart disease is often marked by acute decompensations followed by periods of stability. This unpredictable nature often discourages end of life discussions for children and their families.

Because of the trajectory of acute decompensation alternating with periods of stability, many children with advanced heart disease die in the hospital, most often in an intensive care setting as advanced therapies are used even at the end of life. Little data are available for children with advanced heart disease. Fig. 40-1 shows the data from one large Cardiac Intensive Care Unit with approximately 1000 admissions per year. Overall, the ICU mortality is between 2% and 4% each year, which is approximately 30 to 40 deaths yearly. This percentage may vary between institutions and internationally. Although end of life discussions are happening with these families, there are limited data as to when and where these discussions are occurring.

Despite ongoing challenges, providing palliative care for children with CHD is a critical need. Key aspects include symptom management, promoting psychosocial health and quality of life, and decision making. Each of these areas will be discussed in the sections that follow.

SYMPTOM MANAGEMENT FOR CHILDREN WITH ADVANCED HEART DISEASE

Children with advanced heart disease represent a diverse group with complex cardiac issues that result from either palliated complex CHD or from severe forms of cardiomyopathy or post-transplant care. Symptom management includes a variety of complex medical and psychosocial interventions in order to optimize quality of life. As cardiac function deteriorates, traditional symptoms of heart failure can ensue (Fig. 40-2). Symptom management can be complex and side effects of drugs can worsen symptoms. Some guidelines are offered in Table 40-1.

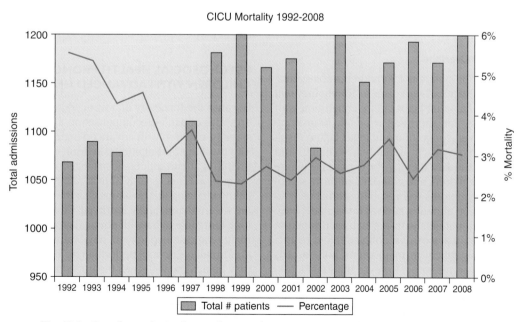

Fig. 40-1 Overall mortality in a large pediatric cardiac intensive care unit. (Data provided by the authors.)

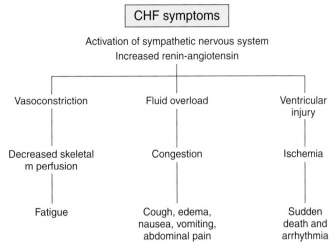

Fig. 40-2 Pathophysiology of cardiac symptoms in children.

Fatigue

The activation of both the renin-angiotensin system and the sympathetic nervous system results in vasoconstriction and poor skeletal muscle perfusion. This often leads to overwhelming fatigue, sometimes out of proportion to the cardiac dysfunction. For patients in the early phases of advanced heart disease, fatigue can be particularly difficult to sort out, as it can often be confused with laziness or depression. Modified physical therapy and cardiac rehabilitation programs can be useful to avoid deconditioning and maintaining muscle tone. In addition, modified exercise programs have been shown to be beneficial to outlook and endurance in patients with CHD.[12] For the more advanced heart disease patients, systemic vasodilators, such as milrinone, can help lower systemic vascular resistance and result in temporary improvement of fatigue. Many children and young adults describe "something lifting off my chest" after a few hours of a milronone infusion. There is some anecdotal evidence that a short infusion holiday of 3 to 5 days can have an improved effect lasting for several weeks. Some patients may benefit from this therapy either intermittently or as a continuous infusion.

Congestion and/or Fluid Overload

Fluid overload is a common symptom for children, adolescents, and young adults with advanced heart disease. Rarely, they will present with the traditional adult heart failure congestion with rales, respiratory distress, and shortness of breath. More commonly in children however, congestion and heart failure result in gastrointestinal symptoms such as nausea, vomiting, and anorexia. Diuretics are the key therapy for congestive symptoms in heart failure in children, and can often improve symptoms rapidly. Often GI symptoms will respond dramatically to diuretic therapy. Many loop diuretics, such as furosemide, have a threshold effect, and if patients with normal renal function are not responding, then doses can be doubled. Fluid restriction for these patients is critical in maintaining homeostasis and decreasing hospital admissions. However, fluid restriction can be very difficult, as the body's response to lower output is secretion of ADH and subsequent thirst. Discussion about the utility of fluid restriction and the understanding that the thirst response is counter-regulatory may help some patients and families. The maintenance of fluid restriction for many families is endless and futile, and increasing diuretics may be the simplest action. In addition, timing of diuretics is critical in maintaining good sleep hygiene. Diuretics before bedtime will obstruct sleep. Diuretics should not be given within 4 hours of bedtime.

Dizziness and/or Syncope

Syncope can be a result of primary ventricular arrhythmia, secondary to myocyte fibrosis. This can be very frightening for families and patients. It may be worsened by electrolyte abnormalities such as hypomagnesemia and hypokalemia, which should be monitored closely. Dizziness can be very disturbing for patients, as it may remind them of the pre-syncopal state. It may be due to low cardiac output. More often, however, it is a symptom related to side effects of the cardiac medications and can limit quality of life. The use of multiple anithypertensives together in the morning can often lead to dizziness and headache. Awareness of the total medical picture can help improve timing of medications for patient comfort. However, vasodilating medication could be given at bedtime, as dizziness is less likely once the patient is lying down.

Pain

Pain is unusual in the ambulatory advanced heart disease population. However, pain associated with medical procedures, including minor ones, is not unusual. Needle-stick pain is a major source of trauma for children in healthcare settings, including children who require frequent needle sticks. For outpatient procedures, it may be helpful to provide a written prescription for topical anesthetic cream and instructions for application for the parents. Managing inpatient needle sticks with pain prevention protocols, which include distraction techniques and topical anesthetic creams, may reduce the trauma. Pain can also result from excessive fluid overload and edema of neck, abdomen, and extremities.

Although chest pain is rare, it is very frightening and carries multiple meaning for the families. Opioids can improve coronary perfusion, and may have a primary cardiac role in patients with ischemic disease. Discussions about pain control should occur early on. Many families and caretakers worry about the cardiac effects of opioids. Most cardiac ICUs are comfortable with opioids in the post-operative period. They are critical for comfort at end of life, even while life-extending measures are still in play.

PSYCHOSOCIAL HEALTH PROMOTION FOR CHILDREN WITH ADVANCED HEART DISEASE

Because the trajectory of advanced heart disease is marked by episodes of acute decompensation alternating with periods of stability, children with advanced heart disease may be community dwelling and attending school, community dwelling, and unable to attend school, hospitalized, or in hospice care. Health promotion is necessarily individualized to each child. However, acknowledging this, awareness of the pervasive impact of CHD on the child and family is critical. Children with CHD may have long-term difficulties with physical growth, gross motor development, exercise capacity, behavioral abnormalities, psychiatric abnormalities, school performance, and quality of life.[13] Parents may be dealing with both the uncertainty of their child's illness and the stress of managing complicated feeding regimens, multiple medications, outpatient visits, and diagnostic procedures. Though evidence is limited, this may result in physical and mental health problems in parents or siblings, attenuated education for mothers, and a negative impact on parent employment.[14,15]

TABLE 40-1   Medication Guidelines

Medication	Indication for use	Dosing	Onset	Side effects	Half-life	Metabolism	Contraindications
Dopamine	To increase cardiac output, blood pressure, and urine output. Volume depletion should be corrected before starting dopamine.	Renal and mesenteric vasodilation: 2–5 mcg/kg/min (beta) effect: 5–10 mcg/kg/min IV infusion	Within 5 min	Tachydysrhythmias, vasoconstriction, at higher doses. Anginal pain, and palpitations	2 min	Metabolized in the plasma, kidneys, and liver	Hypersensitivity to sulfites. Care must be given to ensure that extravasation does not occur. Extravasation causes severe tissue necrosis
Dobutamine	To increase cardiac output and to manage short-term cardiac decompensation. Volume depletion should be corrected before starting dobutamine.	2–20 mcg/kg/min IV infusion Transient hypotension	1–10 min	Ectopic heart beats, increased heart rate, chest pain, headache, nausea and vomiting, dyspnea	2 min	Metabolized in the tissues and liver	Hypersensitivity to sulfites and idiopathic hypertrophic subaortic stenosis
Milrinone	To treat low cardiac output syndrome and congestive heart failure. Increase cardiac output and stroke volume, decrease intracardiac filling pressures, and decrease systemic vascular resistance without changing heart rate or myocardial oxygen consumption. Milrinone has fewer side effects.	Maintenance infusion: 0.2 to 1 mcg/kg	5–15 min	Headache, ventricular dysrhythmias, hypotension, and chest pain	1–5 hrs	Excretion by the kidneys	Severe pulmonary or aortic obstructive disease and hypersensitivity to milrinone
Furosemide	A loop diuretic used to reduce preload. Furosemide as either a continuous drip or intermittent boluses can be given.	IV infusion: 0.05 mg/kg/hr titrated to clinical effect. Intermittent IV: 1–2 mg/kg/dose every 6–12 hrs 2 mg/kg orally 3 times a day	IV: 5 min PO: 30–60 min	Hypotension, dizziness, uticaria, electrolyte imbalances, potential ototoxicity with high doses, jaundice	Normal renal function 30 min; with renal failure—9 hrs	Metabolized by the liver in 80% excreted in the urine	Indomethacin decreases effect
Bumetanide	A loop diuretic is indicated to reduce preload	0.015–0.1mg/kg/dose, given every 6–24 hrs IV/PO	Within a few minutes when given IV	Hypotension, chest pain, dizziness, rash, hyperglycemia, electrolyte imbalance, elevated liver enzymes, ototoxicity, elevated serum creatinine	Ranges from 1 hr to 2½ hrs	Partially metabolized in the liver and excreted in the urine	Hypersensitivity to bumetanide and anuria or increasing azotemia

Continued

TABLE 40-1 Medication Guidelines—cont'd

Medication	Indication for use	Dosing	Onset	Side effects	Half-life	Metabolism	Contraindications
Spironolactone	A potassium-sparing diuretic acting on the distal collecting duct of the nephron. This drug is indicated for treatment of CHF. May be used in conjunction with Lasix and digoxin	1–2 mg/kg/day orally given once a day or divided into 2 doses given every 12 hrs	1 to 3 hrs	Dysrhythmias, lethargy, confusion, ataxia, rash, electrolyte imbalance, dehydration, decreased renal function		Metabolized in the liver and excreted in the urine and biliary tracts	If given with potassium supplements, may increase potassium serum levels. Spironolactone, when given with potassium supplements, may potentiate inotropic affect of digoxin while decreasing digoxin clearance
Prostaglandin E₁	An endogenous fatty acid indicated to maintain the patency of the ductus arteriosus. This is vitally important with ductal dependent lesions such as severe coarctation of the aorta, critical pulmonary stenosis, and transposition of the great arteries	0.05 mcg/kg/min may be doubled every 15–30 min up to a maximum dose of 0.2 mcg/kg/min until desired effect is obtained. The infusion may be decreased to the lowest effective dose once ductal patency is achieved	Relatively short, with immediate effects	Apnea, hypotension, seizures, flushing, elevated temperature		Metabolized rapidly in the pulmonary circulation and excreted by the kidneys	

Adapted from Miller-Hoover, S.R. Pediatric and Neonatal Cardiovascular Pharmacology. Pediatric Nursing 2003; 29(2): 105–115. Reprinted with permission of Janetti Publications, Inc. www.pediatricnursing.net

Very little is known about the subset of children with advanced heart disease and their families in this regard. However, it is likely that their difficulties are even more accentuated.

The evidence that CHD has a pervasive impact on the child and family has resulted in a paradigm shift from survival and managing medical morbidity to proactively maximizing not only the physical health, but also the psychosocial health of both affected children and their families for all children with CHD. Therefore, palliative care provides an ideal framework for the long-term management of children with CHD beginning with diagnosis, recognizing that for some, this means beginning palliative care prenatally.

PSYCHOSOCIAL CARE FOR CHILDREN WITH ADVANCED HEART DISEASE AND THEIR FAMILIES

As with any life-threatening chronic illness, CHD impacts the psychosocial health of affected children and families. The exact nature of the risk is difficult to pinpoint given the complexity of adaptation to chronic illness and inconsistencies in both research methods and findings. However, a body of research is emerging indicating that children with CHD may be at risk for a range of psychosocial issues, including behavioral problems, neurodevelopmental abnormalities, difficulty with social functioning, and psychiatric disorders.[13,16] As healthcare team members evaluate children with CHD, each of these areas should be considered in order to identify areas for intervention to maximize the child's quality of life.

Behavioral Problems

A systematic review of psychological adjustment of children with CHD described parental reports of behavioral difficulties ranging from 5% to 41% and at rates in excess of those occurring in normative samples or control groups.[17] Both internalizing and externalizing problems are described in the literature.[16–19] Further, school-age children who required surgery for CHD in the newborn period were 3 to 4 times more likely to achieve clinically significant scores for inattention and hyperactivity than normative samples.[20] Disease severity was not significantly related to behavior problems in a recent meta-analysis.[17] However, there is evidence that older age,[17,19] deep hypothermic circulatory arrest, cyanosis, older age at repair, and multiple surgical procedures[21] may be risk factors for long-term behavior problems. Despite the technological advances, behavioral outcomes of children repaired recently are not statistically different than those of children repaired in previous eras.[22] Family characteristics have been associated with behavioral problems in children with CHD, including maternal worry and distress, maternal mental health, parenting style, and single parent household.[17,23] Importantly, in a 2007 study,[23] 59% of the variance in behavioral outcomes was explained by parenting style, maternal worry, marital status, maternal mental health, and cyanotic status. Behavioral problems may affect many areas of quality of life, including family dynamics, school success, and social interactions, and are a key area for assessment and intervention when identified.

Neurodevelopmental Abnormalities

Children with CHD have, in general, higher rates of neurodevelopmental abnormalities than healthy peers[13] with a reported incidence as high as 46% of children who require intervention for CHD.[24] These abnormalities are multifactorial, including genetic abnormalities, brain abnormalities, and peri-operative factors such as deep hypothermic circulator arrest.[13,25] Specific areas of concern include developmental and cognitive delays, sensorimotor abnormalities, and social skills delays.[23,24,26–28] Much like behavioral problems, careful evaluation of the neurodevelopment status of children with CHD is very important along with early referral for special services when abnormalities are identified.

Social Functioning

The social milieu of children with CHD is much like that of other children, with an initial focus on the home and family and broadening to an ever-increasing focus on school and peers. Children with CHD and behavioral and/or neurodevelopmental abnormalities may be at particular risk socially because those abnormalities may accentuate differences from their peers. Further, limited exercise capacity may preclude participation in activities with their peers. These factors are critically important because adolescents and young adults with CHD often describe feeling different from their peers[29,30] and report low self-esteem.[31] School-age children who had undergone cardiac transplantation, most of whom had CHD, described the impact of scars, the need for medication, activity restrictions, and decreased physical endurance on their self-perception.[32] Further, they described problems with being bullied and teased by their peers.[32] Children with CHD may be more at risk for social difficulties as they mature, given the increasing importance of peer relationships with age. This may be particularly challenging for children with advanced heart failure because fatigue will decrease their ability to participate in social and recreational activities with peers and accentuate differences from peers.

Family Psychosocial Impact

Life-threatening CHD affects the child's family as well. Parents of children with CHD have higher rates of psychosocial morbidity than parents of either healthy children or those with other chronic medical conditions.[33] Research has identified areas of risk for parents, including high care-giving demand, psychological distress, and psychiatric disorders.[13] Parents describe high care-giving demands, particularly related to feeding and medication regimens.[34] However, they identify psychological stress as their most significant problem[15] and at rates in excess of normative samples.[35] Sources of stress include medical and surgical procedures, activity restrictions, uncertainty, the child's prognosis, the child's behavior, decisions about disclosing medical details to the child, transitioning older children to self-management, and perceptions that their child is different.[34–38] Parents of children with hypoplastic left heart syndrome may be at particular risk[18] as are parents of children with advanced heart failure. Parents also experience significant rates of psychiatric comorbidities, including depression, anxiety, and somatization, and there is evidence that these are chronic in nature.[39] Further, parents of children with CHD may also be at risk for post-traumatic stress disorder given the known incidence in parents of children with life-threatening illness.[40,41] Risk factors for psychiatric comorbidities include the burden of care giving, social isolation, financial issues, and dissatisfaction with medical care.[39] Further, mothers of children with CHD may be at risk for attenuated education and employment.[15]

Less is known about the psychosocial impact of CHD on siblings. However, there is evidence that healthy siblings of children with CHD have an increased incidence of behavior, school and emotional problems, and depression.[16,42] In a 2005 study,[43] 30% of parents indicated that CHD affected their healthy children in a variety of ways including anxiety, depression, anger, jealousy, recreational opportunities, feeling left out, and perceiving that the child with CHD lived under different rules. Parents of transplanted children and those with cyanotic CHD were more likely to report negative sibling effects.[43] Given the described impact of CHD on the psychosocial well-being of the affected child and his or her parents and siblings, palliative care for children with CHD involves attention to the psychosocial health of the entire family.

Promoting Quality of Life for Children and Families

Much of the research describing the quality of life of children with CHD indicates that it is good and/or equivalent to that of healthy children, yet describe abnormalities on both the physical and psychosocial domains of quality of life.[13,17,44,45] Little is known about the quality of life of children with advanced heart failure. However, in a 2008 study, 20% of children with CHD reported significantly impaired quality of life, with similar rates for both mild and severe CHD.[44] In children and adolescents with CHD, parents and healthcare providers were asked to identify quality of life concerns, all groups more frequently identified physical dimensions, most often physical limitations.[46] This is critically important in the subset of children with advanced heart failure who lack the physical stamina to participate in many developmentally appropriate activities. Scarring, medication regimens, receiving special treatment, school issues, and social issues were identified by school-age children and/or their parents as negatively affecting the children's quality of life.[46] While medication regimens were also identified by adolescents and their parents, adolescents also noted the negative impact of feeling different from peers and recognition of their own mortality.[46] Adolescents also noted positive aspects of CHD, including increased strength as a person and not taking life for granted.[46] Research with children with cancer and after heart transplant has demonstrated the utility of asking children a few simple questions to assess quality of life: what makes a good day for you, what makes a bad day for you, and are there some things you would like to do that you cannot?[32,47] Although less is known about the quality of life of parents and siblings of children with CHD, in a 2008 study, parents of children with CHD reported significantly worse quality of life than control parents on all dimensions.[48]

DECISION MAKING IN CHILDREN WITH ADVANCED HEART DISEASE

As summarized previously, many children and families with advanced heart disease have long-standing and complex behavioral, psychosocial, and neurocognitive issues that must be clearly understood and evaluated before or in parallel with the decision-making process. There are, however, limited data surrounding the end-of-life care in pediatric cardiology. There are several issues that are specific to children with advanced heart disease that need to be understood in order to help families with decision-making around end of life. The overall level of palliative care needs is most likely similar between cardiac and oncology patients; that is need for symptom relief, and communication and decision-making issues with intense family support. This is complicated by the highly variable trajectory of advanced heart disease with many patients experiencing acute exacerbations followed by periods of stability. The trigger point to discuss palliative decision making versus curative therapy is often hazy, and caretakers do not always agree on that point in time. Care of children with CHD is interdisciplinary from the beginning. However, the shift from a curative approach to palliative care is a critical time for the interdisciplinary team to work together to address symptom relief and end of life options. While the roles of many team members overlap, such as providing support to the child and family, and communicating with the child, family, and other team members, each team member makes a valued contribution to the palliative care of children with advanced heart disease (Table 40-3).

High Technological Interventions and Advanced Planning

Decisions regarding technological devices are another important component to decision making. The wider acceptance of mechanical support in the form of ventricular assist devices and extracorporeal membrane oxygenation (ECMO) support bring another level of complexity to the decision making process. The acceptance of technology must not be seen as working in contrast with palliative care. These technologies must be incorporated into the spectrum of therapy for advanced heart disease. Families and caretakers can hold on to the hope of recovery or transplant while on a device, while also making preparations and plans for symptom relief and minimizing suffering. This balance is delicate. Reliance on mechanical support strategies will provide an important new area for understanding palliative care needs in advanced heart disease patients, and in children in particular.

Many children who progress to advanced heart disease already have an implantable defibrillator. Again, this technology provides some safety from sudden death, but at the expense of pain and anxiety from defibrillation if the device fires, as well as the possibility of continued firing at end of life. Turning off the defibrillator is a difficult decision for families and patients, and plans should be set in place before end of life. Many families cannot bear to turn it off until the end stage, which can sometimes be disturbing at end of life.

Because of the advanced nature of the heart disease of children who require ECMO or ventricular assist device support, there may be instances when withdrawing mechanical support is a consideration. Because both means of support require anticoagulation, there is a risk of hemorrhagic stroke. Children may develop multi-system organ failure that precludes transplantation. In those settings, many families elect to withdraw support. The difficulties for families with a ventricular assist device (VAD) often revolve around the patient, who may be cognitively aware and neurologically intact, with the heart beating, with severe end-organ dysfunction. This type of withdrawal by terminating the pump function feels different to the medical caretakers and families than withdrawal of an endotracheal tube. In a review of caretakers following the withdrawal of intervention support in two patients, medical caretakers identified significant psychological distress regarding discontinuation of VAD support.[49] Formal institutional policy for VAD patients at end of life may help improve medical caretakers and family stress around this issue. These issues will need to be addressed with the intensive care unit teams and families together, in a sensitive and proactive manner.

Advance planning for children with advanced heart failure should include discussion of high-technology interventions such as ECMO and VAD. Many families choose to do everything possible. It should also include consideration of less technologically intensive interventions such as cardiac catheterizations, non-invasive cardiac imaging studies, and blood draws. Many families choose high-risk surgical or interventional procedures

TABLE 40-2 Interdisciplinary Team Approach to Children with Advanced Heart Disease

Team member	Contribution to care
Child and family	• Head of the team • In-depth knowledge of child, family, and illness experience • Awareness of needs, beliefs, values, and culture • Make decisions in collaboration with team • Communicate with one another and team members • Provide care for child

Cardiology medical team:
  Primary cardiologist
  Pediatric intensivist
  Cardiac surgeon
  Advanced practice nurse
	• Assess child and family
	• Manage the child's advanced heart disease and multi-system effects
	• Manage symptoms
	• Presentation of possible appropriate treatment choices
	• Refer to consultants as appropriate
	• Assist with decision making
	• Provide support to child and family
	• Communicate with child, family, and other team members
	• Communicate with primary care team

Primary care team:
  Pediatrician
  Outpatient therapists
  Teachers
	• Assess child and family
	• Manage primary care issues
	• Provide support to child and family
	• Assist with decision making
	• Communicate with child, family, and other team members

Cardiology nursing team	• Assess child and family • Respond to physical and psychosocial responses to advanced heart disease • Provide bedside nursing care • Coordinate care among disciplines • Advocate for child and family • Provide support and education to child and family • Communicate with child, family, and other team members
Palliative care team	• Assess child and family • Identify goals for care • Assist with decision making • Assist with symptom management • Provide a proactive approach to end-of-life discussions • Identify resources • Provide support to child and family • Communicate with child, family, and other team members
Social worker	• Assess child and family • Respond to child and family psychosocial needs • Advocate for child and family • Assist with coping with illness and hospitalization • Provide support to child and family • Identify resources, including financial, and refer as appropriate • Communicate with child, family, and other team members
Psychologist	• Assess child and family • Respond to psychological needs • Provide support to child and family • Communicate with child, family, and other team members
Respiratory therapist	• Assess child and family • Manage respiratory care • Provide support to child and family • Communicate with child, family, and other team members
Child life specialist	• Assess child and family • Prepare child and family for procedures and provide support during • Provide opportunity for medical play, distraction, and therapeutic play • Assist with coping with illness and hospitalization • Provide support to child and family • Communicate with child, family, and other team members
Physical and occupational therapist	• Assess child and family • Help child maintain function • Coordinate rehabilitation • Provide support to child and family • Communicate with child, family, and other team members
Nutritionist	• Assess child and family • Manage nutritional and growth needs • Provide support to child and family • Communicate with child, family, and other team members
Pharmacist	• Assess child and family • Collaborate with team for safe management of complex medication regimens • Educate child and family regarding medications • Communicate with child, family, and other team members
Chaplain	• Assess child and family • Provide spiritual care and respond to spiritual needs • Provide support to child and family • Provide support for decision making within the context of religious and spiritual beliefs • Communicate with child, family, and other team members

with uncertain outcomes because they do not know what may lie ahead otherwise. Families and medical caretakers need to understand the limitations of doing everything. Cardiologists and cardiac surgeons are not always good at validating the choice some families have to preserve independence and not push forward. We must recognize individual differences in preferences for quality of life vs. survival for these children. Key considerations include: impact of the interventions on the child's survival, impact on the child and family's quality of life, and impact on current management. In collaboration with the interdisciplinary team, families may elect to forego interventions based upon burden and/or ambiguous outcomes.

Clinical Vignette

AB was diagnosed with cardiomyopathy at 1 year of age and underwent cardiac transplantation without complication. His course was uncomplicated for the first 5 years post transplant and he was managed as an outpatient by the multi-disciplinary team. At 5 years of age, he presented to clinic because his mother observed that he "did not look right," had poor appetite, and was uninterested in play. On echocardiogram, his cardiac function was very poor and he had evidence of myocarditis, rejection, and cardiac allograft vasculopathy. He was admitted to the intensive care unit for intravenous inotropes to maintain cardiac output. Because of progressive cardiac allograft vasculopathy, persistent poor cardiac function, and continued need for high-dose inotropes, he was re-listed for transplant. Work-up revealed exposure to parvovirus, a likely cause of his acute decompensation. His mother, who was pregnant, was also exposed to parvovirus and delivered at 33 weeks' gestation. The infant died in the newborn period of viral sepsis and cardiomyopathy. AB's physical condition stabilized on IV inotropes and symptoms were manageable medically. However, AB's and his family's psychosocial care was particularly challenging as the team worked to help the family cope with both AB's need for re-transplant and the loss of the premature infant.

AB underwent his second cardiac transplantation 40 days after admission and had a complicated course, including the need for ECMO on post-operative day 1 for graft failure. Once more, the family required intensive psychosocial support from the multi-disciplinary team as they worked to managed the uncertainty of AB's condition in the context of the recent loss of their newborn. His rejection was managed medically and he was weaned off ECMO after 6 days. His course thereafter was uncomplicated. However, he required intensive rehabilitative physical and occupational therapy to restore function after his lengthy critical illness. He was discharged to home just 3 weeks after transplant with outpatient medical management including physical and occupational therapy.

Two years later, AB presented with respiratory distress and was diagnosed with cytomegalovirus pneumonia and was successfully treated. His hospital stay was less than 2 weeks and he was discharged home for continued outpatient medical management. Within 6 months of this admission, he developed signs of heart failure and evaluation revealed cardiac allograft vasculopathy, which once again progressed rapidly. When he required intravenous inotropes for his decompensated heart failure, treatment options, including ECMO and VAD, were considered. Because he had developed cardiac allograft vas-

culopathy with both his first and second transplant, he was not a candidate for a third transplant. Because AB did not have a long-term option, the family and team elected to forego mechanical support and concentrate on supportive care. AB had a wish to see the Disney princesses, therefore the team and family focused on transitioning AB to oral medications to manage his heart failure. AB was discharged home on oral medications for heart failure and went to Disney World with his family. He rode all the rides and saw all the Disney princesses. On the last day of the trip, he was laughing on the water ride with his mom and sister, "fell asleep," and died.

Future Issues

Although there are descriptive studies that help identify areas for palliative care intervention in children with advanced heart disease, few interventions are described in the literature. Therefore, the next steps in the palliative care of children with advanced heart disease includes the need for development and testing of interventions to improve the multidimensional health and quality of life for children with CHD. Further, very little is known about the spiritual health and end of life issues for children and families, even from a descriptive standpoint.

The role for palliative care for children with advanced heart disease is expanding. Although many issues are similar to other life-threatening chronic illnesses, it is critical to understand the differences in the cardiac population in order to maximize the impact of palliative care for children with advanced heart failure and their families. A critical first step in improving palliative care is gaining understanding of and identifying clear prognostic indicators for children with advanced heart disease. This will help the healthcare team better understand which patients will benefit from an early palliative approach. In addition, it is critical to educate physicians and families that using a palliative care model supports maintaining hope for long-term survival while also providing symptom support and decision-making structure. Lastly, research studies attempting to understand bereavement issues for the families around end of life will aid in developing future interventions for this growing population.

REFERENCES

1. Hoffman JI, Kaplan S, Liberthson RR: Prevalence of congenital heart disease, *Am Heart J* 147:425–439, 2004.
2. Keane J, Lock J, Fyler D, editors: *Nadas' pediatric cardiology*, Philadelphia, 2006, Saunders Elsevier.
3. Nugent AW, Daubeney PE, Chondros P, et al: The epidemiology of childhood cardiomyopathy in Australia, *N Engl J Med* 348(17): 1639–1646, 2003.
4. Lipshultz SE, Sleeper LA, Towbin JA, et al: The incidence of pediatric cardiomyopathy in two regions of the United States, *N Engl J Med* 348(17):1647–1655, 2003.
5. Rosenthal D, Chrisant MR, Edens E, et al: International Society for Heart and Lung Transplantation: Practice guidelines for management of heart failure in children, *J Heart Lung Transplant* 23(12): 1313–1333, 2004.
6. Canter CE, Shaddy RE, Bernstein D, et al: Indications for heart transplantation in pediatric heart disease: a scientific statement from the American Heart Association Council on Cardiovascular Disease in the young; the Councils on Clinical Cardiology, Cardiovascular Nursing, and Cardiovascular Surgery and Anesthesia; and the Quality of Care and Outcomes Research Interdisciplinary Working Group, *Circulation* 115(5):658–676, 2007.

7. Noonan JA: A History of Pediatric Specialties: The development of pediatric cardiology, *Pediatr Res* 56(2):298–306, 2004.

8. Freedom RM, Lock J, Bricker JT: Pediatric cardiology and cardiovascular surgery: 1950–2000, *Circulation* 102:IV-58–IV-68, 2000.

9. Boneva RS, Botto LD, Moore CA, Yang Q, Correa A, Erickson JD: Mortality associated with congenital heart defects in the United States: trends and racial disparities, 1979–1997, *Circulation* 103(19):2376–2381, 2001.

10. O'Leary N: The comparative palliative care needs of those with heart failure and cancer patients, *Curr Opin Support Palliat Care* 3(4):241–246, 2009.

11. Hupcey JE, Penrod J, Fensternmacher K: A model of palliative care for heart failure, *Am J Hospice Palliat Care Med* 26(5):399–404, 2009.

12. Rhodes J, Curran TJ, Camil L, Rabideau NC, Fulton DR, Gauthier NS, Gauvreau K, Jenkins KJ: Impact of cardiac rehabilitation upon the exercise function of children with serious congenital heart disease, *Pediatrics* 116:1339–1345, 2005.

13. Green A: Outcomes of congenital heart disease: a review, *Pediatr Nurs* 30(4):280–284, 2004.

14. Bjornstad PG, Spurkland I, Lindberg HI: The impact of severe congenital heart disease on physical and psychosocial functioning in adolescents, *Cardiol Young* 5:56–62, 1995.

15. Samenek M: Congenital heart malformations: prevalence, severity, survival, and quality of life, *Cardiol Young* 10:179–185, 2000.

16. Mussatto KA: Psychological and social aspects of paediatric heart disease. In Anderson RH, et al. editors: *Paediatric cardiology*, ed 3, Philadelphia, 2009, Elsevier.

17. Latal B, Helfricht S, Fischer JE, et al: Psychological adjustment and quality of life in children and adolescents following open-heart surgery for congenital heart disease: a systematic review, *BMC Pediatr* 9:6, 2009.

18. Brosig CL, Mussatto KA, Kuhn EM, et al: Psychosocial outcomes for preschool children and families after surgery for complex congenital heart disease, *Pediatr Cardiol* 28:255–262, 2007.

19. Karsdrop PA, Everaerd W, Kindt M, et al: Psychological and cognitive functioning in children and adolescents with congenital heart disease: a meta-analysis, *J Pediatr Psychol* 32(5):527–554, 2007.

20. Shillingford AJ, Glanzman MM, Ittenback RF, et al: Inattention, hyperactivity, and school performance in a population of school-age children with complex congenital heart disease, *Pediatrics* 121(4):e759–e767, 2008.

21. Utens EM, Verhults FC, Duivenvoorden HJ, et al: Prediction of behavioural and emotional problems in children and adolescents with congenital heart disease, *Eur Heart J* 19:801–807, 1998.

22. Spijkerboer AW, Utens EM, Bogers AJ, et al: A historical comparison of long-term behavioral and emotional outcomes in children and adolescents after invasive treatment for congenital heart disease, *J Pediatr Surg* 43:534–539, 2008.

23. McCusker CG, Doherty NN, Molloy B, et al: Determinants of neuropsychological and behavioural outcomes in early childhood survivors of congenital heart disease, *Arch Dis Child* 92:137–141, 2007.

24. Weinberg S, Kern J, Weiss K, et al: Developmental screening of children diagnosed with congenital heart defects, *Clin Pediatr (Phila)* 40:49–51, 2001.

25. Newburger JW: Neurodevelopmental outcomes after heart surgery in children. In Allen HD, et al. editors: *Moss and Adams' heart disease in infants, children, and adolescents: including the fetus and young adults*, ed 7 Philadelphia, 2008, Lippincott Williams & Wilkins.

26. Mahle WT: Neurologic and cognitive outcomes in children with congenital heart disease, *Curr Opin Pediatr* 13:482–486, 2001.

27. Forbess JM, Visconti KJ, Hancock-Friessen C, et al: Neurodevelopmental outcome after congenital heart surgery: Results from an institutional registry, *Circulation* 106(Suppl 1):I93–I102, 2002.

28. Limperopoulos C, Mahnemer A, Shevell MJ, et al: Predictors of developmental disabilities after open-heart surgery in young children with congenital heart defects, *J Pediatr* 141(1):51–58, 2002.

29. Horner T, Liberthson R, Jellinek MS: Psychosocial profile of adults with complex congenital heart disease, *Mayo Clin Proc* 75(1):31–36, 2000.

30. Tong EM, Sparacino PS, Messias DK, et al: Growing up with congenital heart disease: the dilemmas of adolescents and young adults, *Cardiol Young* 8:303–309, 1998.

31. Salzer-Muhar U, Herle M, Floquet P, et al: Self-concept in male and female adolescents with congenital heart disease, *Clin Pediatr (Phila)* 41:17–24, 2002.

32. Green A, McSweeney J, Ainley K, et al: In my shoes: children's quality of life after heart transplant, *Prog Transplant* 17(3):199–207, 2008.

33. Lawoko S: Factors Influencing satisfaction and well-being among parents of congenital heart disease children: development of a conceptual model based upon a literature review, *Scand J Caring Sci* 21:106–117, 2007.

34. Morelius E, Lundh U, Nelson N: Parental stress in relation to severity of congenital heart disease in offspring, *Pediatr Nurs* 28(1):28–32, 2002.

35. Uzark K, Jones K: Parenting stress with congenital heart disease, *J Pediatr Health Care* 17:163–168, 2003.

36. Gudmundsdottir M, Gillis CL, Sparacino PS, et al: Congenital heart defects and parent adolescent coping, *Fam Syst Health* 14(2):245–255, 1996.

37. Tak YR, McCubbin M: Family Stress, Perceived social support, and coping following the diagnosis of a child's congenital heart disease, *J Adv Nurs* 39(3):190–198, 2002.

38. Sparacino PSA, Tong EM, Messias DKH, et al: The dilemmas of parents of adolescents and young adults with congenital heart disease, *Heart Lung* 26(3):187–195, 1997.

39. Lawoko S, Soares JJF: Psychosocial morbidity among parents of children with congenital heart disease: a longitudinal study, *Heart Lung* 35:301–314, 2006.

40. Santacroce SJ: Parental uncertainty and post-traumatic stress in serious childhood illness, *J Nurs Scholarsh* 35(1):45–51, 2003.

41. Farley LM, DeMaso DR, D'Angela E, et al: Parenting stress and parental post-traumatic stress disorder in families after pediatric heart transplantation, *J Heart Lung Transplant* 26(2):120–126, 2007.

42. Bellin MH, Kovacs PJ: Fostering resilience in siblings of youths with a chronic condition: a review of the literature, *Health Soc Work* 31(3):209–216, 2006.

43. Wray J, Maynard L: Living with congenital or acquired heart disease in childhood: maternal perceptions of the impact on the child and family, *Cardiol Young* 15:133–140, 2005.

44. Uzark K, Jones K, Slusher J, et al: Quality of life in children with heart disease as perceived by children and families, *Pediatrics* 121(5):e1060–e1067, 2008.

45. Landolt MA, Blechel ER, Latal B: Health-related quality of life in children and adolescents after open-heart surgery, *J Pediatr* 152:349–355, 2008.

46. Marino BS, Tomlinson RS, Drotar D, et al: Quality-of-life concerns differ among patients, parents, and medical providers in children and adolescents with congenital and acquired heart disease, *Pediatrics* 123:e708–e715, 2009.

47. Hinds PS, Gattuso JS, Fletcher A, et al: Quality of life as conveyed by pediatric patients with cancer, *Qual Life Res* 13:761–772, 2004.

48. Arafa MA, Zaher SR, El-Dowaty AA, et al: Quality of life among parents of children with heart disease, *Health Qual Life Outcomes* 6:91, 2008.

49. Thiagarajan R: Personal communication, abstract in submission.

41 Cystic Fibrosis

ELISABETH POTTS DELLON | JEFFREY C. KLICK | WALTER M. ROBINSON

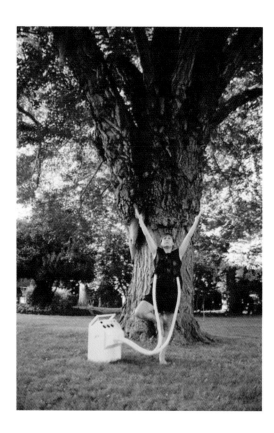

Vrksasana

Magnificent tree

reaching upward toward the sky

grounding me

Miraculous breath

flowing throughout my body

sustaining me

Mind, body, spirit

seeking balance and wholeness

strengthening me

   —Robyn Petras

With permission from "The Breathing Room: The Art of Living with Cystic Fibrosis" at www.thebreathingroom.org (Photo by Stephen Boyer.)

Cystic fibrosis (CF) is a well-known disease to most pediatricians and pediatric palliative care clinicians. Given the degree of familiarity about the disease for the readers of this volume, this chapter intertwines two goals: to provide an updated view of CF in the early twenty-first century and to propose an ideal and somewhat novel model for integrating the pediatric palliative care team into the care of patients and families affected by CF. While the population of adults with CF will soon be larger than that of children,[1] this chapter does not include a comprehensive discussion of the palliative care of adults with CF because most are cared for in adult CF centers with different challenges and resources.

As described further in this chapter, the typical patterns of care for patients with CF have historically presented predictable barriers to the successful integration of palliative care. Understanding of the natural history, the changing epidemiology and cultural understanding, and the perceived and actual physical and psychosocial burden of the disease will help palliative care providers better understand how to integrate their clinical expertise and psychosocial support of the patient and family into the established and successful CF model of clinical care. Further, this can be done without disrupting the typically well-established relationships between patients and their families with the CF care team. While the proposed value added model described later and outlined in Table 41-1, may not seem distinctive to many palliative care providers,[2] it will be seen as a novel approach by most CF care teams.

An Overview

Cystic fibrosis is a life-threatening genetic disease with an incidence of 1 in 3200 live births in the United States. An estimated 30,000 people are now living with CF in North America.[3] CF is a multisystem disease resulting from mutations in the cystic fibrosis transmembrane regulator (CFTR) gene, causing abnormal chloride ion transport across epithelial cells lining the airways, pancreatic ducts, gastrointestinal tract, and reproductive organs. This abnormal transport leads to dehydrated and viscous secretions. Clinical manifestations of this defect include recurrent respiratory infections, nutritional deficiencies related to malabsorption from pancreatic exocrine insufficiency, intestinal obstruction, hepatobiliary disease, diabetes, and male azospermia.[4] The natural history of CF is a progressive decline in lung function caused by recurrent infection, inflammation, and bronchial obstruction leading to bronchiectasis and subsequent ongoing inflammation, infection, and airway damage. Chronic inflammation and infection of the airways accounts for most of the morbidity in CF, and the vast majority of patients with CF eventually die from respiratory failure.[5]

Survival in CF has increased dramatically over time due to advancements in medical care. Additionally, lung transplantation

TABLE 41-1 Help From Palliative Care Teams

How can the pediatric palliative care team help the CF team care for children, adolescents and families with CF throughout the lifespan?

Before the diagnosis is made

Help the CF care team design and implement a supportive and compassionate approach to those who have a positive newborn screen for CF, realizing that a positive screen can be a distressing experience even if the infant is not diagnosed with the disease.

At the time of diagnosis

Help the CF team care develop strategies to mitigate the impact of parental grief following the disclosure of a life-threatening diagnosis in an infant, especially if the infant is apparently healthy.

During routine care

Help the CF care team anticipate and prepare for emotional reactions to the first hospitalization, which can trigger parental anxiety about disease progression and mortality.

Help the CF care team become comfortable with discussions of mortality throughout the patient's life, so that the team is prepared for inevitable questions and discussion with patients and families.

As the disease progresses

Help the CF care team gain expertise in the assessment and treatment of symptoms throughout the lifespan, including expertise in pain management and assessment of non-pulmonary, non-GI symptoms, such as fatigue or anxiety.

Help the CF care team plan a comprehensive roadmap for the decisions, which will be faced by patients, parents, and clinicians in the now rarer instance of a childhood or adolescent death, including anticipatory guidance about the use of aggressive technologies.

Offer the CF care team assistance with planning and carrying out the process of transplant decision making. (See Table 41-3.)

Offer expertise and experience with managing symptoms and end of life care in different settings, such as at home or through pediatric hospice services, if available.

After the death of the child or adolescent

Offer comprehensive bereavement services for the family, siblings, and medical providers.

---

for advanced CF lung disease is an option that may extend life or improve quality of life for select patients. The population of patients with CF is shifting: In 2007, 45% of patients with CF in the United States were adults, and the median predicted survival for patients with CF reached 37.1 years.[1] Despite advancements in care and longer survival, patients with CF and their families endure the challenges associated with a chronic disease, including the burden of numerous therapies and disease exacerbations, the knowledge of a limited lifespan, the responsibility of complex decision making regarding lung transplant and other intensive treatments, and the stigma and reproductive choices associated with a genetic disease.

The Current Approach

From the time of diagnosis, daily therapies are prescribed for maintenance of respiratory health and nutritional status, and emphasis is placed on psychosocial implications of chronic disease. To facilitate management of this complex disease, an interdisciplinary approach to care is believed to be essential. In addition to receiving standard medical care from a primary care provider, many patients attend quarterly or more frequent clinic visits and receive hospital care at specialty CF care centers. CF care teams are composed of multiple providers, including physicians, nurses, social workers, dietitians, physical therapists, and respiratory therapists (Table 41-2).

For patients with CF, basic respiratory care involves a combination of airway clearance techniques to enhance removal of mucus from the lower airways, aerosolized therapies to facilitate mucus clearance by altering its viscosity, various antimicrobial and anti-inflammatory medications, and exercise.[3] Many of these therapies are time-consuming and may prove challenging to maintain. A survey of adults with CF revealed that they spend an average of nearly 2 hours per day on respiratory therapies.[6] Children with CF require close supervision from caregivers, and even older patients often need assistance from caregivers to carry out respiratory therapies and other treatments.[7] With progressive disease, oxygen may be used with exertion, during sleep, and ultimately constantly.[8] Non-invasive positive pressure ventilation may be recommended for patients with hypercarbia and respiratory insufficiency, and has gained favor over time as a bridging therapy for patients awaiting lung transplantation.[9]

Respiratory exacerbations of CF manifest in many ways, with symptoms including increased cough and sputum production, dyspnea, fatigue, fever, chest pain, hemoptysis, sleep disturbance, and weight loss. Concomitant changes in physiologic measures, including chest exam, oxygen saturation, spirometry measures, and weight, may occur. Treatment of respiratory exacerbations involves additional therapies and hospitalization for severe exacerbations for many patients. Intravenous antibiotics are commonly used, often in combination given the challenges of combating virulent and often drug-resistant CF pathogens such as *Pseudomonas aeruginosa*, *oxacillin-resistant Staphylococcus aureus*, and *Burkholderia cepacia*, and therapeutic drug monitoring and surveillance for associated toxicities is necessary. Intensification of aerosolized therapies and airway clearance techniques during exacerbations is also common practice.[5] Complications of progressive CF lung disease, including pneumothorax, hemoptysis, hypercapnia, pulmonary hypertension, and respiratory failure, prompt more extensive evaluation and treatment, sometimes in the intensive care unit.[10]

Patients with pancreatic insufficiency must take pancreatic enzyme supplements with food to enhance digestion and reduce the likelihood of intestinal obstruction, as well as taking fat soluble vitamin supplements to prevent vitamin deficiencies. Anti-reflux medications and laxatives are also commonly prescribed. Because of the established correlation between nutritional status and lung function, great emphasis is placed on appropriate growth for children and weight maintenance in adults.[11] For many patients who struggle to gain weight, nutritional supplements, appetite stimulants, and enteral feedings may become mainstays of therapy. Additionally, approximately one-fifth of adults develop CF-related diabetes, and most of these patients ultimately require frequent glucose monitoring and treatment with insulin injections.[9]

TABLE 41-2 Structure of Outpatient CF Care

Provider	Frequency of visits	Role in CF care
Primary care physician	Variable	Provide routine childhood care Evaluate acute illness Educate and support patients and caregivers
CF physician	At least quarterly	Obtain interval medical and psychosocial history Review multisystem medical issues Perform physical examination Assess physiologic measures Develop and communicate treatment plan Communicate with primary care physician Educate and support patients and caregivers
Nurse	At least quarterly	Assist with medical and psychosocial assessments Coordination Assess understanding of CF and recommended treatments Educate and support patients and caregivers
Dietitian	At least annually	Obtain qualitative dietary history Assess changes in appetite or eating habits Review nutritional status Recommend and assess effects of dietary supplements and other nutritional interventions Educate and support patients and caregivers
Social worker	At least annually	Address psychosocial issues, including coping with chronic disease, family structure, educational issues, financial and insurance concerns Assess understanding of CF and recommended treatments Educate and support patients and caregivers
Physical therapist	At least annually	Educate about airway clearance techniques Assess and educate about exercise Educate and support patients and caregivers
Respiratory therapist	At least quarterly	Lung function testing Assist with obtaining respiratory cultures Educate about airway clearance techniques, aerosolized therapies and oxygen delivery devices
Other consultants*	Variable	Provide services according to discipline and patient need

Adapted from Orenstein DM, Rosenstein BJ, Stern RC. Cystic Fibrosis Medical Care. Lippincott Williams & Williams, Philadelphia, 2000.
*Other specialty areas may include allergy/immunology, anesthesiology, cardiology, endocrinology, gastroenterology, genetics, genetic counseling, infectious disease, neonatology, obstetrics/gynecology, otolaryngology, psychiatry, psychology, pulmonology, radiology, surgery, and urology.

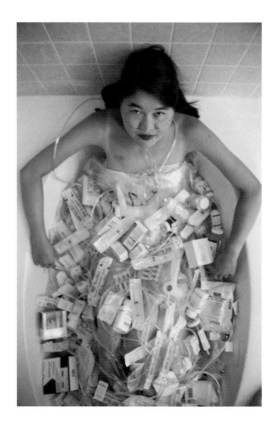

Bathe Me

I want you to bathe me,

cleanse me of this putridity within.

As my body soaks in that which

is meant to remove the foul poison,

I am drowning.

The weight of the tubes,

the pills, the needles, the aerosols pulls me

down like an anchor in a deep sea,

it controls who I am, my time, my life.

I should be floating in a bubble bath

of elegance, luxury, perfection.

Instead, there are no bubbles, they all burst.

It's just me and this bath of disease.

—I. STENZEL

With permission from "The Breathing Room: The Art of Living with Cystic Fibrosis" at www.thebreathingroom.org

Understanding the Goals of Care for the CF Team

When the CFTR gene was initially described in 1989, many believed a cure for the disease was imminent.[12] This hope led to great optimism regarding the approach to care for children with CF. Now, 20 years later, no cure is on the horizon.[13] Widespread and consistent application of chronic treatments by patients and their families has led to increasing life expectancy, and even in the face of the discouraging results of research into a cure from gene transfer, most patients, families, and clinicians maintain an attitude of vigorous optimism toward the disease. CF clinicians generally adopt an enthusiastic approach, becoming cheerleaders for their patients, emphasizing the optimistic increases in life expectancy and vigorously encouraging their patients to keep up hope for improved survival and quality of life. This attitude is in part a response to the outdated image of CF among the general public as a killer of children, in part a strategy to encourage adherence to the increasingly time-consuming daily CF regimen, and in part an antidote to the unpredictable, waxing and waning course of the illness. CF care teams maintain a position of enthusiastic optimism in coaching patients and their families to continue the work associated with a life with CF.

Although there is much to be optimistic about with regard to CF, in some circumstances this optimism may inhibit frank discussion of the reality of life with CF. Despite the ever-expanding life expectancy, people with CF still experience significant suffering.[14-24] The disease burden and physical and psychosocial distress can be seen:

- In the family's distress at the time of diagnosis,
- With the physical symptoms and the emotional suffering during pulmonary exacerbations and intensive care unit stays,
- With the social isolation imposed by the relative rarity of the disease and concerns about transmission of respiratory pathogens between patients, resulting in physical separation from CF peers,
- With the chronic grief that many parents feel as they ponder the effects of a prolonged illness on their child and their family,
- With the physical burden and loss of function associated with symptoms and complications associated with disease progression,
- With the reality that there is still no cure and lung transplant offers only a transient solution to this life-threatening disease.

CF is a lifelong illness that necessitates intense and never-ending therapy. While intensive therapies aimed at maintaining airway clearance and nutrition may stave off exacerbations, patients with CF will invariably experience progressive loss of function; live with the unpredictable risk of exacerbations, worsening lung function and frequent hospitalizations; and, ultimately, suffer a premature death.

Unfortunately, even the most experienced CF medical provider is unable to predict when these episodes of acute illness and loss may occur,[25] and the disease carries a large degree of uncertainty.[26] Many patients with CF experience acute decompensations, recoveries, and periods of relative stability, usually superimposed upon a gradual downward trajectory in lung function (Fig. 41-1). The functional ability of patients over time often mirrors this course. Most patients will have periodic setbacks, and while some of these setbacks will include a complete recovery, others may result in a decline in functional ability. The palliative care provider should recognize how this uncertainty and progressive loss of function will affect children and adults with CF, their families, and their medical providers.

For those with CF and those who care for them, hope and despair are inextricably intertwined. In some circumstances, the hopeful enthusiasm of medical providers and parents can crowd out concerns of the child regarding what he or she has heard about the limited life expectancy in CF. The same enthusiasm may discourage him or her from reporting bothersome symptoms or concerns regarding the burdens of treatment. In these instances, cheerleading is inappropriate, and may even worsen the child's or family's anxiety when a quiet but hopeful discussion might have alleviated their concerns. Cheerleading by medical providers may also prevent the CF care team from recognizing the benefits of collaboration with the palliative care team. What is needed instead is

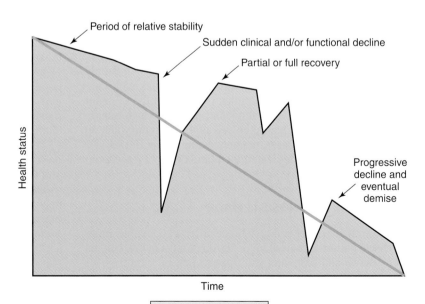

Fig. 41-1 Anticipated trajectory of illness in cystic fibrosis.

a rejection of the either/or attitude toward hope and despair, and a recognition that hope can flourish even in the face of the grim truth of the symptom burden and the limited life expectancy of CF.

Integrating the Palliative Care Team into CF Care

Given this mixed picture of CF, discussing palliative care has been a challenge. In the view of many CF care teams, palliative care is associated only with the medical interventions aimed at providing comfort at the end of life. As a result, specific palliative care interventions, including therapies directed at managing symptoms present in those with mild to moderate disease, are often not introduced until the patient is clearly at the end of life—often too late for the patient and family to derive the benefit of the palliative care team's expertise. Palliative care, clearly differentiated from end of life care and integrated with curative and restorative measures, offers the best chance at limiting the burden of disease, maximizing quality of life at all stages of illness, and providing effective support to children and adults with CF and their families.[27] A value added model, when provided as consulting expertise in a programmatic approach, may succeed in these situations when a more conventional approach has failed and help limit the reluctance of the CF team to involve palliative services.

The model is based on using the expertise of the palliative care team to help the CF team address the grief that often accompanies the diagnosis of a chronic life-threatening illness. It continues by emphasizing the expertise of the palliative care team in assessing and managing symptoms and assessing the burdens of treatment relative to the benefit. As symptoms progress in CF, the palliative care team assists the CF team in responding to the inevitable questions about mortality both from parents and children. The palliative team uses its expertise in discussing these matters to help the CF team be more comfortable with these issues in the context of the generally successful CF routine care. As the disease progresses, the palliative care team should further support the family in the decision making process about lung transplantation, including discussions of mortality and the benefits and burdens of an intensive treatment in pursuing the goals of care, because the current model of care leaves little time for discussion of the use of intensive measures and the goals of care.[28] The palliative care team will then act in a traditional way—it is only during this phase of care that many CF teams traditionally contact the pediatric palliative care team—to assist the CF team in managing end-stage symptoms and providing high quality care at the end of life. Finally, the palliative care team will help in the bereavement process, not only for the family, but also for the long-serving and dedicated members of the CF care team (see Table 41-1).

BEFORE THE DIAGNOSIS IS MADE

CF is a well-characterized genetic disorder with an autosomal recessive pattern of inheritance. Although most living patients were diagnosed following the appearance of symptoms or due to the diagnosis of a sibling, most new diagnoses will now be made through newborn screening programs, which have spread rapidly across the United States in the past few years.[29] The advent of newborn screening using immunoreactive typsinogen and/or DNA analysis has resulted in a population of asymptomatic patients diagnosed in the first month of life. Earlier diagnosis has led to some improved clinical outcomes,[30,31] but does carry some associated risks for families, including psychological impact of false negative and false positive results and implications of diagnosis of a genetic disease.[2,32,33] Because of their experience with breaking bad news and with helping families manage the grief that may accompany the news, palliative care teams are in a good position to help CF care teams design a compassionate program for revealing the diagnosis to those parents of newborns who have a positive screen and then a confirmatory genetic analysis or sweat test.[34]

AT THE TIME OF DIAGNOSIS

As the diagnosis is given, families must process not only the shock of the diagnosis but also the beginning of a complex new care regimen, which must be followed every day if the benefit of newborn screening is to be realized.[35,36] The obvious parallel for the palliative care team is a new and unexpected diagnosis of cancer in a child, with the rapid institution of a complex and toxic therapy. While the side effects of therapy are less in the newly diagnosed child with CF, the shock and grief may be similar. CF care teams are accomplished at helping families with this news, but the advent of newborn screening brings a new group to light in the CF clinic: the largely asymptomatic child with a genetic diagnosis. The change in the experience of the diagnosis may offer an opportunity for the palliative care team to approach the CF care team with an offer to help it do the best possible job in supporting this new type of patient. While we do not recommend the palliative care team have direct contact with the family at the time of diagnosis, the interdisciplinary expertise of the palliative care team may prove to be useful to the CF care team during this time.

DURING ROUTINE CARE

Two events in particular may provide room for the palliative care team to assist the CF care team. The first is preparing it to respond to the patient and family when they bring up the limited life expectancy of someone diagnosed with CF. Many CF clinicians prefer never to talk about this issue, or to brush it aside with discussion of the progress in CF. However, it is clear that patients, especially by adolescence, recognize this issue and may very well want to talk about it.[37,38] In the popular culture, CF is viewed as a progressive killer of children: movies, books, and novels about CF are inevitably tragic and highly melodramatic.[39-43] Popular narratives about CF may be years out of date,[44] and it is a trope that anyone portrayed on television with CF will die before the show ends. Patients and families swim in this cultural sea, and so are exposed to this inaccurate but tight link of CF with childhood death. This may cause them to be reluctant to disclose their disease to others, even friends, and so may cut them off from sources of social support that could have a positive effect of quality of life.[45] Palliative care teams, as outsiders to the CF community, may be able to help the CF care team counter these popular images of CF and replace them with a more accurate portrayal of patients with CF as deeply courageous and dedicated in the face of a difficult but potentially life-affirming situation.

CF medical providers do not want to be surprised when an adolescent asks about mortality, and the palliative care team may be able to develop an educational approach that explores the range of developmentally appropriate responses to a patient's questions.

The palliative care team may also have a window of opportunity to assist the CF care team at the time of the first hospitalization for a pulmonary exacerbation. Even when most children were symptomatic at the time of diagnosis, the first pulmonary exacerbation was a time of substantial stress, during which the reality of disease progression had to be faced.[46,47] Now, in the era of the asymptomatic diagnosis via newborn screening, the first exacerbation can stir up considerable anxiety for parents, and they may interpret it as a sign of more rapid decline of the child. Of course, it is the intensive and preventive approach to CF that is the cause of both the treatment for pulmonary exacerbation and the increase in life expectancy, and habituating the family to the routine of careful surveillance and vigorous treatment of any fall from the pulmonary baseline is an important goal. CF teams may not recognize the increased symbolic meaning of this first exacerbation in the era of newborn screening, as pulmonary exacerbations and their treatment are routine for the teams.

AS THE DISEASE PROGRESSES

There are three general opportunities for integration of palliative care into CF as the disease accelerates: expert assessment and management of CF-related symptoms, assistance with the difficult decisions around lung transplantation, and assistance with advance care planning.

Assessment and Management of CF-Related Symptoms

Distressing symptoms are common in patients with CF[14,16,19,23,24,48] and are known to increase as lung disease progresses,[17,49,50] but little research defines the impact of symptoms on quality of life or on the end of life experience of these patients. General principles of symptom assessment and management can be applied to the CF population, and the interdisciplinary nature of CF care should allow for regular attention to symptoms with both physiologic and non-organic origins. Attention must be paid to the psychological impact of symptoms, particularly respiratory symptoms, as their increasing frequency and intensity typically denotes disease progression.

Respiratory Symptoms Respiratory symptoms, such as cough and dyspnea, may be minimal or only intermittent during infancy and early childhood but in most patients progress steadily, with periods of increased cough and dyspnea occurring during respiratory exacerbations. Cough is necessary for clearance of respiratory secretions, and is encouraged in this setting, but excessive cough may be distressing and disruptive. Aerosolized therapies and airway clearance techniques facilitate cough, and are routinely recommended for maintenance of health and are intensified during respiratory exacerbations. While these treatments are intended to reduce chronic respiratory symptoms, they are thought to be burdensome by many patients.[6] This perception is due in part to the extensive amount of time required to complete such treatments, but clinical experience suggests that they may also cause distressing symptoms such as pain, dyspnea, sleep disturbance, and urinary incontinence. Treatment of increased cough includes use of aerosols and airway clearance therapies, antibiotics for infection, and specific treatments for other common causes of cough, including gastroesophageal reflux disease, sinus disease, asthma, and allergies. While most pulmonologists who treat patients with CF discourage the use of antitussives because of their negative impact on airway clearance, these agents may be helpful in managing distressing cough under certain circumstances.

Hemoptysis may occur in association with cough, particularly with lower respiratory infections. Small-volume hemoptysis is generally managed with antibiotics, correction of bleeding disorders, and cautious use of or temporary suspension of aerosols and airway clearance therapies. Massive hemoptysis, which is more than 240 mL in 24 hours or recurrent bleeding of more than 100 mL per day, occurs in approximately 1% of children with CF and is unrelated to severity of lung disease. It is also associated with other respiratory complications and has a high likelihood of recurrence.[51,52] Bronchial artery embolization is used for acute treatment, but recurrent and unremitting end-stage hemoptysis may require sedation and the use of dark towels and linens to minimize the sight of blood, which may help lessen the anxiety of patients, caregivers, and medical providers.

Dyspnea is commonly reported as CF lung disease progresses[50] and is likely to be the most distressing symptom near the end of life. This complex symptom is related to: increased ventilatory demand due to increased dead space in abnormal CF lungs, increased respiratory effort to move air through dilated and obstructed airways, and increased muscle force required for maintenance of normal ventilation because of abnormal airway resistance and flattening of the diaphragm by hyperinflated lungs.[53] In addition, the interplay between dyspnea and anxiety can be complicated.[54,55] There are many approaches to the treatment of dyspnea. Enhancing airway clearance and treating infection and inflammation with standard CF therapies is a standard strategy, which may reduce acute or subacute dyspnea, ideally returning the patient back to their baseline respiratory status. With disease progression, dyspnea may become less responsive to such treatments.

For those with chronic dyspnea and more advanced lung disease, physical therapy to improve conditioning may be helpful. Respiratory support, including the use of oxygen to support gas exchange, may reduce the sensation of dyspnea. Oxygen may be used with exertion, during sleep, and on a continual basis later in the course of disease. The route of administration is typically nasal cannula, although some patients prefer to use face masks during periods of acute illness. The use of positive airway pressure for management of dyspnea, hypoxemia, and hypercapnia was typically avoided in the past because of poor outcomes of patients receiving these treatments.[56–58] Applying positive pressure to airways that are abnormally dilated and impacted with thick mucus makes airway clearance, which is critical to management of respiratory infection, more difficult. In addition, ventilator modes and settings that combat hypercapnia due to respiratory failure in advanced CF lung disease are uncomfortable and typically necessitate sedative medications that interfere with the patient's ability to communicate. However, the use of non-invasive positive pressure ventilation, typically bi-level positive airway pressure (BiPAP), has gained favor for patients with sleep disturbance and daytime fatigue and as a bridging therapy for patients with respiratory insufficiency awaiting lung transplantation.[59,60] Full respiratory support with intubation and mechanical ventilation may also be considered for some patients with reversible causes of respiratory failure and for transplant candidates.[61,62] The decision to use these treatments must be made with the knowledge that, while they may provide relief of severe dyspnea and may prolong life for those whose goal is to receive a lung transplant, their use has many associated risks that must be understood by patients and caregivers.

Decreasing the sensation of dyspnea using oral and intravenous opioids and benzodiazepines may be considered for patients with advanced lung disease. Opioids decrease respiratory drive and may act locally in the lungs to relieve dyspnea.[63] However, despite evidence that these medications can be used safely in patients with respiratory diseases,[54] concerns about respiratory depression in patients with advanced CF lung disease have been described and may act as barriers to effective palliation of dyspnea.[10,49,53,64] Aerosolized opioids are sometimes offered, but small studies of their use to treat dyspnea do not suggest universal efficacy.[63,65,66] Given the demonstrated efficacy of opioids in relieving dyspnea, concerns about their use may be alleviated by starting with very low oral or intravenous doses and titrating to effect, monitoring closely for undesirable secondary effects. This strategy also allows the patient, caregivers, and medical providers time to become more comfortable with the use of opioids to treat dyspnea. Other supportive and adjunctive therapies, including lowering ambient temperature or blowing cool air with fans, maintaining cooler ambient temperatures, positioning, relaxation techniques, and psychotherapy, may be beneficial for some patients.

Pain Pain, including headache, sinus, chest, back, abdominal, and joint, is common in patients with CF throughout their lives.[14,16,23] Careful investigation for the cause of pain is essential in selecting effective treatments. Headache may be due to cough, sinus disease, or hypercapnia in addition to the numerous other causes of headache in people without CF, and treatment should reflect the cause. Sinus pain may respond to treatment for infection with systemic or nasally instilled antibiotics or the use of intranasal steroids and saline to facilitate drainage. Surgical intervention by an otolaryngologist for severe or persistent pain may be warranted. Chest pain that originates from the lung may be due to infection, hemoptysis or pneumothorax, and is often localized and may be pleuritic. Musculoskeletal chest pain may result from frequent cough, increased thoracic volume,[67] or, in those with osteoporosis related to chronic vitamin D deficiency and/or systemic steroid use, rib fractures or vertebral compression fractures.[22,68] Physical therapy, pharmacologic agents, and orthopedic referral can be considered depending on the etiology of the pain. Joint pain may be due to typical injuries or causes of arthritis in the non-CF population and to quinolone use,[69] but CF arthropathy, which is a diagnosis of exclusion, affects a small proportion of patients. Symptoms are typically episodic and present at times of illness and stress. Treatment may involve analgesics and anti-inflammatory medications, sometimes including disease-modifying antirheumatic drugs.[70,71]

Distressing and/or debilitating pain from any source warrants careful evaluation. Appropriate management involves identifying and, if possible, eliminating underlying causes.

Establishing goals of treatment, selection of medications and other treatments, and monitoring response to and side effects of treatments should follow standard approaches to pain management addressed in previous chapters.

Gastrointestinal Symptoms Gastrointestinal manifestations of CF are numerous and include steatorrhea and malnutrition related to pancreatic exocrine insufficiency, gastroesophageal reflux, and obstructive biliary tract disease. Symptoms related to these problems include abdominal pain, constipation, anorexia, and, for a small percentage of patients, symptoms of progressive hepatobiliary disease. Abdominal pain that is associated with an increase in bowel movements, urgency or distension, should prompt optimization of pancreatic enzyme replacement. Constipation may be acute or chronic, and may be treated with prokinetic agents and oral electrolyte solutions. Distal intestinal obstruction syndrome may occur when excessively viscid intestinal contents become impacted in the distal small intestine and proximal colon, and should be suspected when pain and obstipation occur concomitantly. Treatment involves intestinal lavage and close monitoring for progression to frank bowel obstruction, which warrants surgical intervention.[72,73] Gastroesophageal reflux is managed with standard therapies, including histamine-receptor antagonists and proton pump inhibitors. Surgical treatment of reflux does not appear to confer benefit, but is considered in some cases.[74] Other causes of gastrointestinal symptoms that are not specific to or more common in CF must not be overlooked.

Because of malabsorption and increased metabolic demands, patients with CF require greater caloric intake to achieve and maintain adequate nutritional status. While young patients with pancreatic insufficiency often have hearty appetites, cough and the increased work of breathing may make eating laborious and maintenance of weight difficult or impossible without medical interventions as lung disease progresses. Behavioral interventions around feeding, calorie dense oral supplements, and appetite stimulants are typically offered in a stepwise fashion while other causes of and contributors to anorexia, including gastroesophageal reflux disease, sinus disease, depression, and anxiety are addressed.[75] For those who are unable to maintain acceptable nutritional status, feeding tubes may be used. Patients with advanced disease who choose to pursue lung transplantation are obligated to follow intensive nutritional interventions in order to reduce operative and recovery-related risks. Those for whom transplantation is not desired or is not an option may be offered more choices about the ongoing use of nutritional interventions.

Psychological Symptoms Depression and anxiety are known to be problematic in chronic respiratory diseases,[76] and studies suggest that their prevalence in CF is higher than in the general population.[77] They may adversely impact health outcomes and quality of life, and screening for depression and anxiety might ultimately be recommended as a routine part of CF care.[78–80] For patients and families affected by any chronic illness, disease-specific social support can play a vital role in coping with stress and in managing depression and anxiety. In contrast to past extensive social support available on hospital wards and summer camps, strict guidelines for infection control have led to physical isolation of patients, and thus often their families, leading to social networking and support via the Internet and other media that allow for indirect contact. For some patients and families, this is extremely effective, but for others, it leads to loneliness that may theoretically impact disease-related coping.

Treatment of depression in CF does not differ from standard treatment, apart from recognition of the role of chronic disease as a provocative factor and of the possibility of depression and other mood disorders in family members and other caregivers.[81] Anxiety may be acute or chronic in nature, and in either form may be highly distressing.[16] Anxiety about disease progression is common, suggesting the need for ongoing attention to this symptom. Overlap in symptoms may occur, such that anxiety may be perpetuated by dyspnea, cough, pain and fatigue, thus addressing these symptoms may reduce and indirectly treat anxiety. Medications such as beta-agonists and steroids, which are commonly used to treat CF, may also contribute to anxiety. Treatment of anxiety may initially involve cognitive behavioral therapy, psychotherapy, and complimentary techniques such as biofeedback and relaxation. Pharmacologic agents may be used in select cases, with favor given to selective serotonin reuptake inhibitors (SSRIs) and selective-norepinephrine reuptake inhibitors (SNRIs), with benzodiazepines considered for short-term treatment of acute anxiety[77] but otherwise reserved for those with severe and unremitting symptoms or advanced lung disease.

Fatigue Fatigue is a highly prevalent but often underappreciated symptom in patients with life-threatening illnesses[55] and is common in patients with CF.[16] Fatigue is reported to impact adherence to prescribed treatments[82] and undoubtedly quality of life. This complex symptom is often pervasive, unresponsive to rest, limits functioning, and affects physical, cognitive and emotional stamina.[55] The interaction between fatigue and other symptoms such as cough, dyspnea, pain, and depression is not well described in CF, but is presumably substantial in some patients. Treatment for fatigue is also complex and not well studied in CF, but exercise, psychosocial interventions such as psychotherapy and disease-specific support networks, complimentary and alternative therapies, improving sleep hygiene, and the use of stimulants are possible options. Fatigue may likely also be reduced indirectly by treating other symptoms.

ROLE OF THE PALLIATIVE CARE TEAM IN SYMPTOM MANAGEMENT

While pulmonologists and other CF clinicians are aware of the high symptom burden in CF, many lack specific training in thorough assessment and management of symptoms. Additionally, the focus of routine CF care is often on preservation of health rather than on chronic management of symptoms, even for those symptoms which are more likely to progress than to remit. Concerns about medication side effects and long-term implications of certain symptom-specific treatments, as well as lack of clinical decision support, may lead to under-prescribing of medications and other symptom-specific treatments, particularly in the late stages of CF lung disease. Palliative care clinicians may use their expertise to bring attention to and offer relief from distressing symptoms experienced by patients with CF as their disease progresses.

Lung Transplantation for Advanced CF Lung Disease

Lung transplantation is the most intensive treatment available for advanced CF lung disease, and is considered when a patient's functional status and quality of life are significantly impaired and their anticipated survival is 2 years or less.[83] Transplant may improve survival and quality of life for selected patients.[84,85] Despite its promise as a definitive treatment for advanced CF lung disease, transplant survival outcomes are suboptimal, with a median 5-year survival of about 50% in the United States.[84,86] While some patients have relatively benign operative and post-transplant courses, complications are difficult to predict and are the second leading cause of death among patients with CF.[87] It is important to understand the complexity of the transplant decision, transitions in care that occur when patients decide to pursue transplant, and the interaction between curative and palliative care for patients on the transplant pathway.

Lung Transplant Decision-Making Appropriate timing of transplant referral is difficult to predict, but there is consensus about which disease related and physiologic factors, including lung function, body mass index, functional status, and other organ involvement, should prompt consideration of referral for transplant.[88,89] Because CF is a life-threatening disease with many possible treatment options and substantial uncertainty exists with regard to both survival and quality of life outcomes, it is important that patients and caregivers fully understand the risks and benefits of transplant and alternative treatment options. Informed decision-making is the clinical and ethical practice standard for complex decisions about medical care. The elements of informed decision-making[90] about lung transplant are outlined in Table 41-3.

For a majority of patients who have undergone transplant, the experience of advanced lung disease unfortunately recurs. Bronchiolitis obliterans syndrome (BOS), another chronic progressive lung disease that is believed to be a manifestation of rejection, is the most common cause of death in lung transplant recipients surviving longer than one year after transplant.[91] BOS symptoms and treatments often mirror those of CF,[92] thus similar decisions about treatments to those made pre-transplant may again be faced. Second transplants are offered to and accepted by select patients, but they have poorer survival outcomes and greater associated morbidity.[93]

Discussions about transplant often take place with various providers, including members of the CF care team, the lung transplant team, and the palliative care team. Input from different providers may help patients and caregivers decide about transplant within the context of their own goals and values. Open communication among providers is essential so that patient and caregiver decisions can be supported. In addition, offering peer decision support by means of support groups and mentoring programs may be helpful to patients and caregivers. Issues of caregiver stress and fatigue should also be acknowledged and addressed.[94,95]

Patients who would like to be considered for lung transplant but are deemed ineligible because of medical or psychosocial contraindications deserve thoughtful discussion of their goals for ongoing medical care, which may include continuation of standard CF therapies, incorporation of palliative treatments, and/or transition to hospice care. Palliative care

TABLE 41-3 Elements of Informed Decision Making

Element of informed decision making	Selected important information for patients and caregivers
Discussion of the patient's role in decision making	Shared decision making, including patients, caregivers, and medical providers is ideal Role of young child in deciding about lung transplant is to provide assent for transplant
Clinical issue or nature of the decision	Transplant is considered because lung disease is severe enough that predicted survival may be greater with transplant than without Patient's place on the transplant wait list will be determined by comparison of their physiologic measures to those of others with severe lung disease due to CF and other causes who are waiting for transplants Transplant affords a new set of medical issues, new medications, and ongoing frequent medical care
Discussion of the alternatives	Ongoing medical care and palliative treatments without transplant Transition to hospice care
Discussion of the potential benefits and risks of transplant	Intra-operative morbidities and mortality Post-operative complications, including graft rejection, infection, and toxicities of anti-rejection medications
Discussion of uncertainties associated with the transplant decision	Ideal timing of transplant is difficult to predict; goal is to first transplant those in greatest need and who would likely derive the greatest benefit Up-to-date survival data Quality of life after transplant may be impacted by complications Changes in medical providers, need to move care to another institution if transplant not offered at CF care center
Assessment of the patient's understanding about transplant	Assess understanding and address questions during discussions about transplant Identify deficiencies in understanding by addressing the issue of transplant over the course of several encounters
Exploration of patient and caregiver preferences for or against lung transplant	Identify and explore differences in opinion among patients and caregivers Patient and caregiver preferences may change over time Address concerns about changes in lifestyle, including possible relocation, temporary changes in plans for education or employment, and the impact on extended family, friends, and CF peers

Adapted from Braddock CH, Edwards KA, Hasenberg NM, et al. Informed decision making in outpatient practice: time to get back to basics. JAMA 1999;282(24): 2313–20 and Boyle MP. Adult cystic fibrosis. JAMA 2007;298(15):1787–93.

consultation for discussion of treatment options and further planning may be beneficial for patients, caregivers, and the CF care team.

Transitions in Care Around Lung Transplant CF care teams and transplant teams are often separate entities; there may be some overlap in providers, but in general patients who undergo lung transplants meet a new care team at the time of referral that then assumes care once the transplant takes place. Members of the transplant team may have more experience caring for adults than children, making the transition not only from the CF care team to the transplant team but also from pediatric to adult providers. Team structure, means of accessing care, subspecialty consultants, and locations of both outpatient and inpatient medical care may all change abruptly. Patients and caregivers must understand the roles and responsibilities of their previous and new medical teams with regard to patient care and support throughout the transplant process so as to reduce confusion, mistrust, or concerns about abandonment.

Interaction Between Curative and Palliative Care Patients with advanced CF lung disease are highly symptomatic and must constantly attend to their disease in order to prevent further deterioration in health. Because of the goal of extending survival, the decision to pursue transplant may inherently change the focus of care from restorative and palliative to curative in the eyes of patients, caregivers, and medical providers.[28,64] It is important to recognize that the additional stress of waiting for a transplant, with candidacy for transplant always at risk because of the development of disease complications that might preclude it and risk of dying before receiving a transplant, may have great emotional impact[96] and patients with advanced lung disease remain highly symptomatic and may have little physi-

cal reserve. Discussions about transplant provide a natural opportunity to address wishes for ongoing healthcare, including hopes for survival, goals and expectations for palliation of symptoms, and desired roles of caregivers. While changing medical providers may be an additional stress, palliative care consultation during the transplant decision making process and after transplant, ideally with continuity throughout, may benefit patients, caregivers and the transplant team. Table 41-4 is a summary of ways palliative care consultants may contribute to the care of patients with CF who are making decisions about or who will undergo lung transplant.

Advance Care Planning

Most patients with CF will live to become adults, necessitating a transition of decision making from surrogates to autonomous. Often in this transition, the adult patient may defer decision making to the parent who has carried that burden.[7] For this reason, special care should be taken to assess the role of each patient in the decision making process. Effort should be made to transition decision making to the adolescent and young adult.

The possibility of a premature death will come as a shock to parents. While few patients give any thought to the life-threatening nature of their disease,[97,98] some adolescents and young adults develop certain fantasies or beliefs about their lifespan and may develop symbolic meaning to living past a certain age.[99] These expectations and perceptions may directly influence planning for the future, adherence to the therapeutic regimen, and quality of life. While advance care planning for minor children does not carry legal weight, children with CF should be included in medical decision making in a culturally and developmentally appropriate way with an effort of transition from assent to autonomy. The palliative care team can use the long-term relationships

TABLE 41-4 Contributions of the Palliative Care Team

How can palliative care consultants contribute to the care of patients with CF during the lung transplant decision making process and after lung transplant?

Topic	During decision making process	After transplant
Symptom management	Assessment and recommendations for management, often in the context of need to participate in pulmonary rehabilitation programs despite profound illness and possible restrictions on use of opioids and benzodiazepines while waiting for transplant	Assessment and recommendations for management, including symptoms related to side effects of new medications
Psychosocial support for patient and family	Providing resources to patient and family that are focused on fears about surviving to transplant and transplant outcomes, caregiver stress and fatigue, and impact on other loved ones	Providing resources to patients who experience anxiety and uncertainty after transplant, assist in development of coping skills for those who experience complications and chronic rejection and/or graft failure
Informed consent	Exploring deficiencies in understanding of the transplant process and feeding back information to transplant team	Assisting with understanding of procedures and treatments related to transplant, continuing to advocate for good communication with transplant team
Decision support	Delineating goals of care, exploring other factors in decision making other than informed consent	Delineating goals of care in the context of health related and quality of life outcomes after transplant
Education for transplant team	Didactic sessions and discussions about mortality, focusing on awareness of patients and families of limited lifespan in CF and uncertainties about transplant outcomes. Symptom management skills for patients with high symptom burden who are asked to meet goals for pulmonary rehabilitation and nutrition before transplant	Didactic sessions and discussions about treating patients with poor health related and quality of life outcomes after transplant, importance of ongoing involvement of transplant team when patients are dying after transplant. Symptom management after transplant, focused on recovery from surgery, side effects of new medications, and symptoms related to transplant complications

with CF care team that can facilitate multiple avenues of communication.[100]

A study of adults with CF revealed that most recognize the life-threatening nature of their disease and have considered the type of care they want to have if they became unable to decide for themselves, even developing specific plans about end of life care.[97] While these adults discussed their plans with family members and said they would be comfortable discussing them with the CF care team, only one third had discussed advance care planning with any member of the team. It is unclear if this lack of communication is due to perceptions that these discussions will hinder hope, beliefs that they only need to occur when death is imminent, or a notion that advance care planning tools do not apply to adults with CF.

Existing advance care planning tools are generally based on an oncology model and may not fit the clinical characteristics of CF, given the different trajectory of disease and the less toxic curative and restorative disease-specific therapies. In the attempt to improve advance care planning, some CF care centers have developed CF-specific living wills or have adapted programs such as Five Wishes[101] for use in CF clinical care.[102]

Do not resuscitate (DNR) and do not intubate (DNI) orders appear to be perceived as having limited practical use in advance care planning in CF in the United States because a DNR order is not in place for most patients until the last day or so of life.[28,49] In practice, DNR and DNI orders should not be used as the sole document regarding appropriate interventions near the end of life. Instead, these orders should be used as part of meeting the goals of care of the patient and family and should be consistent with the expected outcome of the intervention.

After Death

Improved survival in CF and ongoing optimism for cure on the part of patients, caregivers, medical providers and society affects attitudes about dying from CF. While death is the inevitable outcome, it is more difficult to accept than in the past. As with many chronic diseases, death may be viewed as failure.[103] Prognostic difficulties and the intensity of treatments offered to patients with CF near the end of life further complicate thinking about and anticipating death. The topics of anticipatory grief and bereavement are covered in detail elsewhere in this text; in the following we address issues specific to bereavement in CF.

CHILDREN WITH CF

Prognostic uncertainty and discussions about life expectancy lead to anticipatory grief in children with CF. This grief is intensified during hospitalization and during times of obvious decline as well as through observation of serious illnesses and deaths of CF peers. Children, caregivers, and medical providers should be encouraged to identify grief as an expected part of life with CF. Much as with other children with chronic life-threatening illnesses,[104] children with CF are often aware they are dying even if never told directly and have concerns about impending death and separation from caregivers, family, and friends. They may also grieve the loss of function, lack of interaction with their family and peers, and changes in body image. Palliative care consultants and other providers with expertise in psychosocial support can help children communicate these concerns and find meaning as the disease progresses. They can also be helpful in educating caregivers and members of the CF care team in how to provide appropriate supports to the child.

CAREGIVERS AND OTHER FAMILY MEMBERS

For caregivers whose lives were irrevocably altered by caring for a child with CF, there may be a loss of identity and external validation related to this parenting role. Healthy siblings who may have received less attention than their siblings with CF often experience feelings of guilt[105] and may be left struggling to understand their new roles within the family and their relationships with their parents. Additionally, families may experience the deaths of more than one child with CF, with each death perhaps impacting family members in different ways. Siblings who also have CF must face their own mortality and may experience anticipatory grief surrounding their own disease. Offering support and location of resources for grieving and bereaved family members can be very helpful.

Ongoing involvement with bereaved families in the period following death is an option for CF care team members. In an unpublished study, bereaved caregivers expressed gratitude toward members of the CF care team who sent cards, attended funerals or memorial services, and welcomed the family back to the care center for a visit after an initial period of grieving. Many described the CF care team as extended family and the care centers as a second home, making communication with team members during the grieving process seem natural. Several mentioned ongoing work with the CF Foundation and other organizations serving families with chronically ill children, such as helping them to cope with their losses. It is important to recognize that there are no standards for bereavement care of CF caregivers, and it is likely that practices vary from one care center to another. Palliative care consultants may be able to provide valuable education to CF care teams about bereavement care.

CF COMMUNITY

As a relatively rare disease with an organized system of care, there is extensive social networking within the CF community. The impact of a child's death on others with CF and their caregivers must not be overlooked. The CF care team, with careful attention to privacy of health information, should explore grief and offer support to those affected by the death.

CF CARE TEAM

The CF care team, whose long-term relationship with a patient suddenly comes to an end, also grieves. An organized debriefing shortly after a patient's death may help team members and hospital staff to cope more effectively with the loss. Some centers hold periodic memorial services to honor patients within a CF care center who have died. Such gatherings provide a forum for expression of sadness and also celebration of the lives of former patients.

Clinical Vignette

Kylie was born beautiful, the second child in a family happy to welcome her to the world. Things were going so well. Then the pediatrician called before the 2-week check-up: could they come in for a talk? The newborn screen was positive for something called cystic fibrosis, and Kylie needed to go to the children's hospital 2 hours away for some sort of test of her sweat to confirm the diagnosis.

At the hospital, they waited in the room after the sweat chloride test. A smiling nurse came in and said, "Wait here, the doctor will see you soon." They knew, right away, that it was bad news. They knew it was serious. And then they heard the news: Kylie had CF.

Although the doctors and nurses were nice and had kind eyes, Kylie's mom could tell they were worried. This was seri-

ous. The nurse said Kylie had to start taking medicine every time she ate to help her absorb fat, and that they would have to come back tomorrow to take some blood, to meet the CF team, and to start their new life with CF.

That night, Kylie's mother said to her husband, "I know they told us not to look it up online, but I just have to see. I have to see what my baby's life will be like." So they looked. Some of the news was good—there was lots of research on CF, but some was very bad—all those memorials to all those people. And they cried the rest of the night.

The next day at the hospital there was a flood of new information. It was like drinking from a firehose. A thousand questions came up all at once. What had caused this? Are we good enough parents to do all this? It's in our genes, so are we responsible? What about Kylie's sister? What about other children? Can Kylie have children? Will we have grandchildren? How will we pay for all of this? Will I have to quit my job? When will the cure come? Will she be sick always? Can she go to school? How will we explain to our parents? Will she be normal?

Things settled down a bit, and with the help of the CF team, and a lot of phone calls, they started to adjust. Kylie got some colds, and they were not a big deal at first. She grew. Her parents got used to seeing the CF team every 3 months. And then, Kylie got sick with lots of coughing; choking and coughing all night. The doctors said she had to be admitted for IV antibiotics. Just when things had seemed to get back to normal, their world fell apart again. Being in the hospital meant Kylie really was sick, really did have CF, and they couldn't pretend that things were going to be completely normal. The family was going to have to get used to a new kind of normal: normal for CF.

But things went along, and they got used to the CF life. They welcomed a baby boy shortly after Kylie's second birthday and were relieved to learn that he did not have CF. They had decided against the prenatal genetic testing, because they could not bear to make the decision about what to do with the results.

As she got older, Kylie had respiratory infections and was hospitalized again for IV antibiotics. She struggled with weight gain, and meal times became a struggle as well. It was frustrating to do all these daily treatments, and yet see only slow progress. It was hard to support a frightened young child through hospitalizations while also caring for two other children and working full time. Kylie's mother decided to take time off to focus on Kylie's health and the well being of the family. This allowed her to administer IV antibiotics at home, to provide airway clearance therapies, and to become comfortable providing supplemental feedings through Kylie's new gastrostomy tube, something Kylie's family previously perceived as a last resort but now relied on. The tube made it easy to make sure she got enough calories every day so there were no more fights at dinner time.

Kylie started school, but she still had so many respiratory exacerbations and she just did not grow. At each clinic visit, Kylie's doctor expressed concern about her below-average lung function, resistant respiratory pathogens, and below par nutrition, but he always seemed to have a new plan or another idea to try. He always focused on returning to her previous baseline when she became ill or achieving

Clinical Vignette—cont'd

a better baseline. If he was optimistic, then they could be optimistic, too.

A few days before her eleventh birthday, Kylie developed a high fever and body aches: influenza. She coughed like never before, with fever and chest pain. For the first time, they had to go to the local ER instead of making the drive to the CF Clinic. In the ER her oxygen saturation was 85%; a chest x-ray showed a pneumothorax. A chest tube was put in, and she was driven by ambulance to the ICU at the CF center. The ICU doctor said, "We need to do everything to avoid putting her on the ventilator. CF patients don't make it off the ventilator." What should they tell Kylie? She always wanted to know every detail. But she was scared enough, and they just held her hand and told her it would all be okay. Then the ICU doctors wanted to try something new call BiPAP, and Kylie was terrified. But she was so weak and out of breath that she let them put the mask on her, and she slept soundly for a few hours. It was all so new, and so unexpected, but after 2 days they got adjusted. After a few days of treatment with high-flow oxygen alternating with BiPAP, Kylie was able to start weaning from the oxygen, her chest tube was removed, and they left the ICU to go to the regular hospital floor. After all that time, it felt wonderful to be back on the regular floor and see the familiar faces of the nurses and the CF team.

But things would be different for Kylie now. Her lung function was much lower than it had been before her severe illness. She needed oxygen to exercise. She even needed oxygen to sleep. Life at home following the hospitalization was rough. Kylie struggled with the CF routine and lost interest in eating. She got frustrated at the drop of a hat. She was scared to go back to school because of all the germs, and she argued with her mother about doing schoolwork at home. Her cough was constant, always productive, and her chest and head hurt most of the time. She seemed unable to make it for more than a few days at a time without antibiotics, and the antibiotics always gave her nausea and diarrhea. She dreaded clinic visits because of the way her parents and her doctor reacted when they saw her weight and lung function results. At the next clinic visit, Kylie and her family heard the word they never said out loud at home: transplant.

They didn't hear the rest of the conversation after that word, and nobody mentioned it on the drive home. Everybody knew about transplant, and everybody knew you didn't bring it up until things were bad. But the next day, Kylie said to her mother, "We have to go see about it. To see what they say." Kylie didn't think she wanted a transplant because she knew it meant more tubes, more ICUs, more stuff to put up with. But she wanted to hear what they had to say. She wanted to take deep breaths, to run, to shout, to laugh—to do everything without coughing. So she wanted to hear what they had to say.

The doctors said that lung transplant was like trading one disease for another because there would still be pills, still be appointments, still be worries. But the whole family felt encouraged by the transplant team's optimistic views of the procedure and outcomes. The transplant team social worker offered to connect them with other patients and families via a support group; they took to this right away, because they knew only a few other people with CF and nobody that had

a transplant. After hearing about personal experiences with transplant, Kylie herself felt uncertain about going through with it, but worried about what would happen to her family after she died. She asked the transplant team a few questions at each visit, and admitted that her biggest concerns were having more tubes in her chest, given her previous experience, and not waking up after the surgery. But she wanted to run, she wanted to shout, she wanted to laugh without coughing.

Kylie underwent double lung transplant on New Year's Day, and she and her family curbed their nervousness by discussing future celebrations of both this holiday and the anniversary of receiving new lungs on the same day. Grandparents and fellow church members agreed to care for Kylie's siblings as their parents were needed at her bedside. After a relatively uncomplicated surgery and recovery, Kylie went home 3 weeks later without oxygen, delighted to shout her goodbyes to the medical staff as she left the hospital.

The next 2 years brought some ups and downs, with long periods of good health interrupted by infections and admission for rejection, with some hospitalizations but primarily outpatient care. Kylie returned to school part time. Her mother returned to work, and encouraged Kylie to become increasingly responsible for managing her medications. Kylie, now 14, disliked the side effects of some of her new medications and began taking them only now and then. She was perfect right before visits to the transplant clinic because she wanted everyone to see her good numbers, but she wasn't perfect the rest of the time.

Over time, Kylie noticed it was harder to carry her backpack at school, especially up the stairs. She started to cough again, but this time a dry cough that she tried hard to hide. A big drop in lung function led to another lung biopsy, with some bad news. It was bronchiolitis obliterans syndrome (BOS), or chronic rejection. Kylie reluctantly admitted to her parents that she often skipped her anti-rejection medications. They were angry, worried, sad, and desperate, all at the same time. What to do now?

Kylie's BOS progressed fairly rapidly. She now needed continuous oxygen again, she lost weight, and she stopped attending school. After developing a contract with the transplant team about taking her medications, Kylie was listed for a second double lung transplant. Now she was short of breath all the time. She began to feel extremely anxious about having another transplant and about the possibility of dying. Her parents worried about her fragile condition, and asked the transplant team to talk with her about the future. Once more, everyone in the family was worried about the same thing, but they just didn't know how to talk about it.

The transplant team enlisted the social worker to address Kylie's fears, but the team didn't directly discuss what might happen in the future. Taking this as a signal not to talk about it, Kylie's parents decided not to ask any more questions.

Kylie now became dependent on BiPAP around the clock. One afternoon, her family returned home from her older sister's high school graduation to find Kylie on the floor, unconscious. The ambulance team came and resuscitated her with a breathing tube and rushed her to the hospital. She was airlifted to the ICU at the transplant center. At first, it looked like she might be able to come off the ventilator quickly. But after

Clinical Vignette—cont'd

2 days, her lungs got worse and her kidneys and her liver began to fail. Privately, the transplant team decided she could no longer be a candidate for the second transplant, and they asked the ICU team to join them to tell the family the bad news.

At the meeting, the transplant doctor said he had to take Kylie off the transplant list. The ICU doctor said he thought Kylie was not going to make it. But Kylie's parents, and her siblings, wanted to keep going. After all, they said, she has pulled through so many times before. They asked, "Didn't you always tell us to be optimistic, to be hopeful?" "Maybe God will give us a miracle?" "Maybe she will get just better enough to go back on the transplant list?" The transplant team and the ICU doctors told the family to think about what they had talked about for the next 24 hours, after which they had to make some decisions.

In the day that followed, Kylie's parents felt comforted by seeing familiar faces from the transplant team and even from her old CF team, but were uncertain who to ask for help in deciding what to do next. They spent time talking and praying with the hospital chaplain, and followed suggestions from the PICU nurses about how to assist in Kylie's care. Fewer people visited as the day passed, and conversations with the medical team grew shorter. When they felt ready to withdraw life support, they were relieved to be offered help for their family to grieve. They knew it might happen, but they never expected it this soon. After all they had been through, they would have to find a way to go home without Kylie.

Summary

In this chapter, we have reviewed CF in the twenty-first century, focusing on the changing epidemiology of the disease, the symptom burden, and the changing conception of CF care resulting from improvement in survival. We have also proposed the value added model for involvement of the pediatric palliative care team in the care of patients and families affected by CF. Application of this model could enhance the quality and comprehensiveness of CF care even as treatments and disease outcomes, including survival, continue to change over time.

REFERENCES

1. Boyle MP: Adult cystic fibrosis, *JAMA* 298(15):1787–1793, 2007.
2. Mack JW, Wolfe J: Early integration of pediatric palliative care: for some children, palliative care starts at diagnosis, *Curr Opin Pediatr* 18(1):10–14, 2006.
3. O'Sullivan BP, Freedman SD: Cystic fibrosis, *Lancet* 373(9678): 1891–1904, 2009.
4. Knowles MR, Durie PR: What is cystic fibrosis? *N Engl J Med* 347(6):439–442, 2002.
5. Flume PA: Pulmonary complications of cystic fibrosis, *Respir Care* 54(5):618–627, 2009.
6. Sawicki GS, Sellers DE, Robinson WM: High treatment burden in adults with cystic fibrosis: challenges to disease self-management, *J Cyst Fibros* 8(2):91–96, 2009.
7. McGuffie K, Sellers DE, Sawicki GS, et al: Self-reported involvement of family members in the care of adults with CF, *J Cyst Fibros* 7(2): 95–101, 2008.
8. Mallory GB, Fullmer JJ, Vaughan DJ: Oxygen therapy for cystic fibrosis, *Cochrane Database Syst Rev* (4):CD003884, 2005.
9. Moran F, Bradley JM, Piper AJ: Non-invasive ventilation for cystic fibrosis, *Cochrane Database Syst Rev* (1):CD002769, 2009.
10. Kremer TM, Zwerdling RG, Michelson PH, et al: Intensive care management of the patient with cystic fibrosis, *J Intensive Care Med* 23(3):159–177, 2008.
11. Conway SP, Morton A, Wolfe S: Enteral tube feeding for cystic fibrosis, *Cochrane Database Syst Rev* (2):CD001198, 2008.
12. Koshland DE Jr: The Cystic Fibrosis Gene Story, *Science* 245(4922):1029, 1989.
13. Couzin-Frankel J: Genetics: The promise of a cure: 20 years and counting, *Science* 1504–1507, 2009.
14. Koh JL, Harrison D, Palermo TM, et al: Assessment of acute and chronic pain symptoms in children with cystic fibrosis, *Pediatr Pulmonol* 40(4):330–335, 2005.
15. Palermo TM, Harrison D, Koh JL: Effect of disease-related pain on the health-related quality of life of children and adolescents with cystic fibrosis, *Clin J Pain* 22(6):532–537, 2006.
16. Sawicki GS, Sellers DE, Robinson WM: Self-reported physical and psychological symptom burden in adults with cystic fibrosis, *J Pain Symptom Manage* 35(4):372–380, 2008.
17. Ravilly S, Robinson W, Suresh S, et al: Chronic pain in cystic fibrosis, *Pediatrics* 98(4 Pt 1):741–747, 1996.
18. Lee A, Holdsworth M, Holland A, et al: The immediate effect of musculoskeletal physiotherapy techniques and massage on pain and ease of breathing in adults with cystic fibrosis, *J Cyst Fibros* 8(1): 79–81, 2009.
19. Sermet-Gaudelus I, De Villartay P, de Dreuzy P, et al: Pain in children and adults with cystic fibrosis: a comparative study, *J Pain Symptom Manage* 38(2):281–290, 2009.
20. Stenekes S, Hughes A, Gregoire M, et al: Frequency and self-management of pain, dyspnea, and cough in cystic fibrosis, *J Pain Symptom Manage* 4(4):2009.
21. Walker LS, Smith CA, Garber J, et al: Testing a model of pain appraisal and coping in children with chronic abdominal pain, *Health Psychol* 24(4):364–374, 2005.
22. Jones AM, Dodd ME, Webb AK, et al: Acute rib fracture pain in CF, *Thorax* 56(10):819, 2001.
23. Festini F, Ballarin S, Codamo T, et al: Prevalence of pain in adults with cystic fibrosis, *J Cyst Fibros* 3(1):51–57, 2004.
24. Hubbard PA, Broome ME, Antia LA: Pain, coping, and disability in adolescents and young adults with cystic fibrosis: a web-based study, *Pediatr Nurs* 31(2):82–86, 2005.
25. Konstan MW, Wagener JS, VanDevanter DR: Characterizing aggressiveness and predicting future progression of CF lung disease, *J Cyst Fibros* 8(Suppl 1):S15–S19, 2009.
26. Hynson JL: The child's journey: transition from health to ill health. In Goldman A, Hain R, Liben S, editors: *Oxford textbook of palliative care for children*, 2006, Oxford University Press.
27. Bourke S, Doe S, Gascoigne A, et al: An integrated model of provision of palliative care to patients with cystic fibrosis, *Palliat Med* 2009.
28. Dellon EP, Leigh MW, Yankaskas JR, et al: Effects of lung transplantation on inpatient end of life care in cystic fibrosis, *J Cyst Fibros* 6(6):396–402, 2007.
29. Southern KW, Merelle MM, Dankert-Roelse JE, et al: Newborn screening for cystic fibrosis, *Cochrane Database Syst Rev* (1):CD001402, 2009.
30. Linnane BM, Hall GL, Nolan G, et al: Lung function in infants with cystic fibrosis diagnosed by newborn screening, *Am J Respir Crit Care Med* 178(12):1238–1244, 2008.
31. Rock MJ: Newborn screening for cystic fibrosis, *Clin Chest Med* 28(2):297–305, 2007.
32. Lewis S, Curnow L, Ross M, et al: Parental attitudes to the identification of their infants as carriers of cystic fibrosis by newborn screening, *J Paediatr Child Health* 42(9):533–537, 2006.
33. Comeau AM, Parad R, Gerstle R, et al: Challenges in implementing a successful newborn cystic fibrosis screening program, *J Pediatr* 147(Suppl 3):S89–S93, 2005.
34. Grob R: Is my sick child healthy? Is my healthy child sick? Changing parental experiences of cystic fibrosis in the age of expanded newborn screening, *Soc Sci Med* 67(7):1056–1064, 2008.
35. Collins MS, Abbott MA, Wakefield DB, et al: Improved pulmonary and growth outcomes in cystic fibrosis by newborn screening, *Pediatr Pulmonol* 43(7):648–655, 2008.

36. Stick SM, Brennan S, Murray C, et al: Bronchiectasis in infants and preschool children diagnosed with cystic fibrosis after newborn Screening, *J Pediatr* 155(5):623–628.e1.Epub 2009.

37. Christian BJ, D'Auria JP, Moore CB: Playing for time: adolescent perspectives of lung transplantation for cystic fibrosis, *J Pediatr Health Care* 13(3 Pt 1):120–125, 1999.

38. Powers PM, Gerstle R, Lapey A: Adolescents with cystic fibrosis: family reports of adolescent health-related quality of life and forced expiratory volume in one second, *Pediatrics* 107(5):E70, 2001.

39. Merullo RA: *Little love story*, New York, 2005, Vintage Books.

40. Mitchell I, Nakielna E, Tullis E, Adair C: Cystic fibrosis: end-stage care in Canada, *Chest* 118(1):80–84, 2000.

41. Woodson M: *Turn it into glory: a mother's moving story of her daughter's last great adventure*, Minneapolis, 1991, Bethany House Publishers.

42. McDaniel LA: *Time to die*, New York, 1992, Laurel Leaf.

43. Pitts D: *Living on borrowed time: life with cystic fibrosis*, Bloomington, Ind, 2007, AuthorHouse.

44. Deford F: *Alex: the life of a child*, Nashville, 1983, Rutledge Hill Press.

45. Lowton K: Only when I cough? Adults' disclosure of cystic fibrosis, *Qual Health Res* 14(2):167–186, 2004.

46. Bluebond-Langner M: *The private worlds of dying children*, Princeton, NJ, 1978, Princeton University Press.

47. Bluebond-Langner M: *In the shadow of illness: parents and siblings of the chronically ill child*, Princeton NJ, 1996, Princeton University Press.

48. Smith JA, Owen EC, Jones AM, et al: Objective measurement of cough during pulmonary exacerbations in adults with cystic fibrosis, *Thorax* 61(5):425–429, 2006.

49. Robinson WM, Ravilly S, Berde C, et al: End-of-life care in cystic fibrosis, *Pediatrics* 100(2 Pt 1):205–209, 1997.

50. Yankaskas JR, Marshall BC, Sufian B, et al: Cystic fibrosis adult care: consensus conference report, *Chest* 125(Suppl 1):1S–39S, 2004.

51. Barben JU, Ditchfield M, Carlin JB, et al: Major haemoptysis in children with cystic fibrosis: a 20-year retrospective study, *J Cyst Fibros* 2(3):105–111, 2003.

52. Flume PA, Strange C, Ye X, et al: Pneumothorax in cystic fibrosis, *Chest* 128(2):720–728, 2005.

53. Orenstein DM, Rosenstein BJ, Stern RC: *Cystic fibrosis medical care*, Philadelphia, 2000, Lippincott Williams & Williams.

54. Luce JM, Luce JA: Perspectives on care at the close of life. Management of dyspnea in patients with far-advanced lung disease: "Once I lose it, it's kind of hard to catch it, *JAMA* 285(10):1331–1337, 2001.

55. Ullrich CK, Mayer OH: Assessment and management of fatigue and dyspnea in pediatric palliative care, *Pediatr Clin North Am* 54(5):735–756, xi, 2007.

56. Berlinski A, Fan LL, Kozinetz CA, et al: Invasive mechanical ventilation for acute respiratory failure in children with cystic fibrosis: outcome analysis and case-control study, *Pediatr Pulmonol* 34(4):297–303, 2002.

57. Davis PB, di Sant'Agnese PA: Assisted ventilation for patients with cystic fibrosis, *JAMA* 239(18):1851–1854, 1978.

58. Texereau J, Jamal D, Choukroun G, et al: Determinants of mortality for adults with cystic fibrosis admitted in intensive care unit: a multicenter study, *Respir Res* 7:14, 2006.

59. Madden BP, Kariyawasam H, Siddiqi AJ, et al: Noninvasive ventilation in cystic fibrosis patients with acute or chronic respiratory failure, *Eur Respir J* 19(2):310–313, 2002.

60. Noone PG: Non-invasive ventilation for the treatment of hypercapnic respiratory failure in cystic fibrosis, *Thorax* 63(1):5–7, 2008.

61. Bartz RR, Love RB, Leverson GE, et al: Pre-transplant mechanical ventilation and outcome in patients with cystic fibrosis, *J Heart Lung Transplant* 22(4):433–438, 2003.

62. Sood N, Paradowski LJ, Yankaskas JR: Outcomes of intensive care unit care in adults with cystic fibrosis, *Am J Respir Crit Care Med* 163(2):335–338, 2001.

63. Brown SJ, Eichner SF, Jones JR: Nebulized morphine for relief of dyspnea due to chronic lung disease, *Ann Pharmacother* 39(6):1088–1092, 2005.

64. Robinson W: Palliative care in cystic fibrosis, *J Palliat Med* 3(2):187–192, 2000.

65. Currow DC, Ward AM, Abernethy AP: Advances in the pharmacological management of breathlessness, *Curr Opin Support Palliat Care* 3(2):103–106, 2009.

66. Graff GR, Stark JM, Grueber R: Nebulized fentanyl for palliation of dyspnea in a cystic fibrosis patient, *Respiration* 71(6):646–649, 2004.

67. Ross J, Gamble J, Schultz A, et al: Back pain and spinal deformity in cystic fibrosis, *Am J Dis Child* 141(12):1313–1316, 1987.

68. Yen D, Hedden D: Multiple vertebral compression fractures in a patient treated with corticosteroids for cystic fibrosis, *Can J Surg* 45(5):383–384, 2002.

69. Sendzik J, Lode H, Stahlmann R: Quinolone-induced arthropathy: an update focusing on new mechanistic and clinical data, *Int J Antimicrob Agents* 33(3):194–200, 2009.

70. Dixey J, Redington AN, Butler RC, et al: The arthropathy of cystic fibrosis, *Ann Rheum Dis* 47(3):218–223, 1988.

71. Schidlow DV, Goldsmith DP, Palmer J, et al: Arthritis in cystic fibrosis, *Arch Dis Child* 59(4):377–379, 1984.

72. Dray X, Bienvenu T, Desmazes-Dufeu N, et al: Distal intestinal obstruction syndrome in adults with cystic fibrosis, *Clin Gastroenterol Hepatol* 2(6):498–503, 2004.

73. Turcios NL: Cystic fibrosis: an overview, *J Clin Gastroenterol* 39(4):307–317, 2005.

74. Boesch RP, Acton JD: Outcomes of fundoplication in children with cystic fibrosis, *J Pediatr Surg* 42(8):1341–1344, 2007.

75. Stallings VA, Stark LJ, Robinson KA, et al: Evidence-based practice recommendations for nutrition-related management of children and adults with cystic fibrosis and pancreatic insufficiency: results of a systematic review, *J Am Diet Assoc* 108(5):832–839, 2008.

76. Shanmugam G, Bhutani S, Khan DA, et al: Psychiatric considerations in pulmonary disease, *Psychiatr Clin North Am* 30(4):761–780, 2007.

77. Cruz I, Marciel KK, Quittner AL, et al: Anxiety and depression in cystic fibrosis, *Semin Respir Crit Care Med* 30(5):569–578, 2009.

78. Havermans T, Colpaert K, Dupont LJ: Quality of life in patients with cystic fibrosis: association with anxiety and depression, *J Cyst Fibros* 7(6):581–584, 2008.

79. Quittner AL, Barker DH, Snell C, et al: Prevalence and impact of depression in cystic fibrosis, *Curr Opin Pulm Med* 14(6):582–588, 2008.

80. Riekert KA, Bartlett SJ, Boyle MP, et al: The association between depression, lung function, and health-related quality of life among adults with cystic fibrosis, *Chest* 132(1):231–237, 2007.

81. Glasscoe C, Lancaster GA, Smyth RL, et al: Parental depression following the early diagnosis of cystic fibrosis: a matched, prospective study, *J Pediatr* 150(2):185–191, 2007.

82. Prasad SA, Cerny FJ: Factors that influence adherence to exercise and their effectiveness: application to cystic fibrosis, *Pediatr Pulmonol* 34(1):66–72, 2002.

83. Yankaskas JR, Knowles MR, editors: *Clinical pathophysiology and manifestations of lung disease: cystic fibrosis in adults*, Philadelphia, 1999, Lippincott-Raven.

84. Egan TM, Detterbeck FC, Mill MR, et al: Long term results of lung transplantation for cystic fibrosis, *Eur J Cardiothorac Surg* 22(4):602–609, 2002.

85. Gee L, Abbott J, Hart A, et al: Associations between clinical variables and quality of life in adults with cystic fibrosis, *J Cyst Fibros* 4(1):59–66, 2005.

86. Egan TM, Murray S, Bistami RT, et al: Development of the new lung allocation system in the United States, *Am J Transplant* 6(5):1212–1227, 2006.

87. *Cystic Fibrosis Foundation Patient Registry: Annual Data Report*. 2006. www.cff.org/research/ClinicalResearch/PatientRegistryReport. Accessed December 2009.

88. Egan TM, Kotloff RM: Pro/Con debate: lung allocation should be based on medical urgency and transplant survival and not on waiting time, *Chest* 128(1):407–415, 2005.

89. Yankaskas JR, Mallory GB Jr: Lung transplantation in cystic fibrosis: consensus conference statement, *Chest* 113(1):217–226, 1998.

90. Braddock CHr, Edwards KA, Hasenberg NM, et al: Informed decision making in outpatient practice: time to get back to basics, *JAMA* 282(24):2313–2320, 1999.

91. Song MK, De Vito Dabbs A, Studer SM, et al: Course of illness after the onset of chronic rejection in lung transplant recipients, *Am J Crit Care* 17(3):246–253, 2008.

92. Song MK, De Vito Dabbs AJ: Advance care planning after lung transplantation: a case of missed opportunities, *Prog Transplant* 16(3):222–225, 2006.

93. Osaki S, Maloney JD, Meyer KC, et al: Redo lung transplantation for acute and chronic lung allograft failure: long-term follow-up in a single center, *Eur J Cardiothorac Surg* 34(6):1191–1197, 2008.

94. Claar RL, Parekh PI, Palmer SM, et al: Emotional distress and quality of life in caregivers of patients awaiting lung transplant, *J Psychosom Res* 59(1):1–6, 2005.

95. Lefaiver CA, Keough VA, Letizia M, et al: Quality of life in caregivers providing care for lung transplant candidates, *Prog Transplant* 19(2):142–152, 2009.

96. Vermeulen KM, Bosma OH, Bij W, et al: Stress, psychological distress, and coping in patients on the waiting list for lung transplantation: an exploratory study, *Transpl Int* 18(8):954–959, 2005.

97. Sawicki GS, Dill EJ, Asher D, et al: Advance care planning in adults with cystic fibrosis, *J Palliat Med* 11(8):1135–1141, 2008.

98. Sawicki GS, Sellers DE, McGuffie K, et al: Adults with cystic fibrosis report important and unmet needs for disease information, *J Cyst Fibros* 6(6):411–416, 2007.

99. Auclair C: The Fog of Math, *SVB: Newsletter of the Adult CF Committee of Quebec* 31:5, 2007.

100. Freyer DR, Kuperberg A, Sterken DJ, Pastyrnak SL, Hudson D, Richards T: Multidisciplinary care of the dying adolescent, *Child Adolesc Psychiatr Clin N Am* 15(3):693–715, 2006.

101. *Five Wishes*, 2007. www.agingwithdignity.org. Accessed December 2009.

102. McCollum AT, Schwartz AH: Social work and the mourning parent, *Soc Work* 17:25–36, 1972.

103. Liben S, Papadatou D, Wolfe J: Paediatric palliative care: challenges and emerging ideas, *Lancet* 371(9615):852–864, 2008.

104. Waechter EH: Children's awareness of fatal illness, *Am J Nurs* 7(6):1168–1172, 1971.

105. Fanos JH: *Sibling loss*, Mahwah, NJ, 1996, Lawrence Earlbaum Associates.

42 Solid Organ Transplant

MICHAEL MCCOWN | DAWN FREIBERGER |
LYNNE HELFAND | DEBRA BOYER

Every obstacle I have overcome
Has made me stronger in some way
And to get the best out of life
I must live it day by day.
So this bump I've now stumbled upon
Is no different from the rest
I must smile, hope, and fight
And try my very best.
As my hair may all fall out
My diabetes out of whack
I will continue to get better
And my hair will grow back
So accept me as I am
While I go around this bend
Cause I'm going to get through this
I'm fighting till the end...
  —Cystic fibrosis patient

Providing palliative care to patients pursuing an intensive, life-extending treatment such as organ transplantation may seem paradoxical. However, the presence of severe underlying disease, inadequate organ availability, and significant morbidity and mortality associated with the transplant process requires the application of palliative care concepts throughout the transplant process. By definition, the involved patient population has severe end-stage disease that carries with it significant morbidity and mortality. The disparity between the number of patients needing organs and donors is significant and leaves listed patients with unpredictable waiting times. During this period, the patient's medical status may worsen and his or her care needs change dramatically. Therefore, transplant medicine is focused on providing life-extending treatments but must always recognize the medical realities and emotional needs of the patients and families involved.

The frequency of organ transplantation has increased dramatically over the past 30 years and has increasingly become a part of patient care. In 2008, there were 27,961 solid organ transplants in the United States, with 1,964 of these procedures occurring in patients less than 18 years old (Table 42-1). Greater experience with the surgical techniques involved with organ transplantation and improved understanding of the etiology of organ rejection will likely lead to increases in the number of patients involved with transplant medicine.

The specific criteria to be listed for organ transplantation will vary depending on which organ is involved, but generally patients are referred when the morbidity and mortality associated with their underlying disease is greater than that associated with transplant. Mortality rates reflect a variety of factors, including the impact of the patient's underlying disease, the technical and medical difficulties associated with the transplant procedure, a variety of post-transplant complications and the availability of other life-extending treatments in the event of transplant failure. Morbidity rates are more difficult to quantify and the impact of transplantation on a patient's quality of life is similarly challenging. Reported morbidity associated with transplant includes complications from the surgery, chronic organ dysfunction due to ischemic injury or rejection, and the complications associated with long-term immunosuppressive medications. Ultimately, all transplantations require a patient and family commitment to continued medical follow-up and evaluation. Transplantation should not be viewed as a complete cure of the underlying disease process, but rather a transition to a different, chronic medical condition.

Solid organ transplantation is offered in many countries, generally in the more developed and financially sound environments. Patients often have to travel great distances and even cross borders to obtain needed services. In addition, patients do come to the United States seeking organ transplantation. While this is permitted as per United Network for Organ Sharing (UNOS) there are limits as to how many international patients each program can transplant each year.

In the United States, transplant centers are not ranked, but there are national survival rates published on www.ustransplant.org. Patients and families are able to access this data to compare the outcomes of various transplant centers.

Transplant Evaluation

Transplantation is an extraordinarily stressful time from every perspective. Careful patient selection is required due to the physical demands involved with the actual procedure, the psychosocial upheaval involved throughout the process, and the extensive financial and social support required after a transplant. Transplant evaluation is a comprehensive review of the patient's medical history, current physical condition, psychological and/or emotional status, and available resources. Evaluation is also a time when the family and patient are introduced to the entire transplant team and the process of transplantation. It is essential that the family learn about all aspects of transplantation, including anticipated time on wait lists, potential risks associated with the procedure, and what

TABLE 42-1 Distribution of Pediatric Solid Organ Transplants in 2008

Organ	Number of pediatric transplants	3-Year survival rates
Kidney	773 (39%)	97%
Liver	613 (31%)	88%
Heart	365 (19%)	81%
Intestine	93 (5%)	64%
Lung	45 (2%)	60%

Data compiled from United Network for Organ Sharing 2008 and www.ustransplant.org.

level of care and lifestyle they can expect post-transplant. The development of stable relationships with the care team during this process can have a lasting impact on patient care throughout the transplant process. At the end of the evaluation process, the patient may be actively listed for transplant, placed on a deferred status until they meet criteria, or be declined for a specific reason. Occasionally, the patient and/or family may elect to not pursue transplantation, may elect to visit other centers, or may decide to postpone becoming listed.

The medical evaluation includes an assessment of the underlying disease process for which the patient was referred, as well as a comprehensive assessment to identify any comorbid conditions that may complicate or preclude transplantation. The substantial risks involved with transplantation and the relative scarcity of available organs mandates an intensive evaluation of the patient's current and past medical history. Each transplant team will have specific requirements for further testing, but in general patients undergo a variety of physical exams, laboratory tests, radiographic procedures, and consultations. Patients are frequently referred to a transplant program from remote locations with little or no preceding contact with the transplant center. Furthermore, this referral often comes at a time of great crisis for the family because the patient may have recently had a dramatic decline in his or her medical condition. It is not uncommon for transplant centers to repeat testing that has already been completed at the referring institution to confirm results and to evaluate for disease progression.

Each patient being referred for solid organ transplantation will be evaluated by an interdisciplinary team including social workers, financial planners, mental health professionals, and pharmacists. Social workers will assess a family's ability to handle post transplant care and identify their practical and emotional means of support. There are numerous psychosocial stressors present throughout the transplant process, including living with chronic disease, frequent medical evaluation and treatment, the uncertainty of an organ's availability, and the substantial requirements for ongoing care after transplantation. In addition to the impact of these stressors on the patient's and family's psyche, there are significant associated financial expenses involved in the process. These include the need for frequent admissions, and clinic visits and procedures that are commonly at centers remote from their home. Families may miss work or have travel and food expenses that they would not normally have. Depending on the patient's insurance, uncovered expenses for office visits and medications can be overwhelming. A social worker will evaluate the family's ability to cope with these stressors and to identify potential

areas of concern that may impact the care of the transplanted patient. Ultimately, the social worker will assist the family in locating and developing the resources and support they will need to successfully navigate this process. A mental health professional will assess the readiness of the patient and family for transplant and evaluate the level of understanding regarding the child's health and prognosis. There are times when a family and medical team are ready to list for transplant, but the child is not ready. In these instances, the psycho-social support team can be very helpful in navigating issues of assent in these young patients.

At the conclusion of the evaluation process, the patient's disposition regarding transplant will be determined. Patients are formally presented to the transplant team for discussion and all factors, medical, psychosocial, financial, developmental, and family resource, are taken into consideration. Both medical and psychosocial factors will play a large role in the ultimate decision about whether to list a patient for transplantation. Prior adherence to medical regimens must also be considered. A decision to list a patient will occur when the benefits of a transplant are greater than the predicted morbidity and mortality. There are no clear criteria as to when this threshold is met and therefore listing can be a complicated decision. Importantly, the patient's quality of life is a vital factor in deciding when to proceed with transplantation. Application of this standard must be tempered by a thorough understanding of the overall health of the patient and care must be taken to not wait too long when comorbid conditions and overall poor health may adversely affect the post-transplant prognosis.

Ethical issues arise when transplant teams are faced with a family with financial and psychosocial limitations. The team must ensure that resources are available to allow the family to overcome these obstacles so that they do not compromise the child's care. It is well documented that proper post-transplant care is essential to allow for a good outcome. Therefore, in some instances, patients are declined for transplant due to insurmountable psychosocial limitations. On rare occasions, issues of medical foster care are raised to provide a safe environment for the child post-transplant (Table 42-2).

Transplant Preparations

Once the determination has been made to list a patient for transplantation, he or she is placed on the national wait list, thus beginning a new period of uncertainty. The waitlist

TABLE 42-2 Transplant Team Members

Transplant team member	Role
Surgeon	Performs transplant surgery
Physician	Provides medical care both pre- and post-transplant
Coordinator	Responsible for pre- and post-transplant care from a nursing perspective, coordination of care, evaluations and patient and/or family education
Social worker	Provides assessment and care around psychosocial needs of family during all phases of transplant process
Psychologist	Performs pre-transplant evaluation to identify any contraindications to transplant. Identifies need for continued therapy pre- and post-transplant

process varies by organ type, with some organs using allocation scores based on disease severity to determine the place on the list. Other organs use pure time on the list, with some preference given to children and adolescents.

Waiting for a transplant can be very stressful for the patient and family. Families are aware that in hoping for a transplant for their child, they are waiting for a tragic event to happen to another family. Understandably, this is very difficult for both older children and their families to process. It is explained that for a donor family, organ donation enables them see some benefit come from their tragic situation.

Waiting times on the list vary depending on the organ, the size of the patient, and region where the patient is listed. This could vary from a day to years. Most families carry a beeper so that the transplant center can reach them quickly when an organ becomes available. Arrangements need to be made in advance for other family responsibilities such as sibling child care, because families need to get to the transplant center in a very short amount of time once an organ is located. Not uncommonly, patients are called in for a transplant only to be sent home without the surgery when complications with the donor arise. Patients can also be listed in more than one region, which may mean double clinic visits and added travel expenses. Certainly, this compounds the time and financial investment for the family.

It can feel as if life is put on hold while a patient is listed for transplant. Because a family needs to be near the transplant center, vacations generally need to be close to home. Activities that have a high exposure to potentially sick contacts should be curtailed. The uncertainty that transplant will occur leads to an extraordinarily stressful time in many patients' and families' lives.

It is during this pre-transplant phase that applying palliative care can be most helpful. The patient will frequently be receiving intensive medical care to optimize his or her overall health for when the transplant occurs. These treatments will frequently occur in the face of a progressive, end-stage disease that has high morbidity and mortality without transplant. Balancing the benefits of intensive continued disease-directed therapy with an acceptable quality of life needs to be continually considered and assessed. Open and frank discussions with the patient and family regarding their views of the process, goals, and wishes should occur regularly between the patient and the transplant team. Similarly, palliative care teams can be very helpful in working with the patient's primary physicians and the transplant teams to ensure that the goals and wishes of the family are continually respected.

It is important to acknowledge that some patients become too ill and no longer remain viable transplant candidates. Furthermore, there are also numbers of waitlist deaths each year, where the appropriate organ is not found in time to save the child. Transplant caregivers then can find themselves in the situation of concurrently managing and maintaining end-stage diseases while simultaneously navigating the dying process. This can feel contradictory to the needs of staying active on a transplant list. It is not uncommon for members of the medical teams to have differing opinions on how to handle these situations. Families are also conflicted with the need to not give up, and yet spare their child any unnecessary pain or discomfort. Discussions about whether a patient can have a DNR order in place and still be active on the transplant list are not infrequent. An example might be a patient with cystic fibrosis who faces potential intubation for progressive end-stage lung

disease yet still desires to reach transplantation. In this situation, some patients and/or families elect to proceed with intubation in the hope that an organ will be located in time. Others will choose to pursue more comfort care measures at this time. The palliative care team can be instrumental in guiding the patient, family, and caregivers through these difficult decisions (Fig. 42-1).

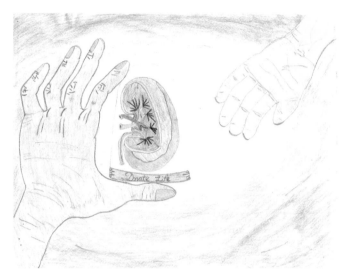

Fig. 42-1 Drawing by a child awaiting an organ transplant at Children's Hospital Boston.

Transplant

The actual transplant procedure is that start of a new experience for the patient and his or her family. While many of these patients have lived their lives with a chronic disease, they are now facing procedures, medications, and complications that are vastly different. Each organ transplant has its own set of immediate surgical risks and subsequent recovery period. Post-operatively, patients may require varying periods of ventilatory support and intensive care unit support. Many solid organ transplant patients will receive induction therapy, which provides intensive immediate immunosuppression in the post-operative period. Depending on the organ and transplant program, this may consist of a few doses of a medication or months of intermittent therapy. This is in contrast with maintenance immunosuppression, which is generally lifelong. Hospitalizations can be brief with discharges within one week or can be prolonged by months should complications arise.

In general, after a transplant, patients will receive immunosuppressive therapy to minimize the chances of rejection. While the degree of immunosuppression differs with each organ, the result is that each patient is at greater risk for infectious complications. For some organs, this risk diminishes over time as immunosuppression is lowered. For others, this risk is significant and lifelong. In general, most solid organ transplant patients are at risk for both acute and chronic rejection. While acute rejection most often occurs in the first few years post transplant and chronic rejection most often after 1 year, these distinctions are not absolute. Therefore, each transplant team will have individualized plans on how to monitor patients for each of these entities. Secondary to these immunosuppressive medications, transplant patients are at risk for long-term complications, including an increased risk of infection, hypertension, renal insufficiency, fluid retention, diabetes, dyslipidemias, seizures, and malignancy. While each patient will have a variable medication regimen, common symptoms experienced by this patient population include gastrointestinal upset, thrush, tremors and headaches, hirsutism, and mood changes (Table 42-3).

A second important consideration after transplant is adequate pain control, both in the immediate post-transplant period and afterward. Patients will generally have multiple lines for intravenous access, often chest tubes or other drains as well as incisions related to their transplant surgery. While most transplant surgeons, physicians, and nurses are well versed in adequate pain control, a palliative care service can be vital at this time to ensure that the patient is receiving the appropriate degree of analgesia. Furthermore, if the palliative care service has a longstanding relationship with the patient and family, they may be aware of differing mechanisms both pharmacologic and nonpharmacologic to help treat a patient's pain and/or anxiety.

After transplant, patients and families are often adjusting to a new care team with physicians, surgeons, nurses, and hospi-

tals. This period of adjustment can be stressful, and having the continuity of their palliative care team can be very beneficial.

Post-Transplant Period

In the period immediately following transplant, patients and families are adjusting not only to new medical issues but to a new lifestyle as well. Many families have experienced years of coping with the illness that brought them to transplant, and they have developed a level of comfort with the way they feel and how they care for themselves or their child. Post-transplant patients are now forced to revisit this and learn about their body and their care in new ways. Patients and families may also feel that they have been given a second chance. When the transplant was received from a cadaveric donation they are aware of this gift being the result of a tragedy. This can lead to tremendous feelings of guilt as patients and families try to reconcile their joy with the tragedy that another family has experienced.

Patient's bodies feel different as they incorporate the new organ and begin to feel that it is truly theirs. Patients often wonder about the identity of the donor and whether they might assume some of their donor's character traits. This can occur

TABLE 42-3   Transplant Immunosuppressive Therapies

Induction Agents

Medication	Mechanism	Adverse effects
Induction medications		
Rabbit anti-thymocyte globulin (Thymoglobulin)	Polyclonal antibody decreases CD4 lymphocytes	Persistent lymphopenia
Horse anti-thymocyte globulin (Atgam)	Polyclonal antibody against T lymphocytes	Persistent lymphopenia Severe thrombocytopenia
Basiliximab (Simulect)	Monoclonal antibody to Il-2 receptor complex	Anaphylactoid and hypersensitivity reactions Development of human automurine antibodies
Alemtuzumab (Campath)	Monoclonal antibody to CD52	Severe cytopenia Hypersensitivity with infusion
Maintenance medications		
Medication	Mechanism	Adverse effects
Tacrolimus (Prograf)	Calcineurin inhibitor	Nephrotoxic Diabetes mellitus Hyperkalemia Hypertension Hepatic toxicity
Cylcosporine (Neoral/Sandimmune)	Inhibition of T-cell activation	Hypertension Nephrotoxicity
Mycophenolate mofetil (Cellcept)	Inhibition of inosine monophosphate dehydrogenase (IMPDH) with decreased T and B cell proliferation	GI disturbance Bone marrow suppression
Mycophenolic acid (Myfortic)	IMPDH inhibition with decreased T- and B-cell proliferation	GI disturbance Bone marrow suppression
Azathioprine (Imuran)	Purine metabolism antagonist	GI toxicity Dose-related hematologic toxicity Hepatotoxicity Mutagenic effects
Sirolimus (Rapamune)	Suppresses cytokine mediated T-cell proliferation	Anaphylaxis and/or angioedema Interstitial lung disease Lymphocele Proteinuria and/or nephro toxicity Impaired wound healing
Prednisone	Inhibits leukocyte migrations and decreases inflamatory response	Hypertension Hyperglycemia Cataracts Osteoporosis Cushing disease

with children of all ages and it might affect them in both positive and negative ways. During this post-transplant period many patients or families may wish to write a letter to the donor family. In general, organ procurement organizations will facilitate the communication of this letter to the donor family if they choose to receive it.

Although patients may think about their donors and feel grateful for the gift, one study[1] showed that none of the study participants "acknowledged any sign of guilt (for surviving the cadaveric donor or for putting a parent/relative/friend through the physical pain of living related donation). Few had considered that they received any of the donor's traits. All believed that their sense of self was stronger after transplant with many respondents emphasizing a new, inner strength during the post-transplant period."[1]

During the evaluation and as they wait for organs to become available, all families and patients discussed with the medical team that transplant essentially trades one disease process for another. Post-transplant, these patients will face a new set of medical issues. Adjusting to these changes can be a challenging process that varies with the patient's developmental level. Young children tend to incorporate their new medical regime into their life and continue to work with their parents to manage their medications and medical appointments. Some adults may adjust easily while others may find their new medical regime difficult to adapt to. However, as they become more comfortable with their post-transplant care, they may become less adherent and less anxious when a problem arises, or feel annoyed when their care needs interfere with work or other activities.

Adolescent patients pose a different set of concerns to the transplant professionals. During this stage of development, children feel invincible and are struggling to assert themselves as autonomous individuals. "Risk-taking behaviors function to fulfill developmental needs for independence, autonomy and self-competence."[2] This is the most difficult developmental period for parents and for medical professionals. A healthy teen would be given increasing autonomy and responsibility. For the teen with a transplant, however, parents need to walk a fine line between helping their child learn to manage their own care while they remain involved to ensure that their child is adhering to the medical regime. Their goal is to prepare their child to become an independent adult able to manage his or her own medical care. The foremost concern certainly is that the adolescent will not adhere to the medication regime. In a transplant patient, this can have life-threatening consequences. Teens often want to test the limits of their bodies and don't fully believe that they need the medications. They may purposefully or subconsciously forget to take their medication for a day or longer. When they realize their error, they may not bring this to the attention of their parents. Additionally, teenagers generally have a strong desire to be like their peers and to feel normal. "During adolescence, a sense of identity and self-understanding is created through social relationships with peers."[3] They may want to feel that they can have days without medications and days just like their healthy friends. Patients whose friends do not know about their transplant may prefer the risk of missing a dose of medication rather than the risk of having a peer ask them about their treatments. There are transplant centers that resist transplanting teens because of these significant concerns about non-adherence.

An additional stressor for the adolescent transplant patient is the eventual transfer of care to an adult center. This is a diffi-cult transition period both medically and psychosocially for the transplant patient. Patients feel abandoned by having to leave a pediatric center, where they may have received care their entire life. Furthermore, adjusting to a new mode of care delivery in an adult center can be challenging to pediatric patients. From a medical standpoint, studies have shown an increased incidence of organ rejection during adolescence.[4]

In adolescence and adulthood, questions regarding pregnancy post-transplant are often asked. Depending on the health of the transplant patient and the particular organ that they received, the risk of pregnancy is variable. For some organs, such as a lung transplant patient, the risk of experiencing significant and potentially life-threatening rejection is quite high.[5] For other patients such as kidney transplant recipients, the risk is likely far less.[6] For all transplant patients, they must be aware of the potential risks to a fetus of all medications they are taking.

For the child undergoing a transplant there are many social stressors. There may be extended periods when they miss school and other activities, as well as the continued restrictions of exposure to ill contacts. There are physical changes due to medications such as hair growth or loss, Cushingoid features, and weight gain. In addition, there is the constant feeling of being different from others. "The threat of rejection or infections is a reminder to the patients of the uncertainly of the transplant course. This uncertainty could be viewed as a threat to the adolescent's sense of self. While some of the patients experienced serious post transplant medical problems, many generally express a determination to focus on the present."[1]

There are financial stressors for families, including lost work time and costs inherent in spending time at the hospital with their child. For siblings there can be a sense of deprivation, as more attention must be paid to the patient, fostering any perception that the sick sibling is more important. They may also harbor feelings of guilt or fear that they have caused or contributed to their sibling's illness. For the patient there may be feelings of guilt as he or she is aware that time spent with them is time away from the sibling.

Children do not perceive death as permanent. This understanding of death gradually develops for children after the age of 5. Children living with life-threatening illness are coping with concerns that are beyond their developmental stage. They must live with the inherent knowledge that death is a reality. "The reality is that children often know much about what is happening to them, regardless of what they have been shielded from or formally told."[7,8] Many of these children and young adults know of other patients who have died and may have experienced a life-threatening event in their own lives.

For the transplant team, there may be judgments that are inherent in having a limited resource with underlying questions about the patients' worthiness to receive this gift, as well as concerns about other patients who may not survive to transplant. This can become apparent if the patient does not adhere to the treatment regime, particularly if there is a rejection episode.

In time, a recipient becomes more comfortable with his or her changed body and the organ becomes a part of the sense of self. For some this level of comfort is challenged with any medical complications.

Patients and their families may be faced with transitioning from end of life disease to post-transplant recovery and, in some instances, to morbidity from post-transplant complications.

Patients can feel well and be more active and then experience complications that quickly reverse these gains. In other instances, there may be gradual post-transplant complications such as living with chronic rejection. Patients and their families may need to shift their mindsets to one of recovery to, once again, facing loss and possibly death.[9]

End of Life

When a transplanted organ begins to fail, many of the issues surrounding end-stage disease and end of life care are again a reality for a patient and their family. This will certainly vary by organ with various salvage therapies available to each. For example, renal transplant recipients may be faced with considering restarting dialysis. When a transplant organ has failed, an organ recipient and his or her caregivers must consider whether re-transplantation is an option. This decision is generally quite difficult for patients and the transplant team for a variety of reasons. One main consideration would be outcomes following a re-transplant. In some cases, outcomes are worse than with the primary transplant, although this varies significantly with the organ involved.[10-12] Additionally, the transplant medications and therapies may have caused problems with other organ systems, such as the kidneys or liver. In some cases, these consequences have resulted in a patient who is not a good re-transplant candidate. Furthermore, it is essential to continue to assess psychological and social factors that could make retransplantation more difficult. Examples would include issues with non-adherence, drug use or poor medical follow up. As each individual transplant center will have its own criteria for primary and for re-transplant patients, it is not uncommon for a patient to be referred to a new program for consideration of re-transplantation. In some cases, this program may be quite a distance from the patient's home.

Families themselves may be ambivalent about re-transplant. If the first transplant went well, then a family is generally more interested in relisting than if there were significant complications. Some ethicists would argue that with all the waitlist deaths that occur each year, it is unfair to list someone for a second transplant when so many have been waiting so long for their first transplant.

When a patient is relisted for transplant and the organ continues to fail, all of the same issue and feelings return that existed while waiting for the first transplant. Again, medical providers are going down two separate paths; addressing end of life issues and optimizing medical care in order to maintain the patient as a re-transplant candidate. Just as in the initial pre-transplant period, these two paths can seem contradictory to each other both for patients and caregivers alike. For example, giving too much pain medication can cause sleepiness and decrease the ability to stay ambulatory. Yet, we are compelled to not allow our patients to suffer discomfort as much as possible. In this scenario, the palliative care team can be very helpful in walking this fine line. Some medical professionals believe that listing for transplant in general disrupts the normal end of life process. Finding a balance between the two positions must be looked at on an individual patient basis.

Transplant patients have challenges in particular when considering hospice care. For young children these challenges can be even greater. Depending on the hospice and the type of insurance that a child has, there could be a set amount of funds that are allocated once a patient goes into hospice care. At times choices have to be made regarding transplant medications, home nursing services and other services normally offered through hospice care.

Because the goal of transplant is giving life, death in transplant patients requires a different focus of care that is often just as difficult for medical providers as it is for families. Healthcare professionals need continued education and support when helping patients through these challenging times. Having a member of the palliative care team at family meetings and rounds assures that all aspects of care are considered for the patient and family. Medical professionals, especially nursing staff, need both the emotional tools and the educational resources to care for the dying patient.

Clinical Vignette

CK is a 17-year-old boy who was diagnosed with cystic fibrosis as a toddler. At age 12 he was referred to the transplant center for evaluation because of declining pulmonary function and was listed for a double lung transplant. CK waited for 2 years before lungs became available. After transplant CK had several admissions for treatment of infection but was healthy overall.

During this period CK returned to school and for the first time had peers that did not know of his medical background. Initially CK took his medications on time, monitored his pulmonary function by home spirometry, exercised, and was followed closely in transplant clinic. He was independent with most of his care because his mother worked full time. Several years after transplant CK missed several doses of his antirejection medications and stopped doing his home spirometry when his friends were around as he struggled to "live like a normal teenager." Three years after his transplant, CK was diagnosed with chronic rejection. He was again evaluated for a double lung transplant. During the re-evaluation period, CK's medical status was reviewed and significant concerns were expressed regarding his previous non-adherence. Ultimately, the transplant team believed that this was an isolated event of adolescence and were confident that CK could continue to adhere to the challenging medical regimen required of him with a re-transplant.

CK's lung function continued to decline rapidly. CK and his father questioned if he would survive long enough to receive a second transplant. His parents were able to discuss procedures and choices around his care with their son but had an increasingly difficult time staying at the hospital during his lengthy admissions. CK worked closely with mental health providers at the transplant center and began to clarify his end of life wishes, which included doing everything possible to receive a transplant but dying peacefully if transplant would no longer be an option. Fortunately, CK did receive a second double lung transplant. The transplant team continues to work closely with CK and his parents around managing his medical regime, discussing changing roles as CK moves toward adulthood and coping with the sadness and anxiety the family has experienced as they have been repeatedly confronted by the fragility of life.

Summary

Outcomes from organ transplantation have improved dramatically since the first organ transplant was performed in 1954. However, as with all patients with complex medical conditions, it remains a process with variable outcomes. Through every step of the transplant process from referral and evaluation to listing, transplant, and the post-transplant period, numerous challenges are faced by patients and caregivers. Palliative care has a role in all of these stages and can help to improve the quality of life for patients in these very challenging situations.

REFERENCES

1. Durst CL, Horn MV, Maclaughlin EF, Bowman CM, Starnes VA, Woo MS: Psychosocial responses of adolescent cystic fibrosis patients to lung transplantation, *Pediatr Transplant* 5:27–31, 2001.
2. Millstein SG, Ingra V: Theoretical models of adolescent risk-taking behavior. In Wallander JL, Siegel IJ, editors: *Adolescent health problems*, New York, 1995, Guilford, pp 52–71.
3. Sroufe LA, Cooper RG, Dehart G: *Child Development: its nature and course*, ed 3, New York, 1996, McGraw Hill.
4. Bell LE, Bartosh SM, Davis CL, Dobbels F, Al-Uzri A, Lotstein D, Reiss J, Dharnidharka VR: Adolescent transition to adult care in solid organ transplantation: a consensus conference report, *Am J Transplant* 8:2230–2242, 2008.
5. Armenti VT, Radomski JS, Moritz MJ, Gaughan WJ, McGrory CH, Coscia LA: Report from the National Transplantation Pregnancy Registry (NTPR): outcomes of pregnancy after transplantation. In Cecka, Terasaki, editors: *Clinical transplants*, Los Angeles, 2003.
6. Zachariah MS, Tornatore KM, Venuto RC: Kidney transplantation and pregnancy, *Curr Opin Organ Transplant* 14:386–391, 2009.
7. Sourkes BM: *Armfuls of time: the psychological experience of the child with a life-threatening illness*, Pittsburgh, 1995, University of Pittsburgh Press.
8. Bluebond Langer M: *Private worlds of dying children, Princeton, NJ*, 1978, Princeton University Press.
9. Berzoff J, Silverman PR, editors: *Living with dying. a handbook for end-of-life healthcare practitioners*, New York, 2004, Columbia University Press.
10. Aurora P, Edwards LB, Christie JD, Dobbels F, Kirk R, Rahmel AO, Stehlik J, Taylor DO, Kucheryavaya AY, Hertz MI: Registry of the International Society for Heart and Lung Transplantation: Twelfth Official Pediatric Lung and Heart/Lung Transplantation Report-2009, *J Heart Lung Transplant* 28:1023–1030, 2009.
11. Kanter KR, Vincent RN, Berg AM, Mahle WTM, Forbess JM, Kirshbom PM: Cardiac retransplantation in children, *Ann Thoracic Surg* 78:644–649, 2004.
12. Shen ZY, Zhu ZJ, Deng YL, Zheng H, Pan C, Zhang YM, Shi R, Jiang WT, Zhang JJ: Liver retransplantation: report of 80 cases and review of the literature, *Hepatobiliary Pancreat Dis Int* 5(2):180-184, 2006.

43

Integration of Therapeutic and Palliative Care in Pediatric Oncology

DEBORAH A. LAFOND | BRIAN R. ROOD |
SHANA S. JACOBS | GREGORY H. REAMAN

If we listen closely, children who are dying, and their families, will tell us everything we need to know to care for them: they want to be loved, to be cared for and cared about, to know that their lives have meaning and purpose, to be remembered as the special people they are. Most of all, they want the people caring for them to appreciate and celebrate their lives.

—Cindy Stutzer

The improved outcome for children with cancer is a success story of modern medicine and one of several examples from the past century of previously untreatable diseases for which effective treatments have now been identified. These treatments have been identified through successive series of randomized controlled trials resulting in a strong evidence base, which has translated into progressively improving standards of care. This success has been accomplished through the integration of clinical research and clinical care of pediatric cancer patients primarily in academic settings, which has been linked tightly within a national clinical trials infrastructure.

The overall five-year survival rates for children younger than 15 years with cancer have increased from less than 60% from 1975 to 1978 to more than 80% from 1999 to 2002.[1] Most notable have been improvements in 5-year survival rates for children with acute lymphoblastic leukemia (ALL) now approaching 90%; non-Hodgkin lymphoma similarly approaching 90%; and Wilm tumor, exceeding 90% since the late 1980s. Overall 5-year survival rates most recently reported by the Surveillance Epidemiology and End Results (SEER) Program of the National Cancer Institute approximate 70% overall for primary central nervous system (CNS) tumors and approach 65% to 75% for sarcomas of soft tissue and bone.

Given the profound heterogeneity in diagnosis, clinical presentation, biologic behavior and outcome in primary tumors of the CNS, survival rates for individual tumor types vary considerably. Similarly, for soft-tissue and bone sarcomas, the likelihood of prolonged survival is highly linked to the initial extent of disease. Therefore, reported overall 5-year survival rates should not be considered predictive of cure for all patients with these diseases.[2] For example, whereas 5-year survival rates for infants with neuroblastoma are extremely favorable and have been relatively stable at 90% to 95% since the early 1980s, until very recently, improvements in older patients with unfavorable biologic features have not shown the same improvement with current five-year survival rates now approaching only 50%.[3]

As survival rates differ depending upon the cancer diagnosis, trajectories of illness and patterns of death also differ. For most pediatric oncology diseases, the trajectory from diagnosis to long-term survival or death is characterized by periods of relative stability interspersed with periods of decline or crisis. Symptoms and the trajectory of illness are dependent upon the underlying malignancy.[4] Leukemias are the most common type of childhood cancer and tumors of the central nervous system are the most frequent type of solid tumor in children.[1] However, specific types of these common childhood malignancies have unique trajectories of illness. For example, a child diagnosed with a brain stem glioma has a poor chance of long-term survival and often presents with multiple neurological deficits, however, a period of symptom improvement may occur with treatment. Unfortunately this period of improvement may be short-lived and is likely followed by exacerbation of symptoms and ultimately death from progressive disease. The timeline from diagnosis to death may be as short as a few months to a couple of years. In contrast, a child with leukemia may initially respond well to treatment and remain in remission. However, if the leukemia returns then the course of illness may be characterized by multiple treatment protocols followed by periods of remission, but may still ultimately end in death due to progressive disease over a period of years. As a further contrast, children undergoing stem cell transplant for a variety of childhood malignancies may die relatively quickly in the trajectory of illness because of sepsis or other side effects of treatment. The palliative care practitioner should be familiar with the symptoms and disease trajectory of the underlying malignancy in order to provide recommendations for effective symptom management.

Despite the impressive record of success in improving survival outcomes, cancer remains the leading cause of death from disease in the pediatric age group. Even cancers such as ALL with high cure rates still account for a significant number of deaths from cancer. Because ALL is the most common cancer of childhood, death related to treatment failure and treatment-related complications in acute leukemia contribute the most to cancer-related mortality statistics in children.[1]

For decades the focus of clinical investigation, translating to standards of clinical care for childhood cancer, has centered on cure. Significant sequelae and late effects associated with the various diagnoses and successful anti-cancer treatments are now well recognized and have become a major area of research. More recently, while not diminishing the importance of cure and quality of survivorship, appropriate attention and clinical research focus on the quality of life during the entirety of the cancer experience has begun to assume a more prominent position, with corresponding attention paid to symptom management using pharmacologic as well as behavioral approaches for children with cancer.

Whereas the concepts of cure and palliation have historically been somewhat competing objectives, recognition that palliation should not be considered exclusively applicable to end of life is paramount to the childhood cancer journey. Understanding and evaluating interventions to address physical, psychological, social, educational, and spiritual needs in children with cancer from the time of diagnosis onward must be considered.[5]

This chapter will address the needs of pediatric cancer patients and their families as well as the requirement for an interdisciplinary approach to providing appropriate palliative care. In addition, we will discuss opportunities for and challenges to the effective integration of appropriate palliative care with both curative disease management and investigational therapies where the potential for clinical benefit may be considerably smaller. A particular emphasis will be on the integration of palliation and symptom management with curative therapy that would appear warranted in patients with specific diagnoses where the prognosis for favorable outcome with current therapy approaches is less optimal. However, approaching every patient and family faced with a potentially life-threatening illness with a recognition of the need to address palliative elements would benefit patients, families, and providers in guiding those important considerations and decisions involving cancer-directed care, quality of life, symptom management, and, if necessary, end of life care and bereavement.

The Need for Palliative Care Services in Pediatric Oncology

Approximately 2300 pediatric patients die of cancer in the United States each year.[6,7] Most of these patients die of recurrent or progressive disease, and most have been battling their cancers for months to years. For pediatric patients with cancer, cure-directed therapy and palliative care needs go hand in hand from the moment of diagnosis throughout therapy. All patients, even patients with a high likelihood of cure, are likely to suffer multiple symptoms from the point of diagnosis onward. These symptoms include physical side effects from chemotherapy, such as nausea and vomiting, mouth sores and pain, and fevers and hospitalizations, as well as spiritual and psychological malaise. On the other side of the spectrum, many patients who reach the point where there are no known cures for their cancers may continue chemotherapy either as part of an experimental protocol or for palliative purposes.[8] Therefore, unlike many other disciplines, pediatric oncology patients are often in need of simultaneous cure-directed and palliative therapies. Effective palliative care services can ease suffering in children with cancer, allowing more hospice referrals and home death, less pain and dyspnea, and better preparation for death compared to families who did not receive palliative care services.[9]

Despite the clear relationship between palliative care and cancer care for children, many pediatric cancer patients do not receive palliative care services. A survey of institutions that are members of the Children's Oncology Group revealed that only 58% have palliative care services available for their patients.[10] Children with cancer are often receiving intense therapies for extended periods, sometimes years. As a result, they form strong relationships with their oncology team. These relationships can be a great asset as patients and families feel supported by members of the healthcare team who care a great deal about them. However, at times the intensity of the relationship may interfere with a patient's ability to get appropriate palliative or end of life care. The healthcare team's members may feel they have failed the patient if cure cannot be offered and may therefore push for cure-directed therapy over comfort care even when the chance of cure is very small.[11] In addition, the healthcare team may overestimate the patients' prognosis in an effort to keep the patient and family hopeful, which affects the families' ability to make informed decisions about care.[6] One study showed that physicians understand that patients have no realistic chance of cure a mean of 101 days before the parents' recognition.[12] Despite the clinicians' worry, an accurate portrayal of prognosis, even bad, makes families more hopeful, not less.[13] Even when parents find the news upsetting, they still derive benefit from hearing the prognosis.[14] Additionally, families who know that a child is dying are more likely to spend their end of life period pain-free at home.[15]

COMMON SYMPTOMS OF CHILDREN WITH ADVANCED CANCERS

Effective pain and symptom management for children with advanced cancers is dependent upon a sound knowledge of these symptoms.[16] Cancer is not unique in the palliative care spectrum in that children often experience multiple symptoms of varying intensities throughout the trajectory of illness. Few studies to date have addressed symptoms or the quality of life experienced by children with advanced cancer or who are dying of cancer.[17] Of particular interest are CNS tumors, which are a life-threatening illness with high morbidity and the second-leading cause of cancer deaths in children.[18] Children with brain tumors experience more severe symptom distress and treatment-related distress than children with other cancers.[19] A variety of symptoms are reported in pediatric patients with advanced cancer. The underlying malignancy impacts the type and severity of symptom distress, however the most common symptoms include pain, fatigue, dyspnea, nausea and vomiting, anxiety, and weight loss and/or cachexia.[16,20–23] In addition to these commonly experienced symptoms, children with hematologic malignancies may experience increased bleeding and coagulopathies and children with solid tumors may experience other symptoms related to compression of vital structures by tumor, such as spinal cord compression. An analysis of 164 children with advanced cancers in the last month of life noted that many symptoms are under-recognized and symptoms vary significantly based on the underlying malignancy[4] (Table 43-1). Palliative care practitioners must have knowledge of the symptoms associated with the specific pediatric malignancies in order to adequately address symptom distress. Symptom distress is significant for children with advanced cancers and affects their quality of life. Healthcare must not merely be vested in tumor outcomes but must instead address quality of life and functional status outcomes.

TUMOR-DIRECTED THERAPY

Palliative care should ideally be pursued from diagnosis, given the high rate of disease-and treatment-associated symptoms experienced by oncology patients. However, the imperative for a focus on the reduction of suffering is most acute in end of life

TABLE 43-1 Major and Minor Symptom Prevalence in Month Before Death

Symptom prevalence (%)	CNS (n=59) M/F (53:47)	Leukemia/lymphoma (n=41) M/F (56:44)	Other solid (n=64) M/F (53:47)	All patients (n=164) M/F (54:46)
Pain	81.4	95.1	98.4	91.5
Weakness	93.2	82.9	93.8	90.9
Anorexia	57.6	56.1	84.4	67.7
Weight loss	52.5	56.1	87.5	67.1
Mobility loss	89.8	36.6	50.0	61.0
Nausea	62.7	48.8	60.9	58.5
Constipation	57.6	46.3	67.2	58.5
Vomiting	64.4	43.9	57.8	56.7
Too much sleep	57.6	36.6	48.4	48.8
Anxiety and/or depression	37.3	43.9	53.1	45.1
Speech	76.3	14.6	26.6	41.5
Dyspnea	39.0	31.7	46.9	40.2
Excess secretions	69.5	14.6	28.1	39.6
Headache	64.4	24.4	26.6	39.6
Anemia	6.8	75.6	45.3	39.0
Pressure areas	39.0	19.5	50.0	38.4
Swallowing difficulties	62.7	17.1	25.0	36.6
Micturition	44.1	22.0	37.5	36.0
Vision and/or hearing loss	62.7	7.3	25.0	34.1
Infection	28.8	58.5	23.4	34.1
Fever	25.4	48.8	28.1	32.3
Bleeding	8.5	65.9	29.7	31.1
Skin problems	15.3	41.5	37.5	30.5
Cough	20.3	31.7	37.5	29.9
Change in behavior	30.5	26.8	31.3	29.9
Sore mouth	27.1	41.5	20.3	28.0
Confusion	23.7	19.5	31.3	25.6
Convulsions	39.0	12.2	12.5	22.0
Edema	13.6	12.2	34.4	21.3
Dizziness	33.9	19.5	7.8	20.1
Too little sleep	8.5	22.0	18.8	15.9
Diarrhea	6.8	22.0	14.1	13.4
Sleep reversal	13.6	14.6	12.5	13.4
Weight gain	23.7	4.9	4.7	11.6

From Goldman A, Hewitt M, Collins GS, Childs M and Hains R. Symptoms in children/young people with progressive malignant disease: United Kingdom children's cancer study group/paediatric oncology nurses' forum palliative care working group. Pediatrics. 2006: 117(6); e1179-e1186.
M, male; F, female.

care when therapies with known, significant curative potential have been exhausted. The means used to relieve symptoms include virtually every modality in modern medical practice, ranging from simple nonpharmacologic means such as massage to invasive procedures such as surgery. The key determinant of whether an intervention is palliative resides in the intent to relieve suffering in order to preserve or enhance the quality of life for the patient. Inherent in making this determination is a consideration of the likelihood that a chosen therapy may carry a risk of inducing a symptom burden.

In the treatment of cancer, reducing the tumor size or mass effect can also result in the alleviation of symptoms. Chemotherapy, radiation, and steroids can be used to this end. However, given that these modalities are often part of therapies used with curative intent, there is a potential for both the practitioner and the patient and his or her family to engage in a tacit shared misperception that cure is still a realistic goal. The power of this misperception lies in

the compassionate desire to avoid a painful focus on the impending death. The dangers of engaging in this delusion are insidious. First, the provider is more likely to propose, and the patient and family is more likely to accept, therapies that run a higher risk of jeopardizing quality of life whether through deleterious side effects or excessive trips to the hospital. Second, by not engaging in the end of life process, the patient and family are robbed of the opportunity to plan important aspects of the child's death. Lastly, the medical establishment is placed in a position where it must necessarily do harm in that it is unable to achieve the goal set before it, cure, and therefore neglects the more important charge, the relief of suffering.

In one study of bereaved parents, more than one third of the patients had received chemotherapy after it was recognized that the child had no realistic chance of cure. Also, 61% of parents felt their child had suffered as a result of the chemotherapy, and most of the parents would not recommend chemotherapy to other parents of children with cancer without realistic chance of cure. This suggests that in some cases physicians may not fully reveal the potential negative impact of continuing chemotherapy.[24] In end of life situations, physicians often use chemotherapy with the goal of reducing symptoms, while many parents believe that the chemotherapy has curative intent.[25] Therefore, it is imperative that therapy aimed at shrinking a tumor for symptom relief is clearly identified as such and that the temptation to allow such efforts to be labeled potentially curative, and thereby avoid an honest engagement with end of life, be resisted.

THE ESSENTIAL ROLE OF HOPE

None of the above considerations is meant to devalue or undermine the role of hope. Hope is a human state of existence and parents in particular cannot help but harbor hope for their children. Hope is not qualitative; there is no good hope or bad hope. False hope is a misnomer for what should be termed unrealistic expectation. Unlike unrealistic expectations, if a hope is unrealized, it does not result in the negative emotions that carry the power to complicate grief. For parents facing their child's death, hope often provides them the strength to continue to be mentally and emotionally present to comfort and parent their child. Hope can be described as having three domains: specific future-directed goals, imagining or planning the steps to realize those goals, and believing in one's own capacity to realize those goals. The degree of hopefulness is the interaction among these three domains.[26] An example of this in the context of pediatric oncology may be that of a hospitalized adolescent with advanced cancer who realizes that he will not recover from his illness and is likely to die from his disease, however, he clearly communicates the goal that he would like to attend his high school graduation ceremony in one month. The adolescent and his family meet with the oncology team and the school counselors to discuss how he may participate in the ceremony either in person with his peers or by having a private ceremony, which is developing a plan to meet that goal. They then continue to discuss the ceremony and plan for the events of the day with confidence that the adolescent will be able to participate in the event with specific modifications they have worked out with the school, which is believing in their own capacity to realize the goal. In this context, the family has hope. The phenomenon of hope is a complex and profoundly personal experience for each patient and family.

The paramount hope of parents of children with cancer is for survival. This is by no means the only meaningful hope that parents possess. It is important to help them to identify the other meaningful things for which they hope such as the minimization of suffering, the ability of their child to interact with loved ones, and their child's ability to feel joy or participation in a meaningful experience as above. The healthcare team often struggles with balancing hope with providing accurate information about the child's disease.[27] The healthcare team should not undermine the family's hope for a miracle but rather provide guidance for the family to identify realistic goals and other meaningful hopes. Providing families with accurate prognostic information and awareness building resources may help them have a healthier bereavement process.[13]

PREPARATIONS FOR END OF LIFE

Part of the process of maintaining hope at the end of life is control over the process for patients and their families. Frank discussions with families when cure becomes extremely unlikely allow families and children to have some control. For example, choosing the location of death has been shown to help families feel prepared for their child's death.[28] Families who know their children are likely to die can make educated decisions about advanced care planning, or about further therapies.

In addition, when families are prepared, they are more likely to be able to talk to their children about the fact that they are likely to die. Children with cancer tend to be very savvy about their conditions, and often surprise their families and caregivers with their insight into their care plans and desire to be involved with their treatment decisions. A study of 20 children and adolescents with refractory cancers showed that children understood they were involved in end of life decisions and were capable of participating in those discussions. This study also found that children, as well as their parents, often cited altruism as a factor in their decision making about care.[25] In addition, another study found that parents were actually less upset about receiving news about their child's cancer and treatment when their children were present for the conversation.[14] Finally, in a follow-up study of parents whose child died of cancer, no parents who talked to their children about death had regrets, while 27% of those who had not had the discussion did have regrets.[29]

Phase I Clinical Trials in the Context of Palliative Care

As parents and children make the emotional and intellectual transition from a therapeutic environment centered on curative intent to one where quality of life and management of symptoms dominate, they often become paralyzed by a feeling that they are giving up. This false perception is rooted in a number of factors, including an unrealistic belief in the power of modern medicine to control the course of disease, the feeling that the hope for survival is the only sustaining hope, and parental fear that they are ill-equipped to help their child. In many cases, the transition is complicated by a sense of suddenness if the provider and family have previously collaborated to avoid the painful acknowledgment of the potential for a fatal outcome. This time of transition is also when many families are offered enrollment in Phase I clinical trials because eligibility for such trials stipulates that no known curative therapies be available. Given the difficulty of this transition and the vulnerability of parents in this position, an inherent trap exists in the presentation of Phase I clinical trial; they can be seen as a continuation of cure-oriented therapy using a new drug. A study of parental reasons for enrollment in a Phase I study showed that two thirds believed that the alternative of no tumor-directed treatment was unacceptable.[30] This perception implies an expectation of therapeutic benefit. It is incumbent upon the clinical researcher to clearly describe the nature of Phase I clinical trials as seeking to determine the safety of new compounds, rather than offering a realistic expectation of disease response.

As has been shown, dying children tend to have higher symptom burdens and a greater need for palliative care.[31] Thus, Phase I clinical research virtually always takes place in a context of palliative care. However, it is important to distinguish palliative therapies intended to reduce tumor burden in an attempt to relieve symptoms from the Phase I clinical trials. Novel agents being given in a research context should not be used with a palliative intent. One large meta-analysis found an objective response rate of only 9.6% in 69 trials.[32] Indeed, the potential exists to induce bothersome symptoms and thereby detrimentally affect quality of life, the antithesis of the goal of the end of life period. The risk of inducing suffering must therefore be carefully weighed in the decision to pursue Phase I clinical trials in each individual case.

However, an admonition to avoid creating an expectation of disease response does not preclude that the patient and family may derive benefit from participation in a clinical research trial. Indeed, objective tumor response is not a good surrogate measure of direct benefit from participation in a trial. In a minority of cases, disease stabilization can provide relief from symptoms and prolong good quality of life. A study of 16 Phase I trials conducted at the NCI found a disease stabilization rate of 17%, although stabilization was modestly defined as completing three cycles of therapy without disease progression.[33] Other potential benefits include the strengthening of hope and the altruistic opportunity to help other children and thereby derive some meaning from their ordeal. In a study of parental decision making around Phase I trials, the provision life-prolonging treatment to allow for the possibility of a new therapy, having more time with their child, the hope for a cure and/or miracle, and the desire to help other children were identified as operative factors; the two main themes represented by these factors are hope and altruism.[25]

A common consequence of trying a new medicine, as families see it, is bolstering hope for survival. This is not unhealthy as long as efforts are taken to differentiate such a hope from an unrealistic expectation for effectiveness. When properly framed, such hope can free parents from the paralytic effects of despair and allow them to actively pursue other quality of life oriented hopes and goals. The mantra hope for the best and plan for the worst places the proper perspective on the events of the end of life experience. "There is nothing more we can do" should be reframed to include the idea that even though the disease is unlikely to be cured, there may be other realistic goals for which the patient and family should strive.[27]

Altruism is a commonly cited reason for participation in clinical trials. A study of informed consent conferences for pediatric Phase I trials found that two-thirds of consent conferences contained broad discourse on the potential benefit to others of participation, but it was raised by the physician in 80% of the cases. There was no correlation between the discussion of altruistic motives and the rate of participation.[34] Another study of the personality characteristics of volunteers for clinical studies found a higher than normal scoring for altruism.[35] When adolescents were studied, the qualitative data suggested that a concern for others is more prevalent in patients facing graver threats to their health.[36] Therefore, while altruism may not be a driving factor in the decision-making process, there is abundant anecdotal evidence for parents and adolescents who verbalize comfort in the concept of helping other children. In this sense, adherence to an altruistic motive, among others, can represent a benefit to participation in Phase I trials in that it allows family's to provide a context of meaning for their suffering.

The transition phase from cure directed to palliative therapy is a difficult one for providers, patients and families. Offering Phase I clinical trials at this juncture can be done in a just and noncoercive way that provides benefit to the child and family without setting up an expectation for tumor response. Further, given the essential nature of hope at this time, it is necessary to lead the family in a discussion to discover their perceptions of the elements of a quality-filled life; these things should become objects of hope.[37] The means to achieve these hopes and goals lies within palliative care and hospice care at the end of life. Therefore, the transition period where Phase I therapies are often discussed makes a natural place for the discussion of palliative and hospice care if it has not already been addressed. Indeed, an argument can be made that the responsible discussion of Phase I therapy should always be preceded by or include a discussion of palliative or hospice care.

Symptoms and Suffering of Children with Cancer

A pivotal study published in 2000 revealed that the majority of children with cancer suffer "a lot" or "a great deal" in their last month of life. Physicians were much less likely to report symptoms compared with parents, and treatments for symptoms were often not deemed effective.[38] The most frequent symptoms reported were fatigue, pain, dyspnea, poor appetite, nausea and vomiting, constipation, and diarrhea (Fig. 43-1, A). A follow-up study in 2008 showed that with the initiation of the principles of palliative care earlier in the disease process, children experienced less suffering with regard to many of these prevalent symptoms and parents felt more prepared for the trajectory of the end of life process[9] (Fig. 43-1, B). In a more recent study of children with cancer in the last day and last week of life, parents reported similar distressing symptoms by answering open-ended questions. In this case, the most frequently reported distressing symptoms included change in behavior, breathing changes, pain, change in appearance, weakness and fatigue, and change in heart rate. These symptoms were the same at a week and a day before death, though the frequency changed over the two time points. The interventions that helped the most were not usually disease-specific, but rather related to the medical team being present, and having good and open communication.[31] The effectiveness of symptoms control at the end of life can have lasting repercussions for parents who watch their children die. In one study, more than half of parents whose children had pain at the end of life or a difficult moment of death were still affected by that memory four to nine years later.[39]

INTEGRATIVE THERAPIES AS PALLIATIVE CARE IN CHILDREN WITH CANCER

Integrative therapy is often used by pediatric oncology patients, generally in addition to cure-directed conventional therapies, and often for supportive care purposes. Studies have reported 59% to 84% of children with cancer use integrative therapies.[40,41] Many of the nation's top pediatric hospitals have created centers for integrative medicine practice and research, particularly for use by pediatric cancer patients.

Of the integrative therapies, massage is one of the more popular with about 30% of children in general[40] and 60% of children with cancer[42] reporting use. There are limited studies of

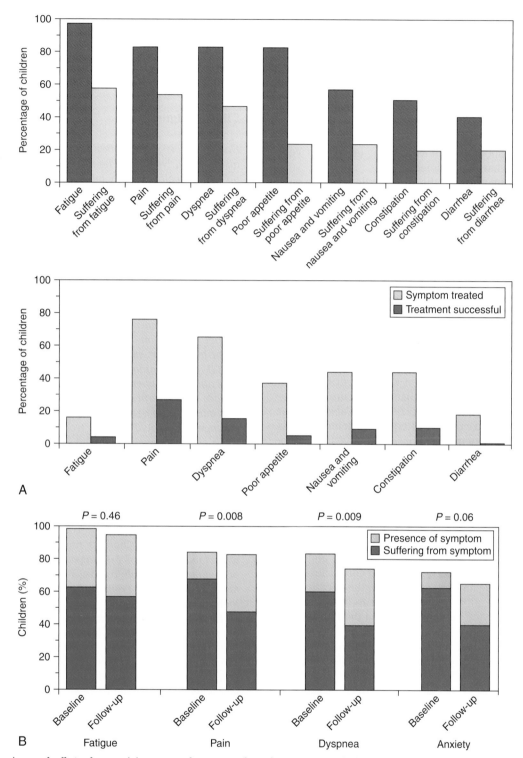

Fig. 43-1   A, The degree of suffering from, and the success of treatment of specific symptoms, in the last month of life. (Wolfe J, Grier HE, Klar N, et al: Symptoms and suffering at the end of life in children with cancer. N Engl J Med 342:326–33, 2000.) **B,** Prevalence and degree of suffering from common symptoms in the last month of life in baseline and follow-up cohorts. (From Wolfe J, Hammel JF, Edwards KE, Duncan J, Comeau M, Breyer J, Aldridge SA, Grier HE, Berde C, Dussel V, Weeks JC. Easing of suffering in children with cancer at the end of life: is care changing? J Clin Oncol, 2008. Apr 1; 26(10): 1717–1723.)

massage in children in general, and only two studies published on massage therapy in pediatric oncology patients. However, the studies consistently demonstrate improvements in anxiety in patients who receive massage, as well as some suggestions of improvement in distress, pain, tension, discomfort, and

mood, indicating that massage can be helpful for palliation of symptoms in children with cancer.[43–46]

Acupuncture is also widely used in pediatric oncology patients. While evidence in pediatric conditions is somewhat lacking due to a paucity of well-designed clinical trials,[47] there is evidence of efficacy in adult cancer patients with symptoms such as nausea and vomiting,[48,49] pain, fatigue, anxiety, and insomnia,[50,51] which are all symptoms that are equally burdensome to pediatric oncology patients. In addition, acupuncture has been shown to be well tolerated in children[52,53] and has been shown to help some children, particularly with pain management.[54–56] Acupuncture has been trialed in one pediatric oncology study of chemotherapy-induced nausea and vomiting where it was found to significantly decrease need for rescue nausea medications as well as vomiting episodes.[57] Very few adverse events have been noted.

This evidence suggests that the best practices for the care of pediatric patients with advanced cancers should include integrative medicine approaches. Integrative therapies can often be an important component of palliative care for oncology patients. The focus on comfort and quality of life is paramount to the philosophy of integrative medicine. Patients and families may have a healthier childhood cancer journey when maximum efforts are directed at controlling symptoms and minimizing suffering, thus maximizing healing.

RESEARCH NEEDS AND OPPORTUNITIES

While the seamless integration of clinical research with clinical care in the approach to children with cancer has had a marked impact on improving the chances for cure, the time has come to provide appropriate focus and to apply similar rigor in the design and conduct of controlled clinical trials evaluating the efficacy of interventions to improve the quality of life during all phases of the cancer experience. Longitudinal investigations of the outcome of children and the associated acute and late sequelae of cancer and its therapy have led to modifications and refinements of subsequent treatment approaches.[58–60] Likewise, both retrospective and prospective studies using patient and family self-reported outcomes must be developed to assess efficacy of symptom management and prevention; interventions for social, psychological, and spiritual health; and end of life and bereavement care. These data can be used to provide a sound rationale for the construction of prospective intervention studies in order to improve quality of life for patients and families, including the minority for whom cure is not possible. Such information is also critical to the development of education and training materials and programs for all levels of caregivers and trainees. It will help to assure that there are no missed opportunities for patients and families if palliative care is conceptualized as integral to all the services provided to a child with cancer and his or her family. It should also be seen as an integral domain with respect to interdisciplinary and multidisciplinary clinical research for which the pediatric oncology community has most definitely demonstrated proof of principle.

The fact that families of children with cancer are fully capable and open to the dual goals of concurrently providing disease-directed and comfort care creates a profound opportunity, and a mandate for early integrated palliative care, rather than an unfortunate and unexpected end result of unsuccessful attempts to provide cure.[25,61,62] The early development of collaborative partnerships among parents, patients, and caregivers has been critical to the success of therapeutic and nontherapeutic research studies in pediatric oncology. These same relationships can and should greatly facilitate the information, trust generation, and consent process for therapeutic research in palliation as well. Meaningful and generally sustainable bonds among caregivers and patients and families can also be effectively used to their full advantage in investigating appropriate interventions at the end of life and even effective supportive measures during bereavement.

Clinical Vignette

Daniel is a 10-year-old boy who presented with a 1-month history of early-morning headaches. Two weeks before diagnosis he developed early morning vomiting associated with headache but no nausea. One week before diagnosis, his mother reported that she noticed "shaking of the eyes." A CT scan of the brain without contrast revealed a large diffuse intrinsic mass in the pons, which was later confirmed with MRI. Daniel was admitted to the local pediatric hospital and started on intravenous steroids. Because of the location of the tumor, there was no surgical option so the patient was referred to the neuro-oncology service for further evaluation and treatment. The family met with the multidisciplinary neuro-oncology team, who informed the family that Daniel had a brain stem glioma, a type of highly aggressive brain tumor. The standard of care for brain stem gliomas (BSG) includes radiation therapy. The family was informed that although somewhat effective in symptom control, the chance of long-term survival was extremely poor. The family was advised that despite the low likelihood of cure, Daniel's management would be directed at trying to achieve cure while simultaneously providing symptom relief and supportive care to Daniel and his family. A recommendation was made to enroll Daniel on a clinical trial using chemotherapy in conjunction with radiation therapy to attempt to improve the rate of cure for this disease. The family, fully informed, gave consent to enroll him in the clinical trial. Daniel did not participate in these initial conversations with the neuro-oncology team, at his parents' request, but the team did meet with Daniel to discuss his diagnosis and the planned course of treatment. Meanwhile, Daniel showed dramatic improvement in his clinical symptoms with the initiation of steroid therapy alone.

Daniel received 6 weeks of focal radiation therapy and adjuvant chemotherapy. Chemotherapy was delivered daily by IV before radiation therapy. He tolerated therapy well and clinically improved. A MRI 6 weeks after completion of radiation therapy revealed significant reduction in the tumor. He had gained a significant amount of weight as a result of the steroid therapy, but he was able to be weaned off the steroids successfully. Over the next few weeks he began to lose weight and was able to return to school. His peers were very supportive and welcomed him back to school. Daniel lived at home with his parents, his 5-year-old sister, and his maternal grandparents, who had emigrated from China 3 years before Daniel's illness. Before the diagnosis, Daniel had many friends and loved to play basketball and video games and played the drum in the school band. Supportive services were in place with social work, child life, art therapy, and pastoral care. A psychologist was introduced, but the family declined these services.

Daniel did well for approximately 9 months when he began to have difficulty playing basketball. He had a mild weakness of the left side and unfortunately a MRI scan revealed tumor progression. He was again started on steroids, with noticeable improvement. The neuro-oncology team offered enrollment on a Phase I clinical trial using a novel oral biologic agent. Daniel tolerated therapy well but unfortunately did not achieve the desired tumor response so this therapy was discontinued. His weakness continued to progress, and he eventually was wheelchair bound. He was unable to be weaned off the steroids and had gained a significant amount of weight. His physical appearance was dramatically altered from initial diagnosis. He was unable to play basketball or attend school and his friends were reluctant to visit. His parents decided to begin treatment with traditional Chinese herbal therapies, which the grandparents had been suggesting to them for some time.

The neuro-oncology team offered participation in another Phase I clinical trial using a novel IV chemotherapy agent given weekly as an outpatient. The family and Daniel decided to stop the herbal therapies and enroll in the clinical trial. Remarkably, over the next year, Daniel had a significant response to therapy and his symptoms improved dramatically. He was able to be weaned off steroids, his strength improved so that he no longer needed a wheelchair and he was able to return to school. Throughout this entire period, he and his family received psychosocial support through social work, child life and art therapy through the hospital, and their own spiritual advisor.

Three months after completing the second Phase I clinical trial, Daniel developed headaches and weakness of his left side. A MRI scan revealed tumor progression. Steroids were started. No clinical trials were available, so the family and neuro-oncology team opted to use metronomic low-dose oral chemotherapy agents, and the family decided to again try the Chinese herbal therapies. Daniel stabilized but shortly thereafter began to deteriorate. His weakness progressed and he developed difficulty swallowing. He became angry at his parents and refused to take the oral chemotherapy agents. His family was distraught. They asked frankly if Daniel was going to die from his tumor. The maternal grandparents had continued to seek traditional Chinese therapies and were now reluctant to support the parents in their quest for continued Western medicine treatments. There was a great deal of tension among all family members.

The team had poignant discussions about the progression and prognosis of his disease and suggested that it was time to add hospice care. The family had previously been resistant to this suggestion. They also asked the team not to tell Daniel that he was dying. The social worker suggested to the family that the psychologist may be able to offer more assistance, so Daniel and his family began to meet regularly with the social worker and psychologist. It became evident that Daniel knew he was dying but did not want to talk to his parents about it because he did not want to burden them. Eventually, the family agreed to transition to hospice care with collaboration of the neuro-oncology team.

Daniel and his parents were able to talk about his illness after working with the hospice team. The family was able to come together and support one another through the remainder of Daniel's illness. Pain and symptom management became the paramount goal. He died peacefully at home with his family and hospice nurse in attendance.

Summary

Clinical research in childhood cancer has and continues to lead to the definition of standard of care; indeed, for some, enrollment on a controlled clinical trial is perceived as the standard of care. The early introduction of the concept of palliative care and its essential integration with the totality of services provided to children and families requires a similar degree of robustness in evaluating the efficacy of specific interventions on the spiritual, emotional, psychological, physical, social, and practical domains of the family and patient impacted by cancer. Enhancing any and all parts of the cancer journey for patients, parents, community, and providers is no less a responsibility for researchers and demands the same degree of scientific and methodological review for merit, validity, need, and feasibility. Furthermore, such research endeavors should experience appropriate public and private support to guarantee that for all children and their families, every effective measure is used to protect and improve the quality of life even if and when cure cannot be assured or even expected.

There are no predictable scenarios in the care of children with cancer. Certainly, children with high-risk cancers should be afforded the opportunities for palliative care and integrative therapies from the time of diagnosis to promote comfort and quality of life. However, all children with cancer should receive care that is focused on integrating these goals in all aspects of the journey. Families must be provided with honest and open communication regarding diagnosis, prognosis, risks and benefits of treatment, and options for integration of palliative care. Together, the healthcare team and patients and families must clarify the goals of care, weighing decisions for pursuit of tumor-directed palliative therapies or Phase I clinical trials against those of comfort and quality of life. Adequate psychosocial support services are imperative to preserve healthy family functioning and to assist the family from diagnosis throughout the childhood cancer journey. Cure is only one object of hope. Hope is always possible, even when cure is not.

REFERENCES

1. United States Department of Health and Human Services: *Surveillance, Epidemiology, and End Results (SEER) Program.* SEER*Stat Database: Incidence SEER 9 RegsLimited-Use, Nov 27Sub (1973–2005) Worldwide website: www.seer.cancer.gov. Accessed Nov.25, 2009.
2. Steliarova-Foucher E, Siller C, Lacour B, Kaatsch P: International Classification of Childhood Cancer, ed 3. *Cancer* 103:1457–1467, 2005.
3. Matthay KK, Reynolds CP, Seeger RC, et al: Long term results for children with neuroblastoma treated on a randomized trial of myeloablative therapy followed by 13-cis-retinoic acid: a Children's Oncology Group study, *J Clin Oncol* 2009.
4. Goldman A, Hewitt M, Collins GS, Childs M, Hains R: Symptoms in children/young people with progressive malignant disease: United Kingdom children's cancer study group/paediatric oncology nurses' forum palliative care working group, *Pediatrics* 117(6):e1179–e1186, 2006.
5. Harris MB: Palliative care in children with cancer: which child and when? *J Natl Cancer Inst Monograph* 32:144–149, 2004.
6. Field M: *When children die: improving palliative and end-of-life care for children and their families*, Washington, DC, 2003, National Academies Press.
7. Klausner R: *Cancer incidence and survival among children and adolescents: United States SEER Program 1975–1995*, Bethesda, Md, 1999, National Cancer Institute.
8. Bluebond-Langner M, Belasco JB, Goldman A, et al: Understanding parents' approaches to care and treatment of children with cancer when standard therapy has failed, *J Clin Oncol* 25:2414–2419, 2007.

9. Wolfe J, Hammel JF, Edwards KE, Duncan J, Comeau M, Breyer J, Aldridge SA, Grier HE, Berde C, Dussel V, Weeks JC: Easing of suffering in children with cancer at the end of life: is care changing? *J Clin Oncol* 26(10):1717–1723, 2008.

10. Johnston DL, Nagel K, Friedman DL, et al: Availability and use of palliative care and end-of-life services for pediatric oncology patients, *J Clin Oncol* 26:4646–4650, 2008.

11. Mack JW, Cook EF, Wolfe J, et al: Understanding of prognosis among parents of children with cancer: parental optimism and the parent-physician interaction, *J Clin Oncol* 25:1357–1362, 2007.

12. Wolfe J, Klar N, Grier HE, et al: Understanding of prognosis among parents of children who died of cancer: impact on treatment goals and integration of palliative care, *JAMA* 284:2469–2475, 2000.

13. Mack JW, Wolfe J, Cook EF, et al: Hope and prognostic disclosure, *J Clin Oncol* 25:5636–5642, 2007.

14. Mack JW, Wolfe J, Grier HE, et al: Communication about prognosis between parents and physicians of children with cancer: parent preferences and the impact of prognostic information, *J Clin Oncol* 24:5265–5270, 2006.

15. Surkan PJ, Dickman PW, Steineck G, Onelov E, Kreicbergs U: Home care of a child dying of a malignancy and parental awareness of a child's impending death, *Palliat Med* 20(3):161–169, 2006.

16. Woodgate RL, Degner LF, Yanofsky R: A different perspective to approaching cancer symptoms in children, *J Pain Symptom Manage* 26(3):800–817, 2003.

17. Hinds PS, Billups CA, Cao X, Guttuso JS, Burghen EA, West N, et al: Health-related quality of life in adolescents at the time of diagnosis with osteosarcoma or acute myeloid leukemia, *Eur J Oncol Nurs* 2009, in press.

18. Lee DP, Skolnik JM, Adamson PC: Pediatric phase I trials in oncology: An analysis of study conduct efficiency, *J Clin Oncol* 23(33):8341–8351, 2005.

19. Meeske K, Katz ER, Palmer SN, Burwinkle T, Varni JW: Parent proxy-reported health-related quality of life and fatigue in pediatric patients diagnosed with brain tumors and acute lymphoblastic leukemia, *Cancer* 101(9):2116–2125, 2004.

20. Hinds P, Quargnenti AG, Wentz TJ: Measuring symptom distress in adolescents with cancer, *J Pediatr Oncol Nurs* 9(2):84–86, 1992.

21. Hongo T, Watanabe C, Okada S, Inoue N, Yajima S, Fuji Y, et al: Analysis of the circumstances at the end of life in children with cancer: symptoms, suffering and acceptance, *Pediatr Int* 45:60–64, 2003.

22. Prichard M, Burghen E, Srivastava DK, Okuma J, Anderson L, Powell B, et al: Cancer-related symptoms most concerning to parents during the last week and last day of their child's life, *Pediatrics* 121(5):e1301–e1309, 2008.

23. Houlahan KE, Branowicki PA, Mack JW, Dinning C, McCabe M: Can end of life care for the pediatric patient suffering with escalating and intractable symptoms be improved? *J Pediatr Oncol Nurs* 23(1):45–51, 2006.

24. Mack JW, Joffe S, Hilden JM, et al: Parents' views of cancer-directed therapy for children with no realistic chance for cure, *J Clin Oncol* 26:4759–4764, 2008.

25. Hinds PS, Drew D, Oakes LL, et al: End-of-life care preferences of pediatric patients with cancer, *J Clin Oncol* 23:9146–9154, 2005.

26. Snyder CR: *Handbook of hope: theories, measures & applications*, San Diego, 2000, Academic Press.

27. Tulsky JA: Beyond advanced directives: the importance of communication skills at the end of life, *JAMA* 294:359–365, 2005.

28. Dussel V, Kreicbergs U, Hilden JM, Watterson J, Moore C, Turner BG, Weeks JC, Wolfe J: Looking beyond where children die: determinants and effects of planning a child's location of death, *J Pain Symptom Manage* 37(1):33–43, 2009.

29. Kreicbergs U, Valdimarsdóttir U, Onelöv E, Henter JI, Steineck G: Talking about death with children who have severe malignant disease, *N Engl J Med* 351(12):1175–1186, 2004.

30. Deatrick JA, Angst DB, Moore C: Parents' views of their children's participation in phase I oncology clinical trials, *J Pediatr Oncol Nurs* 19(4):114–121, 2002.

31. Pritchard M, Burghen E, Srivastava DK, et al: Cancer-related symptoms most concerning to parents during the last week and last day of their child's life, *Pediatrics* 121:e1301–e1309, 2008.

32. Lee DP, Skolnik JM, Adamson PC: Pediatric phase I trials in oncology: an analysis of study conduct efficiency, *J Clin Oncol* 23(33):8431–8441, 2005.

33. Kim A, Fox E, Warren K, et al: Characteristics and outcome of pediatric patients enrolled in phase I oncology trials, *Oncologist* 13(6):679–689, 2008.

34. Simon C, Eder M, Kodish E, Siminoff L: Altruistic discourse in the informed consent process for childhood cancer clinical trials, *Am J Bioeth* 6(5):40–47, 2006.

35. Almeida L, Falcao A, Vaz-da-Silva M, Coelho R, Albino-Teixeira A, Soares-da-Silva P: Personality characteristics of volunteers in Phase 1 studies and likelihood of reporting adverse events, *Int J Clin Pharmacol Ther* 46(7):340–348, 2008.

36. Hinds PS: The hopes and wishes of adolescents with cancer and the nursing care that helps, *Oncol Nurs Forum* 31(5):927–934, 2004.

37. Clayton JM, Butow PN, Arnold RM, et al: Fostering coping and nurturing hope when discussing the future with terminally ill cancer patients and their caregivers, *Cancer* 103:1965–1975, 2005.

38. Wolfe J, Grier HE, Klar N, et al: Symptoms and suffering at the end of life in children with cancer, *N Engl J Med* 342:326–333, 2000.

39. Kreicbergs U, Valdimarsdóttir U, Onelöv E, Björk O, Steineck G, Henter JI: Care-related distress: a nationwide study of parents who lost their child to cancer, *J Clin Oncol* 23(36):9162–9171, 2005.

40. Post-White J, Fitzgerald M, Hageness S, Sencer SF: Complementary and alternative medicine use in children with cancer and general and specialty pediatrics, *J Pediatr Oncol Nurs* 26(1):7–15, 2009a.

41. Kelly KM: Complementary and alternative medicinal therapies for children with cancer, *Eur J Cancer* 40:2041–2046, 2004.

42. McLean TW, Kemper KJ: Complementary and alternative medicine therapies in pediatric oncology patients, *J Soc Integr Oncol* 4(1):40–45, 2006.

43. Post-White J, Fitzgerald M, Savik K, Hooke MC, Hannahan AB, Sencer SF: Massage therapy for children with cancer, *J Pediatr Oncol Nurs* 26(1):16–28, 2009b.

44. Phipps S, Dunavant M, Gray E, Rai SN: Massage therapy in children undergoing hematopoetic stem cell transplantation: results of a pilot trial, *J Cancer Integrative Med* 3(2):62–70, 2005.

45. Beider S, Moyer CA: Randomized controlled trials of pediatric massage: a review, *Evid Based Complement Alternat Med* 4(1):23–34, 2007.

46. Suresh S, Wang S, Porfyris S, Kamasinski-Sol R, Steinhorn DM: Massage therapy in outpatient pediatric chronic pain patients: do they facilitate significant reductions in levels of distress, pain, tension, discomfort, and mood alterations? *Paediatr Anaesth* 18(9):884–887, 2008.

47. Gold JI, Nicolaou CD, Belmont KA, Katz AR, Benaron DM, Yu W: Pediatric acupuncture: a review of clinical research, *Evid Based Complement Alternat Med* 2008, Jan 10.

48. Melchart D, Linde K, Fischer P, Berman B, White A, Vickers A, Allais G: Acupuncture for idiopathic headache, *Cochrane Database Syst Rev* (1):CD001218, 2001.

49. Ernst E: Acupuncture: what does the most reliable evidence tell us? *J Pain Symptom Manage* 37(4):709–714, 2009.

50. Ladas EJ, Post-White J, Hawks R, Taromina K: Evidence for symptom management in the child with cancer, *J Pediatr Hematol Oncol* 28(9):601–615, 2006.

51. Lu W, Dean-Clower E, Doherty-Gilman A, Rosenthal DS: The value of acupuncture in cancer care, *Hematol Oncol Clin North Am* 22(4):631–648, 2008.

52. Kemper KJ, Sarah R, Silver-Highfield E, Xiarhos E, Barnes L, Berde C: On pins and needles? Pediatric pain patients' experience with acupuncture, *Pediatrics* 105(4 Pt 2):941–947, 2000.

53. Wu S, Sapru A, Stewart MA, Milet MJ, Hudes M, Livermore LF, Flori HR: Using acupuncture for acute pain in hospitalized children, *Pediatr Crit Care Med* 10(3):291–296, 2009.

54. Kundu A, Berman B: Acupuncture for pediatric pain and symptom management, *Pediatr Clin North Am* 54(6):885–889, 2007.

55. Tsao JC, Meldrum M, Bursch B, Jacob MC, Kim SC, Zeltzer LK: Treatment expectations for CAM interventions in pediatric chronic pain patients and their parents, *Evid Based Complement Alternat Med* 2(4):521–527, 2005.

56. Lin YC, Lee AC, Kemper KJ, Berde CB: Use of complementary and alternative medicine in pediatric pain management service: a survey, *Pain Med* 6(6):452–458, 2005.

57. Gottschling S, Reindl TK, Meyer S, Berrang J, Henze G, Graeber S, Ong MF, Graf N: Acupuncture to alleviate chemotherapy-induced nausea and vomiting in pediatric oncology—a randomized multicenter crossover pilot trial, *Klin Padiatr* 220(6):365–370, 2008.

58. Friedman DL, Meadows AT: Late effects of childhood cancer therapy, *Pediatr Clin North Am* 49(5):1083–1106, 2002.
59. Institute of Medicine: *Childhood cancer survivorship: improving care and quality of Life*, Washington, DC, 2004, National Academies Press.
60. Green DM: Late effects of treatment for cancer during childhood and adolescence, *Curr Probe Cancer* 27:127–142, 2003.
61. Wolfe J, Friebert S, Hildon J: Caring for children with advanced cancer: integrating palliative care, *Pediatr Clin North Am* 49:1043–1062, 2002.
62. Hurwitz CA, Duncan J, Wolfe J: Caring for the child with cancer at the close of life, *JAMA* 292:2141–2149, 2004.
63. Stutzer C: Pediatric oncology palliative care in British Columbia, *BC Provincial Pediatric Hematology Oncology Network Newsletter* (3):1–4, Fall 2004.

44 Primary and Acquired Immunodeficiency Disorders

ONAJOVWE FOFAH | MARY B. FLECK | NAIMAH CAMPBELL |
SHEILA LENIHAN WALSH | JAMES OLESKE

*A happy birth to 150 million infants born this year. May those
who rule provide the simple gifts of peace: shelter, food and
water, education and health.*

*But alas, though many millions are born, most are birthed alone
with no one there but Mom to hear their cries, no host of angels
calls their name and no kings of Orient travel to give them
precious gifts.*

*Three million of these newborns die, as well as ten million
children under five, most of their deaths could be avoided with
a little food and water, simple gifts to give.*

*In our privileged lands, few children now have AIDS and die,
but where most children live, five million will have AIDS and ten
million more left to live alone, orphans with little hope of care.*

*We must not let another generation be lost nor any child suffer
for lack of care. Health is a fundamental right, a wise gift the
world and each one of us should make!* —J. Oleske

This chapter describes the critical role of palliative care services in improving the quality of life of the immunosuppressed child and his or her family. Primary immunodeficiencies are identified and distinguished from secondary immunodeficiencies, and the clinical features of each category are briefly described to give the reader an appreciation of the prevalence and impact of immunosuppression upon the growth and development of children.

The following pages explore the journey and reflect upon the impact of the devastation that the unanticipated AIDS epidemic brought upon the pediatric community. The need for supportive care to optimize quality of life for these children and their families is addressed and includes details of the initial development of investigative treatment trials, development of effective highly active antiretroviral therapy (HAART) and their role in prevention of perinatally acquired human immunodeficiency virus (HIV) infection, as well as cure of children with primary immunodeficiencies by immune reconstitution, or stem cells.

It is impossible to adequately describe the suffering of HIV-affected children and the impact upon those who care for them.

Response to the lack of effective systems of service delivery has paved the way for the rebirth and evolution of palliative care in the pediatric community. Lessons learned about caring for families of children with HIV serve as a prototype to address the wide range of clinical, developmental medical, social, and political problems encountered by seriously ill children and their families, regardless of the nature of their illnesses. It is hoped that this chapter and others will further stimulate development of evidence-based protocols and practice guidelines to address important areas of palliative and end of life care, especially in underserved populations.

The initial eight cases of pediatric acquired immunodeficiency syndrome (AIDS) were reported in 1983 from the Pediatric Allergy-Immunology and Infectious Disease program in Newark, New Jersey, initially named the Children's Hospital AIDS Program (CHAP).[1] When the children's hospital closed in 1998, the Pediatric HIV/AIDS program was renamed the François-Xavier Bagnoud Children Center. One of the cases from this initial cohort best illustrates the recognition that these infants and children were part of the AIDS epidemic and not a sudden increase in a new form of primary severe combined immunodeficiency disorder (SCID).

Clinical Vignette

A 4-month-old girl presented with chronic diarrhea, leading to failure to thrive and wasting syndrome that was associated with recurrent and severe sino-pulmonary infections anemia, lymphopenia, generalized lymphadenopathy and thrombocytopenia. She was under the supervision of New Jersey's Division of Youth and Family Service (DYFS) by a foster mother, because of abandonment by her chronically ill intravenous drug-using mother. Her initial immunologic laboratory evaluation showed a surprising hypergammaglobulinemia instead of the expected hypogammaglobulinemia, low total T cells and, as was typical for that era, low markers by immunoflorescent microscopy for helper T cells. A lung biopsy was done for chronic infiltrates. During the procedure there was little thymus tissue noted and a small piece was obtained for pathologic evaluation. The lung biopsy demonstrated severe lymphocytic iterstitial pneumonia (LIP) (Fig. 44-1) and the thymus biopsy was reported as showing chronic inflammation,

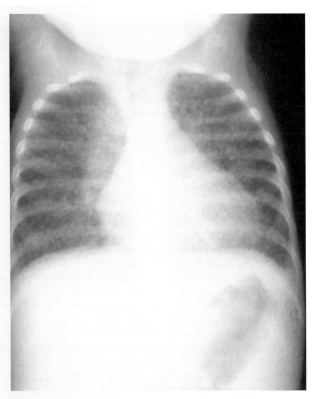

Fig. 44-1 Chest x-ray showing changes of LIP.

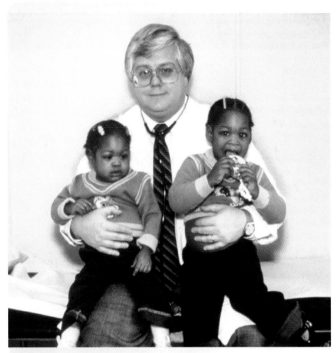

Fig. 44-3 Picture of the two sisters at 18 months of age demonstrating the obvious physical discrepancy.

calcified Hassall bodies with marked reduction in thymus lymphocytes. These changes were unexpected and consistent with a probable chronic perinatal infection (Fig. 44-2). Most importantly, she had an identical second-born twin sister who was and remains healthy (Fig. 44-3). Over time, HIV/AIDS was confirmed in the ill twin while her identical twin sister remained well and thriving with consistently negative HIV assays. Both are now 30 years old and the HIV-infected sibling has survived despite progression of her HIV to AIDS. Until specific HIV diagnostic studies became available, the care team, including one of the coauthors of this chapter (JO), diagnosed differentiated perinatal HIV from the assumed initial diagnosis of SCID, based on the unexpected results of lung and thymus tissue and the discordant clinical course of the twins.

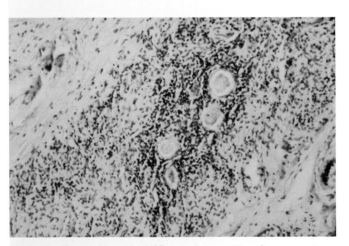

Fig. 44-2 Thymus biopsy by H&E stain demonstrating changes consistent with chronic perinatal infection and not SCID.

Epidemiology of Inherited and Acquired Immunodeficiency Syndromes in Childhood

Approximately 55,000 children, newborn to age 19, die in the United States annually, with nearly half of these deaths being infants, of which two thirds are neonates.[2] These infant mortalities are mostly due to prematurity as well as congenital and/or genetic abnormalities, both having primary or secondary immune dysfunction. Most of these secondary immune problems in the premature infant are related to innate immune dysfunction that include breaks in skin and mucus membrane integrity, nutritional deficiencies, exposure to nosocomial infectious agents and exposure to frequent procedures and broad-spectrum antibiotics. In older children, worldwide mortality has been decreasing, with most deaths attributed to chronic, life-limiting medical conditions. Primary and secondary immunodeficiencies in infants contribute considerably to infant mortality and pose a significant, but often not recognized, threat to the health and well-being of children in the United States.

Primary or inherited immunodeficiencies are almost always genetically determined, often confined to a few rare, familial, monogenic, recessive traits that impair the development or function of one or several leukocyte subsets and result in multiple, recurrent, opportunistic infections during infancy. With improved diagnostic capabilities and an increased understanding of human immune functions, these immunodeficiencies are proving to be more common than previously estimated and may affect a much larger population because of a broadening of the definition of primary immunodeficiencies (PID). Considerable expansion of the understanding of immunological changes is being demonstrated in multiple chronic diseases, as well as improved survival with more effective treatments (Table 44-1).[3] The frequency of PID varies in different

TABLE 44-1, A Classification of Primary Immune Disorders That Manifest in Neonates

Components of the immune disorder	Immune system	Inheritance / associated features
Predominant antibody defects	X-linked agammaglobulinemia Hyper IgM syndrome Transient hypogammaglobulinemia of infancy	XL/recurrent pyogenic infections XL/neutropenia, thrombocytopenia, hemolytic anemia and opportunistic infections (mouth ulcers) Variable/recurrent moderate bacterial infections/common
Predominant defects in cell-mediated immunity	Di-George anomaly MHC class II deficiency Neonatal HIV infection	De novo defect or AD/conotruncal malformation; hypoparathyroidism: cardiac outflow tract malformation; abnormal faces/common AR/failure to thrive and protracted diarrhea/rare Variable frequency-secondary cause of immunodeficiency
Combined antibody and cellular immunodeficiencies	Wiskott-Aldrich Syndrome	XL/thrombocytopenia; small defective platelets, eczema; lymphoreticular malignancies; autoimmune disease Bloody stools, draining ears/rare
Severe combined immunodeficiencies	X-linked SCID Zap—70 deficiency Adenosine deaminase deficiency Omenn syndrome Reticular dysgenesis	XL/symptoms may be similar to GVH disease in neonatal period (maculopapular rash, alopecia, lymphadenopthy)/rare AR/very rare AR/cartilage abnormalities/rare AR (in most cases)/erythroderma, eosinophilia/rare AR/lethal shortly after birth/extremely rare
Defects of phagocytic function	Chronic granulomatous disease of childhood (CDG) Schwachman syndrome Leukocyte adhesion defect	Both XL/AR defective NADPH intravacuole killing of catalase-negative organisms AR/anemia, thrombocytopenia, pancreatic insufficiency, hypogammaglobulinemia AR/delayed umbilical cord detachment, leukocytosis, recurrent infections/very rare
Complement deficiencies	C5, C6, C7, C8a, C8b, C9 deficiency	AR/neisserial infections, SLE/very rare or rare
Auto Inflammatory disorders	Neonatal onset multisystem inflammatory disease (NOMID) or chronic infantile neurologic cutaneous and articular syndrome (CINCA)	AD/Neonatal onset rash, chronic meningitis, and arthropathy with fever and inflammation in response to IL-1R antagonist (Anakinra)/very rare

Notarangelo L et al. International Union of Immunological Societies Expert Committee on Primary Immunodeficiencies: Primary immunodeficiencies: 2009 update. J Allergy Clin Immunol 2009: 124:1162–1178.

XL—X-linked
AD—Autosomal dominant
AR—Autosomal recessive
MHC—major histocompatibility complex

TABLE 44-1, B Classification of Immune Disorders Associated with or Secondary to Other Diseases

Disease	Immune disorder	Inheritance / associated features
Bloom syndrome	Reduced T-cell function and decreased IgM	AR/LBW, retarded growth, facial telangiectasia, sun-sensitive erythemia, increased susceptibility to malignancies, molar hypoplasia, bird-like face/rare
Fanconi anemia	Decreased T lymphocyte and natural killer (NK) cell function, decreased IgA	AR/multiorgan defects, bone marrow failure, café au lait spots, limb defects, abnormal faces, hyperpigmentation
Xeroderma pigmentosa (XP with 7 subgroups A-G and a variant, XPV)	Decrease in CD4+ levels and function due to mutation of the DNA repair gene for ultraviolet (UV) induced damage.	AR/defect in nucleotide excision repair (NER) with mutations of important tumor suppressor genes (e.g., p53 or proto oncogenes) leading to a sixfold increase in metastatic malignant melanoma and squamous cell carcinoma as well as XP being six times more common in Japanese people
Cancers	Bone narrow suppression from tumor infiltration or ablation of marrow from therapy: drugs or radiation	An increasing number of cancers appear to be enhanced by specific genetic characteristics
Malnutrition	Both single nutrient/trace metal impact on specific immune function or generalized wasting	AR/acrodermatitis enteropathica (zinc deficiency)
Infections	Varies with organism and whether localized/systemic or acute/chronic	Chronic, multiorgan system viral infections predominate, penultimate example being HIV/AIDS
Prematurity	Greatest impact on innate host defenses	More profound when gestation <28 weeks because of sharp drop in maternal-to-fetus transfer of immunoglobulins
Chronic organ system diseases: diabetes or renal disease	Like infections, great variations with severity depending on single or multiple organ involvement, timing of onset	Depending on organ systems or specific cause of organ failure, there may be a genetic-linked immuno deficiency syndrome

countries, with certain populations having higher frequency of some specific PID mutations.[4] Progress in medical care has made it possible for many of these children with PID to survive to adulthood with symptoms and complications that may not be recognized by adult primary care providers.[5]

An example of the challenges of caring for a child with PID can be demonstrated by a case of a child with Wiskott-Aldridge syndrome who was cared for by our immunology service from the age of 6 through his death at 24 years. He was one of the initial children enrolled in the Circle of Life Children Centers (COLCC), a palliative and end-of-life care program, established in 2002.

Clinical Vignette

When first seen at age 6 in 1986, the boy had a history of recurrent bacterial sino-pulmonary infections, chronic mild thrombocytopenia, and a palpable spleen. He was brought by his mother, who was concerned about the risk of bleeding recently raised by his pediatrician, who thought the child would outgrow this problem. However, she was concerned that there might be more to his problem. Despite the abnormal history and examination, which revealed the appearance of mild eczema-like rash with scattered petechia and an enlarged spleen, he was a very active child who participated in several physical activities, including karate. The initial blood studies were consistent with Wiskott-Aldridge syndrome (WAS), which was later confirmed by finding the WASP gene mutation on the short arm of his X chromosome. From the outset, the mother wanted do whatever was in her son's best interest. The treating immunologist tried to keep them both informed about latest recommendations in treating WAS. Over time, treatment included starting monthly intravenous gamma globulin replacement therapy, which was later changed to a clinical trial of bi-monthly subcutaneous preparation of gamma globulin to reduce the trauma and pain of finding an IV site. There were long visits to discuss the risk and benefits of splenectomy, cyclic use of rotating courses of antibiotics and always the give and take of negotiating limits of participation in contact sports or traumatic activities for a young adolescent who wanted to be normal, and who, with close medical care was, for the most part, feeling that he was normal. Although we were able to avoid splenectomy and keep him out of the hospital and attending high school, at age 15, he wanted to pursue the option of a cure by stem cell transplantation. After a prolonged search, a partial match was found and both patient and mother wanted to proceed, despite the known risk of failure and possible complications of transplantation, which increased with a less-than-identical match. After transplantation and over the following 5 years, he had only a limited reconstitution of immune function, but also developed all the complications that accompany this procedure, in their most extreme forms and degree. The worse was the need for more hospital stays than days spent at home. Despite his progressive downhill course, both the mother and the young man insisted on trying therapies regardless of significant known toxicities and risks, with little chance that they would help. There were times when he overcame setbacks with his inspiring courage and in so doing, was a positive example to other hospitalized but far less ill children. His love

of life and mother drew the attention of government and civic leadership to focus on the plight of so little access and availability of pediatric palliative and end-of-life care, and helped start support for programs, such as COLCC, in addressing this need. His suffering and forbearance proved too great. Also so remarkable, at his funeral were the statements made by so many people of his impact on advancing the care and programs that will help many others to have the palliative and hospice care that was not allowed him.

Secondary or acquired immunodeficiencies are more common than primary disorders of immune function (Table 44-1, B). By far, the most common secondary immunodeficiency of this era is HIV/AIDS.[6] Based on the original version of the PACTG 219 follow-up study from 1993 through 2000, Table 44-2 lists the most common diagnosis during that period when HAART therapy was not available.[7] Unfortunately, children presenting with these diagnoses at birth through 4 years also experienced the highest mortality rate. In the older age groups, *Pneumocystis jirovecii pneumonia* (PCP) remained associated with a high mortality rate but lymphocytic interstitial pneumonia (LIP) was a marker for prolonged survival before HAART therapy.[8] Sadly, during the early epidemic, despite a high morbidity and mortality rate, most attention was focused on treatment of opportunistic infections with little attention given to palliative and supportive care.

Globally, an estimated 430,000 children younger than 15 were newly infected with HIV in 2008. The vast majority of these children (90%) acquired the virus via perinatal/mother-to-child transmission (MTCT). By the end of 2008, 2 million children were infected with HIV worldwide, with 280,000 children dying of the disease in that same year.[9] In the United States, HIV has become the sixth-leading cause of death among 15-24 year-olds,[10] and continues to disproportionately affect people of color. African Americans, who account for only 13% of the U.S. population, represent 51% of the estimated number of HIV/AIDS diagnoses made through 2007.[11]

HIV is also transmitted via other routes, such as through blood transfusions as evidenced in the hemophilia population. Before the policies for screening HIV in blood supplies were instituted, many people were exposed to the virus through intravenous transfusions of blood or blood products. People with hemophilia routinely need certain blood-clotting components, and receive them through frequent blood transfusions. From 1978 through 1985, many hemophiliacs were inadvertently put at extremely high risk for acquiring HIV through the public blood supply. Hemophiliacs now represent 1% of all people with AIDS in the United States.[12]

The final group of children who acquire HIV are victims of sexual abuse. A small percentage of children (<1%) acquire HIV through sexual abuse by an infected adult male, usually a relative or close friend of the family. Because sexual abuse of children is likely to be under-recognized and under-reported, sexually abused children are not routinely screened for HIV infection, and sexually abused children infected with HIV who have not progressed to AIDS are not reported in many states, the full extent of sexual transmission of HIV among children is not known.[13] It is important to also note that among adolescents ages 15 to 19, the major cause of HIV infection is through high-risk sexual activity.

TABLE 44-2 Most Common HIV Related Diagnoses

Birth to 23 months	2-4 years	5-11 years	12-21 years
Oral candidiasis (OC)	Lymphocytic interstitial pneumonia (LIP)	LIP	Pneumonia
Anemia	Anemia	Pneumonia	OC
Failure to thrive (FTT)	OC	OC	LIP
Pneumonia	Pneumonia	FTT	Varicella zoster
Pneumocystis jirovecii pneumonia (PCP)	FTT	Anemia	PCP

Based on unpublished data from PACTG 219 Long-Term Follow-Up database.

Symptoms, Distress, and Quality of Life in Children and Adolescents with Immunodeficiency Disorders

Clinical manifestations of HIV in children include recurrent bacterial infections; recurrent and intercurrent opportunistic infections; neuro-psychiatric manifestations; gastrointestinal problems, such as diarrhea and malnutrition; weight loss; respiratory problems, such as pneumonia and bronchiectasis; and skin manifestations, such as herpes simplex, seborrhoeic eczema, and molluscum contagiosum. Other problems include lymphadenopathy, hepatosplenomegaly, oral candidiasis, failure to thrive, wasting syndromes, parotitis, malabsorption, and developmental delays and/or loss of developmental milestones.[14] Acute, chronic, and recurrent pain may be related to the disease, to progression, and/or to medications, treatments, and procedures.

Children and adolescents with HIV experience more subjective distress than their uninfected peers, including dysphoria, hopelessness, preoccupation with their illness, and poor body image related to their physical appearance affected by wasting and dermatologic conditions. "Attempting to cope with HIV-positive serostatus may trigger social withdrawal, depression, loneliness, anger, confusion, fear, numbness, and guilt."[10] Children in particular may believe that they did something terrible to deserve HIV, resulting in the development of guilt. "Non-infected siblings are also affected by HIV. Sibling relationships may be damaged by a fear of contagion or feelings of resentment towards the ill child. Because of these multiple difficulties, siblings of infected children also often experience problems in school."[10]

In addition to increased distress, adolescents with HIV often experience greater physical pain, which is a frequent accompaniment to AIDS. Almost 60% of children with HIV experience pain, which may negatively affect their quality of life and sleep patterns. Chest pain, headache, oral cavity pain, abdominal pain, and peripheral neuropathy are commonly reported. As in other chronic illnesses, pain needs to be understood within a developmental context so that preventive and therapeutic intervention strategies can be developed to reduce children's distress.[10]

TREATMENT

Treatments for HIV-1 disease complications that improve quality of life include HAART, prevention of bacterial infections, and the provision of prophylaxis and treatment of opportunistic infections such as *Pneumocystis jirovecii pneumonia (PCP)*, atypical mycobacteria infection (MAC), cryptococcal meningitis, toxoplasmosis, cytomegalovirus, and herpes simplex virus.

Good nutrition is a critical component in health maintenance and quality of life.[15,16] These measures, in addition to good supportive care, have slowed the progression of HIV infection. As a result, many more HIV-infected children are now living longer, well into their teens. Palliative care needs to be integrated with cure-directed therapy and should be available from diagnosis through the entire course of the disease.

Although HAART dramatically changed the outcome for many HIV-infected children in developed countries, problems with adherence to or tolerance of therapy, and the increasing viral resistance rate to multiple antiretroviral drugs suggest that the need for palliative, respite, and hospice care for HIV-infected children will increase. The picture in the resource-poor areas of the world is very different. More than 90% of HIV-infected children who reside in these countries lack access to many therapies such as HAART, PCP, or MAC prophylaxis, that would prevent disease progression and are considered part of the continuum of palliative care.[17,18]

HIV DISEASE-RELATED PAIN

HIV disease-related pain results from both infectious and non-infectious processes in various organ systems that can be acute or chronic. Causes of oropharyngeal pain include candidiasis, dental problems, periodontitis, gingivitis, aphthous ulcers, and herpetic stomatitis.[19] Esophageal pain, or dysphagia, can result from esophageal candidiasis, CMV, or herpetic ulcerative esophagitis. A rare cause of dysphagia may be lymphoma. Common causes of abdominal pain include pancreatitis, hepatitis, cholengitis, MAC enteritis or colitis, CMV colitis, and inflammatory or infectious colitis. Chronic diarrhea, although not classically considered a pain syndrome, is common in HIV disease and is usually associated with abdominal discomfort, including cramping and spasms.[20,21]

The oropharyngeal and gastrointestinal pain syndromes frequently result in poor oral intake and reduced absorption of nutrients, which lead to malnutrition and failure to thrive, and progresses to wasting syndrome. Even in the early stages of HIV disease, the recurrent difficulty with oral intake from various causes may have a significant impact on quality of life. The wasting syndrome is commonly associated with cachexia, fatigue, depression, musculoskeletal pain, abdominal pain, and neuropathy secondary to nutritional deficiencies. The chronic pain and suffering experienced by HIV-infected children with wasting syndrome is one of the most challenging pain syndromes to effectively treat and relieve.[15,19,21]

Neurologic and neuromuscular pain syndromes are relatively common in HIV-infected children. These include hypertonicity; spasticity; encephalitis, including herpes and toxoplasmosis; meningitis, such as *Cryptococcus neoformans*;

primary CNS lymphoma; Guillain-Barre syndrome; and myopathy. Peripheral neuropathies, or the possibility that the neuropathy might be a drug side effect such as to an antiretroviral, should be remembered. Skin and soft tissue complications of HIV, which are associated with both acute and chronic pain and discomfort, include herpes simplex, shingles, and other bacterial or fungal infections, as well as adenitis caused by bacterial or mycobacterial agents. Malignancies such as leukemia, lymphoma, and leimyosarcoma, which seem to be more frequent in HIV-infected children, have cancer-associated pain syndromes in addition to the HIV-associated symptoms.[19,20]

HIV TREATMENT-RELATED PAIN

Some chronic pain experienced by HIV-infected children is related to the side effects and toxicities of the multiple medications used, especially antiretroviral medications. A detailed description of the specific side effects of each antiretroviral is available in published pediatric treatment guidelines.[22] Many of the antiretroviral medications cause abdominal discomfort, nausea, and diarrhea. This is especially true for the protease inhibitors as a class, but is also seen with nucleoside analogues, such as didanosine and zidovudine. Other painful side effects associated with antiretroviral drugs include headache, pancreatitis, and neuropathy. Patients often need to continue the medications causing these symptoms and are asked to live with these side effects or risk development of drug resistance and disease progression. In addition to the pain associated with antiretroviral therapy, the stress of adherence to these complex regimens has its own adverse impact on quality of life.[22]

MANAGEMENT OF PAIN IN THE CHILD WITH HIV

Many physicians are preoccupied with managing the HIV disease and prolonging life, and frequently neglect to alleviate suffering from adverse effects of the disease, treatment interventions, or procedures. One of the major limitations in preventing HIV-infected children from receiving appropriate palliative care is the lack of appreciation of both acute and chronic pain associated with this disease and the multiple painful procedures required in the management of this syndrome.[20] In addition, physicians are not well trained in pain management, particularly in patients with chronic illnesses that result in both somatic and neuropathic pain.

Although great strides have been made in the management of pediatric pain, pain in children with HIV continues to be inadequately treated. Some of the barriers specific to the management of pain in children with HIV include:

- The difficulty of assessing pain in young children,
- The difficulty of assessing pain in children with neurologic impairment, such as encephalopathic or developmentally delayed,
- Parental denial of the child's disease and consequently, his or her pain,
- Physicians' resistance to the use of opioids by families who have a history of drug use,
- Unfounded fears about the addiction potential and the physical dangers of opioids, including respiratory depression,
- Subspecialists who are not trained in assessment of pain and appropriate use of analgesics.[20,23,24]

The goals of pain management in HIV-infected children include:

- Reducing the incidence and severity of acute and chronic pain while providing appropriately aggressive medical therapy,
- Providing adequate pharmacological pain control with minimal side effects,
- Using nonpharmacologic approaches to pain management,
- Educating children and families to communicate about pain,
- Relieving suffering,
- Addressing quality of life issues, especially in terminal illness.

In end-stage disease, pain management often needs to take precedent over other aspects of medical care, including antiretroviral therapy.

Special Considerations Unique to Children and Adolescents with HIV/AIDS

Advances in therapies have led to "survival past 5 years of age for more than 65% of infected children."[10] A majority of these children and adolescents, most of whom contracted HIV via MTCT have lived beyond childhood. With this, caregivers and healthcare providers face the troubling issue of HIV diagnosis disclosure to affected children and adolescents, as well as the array of issues that accompany HIV infection such as stigma and physical and mental signs and symptoms.[10]

COGNITIVE CONCERNS

Although many children are asymptomatic, numerous studies document the occurrence of at least some cognitive and language delays as a result of HIV. These cognitive manifestations, though subtle, do impact the quality of life for children with HIV. The mechanism of brain impairment because of HIV is not completely understood. Three patterns of abnormal neurocognitive development have been described: rapid progressive encephalopathy (PE) with loss of attained milestones, subacute progression of encephalopathy with relatively stable periods, and static encephalopathy with a failure to achieve new milestones.[10]

SOCIAL STIGMA AND OTHER ISSUES

There are major differences in HIV illness that make it difficult to apply evidenced-based knowledge being practiced within other pediatric illness sectors. These differences lie in epidemiology, the multigenerational nature of HIV, and the social stigma surrounding HIV transmission. Pediatric HIV is most prevalent in poor, urban, and ethnic minority populations who have typically suffered years of discrimination and racism. Moreover, HIV infection is associated with stigmatized behaviors such as high-risk sex, same-sex behavior, drug use, and fear of contagion, which have all contributed to a level of stigma beyond that associated with any other disease. "The majority of HIV-infected children acquired the virus from their mothers, and ensuing parental guilt about transmission distinguishes this disease from cancer and other life-threatening pediatric illnesses."[25]

Frequently, children with HIV come from families with a history of substance abuse, which sometimes causes clinicians to fear using opioids to treat these children. Clinical experience has shown that with proper monitoring and systems put in place, the incidence of addicted caregivers using a child's medication is extremely low. Fear of parental misuse is not a reason to withhold opioids from a child in pain.[26]

DISCLOSURE

Unlike disclosing a cancer or other life-limiting disease, disclosure of a child's HIV diagnosis often leads to disclosure of other family secrets, including paternity, parental history of sexual behavior, and substance abuse. "Thus, not only are parents' decisions to disclose affected by their fears about the emotional consequences of disclosure for the child, but also their fears about the child's anger towards the parent, and the potential social consequences associated with the child sharing the diagnosis with others (e.g., ostracism, negative reactions from family, friends, and school, lack of community support)."[25] Disclosure of HIV status to young school-aged children who participate in sports should be addressed while maintaining the confidentiality and well-being of the child.

Fears about potential negative consequences of disclosure are indeed compelling. Neither parents nor health care providers want to inadvertently inflict greater suffering on a child than that which is already present as a result of illness itself. The question still exists of whether knowledge of diagnosis has a significant negative impact on the child. The few studies in literature on children with life-threatening illnesses provide some evidence that diagnosis disclosure helps children cope with their illness. Reasons cited for nondisclosure in published reports include:

- Protecting a child from social rejection,
- Protecting him or her from fear or depression,
- Parental sense of guilt or shame,
- Parental fears of rejection by the child.[27]

As the child with HIV approaches adolescence, disclosure issues emerge related to pubertal development and sexuality, fear of contagion and transmissibility, and a need to promote adherence to complex and often toxic regimens. Adolescence is a time of intense social pressure to fit in and be normal. Adolescence is also a time of increased experimentation with sexual behavior and drug use. "The public health risks of nondisclosure, including non-adherence to medications that may result in drug resistant strains of HIV combined with risky sexual behavior that may result in transmission of the virus (including such drug-resistant strains), add a sense of urgency to the issue of disclosing the HIV diagnosis to youth living with perinatal HIV infection."[25]

For children with HIV who know their diagnosis, the decision to disclose their status to friends, teachers, employers, and especially potential romantic partners has been a primary concern. For those unaware of their diagnosis, ethical and legal conflicts also arise.[25] An example would be when there is a lack of concordance between parent and child readiness for disclosure of the child's status, such as the parents don't want to disclose and the child is beginning to engage in risk behavior, then what are the obligations of the provider? Many providers will not disclose to the child if the parents do not want disclosure to occur out of both respect for parents wishes and concerns that parents will remove the child from treatment.

However, as children age, providers become increasingly uncomfortable with secrecy, particularly when adherence and sexual behavior are issues. At this time, there are limited laws or practice guidelines for providers to consult in these situations.[25]

The process of disclosure should be conceptualized as an ongoing dialogue among the youth, family, and healthcare providers about the impact of HIV infection. The process must reflect the child's developmental understanding of illness and death over time.[25] An important goal throughout is to establish and maintain developmentally appropriate youth participation with the recommended complex medical regimen.[27] A conceptual framework to address the process of disclosure highlights five steps:[28]

1. "Information gathering and trust building, characterized by the establishment and maintenance of a trust-based working relationship between the caregiver and the health care professional.
2. Education, beginning with initial assessments of caregivers and child knowledge and attitudes (including cultural and religious beliefs) and continuing through a gradual full disclosure to the child. This may take weeks to years.
3. Determining when the time is right for disclosure, a process that must include changes in the child's health status, parental health or relationships, and perhaps the initiation of experimental, risky, or more burdensome treatments.
4. The actual disclosure event, which may be accomplished by the caregiver in the presence of the healthcare professional.
5. Monitoring post-disclosure coping and disclosure-related bumps in the road, such as direct or indirect observations of behavior, school performance, and peer relationships, and facilitating acceptance and adjustment with behavioral health professionals' consultation as needed."

There does not appear to be evidence to support the fear that disclosure of HIV infection to children will cause negative consequences. Alternatively, disclosure allows more open involvement in medical care decisions, increased opportunities for peer support, and increased trust of healthcare providers and caregivers.[27]

Interdisciplinary Care of Children with Immunodeficiency Syndromes

Children with immunodeficiency syndromes require complex care from a multitude of providers to manage the acute, chronic and recurrent problems imposed by their underlying disorders. As described previously, they suffer symptoms that range from mild to severe and the course is often unpredictable. Minor problems may evolve into life-threatening events and it is not uncommon for these children to experience frequent life-threatening episodes. There may be a multitude of existing clinical teams with competing priorities that challenge effective communication and care coordination. Successful outcomes for the child and family are ultimately defined as improvement in the quality of life for the child and the family and depend upon the ability of interdisciplinary palliative care teams to work effectively with families, clinicians, multiple subspecialists, school systems, and community agencies.

An example of a core Interdisciplinary Pediatric Palliative Care Team (IPPCT) approach to the care of a children with HIV and family is in Box 44-1.[29]

HIV End Stage and End-of-Life Concerns

End-stage disease in these children is usually characterized by progression to severe clinical disease with marked immune suppression, the CDC classification C-3. Children often have four or more of the following markers that indicate progression to end-stage disease:

- High viral load greater than 100,000 copies/mL despite aggressive antiretroviral therapy,

- Progressive loss of CD4+ lymphocyte cells, below 250 cells /mm^3 with percentages less than 15%,
- Onset of refractory opportunistic infections,
- Progression of weight loss leading to wasting syndrome,
- Progression of HIV encephalopathy,
- Development of HIV malignancy, such as leiomyosarcoma, primary CNS lymphoma, and leukemia,
- Nephropathy, cardiomyopathy, hepatitis.

Judicious use of antiretroviral therapy may improve the quality of life by minimizing the impact of opportunistic infections and sustaining a measure of immunologic health. At the end-stage of HIV disease, decisions relating to the continuation of antiretroviral therapy must be made balancing the limited effect of such treatment versus drug side effects and toxicities. At the end of life, however, aggressive treatment of symptoms is a requisite of good palliative care. For example, the prevention of *Pneumocystis* pneumonia with trimethoprim-sulfamethoxazole prophylaxis provides comfort by avoiding the substantial morbidity of this infection. Clinicians need to recognize when the burden of treatment outweighs the benefits, and when the continuation of curative treatment is not only ineffective, but also a source of greater suffering for the child.[30,31]

Bereavement Needs of Families and Healthcare Providers

CHALLENGES FOR CHILDREN WITH HIV/AIDS

With HIV/AIDS, more rage, shame, fear, and unresolved grief are experienced, often associated with stigmatization, disenfranchisement, and multiple losses, than with other illnesses. In addition, fear of social stigma and fears of contagion can deprive children and their families of critical community and extended family support. Providing care is often complicated by the trans-generational nature of the illness, multiple social and psychological issues, and inadequate financial and community services. In cases where parents have already died from the disease, care of the child transfers to other family members or to foster care, which displaces the child from the family and further complicates the grieving process. By adhering to medication protocols, most children with HIV can live good quality lives for a reasonably long lifespan and can be encouraged to plan for the future. While children and their families are aware that death is a possibility, prognostic uncertainty results in not knowing which course the disease will take or when death will occur.

Little is known from research specifically about the impact of child deaths due to HIV/AIDS or interventions to help families cope with such a loss.[31] As with other chronic, life-threatening illnesses, however, initiating bereavement care before end of life supports both the child and family in important ways, especially by dealing with the child's awareness of his or her own impending death, optimizing the quality of life.[32] Inquiring about and understanding the cultural and spiritual preferences and beliefs of the family are critical. Based on such an understanding, interventions by the palliative care team include:

- Facilitating communication between the family and the healthcare staff in order to ensure that information and options are presented to the family, questions are addressed, information shared is understood, and decisions are made consistent with family values and goals.

BOX 44-1	Interdisciplinary Pediatric Palliative Care Team
Child and family	Participates actively in identifying values, hopes, fears, and dreams, assists clinicians to establish goals that are based upon their wishes; communicates conflicts, identifies evolving needs. The child-family unit is the focus and driving force of team activities.
Physician(s)	Aligns with family to develop a plan that is in the best interests of the child; consults with HIV and other physician specialists; provides expert advice on pain and symptom management, communication, anticipatory guidance, treatment decisions, and end-of-life care.
Advance practice nurse	Evaluates patient and family understanding of illness, symptoms, medication regimens, treatment options, and prognosis. Educates family and assists them to understand decisions to be made, along with consequences, both short and long term. Empowers family to develop effective partnerships with clinicians. Acts independently, with prescriptive privileges in accordance with state statutes, interfaces with physician colleagues, functions as a change agent.*
Nurse clinician	Evaluates patient well-being, monitors patient response to pain and symptom management, and assesses family coping mechanisms. Assesses family realities in relation to adherence. Identifies confusion, fears and barriers to compliance. Reinforces adaptive coping, explores negative consequences of maladaptive coping responses. Acts as clinician, educator, consultant to families, bedside clinicians, and community providers.
Social worker	Identifies family's culture, strengths, challenges, roles, patterns of communication, and ability to adequately care for the child. Assists family to access transportation, address housing needs, reimbursement for equipment and supplies not covered by insurance. Provides emotional support and refers to appropriate social, community, and child protection agencies, when needed.
Bereavement counselor	Provides anticipatory guidance to family and clinicians, coordinates after-death care to parents, siblings, extended family and community groups; develops culturally sensitive systems of follow-up and support; identifies families at risk; provides support for clinicians' grief; provides community outreach services.
Pastoral care	Provides spiritual support and guidance. Assists family to access clergy from a requested denomination. Assists with the implementation of rituals and display of significant symbols. Assists family to explore meaning, resolve guilt, and express forgiveness. Explores beliefs about suffering and existence of afterlife.

*Ferrell B, Coyle N: Textbook of palliative nursing, New York, 2006, Oxford University Press.

- Facilitating communication among family members in order to assure that they understand each other's needs, maintain the integrity of the parent-child relationship, resolve any unfinished business, prepare for the place of death considering the child's preferences and their own values and goals, and share their goodbyes consistent with their cultural and spiritual forms of expression.
- Collecting memories that they can hold onto after the death, including photos, videos, drawings, poetry, music, correspondence, articles of clothing and other personalized keepsakes, and creating a special storage container for these items.
- Helping families, when they are ready, to anticipate planning the funeral or memorial service and talking about the various choices they will need to make. When financial hardship prevents families from having the funeral they want, generating ideas for alternatives and conveying that love for the child is not measured by the ability or lack thereof to provide a funeral, are often helpful.

Following the death of a child with HIV/AIDS, responding appropriately requires sensitivity to individual, familial and cultural differences related to grief and mourning. The death of any child challenges one's assumptive view of the world, including how one engages in meaning making. Making meaning facilitates resilience following a death and has two components.[33] One is making sense of the loss, for example, acknowledging that "she's no longer in pain" or "he won't have to suffer anymore." The other is finding some benefit in the aftermath of the loss, for example, improved family communication, positive change in lifestyle, becoming involved in a social cause. Employing strategies to help families through their personal meaning making process, including using their religious and spiritual bonds, is one way to support their grief journey.

SUPPORTING HEALTHCARE PROVIDERS FOR CHILDREN WITH HIV/AIDS

In research assessing end-of-life care,[34] healthcare professionals who care for children with life threatening conditions were found to themselves suffer not only in grief over the child's circumstances, but also because of role conflicts, or situations that caused moral distress or loss of professional integrity. In some instances they were called upon to act in a manner contrary to personal and professional values causing ethical dilemmas. Additional stressors included communication difficulties with young patients and parents, team conflicts, and the inadequacy of support systems for care providers.[35] Although care providers can experience feelings of being overwhelmed, a commonsense approach to addressing and meeting their basic needs, that is rest, nutrition, and exercise, is obvious but often overlooked. Systemic interventions to address these stressors include building a community to support the work of healthcare providers through regular meetings and intensive training sessions, and implementation of palliative care rounds, patient care conferences, and bereavement debriefings.

Caring for a child with a life-threatening illness has rewards in the nature of the relationship that develops, but when a child with HIV/AIDS dies, it often marks the end of this long-term relationship, leaving healthcare providers to grieve and mourn this loss and what it represents to them. It is important for the healthcare team to have opportunities to grieve over

the death of the child. Healthcare professionals react differently to the dying process and death. Some grieve the loss of their close relationship with the child; while others grieve the loss and pain felt by the family, or grieve their professional failure to save the child. Although the reasons for grieving may be different, a process should be in place to support the various team members to cope with the dying process and death. Such grief is legitimate and deserves recognition. Effective ways of supporting the grief process of health care providers include validating their expressions of loss and grief, helping them to identify methods of personal coping and self care, and encouraging supportive professional relationships through debriefing sessions. The process should be on a regular basis rather than crisis-oriented. To achieve this goal the interdisciplinary team members should continuously exchange information (among themselves and other clinicians) about the dying patient and his/her care and solicit help in the medical and emotional care of this patient. In addition, staff members should share their thoughts and feelings and reflect on the value of their contributions during the child's illness and death. Physicians, who usually experience grieving as a private affair, should participate in these meetings and help in creating a safe and compassionate environment, where commendation about what has been going well and resolution of difficulties will help the team to function as a cohesive unit.

Conclusion

This chapter will hopefully promote the development of evidenced-based guidelines for providing palliative and end-of- life care for infants, children, and adolescents with primary and secondary immuno deficiencies. There is a need to educate healthcare providers across disciplines on how to manage the prognostic uncertainty of severe immuno deficiency disorders whether primary or secondary and the effective management of pain and other symptoms in the context of life-limiting illnesses. In addition, skills of working as an interdisciplinary team are needed to manage complex care as well as to negotiate difficult issues such as resuscitation status and withdrawal of life-sustaining interventions.

The following is offered as a tribute to the millions of infants, children, adolescents, and women from the developing world, who, many times faced alone, the horrors of the epidemic of HIV/AIDS.

REFERENCES

1. Oleske JM, Minnefor AB, Cooper R, Thomas K, de la Cruz A, Ahdieh H, et al: Immune deficiency syndrome in children, *JAMA* 17:2345–2349, 1983.
2. Institute of Medicine, In Field MJ, Behrman RE, editors: *When children die: improving palliative and end-of-life care for children and their families*, Washington, DC, 2003, The National Academies Press.
3. Casanova J, Abel L: Primary immunodeficiencies: a field in its infancy, *Science* 317:617–619, 2007.
4. Notarangelo L, et al: International Union of Immunological Societies Expert Committee on Primary Immunodeficiencies: Primary immunodeficiencies: 2009 update, *J Allergy Clin Immunol* 124:1162–1178, 2009.
5. Casanova J, Fieshi C, Zhang S, Abel L: Revisiting human primary immunodeficiencies, *J Intern Med* 264:115–127, 2008.
6. Centers for Disease Control and Prevention: *HIV AIDS Surveill Rep* 12(2):1–44, 2000.
7. Oleske JM, Ruben-Hale A, Supportive Care Quality of Life Committee: Enhancing supportive care and promoting quality of life: Clinical Practice Guidelines. National Institute of Allergy and Infectious

Diseases (NIAID)-Pediatric AIDS Clinical Trials Group (ACTG), *Pediatric AIDS & HIV infection: fetus to adolescent* 6(4):187–203, 1995.

8. Joshi VV, Oleske JM: Pulmonary lesions in children with AIDS: A reappraisal based on data in additional cases and follow-up of previously reported cases, *Hum Pathol* 17:641–642, 1986.

9. *WHO Global Summary of the HIV/AIDS Epidemic.* Dec. 2009. www.who.int/hiv/data/2009_global_summary.gif Accessed February 17, 2010.

10. Brown LK, Lourie KJ, Pao M: Children and adolescents living with HIV and AIDS: a review, *J Child Psychol Psychiatr* 41:81–96, 2000.

11. Centers for Disease Control and Prevention: *A Glance at the HIV/AIDS Epidemic: CDC HIV/AIDS Fact Sheets*, June 2007. www.cdc.hiv/resources/factsheets/us.htm Accessed February 17, 2010.

12. AIDS.org: *Hemophilia and HIV: A Double Challenge.* http://www.aids.org/atn/a-102–02.html Accessed February 18, 2010.

13. Lindegren ML, Hanson C, Hammett TA, Beil J, Fleming PL, Ward JW: Sexual abuse of children: intersection with the HIV epidemic, *Pediatrics* 102(4):e46, 1998.

14. Norval D, O'Hare B, Matusa R: HIV/AIDS. In Goldman A, Hain R, Liben S, editors: *Oxford textbook of palliative care for children*, New York, 2006, Oxford University Press, pp 467–480.

15. Oleske JM, Rothpletz-Puglia PM, Winter H: Historical perspectives on the evolution in understanding the importance of nutritional care in pediatric HIV infection, *J Nutr* 126:2616S–2619S, 1996.

16. Oleske JM: *Preventing disability and providing rehabilitation for infants, children and youths with HIV/AIDS*, NIH publication no. 95–3850. Bethesda, Md, January 1995, US Department of Health and Human Services/National Institute of Child Health and Human Development.

17. World Health Organization. *The World Health Report 1995—Bridging the Gap.* Report of the Director-General.

18. Oleske JM: The many needs of the HIV-infected child, *Hosp Pract* 29:81–87, 1994.

19. Connolly GM, Hawkins D, Harcourt-Webster JN, et al: Oesophageal symptoms, their causes, treatment and prognosis in patients with acquired immunodeficiency syndrome, *Gut* 30:1033–1039, 1989a.

20. Czarniecki L, Boland M, Oleske JM: Pain in children with HIV disease, *PAAC Notes* 5:492–495, 1993.

21. Hirschfeld S, Moss H, Dragisic K, et al: Pain in pediatric human immunodeficiency virus infection: incidence and characteristics in a single-institution pilot study, *Pediatr* 98:449–456, 1996.

22. The Working Group on Antiretroviral Therapy and Medical Management of HIV-Infected Children: *Guidelines for the Use of Antiretroviral Agents in Pediatric HIV Infection*, 14 December 2001: update available at www.hivatis.org.

23. McGraft PJ, Finley GA: Attitudes and beliefs about medication and pain management in children, *J Palliat Care* 12:46–50, 1996.

24. Zelzer LK, Altman A, Cohen D, et al: Report of the subcommittee on the management of pain associated with procedures in children with cancer, *Pediatr* 86:826–831, 1990.

25. Wiener L, Mellins CA, Marhefka S, Battles HB: Disclosure of an HIV diagnosis to children: history, current research, and future directions, *J Dev Behav Pediatr* 28:155–166, 2007.

26. Schechter NL, Bernstein BA, Beck A, et al: Individual differences in children's response to pain: role of temperament and parental characteristics, *Pediatr* 87:171–177, 1991.

27. Gerson AC, Joyner M, Fosarelli P, Butz A, Wissow L, Lee S, Marks P, Hutton N: Disclosure of HIV diagnosis to children: when, where, why, and how, *J Pediatr Health Care* 15:161–167, 2001.

28. Carter BS, Oleske J, Czarniecki L, Grubman S: The child with HIV infection. In Carter BS, Levetown M, editors: *Palliative care for infants, children, and adolescents: a practical handbook*, Baltimore, 2004, The Johns Hopkins University Press, pp 337–339.

29. Ferrell B, Coyle N: *Textbook of palliative nursing*, New York, 2006, Oxford University Press.

30. Oleske JM, Czarniecki L: Continuum of palliative care: lessons from care for children infected with HIV-1, *Lancet* 354:1287–1291, 1999.

31. Demmer C: Children and infectious diseases. In Corr C, Balk D, editors: *Children's encounters with death bereavement and coping*, New York, 2010, Springer.

32. Stevens M, Rytmeister R, Proctor M, Bolster P: Children living with life-threatening or life-limiting illnesses: a dispatch from the front lines. In Corr C, Balk D, editors: *Children's encounters with death bereavement and coping*, New York, 2010, Springer.

33. Neimeyer R: Meaning and reconstruction and loss. In Neimeyer R, editor: *Meaning reconstruction and the experience of loss*, Washington, DC, 2001, American Psychological Association.

34. Rushton C, Reder E, Hall B, Comello K, Sellers D, Hutton N: Interdisciplinary intervention to improve pediatric palliative care and reduce health care professional suffering, *J Palliat Med* 9:922–933, 2006.

35. Liben S, Papadatou D, Wolfe J: Paediatic palliative care: challenges and emerging ideas, *Lancet* 371:852–864, 2008.

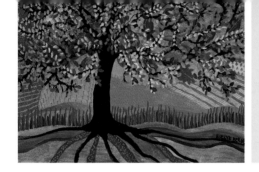

Index

Note: Page numbers followed by *b* indicate boxes; *f*, figures; *t*, tables.

A

Abnormal breathing pattern, 307
Abnormal movements. *See* Movement disorders.
Acetaminophen, guidelines for use, 290–291
ACh-m (muscarinic acetylcholine) receptor antagonists
  antiemetic action of, 314
  dosage recommendations for, 315*t*
Achondroplasia, 404*b*
Acquired immunodeficiency syndrome (AIDS). *See* HIV infection/AIDS, pediatric.
ACT (Association for Children with Life Threatening or Terminal Conditions and their Families), 98, 98*t*
Actigraph monitor, 276
ACT/RCPCH categories, 240, 242*t*
Addiction, to opioids, 289
Adenosine deaminase deficiency, 335, 336*b*. *See also* Primary anemia.
Adherence, use of term, 5
Adjuvant analgesics, 296, 297*t*
Adolescents, in palliative care
  body image of, and reaction to changes, 350
  comfort level of, 205, 205*f*
  and decisions about organ donation, 216–217
  fatigue in, 266, 268
  illness experiences of, 21–22
  role of, 126, 126*b*
  sleep problems in, 275
Adrenoleukodystrophy, 403*t*. *See also* Inherited life-threatening illnesses.
Adult learning, principles of, 104, 105*b*
Advance care planning, 35–36, 81–82
  child or youth participation in, 307
  in cystic fibrosis, 446–447
  in neurologic impairment, 411–412
  of pain management, 81–82
  for respiratory care management, 307
  for symptoms management, 36, 81–82
  treatment goals in, 185, 185*f*
Advanced heart disease, 428
  epidemiology of, 428–429, 429*t*
  mortality rate in, 428–429, 429*f*
  palliative care in, 429–436
    decision making in, 434
    family and child, 433–434
    interdisciplinary, 434, 435*t*
    medication guidelines in, 431*t*
    pain management in, 430
    psychosocial health in, 430–433
  symptoms management in, 429–430
    congestion and fluid overload, 430
    dizziness and syncope, 430
    fatigue, 430
Agitation
  at impending death, 370–371
  management of, in neurologic impairment, 417
Alginate dressings, 363, 361*t*
ALSMT (artificial life sustaining medical treatment), 199. *See also* Resuscitation.
  American Academy of Pediatrics definition of, 199–200

Altered consciousness, at impending death, 370
Aluminum/magnesium trisilicate, 326
Alvimopan, for constipation, 317
Amantadine, 295
Amegakaryocytic thrombocytopenia, 343
Amiodarone, dosage recommendations, in advanced heart disease, 431*t*
Amitriptyline, 297*t*
Analgesia, studies of therapeutic, 290
  results of, 290
Analgesic tolerance, definition of, 289
Analgesics
  adjuvant, 296, 297*t*
  administration routes for, 293
  guidelines for use of, 290–293
    acetaminophen, 290–291
    aspirin and nonsteroidal antiinflammatory drugs, 291
    codeine, 291–292
    fentanyl, 292
    hydromorphone, 292
    meperidine, 292
    methadone, 292–293
    morphine, 292
    opioid dosages, 291*t*
    oxycodone, 292
    tramadol, 292
AND (allow natural death), 199–200
Anemia
  blood product transfusions for
    alternatives to, 339–340
    interdisciplinary management of, 339
    side effects of, 338–339
    specifications for, 337
  causes of, 336*b*
  evaluation and diagnosis of, 337
  primary, 335–337
    chronic side effects of transfusions for, 338–339
    palliative care considerations in, 342–343
    symptoms of, 336
    transfusion guidelines in, 337
    transfusion specifications in, 337
  secondary, 335–336
    palliative care considerations in, 340–341
    symptoms of, 336
    transfusion guidelines in, 337
    transfusion specifications in, 337
  symptoms of, 336, 336*b*
Animal-assisted therapy, 235
Anorexia, and cachexia, 319–321
  causes of, 320
  evaluation and assessment of, 320
  pathogenesis of, 319–320
  treatment of
    integrative and supportive, 320–321
    pharmacologic, 321, 321*t*
Antacids (with or without alginate), 326
Anticholinergics, in dyspnea management, 302*t*
Anticipatory grief, 41, 42*b*, 44–45
  child expression of, 25–26, 25*f*, 26*f*
  current research on, 42

Anticipatory guidance, 33*b*, 34, 35–38, 374–375
  advance care planning in, 35–36. *See also* Advance care planning
  and bereavement care, 38. *See also* Bereavement care
  considerations in
    care coordination and continuity, 37
    emotional, social, spiritual support, 36–37
    ethical and legal, 36
    imminent death, 37–38. *See also* End of life
    resuscitation decision making, 202*b*
    symptom control, 36. *See also* Symptoms, and management
  information sharing in, 35
Anticonvulsants
  indications for, and dosages, 240–242, 241*t*
  in pain management, 296
Antidepressants, 235, 236*t*
  in pain management, 296
Antidiarrheal medications, 318–319
  bismuth subsalicylate, 318
  colestyramine, 318–319
  dosage recommendations for, 319*t*
  loperamide, 318
  octreotide, 319
Antiemetics
  cannabinoids, 314
  corticosteroids, 314
  dopamine (D-2) receptor antagonists, 313–314
  histamine-1 (H-1) receptor antagonists, 314
  5-hydroxytryptamine-3 (5-HT-3) receptor antagonists, 313–314
  muscarinic acetylcholine (ACh-m) receptor antagonists, 314
  neurokinin-1 (NK-1) receptor antagonists, 314
  propofol, 314
Antifibrinolytics, for platelet disorders, 345
Antimicrobial dressings, 363, 361*t*
Antipsychotic agents, for delirium, 260
Anxiety, 229–231, 230*b*
  evaluation of, 231
  interventions for, 233–235
  and respiratory symptoms, 300
Anxiolytic agents, 235, 236*t*
Aplastic anemia, 343
Apnea, management of, 307
Aprepitant, 314
  dosage for, 315*t*
Aranesp. *See* Darbopoetin.
Art therapy, 234–235
Aspirin, guidelines for use, 291
Assessment of needs, in illness experience, 35
Association for Children with Life Threatening or Terminal Conditions and their Families (ACT), 98, 98*t*
Autism, research on, 225
Autopsy and tissue retention, 221, 424
  factors influencing request for, 221–222, 223*b*
  family perspectives on, studies and surveys, 224–225